Electrical Diseases of the Heart

Ihor Gussak and Charles Antzelevitch (Eds)

Arthur A.M. Wilde, Paul A. Friedman, Michael J. Ackerman, and Win-Kuang Shen (Co-Eds)

Electrical Diseases of the Heart

Genetics, Mechanisms, Treatment, Prevention

Springer

Editors
Ihor Gussak MD, PhD, FACC
Deputy Therapeutic Area Head
Cardiovascular
Boehringer Ingelheim Pharmaceuticals
Ridgefield, CT, USA
Clinical Professor of Medicine
University of Medicine and Dentistry of New Jersey
Robert Wood Johnson Medical School
Bridgewater, NJ, USA

Charles Antzelevitch PhD, FACC, FAHA, FHRS
Executive Director and Director of Research
Gordon K. Moe Scholar
Masonic Medical Research Laboratory
Utica, NY, USA
Professor of Pharmacology
Upstate Medical University
Syracuse, NY, USA

Co-Editors
Arthur A.M. Wilde, MD, PhD, FESC, FAHA
Professor
Heart Failure Research Center
Department of Clinical and Experimental Cardiology
Academic Medical Center
Amsterdam, The Netherlands

Paul A. Friedman, MD
Professor of Medicine
Mayo Clinic College of Medicine
Rochester, MN, USA

Michael J. Ackerman, MD, PhD, FACC
Professor of Medicine, Pediatrics and Pharmacology
Consultant
Cardiovascular Disease and Pediatric Cardiology
Director
Long QT Syndrome Clinic and the Mayo Clinic Windland Smith Rice Sudden Death Genomics Laboratory
President
Sudden Arrhythmia Death Syndromes (SADS) Foundation
Mayo Clinic College of Medicine
Rochester, MN, USA

Win-Kuang Shen, MD
Consultant
Division of Cardiovascular Diseases
Professor of Medicine
Mayo Clinic College of Medicine
Rochester, MN, USA

British Library Cataloguing in Publication Data
Electrical diseases of the heart : genetics, mechanisms, treatment, prevention
1. Arrhythmia
I. Gussak, Ihor II. Antzelevitch, Charles III. Wilde, Arthur
616.1′28

ISBN-13: 9781846288531

Library of Congress Control Number: 2007923776

ISBN: 978-1-84628-853-1 e-ISBN: 978-1-84628-854-8

Printed on acid-free paper

9 8 7 6 5 4 3 2 1

Springer Science+Business Media
springer.com

To the pioneers of cardiac electrophysiology whose seminal contributions are depicted in the historical perspectives included in many of the chapters. Our mentors, collaborators, and fellows who have assisted us in advancing the field,

and

last, but not least, to our families, whose understanding and support have permitted us to dedicate the time and effort needed to formulate this text.

I.G.
C.A.

Foreword

She was about 35 years old when she first became my patient in 1975. She had suffered from bouts of a supraventricular tachycardia (SVT) as far back as she could remember. "In the early days," she recalled, "when I was a kid, they would give me something in the emergency room that elevated my blood pressure and damn near tore my head off. What a headache I would get! But a lot of times it didn't work. Then they stuck my head in a bucket of cold water and told me to 'bear down.' Finally, they would give me more digitalis in my vein until I started vomiting. That usually stopped the SVT." But nothing seemed to prevent recurrences. She was on a full dose of digitoxin and was one of the first to try a β blocker (propranolol) in the late 1960s. Her episodes were fast, around 220/min, and frightened her terribly, so much so that she would ride the tractor alongside her farmer-husband all day long just to be near him in case she had a recurrence.

Then came one of the first breakthroughs. Gordon Moe had published a "case report" of a dog with probable atrioventricular node reentry (AVNRT), showing that such a tachycardia could be started and stopped by external stimuli. Clinical studies followed (though somewhat belatedly) and replicated such responses in humans. Medtronic developed an implantable pacemaker (5998 RF unit) that was triggered by an external battery-driven stimulator held over the passive receiver to deliver a burst of rapid stimuli to the epicardial electrodes implanted on her right atrium. Magic! She terminated her own SVT with unerring reliability and never precipitated atrial fibrillation. Now a free woman, she no longer needed tractor rides. But she never left her house without the RF generator and always carried a spare battery in her pocket.

Over time she stopped her medications and gradually stopped coming back for return visits because she had complete control of her SVT. About 15 years later she showed up unannounced because one of the wires in her handheld unit had fractured and she no longer could stop the SVT. Could I get her a replacement or send the broken unit for repairs, she asked. The next day she was in the EP laboratory, had a slow pathway ablation, cure of the AVNRT, and removal of the implanted unit.

My, what a ride the last 30-plus years has provided! From a group of half dozen or so arguing at the American Heart Association Scientific Sessions as to what was the true duration of the H-V interval, to the keynote lecture on pacing I was privileged to give at the very first North American Society of Pacing and Electrophysiology (NASPE) meeting in 1980 attended by maybe 27 people, to the most recent Heart Rhythm Society (HRS) meeting with over 12,500 attendees, there has been excitement at all levels, molecular, ionic, genetic, in vitro, in vivo, and clinical. We have mined the riches offered by the study of cardiac electrical phenomena and that is what this book captures. It offers a true bridge between the basic and clinical, with insights that few texts can claim. To all for whom the squiggles of the electrocardiogram tantalize with further insights into the electrophysiology of the heart, this book offers a wonderful guide—a searchlight—into the incredible electricity that makes us tick. I compliment the editors and the authors for a wonderful job. We've come a long way, baby, and it is awesome to read about it between the covers of this book!

Douglas P. Zipes, MD
Indiana University School of Medicine
Krannert Institute of Cardiology
Indianapolis, IN, USA

Contents

† Deceased.

Part II Clinical Rhythmology: Diagnostic Methods and Tools
Edited by Win-Kuang Shen, Michael J. Ackerman, Paul A. Friedman, Arthur A.M. Wilde, and Ihor Gussak

Part III Heritable Cardiac Channelopathies, Primary Electrical Diseases, and Clinical Syndromes
Edited by Arthur A.M. Wilde, Ihor Gussak, Michael J. Ackerman, Win-Kuang Shen, and Charles Antzelevitch

Part V Iatrongenic (Drug-Induced) Cardiac Channelopathies and Sudden Cardiac Death

Edited by Ihor Gussak, Arthur A.M. Wilde, and Charles Antzelevitch

Part VI Treatment Modalities

Edited by Paul A. Friedman, Win-Kuang Shen, and Michael J. Ackerman

Contributors

Raushan Abdula, MD
Research Attending
Department of Medicine
New York Methodist Hospital
Brooklyn, NY, USA

Michael J. Ackerman, MD, PhD, FACC
Professor of Medicine, Pediatrics and Pharmacology
Consultant
Cardiovascular Disease and Pediatric Cardiology
Director
Long QT Syndrome Clinic and the Mayo Clinic Windland Smith Rice Sudden Death Genomics Laboratory
President
Sudden Arrhythmia Death Syndromes (SADS) Foundation
Mayo Clinic College of Medicine
Rochester, MN, USA

Fadi G. Akar, PhD
Assistant Professor of Medicine
Department of Cardiology
The Johns Hopkins University School of Medicine
Baltimore, MD, USA

Alexey E. Alekseev, PhD
Assistant Professor of Medicine and Pharmacology
Division of Cardiovascular Diseases
Departments of Medicine, Molecular Pharmacology and Therapeutics
Mayo Clinic College of Medicine
Rochester, MN, USA

Charles Antzelevitch, PhD, FACC, FAHA, FHRS
Executive Director and Director of Research
Gordon K. Moe Scholar
Masonic Medical Research Laboratory
Utica, NY
Professor of Pharmacology
Upstate Medical University
Syracuse, NY, USA

Isabelle Baró, PhD
CNRS Senior Research Scientist
Leader of the Team "Cell and Molecular Physiology"
INSERM U533
Nantes France
Université de Nantes
Faculté de médecine
L'institut du thorax
Nantes, France
CHU Nantes
L'institut du thorax
Nantes, France

Cristina Basso, MD, PhD
Professor of Pathological Anatomy
Department of Medico-Diagnostic Sciences and Special Therapies
Pathological Anatomy-Cardiovascular Pathology
University of Padua Medical School
Padua, Italy

Luiz Belardinelli, MD
Senior Vice-President of Pharmacology and Translational Biomedical Research
CV Therapeutics, Inc.
Palo Alto, CA, USA

Bernard Belhassen, MD
Professor
Director
Cardiac Electrophysiology Unit
Department of Cardiology
Tel-Aviv Sourasky Medical Center
Tel-Aviv, Israel

David Benson, MD
Attending Electrophysiologist
Department of Medicine
New York Methodist Hospital
Brooklyn, NY, USA

David H. Birnie, MD, MB, FRCP
Staff Cardiac Electrophysiologist
Division of Cardiology
Department of Medicine
University of Ottawa Heart Institute
Ottawa, ON, Canada

Preben Bjerregaard, MD, DMSc
Professor of Medicine
Director
Electrophysiology and Pacemaker Service
VA Medical Center
Saint Louis, MO, USA

Raffaella Bloise, MD
Medical Genetic Counselor
Molecular Cardiology Laboratories
IRCCS Salvatore Maugeri Foundation
Pavia, Italy

Pierre Bordachar, MD
Hôpital Cardiologique du Haut-Lévêque
Bordeaux-Pessac, France

J. Martijn Bos, MD
Postdoctoral Research Fellow
Department of Medicine
Division of Cardiovascular Diseases
Mayo Clinic College of Medicine
Rochester, MN, USA

Peter R. Brink, PhD
Professor and Chair
Department of Physiology and Biophysics
Stony Brook University
State University of New York
Stony Brook, NY, USA

Alexander Burashnikov, PhD
Research Scientist I
Masonic Medical Research Laboratory
Utica, NY, USA

Brett Burstein, BSc
MD/PhD Student
Pharmacology and Therapeutics
Montreal Heart Institute and McGill University
Montreal, QC, Canada

Alfred E. Buxton, MD
Ruth and Paul Levinger Professor of Medicine
Director
Division of Cardiology
Director
Arrhythmia Services and Electrophysiology Laboratory
The Warren Alpert Medical School of Brown University
Providence, RI, USA

Hugh Calkins, MD
Professor of Medicine
Director of Electrophysiology
Department of Medicine
The Johns Hopkins University School of Medicine
Baltimore, MD, USA

Simona Casini, MSc
PhD Student
Heart Failure Research Center
Department of Clinical and Experimental Cardiology
Academic Medical Center
Amsterdam, The Netherlands

Yong-Mei Cha, MD
Assistant Professor
Consultant
Division of Cardiovascular Diseases
Mayo Clinic College of Medicine
Rochester, MN, USA

Flavien Charpentier, PhD
Researcher
Inserm U533
L'institut du thorax
Nantes, France

Vincent M. Christoffels, PhD
Assistant Professor
Heart Failure Research Center
Department of Anatomy and Embryology
Academic Medical Center
Amsterdam, The Netherlands

Sumeet S. Chugh, MD
Section Chief
Clinical Cardiac Electrophysiology
Associate Professor of Medicine
Oregon Health & Science University
Portland, OR, USA

Jacques Clémenty, MD
Professor
Université Bordeaux II
Hôpital Cardiologique du Haut-Lévêque
Bordeaux-Pessac, France

Ira S. Cohen, MD, PhD
Leading Professor of Physiology and Biophysics
Professor of Medicine
Director
Institute of Molecular Cardiology
Department of Physiology and Biophysics
Stony Brook University
State University of New York
Stony Brook, NY, USA

Philippe Comtois, PhD
Postdoctoral Fellow
Research Center
Montreal Heart Institute
Montreal, QC, Canada

Domenico Corrado, MD
Professor of Medicine
Department of Cardiac, Thoracic and Vascular Science
University of Padua, Italy

Ottorino Costantini, MD
Director
Clinical Trials Program
Heart and Vascular Research Center
MetroHealth Campus
Case Western Reserve University
Cleveland, OH, USA

Lia Crotti, MD
Assistant Professor
Department of Cardiology
Policlinico San Matteo
University of Pavia
Pavia, Italy

Antoine Deplagne, MD
Hôpital Cardiologique du Haut-Lévêque
Bordeaux-Pessac, France

Nicolas Derval, MD
Hôpital Cardiologique du Haut-Lévêque
Bordeaux-Pessac, France

José M. Di Diego, MD
Research Scientist I
Masonic Medical Research Laboratory
Utica, NY, USA

Nabil El-Sherif, MD
Chief
Cardiology Division
Department of Medicine
New York Harbor VA Health Care System
Brooklyn Campus
Brooklyn, NY, USA

Denis Escande, MD, PhD[†]
Director of "L'institut du thorax"
Head of the INSERM U533 Department
Head of the Clinical Physiology Laboratory
Cardiologist
Professor of Physiology and Medicine
University of Nantes, Medical School
INSERM U533
L'institut du thorax
UMR de Médecine
Nantes, France

[†] Deceased.

Tania Ferrer, PhD
Postdoctoral Fellow
Nora Eccles Harrison Cardiovascular Research Institute
University of Utah School of Medicine
Salt Lake City, UT, USA

David M. Ficker, MD
Associate Professor of Neurology
Director
Epilepsy Monitoring Unit and EEG Lab
University Hospital
University of Cincinnati Academic Health Center
Cincinnati, OH, USA

Harry A. Fozzard, MD
Otho SA Sprague Distinguished Service Professor Emeritus
Department of Medicine
The University of Chicago
Chicago, IL, USA

Paul A. Friedman, MD
Professor of Medicine
Mayo Clinic College of Medicine
Rochester, MN, USA

Apoor S. Gami, MD
Assistant Professor of Medicine
Division of Cardiovascular Diseases
Mayo Clinic College of Medicine
Rochester, MN, USA

Yi Gang, MD, PhD
Research Fellow
Department of Cardiac and Vascular Sciences
St George's, University of London
London, UK

Robin E. Germany, MD
Assistant Professor
Cardiovascular Section
Department of Medicine
University of Oklahoma Health Sciences Center
Oklahoma City, OK, USA

Michael Glikson, MD, FACC, FESC
Clinical Professor of Cardiology
Director of Pacing and Electrophysiology Heart Institute
Sheba Medical Center
Tel Aviv University
Tel Hashomer, Israel
Ramat Gan, Israel

Michael H. Gollob, MD, FRCP
Director
Staff Cardiac Electrophysiologist
Arrhythmia Research Laboratory and Division of Cardiology
University of Ottawa Heart Institute
Ottawa, ON, Canada

Robert M. Gow, MD, FRCP
Staff Cardiac Electrophysiologist
Division of Cardiology
Department of Medicine
Children's Hospital of Eastern Ontario
University of Ottawa Heart Institute
Ottawa, ON, Canada

Martin S. Green, MD, FRCP
Staff Cardiac Electrophysiologist
Division of Cardiology
Department of Medicine
University of Ottawa Heart Institute
Ottawa, ON, Canada

Lorne J. Gula, MD, MSc, FRCPC
Assistant Professor of Medicine
University of Western Ontario
Clinical Cardiac Electrophysiologist
Cardiology
Arrhythmia Service
Department of Medicine
Division of Cardiology
London Health Sciences Center
London, ON, Canada

Osnat Gurevitz, MD
Pacing and Electrophysiology Unit
The Heart Institute
Sheba Medical Center and Tel Aviv University
Tel Hashomer, Israel

Hiie M. Gussak, MD
Assistant Professor of Medicine
University of Medicine and Dentistry of New Jersey
Hackensack University Medical Center
Nephrologist
Internal Medicine
Nephrology Associates
Teaneck, NJ, USA

Ihor Gussak, MD, PhD, FACC
Deputy Therapeutic Area Head
Cardiovascular
Boehringer Ingelheim Pharmaceuticals
Ridgefield, CT, USA
Clinical Professor of Medicine
University of Medicine and Dentistry of New Jersey
Robert Wood Johnson Medical School
Bridgewater, NJ, USA

Michel Haïssaguerre, MD
Professor
Université Bordeaux II
Hôpital Cardiologique du Haut-Lévêque
Bordeaux-Pessac, France

Masayasu Hiraoka, MD, PhD
Professor Emeritus
Tokyo Medical and Dental University and Commissioner
Labor Insurance Appeal Committee
Ministry of Health, Labor and Welfare
Shibakouen, Minato-ku, Tokyo, Japan

Siew Yen Ho, PhD
Honorary Consultant Cardiac Morphologist
Cardiac Morphology
Royal Brompton Hospital and National Heart and Lung Institute
London, UK

Mélèze Hocini, MD
Hôpital Cardiologique du Haut-Lévêque
Bordeaux-Pessac, France

Arshad Jahangir, MD
Professor of Medicine
Director
CardioGerontology Research Laboratory
Division of Cardiovascular Diseases
Department of Internal Medicine
Mayo Clinic College of Medicine
Rochester, MN, USA

Pierre Jaïs, MD
Hôpital Cardiologique du Haut-Lévêque
Bordeaux-Pessac, France

Anders Jönsson, MD
Hôpital Cardiologique du Haut-Lévêque
Bordeaux-Pessac, France

Mark E. Josephson, MD
Chief
Cardiovascular Division
Clinical Professor of Medicine
Beth Israel Deaconess Medical Center
Boston, MA, USA

Lilian Joventino, MD
Assistant Professor of Medicine
The Warren Alpert Medical School of Brown University
Department of Medicine
Rhode Island and Miriam Hospitals
Providence, RI, USA

Richard Judson, PhD
National Center for Computational Toxicology
Office of Research and Development
U.S. Environmental Protection Agency
Research Triangle Park, NC, USA

Alan Kadish, MD
Northwestern University
Feinberg School of Medicine
Chicago, IL, USA

Robert S. Kass, PhD
Columbia University Alumnus and David Hoasack Professor and Chairman
Department of Pharmacology
College of Physicians and Surgeons of Columbia University
New York, NY, USA

Anant Khositseth, MD
Department of Pediatrics
Division of Pediatric Cardiology
Faculty of Medicine Ramathibodi Hospital
Mahidol University
Bangkok, Thailand

Robert B. Kleiman, MD
Senior Director
International Cardiology
eResearchTechnology, Inc.
Philadelphia, PA, USA

George J. Klein, MD
Electrophysiology Training Program Director
Professor of Medicine
University of Western Ontario
London, ON, Canada

Peter Kohl, MD, PhD
Senior Fellow
Department of Physiology, Anatomy and Genetics
University of Oxford
Oxford, UK

Andrzej S. Kosinski, PhD
Associate Professor
Department of Biostatistics and Bioinformatics
Duke University
Duke Clinical Research Institute
Durham, NC, USA

John B. Kostis, MD
Chairman
Department of Medicine
Professor of Medicine and Pharmacology
John G. Detwiler Professor of Cardiology
University of Medicine and Dentistry of New Jersey
Robert Wood Johnson Medical School
Chief of Medical Service
Robert Wood Johnson University Hospital
New Brunswick, NJ, USA

Andrew D. Krahn MD, FACC, FRCPC
Electrophysiology Training Program Director
Professor
Division of Cardiology
University of Western Ontario
London, ON, Canada

Yoshihisa Kurachi, MD, PhD
Professor and Chairman
Department of Pharmacology
Osaka University Graduate School of Medicine
Suita, Osaka, Japan

Julien Laborderie, MD
Université Bordeaux II
Hôpital Cardiologique du Haut-Lévêque
Bordeaux-Pessac, France

Dominique Lacroix, MD, PhD
Professor
Hôpital Cardiologique
CHRU De Lille
Lille, France

Hon-Chi Lee, MD, PhD
Professor of Medicine
Mayo Medical School
Consultant
Division of Cardiovascular Diseases
Department of Internal Medicine
Mayo Clinic College of Medicine
Rochester, MN, USA

Hervé Le Marec, MD, PhD
Professor
Head of Cardiovascular Department
Nantes Hospital
L'institut du thorax
Saint-Herblain, France

Nicolas Lindegger, PhD
Postdoctoral Fellow
Department of Pharmacology
Columbia University
New York, NY, USA

Jeffrey S. Litwin, MD
Senior Vice President and Chief Medical Officer
eResearchTechnology, Inc.
Philadelphia, PA, USA

Nian Liu, MD
Research Fellow
Department of Molecular Cardiology
IRCCS Salvatore Maugeri Foundation
Maugeri, Pavia, Italy

David Luria, MD
Senior Cardiologist
Pacing and Electrophysiology Unit
Heart Institute
Sheba Medical Center
Tel Hashomer, Israel

Marek Malik, MD, PhD, DSc (Med), FACC, FESC, FHRS
Professor of Cardiac Electrophysiology
Department of Cardiac and Vascular Sciences
St. George's, University of London
London, UK

Frank I. Marcus, MD
Professor Emeritus
Department of Cardiology
University of Arizona
Sarver Heart Center
Tucson, AZ, USA

Barry J. Maron, MD
Hypertrophic Cardiomyopathy Center
Minneapolis Heart Foundation
Minneapolis, MN, USA

Shaji C. Menon, MD
Fellow
Pediatric Cardiology
Mayo Clinic College of Medicine
Rochester, MN, USA

Paola G. Meregalli, MD
Cardiologist
Heart Failure Research Center
Department of Clinical and Experimental Cardiology
Academic Medical Center
Amsterdam, The Netherlands

Antoon F.M. Moorman, PhD
Professor
Heart Failure Research Center
Department of Anatomy and Embryology
Academic Medical Center
Amsterdam, The Netherlands

Christophe Moreau, PhD
Career Scientist
Biophysique Moléculaire and Cellulaire
CNRS UMR5090
CEA/DRDC
Grenoble, France

Joel Morganroth, MD
Chief Scientist
eResearchTechnology, Inc.
Clinical Professor of Medicine
University of Pennsylvania
Philadelphia, PA, USA

Shingo Murakami, PhD
Assistant Professor
Department of Pharmacology
Osaka University Graduate School of Medicine
Osaka, Japan

Christina M. Murray, MD
Fellow in Cardiovascular Medicine
Department of Medicine
University of Oklahoma Health Sciences Center
Oklahoma City, OK, USA

Carlo Napolitano, MD, PhD
Adjunct Professor
School of Cardiology
University of Pavia
Research Coordinator
Molecular Cardiology Laboratories
Pavia, Italy

Stanley Nattel, MD
Professor
Cardiovascular Electrophysiology
Department of Medicine
Montreal Heart Institute Research Center and Université de Montréal
Montreal, QC, Canada

Jan Nemec, MD, FACC
Assistant Professor of Medicine
Department of Cardiac Electrophysiology
Cardiovascular Institute
University of Pittsburgh Medical Center
Pittsburgh, PA, USA

Timothy M. Olson, MD
Associate Professor of Medicine and Pediatrics
Director
Cardiovascular Genetics
Division of Cardiovascular Diseases
Departments of Medicine, Pediatrics and Adolescent Medicine and Medical Genetics
Mayo Clinic College of Medicine
Rochester, MN, USA

Steve R. Ommen, MD
Associate Professor of Medicine
Cardiovascular Diseases
Mayo Clinic College of Medicine
Rochester, MN, USA

Mark D. O'Neill, MB, BCh, DPhil
Hôpital Cardiologique du Haut-Lévêque
Bordeaux-Pessac, France

Ganiyu O. Oshodi, MD
Heart and Vascular Research Center
MetroHealth Campus
Case Western Reserve University
Cleveland, OH, USA

Mai Ots, MD, ScD (med)
Associate Professor of Medicine
Division of Nephrology
Department of Internal Medicine
Tartu University Clinic
Tartu, Estonia

Antonio Pelliccia, MD
Center of Sports Sciences
Rome, Italy

Yigal M. Pinto, MD, PhD
Professor
Cardiologist
Department of Cardiology
University Hospital Maastricht
Maastricht, The Netherlands

Alex V. Postma, PhD
Department of Anatomy and Embryology
Academic Medical Center
Amsterdam, The Netherlands

Silvia G. Priori, MD, PhD
Professor of Cardiology
University of Pavia
Director of Molecular Cardiology
Department of Molecular Cardiology
IRCCS Salvatore Maugeri Foundation
Pavia, Italy

Sridharan Rajamani, PhD
Scientist
Department of Pharmacology
CV Therapeutics, Inc.
Palo Alto, CA, USA

Robert F. Rea, MD
Associate Professor of Medicine
Cardiovascular Division
Department of Medicine
Mayo Clinic College of Medicine
Rochester, MN, USA

Vikram Reddy, MD
Northwestern University
Feinberg School of Medicine
Chicago, IL, USA

Dwight W. Reynolds, MD
Professor and Chief
Cardiovascular Section
Department of Medicine
University of Oklahoma Health Sciences Center
Oklahoma City, OK, USA

John Jeremy Rice, PhD, MS, BS
Research Staff Member
Department of Functional Genomics and Systems Biology
IBM T.J Watson Research Center
Yorktown Heights, NY, USA

Richard B. Robinson, PhD
Professor of Pharmacology
Associate Dean of Graduate Affairs
Columbia University
New York, NY, USA

Michael R. Rosen, MD
Gustavus A. Pfeiffer Professor of Pharmacology
Professor of Pediatrics
Director, Center for Molecular Therapeutics
Department of Pharmacology
Columbia University
New York, NY, USA

David S. Rosenbaum, MD
Director
Heart and Vascular Center for the MetroHealth System
Professor of Medicine and Biomedical Engineering
MetroHealth Campus
Case Western Reserve University
Cleveland, OH, USA

Yanfei Ruan, MD
Research Fellow
Molecular Cardiology Laboratories
IRCCS Salvatore Maugeri Foundation
Pavia, Italy

Frédéric Sacher, MD
Université Bordeaux II
Hôpital Cardiologique du Haut-Lévêque
Bordeaux-Pessac, France

Jeffrey E. Saffitz, MD, PhD
Mallinckrodt Professor of Pathology
Harvard Medical School Chief
Department of Pathology
Beth Israel Medical Center
Boston, MA, USA

Rafeeq Samie, MD
Fellow
Clinical Electrophysiology
Division of Cardiology
Department of Medicine
University of Ottawa Heart Institute
Ottawa, ON, Canada

Srinivasan Sattiraju, MD
Department of Molecular Pharmacology and Experimental Therapeutics
Mayo Clinic College of Medicine
Rochester, MN, USA

Hartzell V. Schaff, MD
Chair
Division of Cardiovascular Surgery
Stuart W. Harrington Professor of Surgery
Department of Surgery
Mayo Clinic College of Medicine
Rochester, MN, USA

Bas A. Schoonderwoerd, MD, PhD
Department of Cardiology
Thoraxcenter
University Medical Center Groningen
University of Groningen
Groningen, The Netherlands

Jean-Jacques Schott, PhD
Researcher
INSERM U533
L'institut du thorax
Nantes, France

Eric Schulze-Bahr, MD
Professor
Department of Cardiology and Angiology
Molecular Genetics
Hospital of the University of Münster
Münster, Germany

Peter J. Schwartz, MD
Professor of Cardiology
Department of Cardiology
University of Pavia and IRCCS Policlinico San Matteo
Pavia, Italy

Win-Kuang Shen, MD
Consultant
Division of Cardiovascular Diseases
Professor of Medicine
Mayo Clinic College of Medicine
Rochester, MN, USA

Wataru Shimizu, MD, PhD
Senior Staff
Co-Director of Clinical Cardiac Electrophysiology Laboratory
Division of Cardiology
Department of Internal Medicine
National Cardiovascular Center
Suita, Osaka, Japan

John C. Shryock, PhD
Senior Director
Department of Pharmacology
CV Therapeutics, Inc.
Palo Alto, CA, USA

Allan C. Skanes, MD
Director of Electrophysiology Laboratory
University Hospital
University of Western Ontario
London, ON, Canada

Elson L. So, MD
Professor of Neurology
Director
Section of Electroencephalography
Mayo Clinic College of Medicine
Rochester, MN, USA

Virend K. Somers, MD, DPhil
Professor of Medicine
Division of Cardiovascular Diseases
Mayo Clinic College of Medicine
Rochester, MN, USA

Subeena Sood, PhD
Postdoctoral Associate
Department of Molecular Physiology and Biophysics
Baylor College of Medicine
Houston, TX, USA

Marco Stramba-Badiale, MD, PhD
Head
Pediatric Arrhythmias Center
IRCCS Istituto Auxologico Italiano
Milan, Italy

Rajesh N. Subbiah, BSc(Med), MBBS, PhD, FRACP
Electrophysiology Fellow
University of Western Ontario
London, ON, Canada

Yoshihide Takahashi, MD
Hôpital Cardiologique du Haut-Lévêque
Bordeaux-Pessac, France

Hanno L. Tan, MD, PhD
Cardiologist
Heart Failure Research Center
Department of Clinical and Experimental Cardiology
Academic Medical Center
Amsterdam, The Netherlands

Andre Terzic, MD, PhD
Marriott Family Endowed Professor of Cardiovascular Research
Professor of Medicine, Molecular Pharmacology and Experimental Therapeutics
Director
Marriott Heart Disease Research Program
Mayo Clinic Associate Director of Research
Division of Cardiovascular Diseases
Departments of Medicine, Molecular Pharmacology and Experimental
Therapeutics, and Medical Genetics
Mayo Clinic College of Medicine
Rochester, MN, USA

David J. Tester, BS
Senior Research Technologist II
Departments of Medicine, Pediatrics, and Molecular Pharmacology and Experimental Therapeutics
Divisions of Cardiovascular Diseases and Pediatric Cardiology
Mayo Clinic College of Medicine
Rochester, MN, USA

Sergio G. Thal, MD
Staff of Cardiac Electrophysiology
South Arizona VA Health Care System
Assistant Professor of Clinical Medicine
University of Arizona
Tucson, AZ, USA

Gaetano Thiene, MD, FRCPHon
Professor of Pathological Anatomy
Department of Medico-Diagnostic Sciences and Special Therapies
Pathological Anatomy-Cardiovascular Pathology
University of Padua Medical School
Padua, Italy

Gordon F. Tomaselli, MD
David J. Carver Professor of Medicine
The Johns Hopkins University School of Medicine
Baltimore, MD, USA

Jeffrey A. Towbin, MD
Professor of Medicine
Chief
Pediatric Cardiology
Texas Children's Hospital
Baylor College of Medicine
Houston, TX, USA

Martin Tristani-Firouzi, MD
Associate Professor of Pediatrics
Pediatric Cardiology
Nora Eccles Harrison Cardiovascular Research Institute
University of Utah School of Medicine
Salt Lake City, UT, USA

Gioia Turitto, MD
Director
Cardiac Electrophysiology Services
Department of Medicine
New York Methodist Hospital
Brooklyn, NY, USA

Jop H. van Berlo, MD, PhD
Department of Molecular Cardiovascular Biology
Cincinnati Children's Hospital Medical Center
Cincinnati, OH, USA

Isabelle C. van Gelder, MD, PhD
Cardiologist
Department of Cardiology
Thoraxcenter
University Medical Center Groningen
University of Groningen
Groningen, The Netherlands

J. Peter van Tintelen, MD
Clinical Geneticist
Department of Clinical Genetics
University Medical Center Groningen
University of Groningen
Groningen, The Netherlands

Matteo Vatta, PhD
Assistant Professor
Department of Pediatrics (in Cardiology)
Baylor College of Medicine and Texas Children's Hospital
Houston, TX, USA

Richard L. Verrier, MD, PhD, FACC
Associate Professor of Medicine
Harvard Medical School
Beth Israel Deaconess Medical Center
Harvard-Thorndike Electrophysiology Institute
Harvard Institutes of Medicine
Boston, MA, USA

Sami Viskin, MD
Director
Cardiac Hospitalization
Tel Aviv Sourasky Medical Center
Sackler School of Medicine
Tel Aviv University
Tel Aviv, Israel

Michel Vivaudou, PhD
Director of Research
Biophysique Moléculaire and Cellulaire
CNRS UMR5090
CEA/DRDC
Grenoble, France

Marc A. Vos, PhD
Professor
Head of Department
Medical Physiology
Heart and Lung Center Utrecht
University Medical Center Utrecht
Utrecht, The Netherlands

Xander H.T. Wehrens, MD, PhD
Assistant Professor
Department of Molecular Physiology and Biophysics
Department of Medicine (in Cardiology)
Baylor College of Medicine
Houston, TX, USA

Ans C.P. Wiesfeld, MD, PhD
Department of Cardiology
Thoraxcenter
University Medical Center Groningen
University of Groningen
Groningen, The Netherlands

Arthur A.M. Wilde, MD, PhD, FESC, FAHA
Professor
Heart Failure Research Center
Department of Clinical and Experimental Cardiology
Academic Medical Center
Amsterdam, The Netherlands

Bruce L. Wilkoff, MD
Professor of Medicine
Director of Cardiac Pacing and Tachyarrhythmia Devices
Department of Cardiovascular Medicine
Cleveland Clinic Lerner College of Medicine of Case Western Reserve University
Cleveland, OH, USA

Lance D. Wilson, MD
Assistant Professor of Emergency Medicine
Staff Physician
Heart and Vascular Research Center
MetroHealth Campus
Case Western Reserve University
Cleveland, OH, USA

Stephan K.G. Winckels, MD
PhD Student
Medical Physiology
Heart and Lung Center Utrecht
University Medical Center Utrecht
Utrecht, The Netherlands

Satsuki Yamada, MD, PhD
Senior Research Fellow
Division of Cardiovascular Diseases
Department of Medicine, Molecular Pharmacology and Experimental Therapeutics
Mayo Clinic College of Medicine
Rochester, MN, USA

Raymond Yee, MD
Professor of Medicine
Director
Arrhythmia Service
Staff Cardiac Electrophysiologist
London HSC-University Hospital and University of Western Ontario
London, ON, Canada

Leonid V. Zingman, PhD
Assistant Professor of Medicine and Pharmacology
Division of Cardiovascular Diseases
Departments of Medicine, Molecular Pharmacology and Therapeutics
Mayo Clinic College of Medicine
Rochester, MN, USA

Douglas P. Zipes, MD
Distinguished Professor
Professor Emeritus of Medicine, Pharmacology and Toxicology
Director Emeritus
Division of Cardiology and the Krannert Institute of Cardiology
Indiana University School of Medicine
Indianapolis, IN, USA

Part I
Basic Foundations of Normal and Abnormal Cardiac Electrical Activity

The Past and Promise of Basic Cardiac Electrophysiology

Harry A. Fozzard

Introduction

A half-century ago, as an aspiring cardiologist I entered the field of cardiac electrophysiology, frustrated by our inability to intervene successfully in lethal cardiac arrhythmia, and equally frustrated by the paucity of basic understanding of cardiac electricity upon which better treatment could be based. What a remarkable change has occurred since that time; there have been extraordinary advances in both the science and clinical care. I will begin this introduction to the section on *Basic Foundations of Normal and Abnormal Cardiac Electrical Activity* by identifying those basic science steps that I think have contributed to the progress of cardiac electrophysiology. These are the rich historical background for the chapters in this section. Then I will comment on the best strategy for advancing our understanding of cardiac electricity and outline some of the key questions that I think we must address. Although my personal career goal has been how we can now exploit this basic science for clinical care, more than ever basic understanding is the framework for our future advances.

The continuum of science requires that future progress be built on the past. Therefore, before we seek to make judgments about future directions, it is important to examine how we have arrived at the present state of understanding of the cardiac electrical system and of cardiac arrhythmias. Basic scientific development has two very interdependent lines—general electrophysiology and cardiac electrophysiology. Sometimes progress has been motivated by study of heart muscle, sometimes of nerve, sometimes of single cell organisms. The basic features of membrane potential, excitability, and conduction are complementary between these areas, and the field of ion channels is united,[1] albeit with special characteristics to the cardiac system. There is a third line of insight into a basic understanding of cardiac electricity, derived from more clinical studies that have dramatically altered the natural history and the treatment of arrhythymias and that hold important and direct lessons for basic science.

We have no central planning agency to direct cardiac electrophysiological research. Indeed, experience in the last century leads us to believe that individual investigators are the best source of inspiration and direction. In the United States we have been blessed with outstanding financial support from the National Institutes of Health and the National Science Foundation and from private agencies such as the American Heart Association for this investigator-initiated research, and support from the pharmaceutical industry for therapeutically relevant research. Similar support has come from patrons in other countries. However, the success of this nondirective system requires continued lively discussion and debate between investigators in the basic science and with clinicians. Total resources for biomedical research are not infinite and each investigator has limited time and resources. Therefore, we can benefit from some discussion of what the history of our field can teach us and what strategy may be the most efficient direction to lead to greater scientific insight and to further improvement in cardiac care.

Although electrophysiology has greatly increased our scientific understanding, thoughtful reflection leads me to the general impression that in the recent past clinical interventions that reduce or prevent the underlying disease have probably had the greatest impact on lethal arrhythmia. However, this impact has been primarily to delay arrhythmic problems to a later age, rather than to abolish them. Indeed, our success in restoring circulation in ischemia has increased the numbers of people with heart failure, possibly changing the mechanisms of the dominant arrhythmias. Exploitation of genetic methods along with electrophysiology has revealed a small but growing population of primary arrhythmic diseases that provide exciting insights into both normal and abnormal mechanisms.

Historical Landmarks

We can make a strong case that basic science has been an extraordinarily successful contributor to cardiac care. But the insights and tools of biomedical science have expanded so dramatically in the last century that it is daunting to consider what are the most promising directions for cardiac electrophysiologists to follow. The interconnectedness of science means that every approach is potentially valuable. In retrospect, we can perceive that some approaches have been obviously more productive than others, although not always predicted during the basic phase. In the quest for clinically important insight we must not undervalue the progress of general science. The next decades can lead to basic understanding of the cardiac electrical system unimaginable to me when I began my career 50 years ago, and consequently to major advances in clinical care.

The Electrocardiogram

One hundred years ago William Einthoven[2] published a review of the clinical applications of his recordings of cardiac electrical activity, which I take as the beginning of the systematic study of cardiac electrophysiology. The string galvanometer that he developed could reliably measure very small signals, and it provided an invaluable tool not only for the cardiac physiologist but also for the neuroscientist. I will examine three parallel lines of development during the century since Einthoven's publication, jumping between those of basic and cardiac electrophysiology and those of clinical study that have contributed to the development of our basic understanding.

The Action Potential

Rapid advances in electrochemistry and the physics of electricity led logically to the 1902 proposal of Bernstein[3] that excitation of the action potential (AP) resulted from loss of resting membrane selective permeability to *K* (the Nernst potential), and then repolarization from reestablishment of *K* selectivity. The critical all-or-none property of the AP was first shown in the early 1900s by Lucas[4] and Adrian.[5] About this time Mines[6] described the properties of reentry loops, which has been a big factor in understanding cardiac arrhythmias, and in 1912 Herrick[7] described the clinical course of acute myocardial infarction. How the necessary transmembrane ion gradients of high intracellular K and low intracellular Na were achieved and maintained was only gradually resolved by Hodgkin's definition of an Na pump[8] and purification of a K- and Na-dependent ATPase from nerve membrane by Skou.[9] Interestingly, it was early observed that digitalis blocked the Na/K-ATPase and the Na pump, and that this action is likely to be a step in its positive inotropic effect.

Squid Axon and Microelectrodes

The squid giant axon is a 0.5- to1.0-mm-diameter cable-like cell composed of many fused axons. Its rediscovery in 1936 by Young[10] provided a crucial tool for electrophysiological progress. Curtis and Cole[11] quickly demonstrated that the axon membrane resistance fell to a very low value during the peak of the AP, as predicted by the Bernstein hypothesis. Surprisingly, however, Hodgkin and Huxley[12] found the magnitude of the AP exceeded the resting potential (overshoot) and was substantially positive, contrary to the Bernstein proposal. This overshoot was seen as early as 1934 in an attempt to measure the cardiac transmembrane AP,[13] but problems with junction potentials made the measurements uncertain. The existence of an overshoot was finally resolved by Hodgkin and Katz[14] by showing that the overshoot was a function of the Na gradient and that the AP must result from a selective dominance of Na permeability, not simply a loss of selectivity. During this same time period, development by Ling and Gerard[15] in 1949 of a satisfactory glass micropipette that could measure membrane potential in intact cells would revolutionize the study of single cells over the next half-century. As is typical, the development of a new technique precedes major advances in understanding.

Voltage Clamp

Progress by Cole and Marmont now set the stage for a huge advance in 1952. Hodgkin and Huxley[16] used the voltage clamp to determine the voltage and time-dependent properties of Na and K conductances and to build a coherent model of the ionic basis of excitability. It is hard to realize from this distance in time how revolutionary this work was, and how much it required electrophysiologists to change their mindset. One of the Hodgkin-Huxley predictions was that the Na and K channels derived their voltage dependence from movement of tethered charge inherent in their protein structure. This "gating current" was finally recorded in 1973 by Armstrong and Bezanilla,[17] and we now recognize the S4 transmembrane segment as the structural motif of ion channel voltage dependence.

Application to the Cardiac Cell

With the new microelectrodes and the voltage clamp, cardiac electrophysiology entered a period of spectactular growth. Woodbury, having learned the Ling technique, collaborated with his brother and Hans Hecht to record in 1950 the frog heart AP.[18] At about the same time Weidmann and Coraboeuf,[19] fellows in Hodgkin's laboratory, having learned the microelectrode technique brought back from Chicago by Hodgkin, recorded the AP of a dog Purkinje fiber. Weidmann[20,21] in 1956 went on to demonstrate that the ionic basis for excitability was similar in the heart to that in squid nerve, and that the Na channel can be blocked by local anesthetic drugs. Hutter and Trautwein[22] recorded the diastolic depolarization characteristics of the pacemaker AP and showed the dramatic effects of vagal and sympathetic stimulation on the pacemaker rate. Noble[23] then showed in a computer model that a modification of the Hodgkin–Huxley kinetics for the Na channel and an inwardly-rectifying K channel, along with adjustment of Na and K leak paths, could generate an AP with a cardiac-like plateau.

Trautwein and colleagues[24] devised in 1964 a reasonable voltage clamp method for cardiac Purkinje fibers, and Reuter[25] used it to demonstrate for the first time that cardiac cells had excitatory calcium channels and that they were sensitive to adrenergic hormone. The voltage-dependent calcium current was then directly linked to the onset and magnitude of cardiac contraction.[26,27] Earl Sutherland's[28] discovery of the adrenergic signaling cascade via second messenger systems provided the basis for our present understanding of cellular modulation of ion channels. The dramatic dependence of cardiac contraction on both Na and Ca concentrations was solved by discovery of the Na/Ca exchange system.[29] We must remember that the AP exists not only to malfunction in arrhythmias but to activate and regulate cardiac contraction.

Although it was well known that cardiac cells behaved as if they are electrically and chemically coupled, allowing rapid conduction without synapses,[30] the structures responsible for the coupling were identified only much later.[31] These "gap junctions" are composed of clusters of channels that span the extracellular space between cells and allow both electrical and chemical transmission. They are also heavily modulated and influenced by disease, producing various levels of anisotropic conduction that provide some of the substrate for arrhythmia. They also are the structures involved in "healing over", the sealing of cell boundaries so that injury from infarct or a surgical scalpel does not propagate to the entire heart.

Parallel Clinical Advances

During this golden period of basic cardiac electrophysiology, major ideas were emerging on the clinical side. Lown[32] in 1962 helped develop the DC defibrillator, which was markedly better than the earlier AC defibrillator system. Implantable pacemakers began a long course of development into complex clinical tools, meanwhile contributing to our understanding of excitability. Kuller[33] described landmark studies of sudden death, showing that the dominant pathological process is obstructive coronary disease. Coronary Care Units (CCUs) were established because in-hospital mortality of acute myocardial infarction was 30–40%, and this specialized nursing and monitoring concept greatly enhanced our understanding of arrhythmias related to ischemia. Lown's battle cry of "Hearts too good to die!" was true in part, but the fact is that CCU arrhythmic death did not fall immediately with the use of lidocaine, but only gradually diminished as we found ways to relieve ischemia by improving coronary blood flow.[34] Mirowski's[35] idea of an implantable defibrillator began its long journey to standard clinical application. Scherlag and colleagues[36] initiated invasive electrophysiological studies in humas, beginning another long development path to invasive testing and ablation. Early versions of computerized real-time computer systems for arrhythmia monitoring were published.[37] It seems clear in retrospect that most advances in the clinical area were focused on treating very sick patients. They also were the product of medical engineering, rather than basic cardiac electrophysiology, although the background of electrical mechanisms was the essential framework for the engineering applications.

Clinical Trials

Cardiology was slow to employ the invaluable tool of randomized treatment trials, compared to infectious disease and oncology, and the first attempts with cholesterol-lowering strategies in the Coronary Drug Project were abject failures—the treatment arms showed higher mortality. But this was followed by a very successful trial of β-blockers after acute myocardial infarction.[38] It was clear that the mechanism of the β-blocker benefit was not via a direct antiarrhythmic effect, presaging the role of modulators of electrical activity. We also entered a period of great hope that powerful antiarrhythmic drugs would successfully prevent out-of-hospital sudden death, a hope that was dashed by the CAST study.[39] Pharmaceutical research efforts to develop more powerful ion channel-active drugs almost ceased at that point, although some recovery can now be seen.

Molecular Electrophysiology

In 1981 electrophysiology was ready to enter the molecular arena. Improvements to the electronics and use of polished micropipettes led Neher, Sakmann, and colleagues[40] to the ability to record single ion channel openings (gating of single molecules) and to voltage clamp single small cells. Now, it was possible to study single cardiac cells under high-quality voltage clamp. The next step was to determine the amino acid structure of ion channels and express them in heterologous systems. Tetrodotoxin as a high-affinity ligand for the voltage-gated Na channel was essential.[41] Following the lead of purification and cloning of the muscle acetylcholine receptor, the tritiated toxin was then used to purify the tiny amounts of Na channel protein found in eel electroplax (a relatively rich source) and with some amino acid sequencing an Na channel was cloned in 1984.[42] The Numa laboratory subsequently cloned three mammalian Na channels from the brain, and this was followed by the Rogart laboratory's cloning of the cardiac Na channel.[43] Cloning of the Shaker fruit fly potassium channel[44] was challenging, but it set the stage for cloning of the human cardiac KCNQ1 and HERG genes in the context of Long QT syndrome in 1995 by Keating and colleagues.[45,46] Many structural details of ion channels could be inferred from physiological experiments with cloned and mutated channels, providing us with a good picture of ion channel structure, but this is not a substitute for directly obtaining the channel structure from crystallography. This was finally achieved for a bacterial K channel by MacKinnon and colleagues.[47] Basic electrophysiology is now a mature science, with great clinical implications, as presented in this section and throughout this book.

Present Status of Basic Cardiac Electrophysiology

Electrical activity exists because of ion gradients and ion channels, and I think we have probably identified all of the mammalian primary players—the channels and pumps—except for some subunits. Most have been cloned and details of their molecular function are emerging, greatly helped by identification of the disease-related mutations discussed in later chapters. Physical structures of only a few are available, but this is likely to be resolved in the near future. We understand that the difference between normal and abnormal electrical activity is the fine balance between numbers of various ion channels/transporters, their function, and their location in the membrane. The function of these voltage-dependent processes is highly dependent on the interaction between the channels and transporters and their modulation by cytoplasmic systems. We are now experiencing an explosion of information from relating gene mutations in these primary players to cardiac electricity and arrhythmic disease.

In other critical areas our ignorance is immense. We have only tantalizing clues about regulation of transcription and translation of the relevant genes, posttranslational processing, and transport to and from the membrane. We are especially ignorant about the coordination of these processes to create an electrically balanced ensemble or to compensate for changes secondary to disease. Although enough of the cytoplasmic modulatory systems has been identified for us to realize their critical importance, there are likely to be many other modifier systems as yet undiscovered, and their interaction/interdependency challenges our ability to comprehend. This is an area where large-scale computer systems will be required.[48]

Gene therapy, defined as "fixing" a cardiac gene with a disease-producing mutation, is an appealing and logical clinical step. However, it turns out to be a daunting task, and is not likely to be an effective therapeutic tool in the near future. Nor are cardiac electrophysiologists suited to solving this problem. More promising, and more within reach of cardiac electrophysiologists, are approaches to adjust expression levels and to modulate function to restore electrical balance.

What Can the Cardiac Electrophysiology Community Do?

The critical question for cardiac electrophysiology has two components: sudden arrhythmic death in the general population and arrhythmic death in those with specific electrical disease. If we ask how to reduce sudden arrhythmic death in the general population, then the target is mainly those with ischemic heart disease and heart failure from other causes such as hypertension or cardiomyopathy. In spite of great progress managing arrhythmias, the incidence of sudden death continues to approach 20% of deaths in developed countries where adequate data are available, and a large fraction is in people who do not know they have cardiac disease.[49] The successes in the last several decades have come mainly from reduction or delay in onset of the underlying causative diseases, for example with the widespread use of statins and angiotensin-converting enzyme (ACE) inhibitors. Specific electrical diseases are relatively few in number now, and certainly this population will grow some. Clinical interventions such as ablation are often curative, but for potentially lethal arrhythmias the implanted defibrillator is only a stopgap therapy. The cardiac electrophysiology community can address several parts of a continued effort to control arrhythmia.

General Population Questions

This is the broad field of arrhythmias occurring in the course of various nonelectrical diseases:

1. Determine what polymorphisms in the genes of proteins responsible for electrical function predispose certain individuals to life-threatening arrhythmia. It is likely that soon typing of individual genomes will be cheap enough to use for screening, if we can determine what changes are important. The logic of this question is that perhaps half of individuals with these diseases die of arrhythmia before crippling loss of cardiac function. This question will require close cooperation between geneticists and electrophysiologists.
2. Devise simple and inexpensive electrical tests for predisposition to life-threatening arrhythmia. Many are available now, but they are too invasive and too expensive for application to the general population, and are not very accurate. Furthermore, this area does not represent the strength of basic electrophysiology. It is better to leave this to clinicians.
3. It now seems possible to imagine that cardiac cells can be regenerated. Although not directly cardiac electrophysiology, the field has an important role because regeneration must include balanced electrical function, or else the treatment

will terminate in lethal arrhythmia before any improved electrical or contractile function can be achieved.

4. Contribute to the explication of cardiac embryonic development that produces the congenital cardiac defects that predispose to arrhythmia. Although not central to this field of cardiac development, electrophysiologists can resolve mechanisms of these arrhythmias as background for better management or prevention. In particular, understanding the intrinsic genetic control of membrane expression of the array of electrically important molecules and the influence of extrinsic factors could provide the foundation for entirely new therapeutic approaches.

Electrical Disease Questions

The second kind of critical question is how to manage those electrical diseases that we can directly associate with malfunction of electrically important proteins. These include diseases associated with mutations of single genes, such as long QT syndrome, Brugada syndrome, catecholaminergic ventricular tachycardia, right ventricular dysplasia, familial cardiomyopathy, and others soon to be discovered. These monogenetic diseases so far identified represent only a small fraction of individuals at risk for lethal arrythmia, but they have been responsible for a huge increase in our understanding of arrythmic mechanisms.

1. Recognize that only a fraction of individuals with long QT syndrome, familial cardiomyopathy, Brugada syndrome, etc., have had a molecular mechanism identified. The search for causes must be broadened to factors that modulate electrical function. These other mechanisms, probably not mutations of ion channels or pumps, will be another important stimulus to a new understanding of electrical function. This requires a search broader than one focused only on channels and transporters.

2. Understand the complex interactions and functions of all of the molecular players in normal electrical function and the consequences of modification of them, especially those modulating excitability and intracellular calcium.

3. Resolve the structure–function of molecules critical for electrical function, as substrate for their modulation by ligands.

Summary

This brief historical review, with no less than nine Nobelists cited, shows cardiac electrophysiology to be in the mainstream of biomedical science. Progress has been closely tied to the development of new measurement methods and, recently, to our collaboration with the fields of genetics and molecular biology. Conceptual advances in the basic science will continue to depend on avoiding insularity and on exploitation of ideas and methods from the broad range of biomedical and biophysical science. Basic cardiac electrophysiology has also provided the foundation of some major clinical advances, but the shift over the last century from MD investigators to PhD investigators increases the importance of close communication with clinicians.

In spite of remarkable achievements, sudden arrhythmic death remains a massive problem With our new tools, as described in this basic science section, and with colleagues in other areas of science, cardiac electrophysiology has great opportunities for both basic insight and clinical relevance by focusing on the key questions.

Acknowledgment. Supported by RO1 HL65661.

References

1. Hille B. *Ion Channels of Excitable Membranes*, 3rd ed. Sunderland, MA: Sinauer Associates, 2001.
2. Einthoven W. Le télécardiogramme. *Arch Int Physiol* 1906;4:132–164.
3. Bernstein J. Über den zeitlichen Verlauf der negativen Schwankung des nervenstroms. *Arch Physiol* 1902;1:173–207.
4. Lucas K. The "all-or-none" contraction of amphibian skeletal muscle fibre. *J Physiol* 1908;38:113–133.
5. Adrian ED. The all-or-none principle in nerve. *J Physiol* 1913;47:460–474.
6. Mines GR. On dynamic equilibrium in the heart. *J Physiol* 1913;46:349–383.
7. Herrick JB. Clinical features of sudden obstruction of the coronary arteries. *JAMA* 1912;59:2015–2018.
8. Hodgkin AL. The Croonian lecture. Ionic movements and electrical activity in giant nerve fibres. *Proc R Soc Lond B Biol Sci* 1958;148:1–37.

9. Skou JC. The influence of some cations on an adenosine triphosphatase from peripheral nerve. *Biochim Biophys Acta* 1957;23:394–401.
10. Young JZ. Structure of nerve fibres and synapses in some invertebrates. *Cold Spring Harbor Symp Quant Biol* 1936;1:1–6.
11. Curtis HJ, Cole KS. Transverse electric impedance of the squid giant axon. *J Gen Physiol* 1938;21:757–765.
12. Hodgkin AL, Huxley AF Action potentials recorded from inside a nerve fibre. *Nature* 1939;144:710–711.
13. Hogg BM, Goss CM, Cole KS. Potentials in embryo rat heart muscle cultures. *Proc Soc Exp Biol Med* 193;32:304–307.
14. Hodgkin AL, Katz B. The effect of sodium ions on the electrical activity of the giant axon of the squid. *J Physiol* 1949;8:37–77.
15. Ling G, Gerard RW. The normal membrane potential of frog sartorius fibers. *J Cell Comp Physiol* 1949;34:383–396.
16. Hodgkin AL, Huxley AF. A quantitative description of membrane current and its application to conduction and excitation in nerve. *J Physiol* 1952; 117:500–544.
17. Armstrong CM, Bezanilla F. Currents related to movement of the gating particles of sodium channels. *Nature* 1973;242:459–461.
18. Woodbury LA, Woodbury JW, Hecht HH. Membrane resting and action potentials from single cardiac muscle fibers. *Circulation* 1950;1:265–266.
19. Coraboeuf E, Weidmann S. Potentiel de repos et potentiels d'action du muscle cardiaque, mesurés à l'aide d'électrodes intracellulaires. *Compt Rend* 1949;143:1329–1331.
20. Weidmann S. The effect of the cardiac membrane potential on the rapid availability of the sodium-carrying system. *J Physiol* 1955;127:213–224.
21. Weidmann S. Effects of calcium ions and local anesthetics on the electrical properties of Purkinje fibres. *J Physiol* 1955;129:568–582.
22. Hutter O, Trautwein W. Vagal and sympathetic effects on the pacemaker fibers in the sinus venosus of the heart. *J Gen Physiol* 1956;39:715–733.
23. Noble D. A modification of the Hodgkin-Huxley equations applicable to Purkinje fibre action and pace-maker potentials. *J Physiol* 1962;60:317–352.
24. Deck KA, Kern R, Trautwein W. Voltage clamp technique in mammalian cardiac fibres. *Pfluegers Arch* 1964;280:50–62.
25. Reuter H. The dependence of slow inward current in Purkinje fibres on the extracellular calcium concentration. *J Physiol* 1967;192:479–492.
26. Fozzard HA, HellamDC. Relationship between membrane voltage and tension in voltage-clamped cardiac Purkinje fibres. *Nature* 1968;218:588–589.
27. Morad M, Trautwein W. Effect of the duration of the action potential on contraction in the mammalian cardiac muscle. *Pfluegers Arch* 1968;299: 66–82.
28. Sutherland EW. Studies on the mechanism of hormone action. *Science* 1972;177:401–408.
29. Reuter H, Seitz H. The dependence of calcium flux from cardiac muscle on temperature and external ion concentration. *J Physiol* 1968;95:451–470.
30. Engelmann TW. Über die Leitung der Erregung im Herzmuskel. *Pfluegers Arch* 1877;1:465–480.
31. Barr L, Dewey MM, Berger W. Propagation of action potentials and the structure of the nexus in cardiac muscle. *J Gen Physiol* 1965;48:797–823.
32. Lown BR, Amarasingham R, Newman J. New method for terminating cardiac arrhythmias. *JAMA* 1962;182:548–555.
33. Kuller L. Sudden and unexpected non-traumatic deaths in adults: A review of epidemological and clinical studies. *J Chronic Dis* 1966;19:1165–1197.
34. Lie KI, Wellens HJ, van Capalle FJ, Durrer D. Lidocaine in the prevention of primary ventricular fibrillation. *N Engl J Med* 1974;291:1324–1326.
35. Mirowski M, Mower MM, Staewen WS, Tabatznik B, Mendeloff AI. Standby automatic defibrillator. *Arch Intern Med* 1970;126:158–161.
36. Scherlag BJ, Lau SH, Helfant RA, *et al.* Catheter technique for recording His bundle activity in man. *Circulation* 1969;39:13–18.
37. Cox JR, Nolle FM, Fozzard HA, *et al.* AZTEC, a preprocessing program for real-time ECG rhythm analysis. *IEEE Trans Biomed Eng* 1968;15:128–129.
38. Beta-Blocker Heart Attack Trial Research Group. A randomized trial of propranalol in patients with acute myocardial infarction. I. Mortality results. *JAMA* 1982;247:1707–1710.
39. CAST Investigators. Preliminary report: Effect of encainide and flecainide on mortality in a randomized trial of arrhythmia suppression after myocardial infarction. *N Engl J Med* 1989;321:406–412.
40. Hamill OP, Marty A, Neher E, *et al.* Improved patch-clamp techniques for high resolution current recording from cells and cell-free membrane patches. *Pfluegers Arch* 1981;391:85–100.
41. Narahashi T, Moore JW, Scott WR. Tetrodotoxin blockage of sodium conductance increase in lobster giant axons. *J Gen Physiol* 1964;47:965–974.
42. Noda M, Shimizu S, Tanabe T, *et al.* Primary structure of *Electrophorus electricus* sodium channel deduced from cDNA sequence. *Nature* 1984;312: 121–127.

43. Rogart RB, Cribbs LL, Muglia LK, *et al.* Molecular cloning of a putative tetrodotoxin resistant rat heart Na channel isoform. *Proc Natl Acad Sci USA* 1989;86:8170–8174.
44. Tempel BL, Papazian DM, Schwarz TL, *et al.* Sequence of a probable potassium channel component encoded at *Shaker* locus of *Drosophila*. *Science* 1987;237:770–775.
45. Curran ME, Splawski I, Timothy KW, *et al.* A molecular basis for cardiac arrhythmias: HERG mutations cause long QT syndrome. *Cell* 1995;80:795–803.
46. Wang Q, Curran ME, *et al.* Positional cloning of a novel potassium channel gene: KVLQT1 mutations cause cardiac arrhythmias. *Nat Genet* 1996;12:17–23.
47. Doyle DA, Morais Cabrall J, Pfuetzner RA, *et al.* The structure of the potassium channel. *Science* 1998; 280:69–77.
48. Gilman AG, Simon MI, Bourne HR, Harris BA, Long R, Ross EM, Stull JT, Taussig R, Bourne HR, Arkin AP, Cobb MH, Cyster JG, Devreotes PN, Ferrell JE, Fruman D, Gold M, Weiss A, Stull JT, Berridge MJ, Cantley LC, Catterall WA, Coughlin SR, Olson EN, Smith TF, Brugge JS, Botstein D, Dixon JE, Hunter T, Lefkowitz RJ, Pawson AJ, Sternberg PW, Varmus H, Subramaniam S, Sinkovits RS, Li J, Mock D, Ning Y, Saunders B, Sternweis PC, Hilgemann D, Scheuermann RH, DeCamp D, Hsueh R, Lin KM, Ni Y, Seaman WE, Simpson PC, O'Connell TD, Roach T, Simon MI, Choi S, Eversole-Cire P, Fraser I, Mumby MC, Zhao Y, Brekken D, Shu H, Meyer T, Chandy G, Heo WD, Liou J, O'Rourke N, Verghese M, Mumby SM, Han H, Brown HA, Forrester JS, Ivanova P, Milne SB, Casey PJ, Harden TK, Arkin AP, Doyle J, Gray ML, Meyer T, Michnick S, Schmidt MA, Toner M, Tsien RY, Natarajan M, Ranganathan R, Sambrano GR; Participating investigators and scientists of the Alliance for Cellular Signaling. Overview of the Alliance for Cellular Signaling. *Nature* 2002;420:703–706.
49. Myerberg RJ, Kessler KM, Castellanos A. Sudden cardiac death: Structure, function, and time-dependence of risk. *Circulation* 1992;85(Suppl. 1): 2–10.

1
Basic Physiology of Ion Channel Function

Isabelle Baró and Denis Escande†

Introduction

It is a common habit that the first chapter of a book on electrical diseases deals with the basic principle of cardiac cellular electrophysiology. It is also common behavior that readers (almost a rule if they are clinicians) skip this chapter to directly enter what they consider the heart of the matter: clinical rhythmology. However, skipping the first chapter would be a great mistake. In cardiac electrophysiology, there is a continuum of concept between the function of ion channel molecules and the clinical phenotype (Figure 1–1). As an example, it would be almost impossible to understand heritable or iatrogenic cardiac channelopathies without knowing what an action potential is and how it is formed. The beauty of cardiac electrophysiology is that it is the same elementary electrical signal arising from billion of single channel proteins that is summed up at the level of a single cell to generate action potentials and is also summed up in time and space to generate a surface electrocardiogram (EKG) signal. Thus cardiac electrophysiology offers the unique opportunity to obtain different levels of view of the same phenomenon either nanoscopically (at the level of a channel pore) or macroscopically (at the level of the whole organ). The present chapter aims to provide the clinical cardiologist specialized in arrhythmias with the very minimum that should be known about ion channel function to understand serenely the mechanisms generating these either acquired or inherited arrhythmias and the fundamentals of antiarrhythmic drug therapy.

† Deceased.

Basic Principles of Cardiac Electrophysiology: From Ion Channels to Ion Currents, Action Potentials, and EKG

Ion Channels

The cell membrane is made of lipids and as such is a perfectly hydrophobic milieu, which hydrophilic ions cannot directly cross. To penetrate the cell membrane, ions need to find hydrophilic pathways, which are formed by specialized proteins (the ion channels). It happens that the ion channel pathway is not permanently available, but inversely flips between an open and a closed state. Once a hydrophilic pathway is available (the channel is open), ions move passively across the cell membrane depending on their respective electrochemical gradient (Figure 1–2). If the gradient for a given ion species is directed inward then ions enter the cell. If the gradient is outward then ions leave the cell. "Electrochemical" means that two independent forces can move ions across the membrane: the electrical gradient and the chemical gradient. The chemical gradient makes ions move from a compartment of higher concentration to a compartment of lower concentration (according to their chemical gradient K^+ ions are keen to move from the intracellular to the extracellular compartment; inversely Na^+ ions are keen to move from the extracellular to the intracellular compartment). The electrical gradient makes ions move in the direction of their inverse sign (negative for a cation and positive for

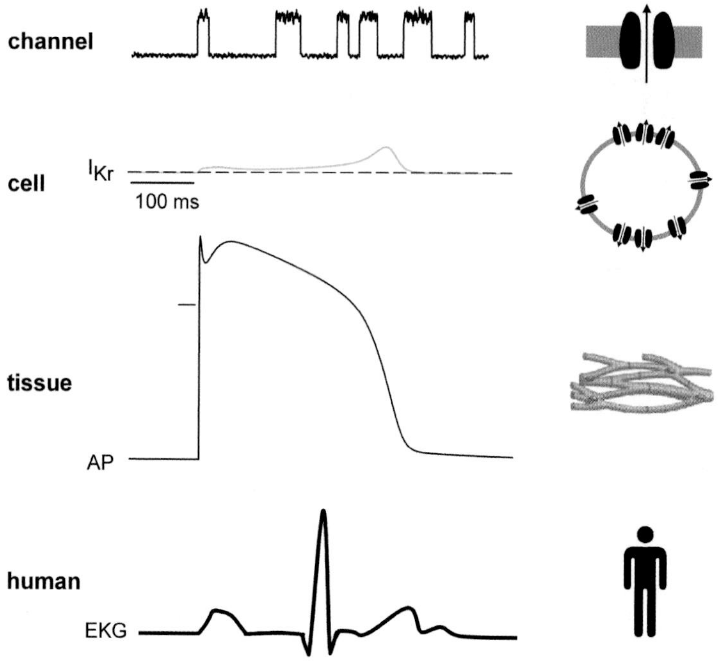

FIGURE 1–1. Schematic cardiac electrical activity, from molecule to patient. Channel: single channel current versus time recorded using the patch-clamp technique; upward inflection of the signal indicates outward current through a single channel. Cell: outward K^+ current through the open K^+ channels present on the cell membrane. Tissue: action potential resulting from the activity of all the different channels of a myocyte, recorded using the voltage-clamp technique. Human: EKG resuming the electrical activity of the different regions of the heart.

an anion). A negatively charged compartment (i.e., a compartment with a deficit in positive charges) will attract cations but reject anions. In some instances, the electrical gradient and the chemical gradient can oppose each other and eventually be equal; in this situation the force promoting the move of an ion in one direction equals that promoting its move in the reverse direction. An equilibrium is so reached. The electrical gradient depends on the transmembrane potential. Therefore, there is a transmembrane potential value for which the electrical gradient perfectly opposes the chemical gradient and permits the equilibrium of an ion species. In a cardiac cell, the equilibrium potential is around −98 mV for K^+ ions, i.e., at −98 mV (inside negative compared to the outside), the force related to the chemical gradient (directed outward) equals the force related to the electrical gradient (directed inward). The equilibrium (or reverse) potential for each ion species is given by the Nernst equation.*

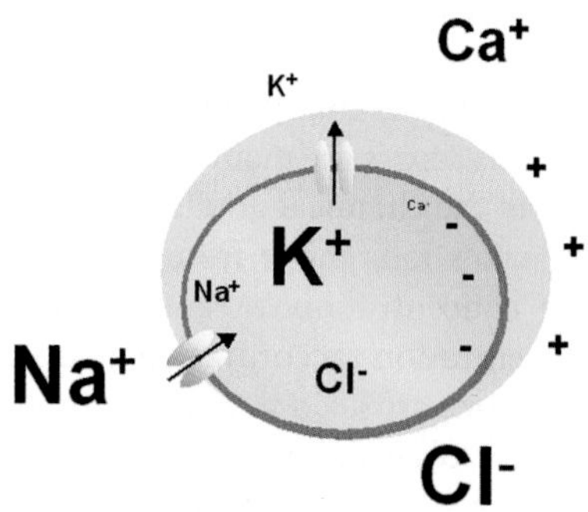

FIGURE 1–2. Schematic representation of the ion and electrical transmembrane gradient of the cardiomyocyte. Pole size is correlated with the ion concentration.

Membrane Resting Potential

A membrane that would exclusively conduct an ion species (i.e., K^+ ions), polarizes at the equilibrium potential for this ion species (i.e., −98 mV for K^+ ions). It happens that in a cardiac cell, the sodium–potassium pump enriches the cell with potassium and depletes the cell with sodium. It also happens that a cardiac cell at rest is

*$Ei = R\ T/zF$ ln(Extra [i]/Intra [i]) where Ei is the equilibrium potential for ion I, R the thermodynamic gas constant, T is the absolute temperature, z is the charge/valence of ion I, F is the Faraday constant (96485.309 C/mol), Extra [i] is the extracellular concentration of ion i, and Intra [i] is the intracellular concentration of ion i.

predominantly permeable to K^+ and thus the resting membrane potential of −80 mV is closed to the K^+ equilibrium potential. In general, a membrane potential depends on its relative permeability to the different ion species. During the action potential (see below), the cardiac membrane potential is no longer exclusively permeable to K^+ ions but is also permeable to other ion species and therefore diverges from −80 mV.

Ohm's Law

One cannot escape Ohm's law: $U = RI$ where U is the voltage, I is the current, and R is the resistance of the cell membrane. It means that currents generated by ion movements through ion channels surrounded by an electrical insulator (the cell membrane) affect the membrane potential depending on the membrane resistance. It happens that most ion channels expressed in the heart are voltage dependent, i.e., they open or close in relation to variations in the membrane voltage. In most cases, channels open when the cell depolarizes (inside less negative in relation to the outside). However, channel opening is not instantaneous but usually takes time (as much as hundreds of milliseconds in instances). Thus, most cardiac ion channels are both voltage and time dependent.

When an ion channel opens, it generates an ion current, which affects the voltage (Ohm's law). This is turn affects channel opening (voltage dependence) but not instantaneously (time dependence). Thus, the electrical activity of the cell should be considered in a tridimensional space: voltage, current, and time. If positively charged ions (i.e., cations) enter the cell, this movement creates an inward current that depolarizes the cell membrane (the inside is less negative). If positively charged ions leave the cell, this movement creates an outward current, which hyperpolarizes or repolarizes the cell membrane if previously depolarized (the inside is more negative).

Activation/Inactivation

Most cardiac ion channels are governed by two independent processes: activation and inactivation. The cardiac sodium channel is a caricature example (Figure 1–3). At the level of the resting

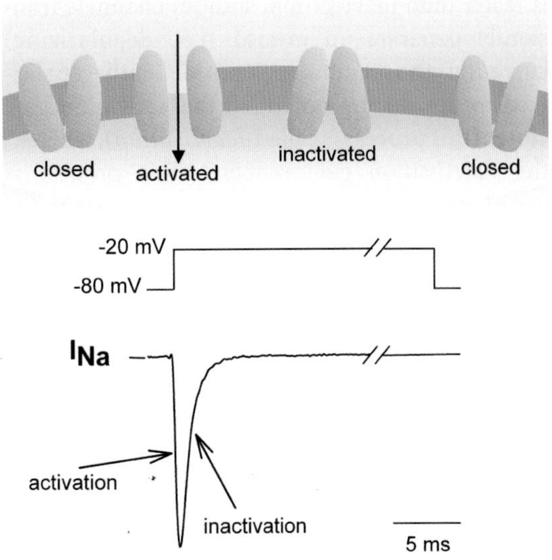

FIGURE 1–3. Activation and inactivation of the Na^+ current linked to the channel conformation. Schematic Na^+ current (bottom) recorded during a voltage pulse (middle). Activation of the current corresponds to an increasing number of Na^+ channels in the open conformation (top) due to the depolarization; inactivation corresponds to an increasing number of channels passed from the open to the inactivated conformation. Repolarization allows the inactivated channels to restore the closed conformation.

potential (−80 mV), the driving force for sodium ions is clearly in the inward direction (both electrical and chemical gradients are inwardly directed; the equilibrium potential for sodium ions is around +70 mV), but because sodium channels are permanently closed, no current is generated. If the transmembrane potential is brought to values more positive than say −60 mV, sodium channels open (voltage dependence). It is said that they *activate* (a current is generated). Activation is not instantaneous but takes a few milliseconds (time dependence). Sodium channel activation creates an inward current that further depolarizes the cell. This in turn further recruits sodium channel activation (positive feedback). The positive feedback loop is interrupted when Na^+ channels *inactivate.* Indeed, if the membrane stays depolarized, sodium channels do not remain open but close spontaneously. It is said they *inactivate,* a process that is independent of activation. Thus, in response to membrane depolarization, sodium channels undergo rapid *activation* and then (less) rapid *inactivation*. Because activation is faster than inactivation, sodium channels transiently generate an inward (i.e., depolarizing) current. If the membrane is subsequently repolarized to the resting potential, the activation gate closes (this process is called *deactivation*), whereas the inactivation gate reopens (this process is called *reactivation* or *removal of inactivation*): the channel is ready to open in response to a new depolarization stimulus.

Action Potential

Suppose that for a very few milliseconds the cell membrane is much more permeable to sodium than to potassium ions (a large number of Na^+ channels activates) (Figure 1–4). In this situation, the membrane potential is immediately attracted toward the equilibrium potential for Na^+ ions (about +70 mV). This occurs during the initial phase of the action potential (phase 0) where the membrane potential is abruptly driven to positive values (inside positive relative to outside). The membrane potential crosses the zero line (this is called an *overshoot*). Depolarization caused by activation of the Na^+ channel in turn activates other ion currents such as Ca^{2+} and K^+ currents (Figure 1–4), which have slower activation kinetics than Na^+ currents. Because the driving force for Ca^{2+} is inward (between 0 mV and the highly positive equilibrium potential for Ca^{2+} ions, chemical gradient attracts more Ca^{2+} into the cell than the electrical gradient limits its entry), activation of Ca^{2+} channels in response to depolarization generates an inward current, which maintains depolarization and (with other currents) creates the plateau phase of the action potential. Meanwhile, K^+ currents are also activated. In this depolarized state, the driving force for K^+ ions is outward (above 0 mV, both chemical and electrical gradients attract K^+ outside the cell). Activation of K^+ channels by membrane depolarization creates an outward current that tentatively repolarizes the cell membrane. During the plateau phase (phase 2), inward currents (mainly Ca^{2+}) equal outward currents (mainly K^+); the membrane potential is stable for a few tens of milliseconds. The Ca^{2+} current then progressively inactivates, whereas K^+ currents progressively activate, inducing the cell membrane to repolarize (between 0 mV and −98 mV the chemical gradient attracts more K^+ outside the cell than the electrical gradient retains it) toward the equilibrium potential of K^+, which is about −98 mV. From what is presented above, it can be understood that if Na^+ channels are made to open (i.e., the membrane potential is brought to values more positive than say −60 mV), an action potential is generated. The membrane potential is brought positive to −60 mV because an adjacent cell electrically connected through gap junctions undergoes its own action

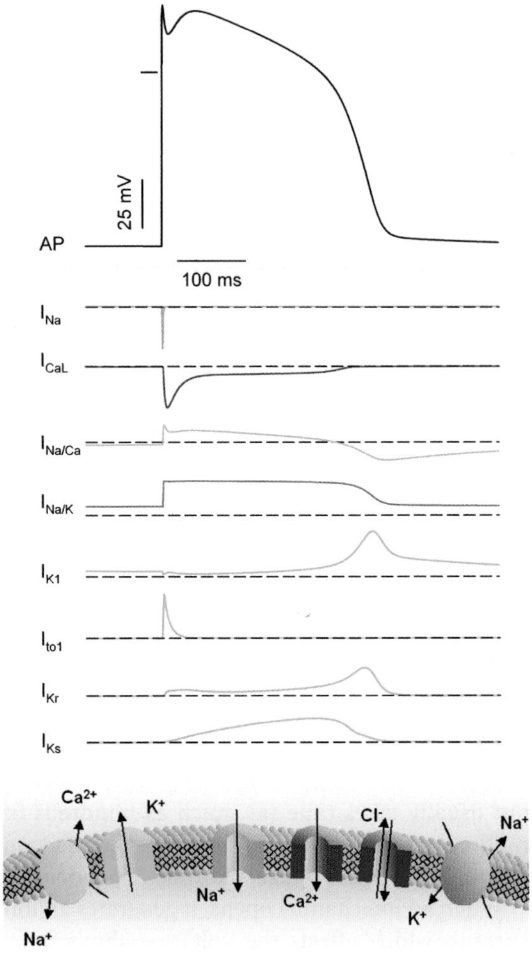

FIGURE 1–4. Schemes of the cardiac action potential and underlying ionic currents (top). This is a dynamic process: activation of the Na^+ channels generates the voltage upstroke, which activates the other ionic currents. In return, the action potential modulates the shape of the different currents. Bottom: the different ion channels and transporter species. Arrows represent the different current directions in the action potential voltage range.

potential process. From action potentials to action potentials in adjacent cells, the electrical signal is conducted from the sinus node down to the ventricular myocardium. The membrane potential can also be brought positive to −60 mV by an external stimulus (e.g., a pacemaker).

Theoretically, generating a cardiac action potential would require an Na^+ current, a Ca^{2+} current, and a K^+ current. This is clearly an oversimplification. Indeed, the cardiac cell expresses much more different ion currents. Concerning K^+ channels, for example, the human genome contains at least 75 genes encoding K^+ channels with different physiological characteristics of which about 35 are expressed in the human heart.[1–3] Thus, the cardiac action potential results from a very complex and finely tuned interplay of an ensemble of ion channels with different relationships to voltage and time. Only sophisticated computerization can approach the complexity of the cardiac action potential (see below).

Excitation–Contraction Coupling

Coupling between the electrical stimulus and contraction is ensured through movement of Ca^{2+} in and out of intracellular stores.[4] The main store for Ca^{2+} in a cardiac cell is the sarcoplasmic reticulum, where Ca^{2+} is buffered on specialized proteins such as calsequestrin. Diastolic free Ca^{2+} in the cytosol is maintained very low, in the order of 10^{-7} M. During the action potential, a small amount of Ca^{2+} entering the cell through L-type Ca^{2+} channels triggers the release of Ca^{2+} from the sarcoplasmic reticulum through Ca^{2+}-release channels (these are intracellular ion channels labeled by their high affinity for the alkaloid ryanodine) located in the sarcoplasmic reticulum membrane (Figure 1–5). This mechanism, called Ca^{2+}-induced Ca^{2+}-released, produces massive release of Ca^{2+} from the sarcoplasmic reticulum and invasion of the cytoplasm with free Ca^{2+}. Increased cytoplasmic Ca^{2+} binds to troponin, opening the myosin binding sites on filamentous actin, and force is produced. Decreased cytoplasmic Ca^{2+} resulting from its recapture in the sarcoplasmic reticulum by Ca^{2+}-ATPase located in the sarcoplasmic reticulum membrane produces relaxation. Because the system is in perfect equilibrium, the exact amount of Ca^{2+} that has entered the cell via L-type channels is now extruded out of the cell through the Na–Ca exchanger.

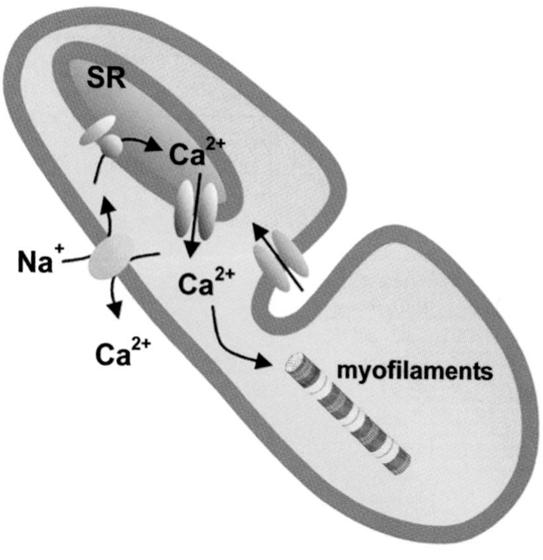

FIGURE 1–5. Schematic representation of the cellular mechanisms relating the action potential to cardiomyocyte contraction. Ca^{2+} enters into the cell when L-type Ca^{2+} channels are activated. The local intracellular Ca^{2+} concentration ($[Ca^{2+}]_i$) increase activates Ca^{2+}-dependent channels localized on the sarcoplasmic reticulum (SR) membrane (ryanodine receptors),which liberate further Ca^{2+} into the cytoplasm. A chain reaction induces a general $[Ca^{2+}]_i$ increase, which induces sarcomeric contraction. At the same time, it induces (1) the Ca^{2+}-dependent inactivation of the sarcolemmal L-type Ca^{2+} channels and (2) the repumping of the intracellular Ca^{2+} toward the sarcoplasmic reticulum (Ca^{2+}-ATPase) and outward to the myocyte (Na–Ca exchanger), resulting in a decrease in $[Ca^{2+}]_i$.

Specialized Tissues

Cardiac cells specialized in automaticity (e.g., nodal cells) or in conduction (e.g., Purkinje fibers) express a different repertoire of ion channels than regular myocardium[5,6] (Table 1–1). Consequently, their action potential has a different shape and characteristics (Figure 1–6). Automatic cells from the sinus node or from the atrioventricular node have a less polarized membrane potential because they express less background K^+ channels. Because of a less negative membrane potential, their Na^+ current is permanently inactivated and the depolarizing phase of their action potential relies on the activation of slow Ca^{2+} currents. As a consequence, the kinetics of the rising phase (a parameter

TABLE 1–1. Principal ionic currents, channels and auxiliary subunits, and genes expressed in the human heart.

		α-subunit or transporter		Auxilary subunit		
Current	Name	Name	Gene	Name	Gene	Remarks
I_{Na}	Na^+ current	Nav1.5	SCN5A	β1–β3	SCN1B–SCN3B	TTX insensitive channel
		Nav1.7	SCN9A			Channel in Purkinje fibers only
		Nav1.3	SCN3A			In atrial cells only
$I_{to\ fast}$	Fast transient outward K^+ current	Kv4.3	KCND3	KChiP2–KChaP	KCNIP2–PIAS3	KChiP2 gradient in ventricle
$I_{to\ slow}$	Slow transient outward K^+ current	Kv1.4	KCNA4	Kvβ1.2–Kvβ2	KCNAB1–KCNAB2	
I_{CaL}	L-type Ca^{2+} current	Cav1.2	CACNA1C	β2–α2δ1 and 2	CACNB2–CACNA2D1 and D2	Channel absent in ventricle
		Cav1.3	CACNA1D			
I_{CaT}	T-type Ca^{2+} current	Cav3.1	CACNA1G			Absent in ventricle
I_{Kr}	Fast delayed rectifier K^+ current	HERG	KCNH2	MiRP1?	KCNE2?	
I_{Ks}	Slow delayed rectifier K^+ current	KvLQT1	KCNQ1	minK (MiRP3)	KCNE1 (KCNE4)	Gradient in ventricle
I_{Kur}	Ultra-rapid outward K^+ current	Kv1.5	KCNA5	Kvβ1.2–Kvβ1.3	KCNAB1	Channel absent in ventricle
I_{K1}	Inward rectifier K^+ current	Kir2.1	KCNJ2			Mostly in ventricle, absent in node cells
		Kir2.2–Kir2.3	KCNJ12–KCNJ4			Absent in node cells
$I_{K,\ Ach}$	Acetylcholine-dependent K^+ current	Kir3.1–Kir3.4	KCNJ3–KCNJ5			Absent in ventricle
$I_{Na/K}$	Na-K pump current	Na-K pump	ATP1A			Responsible for K^+ and Na^+ gradient
$I_{Na/Ca}$	Na-Ca exchanger current	Na-Ca exchanger	SLC8A1			Contributes to Ca^{2+} gradient
I_f	Pacemaker current		HCN2–HCN4			In nodal tissue

that strongly influences conduction velocity) is much slower than in the myocardium. Another consequence of decreased K^+ current is slow depolarization of the cell membrane during diastole, allowing the membrane potential to spontaneously reach the activation voltage for Ca^{2+} current and thereafter to generate an automatic action potential. Inversely, cardiac cells specialized in

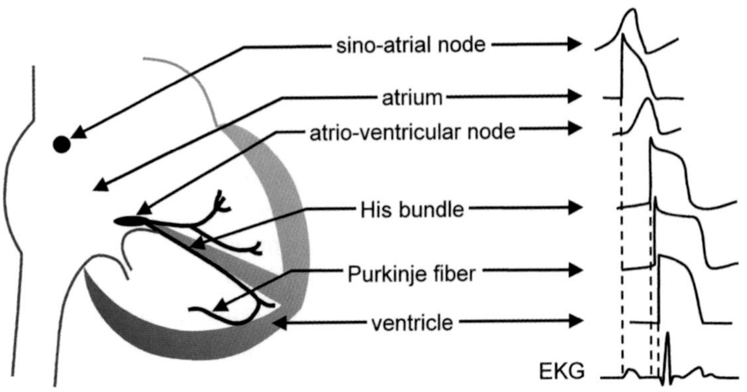

FIGURE 1–6. Schematic shapes of the action potentials of the different regions of the heart. Dotted lines correlate EKG events with the occurrence of different action potentials.

conduction have a faster rate of rise of phase 0 (*dV/dt* max) and a faster conduction velocity.

Surface EKG

As already stated in the introduction, the action potential results from the effects on membrane potential of a summation in time of individual channel opening and closing. Multiple action potentials arising from the different segments of the heart are integrated in time and space to generate the extracellular signal known as the surface EKG. Because of this continuum, it might be expected that an alteration in a channel function traduces itself into an anomaly of the action potential shape and finally in the surface EKG. The long QT syndrome is such a situation where a loss-of-function mutation in a K^+ channel gene involved in cardiac repolarization prolongs the action potential duration (less net outward current is available to repolarize the cell membrane) and prolongs the QT interval.

Gene Correlates for Cardiac Ion Channels

The vast majority of the genes encoding cardiac ion channels have been identified and precisely assigned to a chromosomal region. Most ion channel proteins share a common signature. For example, the large potassium channel protein family has two, four, or six transmembrane segments. Voltage-gated K^+ channels possess six transmembrane segments,[1] whereas inward rectifiers[2,3] (this label refers to their capacity to conduct more easily ions in the inward than in the outward direction), which are considered as time independent, have only two transmembrane segments. Six- and two-transmembrane segment K^+ channels share a common pore structure identified by the canonical GYG signature. In 1998, Rod MacKinnon published the structure of a potassium channel obtained by X-ray diffraction studies of a potassium channel crystal and was awarded the 2003 Nobel price in chemistry for his work.[7,8]

Expression of recombinant foreign channel proteins in host cell systems (see below) as well as genetic invalidation of ion channel genes in the mouse have been instrumental in correlating cardiac ion channels (and ion currents) with their encoding genes. In addition, these investigations have also shown that ion channels are often formed by the assembly of α-subunits (the channel pore itself) and β-subunits (an associated protein encoded by a distinct gene that regulates α-subunits) and in occasion with γ- or δ-subunits (see Table 1–1). In general, it is more and more clear that ion channels are not expressed in isolation in the cell membrane but rather in concert with other regulatory proteins within a channel complex. Identification of missing members of the ion channel complex is the subject of active research in various laboratories with the objective of targeting novel candidate genes for cardiac channelopathies.

Technologies to Explore Cardiac Cellular Electrophysiology

Although the first recording of a cardiac action potential was obtained about 50 years ago,[9] it is the discovery and development of the patch-clamp technique (which brought the Nobel prize of medicine to E. Neher and B. Sakman in 1991) that have been the key to our understanding of cardiac cellular electrophysiology.[10,11] The technique is applied to isolated cells either freshly dissociated from cardiac tissues or maintained in culture. Depending on the configuration used, the patch-clamp technique can record the electrical activity of a single channel molecule (amplitudes of a single channel current are in the order of $1\,pA = 10^{-12}\,A$) or the electrical activity of the ensemble of channel protein expressed in a whole cell (current amplitudes may be in the order of $1\,nA = 10^{-9}\,A$). At the level of a single protein recording, the channel appears in a binary situation either closed or open. Voltage-dependent activation is visible because the channel spends more time in the open configuration and thus less time in the closed configuration in response to a voltage step (usually depolarizing). Inactivation is also visible as a progressive decrease in channel firing with time at a stable voltage (see Figure 1–3). In the current-clamp mode, variations in the voltage (action potentials) are measured, whereas in the voltage-clamp mode, ion currents are measured.

Another major technical step in cardiac electrophysiology has been inherited from molecular biology techniques and relates to our capacity to enable host cells (e.g., COS or HEK cells) maintained in culture to express foreign genes. Cells are transfected with ion channel cDNA using routine nonviral methods and then patch-clamped after 24–48 h in culture. Recombinant ion channel proteins (in particular of human origin) are available for physiological and pharmacological investigations.[12] Site directed mutagenesis permits investigations of mutated constructs shading light into genotype–phenotype relations.[13]

Genetic manipulation of ion channel genes and regulators has been successfully achieved in the mouse with either overexpression[14,15] or invalidation of target channels.[16,17] Development of *in vivo* electrophysiological methods adapted to the very small size of this animal (a mouse heart is about 100 mg) has provided investigation capacities similar to those in humans.[18]

More recently, the genomics of ion channel genes has provided information on ion channel expression at a genome scale in various physiological and physiopathological situations.[19]

Cardiac Cellular Electrophysiology of the Human Heart

The patch-clamp technique applied to single cells dissociated from cardiac biopsies sampled during open-heart surgery in association with molecular biology techniques has provided an impressive body of information on the cellular electrophysiology of the human heart.

At the atrial level, the human action potential is initiated by a fast-activating fast-inactivating Na^+ current carried by Nav1.5 channels (encoded by the *SCN5A* gene) in association with its β1 subunit (*SCN1B*).[20,21] Other Na^+ channel α-subunits including Nav1.3 (*SCN3A*),[22] Nav2.1 (*SCN6A*),[23] and β-subunits (*SCN3B*)[24] are also expressed in the human atrium, although at a much lower level than Nav1.5, which is by far the predominant cardiac Na^+ channel. The Nav1.5-carried Na^+ current is responsible for the upstroke of the action potential (phase 0) and carries energy for fast conduction in the atrium. Fast depolarization triggers the activation of transient outward and inward currents. The transient outward current produces initial repolarization of the action potential and a clearly visible notch inscribed prior to the AP plateau. Transient outward current is made predominantly by the Kv4.3 channel (*KCND3*)[25] in association with its regulatory β-subunit KChiP2.[26] Because inactivation of the transient outward current is fast, this current determines the level of the plateau phase and therefore influences the activation of other currents but does not directly influence phase 3 repolarization kinetics. Transient Ca^{2+} currents provide inward current to maintain the depolarized cell during the plateau. Two types of Ca^{2+} currents are operative: L-type (long lasting), which are targets for calcium channel blockers, and T-type (fast inactivated). L-type Ca^{2+} currents are predominantly carried by Cav1.2 (*CACNA1C*)[27] and to a much lower extent by Cav1.3 (*CACNA1D*)[28] channels in conjunction with their auxiliary subunits: Cavβ2,[27] Cavα2δ2,[29] and Cavα2δ1.[30] T-type Ca^{2+} currents are brought by Cav3.1 channels (*CACNA1G*).[31] Repolarization of the action potential (phase 3) is initiated by the delayed rectifier K^+ current, which has two components: a fast activating component termed I_{Kr}, which is carried by HERG channels,[32] and a slow component I_{Ks}, which is carried by KvLQT1 (*KCNQ1*) channels in association with the regulatory β-subunit minK (*KCNE1*).[33] An ultrarapid K^+ current (activation is 2-fold faster than I_{Kr}) is specific of the atrium in human and is carried by Kv1.5 channels (*KCNA5*).[34,35] Final repolarization is achieved by background time-independent currents (also called inward rectifiers), which are also responsible for maintaining a negative membrane polarization during diastole. Kir2.1 channels (*KCNJ2*) are less abundant than in the ventricle, accounting for the less negative resting potential in the atrium.[36] Atrial myocytes also express Kir2.2 and Kir2.3 channels (*KCNJ12* and *KCNJ4*). Specific to the atrium are Kir3.1 and Kir3.4 channels (*KCNJ3* and *KCNJ5*), which open in response to cholinergic stimulation and shorten the duration of the action potential.[32] Other background K^+ currents include TWIK1 (*KCNK1*)[36] and TASK1 (*KCNK3*)[37] currents. Other currents are related to the Na–K pump (*ATP1A1*),[38] which generates an outward current, and the Na–Ca exchanger (*SLC8A1*), which generates an inward current and helps maintain the plateau. The role of chloride channels in the human heart has still not been ascertained. The electrical connection between cells is ensured by the expression of connexin channel proteins. Connexin 40 (*GJA5*) is specific to the atrium. Cx43 (*GJA1*) and Cx45 (*GJA7*) are also expressed in this tissue.[39]

The ventricular action potential shape differs from that of the atrium. In particular, the initial repolarization phase is less pronounced, the plateau phase is more positive, and phase 3 repolarization is more rapid. As in the atrium, there is no spontaneous depolarization in the contractile myocardium. The ventricle exhibits almost no ultrarapid K^+ current (Kv1.5 channels)[40,41] or T-type Ca^{2+} current.[42] Similarly, Kir3.1 or Kir3.4 channels, which are activated under acetylcholine, are not expressed, whereas the background K^+ current (Kir2.1 channels) is more prominent in comparison with the atrium.[36] Consistent differences are seen between the endocardium and the epicardium with a more pronounced initial repolarization attributed to transient outward current in the epicardium.[43] These differences, which are crucial for the inscription of normal EKG waves, have been linked to a greater KChiP2 expression in the epicardium with no Kv4.3 transmural gradient.[44] Cx40 is not expressed in the regular ventricular myocardium.[39]

Much less information is available on the cellular electrophysiology of specialized regions of the human heart, and most of our knowledge has been obtained from animal models. Action potentials from the sinus node (SAN) have relatively less negative maximum diastolic potential (about −55 mV), a slow rate of rise, and a spontaneous diastolic depolarization than the origin of cardiac automatism. Cholinergic and β-adrenergic stimulations slow and accelerate the spontaneous sinus node, respectively. Many different ion currents are responsible for pacemaking activity with this redundancy being considered as a security system. Cells from the SAN express an inward current that activates when the cell repolarizes. This inward current, sometime called the pacemaker current, is related to the specific expression of HCN channels (*HCN1* and *HCN4* genes).[45,46] Other currents that contribute to depolarizing the cell during diastole including L-type Ca^{2+} currents (*CACNA1D and CACNA1C*), T-type Ca^{2+} current (*CACNA1G*),[6,47] and a delayed rectifier K^+ current that progressively deactivates during diastole (likely made of HERG, KvLQT1, and minK expression).[48–50] Partial depolarization of automatic cells is explained on the basis of the low expression of background Kir2.1 channels (*KCNJ2*).[50,51] Kir3.1 and Kir3.4 channels provide an additional outward current when activated by acetylcholine, leaving less net inward current for diastolic depolarization and thereafter producing bradycardia.[46,52,53] Cholinergic stimulation also decreases the availability of L-type Ca^{2+} channels.[54] β-adrenergic stimulation increases the L-type Ca^{2+} current amplitude[55] and facilitates the activation of HCN channels during repolarization.[56]

The main function of the atrioventricular (AV) node is to slow conduction at the AV junction so as to create a delay between atrium and ventricular contraction. Atrioventricular node cells also have postrepolarization refractoriness, which limits the number of impulses that can activate the ventricle. Finally, AV node cells are the place for accessory pacemaking when the sinus node fails to ensure automatism. These node cells have a faster rate of rise of the action potential than SAN cells, although this value remains much lower in the AV node than in the regular myocardium. As in the SAN, automatism in the AV node is achieved through the expression of specialized channels such as HCN channels.[46] Among delayed rectifiers, I_{Kr} predominates over I_{Ks}.[57] As in the SAN, there is little background K^+ current in the AV node.[58] Also as in the SAN, the AV node expresses more Cav1.3 channels and less KChiP2 and Kv4.x channels than the regular myocardium.[46]

Cardiac cells specialized in conduction belongs to the His-Purkinje system. They have a more negative resting potential than contractile fibers and a greater maximum rate of rise of depolarization. The plateau potential is more negative and the action potential is longer than in the ventricular myocardium.[59] In addition, Purkinje fibers show spontaneous diastolic depolarization responsible for the idioventricular rhythm during atrioventricular dissociation. Human Purkinje fibers express less Cav1.2 (unpublished data), more Cx40, but less Cx43 than regular myocardium.[60] KChiP2 is almost undetectable, whereas Kv4.3 channels are more expressed than in the ventricle (unpublished data). Kir2.1 and Kir2.2 are lower than in the ventricle, whereas TWIK1 is higher (unpublished data).

Cardiac Cellular Electrophysiology in Other Mammalians

Because in the obvious difficulties in obtaining undiseased human myocardial cells, most electrophysiological and electropharmacological studies have been conducted in animal models. However, the human cardiac cell electrophysiology is unique and clearly differs from that of other mammals. This is seen when a comparison is made with the mouse, a model that has became very popular because of the possibilities offered to manipulate its genome. A mouse heart beats 600 times per minutes, i.e., 10 times faster than a human heart. Accordingly, the mouse has a very abbreviated action potential with virtually no plateau phase.[61] A mouse does not express sizable delayed rectifier (I_{Ks} and I_{Kr})[62] but relies mainly on transient outward currents (Kv4.2 in association with KChiP2 but also Kv1.5 and Kv2.1 channels) to ensure repolarization.[63–65] Thus, the mouse is not an adequate model for human pathology when repolarization is concerned. Inversely, depolarization and conduction have comparable characteristics in the mouse and human hearts.[66] I_{Ks} and I_{Kr} are easily recorded in the guinea pig heart with $I_{Ks} > I_{Kr}$ (the reverse than in human).[67,68] Guinea pigs and pigs inversely express almost no transient outward current.[69,70] The dog has a large endocardium-to-epicardium transient outward current gradient similar to humans, although the biophysical characteristics of this current differ significantly between the two species.[71]

As a consequence, there is no single species that can be used as a convincing model of the human heart. Depending on the problem under study, a different model could be chosen. As an example, ventricular transmural differences in ion channel expression and function are convincingly recapitulated in the dog but not in the mouse.[44,72] In spite of the pronounced differences between the human and mouse heart, a tremendous amount of valuable information has been obtained in this latter species. Finally, it should be kept in mind that *Drosophila* has been the key to identifying the multiple families of K^+ channel genes that later appeared as largely conserved during the evolution from *Drosophila* to human.[73]

Computer Models of Cardiac Cellular Electrophysiology

Each ion current is characterized by its amplitude and relation to voltage and time (activation, deactivation, inactivation, reactivation, etc.) and therefore can be fully described by series of equations and parameters. If the equations and parameters for every ion current expressed in the heart are entered into a computer, a normal action potential can be reconstituted that is related to rate or interpolated stimulus very similar to biological data. Such a complex computerization has been achieved for several animal models[74–77] and for the human atrium[78,79] and ventricle.[80–82] These models have proved of tremendous value not only in understanding the role of each single ion channel function in the global electrical activity of a cell but also, and most importantly, in inferring the consequences of subtle changes in ion current characteristics (as produced, for example, by genetically inherited mutations or drugs). As a matter of fact, the impact of alterations in the characteristics from one ion current to other ion channels contributing to generate the action potential is so complex that it cannot be accurately deduced by a humans without the help of a computer. The computerized action potentials from different cells can also be integrated in two- or three-dimensional thin layers approaching the geometry of the normal heart to reconstitute its global activity on a computerized electrocardiogram.[81]

Conclusion

After decades of electrophysiological studies on animal and human cardiac tissues, many aspects of the molecular basis for cardiac electrogenesis have been unveiled. Although much knowledge of human ionic currents has been gathered, data from human cardiac nodes and conducting tissues are still missing and direct extrapolations from animal data may be hazardous. Furthermore, despite the sequencing of the human genome, a function assignment for every predicted protein is far from being achieved. As a consequence, the list of yet identified channel auxiliary proteins is largely incomplete. The quest for the Holy Grail assumes that knowledge of every member of the orchestra would provide access to the global cardiac symphony.

References

1. Nerbonne JM, Guo W. Heterogeneous expression of voltage-gated potassium channels in the heart: Roles in normal excitation and arrhythmias. *J Cardiovasc Electrophysiol* 2002;13:406–409.
2. Dhamoon AS, Jalife J. The inward rectifier current (I_{K1}) controls cardiac excitability and is involved in arrhythmogenesis. *Heart Rhythm* 2005;2:316–324.
3. Kurachi Y, Ishii M. Cell signal control of the G protein-gated potassium channel and its subcellular localization. *J Physiol* 2004;554:285–294.
4. Song LS, Guatimosim S, Gomez-Viquez L, *et al.* Calcium biology of the transverse tubules in heart. *Ann NY Acad Sci* 2005;1047:99–111.
5. Schram G, Pourrier M, Melnyk P, *et al.* Differential distribution of cardiac ion channel expression as a basis for regional specialization in electrical function. *Circ Res* 2002; 90:939–950.
6. Mangoni ME, Couette B, Marger L, *et al.* Voltage-dependent calcium channels and cardiac pacemaker activity: From ionic currents to genes. *Prog Biophys Mol Biol* 2006;90:38–63.
7. Doyle DA, Morais Cabral J, Pfuetzner RA, *et al.* The structure of the potassium channel: Molecular basis of K^+ conduction and selectivity. *Science* 1998;280:69–77.
8. Long SB, Campbell EB, MacKinnon R. Crystal structure of a mammalian voltage-dependent Shaker family K^+ channel. *Science* 2005; 309:897–903.
9. Coraboeuf E, Weidmann S. Potentiel de repos et potentiels d'action du muscle cardiaque, mesurés à l'aide d'électrodes internes. *C R Séances Soc Biol* 1949;143:1329–1331.
10. Neher E, Sakmann B. Single-channel currents recorded from membrane of denervated frog muscle fibres. *Nature* 1976;260:799–802.
11. Hamill OP, Marty A, Neher E, *et al.* Improved patch-clamp techniques for high-resolution current recording from cells and cell-free membrane patches. *Pflügers Arch* 1981;391:85–100.
12. Bellocq C, Wilders R, Schott JJ, *et al.* A common antitussive drug, clobutinol, precipitates the long QT syndrome 2. *Mol Pharmacol* 2004;66:1093–1102.
13. Mohammad-Panah R, Demolombe S, Neyroud N, *et al.* Mutations in a dominant-negative isoform correlate with phenotype in inherited cardiac arrhythmias. *Am J Hum Genet* 1999;64:1015–1023.
14. Nerbonne JM, Nichols CG, Schwarz TL, *et al.* Genetic manipulation of cardiac K^+ channel function in mice: What have we learned, and where do we go from here? *Circ Res* 2001;89:944–956.
15. Royer A, Demolombe S, El Harchi A, *et al.* Expression of human ERG K^+ channels in the mouse heart exerts anti-arrhythmic activity. *Cardiovasc Res* 2005;65:128–137.
16. Papadatos GA, Wallerstein PM, Head CE, *et al.* Slowed conduction and ventricular tachycardia after targeted disruption of the cardiac sodium channel gene Scn5a. *Proc Natl Acad Sci USA* 2002; 99:6210–6215.
17. Royer A, van Veen TA, Le Bouter S, *et al.* Mouse model of SCN5A-linked hereditary Lenègre's disease: Age-related conduction slowing and myocardial fibrosis. *Circulation* 2005;111:1738–1746.
18. Berul CI. Electrophysiological phenotyping in genetically engineered mice. *Physiol Genomics* 2003;13: 207–216.
19. Demolombe S, Marionneau C, Le Bouter S, *et al.* Functional genomics of cardiac ion channel genes. *Cardiovasc Res* 2005;67:438–447.
20. Gellens ME, George AL Jr, Chen LQ, *et al.* Primary structure and functional expression of the human cardiac tetrodotoxin-insensitive voltage-dependent sodium channel. *Proc Natl Acad Sci USA* 1992; 89:554–558.
21. Makita N, Bennett PB Jr, George AL Jr. Voltage-gated Na^+ channel beta 1 subunit mRNA expressed in adult human skeletal muscle, heart, and brain is encoded by a single gene. *J Biol Chem* 1994;269:7571–7578.
22. Thimmapaya R, Neelands T, Niforatos W, *et al.* Distribution and functional characterization of human Nav1.3 splice variants. *Eur J Neurosci* 2005; 22:1–9.
23. George AL Jr, Knittle TJ, Tamkun MM. Molecular cloning of an atypical voltage-gated sodium channel expressed in human heart and uterus: Evidence for a distinct gene family. *Proc Natl Acad Sci USA* 1992;89:4893–4897.
24. Stevens EB, Cox PJ, Shah BS, *et al.* Tissue distribution and functional expression of the human voltage-gated sodium channel beta3 subunit. *Pflügers Arch* 2001; 441:481–488.
25. Wang Z, Feng J, Shi H, *et al.* Potential molecular basis of different physiological properties of the transient outward K^+ current in rabbit and human atrial myocytes. *Circ Res* 1999;84:551–561.

26. Decher N, Uyguner O, Scherer CR, *et al.* hKChIP2 is a functional modifier of hKv4.3 potassium channels: Cloning and expression of a short hKChIP2 splice variant. *Cardiovasc Res* 2001;52:255–264.
27. Schotten U, Haase H, Frechen D, *et al.* The L-type Ca^{2+}-channel subunits alpha1C and beta2 are not downregulated in atrial myocardium of patients with chronic atrial fibrillation. *J Mol Cell Cardiol* 2003;35:437–443.
28. Qu Y, Baroudi G, Yue Y, *et al.* Novel molecular mechanism involving alpha1D (Cav1.3) L-type calcium channel in autoimmune-associated sinus bradycardia. *Circulation* 2005;111:3034–3041.
29. Gao B, Sekido Y, Maximov A, *et al.* Functional properties of a new voltage-dependent calcium channel alpha2delta auxiliary subunit gene (CACNA2D2). *J Biol Chem* 2000;275:12237–12242.
30. Grammer JB, Zeng X, Bosch RF, *et al.* Atrial L-type Ca^{2+}-channel, beta-adrenoreceptor, and 5-hydroxytryptamine type 4 receptor mRNAs in human atrial fibrillation. *Basic Res Cardiol* 2001;96:82–90.
31. Monteil A, Chemin J, Bourinet E, *et al.* Molecular and functional properties of the human alpha1G subunit that forms T-type calcium channels. *J Biol Chem* 2000;275:6090–6100.
32. Brundel BJ, Van Gelder IC, Henning RH, *et al.* Alterations in potassium channel gene expression in atria of patients with persistent and paroxysmal atrial fibrillation: Differential regulation of protein and mRNA levels for K^+ channels. *J Am Coll Cardiol* 2001;37:926–932.
33. Bendahhou S, Marionneau C, Haurogné K, *et al.* In vitro molecular interactions and distribution of KCNE family with KCNQ1 in the human heart. *Cardiovasc Res* 2005;67:529–538.
34. Feng J, Wible B, Li GR, *et al.* Antisense oligodeoxynucleotides directed against Kv1.5 mRNA specifically inhibit ultrarapid delayed rectifier K^+ current in cultured adult human atrial myocytes. *Circ Res* 1997;80:572–579.
35. Bertaso F, Sharpe CC, Hendry BM, *et al.* Expression of voltage-gated K^+ channels in human atrium. *Basic Res Cardiol* 2002;97:424–433.
36. Wang Z, Yue L, White M, *et al.* Differential distribution of inward rectifier potassium channel transcripts in human atrium versus ventricle. *Circulation* 1998;98:2422–2428.
37. Duprat F, Lesage F, Fink M, *et al.* TASK, a human background K^+ channel to sense external pH variations near physiological pH. *EMBO J* 1997;16:5464–5471.
38. Wang J, Schwinger RH, Frank K, *et al.* Regional expression of sodium pump subunits isoforms and Na^+-Ca^{++} exchanger in the human heart. *J Clin Invest* 1996;98:1650–1658.
39. Vozzi C, Dupont E, Coppen SR, *et al.* Chamber-related differences in connexin expression in the human heart. *J Mol Cell Cardiol* 1999;31:991–1003.
40. Li GR, Feng J, Yue L, *et al.* Evidence for two components of delayed rectifier K^+ current in human ventricular myocytes. *Circ Res* 1996;78:689–696.
41. Ordog B, Brutyo E, Puskas LG, *et al.* Gene expression profiling of human cardiac potassium and sodium channels. *Int J Cardiol* 2006;111:386–393
42. Richard S, Leclercq F, Lemaire S, *et al.* Ca^{2+} currents in compensated hypertrophy and heart failure. *Cardiovasc Res* 1998;37:300–311.
43. Antzelevitch C, Fish J. Electrical heterogeneity within the ventricular wall. *Basic Res Cardiol* 2001; 96:517–527.
44. Rosati B, Pan Z, Lypen S, *et al.* Regulation of KChIP2 potassium channel beta subunit gene expression underlies the gradient of transient outward current in canine and human ventricle. *J Physiol* 2001;533: 119–125.
45. Shi W, Wymore R, Yu H, *et al.* Distribution and prevalence of hyperpolarization-activated cation channel (HCN) mRNA expression in cardiac tissues. *Circ Res* 1999;85:e1–6.
46. Marionneau C, Couette B, Liu J, *et al.* Specific pattern of ionic channel gene expression associated with pacemaker activity in the mouse heart. *J Physiol* 2005;562:223–234.
47. Hagiwara N, Irisawa H, Kameyama M. Contribution of two types of calcium currents to the pacemaker potentials of rabbit sino-atrial node cells. *J Physiol* 1988;395:233–253.
48. Brahmajothi MV, Morales MJ, Reimer KA, *et al.* Regional localization of ERG, the channel protein responsible for the rapid component of the delayed rectifier, K^+ current in the ferret heart. *Circ Res* 1997;81:128–135.
49. Wymore RS, Gintant GA, Wymore RT, *et al.* Tissue and species distribution of mRNA for the I_{Kr}-like K^+ channel, ERG. *Circ Res* 1997;80:261–268.
50. Brahmajothi MV, Morales MJ, Liu S, *et al.* In situ hybridization reveals extensive diversity of K^+ channel mRNA in isolated ferret cardiac myocytes. *Circ Res* 1996;78:1083–1089.
51. Satoh H. Sino-atrial nodal cells of mammalian hearts: Ionic currents and gene expression of pacemaker ionic channels. *J Smooth Muscle Res* 2003; 39:175–193.
52. Dobrzynski H, Marples DD, Musa H, *et al.* Distribution of the muscarinic K^+ channel proteins Kir3.1 and Kir3.4 in the ventricle, atrium, and sinoatrial node of heart. *J Histochem Cytochem* 2001;49:1221–1234.

53. Wickman K, Nemec J, Gendler SJ, *et al.* Abnormal heart rate regulation in GIRK4 knockout mice. *Neuron* 1998;20:103–114.
54. Petit-Jacques J, Bois P, Bescond J, *et al.* Mechanism of muscarinic control of the high-threshold calcium current in rabbit sino-atrial node myocytes. *Pflügers Arch* 1993;423:21–27.
55. Mangoni ME, Couette B, Bourinet E, *et al.* Functional role of L-type Cav1.3 Ca^{2+} channels in cardiac pacemaker activity. *Proc Natl Acad Sci USA* 2003;100:5543–5548.
56. DiFrancesco D, Mangoni M. Modulation of single hyperpolarization-activated channels (I_f) by cAMP in the rabbit sino-atrial node. *J Physiol* 1994;474: 473–482.
57. Mitcheson JS, Hancox JC. An investigation of the role played by the E-4031-sensitive (rapid delayed rectifier) potassium current in isolated rabbit atrioventricular nodal and ventricular myocytes. *Pflügers Arch* 1999;438:843–850.
58. Noma A, Nakayama T, Kurachi Y, *et al.* Resting K conductances in pacemaker and non-pacemaker heart cells of the rabbit. *Jpn J Physiol* 1984;34:245–254.
59. Dangman KH, Danilo P Jr, Hordof AJ, *et al.* Electrophysiologic characteristics of human ventricular and Purkinje fibers. *Circulation* 1982;65:362–368.
60. Davis LM, Rodefeld ME, Green K, *et al.* Gap junction protein phenotypes of the human heart and conduction system. *J Cardiovasc Electrophysiol* 1995;6:813–822.
61. Nerbonne JM. Studying cardiac arrhythmias in the mouse–a reasonable model for probing mechanisms? *Trends Cardiovasc Med* 2004;14:83–93.
62. Xu H, Guo W, Nerbonne JM. Four kinetically distinct depolarization-activated K^+ currents in adult mouse ventricular myocytes. *J Gen Physiol* 1999; 113:661–678.
63. Guo W, Li H, Aimond F, *et al.* Role of heteromultimers in the generation of myocardial transient outward K^+ currents. *Circ Res* 2002;90:586–593.
64. Li H, Guo W, Yamada KA, *et al.* Selective elimination of $I_{K,slow1}$ in mouse ventricular myocytes expressing a dominant negative Kv1.5alpha subunit. *Am J Physiol Heart Circ Physiol* 2004;286:H319–328.
65. Xu H, Barry DM, Li H, *et al.* Attenuation of the slow component of delayed rectification, action potential prolongation, and triggered activity in mice expressing a dominant-negative Kv2 alpha subunit. *Circ Res* 1999;85:623–633.
66. Charpentier F, Demolombe S, Escande D. Cardiac channelopathies: From men to mice. *Ann Med* 2004;36(Suppl. 1):28–34.
67. Sanguinetti MC, Jurkiewicz NK. Two components of cardiac delayed rectifier K^+ current. Differential sensitivity to block by class III antiarrhythmic agents. *J Gen Physiol* 1990;96:195–215.
68. Jost N, Virag L, Bitay M, *et al.* Restricting excessive cardiac action potential and QT prolongation: A vital role for I_{Ks} in human ventricular muscle. *Circulation* 2005;112:1392–1399.
69. Inoue M, Imanaga I. Masking of A-type K^+ channel in guinea pig cardiac cells by extracellular Ca^{2+}. *Am J Physiol* 1993;264:C1434–1438.
70. Li GR, Sun H, To J, *et al.* Demonstration of calcium-activated transient outward chloride current and delayed rectifier potassium currents in swine atrial myocytes. *J Mol Cell Cardiol* 2004;36:495–504.
71. Akar FG, Wu RC, Deschênes I, *et al.* Phenotypic differences in transient outward K^+ current of human and canine ventricular myocytes: Insights into molecular composition of ventricular Ito. *Am J Physiol Heart Circ Physiol* 2004;286:H602–609.
72. Brunet S, Aimond F, Guo W, *et al.* Heterogeneous expression of repolarizing, voltage-gated K^+ currents in adult mouse ventricles. *J Physiol* 2004; 559:103–120.
73. Miller C. An overview of the potassium channel family. *Genome Biol* 2000;1:REVIEWS0004.1–5.
74. Luo CH, Rudy Y. A dynamic model of the cardiac ventricular action potential. I. Simulations of ionic currents and concentration changes. *Circ Res* 1994; 74:1071–1096.
75. Silva J, Rudy Y. Subunit interaction determines I_{Ks} participation in cardiac repolarization and repolarization reserve. *Circulation* 2005;112:1384–1391.
76. Bondarenko VE, Szigeti GP, Bett GC, *et al.* Computer model of action potential of mouse ventricular myocytes. *Am J Physiol Heart Circ Physiol* 2004;287: H1378–1403.
77. Winslow RL, Rice J, Jafri S, *et al.* Mechanisms of altered excitation-contraction coupling in canine tachycardia-induced heart failure. II: Model studies. *Circ Res* 1999;84:571–586.
78. Nygren A, Fiset C, Firek L, *et al.* Mathematical model of an adult human atrial cell: The role of K^+ currents in repolarization. *Circ Res* 1998;82:63–81.
79. Courtemanche M, Ramirez RJ, Nattel S. Ionic mechanisms underlying human atrial action potential properties: Insights from a mathematical model. *Am J Physiol* 1998;275:H301–321.
80. Priebe L, Beuckelmann DJ. Simulation study of cellular electric properties in heart failure. *Circ Res* 1998;82:1206–1223.
81. ten Tusscher KH, Noble D, Noble PJ, *et al.* A model for human ventricular tissue. *Am J Physiol Heart Circ Physiol* 2004;286:H1573–1589.
82. Iyer V, Mazhari R, Winslow RL. A computational model of the human left-ventricular epicardial myocyte. *Biophys J* 2004;87:1507–1525.

2
Developmental Aspects of the Electrophysiology of the Heart: Function Follows Form

Alex V. Postma, Vincent M. Christoffels, and Antoon F.M. Moorman

Introduction

The cardiovascular system is the first organ system to form and function in the developing embryo. The function of the system is to continuously pump blood throughout the body for an entire lifetime. The adult heart, as the main pump in this system, performs roughly two thousand million cycles (2.3×10^9) in a typical lifetime. This continuous cycle is necessary to supply the whole body and all of its organs with oxygen and nutrients. Realization of this requires that the heart relaxes so that its chambers, the atria and ventricles, can fill with blood and then contract to propel the blood throughout the body. To achieve this, an intricate and complex organ developed, containing multiple chambers, nodes, valves, and electrical and force-producing components. In contrast, in primitive chordates and early vertebrate embryos the heart merely constitutes a myocardial mantle enfolding a ventral aorta, in which the blood is propelled by peristaltic contractions. The cardiomyocytes of such a primitive heart can be considered as "nodal" cells as they display automaticity and are poorly coupled, resulting in slow propagation of the depolarizing impulse and a matching peristaltic contraction. Eventually, the development of polarity, specifically, dominant pacemaker activity at the intake of the heart, led to the evolution of a one-way pump. Although dominant pacemaker activity implies development of sinus node function, only in mammals does a morphologically distinct node actually develop.[1] The addition of highly localized, fast conducting cardiac chambers to the straight heart tube is an evolutionary novel event, and resulted in the four-chambered hearts of birds and mammals with synchronous contraction for a dual circulation. Interestingly, concomitant with the formation of chambers, an adult type of electrocardiogram (ECG) can already be monitored in the embryo (Figure 2–1).[2] Thus, cardiac design, e.g., the positioning of the atrial and ventricular chambers within the straight heart tube, rather than the invention of nodes, principally explains the coordinated activation of the heart reflected in the ECG. To address the question why some areas of the embryonic heart tube do not participate in the formation of atrial or ventricular working myocardium and mature in a nodal direction, we suggest that the chamber-specific program of gene expression is specifically repressed by T-box factors and by other transcriptional repressors. Consequently, aberrant expression of these factors might be at the basis of ectopic automaticity and congenital malformations of the cardiac conduction system in the formed human heart.

Confusing Terminology

In authoritative work by Davies and colleagues, for which they scrutinized numerous anatomical, developmental, and clinical aspects,[3] the conduction system is defined as the system that initiates and conducts the sinus impulse. In their view it was composed of the sinus node, atrioventricular node, atrioventricular bundle, and the bundle branches and their ramifications. However, the

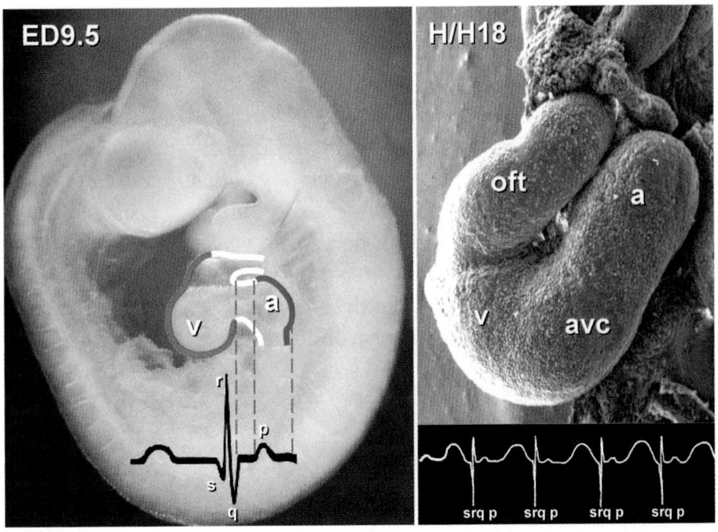

FIGURE 2–1. Concomitant with the formation of chambers (atria, ventricles), an adult type of electrocardiogram (ECG) can already be monitored in the embryo.[2] Scanning electron microscopic photographs of the developing chicken heart with matching electrocardiograms. At H/H 18, locally fast-conducting chamber myocardium has differentiated as reflected in the electrocardiogram. A = atrium; avc = atrioventricular canal; oft = outflow tract; V = ventricle. Note that the ECGs are displayed mirrored to match the position of the chambers in the embryonic heart. The apparent T-wave has not been labeled since it reflects the depolarization of the muscularized outflow tract at this stage rather than the repolarization of the ventricle.

myocardium of the atrial and ventricular chambers were not classified as component parts of the conduction system. This strict dichotomy between conduction system and chamber myocardium was, and still is, the conventional view.

The cardiac electrical impulse of a healthy heart is generated in the sinus node and propagates rapidly through the atrial myocardium toward the atrioventricular node, where the propagation of the depolarizing impulse is delayed. Subsequently, this impulse is then rapidly propagated via the atrioventricular bundle, bundle branches, and their ramifications, finally resulting in the fast depolarization of the ventricular myocardium. The whole sequence of cardiac electrical activity can be registered by ECG, which explicitly includes both the atrial and ventricular chamber myocardium as fast-conducting elements. According to the conventional dichotomy mentioned above, the slow-conducting nodal tissues and the fast-conducting bundle branches belong to the conduction system, while the fast-conducting myocardium of the chambers does not. This division is particularly confusing in the developing heart, in which the separate structures are not yet recognizable, although an adult-like ECG can already be derived from the embryonic heart (Figure 2–1).[2,4]

In the view of the above-mentioned inconsistencies in terminology, it is not surprising that the cardiac conduction system and its development have been surrounded by controversy, and therefore we have tried in this chapter to present in simple terms what we regard as a primer for the design and development of the cardiac conduction system.

Early Peristaltic Hearts

Circulatory systems are composed of pumps and transporting vessels. In practice, nature uses two arrangements to make muscle-pumping devices. One version, also utilized by the intestine, uses peristalsis as a driving force, while the other version, present in adult vertebrates, uses chambers and valves (see the next section). In the peristaltic version, a wave of contractions runs along the muscle mantel enfolding the main blood vessel, and this action pushes ahead the encompassed fluid in either direction. Such a rudimentary system is not particularly efficient, but allows the steady movement of fluids and slurries without interfering or obstructing valves and chambers. During evolution, polarity evolved in this primitive peristaltic chordate heart and this resulted in dominant pacemaker activity at one end of the cardiac tube, transforming such a heart into a one-way pump. It was demonstrated that retinoic acid is involved in this anteroposterior patterning.[5] All regions of peristaltic hearts possess poorly coupled cells and intrinsic automaticity, by which depolarizing impulses propagate slowly along the tube, resulting in matching peristaltic waves of contraction.[6–10] Such slow contractions do not require well-developed contractile structures as are present in the chamber myocardium of higher vertebrates.

Development of Chambered Hearts

It is important to appreciate that the basic characteristics of muscle cells comprising a peristaltic heart are similar to those comprising the nodes of a chambered heart,[11] as this facilitates the understanding that the design of chambered hearts is derived from the peristaltic heart. Though they share design characteristics, the chambered heart and its associated functional requirements are obviously far more complex than a peristaltic heart. Chambered hearts are the more powerful hearts that can cope with the increasing demands imposed by a growing microcirculatory resistance due to the evolutionary development of liver and kidneys. To achieve this, the atria became the drainage pool of the body to allow efficient filling of the ventricles, while the ventricles themselves became the power pumps. Like peristaltic hearts, chambered hearts are directional because dominant pacemaking activity remains localized at the intake of the heart. A logical further addition to chambered hearts involved one-way valves at both the inflow and the outflow of a chamber. Because of this, with relaxation, a chamber could to be prevented from refilling from the downstream compartment, and this prevented, with contraction, backflow into the preceding compartment. Remarkably, the areas in which these valves evolve display many nodal characteristics, and are the same areas that in the vertebrate embryonic heart will not, or will only later develop into chamber myocardium.[12] Thus, cardiac valves are always found in nodal regions. This holds true for the sinoatrial region, the atrioventricular junctional region, and also the myocardial outflow region of the embryonic heart. Interestingly, the outflow tract myocardium in humans can extend as far downstream as the semilunar valves. Spontaneous activity and even tachycardias originating from this area have been reported,[13] underscoring the notion that this myocardium is persisting embryonic nodal-like tissue.

In a broad view, the vertebrate chambered heart can be considered as a tube with nodal-like tissue, which conducts slowly, in which at the dorsal inflow side atria and at the ventral outflow side ventricles have developed (Figure 2–2). These ventricles contain the working myocardium characterized by rapidly conducting components. The expression of a number of genes that can serve as markers for working myocardium, such as the atrial natriuretic factor (*NppA*) and gap-junctional channels (see below) *Connexin 40* and *Connexin 43*, illustrates this process.[14–17] For example, at mouse embryonic day E8–8.5, the expression of these marker genes for ventricular and atrial chamber myocardium can already be observed at the ventral side of the heart tube.[18] This region will expand ("balloon") to form the embryonic left ventricle at the outer curvature.[14] Somewhat later, right-ventricular and atrial expression of the chamber markers is observed at discrete sites of the outer curvatures, these being the regions that will expand to form the respective chamber compartments. Importantly, the sinus venosus, atrioventricular canal, inner curvatures, and the outflow tract do not express chamber markers and will not expand. These structures retain their original embryonic phenotype, and will give rise to the nodal components of the conduction system, except for the outflow tract. This view is supported by the work of both Thompson *et al.*[19,20] and our own laboratory, which demonstrates that these areas indeed do not participate in the formation of the chambers and display low proliferative activity.[21] Moreover, work by Burch and co-workers strongly suggests that the myocardium of the atrioventricular node and atrioventricular bundle share a developmental origin.[22] Additionally, Gourdie and co-workers showed that slowly proliferating myocardium will mature into the nodal lineage with the use of lineage-tracing experiments and birth-dating studies.[23]

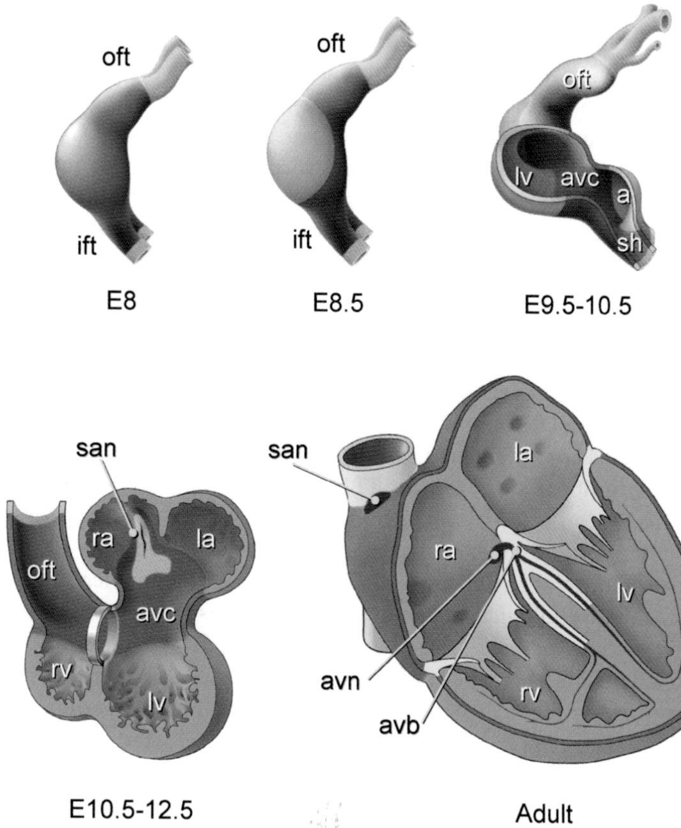

FIGURE 2–2. Schematic overview of heart development in higher vertebrates. Chamber myocardium (blue) expands from the outer curvatures of the primary heart tube, whereas nonchamber myocardium (gray) of the inflow tract (ift), sinus horns (sh), atrioventricular canal (avc), outflow tract (oft), and inner curvatures does not expand. Sinus horn myocardium gives rise to the sinoatrial node (san) and atrioventricular canal myocardium to the atrioventricular node (avn) and atrioventricular junction. The first three panels show a left-lateral view of the heart.

T-Box Transcription Factors Regulate Compartmentalization of the Heart

An important question is why some areas of the (embryonic) heart do not participate in the formation of atrial and ventricular working myocardium and mature in a nodal direction, such as the sinus venosus and the atrioventricular canal. To gain insight into this process we studied the regulation of the *Nppa* gene in more detail. *Nppa* is never expressed in nodal tissues from fish to humans, and in the embryonic heart it marks the developing atrial and ventricular working myocardium.[14] While investigating the mechanism behind the chamber-specific expression of *Nppa*, we established that both a single TBE site (DNA binding/recognition site for T-box transcription factors) and an adjacent NKE site (Nkx2-5 binding element) are present in the *Nppa* promoter and are required for repression of Nppa in the atrioventricular canal[24] and outflow tract.[25] T-box factors are evolutionary highly conserved transcription factors that are important regulators of (cardiac) development. Presently, at least 17 different T-box genes with diverse functions in development and disease are known.[26] In a search for the T-box factors that could act as a repressor for the *Nppa* gene, we observed that *Tbx2* is expressed in inflow, atrioventricular canal, inner curvature, and outflow myocardium. Moreover, expression of *Tbx2* and *Tbx3*, a transcriptional repressor with a similar role, is confined to primary (nonchamber) myocardium, remarkably mutually exclusive to *Nppa*, *Cx40*, *Cx43*, and other chamber-specific genes.[24,27,28] These findings point to a model in which chamber formation (e.g., atria, left and right ventricle) and differentiation are driven by broadly expressed factors, in addition to which a supplementary layer of localized repressors inhibits this process in regions where chambers do not develop.[18] *Tbx2* gain and loss of function experiments have demonstrated that *Tbx2* is indeed able and required to inhibit chamber formation and expression of chamber marker genes.[27,29] *Tbx3* is expressed in a subdomain of the *Tbx2* domain, and whereas it is able to block chamber formation when expressed ectopically, its deficiency does not lead to obvious defects in atrioventricular canal patterning, indicating functional redundancy with *Tbx2* (our unpublished observations).

But how do *Tbx2* and *Tbx3* exert their functions? Both factors act as repressors of transcription and share DNA binding properties and target genes.[30–34] They effectively compete with *Tbx5*, a transcriptional activator, for TBE binding, and for *Nkx2-5* on NKE binding, thereby repressing chamber-specific genes and chamber differentiation.[18,24,28] Interestingly, although lineage data are lacking, morphological analyses and gene expression studies indicate that the sinoatrial node develops from primary myocardium at the junction between the right sinus horn and the right atrium, whereas the atrioventricular node develops from the atrioventricular canal. The node precursors express both *Tbx2* and *Tbx3*, though during development *Tbx2* becomes downregulated. *Tbx3* expression is maintained specifically in the nodes, thereby providing the only transcription factor found to date to be expressed specifically in the nodes (Figure 2–3).[28,29] As mature nodes display many features that resemble primary myocardium in the embryo, it is attractive to hypothesize that their formation is the result of *Tbx2* and *Tbx3* maintaining the primary phenotype.

Concluding, in a generalizing view it may be envisioned that *Tbx2*, *Tbx3*, and/or other transcriptional repressors suppress the chamber-specific program of gene expression, allowing the regions where these factors are expressed to further mature in the nodal direction. Aberrant expression of such factors might thus be at the basis of ectopic automaticity and congenital malformations of the cardiac conduction system in the formed human heart. Obviously, the spatio-

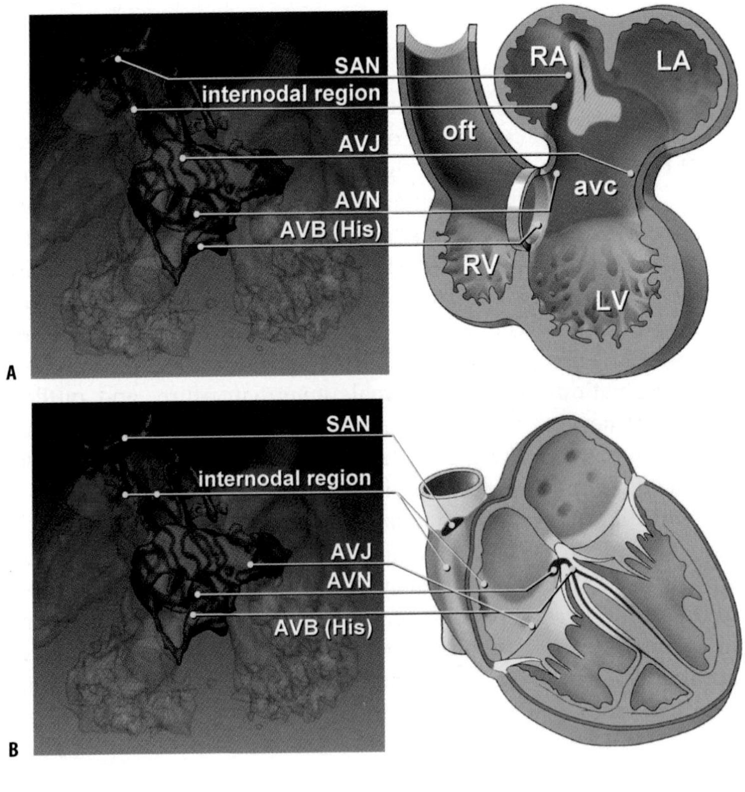

FIGURE 2–3. (A, B) Tbx3 (red) expression visualized in the heart at ED10.5, marking the sinoatrial node (SAN), internodal region, AV junction (AVJ), AV node (AVM), and the AV bundles (AVB) in respect to the location of the atria, the atrioventricular canal, the ventricles, and the outflow tract on ED10.5 and in adult heart.

temporal regulation of these repressors is the next issue to be resolved.

Tbx5 Segregates the Left and Right Ventricle, Implications for Arrhythmias?

Tbx5 is not only of interest because it is a transcriptional activator involved in chamber formation, as mentioned above, but also because *Tbx5* is expressed in an anteroposterior gradient in the heart tube, which is regulated by retinoic acid.[35] As the left and right ventricles are specified along the anteroposterior axis, it is not surprising that the left ventricle expresses more *Tbx5* than the right ventricle.[36] Moreover, ectopic expression of *Tbx5* in the developing ventricles results in interventricular septal defects and a single ventricle with left ventricular identity.[37] This suggests that *Tbx5* is necessary for left ventricular identity, and provides, in part, the boundary between the left and right ventricle. Actually, mutations in *Tbx5* in humans cause, among other things, septal defects (see below). Consequently, target genes of *Tbx5* are likely differentially regulated between the left and right ventricles. Indeed, one such target gene, a connexin (*Cx40*) (see below), is differentially expressed in the adult heart between the right and left ventricles. Interestingly, recent work has shown that transcription factors can directly regulate the expression of ion channels, since the homeodomain transcription factor *Irx5* was demonstrated to establish the cardiac ventricular repolarization gradient.[38] Seeing that the right ventricle, in particular, is prone to the development of various arrhythmias, such as those seen in Brugada syndrome[39] and arrhythmogenic right ventricular dysplasia (ARVD),[40] and given the fact that *Tbx5* is actively involved in segregating the left and right ventricle, it is tempting to speculate that target genes of *Tbx5* might contribute to or oppose arrhythmias. Recent work has shown that numerous genes are influenced by differences in *Tbx5* dosage, including genes expressed during heart development such as transcriptions factors (*Tbx3*, *Irx2*), cell-cell signaling molecules, and ion channels (*Cx40, KCNA5*),[41] thus indicating that further investigation into *Tbx5* and its downstream genes in relation to arrhythmias and ion channel genes is warranted.

Mutations in Transcription Factors Cause Congenital Heart Defects

As the above mentioned transcription factors are essential for proper cardiac (conduction) system development, it is hardly surprising that mutations in these key genes lead to congenital heart defects. Mutations in *Tbx5* in humans lead to the Holt-Oram syndrome (HOS), which is characterized by anterior preaxial limb and cardiac malformations.[42] All affected individuals exhibit upper limb radial ray malformations that range from subtle carpal bone abnormalities to overt proximal defects such as phocomelia. Many have congenital heart disease such as atrial septal defects (ASD) or muscular ventricular septal defects (VSD), or multiple and complex malformations. It has recently been shown that the skeletal defects seen in HOS patients are likely due to disturbed control of *Tbx5* on the expression of *Sox9* (a transcription factor essential for chondrogenesis and skeleton growth) via control of the expression of connexin 40.[43] This underscores the notion that connexins are involved not only in propagation of cardiac impulses but also in morphogenesis (see below). Mutations in *Tbx3* cause ulnar-mammary syndrome characterized by defects in breast development, apocrine gland, limb and genital formation,[44] and as one study reports, ventricular septal defects and pulmonary stenosis.[45] Moreover, mutations in *Tbx5* interacting partners such as *Nkx2-5* and *Gata4*, like *Tbx5* itself, are known to cause septum defects[46] and, in the case of *Nkx2-5*, atrioventricular conduction defects.[47] Presently no diseases are known to be caused by *Tbx2* mutations. A more common congenital disorder called DiGeorge syndrome is caused by a 1.5–3 megabase genomic deletions of the chromosome 22q11 region, which includes the *Tbx1* gene.[48] Patients with DiGeorge syndrome are characterized by a variety of abnormalities including absence/hypoplasia of the thymus, cleft palate, facial dysmorphism, and cardiovascular anomalies such as aortic arch malformation, outflow tract defects, and VSDs. Recently it was postulated that a synergistic interaction between *Tbx1* and

Nkx2-5 might be responsible for the varying heart malformations of DiGeorge syndrome.[49] As *Tbx1*-deficient mice phenocopy important aspects of DiGeorge syndrome including outflow tract abnormalities,[50] it is believed that *Tbx1* might modulate, in part, the outflow tract defects seen in DiGeorge patients.

Development of the Ventricular Conduction System

The final part of the cardiac conduction system not yet discussed is the ventricular conduction system. The ventricular conduction system mainly develops from the localized trabecular ventricular components (bundle branches and their ramifications) and the primary ring (atrioventricular bundle) as we have reviewed previously,[51] which is in line with the lineage study of Burch and co-workers on the development of the atrioventricular canal, atrioventricular node, and atrioventricular bundle,[22] and with the lineage studies on the development of the bundle branches and their ramifications.[52] Generally, ventricular chamber myocardium develops at the ventral side of the anterior part of the heart tube. An intermediate stage of its development is the so-called trabecular myocardium. While the compact myocardium proliferates exteriorly, the interior trabeculations display low proliferative activity[19,20] and differentiate toward the peripheral ventricular conduction system displaying a high abundance of connexin expression (as mentioned earlier).

Although morphological data are available, few molecular markers exists that specifically delineate the ventricular conduction system,[53] so developmental understanding in this area has lagged behind. However, it was recently observed that in both the embryonic mouse and chick, the ventricular conduction system components are in relative proximity to the cardiac endothelium. Neuregulin-1 is expressed by day 8.5 in the ventricular endocardium, whereas its receptors (ErbB2/ErbB4) are present in the underlying myocardium, making this signaling pathway an excellent candidate for regulation of the induction of the ventricular conduction system. Indeed, mice deficient in neuregulin, ErbB2, or ErbB4 die early with a lack of ventricular trabeculae.[54] Moreover, using a mouse model carrying a marker for the conduction system, Rentschler and colleagues established that exposure to neuregulin resulted in upregulation of a conduction system marker, and presumably the ventricular conduction system, in the developing murine heart,[55] indicating that neuregulin-1 indeed plays a role in the formation of the conduction system, possibly in a paracrine manner.

Sarcoplasmic Reticulum and Heart Development

Having discussed the building plan of vertebrate hearts and their conduction system, it is relevant to look at the developmental aspects of their most prominent features, namely contraction and electrical activity. Regular beating is already observed in the very early period of heart development from embryonic day E9 onward,[56] as mentioned above. This implies that an intracellular system of contraction and cardiac automaticity is already established. Interestingly, the atrioventricular canal and the outflow tract are characterized by slow conduction velocity,[12] a low level of gap junction and connexin expression,[57] and low SR activity.[58] This supports the idea that these flanking segments can function as one-way valves, because they fulfill all the requirements needed for a long contraction duration resulting in a peristaltic contraction. However, the radical change from a peristaltic slowly contracting heart tube to one with fast-contracting chambers necessitates proper control on free intracellular calcium ions. This, in turn, requires the regulated movement of calcium ions across both the sarcolemmal and sarcoplasmic membranes. Clearance of intracellular calcium can be obtained in two ways, either by extrusion of the calcium into the extracellular space by the Na^+–Ca^{2+} exchanger (NCX) or by the sarcoplasmic–endoplasmatic Ca^{2+}-ATPase (SERCA2) into the sarcoplasmic reticulum (SR). SERCA2 itself is regulated by the nonphosphorylated form of another protein, phospholamban.[59]

The calcium handling system was the first ionic system to be studied extensively during heart development, although mostly in the late fetal heart stage (embryonic day 16.5 and later).[59] At this stage most calcium required for contraction is derived from the calcium influx through the voltage-dependent calcium channels (L-type and T-type). Although a distinct SR is not morphologically observed in fetal myocytes, calcium influxes nevertheless are capable of triggering calcium releases through the calcium release channels (so-called ryanodine receptors, RYRs).[58] It is thought that in contrast to the mature situation, the calcium store for the RYRs in the fetal myocytes are very small organelles that are located far from the L- and T-type channels on the surface membrane. In this way, calcium flowing through the calcium membrane channels diffuses into the intracellular space, where it stimulates the immature SR. The whole chain of calcium-induced calcium release is thus slowed down, and produces the slow kinetics of calcium signals in fetal myocytes.

In contrast, the expression pattern of the various genes involved in calcium handling has been studied more thoroughly throughout embryonic heart development. SERCA2 and PLB can already be observed as early as the cardiac crest stage (embryonic day 7.5 in the mouse), even before myocardial contraction has begun. At this stage, however, there is already polarity in expression, as SERCA2 is more abundant in the anterior region of the cardiac crest and decreases toward the posterior regions, whereas PLB, in contrast, shows complementary distribution.[60] At the stage of the primitive cardiac tube (E8), several additional calcium-related genes start to be expressed. In correspondence with the previous stage, PLB and SERCA2 are still expressed in opposite gradients, e.g., PLB is expressed more strongly in the posterior regions in comparison to the latter. Interestingly, RYR, NCX, and Na^+–K^+-ATPase are distributed homogeneously over the cardiac tube and remain so throughout further embryonic development of the heart.[60] It thus seems that the control of calcium homeostasis is determined solely by the SERCA/PLB system. At the stage of cardiac looping (E8.5), when the first signs of left/right asymmetry and identity are manifested in the embryo, the calcium-related genes maintain their previous patterns of expression. In the final stage (E16.5), termed fetal heart, SERCA2 is expressed more in atrial myocardium than in ventricular myocardium, whereas PLB is once again expressed in an opposite pattern. Additionally, SERCA2 has low expression in the atrioventricular canal (AVC) and outflow tract (OFT). Interestingly, SERCA2 and PLB display a differential expression between the trabeculated and compact layers of the ventricular myocardium. In contrast, the expression of both genes is very weak in different components of the cardiac conduction system, atrioventricular node, and the bundle of His, which is in line with the nodal-like morphological origin of these components, as discussed earlier. The expression of the other components of the calcium metabolism, RYR, NCX, and Na^+–K^+-ATPase, is homogeneously in the different regions of the fetal heart.

Connexins and Heart Development

The propagation of cardiac impulses is mainly determined by the capacity to rapidly carry changes in the membrane potential of cardiomyocytes. This propagation is mediated by gap junctions, which are aggregates of hydrophobic cell–cell channels that allow the intercellular exchange of ions, metabolites, and second messengers of up to 1 kDa in size.[15] The aqueous pores are formed by serially linked hemichannels (connexons) provided by apposing cell membranes. One connexon hemichannel is composed of six transmembrane proteins called connexins (Cx), which are encoded by 21 connexin genes.[61] Although the main purpose of gap junctions in the heart is the conduction of the depolarizing impulse across the myocardium, evidence exists that connexins also play a role in cardiac morphogenesis, as homozygotic Cx43-knockout mice die shortly after birth from a pulmonary outflow tract stenosis due to cardiac malformation.[62] Analogously, in humans, visceral heterotaxia and hypoplastic left heart syndrome have been found to be associated with mutations of the Cx43 gene.[63,64]

Differences in the expression of the connexins are consistent with a functional myocardium (atria and ventricles) model in which the working myocardium has the capacity to transmit the cardiac impulse more quickly than the adjacent myocardium of the inflow tract, atrioventricular canal, and outflow tract. This guarantees synchronized contraction without the need for a specialized system (as discussed earlier). The expression of the main connexin, Cx43, is detected for the first time in the embryonic heart stage (E10.5). Cx40 has a similar pattern of expression, although more reduced.[60] Cx40 (from ED9.5) and Cx43 mRNA (from 10.5) are detectable in atria and ventricles, but not in their flanking myocardium (inflow tract, AVC, and OFT).[65] Even though Cx40 and Cx43 mRNA eventually become expressed in the inflow tract, they remain undetectable in the sinoatrial node, the AVC (including the atrioventricular node), and the outflow tract.[15] Expression of Cx40 is maximal in the fetal period and declines toward birth. At the stage of the fetal heart (E16.5), Cx43 is restricted to the ventricular myocardium and it is barely detectable in the atrial myocardium in rat, while the mouse atrium expresses much Cx43.[15,60] Analogous to SERCA2 and PLB, Cx43 expression is low in the trabeculated layer and higher in the compact layer.[60] In contrast, Cx40 expression complements Cx43 expression, as Cx40 is expressed mainly in the atrial chambers and shows a transitory differential expression between the right and left ventricles under the influence of Tbx5, as discussed earlier.

It is interesting to note that based on the expression of Cx40 and Cx43 during development, two populations of myocytes can be distinguished, viz. cardiomyocytes that do not express Cx40 and Cx43, and cardiomyocytes that do express both. The first group includes the myocardium of the sinoatrial node, the AVC (including the atrioventricular node), the bundle of His, and the OFT. The second population includes the working myocardium of the atria and the ventricles, and, later in development, the myocardium of the inflow tract (excluding the sinoatrial node), supporting the hypothesis that the structures that do not express Cx40/43 are derived from the embryonic AVC.

Ion Channels and Heart Development

The regulation of the action potential (AP) is determined by a large variety of ion currents. During the depolarization of the myocytes massive amounts of sodium ions are pumped into the cell, whereas the subsequent repolarizations are characterized by a balance of different potassium currents flowing into and out of the myocyte. Many genes are involved in maintaining this dynamic balance, the most prominent being SCN5A, carrying the initial sodium current, and KCNQ1 and KCNH2, carrying the subsequent potassium currents. Several modulator genes, such as KCNE1,2 and SCN1b, also play a role. As much as is known about their function and expression in the adult heart, virtually nothing is known about the different components of the action potential during the various embryonic stages. Attempts to characterize the various individual currents electrophysiologically during development have been hampered by technical difficulties though some studies were published on this topic.[66–68]

In general, the action potentials and resting potentials in cardiomyocytes are altered greatly during development, e.g., both the rate of rise and the overshoot increase along with the duration of the AP. These electrophysiological changes are mainly produced by developmental changes in ion channels, e.g., changes in the amount, the type, and the kinetic properties. The fast sodium current (mainly encoded by SCN5a and SCN1b), which is responsible for the upstroke of the AP, is markedly increased during development. There are few functional sodium channels present at the earliest stage, but the density increases progressively during development. Though the current has a significant sustained component in the earlier stages, this decreases during development, thereby contributing in part to the abbreviation of the AP.[68] The main potassium current in fetal ventricular myocytes is I_{Kr} (mainly encoded by KCNH2 and KCNE2), whereas I_{Ks} (encoded by KCNQ1 and KCNE1) is lacking or very small, though in the early neonate I_{Ks} becomes the dominant repolarizing current. I_f, or the funny current (encoded by the HCN gene family), is the pacemaker current and as such contributes prominently to cardiac rhythm.[69] As it is essential to the function of the sinus node, it is unfortunate that expression studies of HCN during development are scarce. Though recently it was shown that mice lacking HCN4 globally, as well as selectively from cardiomyocytes, die between ED9.5 and 11.5, displaying a strong reduction in I_f and bradycardia.[70] The few studies that investigated I_f electrophysiologically during development did so only in ventricular cells. They show that I_f is prominent at E9.5 in ventricular myocytes and decreases together with loss of regular spontaneous activity of ventricular cells toward the neonatal stage, which is accompanied by a subtype switch from HCN4 to HCN2.[71,72] So while the I_f current of the sinus node type is present in early embryonic mouse ventricular cells, the ventricle tends to lose pacemaker potency during the second half of embryonic development. Moreover, kinetics were found to be changed, as the threshold voltage to evoke I_f significantly lowers from neonatal myocytes to adult ones.[73] The developmental expression pattern of the HCN4 gene shows that it can already be detected in the cardiac crescent at ED7.5, while at ED8 it is symmetrically located in the caudal portion of the heart tube, the sinus venosus, where pacemaker activity has previously been reported.[74] Further in development HCN4 becomes asymmetrically expressed, occupying the dorsal wall of the right atrium, and will eventually be restricted to the junction of the right atrial appendage and the superior vena cava in concordance with the site at which the SA node is located in the postnatal and adult heart.[75] In the adult heart, HCN4 is mostly expressed in the sinoatrial node, while expression of HCN2 is homogeneously low in the sinoatrial node, AV node, and both the atria and ventricles.[72] The molecular pathways underlying the developmental regulation of cardiac HCN channels are not yet known.

A recent study on expression of these ion channels during various developmental stages demonstrates that SCN5A is distributed homogeneously throughout the embryonal heart (E10.5), whereas the expression of KCNQ1 and KCNH2 appears to be homogeneous only in the embryonal myocardium.[60] In contrast, KCNE1 is expressed in a dorsoventral gradient with a greater expression in the outflow tract region, while KCNE2 is confined to the atrial myocardium. Preliminary evidence seems to indicate that at the fetal heart stage (E16.5), SCN5A is principally expressed in the inflow tract, i.e., the myocardium of the caval veins, whereas ventricular expression is low.[60] However, this contrasts with the high expression of SCN5A in the ventricles of the adult heart,[72] indicating the necessity to investigate this important ion channel in more detail during heart development. In addition, SCN5A is located in the sinus node in the adult stage, as heterozygous knockout mice for SCN5A exhibit impaired SA conduction and frequent sinoatrial conduction block.[76] Currently, no data exist regarding the distribution of SCN1B in the fetal heart or the distribution of these channels in the cardiac conduction system. The expression of KCNQ1 and KCNH2 is again homogeneous in the fetal myocardium. However, while KCNQ1 transcripts have similar levels of expression in the cardiac conduction system and working myocardium, there is an increase in the amount of KCNQ1 protein in the conduction system (AV node, bundle of His, and right and left bundle branches), suggesting a posttranscriptional control mechanism specific to the conduction system.[60] KCNH2 is, however, expressed similarly in mRNA and protein in the myocardium. The modulator genes to these ion channels have a dynamic pattern of expression, where KCNE1 remains limited to the ventricular myocardium, and KCNE2 is confined to the atrial myocardium.

Conclusion

The heart evolved from a myocardial tube in primitive chordates to a four-chambered heart with synchronous contraction and dual circulation in higher vertebrates. Each cardiomyocyte of a primitive heart can be considered as a nodal cell because it displays automaticity and is poorly coupled, which, together with slow propagation, give rise to peristaltic contraction. The introduction of dominant pacemaker activity at the intake of the heart perfected this into a one-way pump. Subsequently, highly localized, fast conducting cardiac chambers were added to this nodal tube, resulting in the four-chambered heart. Interestingly, concomitant with the formation of such chambers, an adult type of electrocardiogram (ECG) can already be monitored in the embryo. Thus, cardiac design, e.g., the positioning of the atrial and ventricular chambers within the nodal tube, principally explains the coordinated activation of the heart reflected in the ECG. A crucial question is why some areas of the embryonic heart tube do not participate in the formation of atrial or ventricular working myocardium and mature in a nodal direction. As a generalized hypothesis we propose that the chamber-specific program of gene expression is specifically repressed by T-box factors and by the other transcriptional repressors. Consequently, aberrant expression of these factors might be at the basis of ectopic automaticity, malformations of the conduction system, and congenital heart disease in general.

References

1. Canale ED, Campbell GR, Smolich JJ, *et al. Cardiac Muscle.* Berlin: Springer-Verlag, 1986:318.
2. Seidl W, Schulze M, Steding G, *et al.* A few remarks on the physiology of the chick embryo heart (Gallus gallus). *Folia Morphol (Praha)* 1981;29:237–242.
3. Davies MJ, Anderson RH, Becker AE. Embryology of the conduction tissues. In: Davies MJ, Becker AE, Eds. *The Conduction System of the Heart.* London: Butterworth, 1983:81–94.
4. Paff GH, Boucek RJ, Harrell TC. Observations on the development of the electrocardiogram. *Anat Rec* 1968;160:575–582.
5. Rosenthal N, Xavier-Neto J. From the bottom of the heart: Anteroposterior decisions in cardiac muscle differentiation. *Curr Opin Cell Biol* 2000;12:742–746.
6. Randl DJ, Davie PS. The hearts of urochordates and cephalochordates. In: Bourne GH, Ed. *Hearts and Heart-like Organs.* New York: Academic Press, 1980:41–59.
7. Anderson M. Electrophysiological studies on initiation and reversal of the heart beat in Ciona intestinalis. *J Exp Biol* 1968;49:363–385.
8. Kriebel ME. Wave front analyses of impulses in tunicate heart. *Am J Physiol* 1970;218:1194–1200.
9. Moller PC, Philpott CW. The circulatory system of Amphioxus (Branchiostoma floridae). I. Morphology of the major vessels of the pharyngeal area. *J Morphol* 1973;139:389–406.
10. von Skramlik E. Über den kreislauf bei den niersten chordaten. *Erg Biol* 1938;15:166–309.
11. Moorman AF, Christoffels VM. Cardiac chamber formation: Development, genes, and evolution. *Physiol Rev* 2003;83:1223–1267.
12. de Jong F, Opthof T, Wilde AA, *et al.* Persisting zones of slow impulse conduction in developing chicken hearts. *Circ Res* 1992;71:240–250.
13. Timmermans C, Rodriguez LM, Medeiros A, *et al.* Radiofrequency catheter ablation of idiopathic ventricular tachycardia originating in the main stem of the pulmonary artery. *J Cardiovasc Electrophysiol* 2002;13:281–284.
14. Christoffels VM, Habets PE, Franco D, *et al.* Chamber formation and morphogenesis in the developing mammalian heart. *Dev Biol* 2000;223:266–278.
15. Van Kempen MJ, Vermeulen JL, Moorman AF, *et al.* Developmental changes of connexin40 and connexin43 mRNA distribution patterns in the rat heart. *Cardiovasc Res* 1996;32:886–900.
16. Palmer S, Groves N, Schindeler A, *et al.* The small muscle-specific protein Csl modifies cell shape and promotes myocyte fusion in an insulin-like growth factor 1-dependent manner. *J Cell Biol* 2001;153:985–998.
17. Houweling AC, Somi S, Van Den Hoff MJ, *et al.* Developmental pattern of ANF gene expression reveals a strict localization of cardiac chamber formation in chicken. *Anat Rec* 2002;266:93–102.
18. Christoffels VM, Burch JB, Moorman AF. Architectural plan for the heart: Early patterning and delineation of the chambers and the nodes. *Trends Cardiovasc Med* 2004;14:301–307.
19. Thompson RP, Lindroth JR, Wong YMM. Regional differences in DNA-synthetic activity in the preseptation of myocardium of the chick. In: Clark EB, Takao A, Eds. *Developmental Cardiology: Morphogenesis and Function.* New York: Futura Publishing, 1990:219–234.
20. Thompson RP, Kanai T, Germroth PG. Organization and function of early specialized myocardium. In: Clark EB, Markwald RR, Takao A, Eds. *Developmental Mechanisms of Heart Disease.* New York: Futura Publishing, 1995:269–279.
21. Soufan AT, van den Berg G, Ruijter JM, *et al.* A regionalized sequence of myocardial cell growth and proliferation characterizes early chamber formation. *Circ Res* 2006;99:545–552.
22. Davis DL, Edwards AV, Juraszek AL, *et al.* A GATA-6 gene heart-region-specific enhancer provides a novel means to mark and probe a discrete component of the mouse cardiac conduction system. *Mech Dev* 2001;108:105–119.
23. Cheng G, Litchenberg WH, Cole GJ, *et al.* Development of the cardiac conduction system involves recruitment within a multipotent cardiomyogenic lineage. *Development* 1999;126:5041–5049.
24. Habets PE, Moorman AF, Clout DE, *et al.* Cooperative action of Tbx2 and Nkx2.5 inhibits ANF expression in the atrioventricular canal: Implications for cardiac chamber formation. *Genes Dev* 2002;16:1234–1246.
25. Habets PE, Moorman AF, Christoffels VM. Regulatory modules in the developing heart. *Cardiovasc Res* 2003;58:246–263.

26. Papaioannou VE. T-box genes in development: From hydra to humans. *Int Rev Cytol* 2001;207: 1–70.
27. Harrelson Z, Kelly RG, Goldin SN, *et al.* Tbx2 is essential for patterning the atrioventricular canal and for morphogenesis of the outflow tract during heart development. *Development* 2004;131:5041–5052.
28. Hoogaars WM, Tessari A, Moorman AF, *et al.* The transcriptional repressor Tbx3 delineates the developing central conduction system of the heart. *Cardiovasc Res* 2004;62:489–499.
29. Christoffels VM, Hoogaars WM, Tessari A, *et al.* T-box transcription factor Tbx2 represses differentiation and formation of the cardiac chambers. *Dev Dyn* 2004;229:763–770.
30. Sinha S, Abraham S, Gronostajski RM, *et al.* Differential DNA binding and transcription modulation by three T-box proteins, T, TBX1 and TBX2. *Gene* 2000;258:15–29.
31. He M, Wen L, Campbell CE, *et al.* Transcription repression by Xenopus ET and its human ortholog TBX3, a gene involved in ulnar-mammary syndrome. *Proc Natl Acad Sci USA* 1999;96:10212–10217.
32. Carreira S, Dexter TJ, Yavuzer U, *et al.* Brachyury-related transcription factor Tbx2 and repression of the melanocyte-specific TRP-1 promoter. *Mol Cell Biol* 1998;18:5099–5108.
33. Carlson H, Ota S, Campbell CE, *et al.* A dominant repression domain in Tbx3 mediates transcriptional repression and cell immortalization: Relevance to mutations in Tbx3 that cause ulnar-mammary syndrome. *Hum Mol Genet* 2001;10: 2403–2413.
34. Lingbeek ME, Jacobs JJ, van Lohuizen M. The T-box repressors TBX2 and TBX3 specifically regulate the tumor suppressor gene p14ARF via a variant T-site in the initiator. *J Biol Chem* 2002;277:26120–26127.
35. Niederreither K, Vermot J, Messaddeq N, *et al.* Embryonic retinoic acid synthesis is essential for heart morphogenesis in the mouse. *Development* 2001;128:1019–1031.
36. Bruneau BG, Logan M, Davis N, *et al.* Chamber-specific cardiac expression of Tbx5 and heart defects in Holt-Oram syndrome. *Dev Biol* 1999;211: 100–108.
37. Takeuchi JK, Ohgi M, Koshiba-Takeuchi K, *et al.* Tbx5 specifies the left/right ventricles and ventricular septum position during cardiogenesis. *Development* 2003;130:5953–5964.
38. Costantini DL, Arruda EP, Agarwal P, *et al.* The homeodomain transcription factor Irx5 establishes the mouse cardiac ventricular repolarization gradient. *Cell* 2005;123:347–358.
39. Shimizu W. The Brugada syndrome–an update. *Intern Med* 2005;44:1224–1231.
40. Kies P, Bootsma M, Bax J, *et al.* Arrhythmogenic right ventricular dysplasia/cardiomyopathy: Screening, diagnosis, and treatment. *Heart Rhythm* 2006; 3:225–234.
41. Mori AD, Zhu Y, Vahora I, *et al.* Tbx5-dependent rheostatic control of cardiac gene expression and morphogenesis. *Dev Biol* 2006;297:566–586.
42. Basson CT, Bachinsky DR, Lin RC, *et al.* Mutations in human TBX5 [corrected] cause limb and cardiac malformation in Holt-Oram syndrome. *Nat Genet* 1997;15:30–35.
43. Pizard A, Burgon PG, Paul DL, *et al.* Connexin 40, a target of transcription factor Tbx5, patterns wrist, digits, and sternum. *Mol Cell Biol* 2005;25:5073–5083.
44. Bamshad M, Lin RC, Law DJ, *et al.* Mutations in human TBX3 alter limb, apocrine and genital development in ulnar-mammary syndrome. *Nat Genet* 1997;16:311–315.
45. Meneghini V, Odent S, Platonova N, *et al.* Novel TBX3 mutation data in families with ulnar-mammary syndrome indicate a genotype-phenotype relationship: Mutations that do not disrupt the T-domain are associated with less severe limb defects. *Eur J Med Genet* 2006;49:151–158.
46. Garg V, Kathiriya IS, Barnes R, *et al.* GATA4 mutations cause human congenital heart defects and reveal an interaction with TBX5. *Nature* 2003;424: 443–447.
47. Schott JJ, Benson DW, Basson CT, *et al.* Congenital heart disease caused by mutations in the transcription factor NKX2-5. *Science* 1998;281:108–111.
48. Merscher S, Funke B, Epstein JA, *et al.* TBX1 is responsible for cardiovascular defects in velo-cardio-facial/DiGeorge syndrome. *Cell* 2001;104:619–629.
49. Nowotschin S, Liao J, Gage PJ, *et al.* Tbx1 affects asymmetric cardiac morphogenesis by regulating Pitx2 in the secondary heart field. *Development* 2006;133:1565–1573.
50. Jerome LA, Papaioannou VE. DiGeorge syndrome phenotype in mice mutant for the T-box gene, Tbx1. *Nat Genet* 2001;27:286–291.
51. Moorman AF, de Jong F, Denyn MM, *et al.* Development of the cardiac conduction system. *Circ Res* 1998;82:629–644.
52. Gourdie RG, Mima T, Thompson RP, *et al.* Terminal diversification of the myocyte lineage generates Purkinje fibers of the cardiac conduction system. *Development* 1995;121:1423–1431.

53. Myers DC, Fishman GI. Molecular and functional maturation of the murine cardiac conduction system. *Trends Cardiovasc Med* 2003;13:289–295.
54. Garratt AN, Ozcelik C, Birchmeier C. ErbB2 pathways in heart and neural diseases. *Trends Cardiovasc Med* 2003;13:80–86.
55. Rentschler S, Zander J, Meyers K, *et al.* Neuregulin-1 promotes formation of the murine cardiac conduction system. *Proc Natl Acad Sci USA* 2002;99: 10464–10469.
56. Rentschler S, Vaidya DM, Tamaddon H, *et al.* Visualization and functional characterization of the developing murine cardiac conduction system. *Development* 2001;128:1785–1792.
57. van Kempen MJ, Fromaget C, Gros D, *et al.* Spatial distribution of connexin43, the major cardiac gap junction protein, in the developing and adult rat heart. *Circ Res* 1991;68:1638–1651.
58. Moorman AF, Schumacher CA, de Boer PA, *et al.* Presence of functional sarcoplasmic reticulum in the developing heart and its confinement to chamber myocardium. *Dev Biol* 2000;223:279–290.
59. Kojima M, Sperelakis N, Sada H. Ontogenesis of transmembrane signaling systems for control of cardiac Ca2+ channels. *J Dev Physiol* 1990;14:181–219.
60. Franco D, Dominguez J, de Castro Md Mdel P, *et al.* [Regulation of myocardial gene expression during heart development]. *Rev Esp Cardiol* 2002; 55:167–184.
61. Saffitz JE. Connexins, conduction, and atrial fibrillation. *N Engl J Med* 2006;354:2712–2714.
62. Reaume AG, de Sousa PA, Kulkarni S, *et al.* Cardiac malformation in neonatal mice lacking connexin43. *Science* 1995;267:1831–1834.
63. Britz-Cunningham SH, Shah MM, Zuppan CW, *et al.* Mutations of the connexin43 gap-junction gene in patients with heart malformations and defects of laterality. *N Engl J Med* 1995;332:1323–1329.
64. Dasgupta C, Martinez AM, Zuppan CW, *et al.* Identification of connexin43 (alpha1) gap junction gene mutations in patients with hypoplastic left heart syndrome by denaturing gradient gel electrophoresis (DGGE). *Mutat Res* 2001;479:173–186.
65. Delorme B, Dahl E, Jarry-Guichard T, *et al.* Expression pattern of connexin gene products at the early developmental stages of the mouse cardiovascular system. *Circ Res* 1997;81:423–437.
66. Sperelakis N, Pappano AJ. Physiology and pharmacology of developing heart cells. *Pharmacol Ther* 1983;22:1–39.
67. Wetzel GT, Klitzner TS. Developmental cardiac electrophysiology recent advances in cellular physiology. *Cardiovasc Res* 1996;31(Spec. No.):E52–60.
68. Yokoshiki H, Tohse N. Developmental changes in ion channels. In: Kurachi Y, Terzic A, Cohen MV, *et al.*, Eds. *Heart Physiology and Pathophysiology.* San Diego: Academic Press, 2001:719–735.
69. DiFrancesco D. Serious workings of the funny current. *Prog Biophys Mol Biol* 2006;90:13–25.
70. Stieber J, Herrmann S, Feil S, *et al.* The hyperpolarization-activated channel HCN4 is required for the generation of pacemaker action potentials in the embryonic heart. *Proc Natl Acad Sci USA* 2003;100:15235–15240.
71. Yasui K, Liu W, Opthof T, *et al.* I(f) current and spontaneous activity in mouse embryonic ventricular myocytes. *Circ Res* 2001;88:536–542.
72. Marionneau C, Couette B, Liu J, *et al.* Specific pattern of ionic channel gene expression associated with pacemaker activity in the mouse heart. *J Physiol* 2005;562:223–234.
73. Robinson RB, Yu H, Chang F, *et al.* Developmental change in the voltage-dependence of the pacemaker current, if, in rat ventricle cells. *Pflugers Arch* 1997;433:533–535.
74. Van Mierop LH. Location of pacemaker in chick embryo heart at the time of initiation of heartbeat. *Am J Physiol* 1967;212:407–415.
75. Garcia-Frigola C, Shi Y, Evans SM. Expression of the hyperpolarization-activated cyclic nucleotide-gated cation channel HCN4 during mouse heart development. *Gene Expr Patterns* 2003;3: 777–783.
76. Lei M, Goddard C, Liu J, *et al.* Sinus node dysfunction following targeted disruption of the murine cardiac sodium channel gene Scn5a. *J Physiol* 2005; 567:387–400.

3
Anatomic and Histopathological Characteristics of the Conductive Tissues of the Heart

Cristina Basso, Siew Yen Ho, and Gaetano Thiene

Introduction

The cardiac conduction tissues in the human heart comprise specialized myocytes that can be differentiated from working myocardium with routine histological staining. They are located in specific regions of the heart to form the sinus node and the atrioventricular (AV) node, which then extend into the AV bundle and bundle branches. Both cardiac nodes are sited in the atria with working atrial myocardium in between (so called internodal preferential pathways). Atrial myocardium is separated from ventricular myocardium by fibrofatty tissues at the AV junction and rings. In the normal heart, the continuation of specialized myocytes from the AV node that forms the bundle of His, penetrating the central fibrous body, is the only muscular continuity between atrial and ventricular myocardium, allowing atrial impulses to be conveyed to the ventricles in an orderly fashion. In this chapter, we will deal with normal and pathological features of the conductive tissue of the heart.

Normal Anatomy

Sinus Node: Location, Anatomy, and Histology

Discovered by Keith and Flack a century ago,[1] the sinus node (the cardiac pacemaker) was illustrated as lying in the terminal groove (sulcus terminalis), in the lateral part of the junction between the superior caval vein and the right atrium. This lateral position was endorsed by Koch[2] and by most subsequent investigators.[3–5] A horseshoe arrangement with the node situated anteriorly and draped over the crest of the atrial appendage as described by Hudson[6] is found in approximately 10% of hearts.[7]

The shape of the node, more commonly, is like a tadpole with a head section situated anterosuperiorly and a tapering tail that extends for a variable distance inferiorly toward the entrance of the inferior caval vein (Figure 3–1).[2,8] In the subepicardium, the long axis of the node is parallel to the terminal groove, but the body and tail then penetrate intramyocardially toward the subendocardium. Thus, the fatty tissues of the terminal groove serve as the epicardial landmark, whereas the terminal crest (crista terminalis) in the anterolateral quadrant of the entrance of the superior caval vein is the endocardial landmark for the nodal head. The nodal body and tail lie in the terminal crest and are at varying depths from the endocardium.[8] In the adult the length of the nodal body is approximately 1–2 cm, but the tail portion can extend considerably longer.

The artery supplying the node is a branch from the proximal right coronary artery in 55% of hearts and from the left circumflex coronary artery in the remainder.[7] The nodal artery approaches the node anteriorly in majority of hearts, but can also approach posteriorly or form an arterial circle around the cavoatrial junction.[9] Typically, the nodal artery passes centrally through the length of the nodal body.

The node is a specialized muscular structure composed mainly of small, interlacing myocytes

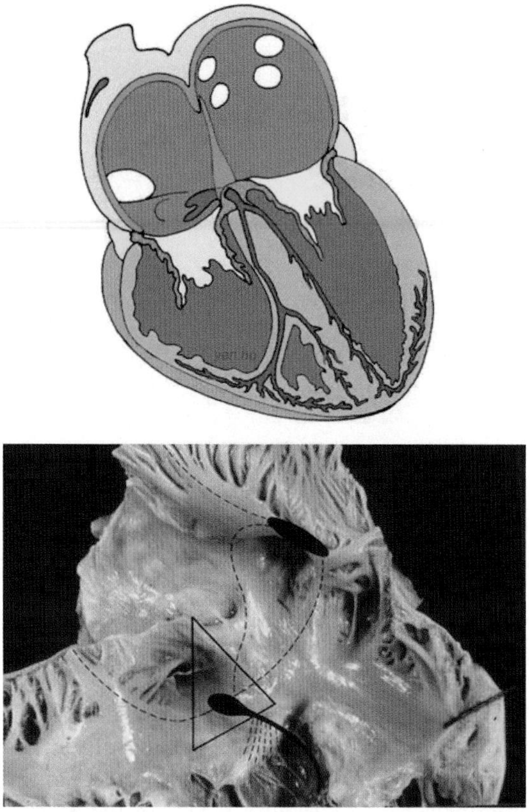

a

b

FIGURE 3–1. (a) Diagram illustrating the topography of the specialized conduction system (red) of the heart; (b) view of the right atrium: the sinus node is located at the root of the superior vena cava, lying over the crista terminalis, and the AV node within the triangle of Koch. Dotted lines depict internodal pathways and left bundle branch.

of no definite orientation within a background of extracellular matrix, surrounded by a parasymphatetic ganglionated plexus accounting for the nerve supply.[10] On histology, the node appears as a dense aggregation and the specialized myocytes (P-cells) appear less darkly stained than the neighboring working atrial myocardium (Figure 3–2). However, the nodal margins may be discrete with fibrous separation from atrial myocardium or interdigitate through a transitional zone. In the latter, prongs of nodal (P) and transitional (T) cells extend into the atrial myocardium but actual cell-to-cell contact is uncertain. Prongs radiating from the nodal body are common.[8] Occasional prongs can be found extending toward the wall of the superior caval vein. In some hearts, the distal part of the nodal tail appears as clusters of specialized myocytes among fibrofatty tissues and atrial myocytes in the subendocardium.[8]

Internodal and Interatrial Myocardium

The transmission of the cardiac impulse from the sinus node to the AV node is often depicted as through three internodal tracts in cardiology texts. These are portrayed as cable-like structures that pass anteriorly, medially, and posteriorly in the right atrium (Figure 3–1b). However, light microscopy and electron microscopy examinations have not revealed specialized bundles in the atrial walls that could satisfy the criteria of conduction tissue tracts. Apart from the occasional caudal extension of the sinus node into the crista terminalis, there are no histologically recognizable specialized pathways. This is also true for the interatrial conduction through the so-called Backman's bundle.[11] Instead, the walls of the atria

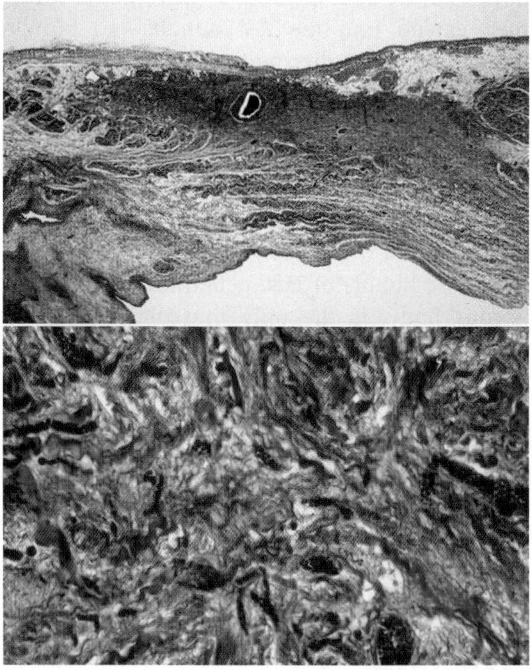

FIGURE 3–2. (a) Longitudinal section of the sulcus and crista terminalis: the sinus node is located subepicardially and centered by the sinus node artery. Note the abundant extracellular matrix (Heidenhain trichrome ×5); (b) at higher magnification, the small, interlacing pale myocytes with P and T cells are visible (Heidenhain trichrome ×40).

are made up of broad bands of working myocardium that are separated by orifices of the veins, foramen ovale, and the AV valves. Parts of the wall, for example, the crista terminalis and the anterior rim around the foramen ovale, show a better alignment of the myocytes than other parts, allowing preferential propagation of the cardiac impulse. Thus, the spread of excitation from pacemaker to AV node as well as to the left atrium is along broad wavefronts within the muscular bands. Through its transitional cell zone, the AV node acts as the "receiver," which then channels the impulse to the ventricles via the specialized conduction bundle and bundle branches.

Atrioventricular Conduction System: Location, Anatomy, and Histology

The pioneering work of Tawara[12] a century ago likened the AV system to a tree, with its roots in the atrial septum and its branches ramifying within the ventricles. He recognized a collection of histologically distinct cells at the base of the atrial septum that he termed the "knoten," and that has subsequently become known as the AV node.

Being the atrial component of the AV conduction system, the AV node receives, slows down, and conveys atrial impulses to the ventricles. It is an interatrial structure located on the right side of the central fibrous body and when considered from the right atrial aspect it is situated within the triangle of Koch (Figure 3–1). The triangle described by Koch[2] is bordered anteriorly by the "annulus" of the septal leaflet of the tricuspid valve, posteriorly by the tendon of Todaro that runs within the sinus septum (Eustachian ridge or crista dividens), and inferiorly by the orifice of the coronary sinus and the atrial vestibule (Figure 3–1). The vestibule is recognized by arrhythmologists as the so-called "septal isthmus." This is the target for ablating the slow pathway in patients with AV nodal reentrant tachycardia.[13] The central fibrous body itself is composed of a thickened area of fibrous continuity between the leaflets of the mitral and aortic valves, termed the right fibrous trigone (Figure 3–3), together with the membranous component of the cardiac septum. The tendon of Todaro inserts into the central fibrous body that lies at the apex of the triangle (Figure 3–4a).[14] The "annulus" of the septal leaflet of the tricuspid valve crosses the membranous septum (Figure 3–5a).

The compact node, approximately 5 mm long, 5 mm wide, and 0.8 mm thick in adults,[15] is adjacent to the central fibrous body on the right side but is uninsulated by fibrous tissue on its other sides, allowing contiguity with the atrial myocardium (Figure 3–3). Due to the lower level of attachment of the tricuspid valve relative to the mitral valve, the AV node "leans" toward the right atrial side and is a few millimeters from the endocardium (Figure 3–3). From the node extends the AV bundle of His that passes through the fibrous core of the central fibrous body (Figure 3–4). The bundle veers leftward as it penetrates the central fibrous body, taking it away from the right atrial endocardium and toward the ventricular septum. In the majority of hearts it emerges to the left of the ventricular septal crest but is insulated from the ventricular myocardium by fibrous tissue and from the atrial myocardium by the membranous septum itself (Figure 3–5b). Viewed from the left ventricle, the hallmark of the AV bundle is the area of fibrous continuity between the aortic and mitral valves that is adjacent to the membranous septum. Viewed from the aorta, the interleaflet fibrous triangle between the right and the noncoronary sinuses adjoins the membranous septum and the AV bundle passes beneath that part of the septum (Figure 3–6).

Progressing forward, the AV bundle divides into left and right bundle branches, still ensheathed by fibrous tissue until the bundle branches have descended approximately half-way down the septum. Descending in the subendocardium, the left bundle branch fans out into interconnecting fascicles as depicted in the original drawings by Tawara (Figure 3–7).[12] The fascicles then ramify into thinner and thinner strands toward the apex. Sometimes its proximal subendocardial course is visible due to the glistening sheen of its fibrous sheath. Due to its fan shape, its proximal portion is considerably more extensive than that of the right bundle branch. The right bundle branch, a cord-like structure, is a direct continuation of the AV bundle. In the majority of hearts, since the AV bundle is usually to the left of the ventricular septal crest instead of being astride the crest, the right bundle branch passes through the septal myocardium before reaching the subendocar-

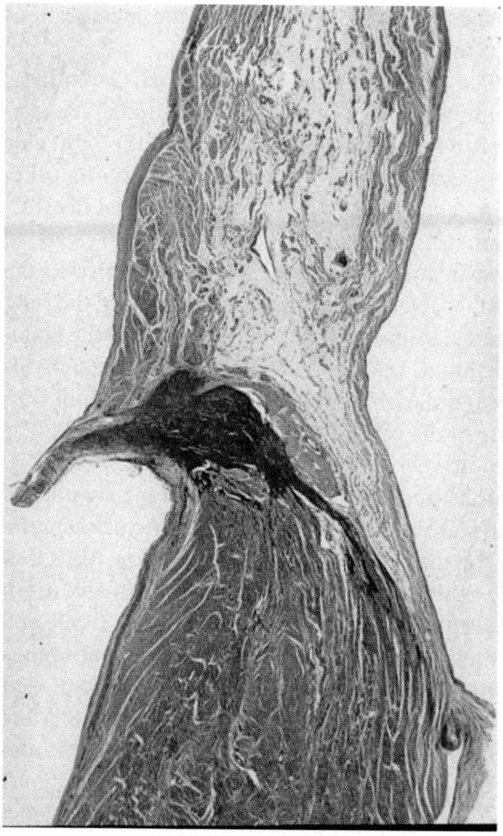

a

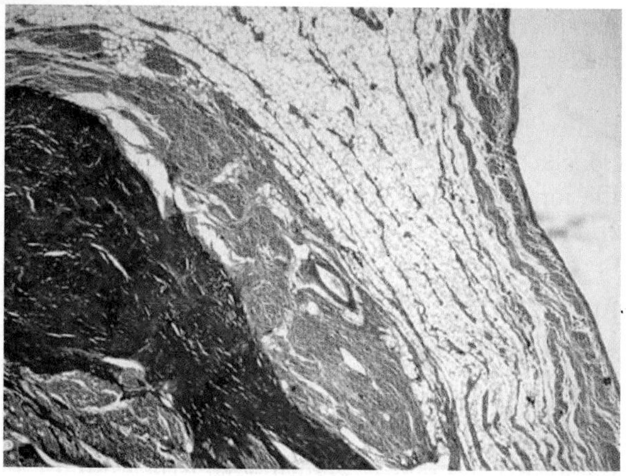

FIGURE 3–3. (a) The AV node is located on the right side of the central fibrous body, which extends to the fibrous mitroaortic continuity (Heidenhain trichrome ×3); (b) close-up of the AV node, with compact and transitional zones, centered by the AV nodal artery (Heidenhain trichrome ×12).

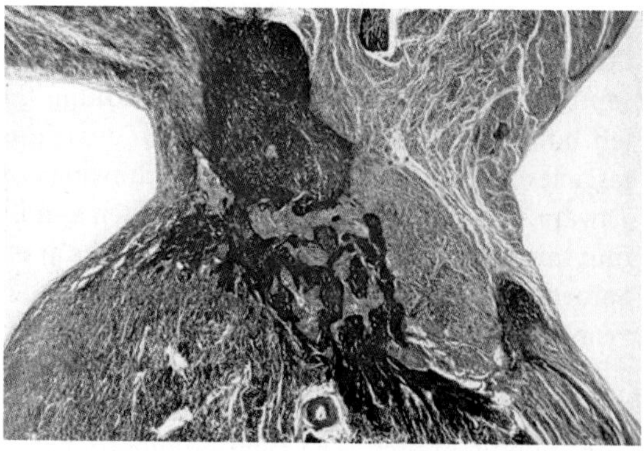

a

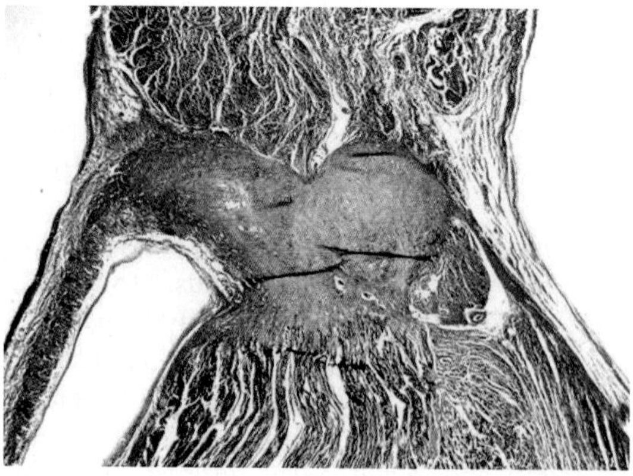

b

FIGURE 3–4. (a) Penetrating AV bundle: note on the top the tendon of Todaro, approximating the central fibrous body (Heidenhain trichrome ×12); (b) common AV bundle running within the fibrous body on the right side and surrounded by a fibrous sheath (Heidenhain trichrome ×12).

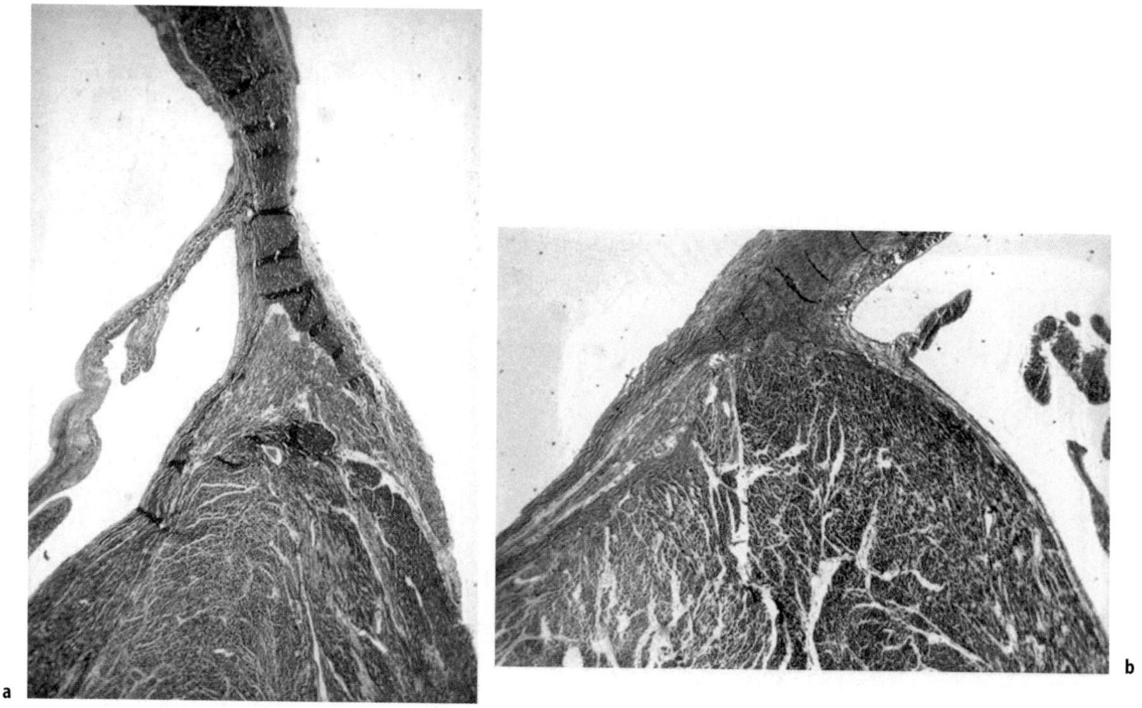

FIGURE 3–5. (a) Bifurcating bundle astride the ventricular septal crest, underneath the membranous septum: note the insertion of the septal leaflet of the tricuspid valve dividing the membranous septum in interventricular and AV components (Heidenhain trichrome ×4); (b) course of the bifurcating bundle on the left side of the ventricular septal crest: note the insulation of the bundle by fibrous tissue and the intramyocardial course of the proximal right bundle branch (Heidenhain trichrome ×8).

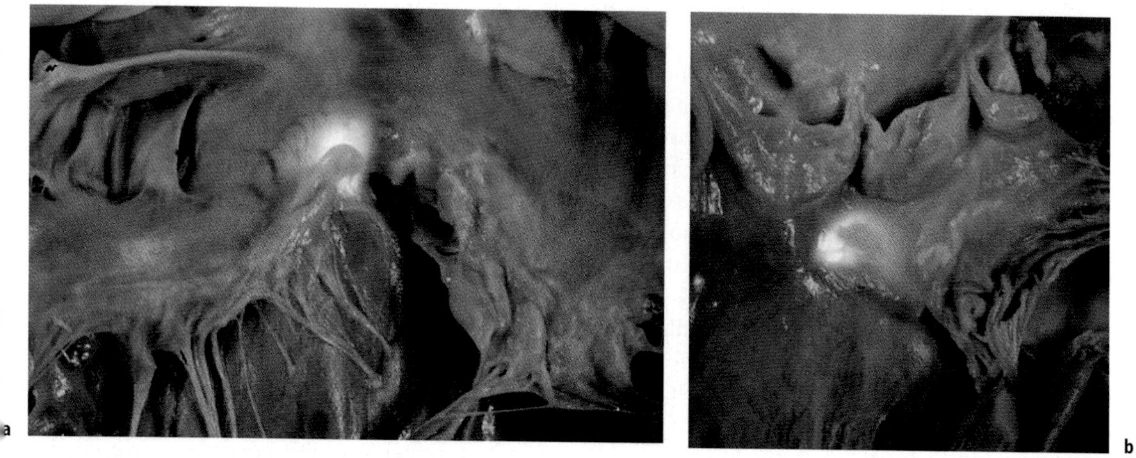

FIGURE 3–6. The "core" of the heart in correspondence to the membranous septum, where the specialized AV junction is located (a, right side view; b, left side view). The hallmark of the AV bundle is the continuity between the aortic and mitral valves, adjacent to the membranous septum, which is located underneath the interleaflet triangle between the right and posterior noncoronary cusps.

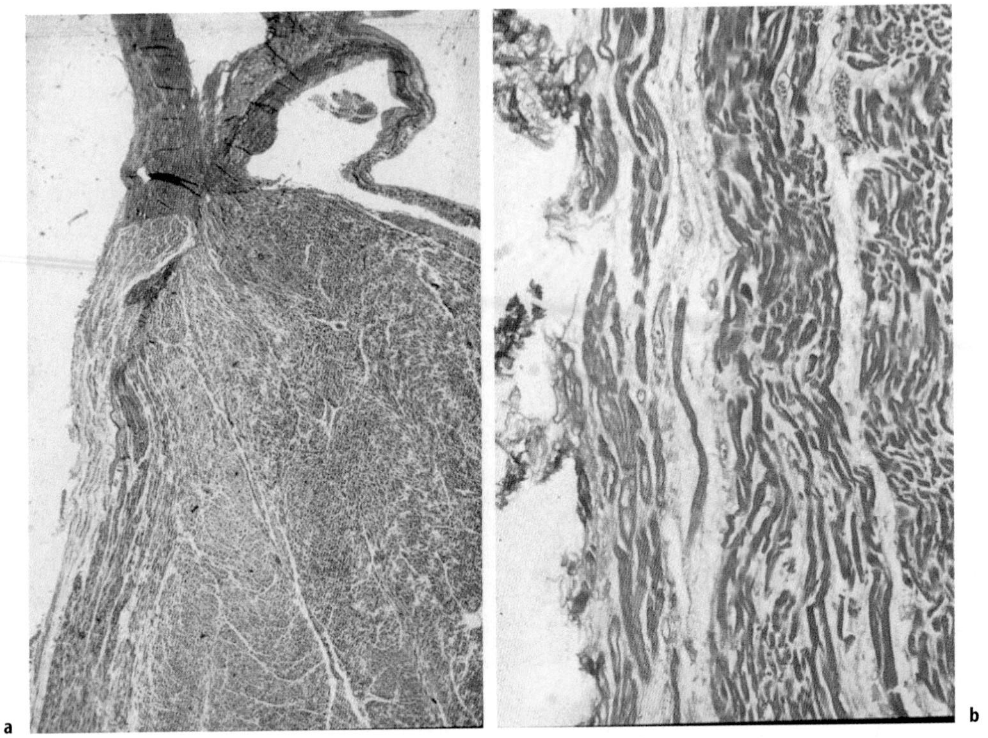

FIGURE 3–7. (a) The course of the left bundle branch under the subendocardium of the left side of the ventricular septum (Heidenhain trichrome ×5); (b) close-up of the Purkinje-like cells of the left bundle branch (Heidenhain trichrome ×25).

dium of the right side of the ventricular septum (Figure 3–5b). The anatomical landmark for its emergence is the base of the medial papillary muscle (Lancisi muscle). From there its proximal portion can often be seen as a white line in the subendocardium of the septomarginal trabeculation where it is still within a fibrous sheath. Distally, ramifications of the right bundle branch extend to the apex of the heart, and are also carried across the ventricular cavity through the moderator band and other muscular bundles (Figure 3–1). In some hearts, an additional bundle arises from the branching bundle, in between the bundle branches, and extends forward. This is described as the "dead end tract" and is more often seen in fetal and infantile hearts than in adult hearts.[16] It continues from the main bundle anterosuperiorly toward the root of the aorta.

Under the microscope, the specialized AV conduction bundle and its main branches are readily identifiable by their encasing fibrous sheaths using basic histological stains. In keeping with Tawara's work,[12] it is the continuity from section to section that serves as the most reliable method for histological localization of the AV conduction system.

Beginning with the AV node, which has the inherent function of delaying the cardiac impulse, the human node has a compact portion and zones of transitional cells (Figure 3–3). The compact node is recognizable, when seen in cross sections, as a half-moon-shaped structure hugging the central fibrous body. The nodal cells are smaller than atrial myocytes. Like the cells of the sinus node, the compact nodal cells are closely grouped and are frequently arranged in an interweaving fashion. In many hearts, the compact node has a stratified appearance with a deep layer overlain by a superficial layer. When traced inferiorly, toward the base of Koch's triangle, the compact area separates into two prongs, usually with the artery supplying the node running in between. The prongs bifurcate toward the tricuspid and mitral annuli, respectively. Their lengths vary from heart to heart and in recent years the rightward prongs have been implicated in so-called slow pathway conduction in AV nodal reentrant tachycardia.[17] Interposing between the compact node and the working atrial myocardium is a zone of transitional cells (Figure 3–3b). These cells are histologically distinct from both the cells of the compact node and the working cells of the atrial myocardium, and are not insulated from the surrounding myocardium. The cells are long, attenuated, and have a wavy appearance. They tend to be separated from one another by thin fibrous strands. According to established definitions, transitional cells do not represent conducting tracts but they provide the crucial bridge between the working and the specialized myocardium. Transitional cells interpose between the left and right margins of the compact node and the myocardium from the left and right sides of the atrial septum. Wider extensions of transitional cells are present inferiorly and posteriorly between the compact node and the mouth of the coronary sinus and into the Eustachian ridge. The right margin of the node faces the vestibule of the right atrium. Here, an overlay of working myocytes in the subendocardium from the atrial wall in front of the fossa ovalis streams over the layer of transitional cells.

When the conduction system is followed distally from the compact node into the penetrating bundle of His, there can be little difference in the cellular composition in the two areas. The specialized cells themselves, however, become aligned in a more parallel fashion distally. Even so, Tawara[12] proposed that the distinction be made on purely anatomical grounds. The key change from node to bundle is that the bundle is insulated by fibrous tissue from the adjacent myocardium (Figure 3–4a), preventing atrial activity from bypassing the node. Thus, all atrial activity must be channeled via the AV node.

Being surrounded by fibrous tissue, the penetrating bundle is the first part of the axis that qualifies as a conducting tract (Figure 3–4b). The cells are marginally larger than compact nodal cells and they increase in size as the penetrating bundle continues into the AV bundle and branching bundle. Here, the cells are very similar in size to ventricular myocytes. Swollen cells or Purkinje cells are not characteristic of specialized myocytes in the human heart and are seldom seen. However, they are typically seen in ungulates.[12,18] The AV bundle, branching bundle, and proximal parts of the bundle branches are recognizable by the fibrous sheaths that encase them, insulating them from the adjacent working ventricular myocardium. When the bundles lose their fibrous sheaths distally, it is no longer possible to distinguish conduction tissues from working myocardium.

Pathology

Sinoatrial Block and Sinus Arrest

The atrial activation may be impaired (atrial standstill) for two main reasons: impulses are not generated from the sinus node (sinus arrest) or their propagation to the atria is impeded (sinus block). In the etiology of sinoatrial block, several lesions of the sinus node and its innervation have been described, in addition to neurovegetative changes (vagal stimulation), drug sensitivity–intoxication, and hyperkalemia.

From a pathological viewpoint, abnormalities of the sinus node artery, of the specialized myocardium of the sinus node, and/or of its connections with the atrial myocardium (nodal approaches), and of the nodal ganglionated plexus have been reported. Myocardial infarction due to occlusion of the right coronary artery, proximal to the origin of the sinus node artery, remains the main cause of sinus node dysfunction, causing severe damage of the node and its atrial approaches in terms of necrosis, leukocytic infiltrates, and hemorrhage. Sinus node artery perfusion can be also altered as a consequence of arteritis (Figure 3–8) embolism (Figure 3–9), amyloid deposition, and connective tissue disorders.[19–22] The recipient sinus node in cardiac transplantation undergoes massive infarction due to nodal artery transection during the surgical procedure and the donor sinus node artery may show obstructive intimal proliferations due to allograft vasculopathy (chronic rejection).[23]

Atrioventricular Block

Any disease, either acute or chronic, that affects the myocardium may produce AV block, which may occur at the level of AV node approaches, the

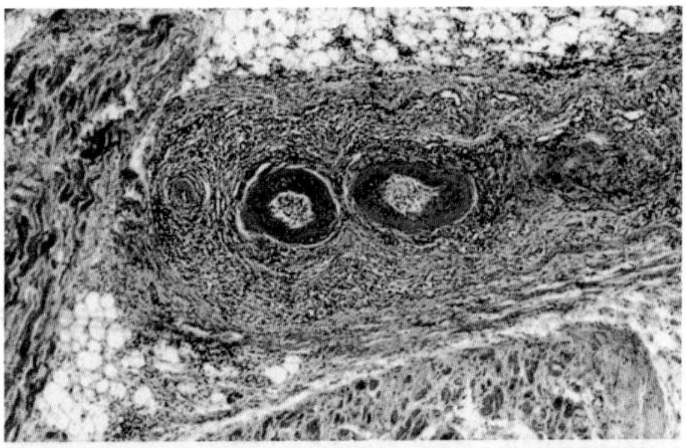
a

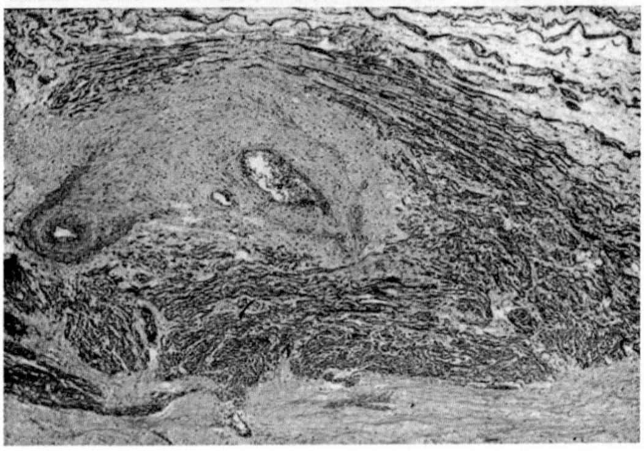
b

Figure 3–8. (a) Arteritis of the sinus node artery in polyarteritis nodosa: note the inflammation extended to the nodal myocardium (hematoxylin–eosin ×15); (b) AV node in polyarteritis nodosa: the AV nodal artery shows aneurysm and recanalized thrombus with extensive fibrotic replacement of conductive cells (hematoxylin–eosin ×15).

AV node itself, the penetrating or branching part of the bundle, and bundle branches.[19–21,24]

Morgagni, Adams, and Stokes share the merit of having individuated the clinical entity of AV block and, after the recognition of the anatomic basis of the AV conduction by His and Tawara, Mahaim did the first clinicopathologic assessment of this entity.[25]

Pathologically, AV block may be classified as being caused by congenital or acquired diseases.[24] The *congenital* AV block in an otherwise normally developed heart is usually a benign condition, mainly due to a lack of connection between the atria and the peripheral conduction system, with fatty replacement of the AV node and nodal approaches.[26] Moreover, the AV bundle may present marked fragmentation and septation. Maternal lupus with an immune mechanism plays a major etiopathogenetic role.[27] Congenital or acquired AV block has been reported in cardiac malformations characterized by the l-loop, like congenitally corrected transposition and single (double-inlet) left ventricle.

Iatrogenic AV block may occur following surgical or interventional manipulation of the conducting system. Surgical (aortic valve replacement, congenital septal defects repair, septal myectomy) or other therapeutic procedures (AV ablation in patients with supraventricular arrhythmias and alcohol septal ablation in patients with obstructive hypertrophic cardiomyopathy) may be complicated by AV block.[26] Patients with perimembranous ventricular septal defects, either isolated or in the setting of various congenital heart diseases (tetralogy of Fallot, truncus arteriosus, or complete transposition of the great arteries), are at risk of postoperative AV block if a stitch crosses the posteroinferior border of the defect. Patients with corrected transposition of the great vessels have anterior displacement of the AV specialized axis and are prone to develop complete heart block during surgical procedures.

Atrioventricular block may be caused by *acute myocardial ischemia or infarction*. Inferior myocardial infarction may be complicated by third-degree AV block due to ischemic injury of the AV node itself. In particular, in posteroseptal myocardial infarction, due to right coronary artery thrombotic occlusion in a right dominant pattern, ischemic damage may involve atrial approaches to the AV node and His bundle. However, since the conducting tissues are resistent to ischemia, pathological changes may be reversible and the AV block transient. Anterior myocardial infarction is usually associated with third-degree AV block

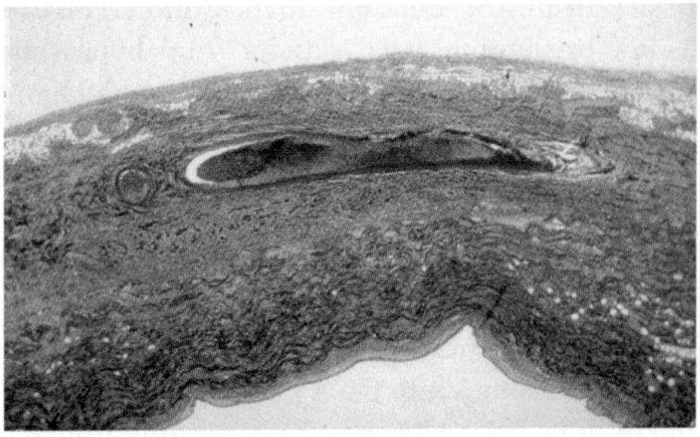

Figure 3–9. Massive infarction of the sinus node and crista terminalis by occlusive thromboembolism of the nodal artery (Heidenhain trichrome ×6).

due to ischemia or infarction of bundle branches; the branching bundle and bundle branches are often involved by the necrotic process and by inflammatory infiltrates of the surrounding working ventricular myocardium.[28] Chronic ischemic heart disease, with or without infarction, may also be characterized by AV block, due to fibrotic changes of the bifurcating bundle and bundle branches, as well as of the crest of the ventricular septum.[24]

The heart may be the target of *angioitides and collagen diseases.* Polyarteritis nodosa is a medium-large vessel vasculitis, with cardiac involvement in up to 80% of cases. It typically manifests as pericarditis, coronary arteritis, myocardial infarction, arrhythmias, and conduction disturbances (Figure 3–8b).[22] Nodal arteries may be of the proper size to be affected and the surrounding conductive tissue may be involved as well.

Cardiac involvement has been reported in 8–44% of cases of Wegener's granulomatosis. It typically manifests as pericarditis, coronary arteritis, and myocarditis with granulomas involving the conduction system.

Similarly, cardiac involvement is seen in up to 70% of cases of systemic lupus erythematosus. The most common findings are pericarditis, myocarditis, and Libman–Sacks endocarditis. As previously mentioned, congenital heart block is a peculiar feature of neonatal lupus syndrome, which is associated with transplacental transfer of anti-Ro and anti-La antibodies.[27] In rheumatoid arthritis, rheumatoid granulomas may affect the myocardium, endocardium, and valves as well as the conductive tissues; conduction disturbances and heart block have been reported.[29]

Myotonic dystrophy, particularly type 1 (Steinert's disease), which is the commonest muscular dystrophy in adults, is characterized by myotonia, muscle weakness, and a variety of other symptoms. Cardiac involvement is a frequent manifestation, the most prominent feature being conduction disturbances and arrhythmias, with risk of sudden death.[30]

Myocarditis, especially in the acute phase, may present with AV block. It is usually transient and relates to inflammatory infiltrates and interstitial edema of the working myocardium surrounding the specialized conducting pathways, although involvement of the sinus node and AV node themselves has been reported. In *acute rheumatic carditis*, all the structures of the heart may be involved by the inflammatory process, including the conduction system. In terms of rhythm disturbance, besides tachyarrhythmias, varying degrees of heart block, mostly first degree, are frequently recorded. Similar features with transient AV block may complicate *acute rejection* of the specialized conducting tissues after cardiac transplantation.[23]

In *infective endocarditis* of the aortic and/or mitral valve, the inflammatory process may extend to the central fibrous body, thereby disrupting the AV node and His bundle to produce AV block.

Complete AV block also occurs in the setting of *hypertensive heart disease*, and it can result from a combination of direct mechanical injury to the origin of the main left bundle branch and ischemic heart disease.

Calcific aortic stenosis has long been recognized as a cause of AV block, and many of the patients originally reported by Stokes correspond to this entity. The His bundle penetrates the central fibrous body in close proximity to both the aortic and mitral valve fibrous continuity, which is the usual site of dystrophic calcification, and extension of calcification can directly involve the His bundle and/or the origin of the left bundle branch (Figure 3–10).

Degenerative changes in the AV node or bundle branches are the most common cause of nonischemic AV block. The term Lenègre–Lev

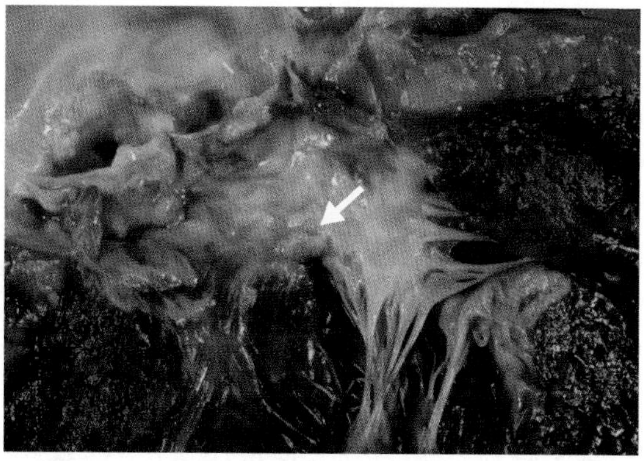

FIGURE 3–10. Calcific aortic stenosis with dystrophic calcification extended to the mitroaortic continuity (arrow), where the His bundle is coming out.

syndrome has been used to indicate an acquired complete heart block due to idiopathic fibrosis and calcification of the AV conduction system of the heart. However, we should keep the two entities distinct.

Lev disease is most commonly seen in the elderly, and is often described as senile degeneration of the conduction system.[31] It may imply, among others, degenerative changes at the summit of the ventricular septum, mitroaortic fibrous continuity, and membranous septum, consisting of fibrosis, hyalinization, and loss of conducting fibers, with or without calcification. The pathological degenerative process, which has been traditionally considered the result of stress and strain, may affect mainly the branching bundle and the proximal right and left bundle branches. In classical Lev disease, the origin of the left bundle branch and the adjacent bifurcating bundle are destroyed with preservation of the peripheral conduction system.

In contrast, AV block due to *Lenègre disease* occurs in younger people and the histopathological features are in keeping with a primary myocardial disease that selectively destroys the right and left bundle branche conduction fibers, extending well down into the periphery (Figure 3–11).[32] It is a form of inherited cardiomyopathy confined to the specialized myocardium and should be classified among cardiomyopathies.[33] In 1999, Lenègre disease with AV block was linked to mutations of the *SCN5A* sodium channel gene, the same gene that may also account for congenital long QT syndrome type 3 and Brugada syndrome.[34]

Among *infiltrative myocardial diseases*, sarcoidosis is frequently associated with AV block due to sarcoid granulomas involving the specialized axis.[35]

Atrioventricular block may complicate *aortic dissection* when the dissecting hematoma infiltrates the atrial septum along with the retrograde extension, thus creating an atrionodal discontinuity.[36]

The term *celothelioma of the AV node*, known also as Tawarioma or cystic tumor of the AV node, refers to a tumor with heterotopic epithelial replacement of the AV node with multicystic appearance (Figure 3–12). It is a rare entity and, thus, an unusual cause of supra-His AV block, at

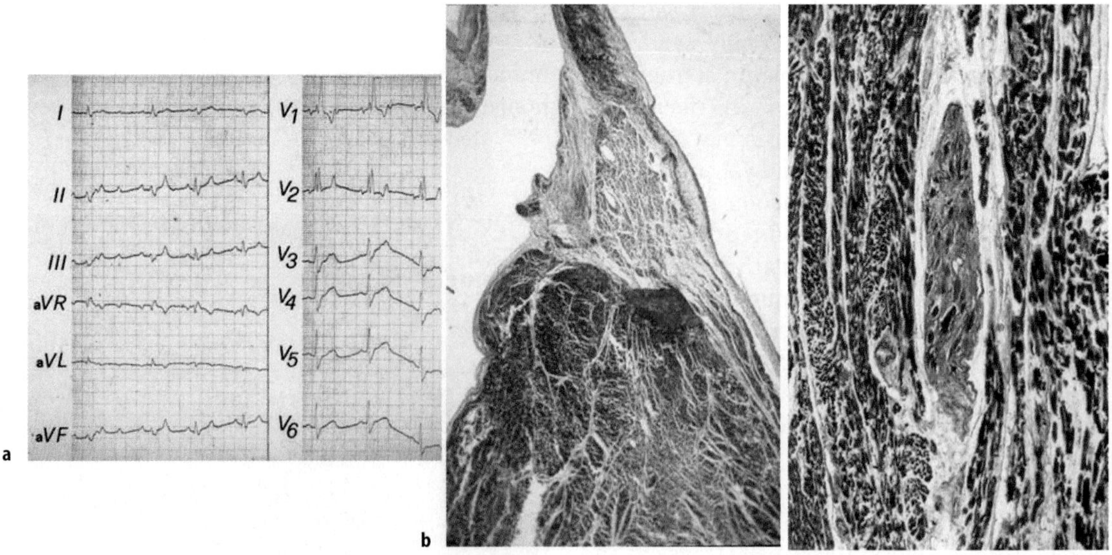

FIGURE 3–11. Lenègre disease with AV block: (a) 12-lead ECG tracing with intermittent AV block; (b) scleroatrophy of the origin of the left bundle branch from the His bundle (Heidenhain trichrome ×6); (c) fibrotic interruption of the intramyocardial tract of the right bundle branch (Heidenhain trichrome ×60).

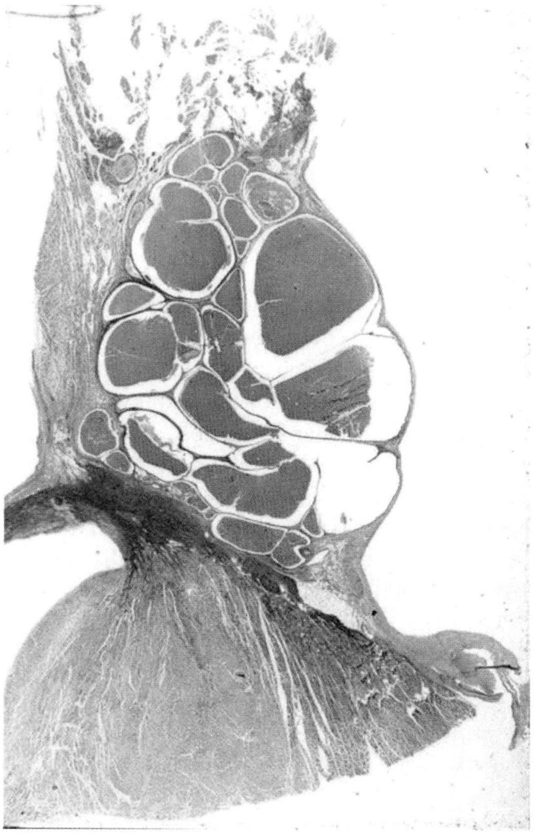

FIGURE 3–12. Cystic tumor of the AV node: note the multicystic neoplasm at the level of the AV node (Heidenhain trichrome ×5).

risk of sudden death. Definitive histological diagnosis is made at autopsy or in explanted hearts from cardiac transplantation.[37,38]

Complete AV block can appear in the setting of other *cardiac tumors*, including metastatic carcinoma of the heart, primary or secondary sarcoma and lymphoma, and by direct infiltration or compression of the conducting tissue.[39]

By studying a series of 177 cases with permanent AV block, Davies[24] showed that idiopathic bilateral bundle branch fibrosis is the commonest single cause (33%), followed by ischemic damage (17%), cardiomyopathies (14%), and calcific AV block (10%). The remaining causes of chronic AV block were individually very rare, and include tumor involvement, congenital defects, collagen diseases, and surgical or traumatic damage.

As far as the site is concerned, according to Rossi[19] the frequency of AV block-producing lesions seems to increase in a downward direction along the AV conducting pathway. Among 400 cases of AV block, which he studied by the serial section histological technique, the AV conduction discontinuity accounting for block could be ascribed to distal lesions of both bundle branches and/or bifurcating bundle in about 70% of cases, of the common His bundle in 15%, of the AV node in 10%, and of the atrio-AV nodal approaches in 5% (Figure 3–13).

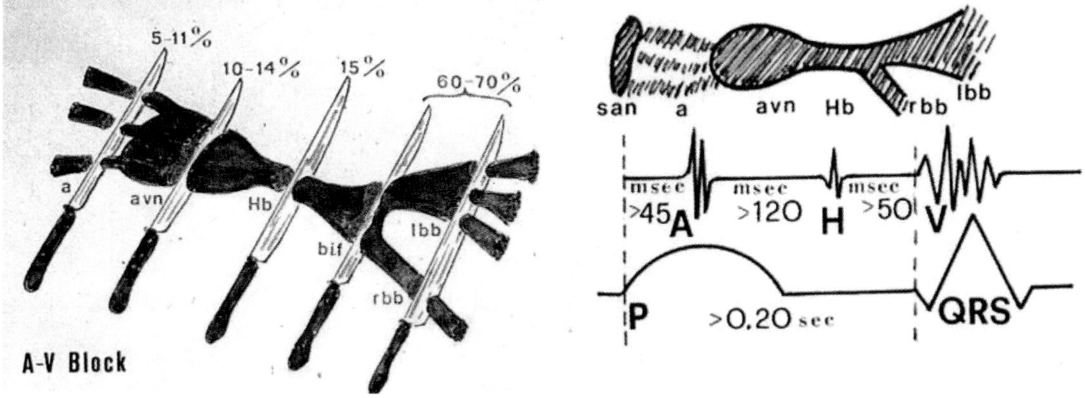

FIGURE 3–13. Site of AV blocking lesions: 60–70% of the interruption of the AV conduction axis is located in the bifurcating proximal bundle branches, accounting for prolongation of the HV interval. (Courtesy of Mito Rossi.)

Ventricular Preexcitation and Enhanced Atrioventricular Conduction

Accessory AV connections accounting for ventricular preexcitation may be "direct" (working-to-working myocardium), when located outside the specialized AV junction and directly connecting the atrial and ventricular myocardium (the so-called "Kent fascicle"), or "mediated" (working-to-specialized myocardium or vice versa), when they involve the specialized AV junction and connect either the septal atrial myocardium with the His bundle (James or Brechenmacher fibers) or the AV conduction axis (Tawarian system) with the ventricular myocardium (Mahaim fibers).[40]

A rare condition that promotes early ventricular excitation is the enhanced AV conduction (so-called Lown–Ganong–Levine syndrome[41]). The impulse runs very quickly through the AV node and His bundle, with a short PR interval and a normal QRS complex. Two histological backgrounds have been reported to explain the missed delay at the specialized AV junction: (1) a congenitally hypoplastic AV node, with a decreased bulk of specialized tissue to slow down impulse transmission from atria to ventricles (Figure 3–14)[42] and (2) the presence of an atrio-Hisian bundle of working myocardium that bypasses the AV node and transmits the activation signal directly to the His bundle without any delay at the nodal level. In both substrates, the onset of atrial fibrillation, with one-to-one AV conduction, may precipitate ventricular fibrillation, as occurs in the Wolff–Parkinson–White syndrome.

In Wolff–Parkinson–White syndrome, an aberrant myocardial fascicle ("Kent fascicle") directly joins the atria to the ventricles out of the specialized AV junction (Figure 3–15).[43,44]

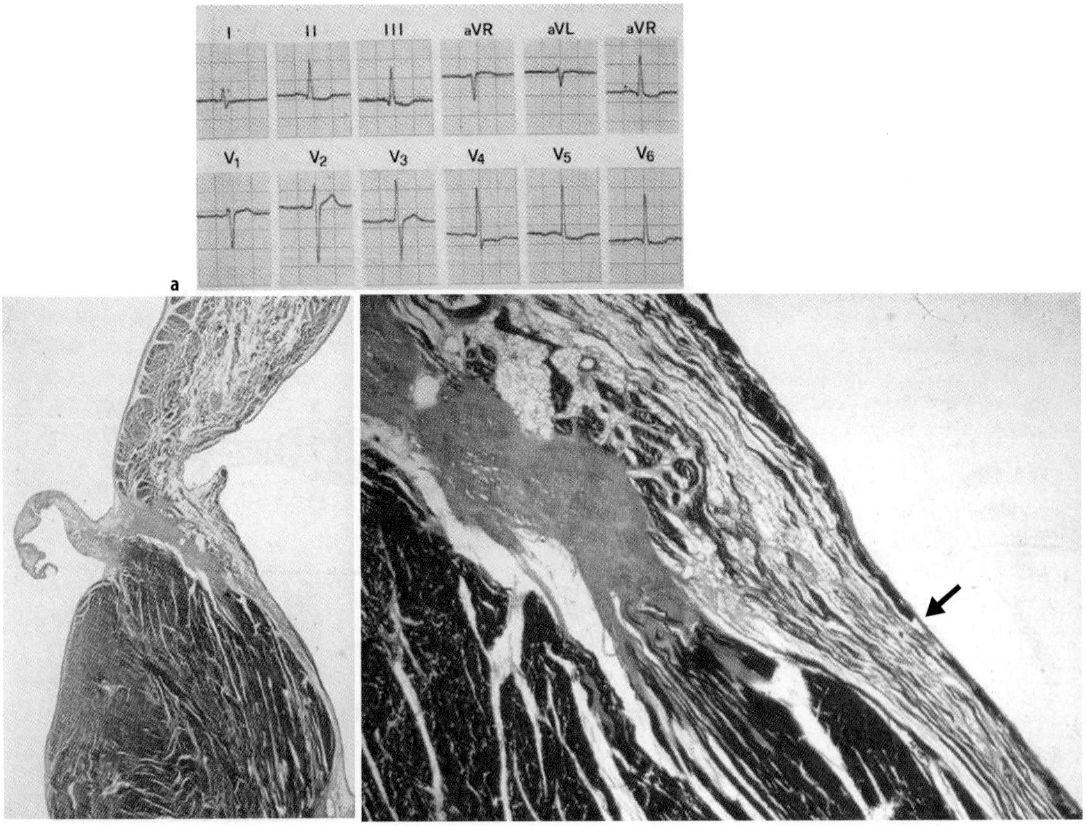

FIGURE 3–14. Lown–Ganong–Levine syndrome: (a) 12-lead ECG tracing with a short PR interval and normal QRS complex; (b) extremely hypoplastic AV node (arrow, Heidenhain trichrome ×6); (c) close-up of (b) (Heidenhain trichrome ×15).

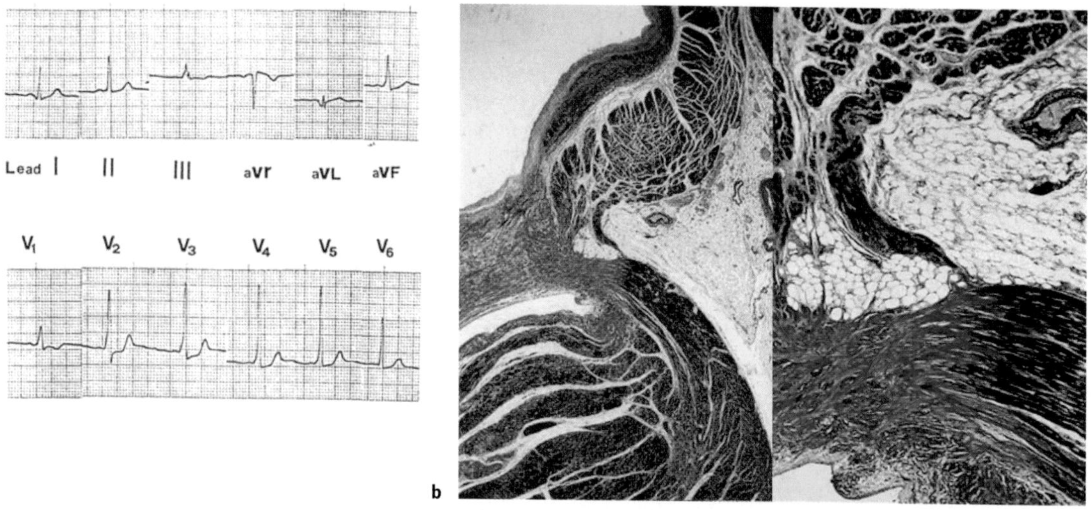

FIGURE 3–15. Wolff–Parkinson–White syndrome: (a) 12-lead ECG tracing with intermittent short PR interval and delta wave; (b) the Kent fascicle, located close to the endocardium, joins the working atrial and ventricular myocardium (Heidenhain trichrome ×6); (c) close-up of (b), with mild fibrosis of the accessory bundle (Heidenhain trichrome ×18).

Such myocardial bridges between atrial and ventricular myocardium, accessory to the normal AV conducting tissue, have been reported either in structurally normal hearts or in hearts with congenital heart diseases, like Ebstein's anomaly[45] and congenitally corrected transposition. This aberrant fascicle of working myocardium can be located all around the left and right AV rings, with the exception of the mitroaortic fibrous continuity area. Accessory pathways in the septal area are less common and are located primarily on the right side. The "Kent fascicle" usually consists of a thin (mean 300 μm in thickness) bundle of working myocardium and, as such, does not possess decremental conduction properties. It may serve not only as a bypass tract for ventricular preexcitation (thus explaining the short PQ interval and the delta wave of the QRS), but also as a limb for an AV reentry circuit, which accounts for a reciprocating supraventricular tachycardia, typical of Wolff–Parkinson–White syndrome. An impedance mismatch between the tiny anomalous fibers and the ventricular muscle bulk, in addition to fibrosis of the accessory fascicle, may explain impaired antegrade conduction and intermittent preexcitation. Preexcitation syndromes are a not so minor cause of sudden death.[44] The mechanism is believed to be paroxysmal atrial fibrillation, with one-to-one conduction, which may degenerate into ventricular fibrillation and cardiac arrest. In these conditions, atrial myocarditis may trigger the onset of life-threatening lone atrial fibrillation.[44] The accessory fascicle along the AV sulcus is always located closer to the endocardium than to the epicardium; size and site are such that "Kent's fascicle" is easily amenable to endocardial transcatheter ablation, which is the current procedure to interrupt the preexcitation and to reestablish the regular electrical connection through the His bundle.

References

1. Keith A, Flack M. The form and nature of the muscular connections between the primary divisions of the vertebrate heart. *J Anat Physiol* 1907;41:172–189.
2. Koch W. *Der Funktionelle Bau des Menschlichen Herzens*. Berlin, Urban und Schwarzenburg, 1922: 92.
3. James TN. Anatomy of the human sinus node. *Anat Rec* 1961;141:109–116.
4. Truex RC, Smythe MQ, Taylor MJ. Reconstruction of the human sinuatrial node. *Anat Rec* 1967;159: 371–378.

5. Lev M, Bharati S. Lesions of the conduction system and their functional significance. *Pathol Annu* 1974;9:157–160.
6. Hudson REB. The human pacemaker and its pathology. *Br Heart J* 1960;22:153–156.
7. Anderson KR, Ho SY, Anderson RH. Location and vascular supply of sinus node in human heart. *Br Heart J* 1979;41:28–32.
8. Sanchez-Quintana D, Cabrera C, Farre J, *et al.* Sinus node revisited in the era of electroanatomical mapping and catheter ablation. *Heart* 2005;91:189–194.
9. Busquet J, Fontan F, Anderson RH, *et al.* The surgical significance of the atrial branches of the coronary arteries. *Int J Cardiol* 1984;6:223–234.
10. James TN. Structure and function of the sinus node, AV node and His bundle of the human heart: Part I-structure. *Prog Cardiovasc Dis* 2002;45:235–267.
11. James TN. The internodal pathways of the human heart. *Prog Cardiovasc Dis* 2001;43:495–535.
12. Tawara S. *Das Reizleitungssystem des Säugetierherzens.* Jena: Gustav Fischer, 1906.
13. Olgin JE, Ursell PC, Kao AK, *et al.* Pathological findings following slow pathway ablation for AV nodal reentrant tachycardia. *J Cardiovasc Electrophysiol* 1996;7:625–631.
14. Ho SY, Anderson RH. How constant anatomically is the tendon of Todaro as a marker of the triangle of Koch? *J Cardiovasc Electrophysiol* 2000;11:83–89.
15. Sanchez-Quintana D, Ho SY, Cabrera JA, *et al.* Topographic anatomy of the inferior pyramidal space: Relevance to radiofrequency ablation. *J Cardiovasc Electrophysiol* 2001;12:210–217.
16. Kurosawa H, Becker AE. Dead-end tract of the conduction axis. *Int J Cardiol* 1985;7:13–18.
17. Inoue S, Becker AE. Posterior extensions of the human compact AV node. A neglected anatomic feature of potential clinical significance. *Circulation* 1998;97:188–193.
18. Ho SY, McCarthy KP, Ansari A, *et al.* Anatomy of the atrioventricular node and atrioventricular conduction system. *J Bifurcation Chaos* 2003;12:3665–3674.
19. Rossi L, Ed. *Histopathology of Cardiac Arrhythmias.* Philadelphia, PA: Lea & Febiger, 1979.
20. Rossi L, Thiene G. *Arrhythmologic Pathology of Sudden Cardiac Death.* Milano: Casa Editrice Ambrosiana, 1983.
21. Davies MJ. *Pathology of Conducting Tissue of the Heart.* Butterworths, London, 1971.
22. Thiene G, Valente M, Rossi L. Involvement of the cardiac conducting system in panarteritis nodosa. *Am Heart J* 1978;95:716–724.
23. Calzolari V, Angelini A, Basso C, *et al.* Histologic findings in the conduction system after cardiac transplantation and correlation with electrocardiographic findings. *Am J Cardiol* 1999;84:756–759.
24. Davies MJ. Pathology of chronic A-V Block. *Acta Cardiol* 1976;21:19–30.
25. Mahaim I. *Maladies Organiques du Faisceau de His-Tawara.* Paris: Masson et Cie, 1931.
26. Bharati S. Pathology of the conduction system. In: Silver MD, Gotlieb AI, Schoen FJ, Eds. *Cardiovascular Pathology*, 3rd ed. Philadelphia, PA: Churchill Livingstone, 2001:607–628.
27. Chameides L, Truex RC, Vetter V, *et al.* Association of maternal systemic lupus erythematosus with congenital complete heart block. *N Engl J Med* 1977; 297:1204–1207.
28. Becker AE, Lie KI, Anderson RH. Bundle-branch block in the setting of acute anteroseptal myocardial infarction. Clinicopathological correlation. *Br Heart J* 1978;40:773–782.
29. James TN. De subitaneis mortibus. XXIII. Rheumatoid arthritis and ankylosing spondylitis. *Circulation* 1977;55:669–677.
30. Nguyen HH, Wolfe JT 3rd, Holmes DR Jr, *et al.* Pathology of the cardiac conduction system in myotonic dystrophy: A study of 12 cases. *J Am Coll Cardiol* 1988;11:662–671.
31. Lev M. Anatomic basis for atrio-ventricular block. *Am J Med* 1964;37:742–748.
32. Lenegre J, Moreau P. Chronic auriculo-ventricular block. Anatomical, clinical and histological study. *Arch Mal Coeur Vaiss* 1963;56:867–888.
33. Maron BJ, Towbin JA, Thiene G, *et al.* Contemporary definitions and classification of the cardiomyopathies: An American Heart Association Scientific Statement from the Council on Clinical Cardiology, Heart Failure and Transplantation Committee; Quality of care and outcomes research and functional genomics and translational biology interdisciplinary working groups, and council on epidemiology and prevention. *Circulation* 2006;113: 1807–1816.
34. Schott JJ, Alshinawi C, Kyndt F, *et al.* Cardiac conduction defects associate with mutations in SCN5A. *Nat Genet* 1999;23:20–21.
35. James TN. Clinicopathologic correlations. De subitaneis mortibus. XXV. Sarcoid heart disease. *Circulation* 1977;56:320–326.
36. Thiene G, Rossi L, Becker AE. The atrioventricular conduction system in dissecting aneurysm of the aorta. *Am Heart J* 1979;98:447–452.
37. James TN, Galakhov I. De subitaneis mortibus. XXVI. Fatal electrical instability of the heart associated with benign congenital polycystic tumor of

the atrioventricular node. *Circulation* 1977;56:667–678.
38. Basso C, Valente M, Poletti A, *et al.* Surgical pathology of primary cardiac and pericardial tumors. *Eur J Cardiothorac Surg* 1997;12:730–737.
39. Thiene G, Miraglia G, Menghetti L, *et al.* Multiple lesions of the conduction system in a case of cardiac rhabdomyosarcoma with complex arrhythmias. An anatomic and clinical study. *Chest* 1976;70:378–381.
40. Anderson RH, Becker AE, Brechenmacher C, *et al.* Ventricular preexcitation. A proposed nomenclature for its substrates. *Eur J Cardiol* 1975;3:27–36.
41. Lown B, Ganong WF, Levine SA. The syndrome of short P-R interval, normal QRS complex and paroxysmal rapid heart action. *Circulation* 1952;5:693–706.
42. Ometto R, Thiene G, Corrado D, *et al.* Enhanced A-V nodal conduction (Lown-Ganong-Levine syndrome) by congenitally hypoplastic A-V node. *Eur Heart J* 1992;13:1579–1584.
43. Becker AE, Anderson RH, Durrer D, *et al.* The anatomical substrates of Wolff-Parkinson-White syndrome. A clinicopathologic correlation in seven patients. *Circulation* 1978;57:870–879.
44. Basso C, Corrado D, Rossi L, *et al.* Ventricular preexcitation in children and young adults: Atrial myocarditis as a possible trigger of sudden death. *Circulation* 2001;103:269–275.
45. Thiene G, Pennelli N, Rossi L. Cardiac conduction system abnormalities as a possible cause of sudden death in young athletes. *Hum Pathol* 1983;14:704–709.

4
Neural Regulation of the Heart in Health and Disease

Richard L. Verrier

Introduction

Neural influences on heart rhythm are not only potent but also diverse. The complexity derives from integration at multiple levels in the brain, a network of intrinsic cardiac nerves, and autonomic reflexes, all of which interact with a cardiac substrate altered by advancing age and disease. In patients with ischemic heart disease, which is the major factor underlying risk for sudden cardiac death (SCD),[1] neural influences can predispose to arrhythmias both directly through effects on excitable properties of the heart and its specialized conducting system and more indirectly by impairing myocardial perfusion through effects on coronary vascular function and platelet aggregability (Figure 4–1). Neural influences may also be arrhythmogenic in patients with channelopathies, including the long QT and Brugada syndromes, as discussed in detail in other chapters.

Integration of Neural Control of Cardiac Electrical Activity

Regulation of cardiac neural activity is highly integrated and is achieved by circuitry at multiple levels[2] (Figure 4–2). Higher brain centers operate through elaborate pathways within the hypothalamus and medullary cardiovascular regulatory sites. Baroreceptor mechanisms have long been recognized as integral to autonomic control of the cardiovascular system, as evidenced by heart rate variability and baroreceptor sensitivity testing of both cardiac patients and normal subjects. The intrinsic cardiac nerves and fat pads provide local neural coordination independent of higher brain centers. Newly recognized is the phenomenon of electrical remodeling attributable to nerve growth and degeneration. At the level of the myocardial cell, autonomic receptors influence G proteins to control ionic channels, pumps, and exchangers. Finally, studies of behavioral states provide evidence that markers of arrhythmia vulnerability can be monitored noninvasively in combination with autonomic parameters during emotional and physical stressors and sleep states to identify individuals at heightened risk of lethal cardiac arrhythmias.

Adrenergic Influences on Cardiac Vulnerability

It is well established that adrenergic inputs constitute the primary neural trigger for arrhythmias. Activation of the sympathetic nerve structures, including the posterior hypothalamus or stellate ganglia, increases susceptibility to ventricular fibrillation. Infusion of epinephrine or norepinephrine is also profibrillatory. A striking surge in sympathetic nerve activity occurs within a few minutes of experimental left anterior descending (LAD) coronary artery occlusion, as documented by direct nerve recording.[3] This enhancement in sympathetic nerve activity is associated with a marked increase in susceptibility to ventricular fibrillation, as evidenced by a fall in the ventricular fibrillation threshold (Figure 4–3), as well as by the spontaneous occurrence of the arrhythmia,

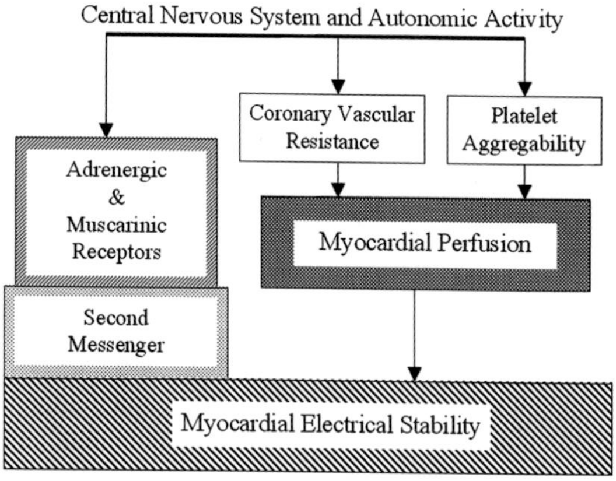

FIGURE 4–1. The interaction between neural triggers and cardiovascular substrate during autonomic activation. Stimulation of β_1-adrenergic receptors can decrease electrical stability directly as a result of changes in second messenger formation and alterations in ion fluxes. This deleterious influence is opposed by muscarinic receptor stimulation, which inhibits presynaptically the release of norepinephrine and opposes its action at the receptor level. Catecholamines may also alter myocardial perfusion by complex means, including α-receptor stimulation of coronary vessels and platelets and by impairing diastolic perfusion time due to adrenergically mediated sinus tachycardia. (From Verrier.[73])

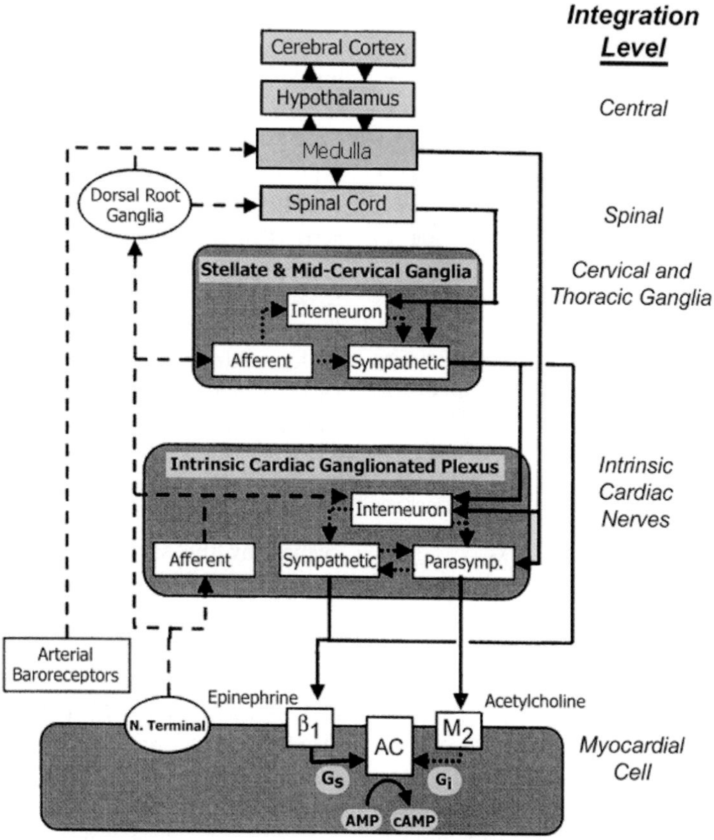

FIGURE 4–2. Synthesis of new and present views on levels of integration important in neural control of cardiac electrical activity. More traditional concepts focused on afferent tracts (dashed lines) arising from myocardial nerve terminals and reflex receptors (e.g., baroreceptors) that are integrated centrally within hypothalamic and medullary cardiostimulatory and cardioinhibitory brain centers and on central modulation of sympathetic and parasympathetic outflow (solid lines) with little intermediary processing at the level of the spinal cord and within cervical and thoracic ganglia. More recent views incorporate additional levels of intricate processing within the extraspinal cervical and thoracic ganglia and within the cardiac ganglionic plexus, where recently described interneurons are envisioned to provide new levels of noncentral integration. Release of neurotransmitters from postganglionic sympathetic neurons is believed to enhance excitation in the sinoatrial node and myocardial cells through norepinephrine binding to β_1-receptors, which enhances adenyl cyclase (AC) activity through intermediary stimulatory G-proteins (G_s). Increased parasympathectomy outflow enhances postganglionic release and binding of acetylcholine to muscarinic (M_2) receptors, and through coupled inhibitory G-proteins (G_i) inhibits cyclic AMP (cAMP) production. The latter alters electrogenesis and pacemaking activity by affecting the activity of specific membrane Na, K, and Ca channels. New levels of integration are shown superimposed on previous views and are emphasized here to highlight new possibilities for intervention. (From Lathrop and Spooner[2] by permission from Blackwell Futura.)

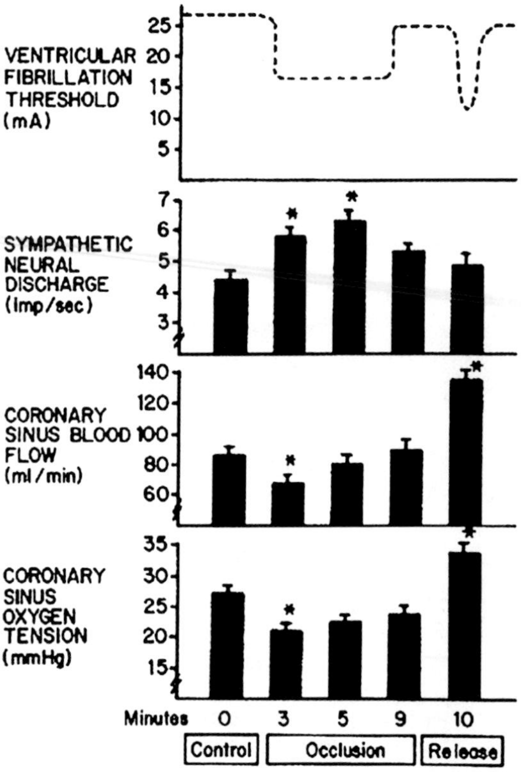

FIGURE 4–3. Effects of a 10-min period of left anterior descending (LAD) coronary artery occlusion and release on neural sympathetic activity, coronary sinus blood flow, and oxygen tension. A schematic representation of the time course of changes in ventricular fibrillation threshold is also displayed. LAD coronary artery occlusion results in a consistent activation of sympathetic preganglionic fibers, which corresponds to the period of maximal increase in vulnerability to ventricular fibrillation (*$p < 0.05$ compared to control period). The concomitant changes in coronary sinus blood flow and reperfusion are also displayed. (From Lombardi *et al.*[3])

and is correlated with an increase in T-wave alternans (TWA) magnitude.[4,5] Upon reperfusion, a second peak in vulnerability occurs, probably due to washout products of cellular ischemia.[3–6] Stellectomy significantly blunts the surge in vulnerability to ventricular fibrillation during occlusion but enhances its magnitude during reperfusion.[4] These findings are consistent with the facts that adrenergic factors play a key role during ischemia,[7] and that stellectomy increases the reactive hyperemic response to release-reperfusion, which in turn probably leads to greater liberation of ischemic byproducts.

Mechanisms Responsible for Arrhythmogenesis during β-Adrenergic Receptor Activation

The mechanisms whereby enhanced sympathetic nerve activity increases cardiac vulnerability in the normal and ischemic heart are complex. The major indirect effects include impairment of the oxygen supply–demand ratio due to increased cardiac metabolic activity, α-adrenergically mediated coronary vasoconstriction, especially in vessels with damaged endothelium, and changes in preload and afterload. The direct arrhythmogenic effects on cardiac electrophysiological function, which are primarily mediated through β_1-adrenergic receptors, are multifold. They include derangements in impulse formation, conduction, repolarization alternans, and heterogeneity of repolarization, with the potential for culmination in ventricular tachycardia and fibrillation (Figure 4–4).[8] Increased levels of catecholamines stimulate β-adrenergic receptors, which in turn alter adenylate cyclase activity and intracellular calcium flux. These effects are probably mediated by the cyclic nucleotide and protein kinase regulatory cascade, which can alter spatial heterogeneity of calcium transients and consequently provoke TWA and dispersion of repolarization. The effect of increased intracellular calcium, with the potential for overload and impaired intracellular calcium cycling by the sarcoplasmic reticulum, may be compounded and become especially arrhythmogenic during concurrent myocardial ischemia, which further predisposes to intracellular calcium excess.[4,9–11] The net effect is an increase in vulnerability to ventricular fibrillation. The converse is also true: reduction of cardiac sympathetic neural drive by stellectomy provides an antifibrillatory influence in animals and humans.

Cardiac β_1-adrenergic receptor blockade is capable of negating the profibrillatory effect of direct sympathetic nerve stimulation[12] by an action at the neurocardiac effector junction. But cardiac β_2-adrenergic receptors do not appear to play a significant role in modulating ventricular excitable properties. The role of cardiac β_3-adrenergic receptors has been enigmatic. Zhou and co-workers[13] have provided evidence that during conditions of sympathetic hyperinnervation, there is a significant and dynamic response in β_3-adrenoreceptor

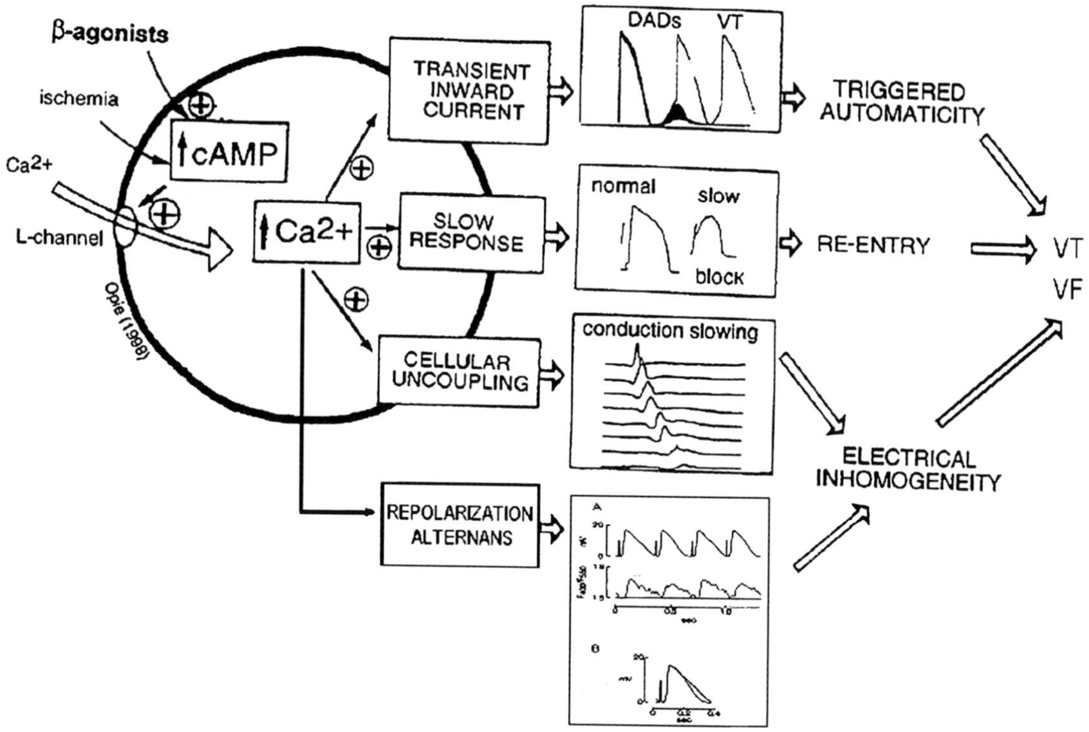

Figure 4–4. The cardiac β-adrenergic signaling system mediating ventricular arrhythmogenesis. The central pathways include links between cyclic adenosine 3′,5′-monophosphate (cAMP), cytosolic calcium, and specific calcium-mediated electrophysiological abnormalities that predispose to ventricular tachycardia (VT) and ventricular fibrillation (VF). The lowest panel is based on a study from Lee *et al.*,[9] indicating that simulated ischemia results in alternation in calcium transients, which appears to underlie action potential alternans. (Adapted from Opie[8] and used with his permission.)

expression. However, it is unknown whether these receptors contribute to the genesis of arrhythmias or whether they serve a rescue function in response to catecholamine excess, as they do with respect to contractility (Figure 4–5).[14]

α-Adrenergic Receptors

Elucidation of the role of α-adrenergic receptors has been challenging because these agents exert direct actions not only on myocardial excitable

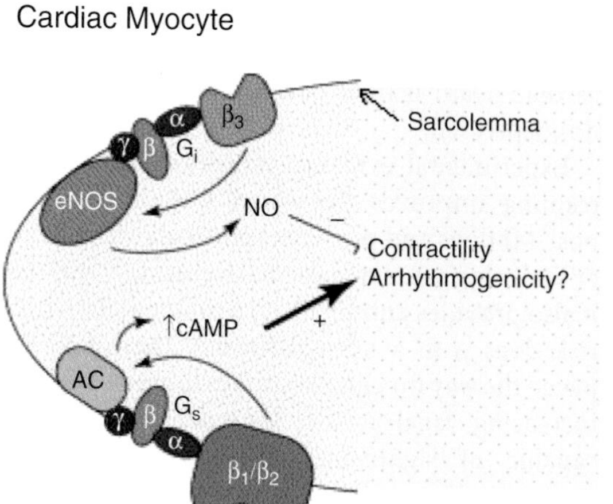

Figure 4–5. Countervailing mechanism proposed by Gauthier and co-workers[74] to account for the interaction between β_1- and β_2-adrenoceptors and the β_3-adrenoceptor subtype. In normal heart, β_1- and β_2-adrenoceptors mediate the classic positive inotropic effect of catecholamines via cAMP. In an opposing manner, stimulation of the β_3-adrenoceptor exerts a negative inotropic response that occurs through activation of a constitutively expressed endothelial nitric oxide synthase (eNOS). It was proposed that the β_3-adrenoceptor can provide a "rescue" function, which occurs particularly in disease conditions associated with hyperadrenergic activity, especially in heart failure. Little is known about the influence of these receptors on susceptibility to arrhythmias. (Adapted from Gauthier *et al.*[74] by permission from Elsevier.)

properties but also on platelet aggregability and coronary hemodynamic function.[15,16] In the normal heart, α-adrenergic receptor stimulation or blockade does not appear to affect ventricular electrical stability, as evidenced by the fact that administration of an α-adrenergic agonist such as phenylephrine or methoxamine does not influence excitable properties when the pressor response is controlled to prevent reflex changes in autonomic tone.[17,18] In the setting of myocardial ischemia, α-adrenergic blockade may alleviate coronary vasoconstriction and reduce platelet aggregability.

Sympathetic–Parasympathetic Interactions

Vagal influences are contingent on the prevailing level of adrenergic tone.[19–23] When sympathetic tone to the heart is augmented by thoracotomy,[20] sympathetic nerve stimulation,[20] myocardial ischemia, or catecholamine infusion,[22] vagal activation exerts a protective effect on ventricular vulnerability. Vagus nerve stimulation is without effect on ventricular vulnerability when adrenergic input to the heart is ablated by β-adrenergic blockade.[20] Levy and co-workers termed this phenomenon "accentuated antagonism." The basis for this antagonism of adrenergic effects is presynaptic inhibition of norepinephrine release from nerve endings[24] and a muscarinically mediated action at the second messenger level, attenuating the response to catecholamines at receptor sites. Also, importantly, vagal influences provide indirect protection against ventricular fibrillation by reducing excess heart rates,[20] which can otherwise critically compromise diastolic perfusion time during acute myocardial ischemia to increase ischemic insult. However, the beneficial effects of vagus nerve activity may be annulled if profound bradycardia and hypotension ensue. Vagus nerve stimulation has been shown in experimental studies to protect against ventricular arrhythmias during myocardial ischemia, but its protection during reperfusion arrhythmias is attributable to decreased heart rate.[25] Finally, myocardial infarction may damage nerve pathways, thereby limiting the potential of the vagus nerve to be activated. Vanoli and colleagues demonstrated the antifibrillatory effect of vagus nerve stimulation during exercise-induced ischemia in canines with a healed myocardial infarction.[26] Direct stimulation of the right cervical vagus through a chronically implanted electrode at 15 sec after onset of exercise-induced acute myocardial ischemia reduced the incidence of ventricular fibrillation by 92%. This effect was only partly due to the attendant heart rate reduction, as in half of the animals, the efficacy of vagal stimulation persisted despite the maintenance of a constant heart rate by atrial pacing.

Baroreflexes and Arrhythmias

The classic studies by Billman, Schwartz, and Stone[27] drew attention to the importance of baroreceptor function on susceptibility to life-threatening arrhythmias associated with myocardial ischemia and infarction. In their initial investigations in canines, they demonstrated that the more powerful the baroreflex response was, the less vulnerable animals were to ventricular fibrillation during myocardial ischemia superimposed on prior myocardial infarction. The protective effect of the baroreceptor mechanism has been linked primarily to the antifibrillatory influence of vagus nerve activity. The latter effect improves diastolic coronary perfusion, minimizing the ischemic insult from coronary artery occlusion. The importance of baroreceptor sensitivity (BRS) was subsequently documented in human subjects in whom baroreceptor function was evaluated with the pressor agent phenylephrine. LaRovere and colleagues[28] demonstrated that patients who experienced a myocardial infarction were less likely to experience sudden cardiac death if their baroreceptor function was not depressed.

Experimental evidence indicates that exercise training improves depressed BRS in high-risk post-MI dogs and prevents ventricular fibrillation (VF) during acute myocardial ischemia,[29] and that it also provides antifibrillatory protection in high-risk dogs with a normal heart.[30] These findings paved the way for clinical studies to assess whether increasing vagal activity by exercise training is capable of significantly improving long-term prognosis. Ninety-five post-myocardial infarction patients, matched for all major variables, were randomized to a 4-week endurance-training period or to no training.[31] During a 10-year follow-up, cardiac mortality among the trained patients who had an exercise-induced increase in baroreflex sensitivity >3 ms/mm Hg was strikingly lower compared to that of the trained patients without such a baroreflex response and to that of the non-trained patients (Figure 4–6).

In the past few years, BRS testing has been pursued by noninvasive monitoring of heart rate turbulence (HRT). This phenomenon refers to fluctuations of sinus-rhythm cycle length after a single ventricular premature beat (VPB) and appears to be mechanistically linked with BRS (Figure 4–7).[32] The basic principle, introduced by Schmidt and co-workers,[33] is that the reaction of the cardiovascular system to a VPB and the subsequent decrease in arterial blood pressure are a direct function of baroreceptor responsiveness, since reflex activation of the vagus nerve controls the pattern of sinus rhythm. Several studies confirm that in low-risk patients, after a VPB, sinus rhythm exhibits a characteristic pattern of early acceleration and subsequent deceleration. By contrast, patients at high risk exhibit essentially a flat, nonvarying response to the VPB, indicating an inability to activate vagal nerves and their cardioprotective effect.[34] The method appears to be a promising independent predictor of total mortality in patients with ischemic heart disease and/or heart failure.[35–37] Heart rate deceleration capacity, a related and even more comprehensive marker of autonomic control than HRT, may be of considerable clinical value in assessing overall autonomic regulation of the heart in patients with diverse types of cardiovascular disease.[38]

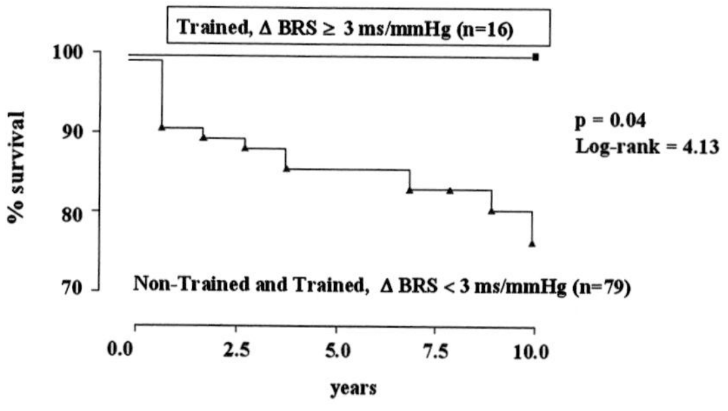

FIGURE 4–6. Cardiac mortality estimated by the Kaplan–Meier method among the patients with a training-induced increase in BRS ≥3 ms/mm Hg and the group including patients who trained without the same BRS increase and nontrained patients. (From La Rovere *et al.*[31] by permission from the American Heart Association.)

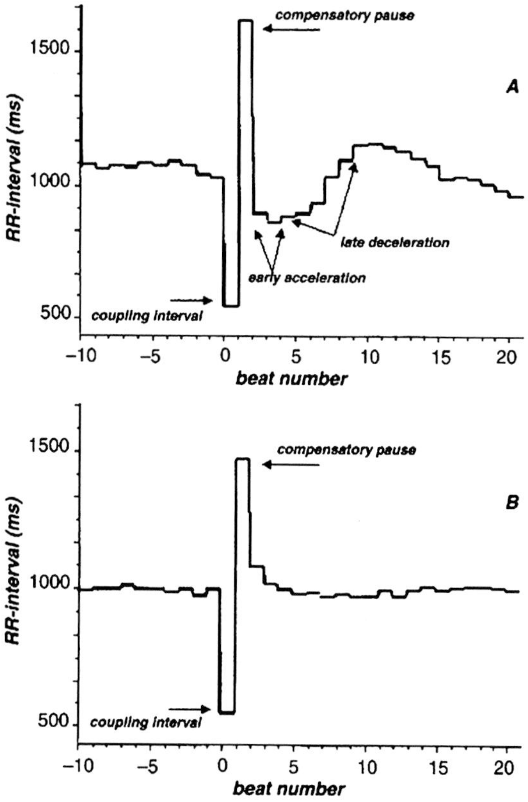

FIGURE 4–7. (A) Heart rate turbulence in a low-risk post-myocardial infarction (post-MI) patient. (B) Blunted heart rate turbulence in a high-risk post-MI patient. (From Guzik and Schmidt[35] by permission from Kluwer Academic Publishers.)

Intrinsic Cardiac Innervation

In the late 1970s, Armour[39] and his colleagues introduced and investigated the elaborate intrinsic neural network within the heart, which provides local, independent heart rhythm control. Randall, Zipes, and their respective co-workers[40–42] subsequently verified this important advance, drawing attention to the fact that components of this innervation system reside within discrete fat pads. Myocardial ischemia can compromise the functional capacity of cardiac intrinsic neurons residing in the fat pad and thus has the potential to increase electrical inhomogeneity and susceptibility to arrhythmias.[43] Intrinsic innervation is also vulnerable to diabetic neuropathy, which accordingly could exacerbate vulnerability to arrhythmias.[44] Surgical incisions through the atrial walls and radiofrequency ablation may isolate SA node pacemaker cells and damage the fat pads and result in proarrhythmia due to iatrogenically induced autonomic imbalance.[45] Heterogeneity of fibers within and without the fat pads contributes to dispersion of electrical activity, which in turn can predispose to arrhythmogenesis in adjacent atrial tissue.[46]

Nerve Growth and Degeneration

Whereas the concept of remodeling has been well established with respect to the heart, the importance of restructuring of cardiac innervation has only recently received due attention, with fundamental contributions from the laboratories of Zipes[47,48] and Chen.[49–52] In particular, in a canine model of atrial fibrillation induced by rapid, prolonged pacing, Jayachandran *et al.*[48] demonstrated that atrial electrical remodeling was associated with spatially heterogeneous uptake of the postganglionic sympathetic indicator hydroxyephedrine into the nerve terminals within the sinus node, crista terminalis, and myocardium. Importantly, increased uptake was accompanied by electrical heterogeneity and augmented norepinephrine tissue levels. Subsequent studies by Chang[50] and Olgin[47] and their respective colleagues provided further evidence in favor of the concept of injury-induced neural repair with selective sympathetic remodeling and the attendant potential for induction and perpetuation of atrial arrhythmias.

Chen and co-workers[51] documented evidence that nerve sprouting could apply to ventricular as well as to atrial arrhythmogenesis and potentially to sudden cardiac death. These investigators demonstrated a significant correlation between increased sympathetic nerve density as reflected in immunocytochemical markers and history of ischemia in native hearts of human transplant recipients. In a canine model, they determined

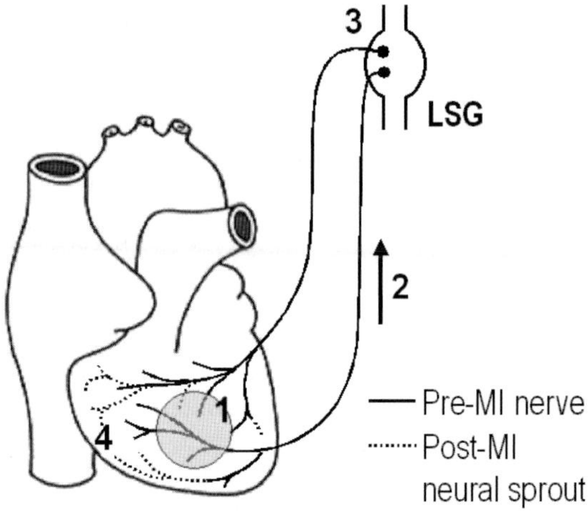

FIGURE 4–8. Signaling of neural remodeling after myocardial infarction. Myocardial injury (shaded area) results in early local nerve growth factor (NGF) release, presumably from damaged cells, followed by upregulated NGF and growth-associated protein 43 (GAP43) expression, especially in the infarct area (1). These signal proteins are then retrogradely transported (2) to the nerve cell bodies in the ganglia (3) where they stimulate the sprouting of new cardiac nerve endings in the heart (4), predominantly in noninfarcted regions, leading to heterogeneous hyperinnervation. (From Verrier and Kwaku[54] by permission from the American Heart Association.)

that induction of nerve sprouting with nerve growth factor resulted in increased incidence of ventricular tachycardias and sudden death, with concomitant TWA, a noninvasive marker of risk for ventricular arrhythmias.[52] Significantly, the predisposition to arrhythmias was linked to immunocytochemical evidence of a heterogeneous pattern of sympathetic nerve reinnervation (Figure 4–8). More recently, Liu and co-workers[53] demonstrated in rabbits that hypercholesterolemia can produce proarrhythmic neural and electrophysiological remodeling that is highly arrhythmogenic and is associated with important changes in ionic currents including I_{Ca}. Collectively, this evidence points to the lability of autonomic innervation and the intricate changes that may be responsible for derangements in neural activity. This adverse effect of heterogeneous remodeling of sympathetic innervation to the heart is likely to play a role in the increased risk for life-threatening arrhythmias.[54] The term "neural remodeling" should be employed alongside "myocardial remodeling" in the conceptual framework of the pathophysiology of acute infarction.

Behavioral State

Stress and Arrhythmogenesis

Behavioral models have been developed to define the impact of behavioral state on cardiac electrical stability.[11,55–57] These have included both aversive behavioral conditioning paradigms and models eliciting natural emotions, notably anger and fear. Aversive conditioning of dogs in a Pavlovian sling with mild chest shock on three consecutive days showed that subsequent exposure to the environment without shock elicited a reduction in the repetitive extrasystole threshold greater than 30%.[55] The same paradigm elicited a 3-fold increase in the occurrence of spontaneous ventricular fibrillation when coronary artery occlusion was carried out in the aversive sling compared to the nonaversive cage environment. In dogs recovering from myocardial infarction, exposure to the aversive environment consistently elicited ventricular tachycardia for several days during the healing process.[56] After this time, the animals continued to exhibit signs of behavioral stress in the aversive environment, but no longer experienced ventricular arrhythmias, indicating that the arousal state required a substrate of cardiac electrical instability for the induction of rhythm disturbances. The stress-induced changes in cardiac excitable properties were largely obtunded by β-adrenergic receptor blockade with propranolol or metoprolol.

In a separate series of experiments, an experimental canine model was developed to emulate anger,[57] which is the emotion most commonly associated with myocardial infarction and sudden death.[58,59] A standardized food-access-denial paradigm provoked intense arousal, which elicited a sizable increase in TWA in precordial V_5 ECG. A 3-min period of coronary artery occlusion potentiated arrhythmia risk, as it more than doubled the magnitude of anger-induced TWA.[11] The stress-related effects were significantly decreased by metoprolol, further implicating a major role of β_1-adrenergic receptors in sympathetic nerve induction of cardiac vulnerability and TWA.

The view that behavioral factors may predispose to malignant arrhythmias has gained strong support in recent years because of batteries of psychometric tests for behavioral testing and indicators of cardiac electrical instability including defibrillator discharge frequency and TWA. In patients with implantable cardioverter defibrillators (ICDs), Lampert and colleagues[60] systematically examined the linkage between emotional and physical stressors in provoking spontaneous ventricular arrhythmias. Subjects completed detailed diaries of mood states and physical activity during two periods preceding spontaneous, appropriate ICD shocks and during control periods 1 week later. A total of 107 documented ICD shocks were reported by 42 patients, the majority of whom had coronary artery disease. In the 15-min period preceding shocks, there was a significant incidence of high levels of anger, with odds ratios of 1.83. Other mood states, notably anxiety, worry, sadness, and happiness, did not trigger ICD discharge. Physical activity was also associated with an increased incidence of shocks. Correlative findings were reported by Fries *et al.*,[61] who found a 7-fold increased risk of ICD shock with high levels of physical activity and a 9-fold increased risk of ICD shock with acute mental stress. These observations are consistent with a recent demonstration in ICD patients that mental stress as well as exercise is capable of significantly increasing TWA, independent of effects on heart rate (Figure 4–9).[62] By contrast, normal matched control subjects did not experience significant exercise- or mental stress-induced increases in TWA. Such surges in TWA indicate electrical instability, as they presage the onset of ventricular tachycardia/ventricular fibrillation (VT/VF).[63–66]

The dynamic influence of mental and physical activity on cardiac electrical function is further supported by results of a recent study of ambulatory ECG-based TWA analysis in post-myocardial infarction patients.[67] Modified moving average analysis[63] was used to measure TWA from 24-h AECGs from patients enrolled in the ATRAMI study obtained at an average of 15 days following the index event. The patients were followed for 21 ± 8 months and were matched for gender, age, site of MI, left ventricular ejection fraction, thrombolysis, and β-adrenergic blockade therapy. Levels of TWA at the 75th percentile of controls or

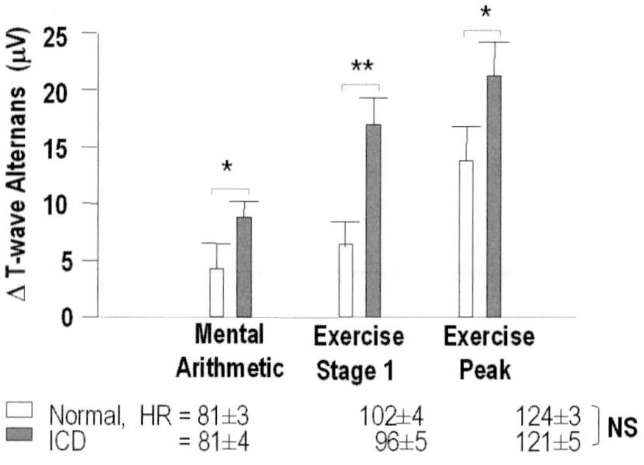

FIGURE 4–9. Comparison of ICD patients with controls in T-wave alternans (TWA) responses to mental stress and exercise (Δ = change from baseline). Although heart rates were not significantly different among the groups, increases in TWA were higher in ICD patients than in controls during mental arithmetic ($p = 0.043$), exercise stage 1 ($p = 0.0004$), and peak exercise ($p = 0.038$). (*$p < 0.05$, **$p < 0.01$, ICD versus control.) (From Kop *et al.*[62] by permission from the American Heart Association.)

approximately 50 μV predicted a 4- to 7-fold higher odds ratio of cardiac arrest or arrhythmic death. Patients who were at increased risk for arrhythmic death showed increased TWA levels at maximum heart rate and at 8:00 am, suggesting that daily mental and physical stress can disclose clinically significant levels of electrical instability. Although the increase in TWA was associated with maximum daily heart rate, elevated heart rate per se does not appear to be the sole factor, as TWA measured at peak heart rate did not correlate with the magnitude of the heart rate change nor did the maximum heart rates differ between patients with and without events. These increases in TWA are likely to reflect the influence of enhanced sympathetic nerve activity, since β-adrenergic receptor blockade reduces TWA magnitude,[68] an effect shown to be independent of heart rate, when this variable was controlled by pacing.[69]

Sleep as an Autonomic Stress Test for the Heart

In healthy individuals, sleep is generally salutary and restorative. Ironically, during sleep in patients with respiratory or heart disease, the brain can precipitate breathing disorders, myocardial ischemia, arrhythmias, and even death. An estimated 250,000 nocturnal myocardial infarctions and 38,000 nocturnal sudden deaths occur annually in the U.S. population, as 20% of myocardial infarctions and 15% of sudden deaths occur during the period from midnight to 6:00 am.[70] This event rate is equivalent to 91% of the number of fatalities due to automobile accidents and is 20% more than the number of deaths due to HIV infection. Thus, sleep is not an entirely protected state. The distribution of deaths and myocardial infarctions during nighttime is nonuniform, a pattern consistent with provocation by pathophysiological triggers. Precise characterization of the precipitating factors for nocturnal cardiac events is incomplete. While death during sleep may be presumed to be painless, in many cases it is premature, as it occurs in infants and adolescents and in adults with ischemic heart disease, for whom the median age is 59 years. High-risk populations for nocturnal cardiorespiratory events include a number of sizable patient groups (Table 4–1).

The two main factors that have been implicated in nocturnal cardiac events are sleep-state-dependent surges in autonomic nervous system activity and depression of respiratory control mechanisms, which impact on a vulnerable cardiac substrate. The brain, in subserving its needs for periodic reexcitation during rapid eye movement (REM) sleep and dreaming, imposes significant demands on the heart by inducing bursts in sympathetic nerve activity, which reaches levels higher than during wakefulness. In susceptible individuals, this degree of sympathetic nerve activity may compromise coronary artery blood flow, as metabolic demand outstrips supply, and may trigger sympathetically mediated life-threatening arrhythmias. Obstructive sleep apnea, which impairs ventilation during sleep and can generate reductions in arterial oxygen saturation, afflicts 5–10 million Americans, or 2–4% of the population.[71] This condition has been strongly implicated, when severe, in the etiology of hypertension, ischemia, arrhythmias, myocardial infarction, and sudden death in individuals with coexisting ischemic heart disease. Autonomic or respiratory disturbances during sleep may trigger atrial fibrillation in certain patient populations. A challenge

TABLE 4–1. Patient groups at potentially increased risk for nocturnal cardiac events.

Indication (U.S. patients/year)	Possible mechanism
Nocturnal angina, ischemia, myocardial infarction (250,000), atrial fibrillation (725,000), ventricular arrhythmias, ischemia, cardiac arrest, sudden death (38,000)	The nocturnal pattern suggests a sleep-state dependent autonomic trigger or respiratory distress. Non-demand ischemia and angina peak between midnight and 6:00 a.m. Nocturnal onset of MI is more frequent in older and sicker patients and carries higher risk of congestive heart failure. Disturbances in sleep, respiration, and autonomic balance may be factors in nocturnal arrhythmogenesis.
Spousal or family report of highly irregular breathing, excessive snoring, or apnea in patients with coronary disease (5 to 10 million U.S. patients with apnea)	Patients with hypertension or coronary artery disease should be screened for the presence of sleep apnea, which conduces to hypertension, ischemia, arrhythmia, and atrial fibrillation, and is a risk factor for lethal daytime cardiac events, including myocardial infarction.
Long QT_3, Brugada syndrome, Sudden Unexplained Nocturnal Death Syndrome (SUNDS)	The profound cycle-length changes associated with sleep may trigger pause-dependent torsade de pointes in these patients.
Near-miss or siblings of sudden infant death (SIDS) victims	Crib death commonly occurs during sleep with characteristic cardiorespiratory symptoms.
Patients on cardiac medications (13.5 million U.S. patients with cardiovascular disease)	Beta-blockers and calcium channel blockers that cross the blood-brain barrier may increase nighttime risk, as poor sleep and violent dreams may be triggered. Medications that increase the QT interval may conduce to pause-dependent torsade de pointes during the profound cycle-length changes of sleep. Because arterial blood pressure is decreased during nonrapid eye movement sleep, additional lowering by antihypertensive agents may induce a risk of ischemia and infarction due to lowered coronary perfusion.

Source: Modified from Verrier and Mittleman.[72]

is also presented by NREM sleep, when malperfusion of the heart and brain may result from hypotension and decreased blood flow in stenosed vessels. These conditions may be confounded by medications that cross the blood–brain barrier, alter sleep structure, and/or provoke nightmares with severe cardiac autonomic discharge. Finally, an insidious component of the problem of nocturnal risk results from the fact that many individuals are unaware of their respiratory or cardiac distress at night and therefore take no corrective action. Thus, sleep presents unique autonomic, hemodynamic, and respiratory challenges to the diseased myocardium that cannot be monitored by daytime diagnostic tests. The importance of monitoring nocturnal arrhythmias extends beyond identifying sleep-state-dependent triggers of cardiac events, as nighttime ischemia, arrhythmias, autonomic activity, and respiratory disturbances carry predictive value for daytime events.[72]

Conclusion

Our understanding of the role of the autonomic nervous system has continued to evolve in a fascinating and productive manner. A number of direct benefits in terms of understanding the function of the autonomic nervous system in health and disease, and quantification of autonomic tone through heart rate variability and through baroreceptor function testing by heart rate turbulence analysis, show considerable promise in terms of sudden death risk stratification, underscoring the crucial role of autonomic reflexes in maintaining cardiac health. Exercise-induced changes in autonomic function also appear capable of disclosing latent cardiac electrical instability, as evidenced by heightened levels of TWA, which is predictive of susceptibility to sudden cardiac death and cardiovascular mortality.[75] From the basic science perspective, there appears to be great promise in understanding the organization and function of the intrinsic nervous system and the dynamic nature of nerve sprouting and neural remodeling. The pattern of local neurocircuitry is likely to play a critical role in influencing heterogeneity of repolarization, a fundamental factor in arrhythmogenesis. A number of promising therapeutic approaches based on pharmacological and electrical targeted neuromodulation to decrease cardiac sympathetic while augmenting vagus nerve tone are being pursued.

Acknowledgment. The authors thank Sandra S. Verrier for her editorial assistance.

References

1. Huikuri HV, Castellanos A, Myerburg RJ. Sudden death due to cardiac arrhythmias. *N Engl J Med* 2001;345:1473–1482.
2. Lathrop DA, Spooner PM. On the neural connection. *J Cardiovasc Electrophysiol* 2001;12:841–844.
3. Lombardi F, Verrier RL, Lown B. Relationship between sympathetic neural activity, coronary dynamics, and vulnerability to ventricular fibrillation during myocardial ischemia and reperfusion. *Am Heart J* 1983;105:958–965.
4. Nearing BD, Huang AH, Verrier RL. Dynamic tracking of cardiac vulnerability by complex demodulation of the T-wave. *Science* 1991;252: 437–440.
5. Nearing BD, Oesterle SN, Verrier RL. Quantification of ischaemia-induced vulnerability by precordial T-wave alternans analysis in dog and human. *Cardiovasc Res* 1994;28:1440–1449.
6. Corbalan R, Verrier RL, Lown B. Differing mechanisms for ventricular vulnerability during coronary artery occlusion and release. *Am Heart J* 1976;92: 223–230.
7. Elharrar V, Zipes DP. Cardiac electrophysiologic alterations during myocardial ischemia. *Am J Physiol* 1977;233:H329–345.
8. Opie LH. *Heart Physiology: From Cell to Circulation*, 4th ed. Philadelphia: Lippincott, Williams & Wilkins, 2004.
9. Lee HC, Mohabir R, Smith N, *et al.* Effect of ischemia on calcium-dependent fluorescence transients in rabbit hearts containing indo 1. Correlation with monophasic action potentials and contraction. *Circulation* 1988;78:1047–1059.
10. Euler DE. Cardiac alternans: Mechanisms and pathophysiological significance. *Cardiovasc Res* 1999; 42:583–590.
11. Kovach JA, Nearing BD, Verrier RL. An angerlike behavioral state potentiates myocardial ischemia-induced T-wave alternans in canines. *J Am Coll Cardiol* 2001;37:1719–1725.
12. Verrier RL, Thompson PL, Lown B. Ventricular vulnerability during sympathetic stimulation: Role of heart rate and blood pressure. *Cardiovasc Res* 1974;8:602–610.
13. Zhou S, Paz O, Cao JM, *et al.* Differential beta-adrenoceptor expression induced by nerve growth factor infusion into the canine right and left stellate ganglia. *Heart Rhythm* 2005;2:1347–1355.
14. Verrier RL. Beta$_3$-adrenoceptors: Friend or foe? *Heart Rhythm* 2005;2:1356–1358.
15. Schwartz PJ, Stone HL. Tonic influence of the sympathetic nervous system on myocardial reactive hyperemia and on coronary blood flow distribution in dogs. *Circ Res* 1977;41:51–58.
16. Mohrman ED, Feigl EO. Competition between sympathetic vasoconstriction and metabolic vasodilation in the canine coronary circulation. *Circ Res* 1978;42:79–86.
17. Verrier RL, Calvert A, Lown B, *et al.* Effect of acute blood pressure elevation on the ventricular fibrillation threshold. *Am J Physiol* 1974;226:893–897.
18. Kowey PR, Verrier RL, Lown B. Effect of alpha-adrenergic receptor stimulation on ventricular electrical properties in the normal canine heart. *Am Heart J* 1983;105:366–371.
19. Lown B, Verrier RL. Neural activity and ventricular fibrillation. *N Engl J Med* 1976;294:1165–1170.
20. Kolman BS, Verrier RL, Lown B. The effect of vagus nerve stimulation upon vulnerability of the canine ventricle. Role of sympathetic-parasympathetic interactions. *Circulation* 1975;52:578–585.
21. Matta RJ, Verrier RL, Lown B. Repetitive extrasystole as an index of vulnerability to ventricular fibrillation. *Am J Physiol* 1976;230:1469–1473.
22. Rabinowitz SH, Verrier RL, Lown B. Muscarinic effects of vagosympathetic trunk stimulation on the repetitive extrasystole (RE) threshold. *Circulation* 1976;53:622–627.
23. Danilo P Jr, Rosen MR, Hordof AJ. Effects of acetylcholine on the ventricular specialized conducting system of neonatal and adult dogs. *Circ Res* 1978;43:777–784.
24. Levy MN, Blattberg B. Effect of vagal stimulation on the overflow of norepinephrine into the coronary sinus during cardiac sympathetic nerve stimulation in the dog. *Circ Res* 1976;38:81–84.
25. Zuanetti G, DeFerrari GM, Priori SG, *et al.* Protective effect of vagal stimulation on reperfusion arrhythmias in cats. *Circ Res* 1987;61:429–435.
26. Vanoli E, De Ferrari GM, Stramba-Badiale M, *et al.* Vagal stimulation and prevention of sudden death in conscious dogs with a healed myocardial infarction. *Circ Res* 1991;68:1471–1481.
27. Billman GE, Schwartz PJ, Stone HL. Baroreceptor reflex control of heart rate: A predictor of sudden cardiac death. *Circulation* 1982;66:874–880.
28. La Rovere MT, Bigger JT Jr, Marcus FI, *et al.* Baroreflex sensitivity and heart-rate variability in prediction of total cardiac mortality after myocardial infarction. ATRAMI (Autonomic Tone and Reflexes After Myocardial Infarction) Investigators. *Lancet* 1998;351:478–484.

29. Billman GE, Schwartz PJ, Stone HL. The effects of daily exercise on susceptibility to sudden cardiac death. *Circulation* 1984;69:1182–1189.
30. Hull SS Jr, Vanoli E, Adamson PB, *et al.* Exercise training confers anticipatory protection from sudden death during acute myocardial ischemia. *Circulation* 1994;89:548–552.
31. La Rovere MT, Bersano C, Gnemmi M, *et al.* Exercise-induced increase in baroreflex sensitivity predicts improved prognosis after myocardial infarction. *Circulation* 2002;106:945–949.
32. Lin LY, Lai LP, Lin JL, *et al.* Tight mechanism correlation between heart rate turbulence and baroreflex sensitivity: Sequential autonomic blockade analysis. *J Cardiovasc Electrophysiol* 2002;13:427–431.
33. Schmidt G, Malik M, Barthel P, *et al.* Heart-rate turbulence after ventricular premature beats as a predictor of mortality after acute myocardial infarction. *Lancet* 1999;353:1390–1396.
34. Ghuran A, Reid F, La Rovere MT, *et al.* Heart rate turbulence-based predictors of fatal and nonfatal cardiac arrest (The Autonomic Tone and Reflexes After Myocardial Infarction substudy). *Am J Cardiol* 2002;89:184–190.
35. Guzik P, Schmidt G. A phenomenon of heart-rate turbulence, its evaluation, and prognostic value. *Card Electrophysiol Rev* 2002;6:256–261.
36. Wichterle D, Melenovsky V, Malik M. Mechanisms involved in heart rate turbulence. *Card Electrophysiol Rev* 2002;6:262–266.
37. Bonnemeier H, Wiegand UK, Friedlbinder J, *et al.* Reflex cardiac activity in ischemia and reperfusion: Heart rate turbulence in patients undergoing direct percutaneous coronary intervention for acute myocardial infarction. *Circulation* 2003;108:958–964.
38. Bauer A, Kantelhardt JW, Barthel P, *et al.* Deceleration capacity of heart rate as a predictor of mortality after myocardial infarction: Cohort study. *Lancet* 2006;367:1674–1681.
39. Armour JA. Intrinsic cardiac neurons. *J Cardiovasc Electrophysiol* 1991;2:331–341.
40. Randall WC, Ardell JL. Selective parasympathectomy of automatic and conductile tissues of the canine heart. *Am J Physiol* 1985;248:H61–68.
41. Chiou CW, Eble JN, Zipes DP. Efferent vagal innervation of the canine atria and sinus and atrioventricular nodes. The third fat pad. *Circulation* 1997;95:2573–2584.
42. Verrier RL, Zhao SX. The enigmatic cardiac fat pads: Critical but underappreciated neural regulatory sites. *J Cardiovasc Electrophysiol* 2002;13:902–903.
43. Armour JA. Myocardial ischaemia and the cardiac nervous system. *Cardiovasc Res* 1999;41:41–54.
44. Stevens MJ, Raffel DM, Allman KC, *et al.* Cardiac sympathetic dysinnervation in diabetes: Implications for enhanced cardiovascular risk. *Circulation* 1998;98:961–968.
45. Randall WC, Wurster RD, Duff M, *et al.* Surgical interruption of postganglionic innervation of the sinoatrial nodal region. *J Thorac Cardiovasc Surg* 1991;101:66–74.
46. Nakajima K, Furukawa Y, Kurogouchi F, *et al.* Autonomic control of the location and rate of the cardiac pacemaker in the sinoatrial fat pad of parasympathetically denervated dog hearts. *J Cardiovasc Electrophysiol* 2002;13:896–901.
47. Olgin JE, Sih HJ, Hanish S, *et al.* Heterogeneous atrial denervation creates substrate for sustained atrial fibrillation. *Circulation* 1998;98:2608–2614.
48. Jayachandran JV, Sih HJ, Winkle W, *et al.* Atrial fibrillation produced by prolonged rapid atrial pacing is associated with heterogeneous changes in atrial sympathetic innervation. *Circulation* 2000;101:1185–1191.
49. Cao JM, Fishbein MC, Han JB, *et al.* Relationship between regional cardiac hyperinnervation and ventricular arrhythmia. *Circulation* 2000;101:1960–1969.
50. Chang CM, Wu TJ, Zhou S, *et al.* Nerve sprouting and sympathetic hyperinnervation in a canine model of atrial fibrillation produced by prolonged right atrial pacing. *Circulation* 2001;103:22–25.
51. Chen PS, Chen LS, Cao JM, *et al.* Sympathetic nerve sprouting, electrical remodeling and the mechanisms of sudden cardiac death. *Cardiovasc Res* 2001;50:409–416.
52. Tsai J, Cao JM, Zhou S, *et al.* T wave alternans as a predictor of spontaneous ventricular tachycardia in a canine model of sudden cardiac death. *J Cardiovasc Electrophysiol* 2002;13:51–55.
53. Liu YB, Wu CC, Lu LS, *et al.* Sympathetic nerve sprouting, electrical remodeling, and increased vulnerability to ventricular fibrillation in hypercholesterolemic rabbits. *Circ Res* 2003;92:1145–1152.
54. Verrier RL, Kwaku KF. Frayed nerves in myocardial infarction: The importance of rewiring. *Circ Res* 2004;94:5–6.
55. Lown B, Verrier RL, Corbalan R. Psychologic stress and threshold for repetitive ventricular response. *Science* 1973;182:834–836.
56. Corbalan R, Verrier RL, Lown B. Psychological stress and ventricular arrhythmias during myocardial infarction in the conscious dog. *Am J Cardiol* 1974;34:692–696.

57. Verrier RL, Hagestad EL, Lown B. Delayed myocardial ischemia induced by anger. *Circulation* 1987; 75:249–254.
58. Mittleman MA, Maclure M, Sherwood JB, *et al.* Triggering of acute myocardial infarction onset by episodes of anger. *Circulation* 1995;92:1720–1725.
59. Verrier RL, Mittleman MA. Life-threatening cardiovascular consequences of anger in patients with coronary heart disease. *Cardiol Clinics* 1996;14: 289–307.
60. Lampert R, Joska T, Burg MM, *et al.* Emotional and physical precipitants of ventricular arrhythmia. *Circulation* 2002;106:1800–1805.
61. Fries R, Konig J, Schafers HJ, *et al.* Triggering effect of physical and mental stress on spontaneous ventricular tachyarrhythmias in patients with implantable cardioverter-defibrillators. *Clin Cardiol* 2002; 25:474–478.
62. Kop WJ, Krantz DS, Nearing BD, *et al.* Effects of acute mental and exercise stress on T-wave alternans in patients with implantable cardioverter defibrillators and controls. *Circulation* 2004;109:1864–1869.
63. Nearing BD, Verrier RL. Modified moving average method for T-wave alternans analysis with high accuracy to predict ventricular fibrillation. *J Appl Physiol* 2002;92:541–549.
64. Nearing BD, Verrier RL. Progressive increases in complexity of T-wave oscillations herald ischemia-induced VF. *Circ Res* 2002;91:727–732.
65. Nearing BD, Verrier RL. Tracking heightened cardiac electrical instability by computing interlead heterogeneity of T-wave morphology. *J Appl Physiol* 2003;95:2265–2272.
66. Shusterman V, Goldberg A, London B. Upsurge in T-wave alternans and nonalternating repolarization instability precedes spontaneous initiation of ventricular tachyarrhythmias in humans. *Circulation* 2006;113:2880–2887.
67. Verrier RL, Nearing BD, LaRovere MT, *et al.* Ambulatory ECG-based tracking of T-wave alternans in post-myocardial infarction patients to assess risk of cardiac arrest or arrhythmic death. *J Cardiovasc Electrophysiol* 2003;14:705–711.
68. Klingenheben T, Gronefeld G, Li YG, *et al.* Effect of metoprolol and d,l-sotalol on microvolt-level T-wave alternans. Results of a prospective, double-blind, randomized study. *J Am Coll Cardiol* 2001; 38:2013–2019.
69. Rashba EJ, Cooklin M, MacMurdy K, *et al.* Effects of selective autonomic blockade on T-wave alternans in humans. *Circulation* 2002;105:837–842.
70. Lavery CE, Mittleman MA, Cohen MC, *et al.* Non-uniform nighttime distribution of acute cardiac events: A possible effect of sleep states. *Circulation* 1997;96:3321–3327.
71. Young T, Palta M, Dempsey J, *et al.* The occurrence of sleep-disordered breathing among middle-aged adults. *N Engl J Med* 1993;328:1230–1235.
72. Verrier RL, Mittleman MA. Sleep-related cardiac risk. In: Kryger MH, Roth T, Dement WC, Eds. *Principles and Practice of Sleep Medicine*, 4th ed. Philadelphia: WB Saunders, 2005:1161–1170.
73. Verrier RL. Central nervous system modulation of cardiac rhythm. In: Rosen MR, Palti Y, Eds. *Lethal Arrhythmias Resulting from Myocardial Ischemia and Infarction*. Boston: Kluwer Academic Publishers, 1988:149–164.
74. Gauthier C, Langin D, Balligant J-L. Beta$_3$-adrenoceptors in the cardiovascular system. *Trends Pharmacol Sci* 2000;21:426–431.
75. Nieminen T, Lehtimäki T, Viik J, *et al.* T-wave alternans predicts mortality in a population undergoing a clinically indicated exercise test. *Eur Heart J*, in press.

5
Mechanisms of Cardiac Arrhythmia

Charles Antzelevitch, Alexander Burashnikov, and José M. Di Diego

Introduction

A cardiac arrhythmia can be defined as a variation from the normal heart rate and/or rhythm that is not physiologically justified. An arrhythmia may be regular, as in the case of monomorphic tachycardia or flutter, or irregular, as in the case of fibrillation or polymorphic tachycardia. Some rhythm disturbances may be relatively benign, as in the case of premature ventricular contractions (PVC), whereas others are malignant, as in the case of ventricular fibrillation, capable of leading to sudden death. The most prevalent sustained arrhythmia in the clinic is atrial fibrillation.

In recent years there have been important advances in our understanding of both the molecular, genetic, and electrophysiological mechanisms underlying the development of a wide variety of cardiac arrhythmias (Table 5–1) and conduction disturbances. Progress in our understanding of these phenomena has been fueled by innovative advances in our understanding of the genetic basis and predisposition for electrical dysfunction of the heart. These advances notwithstanding, our appreciation of the basis for many rhythm disturbances is incomplete. This chapter reviews our current understanding of cellular, ionic, genetic, and molecular mechanisms responsible for cardiac arrhythmias, placing them in historical perspective whenever possible.

Cardiac arrhythmic activity can be categorized as passive [e.g., atrioventricular (AV) block] or active. The mechanisms responsible for active cardiac arrhythmias are generally divided into two major categories: (1) enhanced or abnormal impulse formation and (2) reentry (Figure 5–1). Reentry occurs when a propagating impulse fails to die out after normal activation of the heart and persists to reexcite the heart after expiration of the refractory period. Evidence implicating reentry as a mechanism of cardiac arrhythmias stems back to the turn of the century.[1–16] Phase 2 reentry[17–21] is an interesting new concept of reentrant activity advanced to explain the development of extrasystolic activity. Mechanisms responsible for abnormal impulse formation include enhanced automaticity and triggered activity. Automaticity can be further subdivided into normal and abnormal and triggered activity, consisting of (1) early afterdepolarizations (EADs) and (2) delayed afterdepolarizations (DADs). Recent studies have identified a novel mechanism, termed late phase 3 EAD, representing a hybrid between those responsible for EAD and DAD activity.[22–24] A pivotal distinction between automaticity and triggered activity is that the former can appear *de novo* and the latter needs a preceding activation to appear (therefore the term "triggered activity").

Abnormal Impulse Formation

Normal Automaticity

Automaticity is the ability of cardiac cells to generate spontaneous action potentials. Spontaneous activity is the result of diastolic depolarization caused by net inward current flow during phase 4 of the action potential, bringing the membrane potential to threshold (Figure 5–2, left panel). The

Table 5–1. Mechanisms of atrial and ventricular tachyarrhythmias.[a]

Tachyarrhythmia	Mechanism	Rate range (bpm)
Sinus tachycardia	Automatic (normal)	≥100
Sinus node reentry	Reentry	110–180
Atrial tachycardia	Reentry, automatic or triggered (DADs—secondary to digitalis toxicity)	150–240
Atrial flutter	Reentry	240–350 more commonly 300 ± 20
Atrial fibrillation	Reentry Fibrillatory conduction of triggered impulses from pulmonary veins or SVC	260–450
Supraventricular tachycardia—AV nodal reentry	Reentry	120–250 more commonly 150–220
Supraventricular tachycardia—accessory pathway (WPW)	Reentry	140–250 more commonly 150–220
Accelerated idioventricular rhythm	Abnormal automaticity	>60
Ventricular tachycardia	Reentry automatic (rare)	120–300 more commonly 140–240
Right ventricular outflow tract tachycardia	? Triggered (DADs)	120–220
Bundle branch reentry	Reentry	160–250 more commonly 190–240
Torsade de pointes	Precipitated by an EAD-induced triggered beat Maintained by reentry	>200

[a]AV, atrioventricular; bpm, beats per minute; DAD, delayed afterdepolarization; EAD, early afterdepolarization; SVC, superior vena cava; WPW, Wolff–Parkinson–White syndrome.

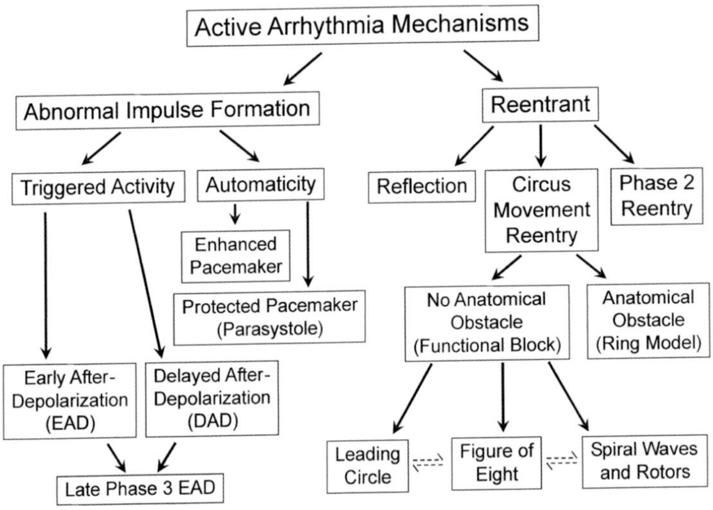

Figure 5–1. Classification of active cardiac arrhythmias.

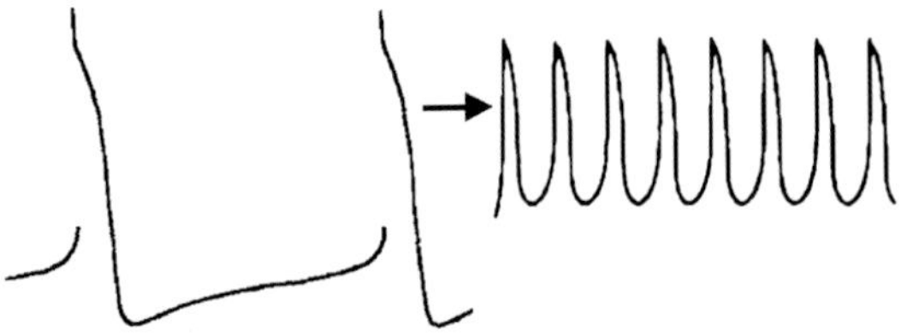

Figure 5–2. Transition of normal to abnormal automaticity (depolarization-induced low voltage activity) in a Purkinje fiber.

sinoatrial (SA) node normally displays the highest intrinsic rate. All other pacemakers are referred to as subsidiary or latent pacemakers, since they take over the function of initiating excitation of the heart only when the SA node is unable to generate impulses or when these impulses fail to propagate. There is a hierarchy of intrinsic rates of subsidiary pacemakers that have normal automaticity: atrial pacemakers have faster intrinsic rates than AV junctional pacemakers and AV junctional pacemakers have faster rates than ventricular pacemakers.[25,26]

The ionic mechanism underlying normal SA and AV nodes and Purkinje system automaticity includes (1) a hyperpolarization-activated inward current (I_f)[27,28] and/or (2) decay of outward potassium current (I_K).[29,30] The contribution of I_f and I_K differs in SA/AV nodes and Purkinje fiber because of the different potential ranges of these two pacemaker types (i.e., −70 to −35 mV and −90 to −65 mV, respectively). The contribution of other voltage-dependent currents may also differ among the different cardiac cell types. For example, L-type I_{Ca} participates in the late phase of diastolic depolarization in SA and AV nodes, but not in Purkinje fibers. In atrial pacemaker cells, low-voltage-activated T-type I_{Ca} has been shown to contribute by SR calcium release, which, in turn, stimulates the inward $I_{Na\text{-}Ca}$.[31] Genetic disruption of the T-type Ca^{2+} channel pore-forming subunit (Cav3.1/α_{1G}) has been shown to slow SA and AV node automativity.[32] The action potential upstroke is provided largely by the fast sodium current in the His–Purkinje system and predominantly by the slow calcium current in SA and AV nodes. A role for sustained inward current (I_{st}) as well as for Ca^{2+} release from the sarcoplasmic reticulum (SR) has recently been proposed.[31,33] Despite extensive electrophysiological study, the ionic mechanisms of SA node pacemaker activity remain unclear and increasingly complex.

The rate at which pacemaking cells initiate impulses is determined by the interplay of the following three factors[34]: (1) maximum diastolic potential, (2) threshold potential, and (3) slope of phase 4 depolarization. A change in any one of these factors will alter the time required for phase 4 depolarization to carry the membrane potential from its maximum diastolic level to threshold and thus alter the rate of impulse initiation. If the maximum diastolic potential increases (becomes more negative), spontaneous depolarization to the threshold potential will take longer and the rate of impulse initiation will slow.

Parasympathetic and sympathetic influences as well as extracellular potassium levels can alter one or more of these three parameters and thus modulate the intrinsic rate of discharge of biological pacemakers. In general, β-adrenergic receptor stimulation increases, whereas muscarinic receptor stimulation reduces, the rate of phase 4 depolarization. Parasympathetic agonists such as acetylcholine exert these actions by activating a K current, $I_{K\text{-}ACh}$, reducing the inward Ca^{2+} current (I_{Ca}) as well as reducing the pacemaker current (I_f).[35] β-Adrenergic agonists such as norepinephrine or isoproterenol increase the spontaneous rate largely through an augmentation of I_{Ca} and the pacemaker current (I_f). Acetylcholine also hyperpolarizes the cell leading to an increase in maximum diastolic potential. Vagal-induced hyperpolarization and slowing of phase 4 depolarization act in concert to reduce the sinus rate and are the principal causes of sinus bradycardia. The prevalence of the sympathetic system over the parasympathetic system during physical exercises or stress largely accounts for an increase in heart rate during these conditions. The opposite takes place during sleep.

Subsidiary atrial pacemakers with diastolic potentials more negative (−75 to −70 mV) than SA nodal cells are located at the junction of the inferior right atrium and the inferior vena cava, near or on the eustachian ridge.[36–38] Other atrial pacemakers have been identified in the crista terminalis[39] as well as at the orifice of the coronary sinus[40] and in the atrial muscle that extends into the tricuspid and mitral valves.[41–43] The cardiac muscle sleeves that extend into the cardiac veins (vena cavae and pulmonary veins) may also have normal automaticity.[44–46] However, a number of investigators report failure to observe any sign of automaticity in pulmonary vein muscular sleeves.[47,48] Latent pacemaking cells in the AV junction are responsible for AV junctional rhythms.[49,50] Both atrial and AV junctional subsidiary pacemakers are under autonomic control, with the sympathetic system increasing and parasympathetic system slowing the pacing rate.

The His–Purkinje system in the ventricles of the heart contain the slowest subsidiary pacemakers.[25,34,51] In the His–Purkinje system, parasympathetic effects are less apparent than those of the sympathetic system. Although acetylcholine produces little in the way of a direct effect, it can significantly reduce Purkinje automaticity via inhibition of the sympathetic influence, a phenomenon termed accentuated antagonism.[52] As in the atria, sympathetic stimulation increases the rate of firing. In the His–Purkinje system, as in all pacemaker cells, an increase of extracellular potassium concentration reduces the rate of diastolic depolarization, while a decrease of extracellular potassium has the opposite effect. This effect of $[K^+]_o$ is due largely to modulation of the inward rectifier current, I_{K1}. A reduction in I_{K1} can also occur secondary to a mutation in KCNJ2, the gene that encodes for this channel, leading to increased automaticity and extrasystolic activity presumably arising from the Purkinje system.[53–55] Interestingly, because β-adrenergic stimulation is effective in augmenting I_{K1},[56] sympathetic stimulation may produce a paradoxical slowing of automaticity and ectopy in this setting.

Abnormal Automaticity

Abnormal automaticity or depolarization-induced automaticity is observed under conditions of reduced resting membrane potential, such as ischemia, infarction, or other depolarizing influences (i.e., current injection) (Figure 5–2, right panel). Abnormal automaticity is experimentally observed in tissues that normally develop diastolic depolarization (i.e., Purkinje fiber), as well as those that normally do not display this feature (e.g., ventricular or atrial myocardium). The membrane potential at which abnormal automaticity develops ranges between −70 and −30 mV.[57] Compared to normal automaticity, abnormal automaticity in Purkinje fibers or ventricular and atrial myocardium is more readily suppressed by calcium channel blockers and shows little or no overdrive suppression.[58,59] The rate of abnormal automaticity is substantially higher than that of normal automaticity and is a sensitive function of resting membrane potential (i.e., the more depolarized resting potential the faster rate). Similar to normal automaticity, abnormal automaticity is enhanced by β-adrenergic agonists and by reduction of external potassium.[58,60]

The ionic basis for diastolic depolarization in abnormal automaticity may be similar to that of normal automaticity, consisting of a time-dependent activation of sodium current[61] and pacemaker current I_f as well as decay of I_K.[60,62] Experiments on depolarized human atrial myocardium from dilated atria indicate that Ca^{2+}-dependent processes also may contribute to abnormal pacemaker activity at low membrane potentials.[63,64] It has been suggested that release of Ca^{2+} from the SR may activate sodium–calcium exchanger current, $I_{Na\text{-}Ca}$, leading to spontaneous diastolic depolarization and abnormal automaticity. This mechanism is similar to that responsible for the generation of DADs (discussed below).

Action potential upstrokes associated with abnormal automaticity may be mediated either by I_{Na} or I_{Ca}, depending on the takeoff potential. In the range of takeoff potentials between approximately −70 and −50 mV, repetitive activity is dependent on I_{Na} and may be depressed or abolished by sodium channel blockers. In a takeoff potential range of −50 to −30 mV, repetitive activity depends on I_{Ca} and may be abolished by calcium channel blockers.

Depolarization of membrane potential associated with disease states is most commonly a result of either (1) an increase in extracellular K^+, which reduces the reversal potential for I_{K1}, the outward current that largely determines the resting membrane or maximum diastolic potential; (2) a reduced number of I_{K1} channels; (3) a reduced ability of I_{K1} channels to conduct potassium ions; or (4) the electrotonic influence of the neighboring depolarized zone. An increase in $[K^+]_o$ reduces membrane potential, but does not induce abnormal automaticity. Indeed, raising $[K^+]_o$ is effective in suppressing abnormal automaticity in atrial, ventricular, and Purkinje fibers.[65,66] This argues against abnormal automaticity being responsible for arrhythmias arising in acutely ischemic myocardium, where cells are partially depolarized by increased extracellular K^+.[67–69] As will be discussed later in this chapter, abnormal automaticity may arise in the border zone of an ischemic region, where electrotonic depolarization may occur in the absence of an increase in $[K^+]_o$.

Membrane depolarization may also occur as a result of a decrease in $[K]_i$, which has been shown to occur in Purkinje fibers surviving an infarct and to persist for at least 24h after coronary occlusion.[70] The reduction in $[K]_i$ contributes to the low membrane potential[70] and the accompanying abnormal automaticity.[71,72] Human tissues isolated from diseased atrial and ventricular myocardium show phase 4 depolarization and abnormal automaticity at membrane potentials in the range of −50 to −60mV.[73–75] It has been proposed that a decrease in membrane potassium conductance is an important cause of the low membrane potentials in the atrial fibers.[74] It is known now that I_{K1} is much smaller in atrial compared to ventricular cells.

Because the conductance of I_{K1} channels is a sensitive function of $[K^+]_o$, hypokalemia can lead to a major reduction in inward rectifier current, leading to depolarization and the development of enhanced or abnormal automaticity, particularly in Purkinje pacemakers.

An example of an inherited disease involving a reduction in I_{K1} is Andersen–Tawil syndrome. A loss of function of I_{K1} occurs secondary to mutations in KCNJ2, the gene that encodes Kir2.1, the protein that forms the I_{K1} channel. Andersen–Tawil syndrome is associated with a very high level of ectopy thought to arise from enhanced pacemaker activity within the Purkinje system as a result of a reduced level of I_{K1}.[53–55,76,77]

Automaticity as a Mechanism of Cardiac Arrhythmias

Arrhythmias caused by abnormal automaticity may result from diverse mechanisms. Sinus bradycardia and tachycardia are caused by a simple alteration in the rate of impulse initiation by the normal SA node pacemaker (Table 5–1). Alterations in sinus rate may be accompanied by shifts in the origin of the dominant pacemaker within the sinus node[34,78] or to subsidiary pacemaker sites elsewhere in the atria. Impulse conduction out of the SA mode may be impaired or blocked as a result of disease or increased vagal activity[79,80] leading to the development of bradycardia.

Atrioventricular (AV) junctional rhythms occur when atrioventricular junctional pacemakers located either in the AV node or in the His bundle take control of the heart, usually in the presence of AV block.[50] When an idioventricular rhythm arises from the Purkinje system during complete heart block, the rate is usually slower and the ECG is characterized by a wide, aberrant QRS complex.[81]

Normal or subsidiary pacemaker activity also may be enhanced, leading to sinus tachycardia or a shift to ectopic sites within the atria, giving rise to atrial tachycardia. One cause may be enhanced sympathetic nerve activity. Another may be the flow of injury current between partially depolarized myocardium and normally polarized latent pacemaker cells.[82] This mechanism is thought to be responsible for ectopic beats that arise at the borders of ischemic zones.[83] Other causes of enhanced pacemaker activity include a decease in the extracellular potassium levels as well as acute stretch.[84,85] Stretch of the Purkinje system may occur in akinetic areas after acute ischemia or in ventricular aneurysms in hearts with healed infarcts. Accelerated idioventricular rhythms have been attributed to enhanced normal automaticity in the His–Purkinje system.[86] Although experimental and clinical three-dimensional mapping studies have shown that ventricular arrhythmias arising under conditions of acute ischemia, infarction, heart failure, and other cardiomyopathies can be ascribed to focal mechanisms,[87–91] it is often difficult to differentiate between automatic and focal reentrant (reflection, phase 2 reentry, and microreentry) mechanisms. It is noteworthy that myocytes isolated from failing and hypertrophied animal and human hearts have been shown to manifest diastolic depolarization[92,93] and to possess enhanced I_f pacemaker current,[94,95] suggesting that these mechanism contribute to extrasystolic and tachyarrhythmias arising with these pathologies.

Although automaticity is not responsible for most rapid tachyarrhythmias, it can precipitate or trigger reentrant arrhythmias. Haissaguerre and co-workers have shown that atrial fibrillation can be triggered by rapid automaticity arising in the pulmonary veins.[96] It is noteworthy that atrial tissues isolated from patients with atrial fibrillation exhibit increased I_f mRNA levels.[97]

The normal automaticity of all subsidiary pacemakers within the heart is inhibited when overdrive paced.[26,98] This inhibition is called *overdrive suppression*. In contrast, sustained activity caused by abnormal automaticity usually displays little or no response to overdrive pacing.[58,59] Under normal physiological conditions, all subsidiary pacemakers are overdrive suppressed by SA nodal activity. Overdrive suppression is largely mediated by intracellular accumulation of Na^+, leading to enhanced activity of the sodium pump (Na^+-K^+-ATPase), which generates a hyperpolarizing electrogenic current that opposes phase 4 depolarization.[98–100] The faster the overdrive rate or the longer the duration of overdrive, the greater the enhancement of sodium pump activity, so that the period of quiescence after cessation of overdrive is directly related to the rate and duration of overdrive.[98] The sinus node itself can be overdrive suppressed if it is stimulated at a rate more rapid than its intrinsic rate, although the degree of overdrive suppression is less than that of subsidiary pacemakers driven at comparable rates.[36,101] This differential may be due to the fact that the sinus node action potential upstroke is largely dependent on L-type Ca^{2+} channel current and less Na^+ accumulates intracellulary to stimulate the sodium pump. Interestingly, spontaneous automaticity in the center of the sinus node can be well preserved during atrial fibrillation due to a minimal degree of overdrive suppression as well as a high degree of sinoatrial entrance block.[102]

Parasystole and Modulated Parasystole

Latent pacemakers throughout the heart are generally reset by the propagating wavefront initiated by the dominant pacemaker and are therefore unable to activate the heart. An exception to this rule occurs when the pacemaking tissue is protected from the impulse of sinus origin. A region of entrance block arises when cells exhibiting automaticity are surrounded by a high resistance barrier due to ischemia, infarction, or otherwise compromised cardiac tissue, which prevents the propagating wave from invading the focus, but which permits the spontaneous beat generated within the automatic focus to exit and activate the rest of the myocardium. A pacemaker region exhibiting entrance block and exit conduction defines a parasystolic focus (Figure 5–3).[103] The ectopic activity generated by a parasystolic focus is characterized by premature ventricular complexes with variable coupling intervals, fusion beats, and interectopic intervals that are multiples of a common denominator. This rhythm is fairly rare. While it is usually considered benign, any premature ventricular activation can induce malignant ventricular rhythms in the ischemic myocardium or in the presence of a suitable myocardial substrate.

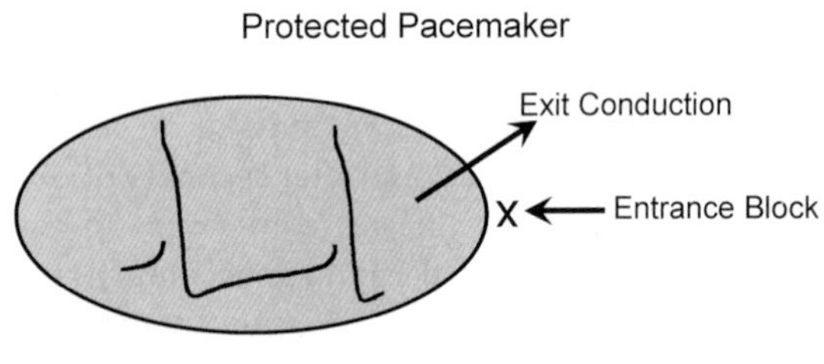

FIGURE 5–3. Classical parasystole. The ectopic pacemaker is protected from invasion by activity outside the focus (entrance block), but when the pacemaker fires, the impulse generated is able to propagate out of the focus to excite the rest of the myocardium (exit conduction).

In the late 1970s and early 1980s Moe and co-workers described a variant of classical parasystole, which they termed modulated parasystole.[104–106] This variant of the arrhythmia was suggested to result from incomplete entrance block of the parasystolic focus. Electrotonic influences arriving early in the pacemaker cycle delayed and those arriving late in the cycle accelerated the firing of the parasystolic pacemaker, so that ventricular activity could entrain the partially protected pacemaker (Figure 5–4). As a consequence, at selected heart rates, extrasystolic activity generated by the entrained parasystolic pacemaker can mimic reentry, generating extrasystolic activity with fixed coupling (Figures 5–5 and 5–6).[104–115] A recent study suggests that bidirectional modulated parasystole can also account for cyclic bursts of ventricular premature contractions.[116]

Afterdepolarizations and Triggered Activity

Oscillatory depolarizations that attend or follow the cardiac action potential and depend on preceding transmembrane activity for their manifestation are referred to as afterdepolarizations.[117] Two subclasses are traditionally recognized: (1) early and (2) delayed. The EADs interrupt or retard repolarization during phase 2 and/or

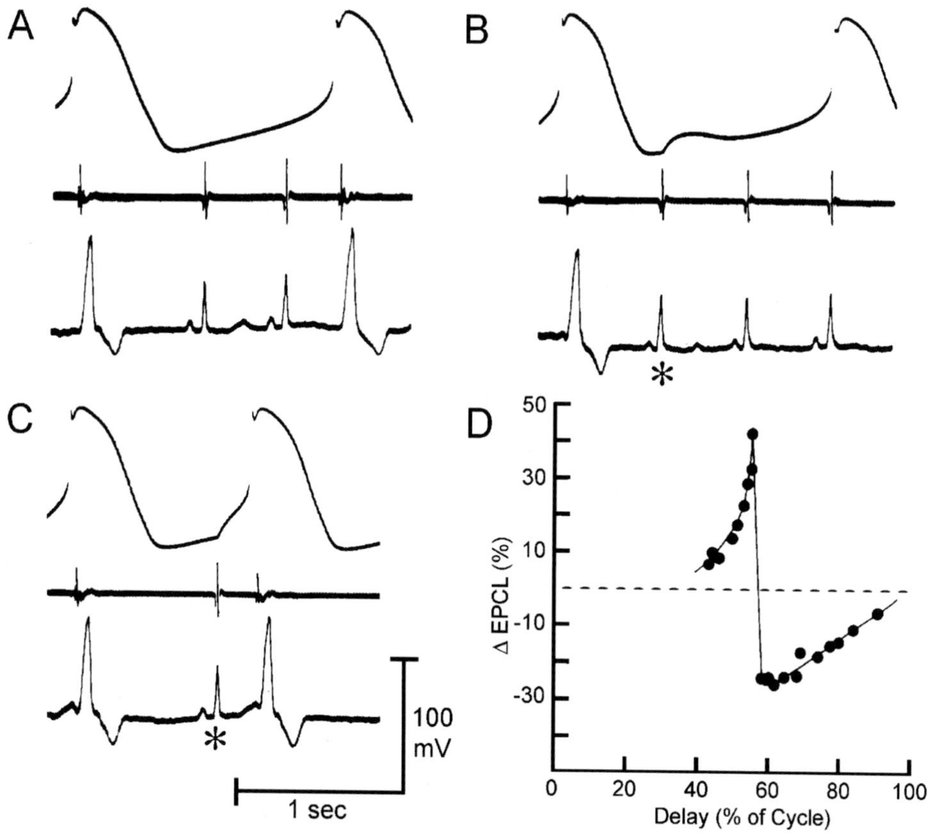

FIGURE 5–4. Electrotonic modulation of a parasystolic pacemaker. Traces were recorded from an experimental model consisting of a sucrose gap preparation *in vitro* coupled to the heart of an open chest dog. Traces (top to bottom): transmembrane potentials recorded from a distal segment of a Purkinje fiber-sucrose gap preparation, and a right ventricular electrogram and lead II ECG from the *in vivo* preparation. (A) The Purkinje pacemaker was allowed to beat free of any influence from ventricular activation. (B and C) Pacemaker activity of the Purkinje is electrotonically influenced by ventricular activation. An electrotonic influence arriving early in the pacemaker cycle delays the next discharge, whereas that arriving late accelerates the next discharge. (D) The electrotonic modulation of pacemaker discharge is described in the form of a phase–response curve. The percentage change in ectopic pacemaker cycle length (EPCL) is plotted as a function of the temporal position of the electrotonic influence in the pacemaker cycle. (From Antzelevitch *et al.*,[110] with permission.)

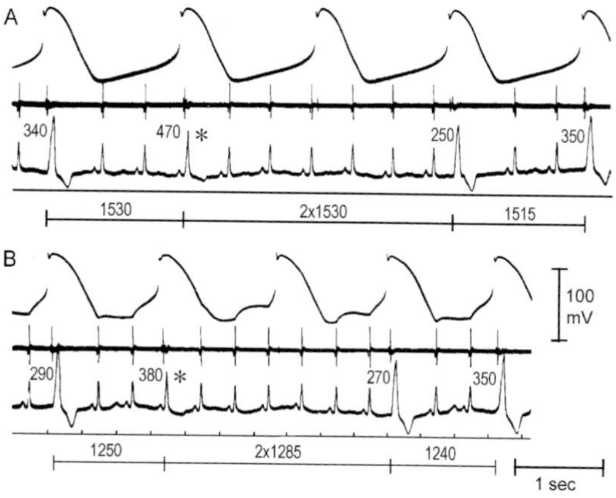

FIGURE 5–5. Patterns of classical parasystole generated by the experimental model described in Figure 5–16 in the absence (A) and presence (B) of modulating influence from the ventricles. The lowest trace is a stimulus marker. Numbers denote the coupling intervals of the ectopic responses to the preceding normal beats (in milliseconds). Asterisks denote fusion beats. Classical parasystolic features are apparent in both cases. (From Antzelevitch *et al.*,[110] with permission.)

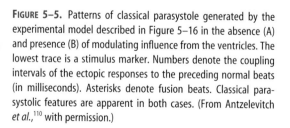

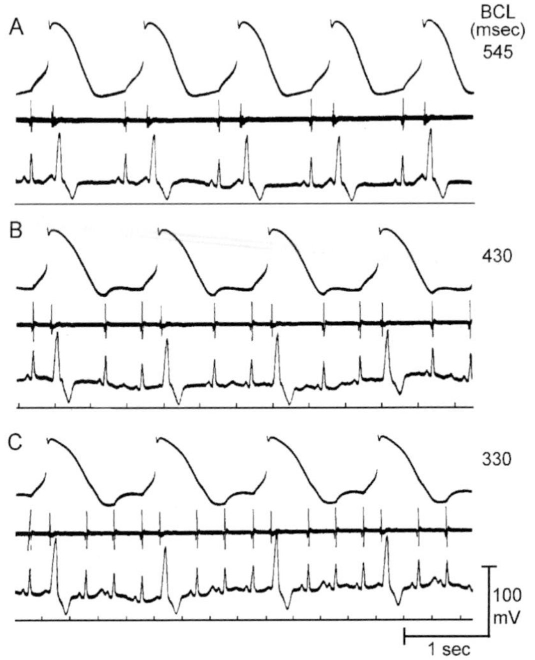

FIGURE 5–6. Records were obtained from the same preparation as in Figure 5–17 but at different cycle lengths. At the basic cycle lengths (BCL) shown, the activity generated was characteristic of reentry (fixed coupling of the premature beats to the basic beats). (A) Bigeminy, (B) trigeminy, and (C) quadrigeminy. (From Antzelevitch *et al.*,[110] with permission.)

phase 3 of the cardiac action potential, whereas DADs arise after full repolarization (Figures 5–7A and B and 5–8). Recent studies from our laboratory have uncovered a novel mechanism giving rise to triggered activity termed "late phase 3 EAD," which combines properties of both EAD and DAD, but has its own unique character (Figure 5–7C).[23,118] When EAD or DAD amplitude suffices to bring the membrane to its threshold potential, a spontaneous action potential referred to as a triggered response is the result.[119] These triggered events may be responsible for extrasystoles and tachyarrhythmias that develop under conditions predisposing to the development of afterdepolarizations.

Early Afterdepolarizations and Triggered Activity

Characteristics of Early Afterdepolarizations and Early Afterdepolarization-Induced Triggered Beats

Early afterdepolarizations are observed in isolated cardiac tissues exposed to injury,[120] altered electrolytes, hypoxia, acidosis,[121,122] catecholamines,[123,124] and pharmacological agents,[125] including antiarrhythmic drugs.[126–130] Ventricular hypertrophy and heart failure also predispose to the development of EADs.[93,131,132] Hyperthermia

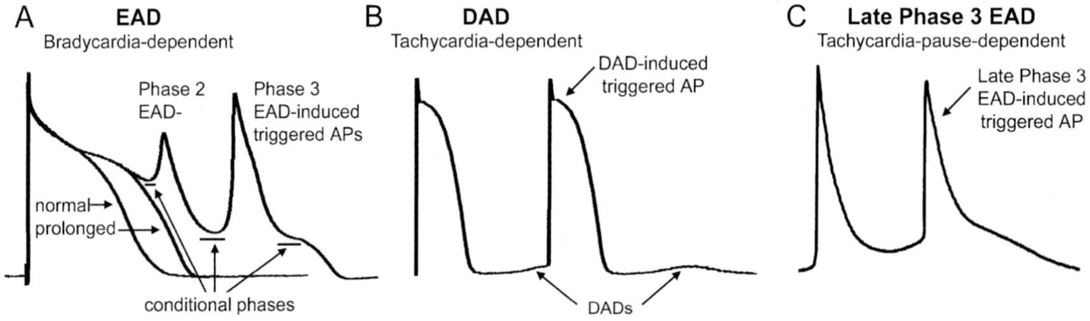

FIGURE 5–7. Early (EAD) and delayed (DAD) afterdepolarizations and EAD- and DAD-induced triggered action potentials (AP). (A) Phase 2 EAD and phase 3 EAD-induced APs in canine isolated Purkinje fiber preparation treated with *d*-sotalol (I_{Kr} block). The conditional phase of EAD is defined as the time interval spanning from the moment when the membrane potential starts to deviate from a normal coarse to the moment that immediately precedes the EAD upstroke or downstroke. (B) DAD- and DAD-induced triggered activity in a canine ventricular preparation induced by rapid pacing in the presence of isoproterenol (β-adrenergic agonist, augmenting intracellular calcium activity). (C) Late phase 3 EAD-induced triggered beat in canine right atrium under conditions of abbreviated repolarization (in the presence of acetylcholine). Shown are the first beat of sinus origin following a period of rapid activation and the late phase 3 EAD-induced triggered beat. [(A and B) Reproduced from Burashnikov *et al.*[23] and (C) Reproduced from Burashnikov *et al.*,[22] with permission.]

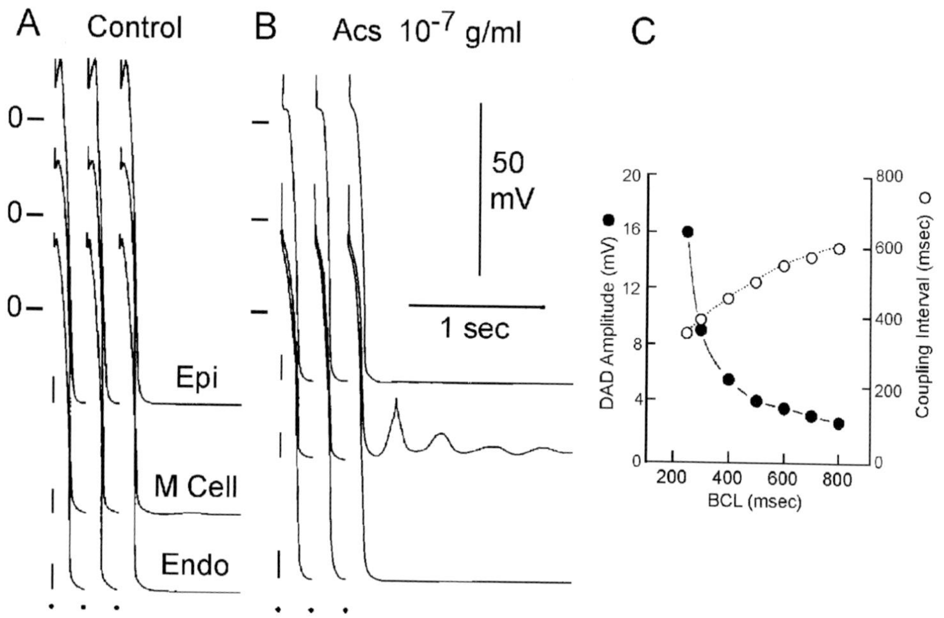

FIGURE 5–8. Digitalis-induced delayed afterdepolarizations (DADs) in M cells but not epicardium or endocardium. Effects of acetylstrophanthidin (AcS) on transmembrane activity of an epicardial (Epi), endocardial (Endo), and M cell preparation. $[K^+]_o = 4$ mM. (A) Control. (B) Recorded after 90 min of exposure to 10–7 g/ml AcS. Each panel shows the last three beats of a train of 10 basic beats elicited at a basic cycle length (BCL) of 250 msec. Each train is followed by a 3 sec pause. AcS induced prominent DADs in the M cell preparation but not in epicardium or endocardium. (C) Rate dependence of coupling interval and amplitude of the AcS-induced DADs. Measured is the first DAD recorded from the M cell. (From Sicouri and Antzelevitch,[142] with permission.)

promotes and hypothermia depresses the appearance of EAD.[133]

The characteristics of the EAD vary as a function of animal species, tissue or cell type, and the method by which it is elicited. Although specific mechanisms of EAD induction may differ, a critical prolongation of repolarization accompanies most, but not all, EADs. Figure 5–7A illustrates the two types of EAD generally encountered in Purkinje fiber. Oscillatory events appearing at potentials positive to –30 mV are generally referred to as phase 2 EADs. Those occurring at more negative potentials are termed phase 3 EADs. Phase 2 and phase 3 EADs sometimes appear in the same preparation (Figure 5–7A). In contrast to Purkinje fibers, EAD activity recorded in ventricular preparations is always a phase 2 EAD.[134]

The EAD-induced triggered activity is a sensitive function of stimulation rate. Agents with Class III action generally induce EAD activity at slow stimulation rates and totally suppress EADs at rapid rates.[129,135] In contrast, β-adrenergic agonist-induced EADs develop at physiologically normal heart rates.[123,124] Recent studies have shown that in the presence of I_{Kr} block, β-adrenergic agonists and/or acceleration from an initially slow rate transiently facilitate the induction of EAD activity in ventricular M cells, but not in epicardium or endocardium and rarely in Purkinje fibers.[136] This biphasic effect is thought to be due to an initial priming of the sodium-calcium exchanger, which provides an electrogenic inward current ($I_{Na\text{-}Ca}$) that facilitates EAD development and prolongs action potential duration (APD). This early phase is followed by recruitment of I_{Ks}, which abbreviates APD and suppresses EAD activity.

Cellular Origin of Early Afterdepolarizations

Before the 1990s, our understanding of the EAD was based largely on data obtained from studies involving Purkinje fiber preparations. With few exceptions,[137,138] EADs were not observed in early experiments involving tissues isolated from the surfaces of the mammalian ventricle.[127,139–141] More recent studies have demonstrated that although canine epicardial and endocardial tissues generally fail to develop EADs when exposed to APD-prolonging agents, midmyocardial M cells readily develop EAD activity under these conditions.[142] Failure of epicardial and endocardial tissues to develop EADs has been ascribed to the presence of a strong I_{Ks} in these cells.[143] M cells have a weak I_{Ks},[143] predisposing them to the development of EADs in the presence of I_{Kr} block. In the presence of chromanol 293B to block I_{Ks}, I_{Kr} blockers such as E-4031 or sotalol induce EAD activity in canine isolated epicardial and endocardial tissues, as well as in M cells.[144] The predisposition of cardiac cells to the development of EADs depends principally on the reduced availability of I_{Kr} and I_{Ks}, as occurs in many forms of cardiomyopathy. Under these conditions, EADs can appear in any part of the ventricular myocardium.

Three-dimensional mapping of torsade de pointes (TdP) arrhythmias in canine experimental models suggests that the extrasystole that initiates TdP can originate from subendocardial, midmyocardial, or subepicardial regions of the left ventricle.[145,146] These data point to Purkinje fibers and M cells as the principal sources of EAD-induced triggered activity *in vivo*. In the presence of combined I_{Kr} and I_{Ks} block, epicardium is often the first to develop an EAD. While EAD-induced extrasystoles are capable of triggering TdP, the arrhythmia is considered by many, but not all, to be maintained by a reentrant mechanism.[147–149]

Ionic Mechanisms Responsible for the Early Afterdepolarization

Early afterdepolarizations are commonly associated with a prolongation of the repolarization phase due to a reduction of net outward current secondary to an increase in inward currents and/or a decrease in outward currents. An EAD occurs when the balance of current active during phase 2 or 3 of the action potential shifts in the inward direction. If the change in the current–voltage relationship results in a region of net inward current during the plateau range of membrane potentials,[150] it leads to a depolarization or EAD. Most pharmacological interventions or pathophysiological conditions associated with EADs can be categorized as acting predominantly through one of four different mechanisms: (1) a reduction of repolarizing potassium currents (I_{Kr}, class IA and III antiarrhythmic agents; I_{Ks}, chromanol 293B, or I_{K1}); (2) an increase in the availability of calcium current (Bay K 8644, catecholamines); (3) an increase in the sodium–calcium exchange current due to augmentation of intracellular calcium activity or upregulation of the exchanger; and (4) an increase in late sodium current (late I_{Na}) (aconitine, anthopleurin-A, and ATX-II). Combinations of these interventions (i.e., calcium loading and I_{Kr} reduction) or pathophysiological states may act synergistically to facilitate the development of EADs.[136,141,147,151–153] While a reduction of I_{Kr} or augmentation of late I_{Na} alone is capable of inducing EAD in ventricular muscles and Purkinje fibers, a reduction of I_{Ks} alone does not induce EAD.[154] However, I_{Ks} greatly facilitates EAD induction in response to reduction of I_{Kr}, augmentation of late I_{Na}, or sympathetic stimulation.[144,155] The EADs can appear without the involvement of intracellular calcium activity (Ca_i); however, augmentation of Ca_i under conditions of APD prolongation greatly facilitates the development of EADs.[136,152]

The upstroke of the EAD is generally carried by L-type calcium. There is less agreement on the ionic basis for the critically important conditional phase of the EAD, defined as the period just before the EAD upstroke. Intracellular calcium levels and Na/Ca exchange current play pivotal roles in the conditional phase of isoproterenol-induced EADs.[123,124,156] Data from several laboratories suggest that intracellular calcium levels do not influence the formation of these phase 2 EADs,[138,157–159] whereas others have presented strong evidence in support of the influence of intracellular calcium levels on the formation of at least the conditional phase of the EAD.[136,160] This discrepancy is in part due to the type of tissues or cells studied. There are important differences in the ionic mechanisms of EAD generation in canine Purkinje fibers and ventricular M cells. Early afterdepolarizations induced in canine M cells are exquisitely sensitive to changes in intracellular calcium levels, whereas EADs elicited in

Purkinje fibers are largely insensitive.[136] Ryanodine, an agent known to block calcium release from the SR, abolishes EAD activity in canine M cells, but not in Purkinje fibers.[136] These distinctions may reflect differences in intracellular calcium handling in M cells, where the SR is well developed, versus Purkinje fibers where the SR is poorly developed.

A sustained component of I_{Na} active during the action potential plateau, originating from channels that fail to inactivate and a nonequilibrium component arising from channels recovering from inactivation during phases 2 and 3, has been shown to contribute prominently to the action potential duration and induction of EADs.[161–163] Calmodulin kinase (CaMK) II has been linked to the development of EAD and TdP in cellular models where repolarization is prolonged.[164–167] Interestingly and somewhat unexpectedly, calmodulin binding to KCNQ1 was recently shown to be required for delivery of the channel protein to the cell surface; this chaperone effect is not dependent on calcium binding to calmodulin.[168–170] Failure of KvLQT1 (protein product of KCNQ1) to traffic to the membrane can prolong QT and facilitate the development of EADs. Agents that inhibit I_{Ca}, CaMK, and late I_{Na} have been shown to be effective in suppressing EAD activity.[171,172] The action of late I_{Na} blockers such as ranolazine and RSD1235 may be mediated by both a direct effect on the late inward current and indirectly by modulating calcium homeostasis.[173–177]

Role of Early Afterdepolarizations in the Development of Cardiac Arrhythmias

As previously discussed, EAD-induced extrasystoles are thought to be involved in precipitating TdP under conditions of congenital and acquired long QT syndromes.[178,179] The EAD-like deflections have been observed in ventricular MAP recordings immediately preceding TdP arrhythmias in the clinic as well as in experimental models of LQTS.[140,180–183] While EAD is most likely to initiate TdP in the congenital LQT2/LQT6 (reduction of I_{Kr}) and LQT3 (augmentation $I_{Na(late)}$) forms of the long QT syndrome, recent experimental evidence points to DAD-induced activity as the trigger in LQT1/LQT5-related TdP (reduction in I_{Ks}).[154]

Early afterdepolarization activity may also be involved in the genesis of cardiac arrhythmias in cases of hypertrophy and heart failure. These syndromes are commonly associated with prolongation of the ventricular action potential, which predisposes to the development of EADs.[85,92,93,131,132,184,185]

It is noteworthy that EADs developing in select transmural subtypes (such as M cells) can exaggerate transmural dispersion of repolarization (TDR), thus setting the stage for reentry. As will be discussed in more detail below, transmural dispersion of repolarization is thought to be the principal substrate permitting the development of TdP.[186–189]

In contrast to ventricular myocardial and Purkinje cells, atrial cells generally do not develop conventional EADs in response to agents that prolong cardiac repolarization.[190,191] These experimental data are consistent with clinical observations that APD-prolonging agents can be associated with EAD-related ventricular arrhythmias (i.e., TdP), but not atrial arrhythmias.[192]

Delayed Afterdepolarization-Induced Triggered Activity

Causes and Origin of Delayed Afterdepolarization-Induced Triggered Activity

DADs and DAD-induced triggered activity are observed under conditions that increase intracellular calcium, $[Ca^{2+}]_i$, such as after exposure to toxic levels of cardiac glycosides (digitalis)[193–195] or catecholamines.[37,40,123,196] This activity is also manifest in hypertrophied and failing hearts[92,131] as well as in Purkinje fibers surviving myocardial infarction.[72] In contrast to EADs, DADs are always induced at relatively rapid rates.

Digitalis-induced DADs and triggered activity have been well characterized in isolated Purkinje fibers.[119] In the ventricular myocardium, they are less commonly observed in epicardial or endocardial tissues, but readily induced in cells and tissues from the M region.[142] However, DADs are frequently observed in myocytes enzymatically dissociated from ventricular myocardium.[197–199] Digitalis, isoproterenol, high $[Ca^{2+}]_o$, and Bay K 8644, a calcium agonist, have been shown to cause DADs and triggered activity in tissues isolated from the M region but not in epicardial or endocardial tissues (Figure 5–8B).[142,154,200,201] The failure of epicardial and endocardial cells to develop DADs has been ascribed to a high density of I_{Ks} in these tissues[143] as compared to M cells where I_{Ks} is small.[143] In support of this hypothesis, reduction of I_{Ks} can promote isoproterenol-induced DAD activity in canine and guinea pig endocardium and epicardium.[154,202]

Interventions capable of altering intracellular calcium, either by modifying transsarcolemmal calcium current or by inhibiting SR storage or release of calcium, can affect the manifestation of DADs, which can also be modified by interventions capable of directly inhibiting or enhancing the transient inward current, I_{ti}. They are modified by extracellular K^+, Ca^{2+}, lisophosphoglycerides, and metabolic factors such as ATP, hypoxia, and pH. Lowering extracellular K^+ (<4 mM) promotes DADs, while increasing K^+ attenuates or totally suppresses DADs.[119,203] Lisophosphatidylcholine, in concentrations similar to those that accumulate in ischemic myocardium, has been shown to induce DAD activity.[204] Elevating extracellular Ca^{2+} promotes DADs[119] and an increase of extracellular ATP potentiates isoproterenol-induced DAD.[205]

Agents that prolong action potential duration, such as quinidine and clofilium, facilitate the induction of DAD activity by augmenting calcium entry. Recent work indicates that calcium calmodulin (CaM) kinase can facilitate the induction of DADs by augmenting I_{Ca}.[171]

Under some pathophysiological conditions, particularly those that predispose to the development of catecholaminergic ventricular tachycardia (VT), DAD activity may be observed to arise from epicardium.[206]

Delayed afterdepolarizations and triggered activity also may occur in the absence of pharmacological agents, catecholamines, or an increase in extracellular Ca^{2+}. DAD-induced triggered activity has been found in the upper pectinate muscles bordering the crista terminalis in the rabbit heart, branches of the sinoatrial ring bundle, or transitional fibers between the ring bundle and ordinary pectinate muscle, apparently normal fibers in human atrial myocardium,[207] rat ventricular muscle that is hypertrophic secondary to renovascular hypertension,[131] and ventricular myocardium from diabetic rats.[208] Abnormal SR function, in which the ability of the SR to sequester calcium during diastole is compromised, may lead to DADs. Such abnormal SR function may result from genetically based alterations in SR proteins and may be the cause of certain inherited ventricular tachyarrhythmias.[209]

Pharmacological agents that affect the release and reuptake of calcium by the SR, including caffeine and ryanodine, can also influence the manifestation of DADs and triggered activity. Low concentrations of caffeine facilitate Ca^{2+} release from the SR and thus contribute to augmentation of DAD and triggered activity. High concentrations of caffeine prevent Ca^{2+} uptake by the SR and thus abolish I_{ti}, DADs, aftercontractions, and triggered activity. Doxorubicin, an anthracycline antibiotic, has been shown to be effective in suppressing digitalis-induced DADs, possibly through inhibition of the Na–Ca exchange mechanism.[210] Potassium channel activators, like pinacidil, can also suppress DAD and triggered activity by activating ATP-regulated potassium current ($I_{K\text{-}ATP}$).[198,201] Flunarizine is another agent shown to suppress DAD and triggered activity, in part through inhibition of both L-type and T-type calcium current.[211–215] Other L-type calcium channel blockers, like verapamil, are effective in suppressing DADs.[119] Ranolazine, an antianginal agent with potent late sodium channel blocking action, has also been shown to reduce the amplitude of DADs induced by isoproterenol, forskolin, and ouabain.[174,216,217] All sodium channel blockers suppress DADs, apparently due to a reduction in Ca_i loading secondary to a reduction in Na_i accumulation.[119,218]

Ionic Mechanisms Responsible for the Development of Delayed Afterdepolarizations

Delayed afterdepolarizations and accompanying aftercontractions are caused by spontaneous release of calcium from the SR under calcium overload conditions. The afterdepolarization is believed to be induced by a transient inward current (I_{ti}) generated either by (1) a nonselective cationic current, I_{ns},[219,220] (2) the activation of an electrogenic Na/Ca exchanger,[219,221–223] or (3) calcium-activated Cl^- current.[222,223] All are secondary to the release of Ca^{2+} from the overloaded SR.

Role of Delayed Afterdepolarization-Induced Triggered Activity in the Development of Cardiac Arrhythmias

Although studies performed in isolated tissues and cells suggest an important role for DAD-induced triggered activity in the genesis of cardiac arrhythmias, especially bigeminal rhythms and tachyarrhythmias observed in the setting of digitalis toxicity,[119] little direct evidence of DAD-induced triggered activity is available *in vivo*. Consequently, even when triggered activity appears a likely mechanism, it is often not possible to completely rule out other mechanisms (e.g., reentry or enhanced automaticity).

Clinical arrhythmias suggested to be caused by DAD-induced triggered activity include (1) *idiopathic ventricular tachyarrhythmias*[224–227] and (2) *idioventricular rhythms*—accelerated AV junctional escape rhythms that occur as a result of digitalis toxicity or in a setting of myocardial infarction. Other possible "DAD-mediated" arrhythmias include exercise-induced adenosine-sensitive ventricular tachycardia as described by Lerman and Belardinelli;[228] repetitive monomorphic ventricular tachycardia caused presumably by cAMP-mediated triggered activity;[229] supraventricular tachycardias, including arrhythmias originating in the coronary sinus;[230] and some heart failure-related arrhythmias.[85,91,92] In a recent study, Iwai and co-workers suggested that most cases of clinical atrial tachycardia are caused by DAD, and the majority of these tachycardias originate from the crista terminalis and tricuspid annulus.[231] Atrial tachycardia in a canine pacing-induced heart failure model is also caused by DAD-mediated triggered activity.[232]

Pogwizd and co-workers demonstrated that ventricular arrhythmias in patients associated with nonischemic cardiomyopathy and healed myocardial infarction are initiated and can be maintained in some cases by apparently non-reentrant mechanisms, including DADs.[91,87] Ventricular arrhythmias associated with ischemic cardiomyopathy may also be initiated by DAD-induced triggered beats.[233] In addition, DADs have been implicated in the reinitiation of ventricular fibrillation (VF) following failed defibrillation attempts. Flunarizine, a DAD inhibitor, significantly improved defibrillation efficacy.[215]

It is thought that DADs play a prominent role in catecholaminergic or familial polymorphic ventricular tachycardia, a rare, autosomal dominant inherited disorder, predominantly affecting children or adolescents with structurally normal hearts. It is characterized by bidirectional ventricular tachycardia (BVT), polymorphic VT (PVT), and a high risk of sudden cardiac death (30–50% by the age of 20–30 years).[234,235] Recent molecular genetic studies have identified mutations in genes encoding for the cardiac ryanodine receptor 2 (RyR2) or calsequestrin 2 (CASQ2) in patients with this phenotype.[209,235–238] Several lines of evidence point to DAD-induced triggered activity (TA) as the mechanism underlying monomorphic or bidirectional VT in these patients. These include the identification of genetic mutations involving Ca^{2+} regulatory proteins, a similarity of the ECG features to those associated with digitalis toxicity, and the precipitation by adrenergic stimulation. A recent model of catecholaminergic polymorphic ventricular tachycardia (CPVT) developed using the left ventricular coronary-perfused wedge preparation was shown to recapitulate the electrocardiographic and arrhythmic manifestations of the disease, most of which were secondary to DAD-induced triggered activity.[206] The DAD-induced extrasystolic activity arising from epicardium was also shown to provide the substrate for the development of reentrant tachyarrhythmias due to reversal of the direction of activation of the ventricular wall.[206]

Late Phase 3 Early Afterdepolarizations and Their Role in Initiation of Atrial Fibrillation

Recent studies have uncovered a novel mechanism giving rise to triggered activity, termed "late phase 3 EAD," which combines properties of both EAD and DAD, but has its own unique character (Figures 5–7C and 5–9).[22,23] Late phase 3 EAD-induced triggered extrasystoles represent a new concept of arrhythmogenesis in which abbreviated repolarization permits "normal SR calcium release" to induce an EAD-mediated closely coupled triggered response, particularly under conditions permitting intracellular calcium loading.[22,23] These EADs are distinguished by the fact that they interrupt the final phase of repolarization of the action potential (late phase 3). In

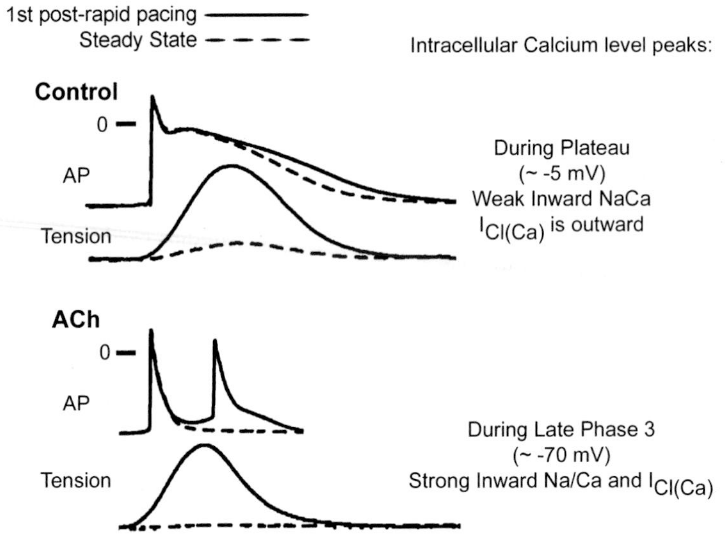

FIGURE 5–9. Proposed mechanism for the development of late phase 3 EADs. Shown are superimposed action potential (AP) and phasic tension recordings obtained under steady-state conditions and during the first regular postrapid pacing beat in control and in the presence of acetylcholine. See the text for further discussion. (Reproduced with permission from Burashnikov *et al.*[22])

contrast to previously described DAD or intracellular calcium (Ca_i)-dependent EAD, it is *normal*, not spontaneous SR calcium release that is responsible for the generation of the EAD. Two principal conditions are required for the appearance of late phase 3 EAD: an APD abbreviation and a strong SR calcium release.[22] These conditions may exist following termination of a period of rapid activation. In coronary-perfused canine right atrial preparations, late phase 3 EADs are observed only when APD is markedly abbreviated as with acetylcholine. Figure 5–9 describes a proposed mechanism for the late phase 3 EAD. Based on the time course of contraction, levels of Ca_i would be expected to peak during the plateau of the action potential (membrane potential of approximately −5 mV) under control conditions, but during the late phase of repolarization (membrane potential of approximately −70 mV) in the presence of acetylcholine. As a consequence, the two principal calcium-mediated currents, $I_{Na\text{-}Ca}$ and $I_{Cl(Ca)}$, would be expected to be weakly inward or even outward ($I_{Cl(Ca)}$) when APD is normal (control), but strongly inward when APD is very short (acetylcholine). Thus, abbreviation of the atrial APD allows for a much stronger recruitment of both $I_{Na\text{-}Ca}$ and $I_{Cl(Ca)}$ in the generation of late phase 3 EADs. It is noteworthy that the proposed mechanism is similar to that thought to underlie the development of DADs and conventional Ca_i-dependent EAD.[223,239] The principal difference is that in the case of these DADs/EADs, $I_{Na\text{-}Ca}$ and $I_{Cl(Ca)}$ are recruited secondary to a *spontaneous* release of calcium from the SR, whereas in the case of late phase 3 EADs, these currents are accentuated as a consequence of the *normal* SR release mechanisms.

In the isolated canine atria, late phase 3 EAD-induced extrasystoles have been shown to initiate atrial fibrillation (AF), particularly following spontaneous termination of the arrhythmia (IRAF, immediate reinduction of AF).[22] The appearance of late phase 3 EAD immediately following termination of AF or rapid pacing has been reported in the canine atria *in vivo*.[240] Patterson *et al.*[241] described "tachycardia-pause"-induced EAD in isolated superfused canine pulmonary vein muscular sleeve preparations in the presence of both simultaneous parasympathetic (to decrease APD) and sympathetic (to augment Ca_i) nerve stimulation. This EAD also appears during late phase 3 of the action potential and a similar mechanism has been proposed.[241] A similar mechanism has recently been invoked to explain catecholamine-induced afterdepolarizations and ventricular tachycardia in mice.[242]

Role for Late Phase 3 Early Depolarizations in Clinical Arrhythmia

Late phase 3 EAD-induced triggered beats are thought to be responsible for the immediate reinitiation of AF following termination of paroxysmal episodes of the arrhythmia. A transient period of post-AF hypercontractility (i.e., strong SR calcium release) takes place following termination of short episodes, but not long lasting AF.[243] Consistent with this fact is the observation that the highest incidence of immediate reinduction of AF occurs following termination of a short-lasting AF (<1–3 hours).[244,245] Early AF reinitiation most often occurs within 1–2 min after successful cardioversion of AF of any duration.[244–246]

The conditions that give rise to late phase 3 EADs may also occur immediately following termination of other tachyarrhythmias (atrial flutter or tachycardia, ventricular tachycardia, or fibrillation). All of these are known to decrease repolarization and induce a transient potentiation of SR calcium release upon return to normal (sinus) rhythm.[247] Extrasystolic activity or bigeminy can also lead to postextrasystolic potentiation of SR calcium release. Bigeminal pacing protocols are known to promote the appearance of premature beats and increase atrial vulnerability.[248] It remains to be determined if this mechanism may be involved in the initiation of arrhythmias in the short QT or Brugada syndromes, as well as the other conditions associated with abbreviated repolarization.

Reentrant Arrhythmias

Circus Movement Reentry

The circuitous propagation of an impulse around an anatomical or functional obstacle leading to reexcitation of the heart describes a circus movement reentry. Four distinct models of this form of reentry have been described: (1) the ring model, (2) the leading circle model, (3) the figure-of-eight model, and (4) the spiral wave model. The ring model of reentry differs from the other three in that an anatomical obstacle is required. The leading circle, figure-of-eight and spiral wave models of reentry require only a functional obstacle.

Electrical heterogeneity and the wavelength are pivotal concepts for understanding the development of circus movement reentry. The wavelength, the distance along the reentrant path occupied by the active response, is calculated as the product of conduction velocity and refractory period. The wavelength must be shorter than the pathlength for reentry to be maintained. In healthy hearts, conduction velocity in most areas of the heart is too rapid and the refractory period is too long to accommodate a reentrant circuit within the atria or ventricles. A structurally and electrically normal heart does not commonly develop reentrant arrhythmias. Slowing conduction velocity and/or abbreviating repolarization generally promote the appearance of reentrant arrhythmias by reducing the wavelength. Augmentation of electrical heterogeneity greatly predisposes the heart for the appearance of reentry as well, by increasing the probability of conduction block (i.e., wavebreak). Complex interactions of electrical dispersion, conduction velocity, and the duration of the refractory period largely determine the propensity of atria and ventricles for the development of reentrant arrhythmias. Cardiac disease is commonly associated with an increase in electrical heterogeneity, slowing of conduction velocity, and changes in refractory period, explaining the predisposition of the abnormal heart to reentrant arrhythmias.

The development of reentry typically requires a trigger as well as a substrate. The precipitating extrasystole or trigger may be automatic, triggered, or reentrant (reflection or phase 2 reentry). The substrate is generally due to electrical and/or structural heterogeneities. For a reentry to be initiated, a trigger must be in the right place (where repolarization gradients are steepest) at the right time (during the vulnerable window). The vulnerable window is that period in time during repolarization when heterogeneity is sufficiently amplified to permit reentry to be established.

Ring Model

The simplest form of reentry is the ring model (Figure 5–10). It first emerged as a concept shortly after the turn of the century when A.G. Mayer reported the results of experiments involving the subumbrella tissue of a jellyfish (*Sychomedusa cassiopea*).[1,2] The muscular disk did not contract until ring-like cuts were made and pressure and a stimulus applied. This caused the disk to "spring into rapid rhythmical pulsation so regular and sustained as to recall the movement of clockwork."[1] Mayer demonstrated similar circus

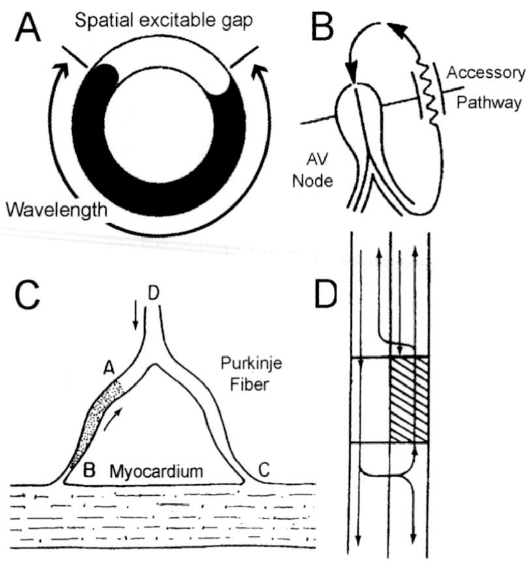

FIGURE 5–10. Ring models of reentry. (A) Schematic of a ring model of reentry. (B) Mechanism of reentry in the Wolf–Parkinson–White syndrome involving the AV node and an atrioventricular accessory pathway (AP). (C) A mechanism for reentry in a Purkinje muscle loop proposed by Schmitt and Erlanger.[251] The diagram shows a Purkinje bundle (D) that divides into two branches, both connected distally to ventricular muscle. Circus movement was considered possible if the stippled segment, A → B, showed unidirectional block. An impulse advancing from D would be blocked at A, but would reach and stimulate the ventricular muscle at C by way of the other terminal branch. The wavefront would then reenter the Purkinje system at B traversing the depressed region slowly so as to arrive at A following expiration of refractoriness. (D) Schematic representation of circus movement reentry in a linear bundle of tissue as proposed by Schmitt and Erlanger.[251] The upper pathway contains a depressed zone (shaded) that serves as a site of unidirectional block and slow conduction. Anterograde conduction of the impulse is blocked in the upper pathway but succeeds along the lower pathway. Once beyond the zone of depression, the impulse crosses over through lateral connections and reenters through the upper pathway. [(C and D) From Schmitt and Erlanger.[251]]

movement excitation in rings cut from the ventricles of turtle hearts, but he did not consider this to be a plausible mechanism for the development of cardiac arrhythmias. His experiments proved valuable in identifying two fundamental conditions necessary for the initiation and maintenance of circus movement excitation: (1) unidirectional block—the impulse initiating the circulating wave must travel in one direction only, and (2) in order for the circus movement to continue, the circuit must be long enough to allow each site in the circuit to recover before the return of the circulating wave.

Mines,[249] in 1914, was the first to develop the concept of circus movement reentry as a mechanism responsible for cardiac arrhythmias.[3] He confirmed Mayer's observations and suggested that the recirculating wave could be responsible for clinical cases of tachycardia.[249] This concept was reinforced with the discovery by Kent of an extra accessory pathway connecting the atrium and ventricle of a human heart.[250] The criteria developed by Mines for identification of circus movement reentry remains in use today: (1) an area of unidirectional block must exist; (2) the excitatory wave progresses along a distinct pathway, returning to its point of origin and then following the same path again; and (3) interruption of the reentrant circuit at any point along its path should terminate the circus movement.

In 1928, Schmitt and Erlanger[251] suggested that coupled ventricular extrasystoles in mammalian hearts could arise as a consequence of circus movement reentry within loops composed of terminal Purkinje fibers and ventricular muscle. Using a theoretical model consisting of a Purkinje bundle that divides into two branches that insert distally into ventricular muscle (Figure 5–10), they suggested that a region of depression within one of the terminal Purkinje branches could provide for unidirectional block and conduction slow enough to permit successful reexcitation within a loop of limited size (i.e., 10–30 mm).

It was recognized that successful reentry could occur only when the impulse was sufficiently delayed in an alternate pathway to allow for expiration of the refractory period in the tissue proximal to the site of unidirectional block. Both conduction velocity and refractoriness determine the success or failure of reentry and the general rule is that the length of the circuit (*pathlength*) must exceed or equal that of the *wavelength*. The theoretical minimum path length required for development of reentry was initially thought to be quite long. In the early 1970s, microreentry within narrowly circumscribed loops was suggested to be within the realm of possibility. Cranefield, Hoffman, and co-workers[252,253] demonstrated that segments of canine Purkinje fibers that normally display impulse conduction velocities of 2–4 m/sec can conduct impulses with apparent velocities of 0.01–0.1 m/sec when encased in high K^+ agar. This finding and the demonstration by Sasyniuk and Mendez in 1971[254] of a marked abbreviation of action potential duration and refractoriness in terminal Purkinje fibers just proximal to the site of block greatly reduced the theoretical limit of the pathlength required for the development of reentry. Soon after, single and repetitive reentry was reported by Wit and co-workers[255] in small loops of canine and bovine conducting tissues bathed in a high K^+ solution containing catecholamines, thus demonstrating reentry over a relatively small path. In some experiments, they used linear unbranched bundles of Purkinje tissue to demonstrate a phenomenon similar to that observed by Schmitt and Erlanger in which slow anterograde conduction of the impulse was at times followed by a retrograde wavefront that produced a "return extrasystole."[256] They proposed that the nonstimulated impulse was caused by a circus movement reentry made possible by longitudinal dissociation of the bundle, as in the Schmitt and Erlanger model (see Figure 5–10). Noting that in many of their experiments "the rapid upstroke within the depressed segment arises after the rapid upstroke of the normal fiber," Wit and co-workers also considered the possibility[256,257] that "the reflected impulse that travels slowly backward through the depressed segment is evoked by retrograde depolarization of the cells within the depressed segment by the rapid upstrokes of the cells beyond."[257] Thus arose the suggestion that reexcitation could occur in a single fiber through a mechanism other than circus movement, namely reflection. While both explanations appeared plausible, proof for either was lacking at the time. Direct evidence in support of reflection as a mechanism of reentrant activity did not emerge until the early 1980s, as discussed later.

These early pioneering studies led to our understanding of how anatomical obstacles such as the openings of the venae cava in the right atrium, an aneurysm in the ventricles, or the presence of bypass tracts between atria and ventricles (Kent bundle) can form a ring-like path for the development of extrasystoles, tachycardia, and flutter.

Leading Circle Model

In 1924, Garrey suggested that reentry could be initiated without the involvement of anatomical obstacles and that "natural rings are not essential for the maintenance of circus contractions."[258] Nearly 50 years later, Allessie and co-workers[259–261] were the first to provide direct evidence in support of this hypothesis in experiments in which they induced a tachycardia in isolated preparations of rabbit left atria by applying properly timed premature extrastimuli. Using multiple intracellular electrodes, they showed that although the basic beats elicited by stimuli applied near the center of the tissue spread normally throughout the preparation, premature impulses propagate only in the direction of shorter refractory periods. An arc of block thus develops around which the impulse is able to circulate and reexcite the tissue. Recordings near the center of the circus movement showed only subthreshold responses. Thus arose the concept of the leading circle,[261] a form of circus movement reentry occurring in structurally uniform myocardium, requiring no anatomic obstacle (Figure 5–11). The functionally refractory region that develops at the vortex of the circulating wavefront prevents the centripetal waves from short circuiting the circus movement and thus serves to maintain the reentry. Since the head of the circulating wavefront usually travels on relatively refractory tissue, a fully excitable gap of tissue may not be present; unlike other forms of reentry the leading circle model may not be readily influenced by extraneous impulses initiated in areas outside the reentrant circuit and thus may not be easily entrained. Subsequent studies showed that the leading circle mechanism could mediate tachycardia induced in isolated ventricular tissues.[262] Allessie and co-workers[263] also described the development of circus movement reentry without the involvement of an anatomic obstacle in a two-dimensional model of ventricular epicardium created by freezing the endocardial layers of a Langendorf perfused rabbit heart.

Lines or functional arcs of block attending the development of a circus movement reentry were shown to develop in *in vivo* models of canine infarction in which a thin surviving epicardial rim overlies the infarcted ventricle.[8,264–269] The lines of block observed during tachycardia are usually oriented parallel to the direction of the myocardial fibers, suggesting that anisotropic conduction properties (faster conduction in the direction

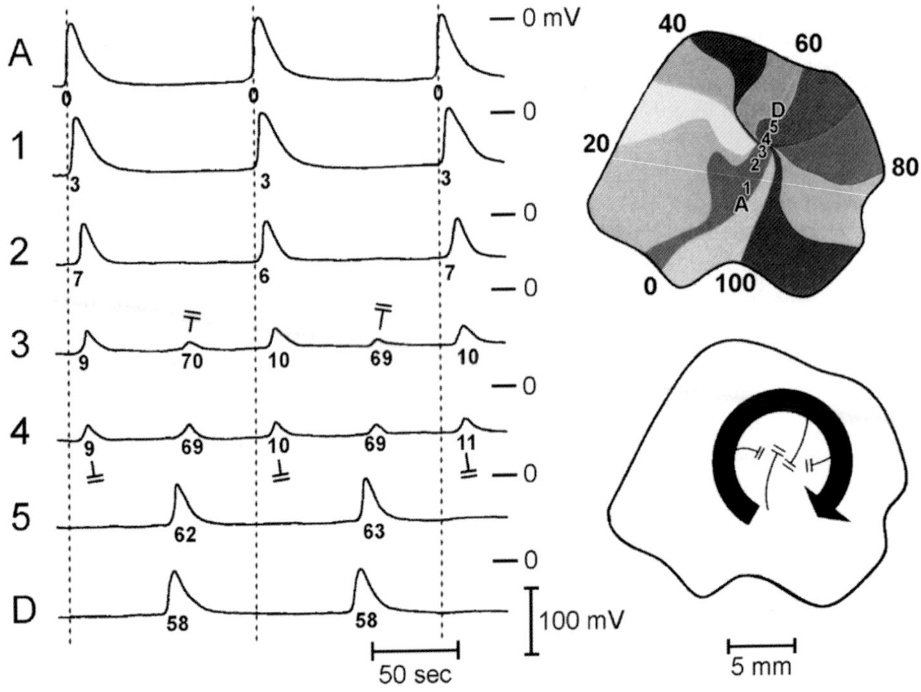

FIGURE 5–11. Leading circle model of reentry. Activation maps during steady-state tachycardia induced by a premature stimulus in an isolated rabbit atrium (upper right). On the left are transmembrane potentials recorded from seven fibers located on a straight line through the center of the circus movement. Note that the central area is activated by centripetal wavelets and that the fibers in the central area show double responses of subnormal amplitude. Both responses are unable to propagate beyond the center, thus preventing the impulse from short-cutting the circuit. Lower right: the activation pattern is schematically represented, showing the leading circuit and the converging centripetal wavelets. Block is indicated by double bars. (From Allessie *et al.*,[261] with permission.)

parallel to the long axis of the myocardial cells)[270–272] also play an important role in defining the functionally refractory zone. Dillon and co-workers[269] subsequently showed that the long lines of functional block that sustain reentry in the epicardial rim overlying canine infarction may represent zones of very slow conduction, implying that the dimensions of the area of functional block may in fact be relatively small and may even approach that of the vortex of functional block described by Allessie and co-workers.[263]

Figure-of-Eight Model

A figure-of-eight model of reentry was first described by El-Sherif and co-workers in the surviving epicardial layer overlying infarction produced by occlusion of the left anterior descending artery in canine hearts in the late 1980s.[13,264–266,273] In the figure-of-eight model, the reentrant beat produces a wavefront that circulates in both directions around a long line of functional conduction block (Figure 5–12) rejoining on the distal side of the block. The wavefront then breaks through the arc of block to reexcite the tissue proximal to the block. The single arc of block is thus divided into two and the reentrant activation continues as two circulating wavefronts that travel in clockwise and counterclockwise directions around the two arcs in a pretzel-like configuration. The diameter of the reentrant circuit in the ventricle may be as small as a few millimeters or as large as several centimeters. In 1999, Lin and co-workers[274] described a novel quatrefoil-shaped reentry induced by delivering long stimuli during the vulnerable phase in rabbit ventricular myocardium. This pattern, a variant of figure-of-eight reentry, consists of two pairs of opposing rotors with all four circuits converging in the center.

Spiral Waves and Rotors

In 1946, Rosenblueth and Weiner[275] first introduced the concept of spiral waves, which has attracted a great deal of interest over the past decade. Originally used to describe reentry around an anatomical obstacle,[275] the term spiral wave reentry was later adopted to describe circulating waves in the absence of an anatomical obstacle,[276,277] similar to the circulating waves of the leading circle mechanism described by Allessie and colleagues.[259,261] Apart from cardiac tissues, spiral wave phenomena have been described in a number of systems, including chemical autocatalytic reactions (i.e., Belousov–Zhabotinsky chemical reaction)[278] as well as intracellular milieu (calcium waves may spread in the form of spiral waves in the cytosol).[279] The spiral wave theory has advanced our understanding of the mechanisms responsible for the functional form of reentry. Although leading circle and spiral wave reentry are considered by some to be similar, a number of distinctions have been suggested.[261,280–282] The curvature of the spiral wave is the key to the formation of the core.[282] The curvature of the wave forms a region of high impedance mismatch (sink-source mismatch), where the current provided by the reentering wavefront (source) is insufficient to charge the capacity and thus excite a larger volume of tissue ahead (sink). A prominent curvature of the spiral wave is generally encountered following a wave break, a situation in which a planar wave encounters an obstacle and breaks up into two or more daughter waves. Because it has the greatest curvature, the broken end of the wave moves most slowly. As curvature decreases along the more distal parts of the spiral, propagation speed increases. Another difference between the leading circle and spiral wave is the state of the core; in the former it is kept permanently refractory, whereas in the latter the core is excitable but not excited.

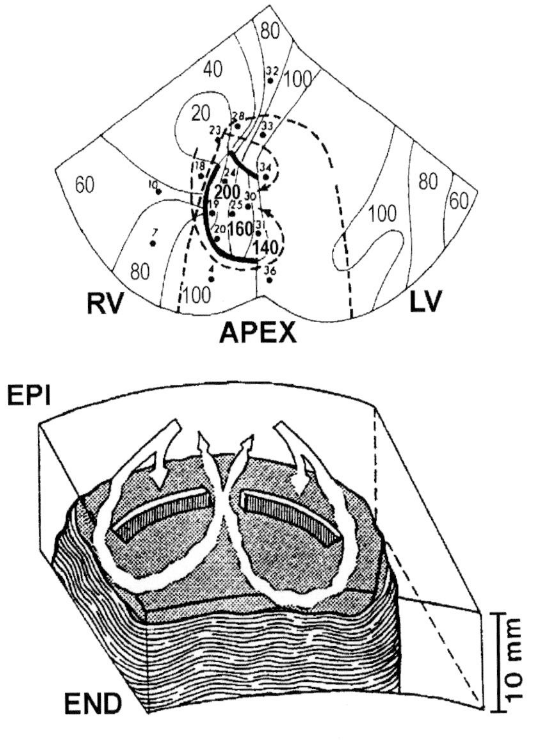

FIGURE 5–12. Figure-of-eight model of reentry. Isochronal activation map during monomorphic reentrant ventricular tachycardia occurring in the surviving epicardial layer overlying an infarction. Recordings were obtained from the epicardial surface of a canine heart 4 days after ligation of the left anterior descending coronary artery. Activation isochrones are drawn at 20 msec intervals. The reentrant circuit has a characteristic figure of eight activation pattern. Two circulating wavefronts advance in clockwise and counterclockwise directions, respectively, around two zones (arcs) of conduction block (represented by heavy solid lines). The epicardial surface is depicted as if the ventricles were unfolded following a cut from the crux to the apex. A three-dimensional diagrammatic illustration of the ventricular activation pattern during the reentrant tachycardia is shown in the lower panel. RV, right ventricle; LV, left ventricle; EPI, epicardium; END, endocardium. (From El-Sherif,[13] with permission.)

The term spiral wave is typically used to describe reentrant activity in two dimensions. The center of the spiral wave is called the core and the distribution of the core in three dimensions is referred to as the filament (Figure 5–13). The three-dimensional form of the spiral wave forms a scroll wave.[283] In its simplest form, the scroll wave has a straight filament spanning the ventricular wall (i.e., from epicardium to endocardium). Theoretical studies have described three major scroll wave configurations with curved filaments (L-, U-, and O-shaped),[283] although numerous variations of these three-dimensional filaments in space and time are assumed to exist during cardiac arrhythmias.[283] Anisotropy and anatomical obstacles can substantially modify the characteristics and spatiotemporal behavior of the vortex-like reentries. As anatomical obstacles are introduced approaching a ring model of reentry, the curvature of the

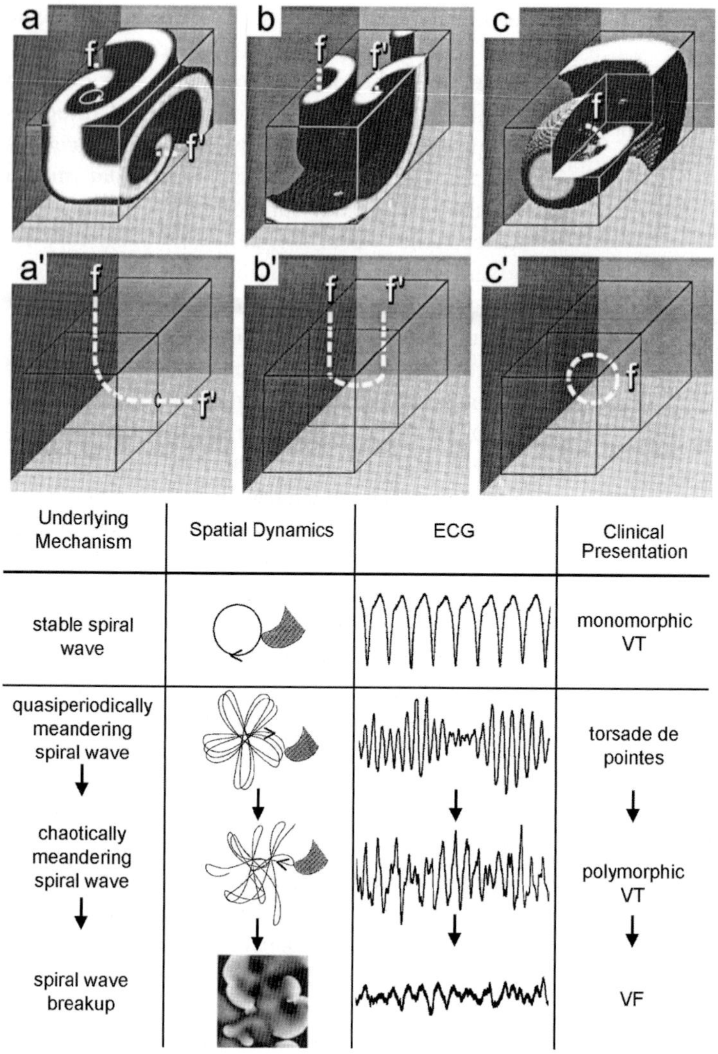

a
b
c
a'
b'
c'
Underlying Mechanism
Spatial Dynamics
ECG
Clinical Presentation
stable spiral wave
monomorphic VT
quasiperiodically meandering spiral wave
torsade de pointes
chaotically meandering spiral wave
polymorphic VT
spiral wave breakup
VF

FIGURE 5–13. Schematic representation of basic scroll-type reentry in three-dimensional and spiral wave phenotypes with their possible clinical manifestations. Upper panel: Basic configurations of vortex-like reentry in three dimensions. a and a′, L-shaped scroll wave and filament, respectively. The scroll rotates in a clockwise direction (on the top) about the L-shaped filament (f,f′) shown in a′. b and b′, U-shaped scroll wave and filament, respectively. c and c′, O-shaped wave and filament, respectively. (From Pertsov and Jalife,[283] with permission.) Bottom panel: Four types of spiral wave phenotypes and associated clinical manifestations. A stable spiral wave mechanism gives rise to monomorphic ventricular tachycardia (VT) on the ECG. A quasiperiodic meandering spiral wave is responsible for torsade de pointes, whereas a chaotically meandering spiral wave is revealed as polymorphic VT. A ventricular fibrillation (VF) pattern is caused by spiral wave breakup. Second column: spiral waves are shown in gray; the paths of their tip are shown as solid lines. (From Garfinkel and Qu,[285] with permission.)

wave becomes less of a determinant of the characteristics of the arrhythmia.

Spiral wave activity has been used to explain the electrocardiographic patterns observed during monomorphic and polymorphic cardiac arrhythmias as well as during fibrillation (Figure 5–13, bottom panel).[277,284,285] Monomorphic VT results when the spiral wave is anchored and not able to drift within the ventricular myocardium. In contrast, a polymorphic VT such as that encountered with long QT syndrome-induced TdP is due to a meandering or drifting spiral wave. Ventricular fibrillation seems to be the most complex representation of rotating spiral waves in the heart. It is often preceded by VT. One of the theories suggests that VF develops when a single spiral wave responsible for VT breaks up, leading to the development of multiple spirals that are continuously extinguished and recreated.

Role of Reentry in the Development of Cardiac Arrhythmias

Reentrant mechanisms are thought to underlie the maintenance of most rapid cardiac arrhythmias. The role of the reentrant models in the generation of these arrhythmias is discussed in this section. Some specific arrhythmogenic conditions where reentry plays a pivotal role (such as long QT, short QT, and Brugada syndrome as well as arrhythmias occurring during ischemia/infarct) are discussed in detail in the following sections. Some specific manifestations of the reentrant mechanism, such as reflection and phase 2 reentry, will be discussed separately as well.

Among the most representative clinical reentrant ring model equivalents are various forms of atrial flutter, involving superior or inferior venae cavae, tricuspid annulus, etc., as anatomical barriers to circulate around. Bundle branch reentry and reentrant tachyarrhythmias in Wolff–Parkinson–White (WPW) preexcitation syndrome are also caused by the anatomically determined pathway. Many forms of ventricular tachycardia occurring under conditions of structural heart diseases are often maintained by anatomically predetermined reentrant pathways.[286,287] Ventricular Purkinje fiber networks are thought to provide anatomical reentrant circuits as well.[288] The figure-of-eight reentrant model may underlie ventricular arrhythmias originating from a thin surviving epicardial layer overlying infarction.

While the leading circle and spiral wave models have some conceptual differences (discussed above), it is difficult to determine which of these is more likely to underlie given functional reentrant arrhythmias in the heart. Comptois and colleagues[289] recently analyzed these two concepts of functional reentry and arrived at the conclusion that the spiral wave concept better explains functional reentrant cardiac arrhythmia and its pharmacological responses than the leading circuit concept, both in clinical and experimental settings.[289] The functional reentrant mechanisms can underlie many forms of tachyarrhythmias in ischemic or infarcted hearts[290] and in structurally normal ventricles, as in the long QT and Brugada syndromes.

A role for spiral waves in AF and VF is likely to be most common. Both AF and VF are considered to have similar spatiotemporal mechanisms. There are two major theories to explain AF/VF generation. The first, originally suggested by Gordon Moe and colleagues, proposes that cardiac fibrillation is maintained by the continuing development of multiple unstable reentrant wavelets.[291] This "multiple wavelet hypothesis" has been the dominating concept of AF and VF for more than three decades. In recent years there has been a revival of another theory for the maintenance of VF/AF known as the "single source hypothesis."[292,293] This theory proposes that AF/VF can be maintained by a single high-frequency source, giving rise to impulse propagation with variable conduction block in the remainder of the ventricle (i.e., fibrillatory conduction), which accounts for the AF/VF pattern in the ECG.[292,294–297] It was first proved to occur in cardiac muscle in 1948.[292] A number of recent studies provide further proof of this concept.[294–297] A reentrant mechanism is believed to underlie a single source maintaining AV/VF in most cases (the so-called "mother rotor").[293] However, a rapidly activating focal source (automatic or triggered activity) can cause some forms of AF/VF as well.[96,298,299]

Whether AF/VF is caused by single or multiple reentrant sources, wavebreak (i.e., conduction block) is an indispensable requirement for reentry to develop. Wavebreak occurs when a propagated activating waveform encounters an anatomical or functional (i.e., refractory state) obstacle. Anatomical heterogeneity is well known to promote wavebreak, reentry, and AF/VF in healthy and particularly in structurally abnormal ventricles and atria.[300–303] Indeed, it has been shown that even in structurally normal ventricles, phase singularities (i.e., wavebreak) during VF occur in a nonrandom spatial distribution, often colocalizing with normal anatomical heterogeneities.[301,304] It is well known that most cases of clinical VF take place in structurally damaged ventricles. Many cases of clinical VF, however, occur in ostensibly normal hearts. Experimental studies have shown that VF can develop spontaneously or may be readily induced in ischemic or infarcted ventricles.[290] In contrast, in healthy ventricles, VF rarely appears spontaneously and can be induced only with very aggressive electrical stimulation protocols, such as burst pacing and direct current of high intensity and long duration. Normal structural heterogeneities present in atria (such as pectinate muscles or the junctions between pulmonary vein muscular sleeve and left atrial body) promote wavebreak and reentry.[305,306] Structural heterogeneities may be greatly augmented in electrically remodeled atria susceptible to AF, secondary to atrial enlargement, an increase in interstitial fibrosis, etc.

Anatomical obstacles and spiral waves interact in a number of interesting ways.[300,303] It is noteworthy that the initial description of the spiral wave involved an anatomical obstacle.[275] Mathematical simulation and experimental studies have shown that an anatomical barrier may serve as a point/line of a wavebreak leading to the initiation of a spiral wave, which subsequently can detach from the barrier and revolve independently of the barrier.[300] Another scenario is one in which the anatomical obstacle may serve as an anchor to stabilize a spiral wave.[303]

Two fundamental hypotheses have been advanced to explain wavebreak occurring in the absence of anatomical obstacles. The first involves spatial refractory period heterogeneity. Gordon Moe's multiple-wavelet concept is fundamentally based on spatial inhomogeneity of refractory periods, providing the substrate for conduction block and wavefront fragmentation (wavebreaks), leading to the continuous appearance and disappearance of multiple wandering reentrant wavelets. The other concept of the spiral breakup, referred to as the "Restitution Hypothesis," was formulated less than a decade ago. It invokes temporal dynamic electrical heterogeneity (which is essentially determined by electrical restitution properties of the myocardium) to explain spiral wave instability and breakup during AF/VF. The original restitution hypothesis stipulates that the wavebreak occurs when the slope of the APD restitution curve (determined as the change in APD as a function of the preceding diastolic interval) exceeds a value of one. In its later versions, the restitution hypothesis includes the restitution of conduction velocity as well as other dynamic factors such as intracellular calcium cycling.[303,307] It has been shown that a steep relationship between conduction time and interstimulus interval might account for wavebreak and VF, particularly under conditions of depressed excitability.[308] Desynchronization of voltage and intracellular calcium cycling, occurring during VF, can affect wavebreak.[303,309] In addition to APD/conduction velocity restitution, a number of other factors have been shown to contribute to wave breakup during VF/AF, including cardiac memory, anatomical obstacles, and anisotropy.[302,303]

The role of spatial versus temporal electrical heterogeneity in wavebreak and the development of VF/AF is a topic of active debate.[302,303] The applicability of the restitution hypothesis is less obvious in the case of AF than in the case of VF. Indeed, most atria susceptible to AF, both in patients and experimental animal models, are associated with an abbreviation of refractoriness, loss of APD rate adaptation, and flattening of the APD restitution curve.[310–312] Many variations on these themes are possible. For example, it has been suggested that a single meandering spiral wave could underlie VF,[313–315] as in the case of the Brugada syndrome.[315] All these concepts of VF/AF maintenance are not mutually exclusive. There are experimental and theoretical data supporting both the multiple wavelet and single source hypotheses.[294,296,297,316–321] It is possible that different mechanisms and manifestations of AF/VF may be operative depending on the prevailing conditions (species, size of the heart, ischemia, time after the start of AF/VF, etc.).[295,299,303,312,322] There are experimental data indicating that early stages of VF/AF are maintained by multiple wavelets and late stages of the arrhythmias by a single stable reentrant source.[295,322] It is thought that the functional spatial and temporal heterogeneities as well as anatomical structures interact synergistically to form a wavebreak, thus contributing to the maintenance of AF/VF.[302,303] An increase in structural heterogeneity greatly promotes the probability of wavebreak and reentry, reducing "the amount" of functional spatial and temporal heterogeneities required for VF appearance (Figure 5–14).[303]

Recent studies have advanced our understanding of the ionic basis for the spatiotemporal behavior of reentrant rotor during VF, although our knowledge remains incomplete. It was recently shown by Samie *et al.*[297] that the anterior left ventricular region of the guinea pig heart displays earlier repolarization than the right ventricle (RV) free wall during VF and that this region is the usual location of a stable rotor underlying VF in isolated guinea pig heart. Based on measurement of a higher density of background outward current, I_{K1}, in left ventricle (LV) versus RV isolated myocytes, Samie *et al.*[297] proposed that the mechanism underlying the primary rotor and wavefront fragmentation may be related to gradients of refractoriness imposed by gradients in I_{K1}. Another recent study suggests a dominant role for I_{Kr} in wavebreak dynamics during VF in guinea

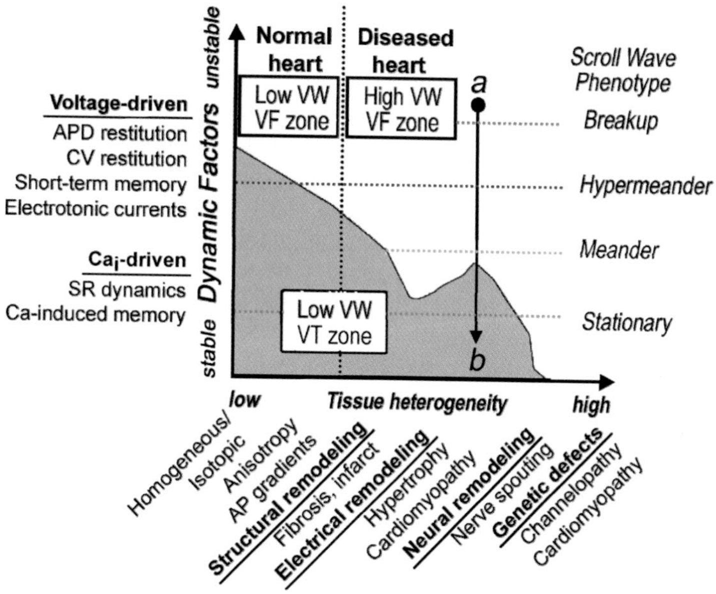

Figure 5–14. Hypothetical interaction between dynamic factors (*y* axis) and tissue heterogeneity (*x* axis) in determining the risk of ventricular fibrillation. (From Weiss *et al.*,[303] with permission.)

pig.[321] In larger animals (like pigs), the region where the posterior free wall of LV intersects with the septum is believed to be the most probable location of the mother rotor.[302] Higher levels of I_{Kr} and/or $I_{K(ACh)}$ in the left atrium, compared to the right atrium, are thought to account for a shorter repolarization and left atrial location of rotor(s) during acute AF.[323,324]

Reflection

Direct evidence in support of reflection as a mechanism of arrhythmogenesis was first provided by Antzelevitch and co-workers in the early 1980s.[107,325] The concept of reflection was first suggested by studies of the propagation characteristics of slow action potential responses in K$^+$-depolarized Purkinje fibers.[252,253,255,257] Using strands of Purkinje fiber, Wit and co-workers demonstrated a phenomenon similar to that observed by Schmitt and Erlanger in which slow anterograde conduction of the impulse was at times followed by a retrograde wavefront that produced a "return extrasystole."[256] They proposed that the nonstimulated impulse was caused by circuitous reentry at the level of the syncytial interconnections, made possible by longitudinal dissociation of the bundle, as the most likely explanation for the phenomenon, but also suggested the possibility of reflection.[107,325]

Several models of reflection have been developed.[107,110,325,326] The first of these involved use of an "ion-free" isotonic sucrose solution to create a narrow (1.5–2 mm) central inexcitable zone (gap) in unbranched Purkinje fibers mounted in a three-chamber tissue bath (Figure 5–15).[107] In this model, stimulation of the proximal (P) segment elicits an action potential that propagates to the proximal border of the sucrose gap. Active propagation across the sucrose gap is not possible

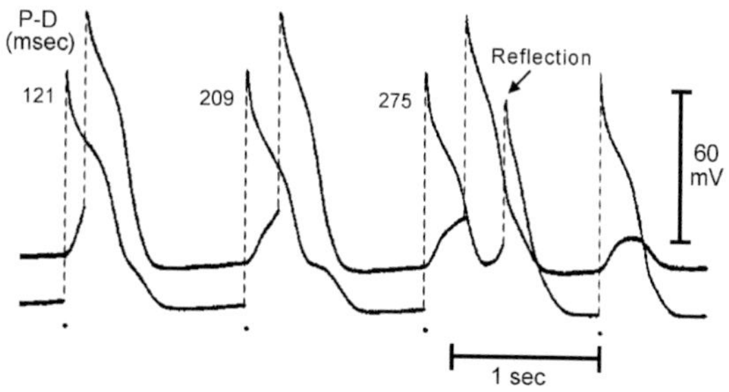

Figure 5–15. Delayed transmission and reflection across an inexcitable gap created by superfusion of the central segment of a Purkinje fiber with an "ion-free" isotonic sucrose solution. The two traces were recorded from proximal (P) and distal (D) active segments. P–D conduction time (indicated in the upper portion of the figure, in milliseconds) increased progressively with a 4:3 Wenckebach periodicity. The third stimulated proximal response was followed by a reflection. (From Antzelevitch,[109] with permission.)

because of the ion-depleted extracellular milieu, but local circuit current continues to flow through the intercellular low resistance pathways (an Ag/AgCl extracellular shunt pathway is provided). This local circuit or electrotonic current, much reduced upon emerging from the gap, slowly discharges the capacity of the distal (D) tissue, thus giving rise to a depolarization that manifests as either a subthreshold response (last distal response) or a foot potential that brings the distal excitable element to its threshold potential (Figure 5–16). Active impulse propagation stops and then resumes after a delay that can be as long as several hundred milliseconds. When anterograde (P → D) transmission time is sufficiently delayed to permit recovery of refractoriness at the proximal end, electrotonic transmission of the impulse in the retrograde direction is able to reexcite the proximal tissue, thus generating a closely coupled reflected reentry. Reflection therefore results from the back and forth electrotonically mediated transmission of the impulse across the same inexcitable segment; neither longitudinal dissociation nor circus movement needs be invoked to explain the phenomenon.

A second model of reflection involves the creation of an inexcitable region permitting delayed conduction by superfusion of a central segment of a Purkinje bundle with a solution designed to mimic the extracellular milieu at a site of ischemia.[325] When the K^+ concentration was increased to between 15 and 20 mM, the "ischemic" solution induced major delays in conduction, as long as 500 msec across the 1.5-mm-wide "ischemic" central gap. The gap was shown to be largely comprised of an inexcitable cable across which conduction of impulses was electrotonically mediated. The long delays of impulse conduction across the "ischemic" gap permit the development of reflection. When propagation across the gap was mediated by "slow responses," transmission was relatively prompt and reflection did not occur.[325]

Reflection has been demonstrated in isolated atrial and ventricular myocardial tissues as

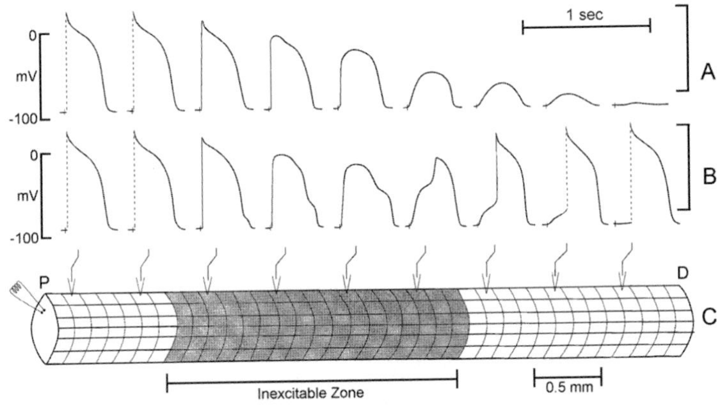

FIGURE 5–16. Conduction block (A) and discontinuous conduction (B) in a Purkinje strand with a central inexcitable zone (C). The schematic illustration is based on transmembrane recordings obtained from canine Purkinje fiber-sucrose gap preparations. An action potential elicited by stimulation of the proximal (P) side of the preparation conducts normally up to the border of the inexcitable zone. Active propagation of the impulse stops at this point, but local circuit current generated by the proximal segment continues to flow through the preparation encountering a cumulative resistance (successive gap junctions). Transmembrane recordings from the first few inexcitable cells show a response not very different from the action potentials recorded in the neighboring excitable cells, in spite of the fact that no ions may be moving across the membrane of these cells. The responses recorded in the inexcitable region are the electrotonic images of activity generated in the proximal excitable segment. The resistive-capacitive properties of the tissue lead to an exponential decline in the amplitude of the transmembrane potential recorded along the length of the inexcitable segment and to a slowing of the rate of change of voltage as a function of time. If, as in (B), the electrotonic current is sufficient to bring the distal excitable tissue to its threshold potential, an action potential is generated after a step delay imposed by the slow discharge of the capacity of the distal (D) membrane by the electrotonic current (foot-potential). Active conduction of the impulse therefore stops at the proximal border of the inexcitable zone and resumes at the distal border after a step delay that may range from a few to tens or hundreds of milliseconds. (Modified from Antzelevitch,[506] with permission.)

well.[326–328] Reflected reentry has also been demonstrated in Purkinje fibers in which a functionally inexcitable zone is created by focal depolarization of the preparation with long duration constant current pulses.[329] This phenomenon is also observed in isolated canine Purkinje fibers homogeneously depressed with high K^+ solution as well as in branched preparations of "normal" Purkinje fibers.[330]

Whether reflection will succeed depends critically on the degree to which conduction is delayed in both directions across the functionally inexcitable zone. These transit delays in turn depend on the width of the blocked segment, the intracellular and extracellular resistance to the flow of local circuit current across the inexcitable zone, and the excitability of the distal active site (sink). Because the excitability of cardiac tissues continues to recover for hundreds of milliseconds after an action potential, impulse transmission across the inexcitable zone is a sensitive function of frequency.[107,331–333] Consequently, the incidence and patterns of manifest ectopic activity encountered in models of reflection are highly rate dependent.[109,110,328,332,334] Similar rate-dependent changes in extrasystolic activity have been reported in patients with frequent extrasystoles evaluated with Holter recordings[335] and in patients evaluated by atrial pacing.[109,336] Because reflection can occur within areas of tissue of limited size (as small as 1–2 mm^2), it is likely to appear as focal in origin. Its identification as a mechanism of arrhythmia may be difficult even with very high spatial resolution mapping of the electrical activity of discrete sites. The delineation of delayed impulse conduction mechanisms at discrete sites requires the use of intracellular microelectrode techniques in conjunction with high- resolution extracellular mapping techniques. These limitations considered, reflection has been suggested as the mechanism underlying reentrant extrasystolic activity in ventricular tissues excised from a 1-day-old infarcted canine heart[337] and in a clinical case of incessant ventricular bigeminy in a young patient with no evidence of organic heart disease.[338]

Phase 2 Reentry

Phase 2 reentry is another example of a reentrant mechanism that can appear to be of focal origin. Phase 2 reentry occurs when the dome of the epicardial action potential propagates from sites at which it is maintained to sites at which it is abolished, causing local reexcitation of the epicardium and the generation of a closely coupled extrasystole. A more rigorous discussion of phase 2 reentry and its role in the precipitation of VT/VF will follow in the next section.

The Role of Ventricular Heterogeneity

It is now well established that ventricular myocardium is composed of at least three electrophysiologically and functionally distinct cell types: epicardial, M, and endocardial cells. These three ventricular myocardial cell types differ principally with respect to phase 1 and phase 3 repolarization characteristics (Figure 5–17). Ventricular epicardial and M, but not endocardial, cells generally display a conspicuous phase 1, due to a prominent 4-aminopyridine (4-AP)-sensitive transient outward current (I_{to}), giving the action potential a spike and dome or notched configuration. These regional differences in I_{to}, first suggested on the basis of action potential data,[339] have now been directly demonstrated in canine,[340] feline,[341] rabbit,[342] rat,[343] and human [344,345] ventricular myocytes.

Differences in the magnitude of the action potential notch and corresponding differences in I_{to} have also been described between right and left ventricular epicardial and M cells.[346,347] This distinction is thought to form the basis for why the Brugada syndrome, a channelopathy-mediated form of sudden death, is a right ventricular disease.

Epicardial cells isolated from the left ventricular wall of the rabbit show a higher density of cAMP-activated chloride current when compared to endocardial myocytes.[348] I_{to2}, initially ascribed to a K^+ current, is now thought to be primarily due to the calcium-activated chloride current ($I_{Cl(Ca)}$); it is also thought to contribute to the action potential notch, but it is not known whether this current differs among the three ventricular myocardial cell types.[349]

Studies conducted in canine ventricular myocytes have failed to detect any difference in I_{Ca} among cells isolated from epicardium, M, and endocardial regions of the left ventricular wall.[350,351]

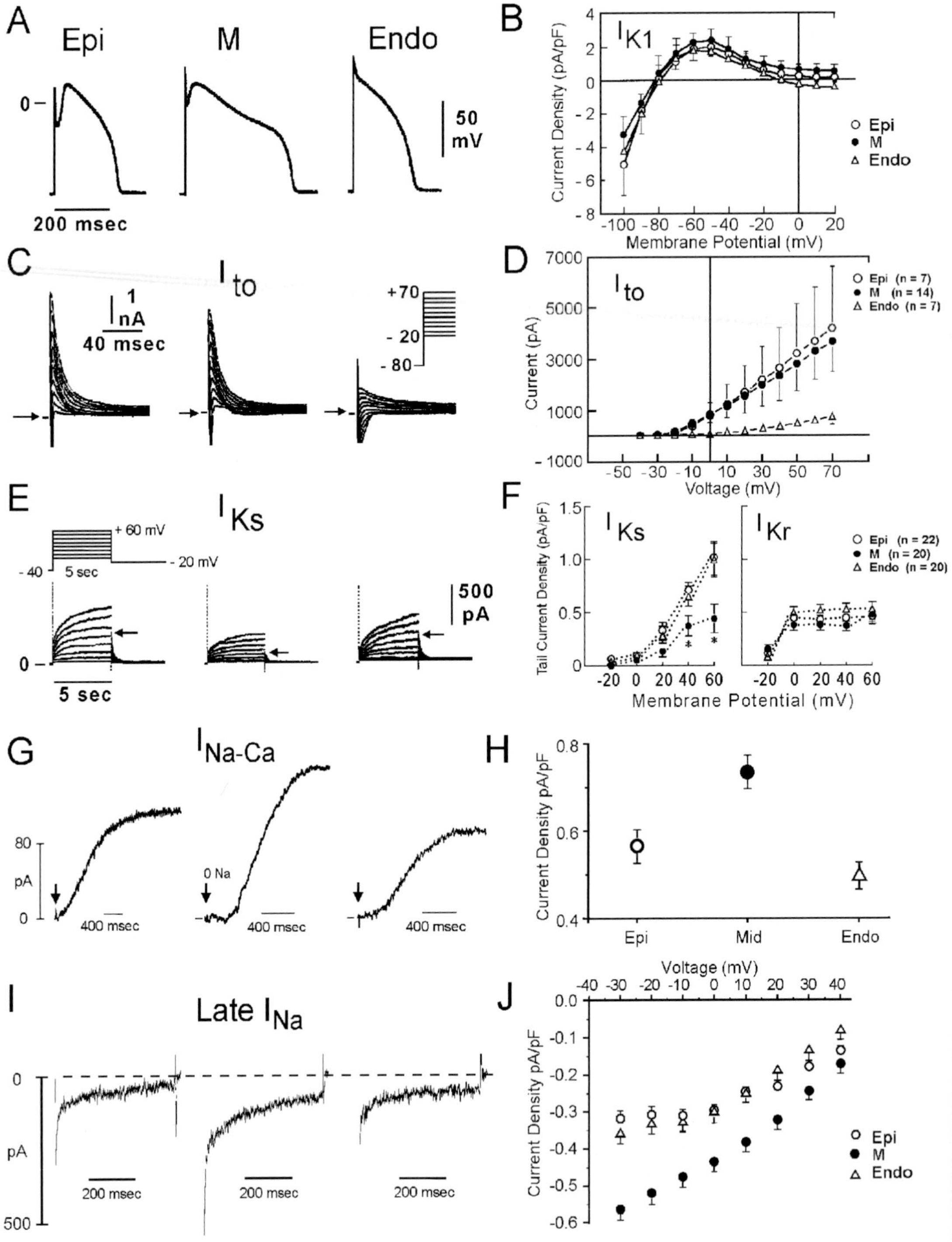
A
Epi
M
Endo
0
50 mV
200 msec
B
I_{K1}
Current Density (pA/pF)
Membrane Potential (mV)
Epi
M
Endo
C
I_{to}
1 nA
40 msec
+70
-20
-80
D
I_{to}
Current (pA)
Voltage (mV)
Epi (n = 7)
M (n = 14)
Endo (n = 7)
E
I_{Ks}
+60 mV
-40
5 sec
-20 mV
500 pA
0
5 sec
F
I_{Ks}
I_{Kr}
Tail Current Density (pA/pF)
Membrane Potential (mV)
Epi (n = 22)
M (n = 20)
Endo (n = 20)
G
$I_{Na\text{-}Ca}$
80
pA
0
0 Na
400 msec
400 msec
400 msec
H
Current Density pA/pF
Epi
Mid
Endo
I
Late I_{Na}
0
pA
500
200 msec
200 msec
200 msec
J
Voltage (mV)
Current Density pA/pF
Epi
M
Endo

One study, however, reported two differences in Ca^{2+} channel properties between epicardial and endocardial canine ventricular cells. I_{Ca} was found to be larger in endocardial than in epicardial myocytes (3.4 ± 0.2 vs. 2.3 ± 0.1 pA/pF). A low-threshold, rapidly activating and inactivating Ca^{2+} current that resembled the T-type current was recorded in all endocardial myocytes, but was small or absent in epicardial myocytes. The T-like current was composed of two components: an Ni^{2+}-sensitive T-type current and a tetrodotoxin-sensitive Ca^{2+} current.[352]

Separating the surface epicardial and endocardial layers are transitional and M cells. M cells are distinguished by the ability of their action potential to prolong disproportionately relative to the action potential of other ventricular myocardial cells in response to a slowing of rate and/or in response to APD-prolonging agents (Figure 5–18).[200,353,354] In the dog, the ionic basis for these features of the M cell includes the presence of a smaller slowly activating delayed rectifier current (I_{Ks}),[143] a larger late sodium current (late I_{Na}),[161] and a larger Na–Ca exchange current ($I_{Na\text{-}Ca}$).[355] In the canine heart, the rapidly activating delayed rectifier (I_{Kr}) and inward rectifier (I_{K1}) currents are similar in the three transmural cell types. Transmural and apicobasal differences in the density of I_{Kr} channels have been described in the ferret heart.[356] I_{Kr} message and channel protein are much larger in the ferret epicardium. I_{Ks} is larger in M cells isolated from the right versus left ventricles of the dog.[347]

Histologically, M cells are similar to epicardial and endocardial cells. Electrophysiologically and pharmacologically, they appear to be a hybrid between Purkinje and ventricular cells.[357] Like Purkinje fibers, M cells show a prominent APD prolongation and develop EADs in response to I_{Kr} blockers, whereas epicardium and endocardium do not. Like Purkinje fibers, M cells develop DADs in response to agents that calcium load or overload the cardiac cell; epicardium and endocardium do not. Unlike Purkinje fibers, M cells display an APD prolongation in response to I_{Ks} blockers; epicardium and endocardium also show an increase in APD in response to I_{Ks} blockers. Purkinje and M cells also respond differently to α-adrenergic agonists. α_1-Adrenoceptor stimulation produces APD prolongation in Purkinje fibers, but abbreviation in M cells, and little or no change in endocardium and epicardium.[358]

The distribution of M cells within the ventricular wall has been investigated in greatest detail in the left ventricle of the canine heart. Although transitional cells are found throughout the wall in the canine left ventricle, M cells displaying the longest action potentials (at BCLs ≥ 2000 msec) are often localized in the deep subendocardium to midmyocardium in the anterior wall,[359] deep subepicardium to midmyocardium in the lateral wall,[353] and throughout the wall in the region of the RV outflow tracts.[360] M cells are also present in the deep cell layers of endocardial structures, including papillary muscles, trabeculae, and the interventricular septum.[361] Unlike Purkinje fibers,

FIGURE 5–17. (A) Ionic distinctions among epicardial (Epi), M, and endocardial (Endo) cells. Action potentials recorded from myocytes isolated from the epicardial, endocardial, and M regions of the canine left ventricle. (B) I–V relations for I_{K1} in epicardial, endocardial, and M region myocytes. Values are mean ± SD. (C) Transient outward current (I_{to}) recorded from the three cell types (current traces recorded during depolarizing steps from a holding potential of −80 mV to test potentials ranging between −20 and +70 mV). (D) The average peak current–voltage relationship for I_{to} for each of the three cell types. Values are mean ± SD. (E) Voltage-dependent activation of the slowly activating component of the delayed rectifier K^+ current (I_{Ks}) (currents were elicited by the voltage pulse protocol shown in the inset; Na^+-, K^+-, and Ca^{2+}-free solution). (F) Voltage dependence of I_{Ks} (current remaining after exposure to E-4031) and I_{Kr} (E-4031-sensitive current). Values are mean ± SE. $*p < 0.05$ compared with Epi or Endo. (From Liu and Antzelevitch,[143] Liu *et al.*,[340] and Zygmunt *et al.*,[355] with permission.) (G) Reverse-mode Na–Ca exchange currents recorded in potassium- and chloride-free solutions at a voltage of −80 mV. $I_{Na\text{-}Ca}$ was maximally activated by switching to a sodium-free external solution at the time indicated by the arrow. (H) Midmyocardial Na–Ca exchanger density is 30% greater than endocardial density, calculated as the peak outward $I_{Na\text{-}Ca}$ normalized by cell capacitance. Endocardial and epicardial densities were not significantly different. (I) TTX-sensitive late sodium current. Cells were held at −80 mV and briefly pulsed to −45 mV to inactivate fast sodium current before stepping to −10 mV. (J) Normalized late sodium current measured 300 msec into the test pulse was plotted as a function of test pulse potential. (Modified from Zygmunt *et al.*,[355] with permission.)

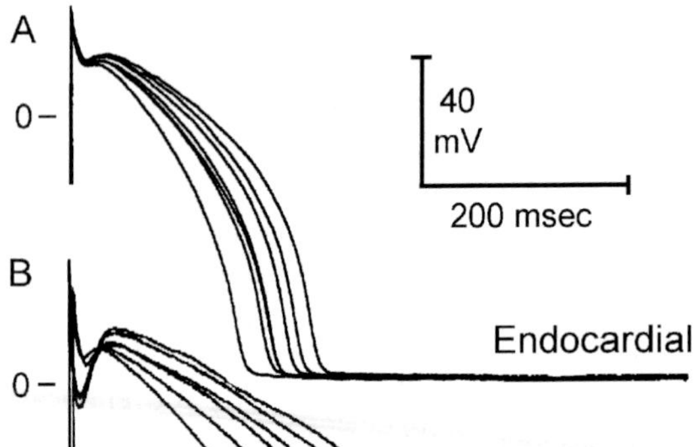

FIGURE 5–18. Transmembrane activity recorded from cells isolated from the epicardial (Epi) (D), M (C), and endocardial (Endo) (A) regions of the canine left ventricle at basic cycle lengths (BCL) of 300–5000 msec (steady-state conditions). The M and transitional (B) cells were enzymatically dissociated from the midmyocardial region. Deceleration-induced prolongation of APD in M cells is much greater than in epicardial and endocardial cells. The spike and dome morphology is also more accentuated in the epicardial cell.

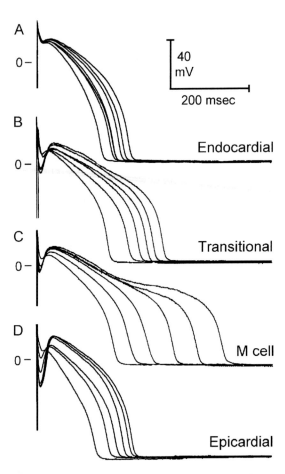

M cells are not found in discrete bundles or islets,[361,362] although there is evidence that they may be localized in discrete muscle layers. Cells with the characteristics of M cells have been described in the canine, guinea pig, rabbit, pig, and human ventricles.[134,136,143,145,201,340,353,354,359,361–376]

Amplification of transmural heterogeneities normally present in the early and late phases of the action potential can lead to the development of a variety of arrhythmias, including the Brugada, long QT, and short QT syndromes (Figure 5–19), as well as heart failure and ischemic and catecholaminergic arrhythmias.

Brugada Syndrome

Sudden cardiac death occurring in individuals with structurally normal hearts accounts for an estimated 3–9% of out-of-hospital cases of VF.[377] Many of these cases are thought to be due to a primary electrical disease. Prominent among these is the Brugada syndrome, a syndrome characterized by an ST segment elevation in right precordial leads (V_1 to V_3) unrelated to ischemia, electrolyte disturbances, or obvious structural heart disease, displaying a right bundle branch block (RBBB) QRS morphology. This electrocardiographic signature was reported as early 1953, but was first described as a distinct clinical entity associated with a high risk of sudden cardiac death by Pedro and Josep Brugada in 1992.[378]

The concept of phase 2 reentry, the mechanism thought to underlie the development of arrhythmogenesis associated with the Brugada syndrome, was first reported in 1991.[379,380] The clinical definition and mechanistic understanding of the disease developed along parallel tracks in the years that followed. A review of the clinical aspects of the Brugada syndrome and discussion of basic mechanisms and approaches to therapy can be found in Part II of this book. Additional reviews are available.[188,381–385]

The Brugada syndrome is more commonly diagnosed in males (8:1 ratio of males:females) of Southeast Asian origin. The syndrome is familial, displaying an autosomal dominant mode of transmission with incomplete penetrance. Arrhythmic events are observed at an average age of approximately 40, but have been reported in infants as well as patients in their 80s (<1 to 84 years of age). The electrocardiographic signature of the Brugada syndrome is dynamic and often concealed, but can be unmasked by potent sodium channel blockers such as flecainide, ajmaline, procainamide, and psilicainide.[386] Although intravenous administration of these agents is most effective in unmasking the syndrome, oral formulations of flecainide have been reported to be effective as well. The specificity of these effects of sodium channel blockers to uncover the syndrome and the prognostic significance of this finding remain to be fully elucidated.

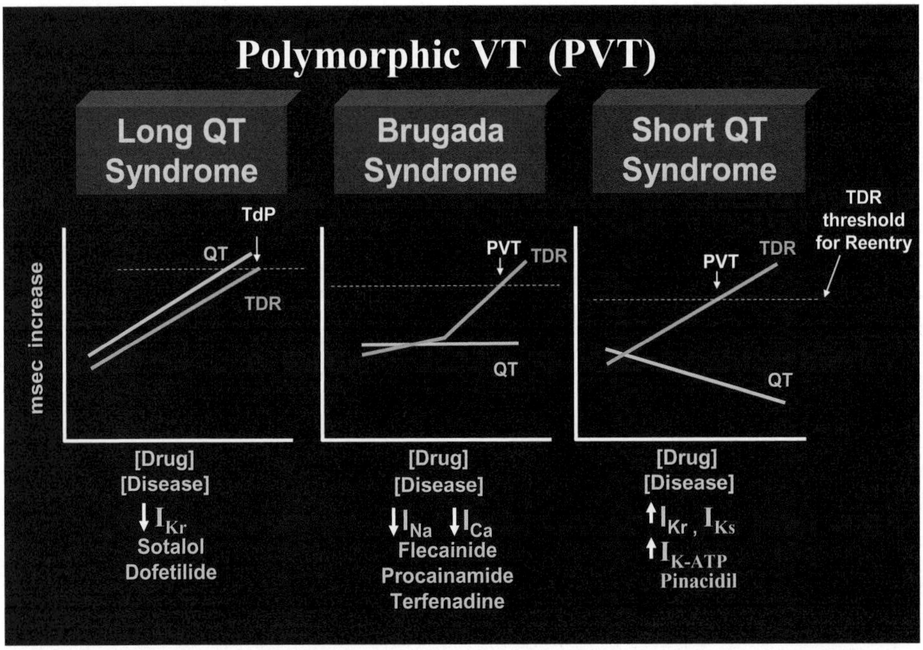

FIGURE 5–19. Relationship between transmural dispersion of repolarization (TDR) and reentrant arrhythmias in long QT, short QT, and Brugada syndromes. (Modified from Antzelevitch,[188] with permission.)

The cellular basis for the Brugada syndrome is thought to be due to an outward shift in the ionic current active during phase 1 of the right ventricular epicardial action potential.[387,388] A rebalancing of the currents contributing to the early phases of the action potential can accentuate the action potential notch or lead to all-or-none repolarization at the end of phase 1, causing loss of the epicardial action potential dome and marked abbreviation of the action potential at that site. A variety of pathophysiological conditions (e.g., ischemia, metabolic inhibition, hypothermia, pressure) and some pharmacological interventions are known to effect these changes in cells in which I_{to} is prominent. Under these pathophysiological conditions or in response to agents that reduce I_{Na} or I_{Ca} or agents that activate $I_{K\text{-}ATP}$ or augment I_{Kr}, $I_{Cl(Ca)}$, or I_{to}, canine ventricular epicardial cells exhibit an accentuation of the spike and dome morphology of the action potential, resulting in a delay in the development of the dome, secondary to widening of the action potential notch. A further shift in the balance of current leads to loss of the action potential dome and marked abbreviation of the epicardial response. The dome fails to develop because the outward currents flowing at the end of phase 1 overwhelm the inward currents that normally give rise to the secondary upstroke and action potential plateau.

Genetic mutations that affect these same currents are capable of producing the Brugada syndrome. The first gene linked to the syndrome is the α subunit of the cardiac sodium channel gene, SCN5A,[389–394] the same gene implicated in the LQT3 form of the long QT syndrome (Figure 5–20). In fact, Bezzina and co-workers[394] recently reported a mutation in SCN5A (1795InsD) capable of producing both the Brugada and LQT3 phenotypes. Three types of mutations in SCN5A have been uncovered thus far, and have been shown to result in (1) failure of the sodium channel to express, (2) reduced current due to a shift in the voltage and time dependence of I_{Na} activation, inactivation, or reactivation, and (3) reduced contribution of I_{Na} during the early phases of the action potential due to accelerated inactivation of the sodium channel.

Insertion of two nucleotides (AA) at the 5′ end, deletion of a single nucleotide (A) at codon 1397 leading to an in-frame stop codon,[390] and some missense mutations (R1432G)[392] result in disruption of protein formation and failure of channel

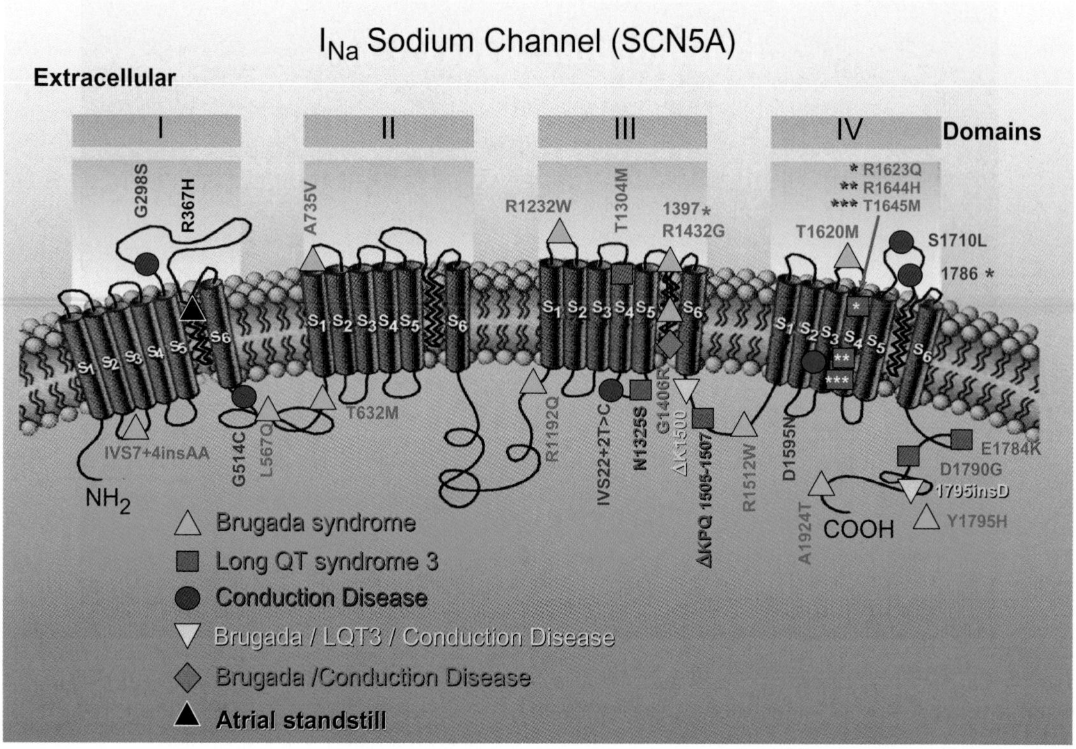

FIGURE 5–20. Schematic of SCN5A, the gene that encodes the α subunit of the sodium channel, illustrating mutations linked to Brugada syndrome, long QT3 syndrome, conduction disease, and atrial standstill. Some mutations are associated with combined phenotypes. (Modified from Antzelevitch, with permission.)

expression. Other insertion mutations (1795InsD) cause a positive shift of activation and negative shift of inactivation curves resulting in a reduction in I_{Na}.[394] In the case of the T1620M missense mutation, inactivation of I_{Na} is accelerated such that I_{to} is left unopposed during phase 1 of the action potential, resulting in a strong predominance of the outward repolarizing current at the end of phase 1, thus providing the substrate for the Brugada syndrome.[389] This change in the function of the sodium channel is observed at physiological temperatures, but not at room temperature, typically used in studies of function involving heterologous expression systems.

Because the accelerated inactivation of this mutant channel was exaggerated at temperatures above the physiological range, it was suggested that patients with the Brugada syndrome may be at more risk during a febrile state.[389] Several Brugada patients displaying fever-induced polymorphic VT have been identified since the publication of this report.[395–405] Other mutations such as L567Q, reported by Priori *et al.* to be responsible for the Brugada syndrome in children, also act by importantly accelerating inactivation of I_{Na}. In comparison with T1620M, the dysfunction of the sodium channel with this missense mutation located in the DI–DII linker of SCN5A is less temperature sensitive (R. Dumaine, S. G. Priori, and C. Antzelevitch, unpublished observations).

A second locus on chromosome 3, close to but distinct from SCN5A, has recently been linked to the syndrome[406] in a large pedigree in which the syndrome is associated with progressive conduction disease, a low sensitivity to procainamide, and a relatively good prognosis. The gene was recently identified as the glycerol-3-phosphate dehydrogenase 1-like gene (GPD1L). A mutation in GPD1L has been shown to result in a reduction of I_{Na}.[407]

In addition to SCN5A and GPD1L, gene mutations that alter the intensity or kinetics of either

I_{to}, I_{Kr}, I_{Ks}, $I_{K\text{-}ATP}$, I_{Ca}, or $I_{Cl(Ca)}$ so as to increase the activity of the outward currents and/or diminish that of the inward currents are candidates for the Brugada syndrome. Other candidate genes include those encoding for autonomic receptors that directly modulate ion current density and/or alter the expression of channels in the membrane (e.g., sympathetic control of I_{to}).

The cellular changes believed to underlie the Brugada phenotype are shown in Figure 5–21. The presence of an I_{to}-mediated spike and dome morphology or notch in ventricular epicardium, but not endocardium, of larger mammals creates a transmural voltage gradient responsible for the inscription of the electrocardiographic J wave (Osborn wave).[408] Under normal conditions, the J wave is relatively small, in large part reflecting the left ventricular action potential notch, since that of right ventricular epicardium is usually buried in the QRS. The ST segment is isoelectric because of the absence of transmural voltage gradients at the level of the action potential plateau (Figure 5–21A). Accentuation of the right ventricular notch under pathophysiological conditions is attended by exaggeration of transmural voltage gradients and thus exaggeration of the J wave or J point elevation and/or the appearance of a saddleback configuration of the repolarization waves (Figure 5–21B). The development of a prominent J wave can also be construed as an ST segment elevation. Under these conditions, the T wave remains positive because epicardial repolarization precedes repolarization of the cells in the M and endocardial regions. Further accentuation of the notch may be accompanied by a prolongation of the epicardial action potential such that the direction of repolarization across the right ventricular wall and transmural voltage gradients is reversed, thus leading to the development of a coved type of ST segment elevation and inversion of the T wave (Figure 5–21C), typically observed in the ECG of Brugada patients. A delay

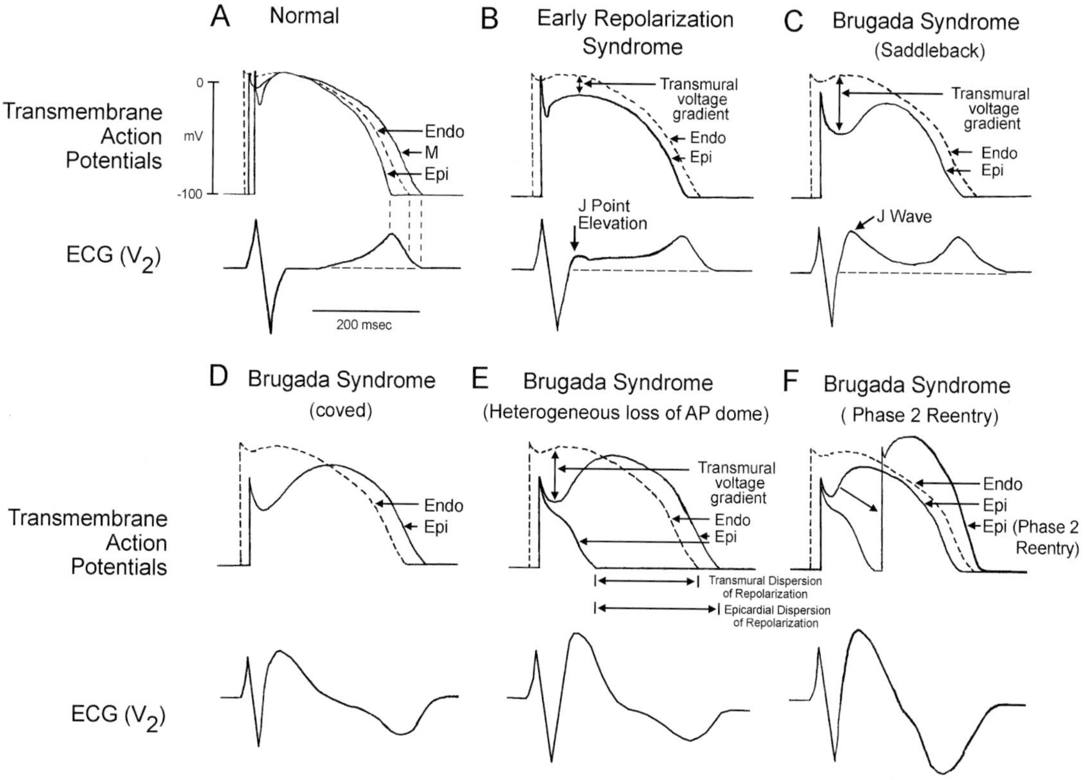

FIGURE 5–21. (A–F) Schematic representation of right ventricular epicardial action potential changes proposed to underlie the electrocardiographic manifestation of early repolarization and Brugada syndromes. (From Antzelevitch *et al.*,[118] with permission.)

in epicardial activation may also contribute to inversion of the T wave.

The downsloping ST segment elevation or accentuated J wave observed in the experimental wedge models often appears as an R′, suggesting that the RBBB morphology often encountered in the Brugada ECG may be due to early repolarization of RV epicardium and not to conduction block in the right bundle. Indeed a rigorous application of RBBB criteria reveals that a large majority of RBBB-like morphologies encountered in cases of Brugada syndrome do not fit the criteria.[409] Moreover, attempts by Miyazaki and coworkers to record delayed activation of the RV in Brugada patients met with failure.[410]

It is interesting to note that although the typical Brugada morphology is present in Figure 5–21B and C, the substrate for reentry is not. A further shift in the balance of current leads to loss of the action potential dome at some epicardial sites, which would manifest in the ECG as a further ST segment elevation (Figure 5–21D). The loss of the action potential dome in epicardium but not endocardium results in the development of a marked transmural dispersion of repolarization and refractoriness, responsible for the development of a vulnerable window during which a premature impulse or extrasystole can induce a reentrant arrhythmia. Because loss of the action potential dome in epicardium is generally not spatially uniform, we see the development of a striking epicardial dispersion of repolarization (Figure 5–21D). Support for these hypotheses derives from experiments involving the arterially perfused right ventricular wedge preparation.[388]

Propagation of the action potential dome from sites at which it is maintained to sites at which it is lost causes local reexcitation via a *phase 2 reentry* mechanism, leading to the development of a closely coupled extrasystole, capable of triggering a circus movement reentry (Figure 5–22)[17,388] The phase 2 reentrant beat fuses with the negative

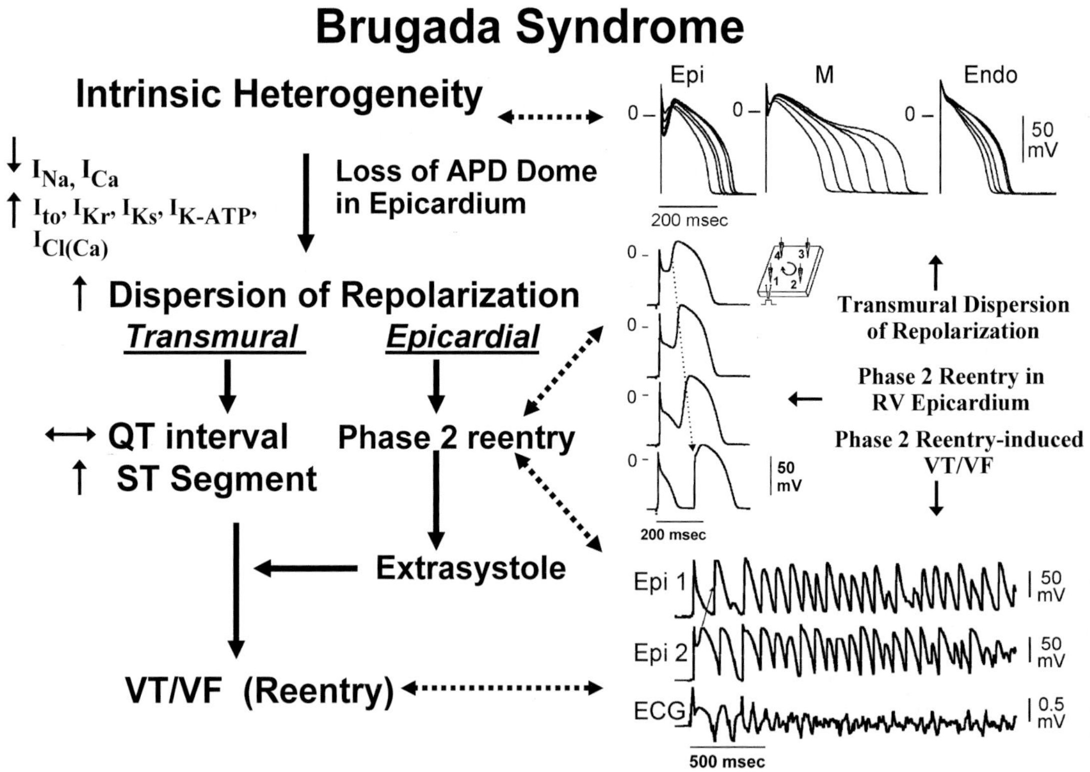

Figure 5–22. Cellular mechanisms proposed to underlie arrhythmogenesis in the Brugada syndrome. (Modified from Antzelevitch,[507] with permission.)

T wave of the basic response. Because the extrasystole originates in epicardium the QRS is largely composed of a Q wave, which serves to accentuate the negative deflection of the inverted T wave, thus giving the ECG a more symmetrical appearance. This morphology is often observed in the clinic preceding the onset of polymorphic VT. Phase 2 reentry is observed in canine epicardium exposed to (1) K^+ channel openers, (2) sodium channel blockers, (3) increased $[Ca_{2+}]_o$, (4) metabolic inhibition, (5) simulated ischemia, and (6) local pressure applied to RV epicardium.[357] Phase 2 reentry has been shown to trigger circus movement reentry in isolated sheets of right ventricular epicardium[17] as well as in the intact wall of the canine right ventricle.[315,408] The arrhythmia commonly takes the form of a polymorphic VT, resembling a rapid TdP, often indistinguishable from VF. In other cases, the experimental model displays monomorphic VT. Both are observed in patients with the Brugada syndrome, although the polymorphic form is much more common.

Pressure applied to a discrete RV site can also produce loss of the action potential, ST segment elevation, phase 2 reentry, and VT/VF in the arterially perfused RV wedge preparation.[388] This mechanism may be responsible for the Brugada-like syndrome caused by a mediastinal tumor compressing the right ventricular outflow tract.[411]

The mechanism proposed to underlie the Brugada syndrome is one that provides the substrate for the development of circus movement reentry in the form of epicardial and transmural dispersion of repolarization, as well as the trigger for VT/VF in the form of a phase 2 reentrant extrasystole.

The experimental findings suggest an accentuated action potential notch and/or depressed right ventricular epicardial action potential dome as the basis for the accentuated J wave or ST segment elevation and to phase 2 reentry as a trigger for episodes of circus movement reentry responsible for VT and VF in Brugada patients. There are a number of similarities between the conditions that give rise to ST segment elevation and phase 2 reentry in the experimental models and those that attend the appearance of the Brugada syndrome. Accentuation of the action potential notch or loss of the action potential dome in epicardium but not endocardium leads to elevation of the ST segment with either a saddleback or coved appearance, similar to those recorded in patients with the Brugada syndrome.[408–410] In Brugada patients , as in the wedge preparation, VT/VF is inducible in the majority of cases. In the wedge preparation, VT/VF is most easily induced by the application of an extrastimulus to the site of briefest refractoriness, always located on the epicardial side. In the clinic, programmed stimulation is most commonly applied to RV endocardium. An epicardial approach is possible via the coronary sinus and it is of interest that in a recent case report VT/VF was shown to be noninducible with endocardial extrastimulation, but readily inducible using an electrode placed deep within the coronary sinus.[412]

In isolated epicardial tissues as well as in wedge preparations, loss of the action potential dome and phase 2 reentry are readily induced in right ventricular preparations, but are more difficult to induce in the left ventricle. These findings are due to the presence of a much more prominent I_{to} in right versus left ventricular epicardium and are consistent with the appearance of the ST segment elevation only in right precordial leads in patients with the Brugada syndrome. Normalization of the ST segment in response to an increase in rate is observed in the wedge model as well as in some Brugada patients,[410] and is consistent with a decreased availability of I_{to} (due to the relatively slow recovery from inactivation), which diminishes the notched configuration of the epicardial action potential. Not all Brugada patients display rate-dependent changes in ST. With some mutations, such as those involving a slowing of reactivation of the sodium channel, or in the presence of sodium channel blockers with strong use dependence, acceleration may be attended by an ST segment elevation.

Because accentuation of the notch and/or loss of the dome are caused by an outward shift in the balance of currents active at the end of phase 1 (principally I_{to} and I_{Ca}), autonomic neurotransmitters like acetylcholine facilitate these changes in the action potential[413] by suppressing I_{Ca} and/or augmenting potassium current, whereas β-adrenergic agonists restore the dome by augmenting I_{Ca}. As a consequence, in the arterially perfused wedge, vagal and sympathetic influences exaggerate and reduce ST segment elevation, respectively.[408] Accentuation of the ST segment elevation in patients with the Brugada syndrome following vagal maneuvers and normalization of the ST segment following β-adrenergic agents are consistent with these findings.[410]

The effect of sodium channel blockers to facilitate loss of the RV epicardial action potential dome in the wedge and in isolated tissues[380] is consistent with their ability[408] to unmask the Brugada syndrome in the clinic.[386] Moreover, the linkage of the Brugada syndrome with mutations in SCN5A is consistent with the conduction disturbances that sometimes accompany the Brugada syndrome.[414]

While augmentation of I_{to} may precipitate phase 2 reentry and the Brugada syndrome, it is not a prerequisite. However, the presence of a prominent I_{to} is essential. Because of the pivotal role of I_{to}, agents that inhibit I_{to}, including 4-AP and quinidine, restore the action potential dome and electrical homogeneity, thus suppressing all arrhythmic activity.[315,388] Agents that potently block I_{Na}, but not I_{to} (flecainide, ajmaline, and procainamide) exacerbate or unmask the Brugada syndrome, whereas those with actions to block both I_{Na} and I_{to} (e.g., quinidine and disopyramide) may exert an ameliorative effect.[388] The anticholinergic effects of quinidine and disopyramide may also contribute to their effectiveness. An experimental drug that may be useful in the treatment of the Brugada syndrome and other syndromes associated with an ST segment elevation is tedisamil, an agent that blocks a variety of outward potassium currents, including I_{to}.

The Long QT Syndrome

Exaggeration of intrinsic heterogeneities of ventricular repolarization also contributes to the development of the long QT syndrome (LQTS). In this case, amplification of differences in final repolarization of the action potential of cells spanning the ventricular wall provides the arrhythmogenic substrate. The congenital and acquired (drug-induced) LQTS are characterized by the development of long QT intervals in the ECG, abnormal T waves, and an atypical polymorphic tachycardia known as TdP.[178,415–418]

The LQTSs are phenotypically and genotypically diverse, but have in common the appearance of a long QT interval in the ECG, an atypical polymorphic ventricular tachycardia known as TdP, and, in many but not all cases, a relatively high risk for sudden cardiac death.[417,419,420] Congenital LQTS is subdivided into 10 genotypes distinguished by mutations in at least seven different ion genes and a structural anchoring protein located on chromosomes 3, 4, 6, 7, 11, 17, and 21 (Table 33–2).[421–428] Timothy syndrome, also referred to as LQT8, is a rare congenital disorder characterized by multiorgan dysfunction including prolongation of the QT interval, lethal arrhythmias, webbing of fingers and toes, congenital heart disease, immune deficiency, intermittent hypoglycemia, cognitive abnormalities, and autism. Timothy syndrome has been linked to loss of voltage-dependent inactivation due to mutations in Cav1.2, the gene that encodes for an α subunit of the calcium channel.[429] The most recent genes associated with LQTS are *CAV3*, which encodes caveolin-3, and *SCN4B*, which encodes NaV β4, an auxiliary subunit of the cardiac sodium channel. Mutations in both genes produce a gain of function in late I_{Na}, causing an LQT3-like phenotype.[427,428]

Inheritance follows two patterns: (1) a rare autosomal recessive disease associated with deafness (Jervell and Lange-Nielsen), caused by two genes that encode for the slowly activating delayed rectifier potassium channel (KCNQ1 and KCNE1), and (2) a much more common autosomal dominant form known as the Romano Ward syndrome, caused by mutations in 10 different genes, including *KCNQ1* (KvLQT1; LQT1); *KCNH2* (HERG;LQT2); *SCN5A* (Nav1.5; LQT3); *ANKB* (LQT4); *KCNE1* (minK; LQT5); *KCNE2* (MiRP1; LQT6); *KCNJ2* (LQT7; Andersen's syndrome), *CACNA1C* (Cav1.2; LQT8; Timothy syndrome), *CAV3* (caveolin-3; LQT9), and *SCN4B* (NaV β4, LQT10). Six of the 10 genes encode for cardiac potassium channels, one for the cardiac sodium channel (*SCN5A*), one for the β subunit of the sodium channel, one for caveolin-3, and one for a protein called ankyrin B (*ANKB*), which is involved in anchoring of ion channels to the cellular membrane.

The prevalence of this disorder is estimated at 1–2:10,000. The ECG diagnosis is based on the presence of prolonged repolarization (QT interval) and abnormal T wave morphology.[430] In the different genotypes, cardiac events may be precipitated by physical or emotional stress (LQT1), a startle (LQT2), or may occur at rest or during sleep (LQT3). Antiadrenergic intervention with β blockers is the mainstay of therapy. For patients unresponsive to this approach, an implantable cardiac defibrillator (ICD) and/or cardiac sympathetic denervation may be therapeutic alternatives.[431,432]

Acquired LQTS refers to a syndrome similar to the congenital form but caused by exposure to drugs that prolong the duration of the ventricular action potential[433] or QT prolongation secondary to cardiomyopathies such as dilated or hypertrophic cardiomyopathy, as well as to abnormal QT prolongation associated with bradycardia or electrolyte imbalance.[162,434–437] The acquired form of the disease is far more prevalent than the congenital form, and in some cases may have a genetic predisposition.

Amplification of spatial dispersion of repolarization within the ventricular myocardium is the principal arrhythmogenic substrate in both acquired and congenital LQTS. The accentuation of spatial dispersion, typically secondary to an increase of transmural, transseptal, or apicobasal dispersion of repolarization, and the development of EAD-induced triggered activity underlie the substrate and trigger for the development of TdP arrhythmias observed under LQTS conditions.[147,438] Models of the LQT1, LQT2, LQT3, and LQT7 forms of the long QT syndrome have been developed using the canine arterially perfused left ventricular wedge preparation (Figure 5–23).[55,439,440] These models suggest that in these three forms of LQTS, preferential prolongation of the M cell APD leads to an increase in the QT interval as well as an increase in TDR, which contributes to the development of spontaneous as well as stimulation-induced TdP (Figure 5–24).[156,369,372] The unique characteristics of the M cells are at the heart of the LQTS. The hallmark of the M cell is the ability of its action potential to prolong more than that of epicardium or endocardium in response to a slowing of rate.[353,360,441] As previously discussed, this feature of the M cell is due to weaker repolarizing current during phases 2 and 3 secondary to a smaller I_{Ks} and a larger late I_{Na} and $I_{Na\text{-}Ca}$[143,161,355] compared to epicardial and endocardial cells.

These ionic distinctions also sensitize the M cells to a variety of pharmacological agents. Agents that block I_{Kr} or I_{Ks} or increase I_{Ca} or late I_{Na} generally produce a much greater prolongation of the APD of the M cell than of epicardial or endocardial cells. Differences in the time course of repolarization of the three predominant myocardial cell types have been shown to contribute prominently to the inscription of the T wave of the ECG. Voltage gradients developing as a result of the different time course of repolarization of phases 2 and 3 in the three cell types give rise to opposing voltage gradients on either side of the M region, which are in large part responsible for the inscription of the T wave.[374] In the case of an upright T wave, the epicardial response is the earliest to repolarize and the M cell action potential is the latest. Full repolarization of the epicardial action potential coincides with the peak of the T wave and repolarization of the M cells is coincident with the end of the T wave. The duration of the M cell action potential therefore determines the QT interval, whereas the duration of the epicardial action potential determines the QTpeak interval.

Experimental models that mimic the clinical congenital syndromes with respect to prolongation of the QT interval, T wave morphology, and the rate dependence of QT have been helpful in elucidating the basis for sympathetic nervous system influences (Figure 5–23).[359,369,372–374]

The I_{Ks} blocker, chromanol 293B, has been used to mimic LQT1. I_{Ks} block alone produces a homogeneous prolongation of repolarization and refractoriness across the ventricular wall and does not induce arrhythmias. The addition of isoproterenol causes an abbreviation of epicardial and endocardial APD but a prolongation or no change in the APD of the M cell, resulting in a marked augmentation of TDR and the development of spontaneous and stimulation-induced TdP.[372] These changes give rise to a broad based T wave and the long QT interval characteristic of LQT1. The development of TdP in the model requires β-adrenergic stimulation, consistent with a high sensitivity of congenital LQTS, in particular LQT1, to sympathetic stimulation.[417,419,420,442,443]

The I_{Kr} blocker *d*-sotalol mimics LQT2 and provides a model of the most common form of acquired (drug-induced) LQTS. A greater prolongation of the M cell action potential and slowing

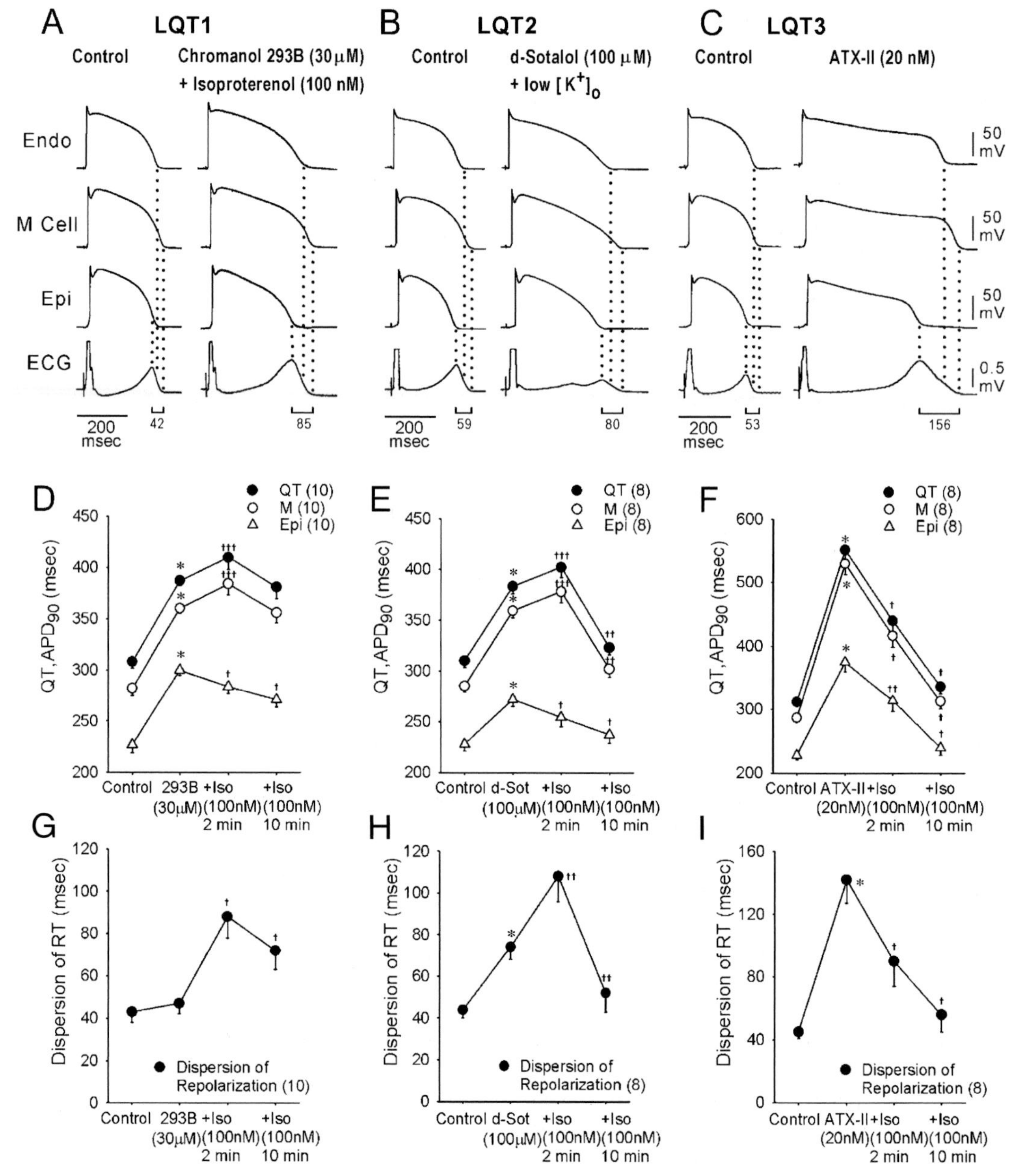

FIGURE 5–23. Transmembrane action potentials and transmural electrocardiograms (ECG) in the LQT1 (A and B), LQT2 (C and D), and LQT3 (E and F) models (arterially perfused canine left ventricular wedge preparations) and clinical ECG lead V5 of patients with LQT1 (*KvLQT1* defect) (G), LQT2 (*HERG* defect) (H), and LQT3 (*SCN5A* defect) (I) syndromes. Isoproterenol + chromanol 293B—an I_{Ks} blocker, *d*-sotalol + low $[K^+]_o$, and ATX-II—an agent that slows inactivation of late I_{Na} are used to mimic the LQT1, LQT2, and LQT3 syndromes, respectively. (A–F) Action potentials simultaneously recorded from endocardial (Endo), M, and epicardial (Epi) sites together with a transmural ECG. BCL = 2000 msec. In all cases, the peak of the T wave in the ECG is coincident with the repolarization of the epicardial action potential, whereas the end of the T wave is coincident with the repolarization of the M cell action potential. Repolarization of the endocardial cell is intermediate between that of the M cell and epicardial cell. Transmural dispersion of repolarization across the ventricular wall, defined as the difference in the repolarization time between M and epicardial cells, is denoted below the ECG traces. (B) Isoproterenol (100 nM) in the presence of chromanol 293B (30 μM) produced a preferential prolongation of the APD of the M, resulting in an accentuated transmural dispersion of repolarization and broad-based T waves as commonly seen in LQT1 patients (G). (D) *d*-Sotalol (100 μM) in the presence of low potassium (2 mM) gives rise to low-amplitude T waves with a notched or bifurcated appearance due to a very significant slowing of repolarization as commonly seen in LQT2 patients (H). (F) ATX-II (20 nM) markedly prolongs the QT interval, widens the T wave, and causes a sharp rise in the dispersion of repolarization. ATX-II also produces a marked delay in onset of the T wave due to relatively large effects of the drug on the APD of epicardium and endocardium, consistent with the late-appearing T wave pattern observed in LQT3 patients (I). (Modified from Shimizu and Antzelevitch[369] and Shimizu *et al.*,[372] with permission.)

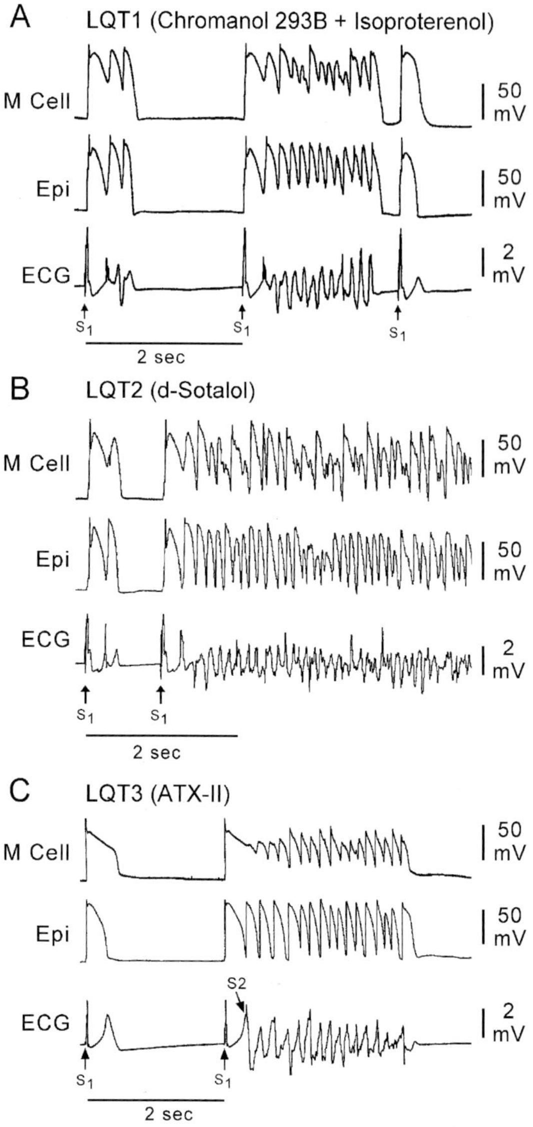

FIGURE 5–24. Polymorphic ventricular tachycardia displaying features of torsade de pointes (TdP) in the LQT1 (A), LQT2 (B), and LQT3 (C) models (arterially perfused canine left ventricular wedge preparations). Isoproterenol + chromanol 293B, *d*-sotalol, and ATX-II are used to mimic the three LQTS syndromes, respectively. Each trace shows action potentials simultaneously recorded from M and epicardial (Epi) cells together with a transmural ECG. The preparation was paced from the endocardial surface at a BCL of 2000 msec (S1). (A and B) Spontaneous TdP induced in the LQT1 and LQT2 models, respectively. In both models, the first groupings show spontaneous ventricular premature beats (or couplets) that fail to induce TdP, and a second grouping that shows spontaneous premature beats that succeed. The premature response appears to originate in the deep subendocardium (M or Purkinje). (C) Programmed electrical stimulation induces TdP in the LQT3 model. ATX-II produced very significant dispersion of repolarization (first grouping). A single extrastimulus (S2) applied to the epicardial surface at an S1–S2 interval of 320 msec initiates TdP (second grouping). (Modified from Shimizu and Antzelevitch[369] and Shimizu *et al.*,[372] with permission.)

of phase 3 of the action potential of all three cell types result in a low-amplitude T wave, long QT interval, large transmural dispersion of repolarization, and the development of spontaneous as well as stimulation-induced TdP. The addition of hypokalemia gives rise to low-amplitude T waves with a deeply notched or bifurcated appearance, similar to those commonly seen in patients with the LQT2 syndrome.[369,374] Isoproterenol further exaggerates transmural dispersion of repolarization, thus increasing the incidence of TdP.[156]

ATX-II, an agent that increases late I_{Na}, has been useful in mimicking LQT3.[369] ATX-II markedly prolongs the QT interval, delays the onset of the T wave, in some cases also widening it, and produces a sharp rise in transmural dispersion of repolarization as a result of a greater prolongation of the APD of the M cell. The differential effect of ATX-II to prolong the M cell action potential is likely due to the presence of a larger late sodium current in the M cell.[161] ATX-II produces a marked delay in onset of the T wave because of a relatively large effect of the drug on epicardial and endocardial APD. This feature is consistent with the late-appearing T wave (long isoelectric ST segment) observed in patients with the LQT3 syndrome.

Also in agreement with the clinical presentation of LQT3, the model displays a steep rate dependence of the QT interval and develops TdP at slow rates. Interestingly, the β-adrenergic influence in the form of isoproterenol *reduces* transmural dispersion of repolarization by abbreviating the APD of the M cell more than that of epicardium or endocardium, and thus reducing the incidence of TdP. While the β- adrenergic blocker propranolol is protective in LQT1 and LQT2 wedge models, it has the opposite effect in LQT3, acting to amplify transmural dispersion and promoting TdP.[156]

The time course of the response to sympathetic stimulation is very different in the case of LQT1 and LQT2, both in experimental models (Figure 5–23) and in the clinic.[438,444] In LQT1, β-adrenergic stimulation induces an increase in TDR that is most prominent during the first 2 min, but that persists, although to a lesser extent, during steady state. The incidence of TdP is enhanced during the initial period as well as during steady state. In LQT2, isoproterenol produces only a transient increase in TDR that persists for less than 2 min. It is therefore enhanced for only a brief period of time. These differences in time course may explain the important differences in autonomic activity and other gene-specific triggers that contribute to events in patients with different LQTS genotypes.[438,443,445]

β-Blockers are first-line therapy in LQT1 and LQT2, although they have not been shown to be of benefit in LQT3. Preliminary data suggest that LQT3 patients might benefit from Na^+ channel blockers, such as mexiletine and flecainide, but long-term data are not yet available.[446,447] Experimental data have shown that mexiletine reduces transmural dispersion and prevents TdP in LQT3 as well as LQT1 and LQT2, suggesting that agents that block the late sodium current may be effective in all forms of LQTS.[369,372] These observations suggest that a combination of β-blockers and late sodium channel blockers may confer more protection in LQT1 and LQT2 than β-blockade alone. Clinical data are not available as yet.

The $T_{peak}-T_{end}$ interval has been shown to provide an index of transmural dispersion of repolarization.[360] The available data suggest that $T_{peak}-T_{end}$ measurements might best be limited to precordial leads (V1–V6) since these leads more accurately reflect transmural dispersion of repolarization. Recent studies have also provided guidelines for the estimation of transmural dispersion of repolarization in the case of more complex T waves, including negative, biphasic, and triphasic T waves.[155] In these cases, the interval from the nadir of the first component of the T wave to the end of the T wave provides an accurate electrocardiographic approximation of transmural dispersion of repolarization.

Although further studies are needed to evaluate the utility of this noninvasive index of electrical heterogeneity and its prognostic value in the assignment of arrhythmic risk, evidence is accumulating in support of the hypothesis that TDR rather than QT prolongation underlies the substrate responsible for the development of TdP.[147,173,448–450] While the clinical applicability of this concept remains to be carefully validated, significant progress toward validation of the $T_{peak}-T_{end}$ interval as an index of transmural dispersion has been achieved in recent studies.[451–457] Direct evidence in support of $T_{peak}-T_{end}$ as an index to predict TdP in patients with long QT syndrome was provided by Yamaguchi and co-workers.[458] They concluded that $T_{peak}-T_{end}$ is more valuable than QTc and QT dispersion as a predictor of TdP in patients with acquired LQTS. Shimizu *et al.* demonstrated that $T_{peak}-T_{end}$, but not QTc, predicted sudden cardiac death in patients with hypertrophic cardiomyopathy.[455] Watanabe *et al.*[457] demonstrated that prolonged $T_{peak}-T_{end}$ is associated with inducibility as well as spontaneous development of VT in high-risk patients with organic heart disease.

Figure 5–25 presents a working hypothesis for our understanding of the mechanisms underlying LQTS-related TdP based on available data. The hypothesis presumes the presence of electrical heterogeneity in the form of transmural dispersion of repolarization under baseline conditions and the amplification of TDR by agents that reduce net repolarizing current via a reduction in I_{Kr} or I_{Ks} or augmentation of I_{Ca} or late I_{Na}. Conditions leading to a reduction in I_{Kr} or augmentation of late I_{Na} lead to a preferential prolongation of the M cell action potential. As a consequence, the QT interval prolongs and is accompanied by a dramatic increase in transmural dispersion of repolarization, thus creating a vulnerable window for the development of reentry. The reduction in net

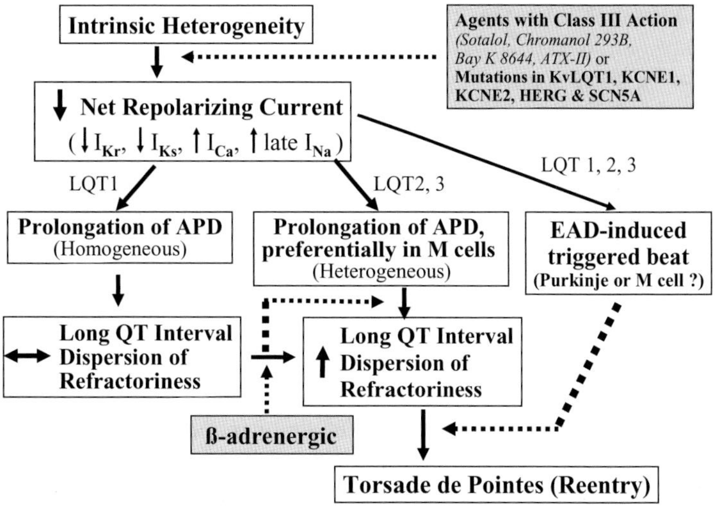

FIGURE 5–25. Proposed cellular and ionic mechanisms for the long QT syndrome.

repolarizing current also predisposes to the development of EAD-induced triggered activity in M and Purkinje cells, which provide the extrasystole that triggers TdP when it falls within the vulnerable period. β-Adrenergic agonists further amplify transmural heterogeneity (transiently) in the case of I_{Kr} block, but reduce it in the case of I_{Na} agonists.[156,367]

Not all agents that prolong the QT interval increase TDR. Amiodarone, a potent antiarrhythmic agent used in the management of both atrial and ventricular arrhythmias, is rarely associated with TdP.[149] Chronic administration of amiodarone produces a greater prolongation of APD in epicardium and endocardium, but less of an increase, or even a decrease at slow rates, in the M region, thereby reducing TDR.[459] In a dog model of chronic complete AV block and acquired LQTS, 6 weeks of amiodarone was shown to produce a major QT prolongation without producing TdP. In contrast, after 6 weeks of dronedarone, TdP occurred in four of eight dogs with the highest spatial dispersion of repolarization (105 ± 20 msec).[460] Sodium pentobarbital is another agent that prolongs the QT interval but reduces TDR. Pentobarbital has been shown to produce a dose-dependent prolongation of the QT interval, accompanied by a reduction in TDR from 51 to 27 msec.[371] Under these conditions TdP is never seen nor can it be induced with programmed stimulation. Amiodarone and pentobarbital have in common the ability to block I_{Ks}, I_{Kr}, and late I_{Na}. This combination produces a preferential prolongation of the APD of epicardium and endocardium so that the QT interval is prolonged, but TDR is actually reduced and TdP does not occur. Another agent that blocks both inward and outward currents is cisapride. Cisapride produces a biphasic dose-dependent prolongation of the QT interval. A parallel biphasic dose–response relationship is seen for TDR, peaking at 0.2 μmol/liter, and it is only at this concentration that TdP is observed. At higher concentrations of cisapride, QT is further prolonged but TDR was diminished, and TdP could no longer be induced.[448] This finding suggests that the spatial dispersion of repolarization is more important than the prolongation of the QT interval in determining the substrate for TdP.

Chromanol 293B, an I_{Ks} blocker, is another example of an agent that increases QT without augmenting TDR. Chromanol 293B prolongs APD of the three cell types homogeneously, neither increasing TDR nor widening the T wave; TdP is never observed under these conditions. This changes very quickly in the presence of β-adrenergic stimulation. Isoproterenol abbreviates the APD of epicardial and endocardial cells but not that of the M cell, resulting in a marked accentuation of TDR[156]; TdP develops under these conditions.

These findings provide further evidence in support of the hypothesis that the risks associated with LQTS are not due to the prolongation of the

QT interval but rather to the increase in spatial dispersion of repolarization that usually, but not always, accompanies the prolongation of the QT interval.

The Short QT Syndrome

First proposed as a clinical entity by Gussak *et al.* in 2000,[461] the short QT syndrome (SQTS) is an inherited syndrome characterized by a QTc ≤ 300–340 msec and a high incidence of VT/VF in infants, children, and young adults.[462] The familial nature of this sudden death syndrome was highlighted by Gaita *et al.* in 2003.[463] The first genetic defect responsible for the short QT syndrome (SQTS1), reported by Brugada *et al.* [464] in 2004, involved two different missense mutations (substitution of one amino acid for another) resulting in the same amino acid substitution in HERG (N588K), which caused a gain of function in the rapidly activating delayed rectifier channel, I_{Kr}. A second gene reported by Bellocq *et al.* (SQTS2)[465] involved a missense mutation in KCNQ1 (KvLQT1), causing a gain of function in I_{Ks}. A third gene (SQT3), identified in 2005, involves KCNJ2, the gene that encodes for the inward rectifier channel. Mutations in KCNJ2 caused a gain of function in I_{K1}, leading to an abbreviation of the QT interval. SQT3 is associated with QTc intervals <330 msec, not quite as short as SQT1 and SQT2.

In addition to an abbreviated QT interval, SQTS is characterized by the appearance of tall peaked often symmetrical T waves in the ECG. The augmented T_{peak}–T_{end} interval associated with this electrocardiographic feature of the syndrome suggests that TDR is significantly increased. Studies employing the left ventricular wedge model of the short QT syndrome have provided evidence in support of the hypothesis that an increase in outward repolarizing current can preferentially abbreviate endocardial/M cells thus increasing TDR and creating the substrate for reentry.[466] The potassium channel opener pinacidil used in this study caused a heterogeneous reduction of APD among the different cell types spanning the ventricular wall, thus creating the substrate for the genesis of VT under conditions associated with short QT intervals. Polymorphic VT could be readily induced with programmed electrical stimulation. The increase in TDR was further accentuated by isoproterenol, leading to easier induction and more persistent VT/VF. It is noteworthy that an increase in TDR to values greater than 55 msec was associated with the inducibility of VT/VF. In LQTS models, a TDR of >90 msec is required to induce TdP. The easier inducibility in SQTS is due to the reduction in the wavelength (the product of the refractory period and conduction velocity) of the reentrant circuit, which reduces the pathlength required for maintenance of reentry.[466]

Catecholaminergic Polymorphic Ventricular Tachycardia

Catecholaminergic polymorphic ventricular tachycardia (CPVT) is a rare, autosomal dominant or recessive inherited disorder, predominantly affecting children or adolescents with structurally normal hearts. It is characterized by BVT, PVT, and a high risk of sudden cardiac death (30–50% by the age of 20–30 years).[234,235] Recent molecular genetic studies have identified mutations in genes encoding for the cardiac ryanodine receptor 2 (RyR2) or calsequestrin 2 (CASQ2) in patients with this phenotype.[209,236–238] Mutations in RyR2 cause autosomal dominant CPVT, whereas mutations in CASQ2 are responsible for either an autosomal recessive or dominant form of CPVT.

Numerous studies point to DAD-induced TA as the mechanism underlying monomorphic or bidirectional VT in patients with this syndrome. The cellular mechanisms underlying the various ECG phenotypes, and the transition of monomorphic VT to polymorphic VT or VF, were recently elucidated with the help of the coronary-perfused left ventricular wedge preparation (Figures 5–26 and 5–27).[206] The wedge was exposed to low dose caffeine to mimic the defective calcium homeostasis encountered under conditions that predispose to CPVT. The combination of isoproterenol and caffeine led to the development of DAD-induced triggered activity arising from the epicardium, endocardium, or M region. Migration of the source of ectopic activity was responsible for the transition from monomorphic to slow polymorphic VT. Alternation of the epicardial and endocardial source of ectopic activity gave rise to a bidirectional VT. The triggered activity-induced monomorphic, bidirectional, and slow polymorphic VT would be expected to be hemodynami-

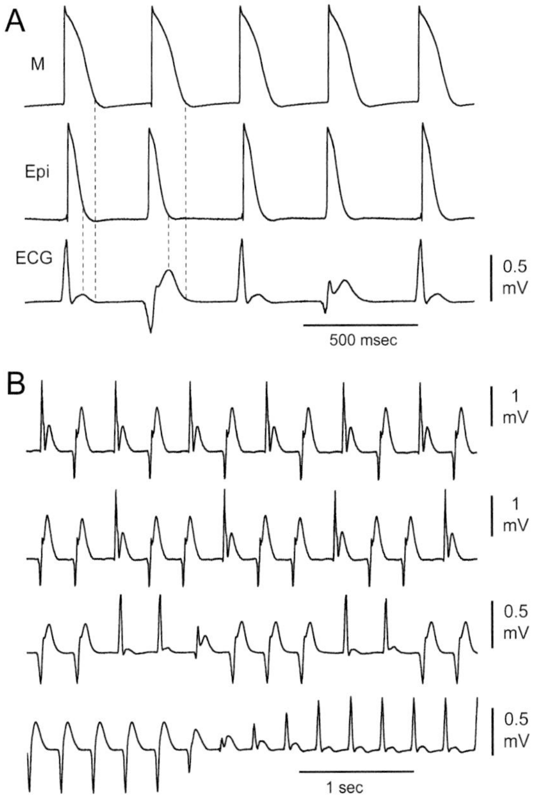

FIGURE 5–26. Experimental model of catecholaminergic VT. Bidirectional VT. (A) Action potentials were simultaneously recorded from epicardial (Epi) and M cells together with a transmural ECG in a left ventricular wedge preparation. Perfusion of isoproterenol (100 nmol/liter) in the presence of caffeine (300 μmol/liter) produced a bidirectional ventricular rhythm as a consequence of alternation in the origin of ectopic activity between endocardium and epicardium. A marked change in the T_{peak}–T_{end} interval (from 53 to 75 msec) and transmural dispersion of repolarization (from 51 to 73 msec) are observed. (B) Bidirectional tachycardias displaying different patterns of alternations in the origin of the ectopic beat. This activity, presumably due to DAD-induced triggered beats, could be observed to generate a slow polymorphic VT. Because of their slow rates, these arrhythmias are unlikely to create hemodynamic compromise or to be responsible for sudden cardiac death. (Modified from Nam *et al.*,[206] with permission.)

cally well tolerated because of the relatively slow rate of these rhythms and are unlikely to be the cause of sudden death in these syndromes.

Epicardial ectopy and VT were associated with an increased T_{peak}–T_{end} interval and transmural dispersion of repolarization due to reversal of the normal transmural activation sequence. The increase in TDR was sufficient to create the substrate for reentry and programmed electrical stimulation induced a rapid polymorphic VT that would be expected to lead to hemodynamic compromise.[206] Thus, even in a syndrome in which arrhythmogenesis is traditionally ascribed to triggered activity, sudden death may be due to amplification of TDR, giving rise to reentrant VT/VF.

Acute Myocardial Ischemia-Induced ST-Segment Elevation and Tachyarrhythmias

Acute myocardial ischemia is linked to life-threatening ventricular arrhythmias. Ischemia-induced disturbances of ionic homeostasis, ion channel dysfunction, and perturbed intercellular communication contribute to the slowing of impulse propagation and increased dispersion of repolarization, which underlie the increased vulnerability to life-threatening arrhythmias. Increased dispersion of repolarization is secondary to differences in repolarization between ischemic and normal zones as well as to accentuation of intrinsic transmural heterogeneities of repolarization. Heterogeneity in the recovery of excitability within the ischemic myocardium and border zone also contributes to the electrophysiological substrate responsible for the development of reentrant excitation underlying VT/VF. The initial beat of VT or VF appears to emerge from small reentrant circuits and/or to be secondary to focal sources.[467] Flow of injury current due to voltage gradients present across the border zone has been proposed as a mechanism for generation of extrasystolic activity.[83,316,467]

Another mechanism suggested to be responsible for the generation of premature beats is epicardial phase 2 reentry. Ischemia-induced heterogeneous loss of the epicardial action potential dome in isolated ventricular preparations has been shown to generate extrasystoles that can precipitate monomorphic or polymorphic VT.[17,468,469]

It is well recognized that despite similar transmural changes in resting membrane potential, ischemia decreases action potential amplitude and duration more in epicardium than in endocardium.[468,470,471] Factors believed to contribute to this differential action potential response include differences in membrane responsiveness,[470] a greater epicardial sensitivity of $I_{K\text{-}ATP}$ to ATP depletion,[472] a greater epicardial depression of the

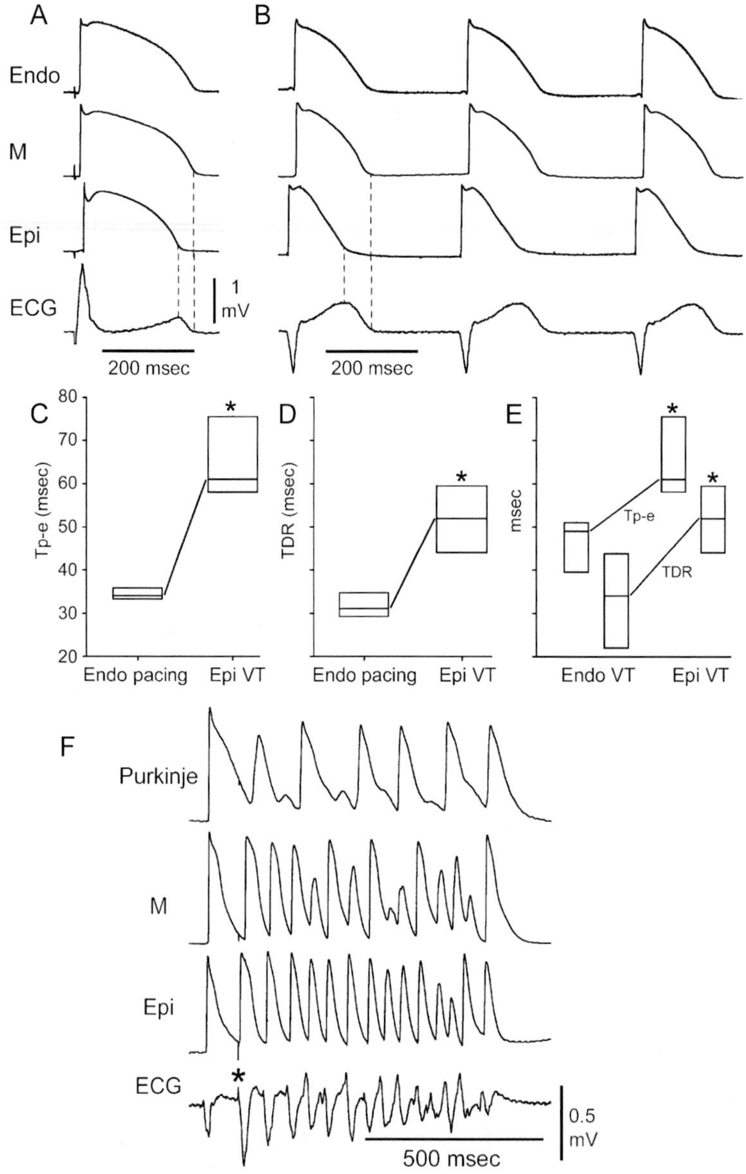

Figure 5–27. Experimental models of catecholaminergic VT. Development of epicardial VT is associated with an increase in transmural dispersion of repolarization (TDR). (A) T_{peak}–T_{end} interval ($T_{p\text{-}e}$) and TDR in a left ventricular wedge preparation during endocardial pacing at a BCL of 2000 msec are 36 and 34 msec, respectively. (B) Reversal of the transmural sequence of activation as a consequence of the focal ventricular rhythm arising from epicardium causes $T_{p\text{-}e}$ and TDR to increase to 57 and 52 msec, respectively. (C–E) Comparison of $T_{p\text{-}e}$ and TDR values during endocardial pacing (caffeine only) and during VT (caffeine + isoproterenol). $T_{p\text{-}e}$ and TDR increased significantly during epicardial VT compared with those recorded during endocardial pacing at 2000 msec (C, D) or during endocardial VT (E). Data are expressed as median (25, 75 percentile) ($n = 7$) $*p < 0.05$. (F) Rapid polymorphic VT induced by single extrastimulus during a sustained episode of slow epicardial VT. Action potentials were recorded simultaneously from subendocardial Purkinje, M, and epicardial (Epi) cells together with a transmural ECG. Perfusion of isoproterenol (100 nmol/liter) in the presence of caffeine (300 μmol/liter) produced a slow monomorphic epicardial VT. A single extrastimulus (S_2, *) applied to the epicardial surface at an S_1–S_2 interval of 100 msec initiated a rapid polymorphic VT. (Modified from Nam *et al.*,[206] with permission.)

calcium current,[472] the presence of a prominent transient outward current (I_{to})-mediated spike and dome configuration in epicardium but not in endocardium,[468] and intrinsic transmural differences in fast I_{Na}.[473]

Under ischemic conditions, changes in the surface ECG are thought to be related to changes in the resting potential, action potential morphology, action potential duration, and conduction characteristics of the injured myocardial region.[474–476] Nevertheless, current thinking regarding the pathophysiological mechanisms of myocardial ischemia-induced changes in the ECG derive principally from theoretical models since attempts to record simultaneously transmembrane action potentials from the ischemic myocardium *in vivo* are limited to the epicardial surface.[477–479] ST-segment elevation is a characteristic ECG manifestation of transmural myocardial ischemia in leads facing the injury.[480] Although the mechanisms responsible for such changes have not been experimentally identified, several theoretical models have predicted their correlation with action potential morphology changes.[474,476]

In the canine ventricular wedge preparation, in which transmembrane action potentials can be simultaneously recorded from endocardium and epicardium along with a transmural ECG, interruption of coronary flow leads to electrocardiographic alterations that reproduce the patterns of acute transmural myocardial ischemia observed clinically. The results of these studies indicate that two distinctly different mechanisms involving (1) loss of the epicardial action potential dome and (2) markedly delayed transmural conduction underlie the apparent ST segment elevation encountered during acute ischemia.[481]

Atrial Electrical Heterogeneity

As with electrical heterogeneity in the ventricle, electrical heterogeneity in the atria plays a pivotal role in the genesis of atrial reentrant arrhythmias. Intrinsic dispersion of action potential duration has been demonstrated in maps generated in the coronary-perfused right atrium.[191] In the coronary-perfused atrial preparation, atrial action potentials have a well-developed plateau morphology (Figure 5–28) very different from those recorded from superfused preparations (Figure 5–29). The triangular action potential morphology observed in the superfused preparations is likely an electrical manifestation of "ischemic" atrial myocardium (Figure 5–29).

Dispersion of APD, V_{max}, spike, and dome morphology is observed along the surface and transmurally in the canine right atrium (Figure 5–28).[191] The longest APDs are observed in the endocardial crista terminalis and the shortest in the AV ring, with all other regions displaying intermediate values. Distribution of APD along the epicardial surface is relatively homogeneous, with the exception of Bachmann's bundle where APD is longest. The APD_{90} differences in the right atrium averaged 37 ± 11 msec between the longest (endocardial upper crista terminalis) and shortest (endocardial AV ring) action potentials. Dispersion of APD at the epicardial surface is 24 ± 8 msec (between Bachmann's bundle and pectinate muscles). Transmural dispersion of APD averages

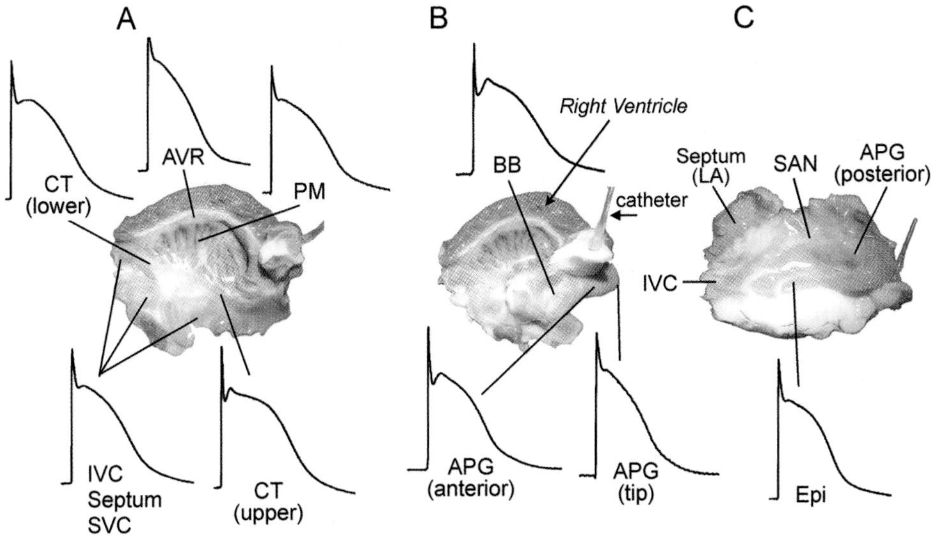

FIGURE 5–28. Regional differences in action potential morphology in the arterially perfused canine right atrium. Recorded during sinus rhythm (cycle length range = 630–800 msec). (A) Endocardial surface. (B) Epicardium in regions of Bachmann's bundle and anterior appendage. (C) Epicardial surface. LA, left atrium. Atrioventricular ring (AVR), pectinate muscle (PM), crista terminalis (CT), Bachmann's bundle (BB), the right atrial appendage (APG), sinoatrial node, about 1 cm of both inferior and superior vena cava (IVC and SVC), and a rim of right ventricular tissue containing the right coronary artery. (From Burashnikov *et al.*,[191] with permission.)

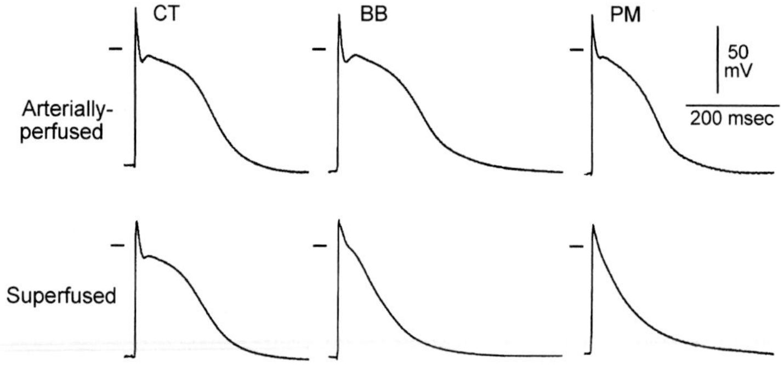

FIGURE 5–29. Conversion of plateau-shaped into triangular-shaped action potentials by switching from perfusion to superfusion mode in endocardial pectinate muscles (PM) and Bachmann's bundle (BB), but not crista terminalis (CT) regions of the right atrial preparation. Action potentials were recorded before and 20 min after the stop of perfusion (with continuous superfusion). (From Burashnikov *et al.*,[191] with permission.)

20 ± 7 msec in the upper crista terminalis and is much smaller (10 ± 5 msec in low crista terminalis) or practically nonexistent in the rest of the right atria.

A spike and dome morphology is consistently recorded in the endocardial crista terminalis, Bachmann's bundle, superior (SVC) and inferior (IVC) vena cava, septum, as well as epicardial Bachmann's bundle, SVC, IVC, and anterior appendage. The action potential notch is less consistently observed in the epicardial crista terminalis, pectinate muscles, posterior appendage, as well as endocardial AV ring.

Average V_{max} values vary by as much as 122 V/sec at different right atrial sites.[191] Endocardial crista terminalis as well as epicardial and endocardial Bachmann's bundle and SVC and IVC show a similarly large V_{max} value. The epicardial posterior and anterior appendage, epicardial and endocardial pectinate muscles, endocardial AV ring, and epicardial crista terminalis have a smaller V_{max}. The crista terminalis and adjacent regions have the largest APD, V_{max}, and spike and dome morphology difference gradients, including transmural ones.[191] Interestingly, the crista terminalis has been shown to be a major region involved in the generation of atrial reentrant arrhythmias.[482]

A detailed map of the electrical distribution of action potentials throughout the left atrium is not available. However, the electrophysiology of pulmonary vein (PV) muscular sleeves and the surrounding left atrial area has been relatively well studied in isolated single cells and superfused preparations. Clinically, it has been shown that PV muscular sleeves are primarily involved in the generation of paroxysmal of atrial fibrillation.[96] A shorter APD in the distal than in the proximal PV muscular sleeves or body of the left atrium has been reported.[47,483] V_{max} values do not differ in PV muscular sleeves and surrounding left atrial areas.[484] As in the right atrium, action potentials recorded in the appendage and Bachmann's bundle of canine coronary-perfused left atrial preparations display a well-developed plateau morphology (A. Burashnikov and C. Antzelevitch, unpublished observations).

Electrical heterogeneity in the atria is amplified under conditions associated with AF. Parasympathetic influences decrease atrial APD inhomogeneously causing an augmentation of electrical dispersion (Figure 5–30), which underlies the ability of parasympathetic influences to promote AF.[312,485,486] Acute ischemia also strongly accentuates electrical atrial heterogeneity.[487] Patients susceptible to AF have a shorter event-related potential (ERP) in PV muscular sleeves than in the left atrial muscle.[488] In contrast, in control patients ERP in PV muscular sleeves is longer than in left atrial muscles. Significant electrical and structural heterogeneities have also been demonstrated in the junctional areas of PV muscular sleeves and left atrial body, leading to a higher propensity for development of reentrant arrhythmias.[306,489,490]

An important distinction between atria and ventricles in response to I_{Kr} and I_{Na} blockers has been described.[191,491] While reduction of I_{Kr} is well known to accentuate dispersion of repolarization in ventricular myocardium, promoting TdP arrhythmias (Figure 5–23), I_{Kr} block prolongs atrial repolarization uniformly, without increasing APD dispersion in the atria (Figure 5–31).[191] This observation may help us understand why I_{Kr} blockers are largely antiarrhythmic in the atria, but often proarrhythmic in the ventricle.[492]

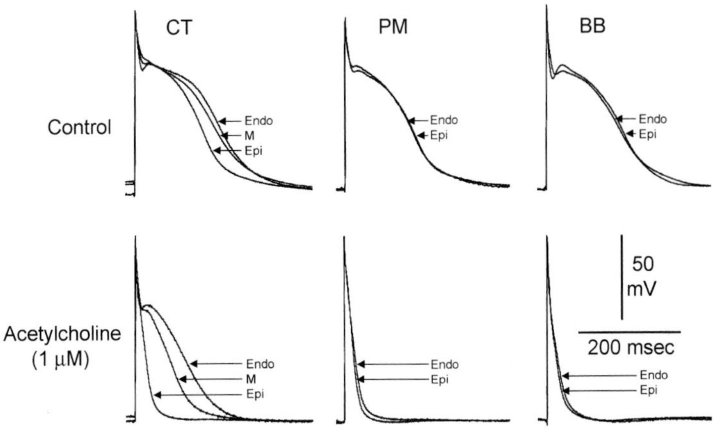

FIGURE 5–30. Acetylcholine abbreviates atrial repolarization inhomogeneously, thus augmenting dispersion of repolarization in the atria. The transmembrane action potentials were obtained from an isolated coronary-perfused right atrium at a pacing cycle length of 700 msec. Endo and Epi, endocardial and epicardial surfaces, respectively; M, midmyocardium; CT, crista terminalis; PM, pectinate muscles; BB, Bachmann's bundle. (From Burashnikov *et al.*,[191] with permission.)

Another recent study compared the electrophysiological effects of ranolazine, a novel antiarrhythmic agent, on canine atrial and ventricular preparations.[491] The findings demonstrated a striking atrial selectivity in the actions of ranolazine to induce potent use-dependent effects on V_{max}, diastolic threshold of excitation, postrepolarization refractoriness, and conduction velocity, parameters dependent on the sodium channels underlying early I_{Na}. Associated with

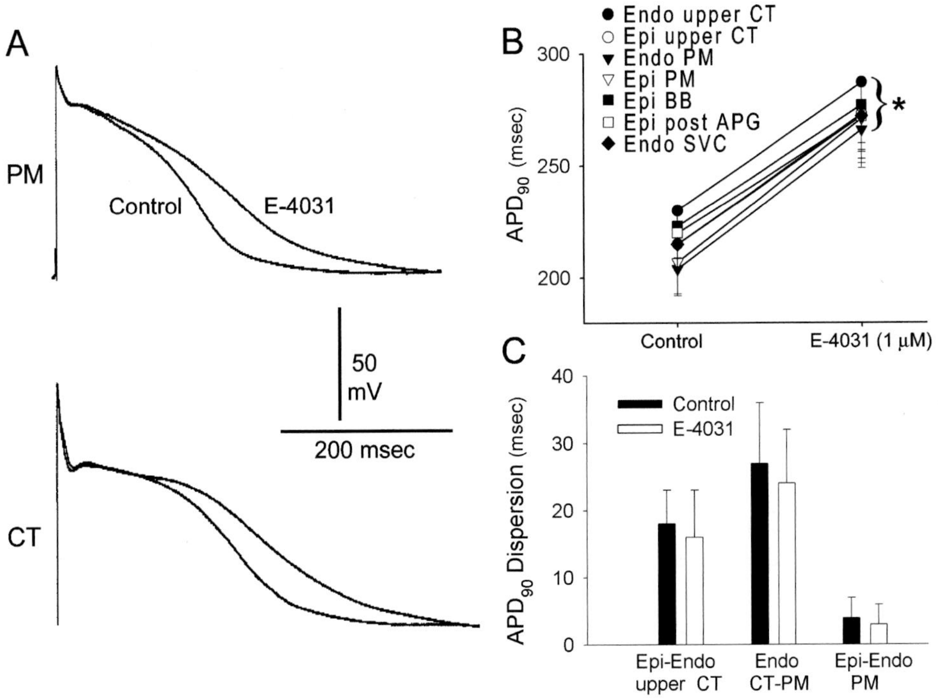

FIGURE 5–31. Effect of I_{Kr} reduction on the regional action potential duration (APD) and dispersion of repolarization in the perfused canine right atrium. (A) Typical superimposed TAPs recorded from endocardial crista terminalis (CT) and pectinate muscle (PM) before and after addition of E-4031 (1.0 μM) in perfusion solution at a pacing cycle length of 1000 msec. (B and C) Graphs summarizing the effect of I_{Kr} block on APD of seven right atrial regions and APD dispersion. *$p < 0.05$. Reduction of I_{Kr} produces a homogeneous APD prolongation, without aggravation of APD dispersion. (From Burashnikov *et al.*,[191] with permission.)

these actions of ranolazine is its ability to suppress and/or prevent the induction of AF in two experimental models. These results point to atrial-selective sodium channel block as a novel strategy for the management of AF.[491]

Slow Conduction and Reentry

Slow or delayed conduction of the impulse can facilitate the development of reentrant arrhythmias by reducing the wavelength of the reentering wavefront so that it can be accommodated by the available pathlength. Several factors determine the velocity at which an action potential propagates through cardiac tissue. Among these is the intensity of the fast inward sodium current that flows during the upstroke of the action potential and the axial resistance to the flow of local circuit current.

Discontinuities in conduction can give rise to apparently very slow conduction and reentry in cardiac tissues by allowing for the development of prominent step delays in the transmission of impulses at discrete sites. Any agent or agency capable of suppressing the active generator properties of cardiac tissues may diminish excitability to the point of rendering a localized region functionally inexcitable and thus creating a discontinuity in the propagation of the advancing wavefront. Examples include an ion-free, ischemic, or high K^+ environment [107,325,326,331,332] as discussed earlier, as well as electrical blocking current,[329,493,494] localized pressure, [331,495] and localized cooling.[495] Inhibition of the inward sodium and calcium currents using blockers of these currents can also create discontinuities in conduction when applied to localized segments.[325] Very slow conduction encountered under these conditions is generally the result of major step delays caused by electrotonically mediated (saltatory) transmission of impulses across a functionally inexcitable zone (i.e., across a large cumulative axial resistance imposed between two excitable regions) rather than of a uniform or homogeneous slowing of impulse propagation (Figure 5–16).[496] The functionally inexcitable zone effectively serves to diminish the electrical coupling between the excitable regions participating in the conduction of the impulse. The decay of the wavefront as it travels across the inexcitable or refractory zone leads to slow activation of the tissue beyond and thus to a step delay in the conduction of the impulse. The resistive barriers created are similar to those encountered with anisotropy.[497] With either condition, small changes in the effective impedance to the flow of local circuit current from one excitable element to the next can give rise to major delays in conduction.

Conduction delays on the order of tens or hundreds of milliseconds occur when the electrotonic communication between the region already activated (source) and the region awaiting activation (sink) is weak. With progressive electrical uncoupling of source and sink, conduction characteristics become progressively more sensitive to changes in the active and passive membrane properties of both the source and sink.[333] Although the importance of the intensity of the source current, as reflected by the action potential amplitude, duration, or maximum rate of rise, $(dV/dt)_{(max)}$, is well appreciated,[72,333,498,499] a number of studies suggest that under a variety of conditions the threshold current requirement of the sink (i.e., changes in excitability) [331,333,499] may be a more critical determinant of conduction delay (or block). Discrete step delays of impulse conduction, associated with electrotonic prepotentials, have been observed in intracellular recordings obtained from human and animal infarcted myocardium.[9,337,500,501] Extracellular mapping experiments also have uncovered step delays in the propagation of impulses in canine hearts subjected to acute regional myocardial ischemia.[83] These studies lend support to an electrotonic interaction across a high impedance barrier as a mechanism responsible for apparently slow conduction. Nonuniform recovery of refractoriness and geometric factors also play an important role in determining impulse conduction velocity as well as the success or failure of conduction. The disparity in the recovery of refractoriness has already been discussed as the basis for unidirectional block or the lines of block that develop in response to premature extrasystoles. The disparity in local refractoriness can also contribute to a major slowing of impulse propagation and thus to reentry.[360,387,496,502]

The geometry plays a critically important role as well. Regions at which the cross-sectional area of interconnected cells increases abruptly are known to be potential sites for the development of unidirectional block or delayed conduction due to an impedance mismatch. Slowing or block of conduction occurs when the impulse propagates in the direction of increasing diameter because the local circuit current provided by the advancing wavefront is insufficient or barely sufficient to charge the capacity of the larger volume of tissue ahead and thus bring the larger mass to its threshold potential. The Purkinje–muscle junction is an example of a site at which unidirectional block and conduction delays are observed.[503–505] The preexcitation (WPW) syndrome is another example, where a thin bundle of tissue (Kent bundle) inserts into a larger ventricular mass.

Acknowledgments. Supported by grants from the National Institutes of Health (HL 47678), the American Heart Association, the New York State Affiliate, and the Masons of New York State and Florida.

References

1. Mayer AG. Rhythmical pulsations in scyphomedusae. *Publication 47 of the Carnegie Institute.* 1906:1–62.
2. Mayer AG. Rhythmical pulsations in Scyphomedusae. II. *Publication 102 of the Carnegie Institute.* 1908;115–131.
3. Mines GR. On circulating excitations in heart muscles and their possible relation to tachycardia and fibrillation. *Trans R Soc Can* 1914;8:43–52.
4. Lewis T. The broad features and time-relations of the normal electrocardiogram. Principles of interpretation. In: *The Mechanism and Graphic Registration of the Heart Beat*, 3rd ed. London: Shaw & Sons, Ltd., 1925:44–77.
5. Moe GK. Evidence for reentry as a mechanism for cardiac arrhythmias. *Rev Physiol Biochem Pharmacol* 1975;72:55–81.
6. Kulbertus HE. In: Kulbertus HE, Ed. *Reentrant Arrhythmias, Mechanisms and Treatment.* Baltimore: University Park Press, 1977.
7. Wit AL, Cranefield PF. Re-entrant excitation as a cause of cardiac arrhythmias. *Am J Physiol* 1978; 235:H1–H17.
8. Wit AL, Allessie MA, Fenoglic JJ Jr, Bonke FIM, Lammers W, Smeets J. Significance of the endocardial and epicardial border zones in the genesis of myocardial infarction arrhythmias. In: Harrison D, Ed. *Cardiac Arrhythmias: A Decade of Progress.* Boston: GK Hall, 1982:39–68.
9. Spear JF, Moore EN. Mechanisms of cardiac arrhythmias. *Annu Rev Physiol* 1982;44:485–497.
10. Janse MJ. Reentry rhythms. In: Fozzard HA, Haber E, Jennings RB, Katz AM, Morgan HE, Eds. *The Heart and Cardiovascular System.* New York: Raven Press, 1986:1203–1238.
11. Hoffman BF, Dangman KH. Mechanisms for cardiac arrhythmias. *Experientia* 1987;43:1049–1056.
12. Antzelevitch C. Reflection as a mechanism of reentrant cardiac arrhythmias. *Prog Cardiol* 1988;1: 3–16.
13. El-Sherif N. Reentry revisited. *Pacing Clin Electrophysiol* 1988;11:1358–1368.
14. Lazzara R, Scherlag BJ. Generation of arrhythmias in myocardial ischemia and infarction. *Am J Cardiol* 1988;61:20A–26A.
15. Rosen MR. The links between basic and clinical cardiac electrophysiology. *Circulation* 1988;77:251–263.
16. Waldo AL, Wit AL. Mechanisms of cardiac arrhythmias and conduction disturbances. In: Alexander RW, Schlant RC, Fuster V, O'Rourke RA, Roberts R, Sonnenblick EH, Eds. *The Heart*, 9th ed. New York: McGraw-Hill, 1998:825–872.
17. Lukas A, Antzelevitch C. Phase 2 reentry as a mechanism of initiation of circus movement reentry in canine epicardium exposed to simulated ischemia. *Cardiovasc Res* 1996;32:593–603.
18. Antzelevitch C. Basic mechanisms of reentrant arrhythmias. *Curr Opin Cardiol* 2001;16:1–7.
19. Antzelevitch C. *In vivo* human demonstration of phase 2 reentry. *Heart Rhythm* 2005;2:804–806.
20. Thomsen PE, Joergensen RM, Kanters JK, Jensen TJ, Haarbo J, Hagemann A, Vestergaard A, Saermark K. Phase 2 reentry in man. *Heart Rhythm* 2005;2:797–803.
21. Yan GX, Joshi A, Guo D, Hlaing T, Martin J, Xu X, Kowey PR. Phase 2 reentry as a trigger to initiate ventricular fibrillation during early acute myocardial ischemia. *Circulation* 2004;110:1036–1041.
22. Burashnikov A, Antzelevitch C. Reinduction of atrial fibrillation immediately after termination of the arrhythmia is mediated by late phase 3 early afterdepolarization-induced triggered activity. *Circulation* 2003;107:2355–2360.
23. Burashnikov A, Antzelevitch C. Late-phase 3 EAD. A unique mechanism contributing to initiation of atrial fibrillation. *Pacing Clin Electrophysiol* 2006; 29:290–295.
24. Patterson E, Lazzara R, Szabo B, Liu H, Tang D, Li YH, Scherlag BJ, Po SS. Sodium-calcium exchange

initiated by the Ca2+ transient: An arrhythmia trigger within pulmonary veins. *J Am Coll Cardiol* 2006;47:1196–1206.
25. Hope RR, Scherlag BJ, El-Sherif N, Lazzara R. Hierarchy of ventricular pacemakers. *Circ Res* 1976;39:883–888.
26. Vassalle M. The relationship among cardiac pacemakers. Overdrive suppression. *Circ Res* 1977;41: 269–277.
27. DiFrancesco D. The cardiac hyperpolarizing-activated current, If. Origins and developments. *Prog Biophys Mol Biol* 1985;46:163–183.
28. DiFrancesco D. The pacemaker current (I(f)) plays an important role in regulating SA node pacemaker activity. *Cardiovasc Res* 1995;30:307 308.
29. Vassalle M. Analysis of cardiac pacemaker potential using a "voltage clamp" technique. *Am J Physiol* 1966;210:1335–1341.
30. Vassalle M. The pacemaker current (I(f)) does not play an important role in regulating SA node pacemaker activity. *Cardiovasc Res* 1995;30:309–310.
31. Huser J, Blatter LA, Lipsius SL. Intracellular Ca2+ release contributes to automaticity in cat atrial pacemaker cells. *J Physiol* 2000;524(Pt. 2):415–422.
32. Mangoni ME, Traboulsie A, Leoni AL, Couette B, Marger L, Le QK, Kupfer E, Cohen-Solal A, Vilar J, Shin HS, Escande D, Charpentier F, Nargeot J, Lory P. Bradycardia and slowing of the atrioventricular conduction in mice lacking CaV3.1/alpha1G T-type calcium channels. *Circ Res* 2006; 98:1422–1430.
33. Mitsuiye T, Shinagawa Y, Noma A. Sustained inward current during pacemaker depolarization in mammalian sinoatrial node cells. *Circ Res* 2000;87:88–91.
34. Hoffman BF, Cranefield PF. *Electrophysiology of the Heart.* New York: McGraw-Hill, 1960.
35. DiFrancesco D, Tromba C. Inhibition of the hyperpolarization-activated current (If) induced by acetylcholine in rabbit sino-atrial node myocytes. *J Physiol* 1988;405:477–491.
36. Jones SB, Euler DE, Hardie E, Randall WC, Brynjolfsson G. Comparison of SA nodal and subsidiary atrial pacemaker function and location in the dog. *Am J Physiol* 1978;234:H471–H476.
37. Rozanski GJ, Lipsius SL. Electrophysiology of functional subsidiary pacemakers in canine right atrium. *Am J Physiol* 1985;249:H594–H603.
38. Rozanski GJ, Lipsius SL, Randall WD. Functional characteristics of sinoatrial and subsidiary pacemaker activity in the canine right atrium. *Circulation* 1983;67:1378–1387.
39. Hogan PM, Davis LD. Evidence for specialized fibers in the canine right atrium. *Circ Res* 1968;23: 387–396.
40. Wit AL, Cranefield PF. Triggered and automatic activity in the canine coronary sinus. *Circ Res* 1977;41:435–445.
41. Wit AL, Fenoglio JJ Jr, Wagner BM, Bassett AL. Electrophysiological properties of cardiac muscle in the anterior mitral valve leaflet and the adjacent atrium in the dog. Possible implications for the genesis of atrial dysrhythmias. *Circ Res* 1973;32: 731–745.
42. Bassett AL, Fenoglio JJ Jr, Wit AL, Myerburg RJ, Gelband H. Electrophysiologic and ultrastructural characteristics of the canine tricuspid valve. *Am J Physiol* 1976;230:1366–1373.
43. Rozanski GJ. Electrophysiological properties of automatic fibers in rabbit atrioventricular valves. *Am J Physiol* 1987;253:H720–H727.
44. Chen YJ, Chen SA, Chang MS, Lin CI. Arrhythmogenic activity of cardiac muscle in pulmonary veins of the dog: Implication for the genesis of atrial fibrillation. *Cardiovasc Res* 2000;48:265–273.
45. Chen YJ, Chen SA, Chen YC, Yeh HI, Chan P, Chang MS, Lin CI. Effects of rapid atrial pacing on the arrhythmogenic activity of single cardiomyocytes from pulmonary veins: Implication in initiation of atrial fibrillation. *Circulation* 2001;104: 2849–2854.
46. Chen YJ, Chen YC, Yeh HI, Lin CI, Chen SA. Electrophysiology and arrhythmogenic activity of single cardiomyocytes from canine superior vena cava. *Circulation* 2002;105:2679–2685.
47. Ehrlich JR, Cha TJ, Zhang L, Chartier D, Melnyk P, Hohnloser SH, Nattel S. Cellular electrophysiology of canine pulmonary vein cardiomyocytes: Action potential and ionic current properties. *J Physiol* 2003;551:801–813.
48. Wang TM, Luk HN, Sheu JR, Wu HP, Chiang CE. Inducibility of abnormal automaticity and triggered activity in myocardial sleeves of canine pulmonary veins. *Int J Cardiol* 2005;104:59–66.
49. Kokobun S, Nishimura M, Noma A, Irisawa H. The spontaneous action potential of rabbit atrioventricular node cells. *Jpn J Physiol* 1980;30:529–540.
50. James TN, Isobe JH, Urthaler F. Correlative electrophysiological and anatomical studies concerning the site of origin of escape rhythm during complete atrioventricular block in the dog. *Circ Res* 1979;45:108–119.
51. Weidmann S. *Elektrophysiologie Der Herzmuskelfaser.* Medizinischer Verlag Hans Huber, 1956.

52. Levy MN. Sympathetic-parasympathetic interactions in the heart. *Circ Res* 1971;29:437–445.
53. Donaldson MR, Yoon G, Fu YH, Ptacek LJ. Andersen-Tawil syndrome: A model of clinical variability, pleiotropy, and genetic heterogeneity 5. *Ann Med* 2004;36(Suppl. 1):92–97.
54. Zhang L, Benson DW, Tristani-Firouzi M, Ptacek LJ, Tawil R, Schwartz PJ, George AL, Horie M, Andelfinger G, Snow GL, Fu YH, Ackerman MJ, Vincent GM. Electrocardiographic features in Andersen-Tawil syndrome patients with KCNJ2 mutations: Characteristic T-U-wave patterns predict the KCNJ2 genotype. *Circulation* 2005; 111:2720–2726.
55. Tsuboi M, Antzelevitch C. Cellular basis for electrocardiographic and arrhythmic manifestations of Andersen-Tawil syndrome (LQT7). *Heart Rhythm* 2006;3:328–335.
56. Zitron E, Kiesecker C, Luck S, Kathofer S, Thomas D, Kreye VA, Kiehn J, Katus HA, Schoels W, Karle CA. Human cardiac inwardly rectifying current IKir2.2 is upregulated by activation of protein kinase A. *Cardiovasc Res* 2004;63:520–527.
57. Hauswirth O, Noble D, Tsien RW. The mechanism of oscillatory activity at low membrane potentials in cardiac Purkinje fibres. *J Physiol* 1969;200:255–265.
58. Imanishi S, Surawicz B. Automatic activity in depolarized guinea pig ventricular myocardium. Characteristics and mechanisms. *Circ Res* 1976; 39:751–759.
59. Dangman KH, Hoffman BF. Studies on overdrive stimulation of canine cardiac Purkinje fibers: Maximal diastolic potential as a determinant of the response. *J Am Coll Cardiol* 1983;2:1183–1190.
60. Katzung BG, Morgenstern JA. Effects of extracellular potassium on ventricular automaticity and evidence for a pacemaker current in mammalian ventricular myocardium. *Circ Res* 1977;40:105–111.
61. Rota M, Vassalle M. Patch-clamp analysis in canine cardiac Purkinje cells of a novel sodium component in the pacemaker range. *J Physiol* 2003;548:147–165.
62. Pappano AJ, Carmeliet EE. Epinephrine and the pacemaking mechanism at plateau potentials in sheep cardiac Purkinje fibers. *Pflugers Arch* 1979;382:17–26.
63. Escande D, Coraboeuf E, Planche C. Abnormal pacemaking is modulated by sarcoplasmic reticulum in partially-depolarized myocardium from dilated right atria in humans. *J Mol Cell Cardiol* 1987;19:231–241.
64. Kimura T, Imanishi S, Arita M, Hadama T, Shirabe J. Two differential mechanisms of automaticity in diseased human atrial fibers. *Jpn J Physiol* 1988; 38:851–867.
65. Carmeliet EE. Chloride and potassium in cardiac Purkinje fibers. *J Physiol* 1961;156:375–388.
66. Gadsby DC, Cranefield PF. Two levels of resting potential in cardiac Purkinje fibers. *J Gen Physiol* 1977;70:725–746.
67. Hill JL, Gettes LS. Effect of acute coronary artery occlusion on local myocardial extracellular K+ activity in swine. *Circulation* 1980;61:768–778.
68. Hirche H, Franz C, Bos L, Bissig R, Lang R, Schramm M. Myocardial extracellular K+ and H+ increase and noradrenaline release as possible cause of early arrhythmias following acute coronary artery occlusion in pigs. *J Mol Cell Cardiol* 1980;12:579–593.
69. Kleber AG. Resting membrane potential, extracellular potassium activity, and intracellular sodium activity during acute global ischemia in isolated perfused guinea pig hearts. *Circ Res* 1983;52: 442–450.
70. Dresdner KP Jr, Kline RP, Wit AL. Intracellular K^+ activity, intracellular Na^+ activity and maximum diastolic potential of canine subendocardial Purkinje cells from one-day-old infarcts. *Circ Res* 1987;60:122–132.
71. Friedman PL, Stewart JR, Wit AL. Spontaneous and induced cardiac arrhythmias in subendocardial Purkinje fibers surviving extensive myocardial infarction in dogs. *Circ Res* 1973;33:612–626.
72. Lazzara R, El-Sherif N, Scherlag BJ. Electrophysiological properties of canine Purkinje cells in one-day-old myocardial infarction. *Circ Res* 1973; 33:722–734.
73. Hordof AJ, Edie R, Malm JR, Hoffman BF, Rosen MR. Electrophysiologic properties and response to pharmacologic agents of fibers from diseased human atria. *Circulation* 1976;54:774–779.
74. Ten Eick RE, Singer DH. Electrophysiological properties of diseased human atrium. I. Low diastolic potential and altered cellular response to potassium. *Circ Res* 1979;44:545–557.
75. Singer DH, Baumgarten CM, Ten Eick RE. Cellular electrophysiology of ventricular and other dysrhythmias: Studies on diseased and ischemic heart. *Prog Cardiovasc Dis* 1981;24:97–156.
76. Tristani-Firouzi M, Jensen JL, Donaldson MR, Sansone V, Meola G, Hahn A, Bendahhou S, Kwiecinski H, Fidzianska A, Plaster N, Fu YH, Ptacek LJ, Tawil R. Functional and clinical characterization of KCNJ2 mutations associated with

LQT7 (Andersen syndrome). *J Clin Invest* 2002; 110:381–388.
77. Tawil R, Ptacek LJ, Pavlakis SG, DeVivo DC, Penn AS, Ozdemir C, Griggs RC. Andersen's syndrome: Potassium-sensitive periodic paralysis, ventricular ectopy, and dysmorphic features. *Ann Neurol* 1994;35:326–330.
78. Boineau JP, Schuessler RB, Mooney CR, Wylds AC, Miller CB, Hudson RD, Borremans JM, Brockus CW. Multicentric origin of the atrial depolarization wave: The pacemaker complex. Relation to dynamics of atrial conduction, P-wave changes and heart rate control. *Circulation* 1978; 58:1036–1048.
79. Toda N, West TC. Changes in sino-atrial node transmembrane potentials on vagal stimulation of the isolated rabbit atrium. *Nature* 1965;205:808–809.
80. Ferrer MI. *The Sick Sinus Syndrome*. Mount Kisco, NY: Futura, 1974.
81. Klein HO, Lebson R, Cranefield PF, Hoffman BF. Effect of extrasystoles on idioventricular rhythm. Clinical and electrophysiologic correlation. *Circulation* 1973;47:758–764.
82. Katzung BG, Hondeghem LM, Grant AO. Letter: Cardiac ventricular automaticity induced by current of injury. *Pflugers Arch* 1975;360:193–197.
83. Janse MJ, Van Capelle FJL. Electrotonic interactions across an inexcitable region as a cause of ectopic activity in acute regional myocardial ischemia. A study in intact porcine and canine hearts and computer models. *Circ Res* 1982;50: 527–537.
84. Deck KA. Aenderungen des Ruhepotentials und der kabeleigenschaften von Purkinje-Faden bei der Dehnung. *Pflugers Arch Gesamte Physiol Menschen Tiere* 1964;280:131–140.
85. Vermeulen JT. Mechanisms of arrhythmias in heart failure. *J Cardiovasc Electrophysiol* 1998;9: 208–221.
86. Katz LN, Pick A. *Clinical Electrocardiography. Part 1. The Arrhythmias*. Philadelphia: Lea & Febiger, 1956:224–236.
87. Pogwizd SM, Hoyt RH, Saffitz JE, Corr PB, Cox JL, Cain ME. Reentrant and focal mechanisms underlying ventricular tachycardia in the human heart. *Circulation* 1992;86:1872–1887.
88. Arnar DO, Bullinga JR, Martins JB. Role of the Purkinje system in spontaneous ventricular tachycardia during acute ischemia in a canine model. *Circulation* 1997;96:2421–2429.
89. Pogwizd SM. Focal mechanisms underlying ventricular tachycardia during prolonged ischemic cardiomyopathy. *Circulation* 1994;90:1441–1458.
90. Pogwizd SM. Nonreentrant mechanisms underlying spontaneous ventricular arrhythmias in a model of nonischemic heart failure in rabbits. *Circulation* 1995;92:1034–1048.
91. Pogwizd SM, McKenzie JP, Cain ME. Mechanisms underlying spontaneous and induced ventricular arrhythmias in patients with idiopathic dilated cardiomyopathy. *Circulation* 1998;98:2404–2414.
92. Vermeulen JT, McGuire MA, Opthof T, Coronel R, de Bakker JM, Klopping C, Janse MJ. Triggered activity and automaticity in ventricular trabeculae of failing human and rabbit hearts. *Cardiovasc Res* 1994;28:1547–1554.
93. Nuss HB, Kaab S, Kass DA, Tomaselli GF, Marban E. Cellular basis of ventricular arrhythmias and abnormal automaticity in heart failure. *Am J Physiol* 1999;277:H80–H91.
94. Hoppe UC, Jansen E, Sudkamp M, Beuckelmann DJ. Hyperpolarization-activated inward current in ventricular myocytes from normal and failing human hearts. *Circulation* 1998;97:55–65.
95. Cerbai E, Barbieri M, Mugelli A. Occurrence and properties of the hyperpolarization-activated current If in ventricular myocytes from normotensive and hypertensive rats during aging. *Circulation* 1996;94:1674–1681.
96. Haissaguerre M, Jais P, Shah DC, Takahashi A, Hocini M, Quiniou G, Garrigue S, Le Mouroux A, Le Metayer P, Clementy J. Spontaneous initiation of atrial fibrillation by ectopic beats originating in the pulmonary veins. *N Engl J Med* 1998;339: 659–666.
97. Lai LP, Su MJ, Lin JL, Tsai CH, Lin FY, Chen YS, Hwang JJ, Huang SK, Tseng YZ, Lien WP. Measurement of funny current (I(f)) channel mRNA in human atrial tissue: Correlation with left atrial filling pressure and atrial fibrillation. *J Cardiovasc Electrophysiol* 1999;10:947–953.
98. Vassalle M. Electrogenic suppression of automaticity in sheep and dog Purkinje fibers. *Circ Res* 1970;27:361–377.
99. Glitsch HG. Characteristics of active Na transport in intact cardiac cells. *Am J Physiol* 1979;236:H189–H199.
100. Gadsby DC, Cranefield PF. Electrogenic sodium extrusion in cardiac Purkinje fibers. *J Gen Physiol* 1979;73:819–837.
101. Jordan J, Yamaguchi I, Mandel WJ, McCullen AE. Comparative effects of overdrive on sinus and subsidiary pacemaker function. *Am Heart J* 1977;93:367–374.
102. Kirchhof CJ, Allessie MA. Sinus node automaticity during atrial fibrillation in isolated rabbit hearts. *Circulation* 1992;86:263–271.

103. Scherf D, Boyd LJ. Three unusual cases of parasystole. *Am Heart J* 1950;39:650–663.
104. Jalife J, Moe GK. A biological model of parasystole. *Am J Cardiol* 1979;43:761–772.
105. Jalife J, Antzelevitch C, Moe GK. The case for modulated parasystole. *Pacing Clin Electrophysiol* 1982;5:911–926.
106. Moe GK, Jalife J, Mueller WJ, Moe B. A mathematical model of parasystole and its application to clinical arrhythmias. *Circulation* 1977;56:968–979.
107. Antzelevitch C, Jalife J, Moe GK. Characteristics of reflection as a mechanism of reentrant arrhythmias and its relationship to parasystole. *Circulation* 1980;61:182–191.
108. Nau GJ, Aldariz AE, Acunzo RS, Halpern MS, Davidenko JM, Elizari MV, Rosenbaum MB. Modulation of parasystolic activity by nonparasystolic beats. *Circulation* 1982;66:462–469.
109. Antzelevitch C. Clinical applications of new concepts of parasystole, reflection, and tachycardia. *Cardiol Clin* 1983;1:39–50.
110. Antzelevitch C, Bernstein MJ, Feldman HN, Moe GK. Parasystole, reentry, and tachycardia: A canine preparation of cardiac arrhythmias occurring across inexcitable segments of tissue. *Circulation* 1983;68:1101–1115.
111. Castellanos A, Melgarejo E, Dubois R, Luceri RM. Modulation of ventricular parasystole by extraneous depolarizations. *J Electrocardiol* 1984;17:195–198.
112. Jalife J, Moe GK. Effect of electrotonic potentials on pacemaker activity of canine Purkinje fibers in relation to parasystole. *Circ Res* 1976;39:801–808.
113. Moe GK, Jalife J, Antzelevitch C. Models of parasystole and reentry in isolated Purkinje fibers. *Mayo Clin Proc* 1982;57(Suppl.):14–19.
114. Oreto G, Luzza F, Satullo G, Schamroth L. Modulated ventricular parasystole as a mechanism for concealed bigeminy. *Am J Cardiol* 1986;58:954–958.
115. Oreto G, Luzza F, Satullo G, Coglitore S, Schamroth L. Sinus modulation of atrial parasystole. *Am J Cardiol* 1986;58:1097–1099.
116. Ikeda N, Takeuchi A, Hamada A, Goto H, Mamorita N, Takayanagi K. Model of bidirectional modulated parasystole as a mechanism for cyclic bursts of ventricular premature contractions. *Biol Cybern* 2004;91:37–47.
117. Cranefield PF. Action potentials, afterpotentials and arrhythmias. *Circ Res* 1977;41:415–423.
118. Antzelevitch C, Burashnikov A, Di Diego JM. Cellular and ionic mechanisms underlying arrhythmogenesis. In: Gussak I, Antzelevitch C, Eds. *Cardiac Repolarization. Bridging Basic and Clinical Sciences*. Totowa, NJ: Humana Press, 2003:201–251.
119. Wit AL, Rosen MR. Afterdepolarizations and triggered activity: Distinction from automaticity as an arrhythmogenic mechanism. In: Fozzard HA, Haber E, Jennings RB, Eds. *The Heart and Cardiovascular System*. New York: Raven Press, 1992: 2113–2164.
120. Lab MJ. Contraction-excitation feedback in myocardium: Physiologic basis and clinical relevance. *Circ Res* 1982;50:757–766.
121. Adamantidis MM, Caron JF, Dupuis BA. Triggered activity induced by combined mild hypoxia and acidosis in guinea pig Purkinje fibers. *J Mol Cell Cardiol* 1986;18:1287–1299.
122. Coraboeuf E, Deroubaix E, Coulombe A. Acidosis-induced abnormal repolarization and repetitive activity in isolated dog Purkinje fibers. *J Physiol (Paris)* 1980;76:97–106.
123. Priori SG, Corr PB. Mechanisms underlying early and delayed afterdepolarizations induced by catecholamines. *Am J Physiol* 1990;258:H1796–H1805.
124. Volders PGA, Kulcsar A, Vos MA, Sipido KR, Wellens HJ, Lazzara R, Szabo B. Similarities between early and delayed afterdepolarizations induced by isoproterenol in canine ventricular myocytes. *Cardiovasc Res* 1997;34:348–359.
125. Brachmann J, Scherlag BJ, Rosenshtraukh LV, Lazzara R. Bradycardia-dependent triggered activity: Relevance to drug-induced multiform ventricular tachycardia. *Circulation* 1983;68:846–856.
126. Damiano BP, Rosen MR. Effects of pacing on triggered activity induced by early afterdepolarizations. *Circulation* 1984;69:1013–1025.
127. El-Sherif N, Zeiler RH, Craelius W, Gough WB, Henkin R. QTU prolongation and polymorphic ventricular tachyarrhythmias due to bradycardia-dependent early afterdepolarizations. Afterdepolarizations and ventricular arrhythmias. *Circ Res* 1988;63:286–305.
128. January CT, Riddle JM, Salata JJ. A model for early afterdepolarizations: Induction with the Ca^{2+} channel agonist BAY K 8644. *Circ Res* 1988;62:563–571.
129. Davidenko JM, Cohen L, Goodrow RJ, Antzelevitch C. Quinidine-induced action potential prolongation, early afterdepolarizations, and triggered activity in canine Purkinje fibers. Effects of stimulation rate, potassium, and magnesium. *Circulation* 1989;79:674–686.
130. Carmeliet E. Electrophysiologic and voltage clamp analysis of the effects of sotalol on isolated cardiac

muscle and Purkinje fibers. *J Pharmacol Exp Ther* 1985;232:817–825.
131. Aronson RS. Afterpotentials and triggered activity in hypertrophied myocardium from rats with renal-hypertension. *Circ Res* 1981;48:720–727.
132. Volders PG, Sipido KR, Vos MA, Kulcsar A, Verduyn SC, Wellens HJ. Cellular basis of biventricular hypertrophy and arrhythmogenesis in dogs with chronic complete atrioventricular block and acquired torsade de pointes. *Circulation* 1998; 98:1136–1147.
133. Burashnikov A, Shimizu W, Antzelevitch C. Can a febrile state contribute to the development of the long QT syndrome? Results of studies conducted in tissues and perfused wedge preparations isolated from the canine left ventricle. *Pacing Clin Electrophysiol* 1997;20:II-1115 (abstract).
134. Antzelevitch C, Sicouri S. Clinical relevance of cardiac arrhythmias generated by afterdepolarizations. Role of M cells in the generation of U waves, triggered activity and torsade de pointes. *J Am Coll Cardiol* 1994;23:259–277.
135. Roden DM, Hoffman BF. Action potential prolongation and induction of abnormal automaticity by low quinidine concentrations in canine Purkinje fibers: Relationship to potassium and cycle length. *Circ Res* 1986;56:857–867.
136. Burashnikov A, Antzelevitch C. Acceleration-induced action potential prolongation and early afterdepolarizations. *J Cardiovasc Electrophysiol* 1998;9:934–948.
137. Bril A, Faivre JF, Forest MC, Cheval B, Gout B, Linee P, Ruffolo RR, Poyser RH. Electrophysiological effect of BRL-32872, a novel antiarrhythmic agent with potassium and calcium channel blocking properties, in guinea pig cardiac isolated preparations. *J Pharmacol Exp Ther* 1995;273:1264–1272.
138. Marban E, Robinson SW, Wier WG. Mechanism of arrhythmogenic delayed and early afterdepolarizations in ferret muscle. *J Clin Invest* 1986; 78:1185–1192.
139. Boutjdir M, El-Sherif N. Pharmacological evaluation of early afterdepolarisations induced by sea anemone toxin (ATXII) in dog heart. *Cardiovasc Res* 1991;25:815–819.
140. Carlsson L, Abrahamsson C, Drews C, Duker GD. Antiarrhythmic effects of potassium channel openers in rhythm abnormalities related to delayed repolarization in the rabbit. *Circulation* 1992;85:1491–1500.
141. Nattel S, Quantz MA. Pharmacological response of quinidine induced early afterdepolarizations in canine cardiac Purkinje fibers: Insights into underlying ionic mechanisms. *Cardiovasc Res* 1988;22:808–817.
142. Sicouri S, Antzelevitch C. Afterdepolarizations and triggered activity develop in a select population of cells (M cells) in canine ventricular myocardium: The effects of acetylstrophanthidin and Bay K 8644. *Pacing Clin Electrophysiol* 1991;14: 1714–1720.
143. Liu DW, Antzelevitch C. Characteristics of the delayed rectifier current (IKr and IKs) in canine ventricular epicardial, midmyocardial, and endocardial myocytes. *Circ Res* 1995;76:351–365.
144. Burashnikov A, Antzelevitch C. Prominent IKs in epicardium and endocardium contributes to development of transmural dispersion of repolarization but protects against development of early afterdepolarizations. *J Cardiovasc Electrophysiol* 2002;13:172–177.
145. El-Sherif N, Caref EB, Yin H, Restivo M. The electrophysiological mechanism of ventricular arrhythmias in the long QT syndrome: Tridimensional mapping of activation and recovery patterns. *Circ Res* 1996;79:474–492.
146. Murakawa Y, Sezaki.K., Yamashita T, Kanese Y, Omata M. Three-dimensional activation sequence of cesium-induced ventricular arrhythmias. *Am J Physiol* 1997;273:H1377–H1385.
147. Belardinelli L, Antzelevitch C, Vos MA. Assessing predictors of drug-induced torsade de pointes. *Trends Pharmacol Sci* 2003;24:619–625.
148. Lankipalli RS, Zhu T, Guo D, Yan GX. Mechanisms underlying arrhythmogenesis in long QT syndrome. *J Electrocardiol* 2005;38(Suppl.):69–73.
149. Antzelevitch C. Role of transmural dispersion of repolarization in the genesis of drug-induced torsades de pointes. *Heart Rhythm* 2005;2:S9–S15.
150. Trautwein W. Mechanisms of tachyarrhythmias and extrasystoles. In: Sandoe E, Flensted-Jensen E, Olesen K, Eds. *Symposium on Cardiac Arrhythmias.* Sodertalje, Sweden: Astra, 1970:53.
151. Szabo B, Kovacs T, Lazzara R. Role of calcium loading in early afterdepolarizations generated by Cs in canine and guinea pig Purkinje fibers. *J Cardiovasc Electrophysiol* 1995;6:796–812.
152. Patterson E, Scherlag BJ, Szabo B, Lazzara R. Facilitation of epinephrine-induced afterdepolarizations by class III antiarrhythmic drugs. *J Electrocardiol* 1997;30:217–224.
153. Antzelevitch C. Cardiac repolarization. The long and short of it. *Europace* 2005;7(Suppl.)2:3–9.
154. Burashnikov A, Antzelevitch C. Block of I(Ks) does not induce early afterdepolarization activity but promotes beta-adrenergic agonist-induced

delayed afterdepolarization activity. *J Cardiovasc Electrophysiol* 2000;11:458–465.
155. Emori T, Antzelevitch C. Cellular basis for complex T waves and arrhythmic activity following combined I(Kr) and I(Ks) block. *J Cardiovasc Electrophysiol* 2001;12:1369–1378.
156. Shimizu W, Antzelevitch C. Differential effects of beta-adrenergic agonists and antagonists in LQT1, LQT2 and LQT3 models of the long QT syndrome. *J Am Coll Cardiol* 2000;35:778–786.
157. January CT, Riddle JM. Early afterdepolarizations: Mechanism of induction and block: A role for L-type Ca^{2+} current. *Circ Res* 1989;64:977–990.
158. Zeng J, Rudy Y. Early afterdepolarizations in cardiac myocytes: Mechanism and rate dependence. *Biophys J* 1995;68:949–964.
159. Ming Z, Nordin C, Aronson MD. Role of L-type calcium channel window current in generating current-induced early afterdepolarizations. *J Cardiovasc Electrophysiol* 1994;5:323–334.
160. Patterson E, Scherlag BJ, Lazzara R. Early afterdepolarizations produced by d,l-sotalol and clofilium. *J Cardiovasc Electrophysiol* 1997;8:667–678.
161. Zygmunt AC, Eddlestone GT, Thomas GP, Nesterenko VV, Antzelevitch C. Larger late sodium conductance in M cells contributes to electrical heterogeneity in canine ventricle. *Am J Physiol* 2001;281:H689–H697.
162. Maltsev VA, Sabbah HN, Higgins RS, Silverman N, Lesch M, Undrovinas AI. Novel, ultraslow inactivating sodium current in human ventricular cardiomyocytes. *Circulation* 1998;98:2545–2552.
163. Clancy CE, Tateyama M, Liu H, Wehrens XH, Kass RS. Non-equilibrium gating in cardiac Na+ channels: An original mechanism of arrhythmia. *Circulation* 2003;107:2233–2237.
164. Anderson ME. Calmodulin and the philosopher's stone: Changing Ca2+ into arrhythmias. *J Cardiovasc Electrophysiol* 2002;13:195–197.
165. Gbadebo TD, Trimble RW, Khoo MS, Temple J, Roden DM, Anderson ME. Calmodulin inhibitor W-7 unmasks a novel electrocardiographic parameter that predicts initiation of torsade de pointes. *Circulation* 2002;105:770–774.
166. Wu Y, MacMillan LB, McNeill RB, Colbran RJ, Anderson ME. CaM kinase augments cardiac L-type Ca2+ current: A cellular mechanism for long Q-T arrhythmias. *Am J Physiol* 1999;276:H2168–H2178.
167. Anderson ME. QT interval prolongation and arrhythmia: An unbreakable connection? *J Intern Med* 2006;259:81–90.
168. Ghosh S, Nunziato DA, Pitt GS. KCNQ1 assembly and function is blocked by long-QT syndrome mutations that disrupt interaction with calmodulin. *Circ Res* 2006;98:1048–1054.
169. Shamgar L, Ma L, Schmitt N, Haitin Y, Peretz A, Wiener R, Hirsch J, Pongs O, Attali B. Calmodulin is essential for cardiac IKS channel gating and assembly: Impaired function in long-QT mutations. *Circ Res* 2006;98:1055–1063.
170. Roden DM. A new role for calmodulin in ion channel biology. *Circ Res* 2006;98:979–981.
171. Wu Y, Roden DM, Anderson ME. Calmodulin kinase inhibition prevents development of the arrhythmogenic transient inward current. *Circ Res* 1999;84:906–912.
172. Anderson ME, Braun AP, Wu Y, Lu T, Wu Y, Schulman H, Sung RJ. KN-93, an inhibitor of multifunctional Ca++/calmodulin-dependent protein kinase, decreases early afterdepolarizations in rabbit heart. *J Pharmacol Exp Ther* 1998;287:996–1006.
173. Antzelevitch C, Belardinelli L, Zygmunt AC, Burashnikov A, Di Diego JM, Fish JM, Cordeiro JM, Thomas GP. Electrophysiologic effects of ranolazine: A novel anti-anginal agent with antiarrhythmic properties. *Circulation* 2004;110:904–910.
174. Antzelevitch C, Belardinelli L, Wu L, Fraser H, Zygmunt AC, Burashnikov A, Di Diego JM, Fish JM, Cordeiro JM, Goodrow RJ, Scornik FS, Perez GJ. Electrophysiologic properties and antiarrhythmic actions of a novel anti-anginal agent. *J Cardiovasc Pharmacol Therapeut* 2004;9(Suppl. 1): S65–S83.
175. Undrovinas AI, Belardinelli L, Undrovinas NA, Sabbah HN. Ranolazine improves abnormal repolarization and contraction in left ventricular myocytes of dogs with heart failure by inhibiting late sodium current. *J Cardiovasc Electrophysiol* 2006; 17:S161–S177.
176. Wu L, Shryock JC, Song Y, Li Y, Antzelevitch C, Belardinelli L. Antiarrhythmic effects of ranolazine in a guinea pig in vitro model of long-QT syndrome. *J Pharmacol Exp Ther* 2004;310:599–605.
177. Orth PM, Hesketh JC, Mak CK, Yang Y, Lin S, Beatch GN, Ezrin AM, Fedida D. RSD1235 blocks late I(Na) and suppresses early afterdepolarizations and torsades de pointes induced by class III agents. *Cardiovasc Res* 2006;70:486–496.
178. Roden DM, Lazzara R, Rosen MR, Schwartz PJ, Towbin JA, Vincent GM, The SADS Foundation Task Force on LQTS, Antzelevitch C, Brown AM, Colatsky TJ, Crampton RS, Kass RS, Moss AJ, Sanguinetti MC, Zipes DP. Multiple mechanisms in the long-QT syndrome: Current knowledge, gaps,

and future directions. *Circulation* 1996;94:1996–2012.

179. Antzelevitch C, Yan GX, Shimizu W, Sicouri S, Eddlestone GT, Zygmunt AC. Electrophysiologic characteristics of M cells and their role in arrhythmias. In: Franz MR, Ed. *Monophasic Action Potentials: Bridging Cell and Bedside.* Armonk, NY: Futura, 2000:583–604.
180. Ben-David J, Zipes DP. Differential response to right and left ansae subclaviae stimulation of early afterdepolarizations and ventricular tachycardia induced by cesium in dogs. *Circulation* 1988;78: 1241–1250.
181. Jackman WM, Friday KJ, Anderson JL, Aliot EM, Clark MA, Lazzara R. The long QT syndromes: A critical review, new clinical observations and a unifying hypothesis. *Prog Cardiovasc Dis* 1988; 31:115–172.
182. Shimizu W, Ohe T, Kurita T, Takaki H, Aihara N, Kamakura S, Matsuhisa M, Shimomura K. Early afterdepolarizations induced by isoproterenol in patients with congenital long QT syndrome. *Circulation* 1991;84:1915–1923.
183. Asano Y, Davidenko JM, Baxter WT, Gray RA, Jalife J. Optical mapping of drug-induced polymorphic arrhythmias and torsade de pointes in the isolated rabbit heart. *J Am Coll Cardiol* 1997;29: 831–842.
184. Ben-David J, Zipes DP, Ayers GM, Pride HP. Canine left ventricular hypertrophy predisposes to ventricular tachycardia induction by phase 2 early afterdepolarizations after administration of BAY K 8644. *J Am Coll Cardiol* 1992;20(7):1576–1584.
185. Beuckelmann DJ, Nabauer M, Erdmann E. Alterations of K^+ currents in isolated human ventricular myocytes from patients with terminal heart failure. *Circ Res* 1993;73:379–385.
186. Antzelevitch C. Heterogeneity and cardiac arrhythmias: An overview. *Heart Rhythm* 2007; in press.
187. Yan GX, Rials SJ, Wu Y, Liu T, Xu X, Marinchak RA, Kowey PR. Ventricular hypertrophy amplifies transmural repolarization dispersion and induces early afterdepolarization. *Am J Physiol* 2001;281: H1968–H1975.
188. Antzelevitch C, Oliva A. Amplification of spatial dispersion of repolarization underlies sudden cardiac death associated with catecholaminergic polymorphic VT, long QT, short QT and Brugada syndromes. *J Intern Med* 2006;259:48–58.
189. Liu J, Laurita KR. The mechanism of pause-induced torsade de pointes in long QT syndrome. *J Cardiovasc Electrophysiol* 2005;16:981–987.
190. Baskin EP, Lynch JJ Jr. Differential atrial versus ventricular activities of class III potassium channel blockers. *J Pharmacol Exp Ther* 1998;285:135–142.
191. Burashnikov A, Mannava S, Antzelevitch C. Transmembrane action potential heterogeneity in the canine isolated arterially-perfused atrium: Effect of IKr and Ito/IKur block. *Am J Physiol* 2004;286: H2393–H2400.
192. Vincent GM. Atrial arrhythmias in the inherited long QT syndrome. *J Cardiovasc Electrophysiol* 2003;14:1034–1035.
193. Ferrier GR, Saunders JH, Mendez C. A cellular mechanism for the generation of ventricular arrhythmias by acetylstrophanthidin. *Circ Res* 1973;32:600–609.
194. Rosen MR, Gelband H, Merker C, Hoffman BF. Mechanisms of digitalis toxicity—effects of ouabain on phase four of canine Purkinje fiber transmembrane potentials. *Circulation* 1973;47: 681–689.
195. Saunders JH, Ferrier GR, Moe GK. Conduction block associated with transient depolarizations induced by acetylstrophanthidin in isolated canine Purkinje fibers. *Circ Res* 1973;32:610–617.
196. Marchi S, Szabo B, Lazzara R. Adrenergic induction of delayed afterdepolarizations in ventricular myocardial cells: Beta-induction and alpha-modulation. *J Cardiovasc Electrophysiol* 1991;2:476–491.
197. Matsuda H, Noma A, Kurachi Y, Irisawa H. Transient depolarizations and spontaneous voltage fluctuations in isolated single cells from guinea pig ventricles. *Circ Res* 1982;51:142–151.
198. Spinelli W, Sorota S, Siegel MB, Hoffman BF. Antiarrhythmic actions of the ATP-regulated K^+ current activated by pinacidil. *Circ Res* 1991;68: 1127–1137.
199. Belardinelli LL, Isenberg G. Actions of adenosine and isoproterenol on isolated mammalian ventricular myocytes. *Circ Res* 1983;53(3):287–297.
200. Antzelevitch C, Sicouri S, Litovsky SH, Lukas A, Krishnan SC, Di Diego JM, Gintant GA, Liu DW. Heterogeneity within the ventricular wall. Electrophysiology and pharmacology of epicardial, endocardial, and M cells. *Circ Res* 1991;69: 1427–1449.
201. Sicouri S, Antzelevitch C. Drug-induced afterdepolarizations and triggered activity occur in a discrete subpopulation of ventricular muscle cell (M cells) in the canine heart: Quinidine and digitalis. *J Cardiovasc Electrophysiol* 1993;4: 48–58.

202. Schreieck J, Wang YG, Gjini V, Korth M, Zrenner B, Schomig A, Schmitt C. Differential effect of beta-adrenergic stimulation on the frequency-dependent electrophysiologic actions of the new class III antiarrhythmics dofetilide, ambasilide, and chromanol 293B. *J Cardiovasc Electrophysiol* 1997;8:1420–1430.
203. Coetzee WA, Opie LH. Effects of components of ischemia and metabolic inhibition on delayed afterdepolarizations in guinea pig papillary muscle. *Circ Res* 1987;61:157–165.
204. Pogwizd SM, Onufer JR, Kramer JB, Sobel BE, Corr PB. Induction of delayed afterdepolarizations and triggered activity in canine Purkinje fibers by lysophosphoglycerides. *Circ Res* 1986;59:416–426.
205. Song Y, Belardinelli L. ATP promotes development of afterdepolarizations and triggered activity in cardiac myocytes. *Am J Physiol* 1994;267: H2005–H2011.
206. Nam G-B, Burashnikov A, Antzelevitch C. Cellular mechanisms underlying the development of catecholaminergic ventricular tachycardia. *Circulation* 2005;111:2727–2733.
207. Mary-Rabine L, Hordof AJ, Danilo P, Malm JR, Rosen MR. Mechanisms for impulse initiation in isolated human atrial fibers. *Circ Res* 1980;47: 267–277.
208. Nordin C, Gilat E, Aronson RS. Delayed afterdepolarizations and triggered activity in ventricular muscle from rats with streptozotocin-induced diabetes. *Circ Res* 1985;57:28–34.
209. Priori SG, Napolitano C, Memmi M, Colombi B, Drago F, Gasparini M, DeSimone L, Coltorti F, Bloise R, Keegan R, Cruz Filho FE, Vignati G, Benatar A, DeLogu A. Clinical and molecular characterization of patients with catecholaminergic polymorphic ventricular tachycardia. *Circulation* 2002;106:69–74.
210. Caroni P, Villani F, Carafoli E. The cardiotoxic antibiotic doxorubicin inhibits the Na+/Ca2+ exchange of dog heart sarcolemmal vesicles. *FEBS Lett* 1981;130:184–186.
211. Gorgels APM, Vos MA, Smeets JL, Kriek E, Brugada P, Wellens HJ. Delayed afterdepolarizations and atrial and ventricular arrhythmias. In: Rosen MR, Janse MJ, Wit AL, Eds. *Cardiac Electrophysiology: A Textbook*. Mount Kisco, NY: Futura Publishing Company, Inc., 1990:341.
212. Tytgat J, Vereecke J, Carmeliet E. Differential effects of verapamil and flunarizine on cardiac L-type and T-type Ca channels. *Naunyn Schmiedebergs Arch Pharmacol* 1988;337(6):690–692.
213. Vos MA, Gorgels APM, Leunissen JDM, Wellens HJ. Flunarizine allows differentiation between mechanisms of arrhythmias in the intact heart. *Circulation* 1990;81:343–349.
214. Park JK, Danilo P, Rosen MR. Effects of flunarizine on impulse formation in canine Purkinje fibers. *J Cardiovasc Electrophysiol* 1992;3:306–314.
215. Chattipakorn N, Ideker RE. Delayed afterdepolarization inhibitor: A potential pharmacologic intervention to improve defibrillation efficacy. *J Cardiovasc Electrophysiol* 2003;14:72–75.
216. Letienne R, Vie B, Puech A, Vieu S, Le Grand B, John GW. Evidence that ranolazine behaves as a weak beta1- and beta2-adrenoceptor antagonist in the cat cardiovascular system. *Naunyn Schmiedebergs Arch Pharmacol* 2001;363:464–471.
217. Belardinelli L, Antzelevitch C, Fraser H. Inhibition of late (sustained/persistent) sodium current: A potential drug target to reduce intracellular sodium-dependent calcium overload and its detrimental effects on cardiomyocyte function. *Eur Heart J Suppl* 2004;6:i3–i7.
218. Takahara A, Sugiyama A, Hashimoto K. Effects of class I antiarrhythmic drugs on the digitalis-induced triggered activity arrhythmia model: A rationale for the short-term use of class I drugs against triggered arrhythmias. *Heart Vessels* 2004;19:43–48.
219. Kass RS, Tsien RW, Weingart R. Ionic basis of transient inward current induced by strophanthidin in cardiac Purkinje fibres. *J Physiol (Lond)* 1978;281:209–226.
220. Cannell MB, Lederer WJ. The arrhythmogenic current I_{TI} in the absence of electrogenic sodium-calcium exchange in sheep cardiac Purkinje fibres. *J Physiol (Lond)* 1986;374:201–219.
221. Fedida D, Noble D, Rankin AC, Spindler AJ. The arrhythmogenic transient inward current I_{ti} and related contraction in isolated guinea-pig ventricular myocytes. *J Physiol (Lond)* 1987;392:523–542.
222. Laflamme MA, Becker PL. Ca2+-induced current oscillations in rabbit ventricular myocytes. *Circ Res* 1996;78:707–716.
223. Zygmunt AC, Goodrow RJ, Weigel CM. I_{NaCa} and $I_{Cl(Ca)}$ contribute to isoproterenol-induced delayed afterdepolarizations in midmyocardial cells. *Am J Physiol* 1998;275:H1979–H1992.
224. Ritchie AH, Kerr CR, Qi A, Yeung-Lai-Wah JA. Nonsustained ventricular tachycardia arising from the right ventricular outflow tract. *Am J Cardiol* 1989;64:594–598.
225. Wilber DJ, Blakeman BM, Pifarre R, Scanlon PJ. Catecholamine sensitive right ventricular outflow tract tachycardia: Intraoperative mapping and

ablation of a free-wall focus. *Pacing Clin Electrophysiol* 1989;12:1851–1856.
226. Cardinal R, Scherlag BJ, Vermeulen M, Armour JA. Distinct activation patterns of idioventricular rhythms and sympathetically-induced ventricular tachycardias in dogs with atrioventricular block. *Pacing Clin Electrophysiol* 1992;15:1300–1316.
227. Cardinal R, Savard P, Armour JA, Nadeau RA, Carson DL, LeBlanc AR. Mapping of ventricular tachycardia induced by thoracic neural stimulation in dogs. *Can J Physiol Pharmacol* 1986;64: 411–418.
228. Lerman BB, Belardinelli LL, West GA, Berne RM, DiMarco JP. Adenosine-sensitive ventricular tachycardia: Evidence suggesting cyclic AMP-mediated triggered activity. *Circulation* 1986;74: 270–280.
229. Lerman BB, Stein K, Engelstein ED, Battleman DS, Lippman N, Bei D, Catanzaro D. Mechanism of repetitive monomorphic ventricular tachycardia. *Circulation* 1995;92:421–429.
230. Ter Keurs HE, Schouten VJA, Bucx JJ, Mulder BM, De Tombe PP. Excitation-contraction coupling in myocardium: Implications of calcium release and Na+-Ca2+ exchange. *Can J Physiol Pharmacol* 1987;65:619–626.
231. Iwai S, Markowitz SM, Stein KM, Mittal S, Slotwiner DJ, Das MK, Cohen JD, Hao SC, Lerman BB. Response to adenosine differentiates focal from macroreentrant atrial tachycardia: Validation using three-dimensional electroanatomic mapping. *Circulation* 2002;106:2793–2799.
232. Fenelon G, Shepard RK, Stambler BS. Focal origin of atrial tachycardia in dogs with rapid ventricular pacing-induced heart failure. *J Cardiovasc Electrophysiol* 2003;14:1093–1102.
233. Rubart M, Zipes DP. Mechanisms of sudden cardiac death. *J Clin Invest* 2005;115:2305–2315.
234. Leenhardt A, Lucet V, Denjoy I, Grau F, Ngoc DD, Coumel P. Catecholaminergic polymorphic ventricular tachycardia in children: A 7-year follow-up of 21 patients. *Circulation* 1995;91:1512–1519.
235. Swan H, Piippo K, Viitasalo M, Heikkila P, Paavonen T, Kainulainen K, Kere J, Keto P, Kontula K, Toivonen L. Arrhythmic disorder mapped to chromosome 1q42-q43 causes malignant polymorphic ventricular tachycardia in structurally normal hearts. *J Am Coll Cardiol* 1999;34:2035–2042.
236. Priori SG, Napolitano C, Tiso N, Memmi M, Vignati G, Bloise R, Sorrentino V, Danieli GA. Mutations in the cardiac ryanodine receptor gene (hRyR2) underlie catecholaminergic polymorphic ventricular tachycardia. *Circulation* 2001;103: 196–200.
237. Laitinen PJ, Brown KM, Piippo K, Swan H, Devaney JM, Brahmbhatt B, Donarum EA, Marino M, Tiso N, Viitasalo M, Toivonen L, Stephan DA, Kontula K. Mutations of the cardiac ryanodine receptor (RyR2) gene in familial polymorphic ventricular tachycardia. *Circulation* 2001;103:485–490.
238. Postma AV, Denjoy I, Hoorntje TM, Lupoglazoff JM, Da Costa A, Sebillon P, Mannens MM, Wilde AA, Guicheney P. Absence of calsequestrin 2 causes severe forms of catecholaminergic polymorphic ventricular tachycardia. *Circ Res* 2002;91: e21–e26.
239. Volders PG, Vos MA, Szabo B, Sipido KR, De Groot SH, Gorgels AP, Wellens HJ, Lazzara R. Progress in the understanding of cardiac early afterdepolarizations and torsades de pointes: Time to revise current concepts. *Cardiovasc Res* 2000;46:376–392.
240. Watanabe I, Okumura Y, Ohkubo K, Kawauchi K, Takagi Y, Sugimura H, Shindo A, Nakai T, Ozawa Y, Saito S. Steady-state and nonsteady-state action potentials in fibrillating canine atrium: Alternans of action potential and late phase 3 early afterdepolarization as a precursor of atrial fibrillation. *Heart Rhythm* 2005;2:S259 (abstract).
241. Patterson E, Po SS, Scherlag BJ, Lazzara R. Triggered firing in pulmonary veins initiated by in vitro autonomic nerve stimulation *Heart Rhythm* 2005;2:624–631.
242. Kirchhof P, Klimas J, Fabritz L, Zweiner M, Jones LR, Schafers M, Hermann S, Boknik P, Neumann J, Schmitz W. Mechanism of catecholamine-induced ventricular tachycardias in mice with heart-directed expression of junctin and triadin: Shortening of action potentials and prolonging calcium transients. *Heart Rhythm* 2005;2:S69 (abstract).
243. Leistad E, Christensen G, Ilebekk A. Atrial contractile performance after cessation of atrial fibrillation. *Am J Physiol* 1993;264:H104–H109.
244. Oral H, Ozaydin M, Sticherling C, Tada H, Scharf C, Chugh A, Lai SW, Pelosi F Jr, Knight BP, Strickberger SA, Morady F. Effect of atrial fibrillation duration on probability of immediate recurrence after transthoracic cardioversion. *J Cardiovasc Electrophysiol* 2003;14:182–185.
245. Schwartzman D, Musley SK, Swerdlow C, Hoyt RH, Warman EN. Early recurrence of atrial fibrillation after ambulatory shock conversion. *J Am Coll Cardiol* 2002;40:93–99.
246. Timmermans C, Rodriguez LM, Smeets JL, Wellens HJ. Immediate reinitiation of atrial fibrillation fol-

lowing internal atrial defibrillation. *J Cardiovasc Electrophysiol* 1998;9:122–128.
247. Bers DM. *Excitation-Contraction Coupling and Cardiac Contractile Force*, 2nd ed. Dordrecht, The Netherlands: Kluwer Academic Publishers, 2001.
248. Attuel P, Leclercq JF, Halimi F, Fiorello P, Stiubei M, Seing S. Bigeminy pacing: A new protocol to unmask atrial vulnerability. *J Cardiovasc Electrophysiol* 2003;14:10–15.
249. Mines GR. On dynamic equilibrium in the heart. *J Physiol (Lond)* 1913;46:350–383.
250. Kent AFS. Observation on the auriculo-ventricular junction of the mammalian heart. *Q J Exp Physiol* 1913;7:193–197.
251. Schmitt FO, Erlanger J. Directional differences in the conduction of the impulse through heart muscle and their possible relation to extrasystolic and fibrillary contractions. *Am J Physiol* 1928;87: 326–347.
252. Cranefield PF, Hoffman BF. Conduction of the cardiac impulse. II. Summation and inhibition. *Circ Res* 1971;28:220–233.
253. Cranefield PF, Klein HO, Hoffman BF. Conduction of the cardiac impulse. I. Delay, block and one-way block in depressed Purkinje fibers. *Circ Res* 1971;28:199–219.
254. Sasyniuk BI, Mendez C. A mechanism for reentry in canine ventricular tissue. *Circ Res* 1971;28: 3–15.
255. Wit AL, Cranefield PF, Hoffman BF. Slow conduction and reentry in the ventricular conducting system. II. Single and sustained circus movement in networks of canine and bovine Purkinje fibers. *Circ Res* 1972;30:11–22.
256. Wit AL, Hoffman BF, Cranefield PF. Slow conduction and reentry in the ventricular conducting system. I. Return extrasystoles in canine Purkinje fibers. *Circ Res* 1972;30:1–10.
257. Cranefield PF. *The Conduction of the Cardiac Impulse.* Mount Kisco, NY: Futura, 1975.
258. Garrey WE. Auricular fibrillation. *Physiol Rev* 1924;4:215–250.
259. Allessie MA, Bonke FIM, Schopman JG. Circus movement in rabbit atrial muscle as a mechanism of tachycardia. *Circ Res* 1973;33:54–62.
260. Allessie MA, Bonke FIM, Schopman JG. Circus movement in rabbit atrial muscle as a mechanism of tachycardia: II. The role of nonuniform recovery of excitability in the occurrence of unidirectional block as studied with multiple microelectrodes. *Circ Res* 1976;39:168–177.
261. Allessie MA, Bonke FIM, Schopman JG. Circus movement in rabbit atrial muscle as a mechanism of tachycardia. III. The "leading circle" concept: A new model of circus movement in cardiac tissue without the involvement of an anatomical obstacle. *Circ Res* 1977;41:9–18.
262. Kamiyama A, Eguchi K, Shibayama R. Circus movement tachycardia induced by a single premature stimulus on the ventricular sheet: Evaluation of the leading circle hypothesis in the canine ventricular muscle. *Jpn Circ J* 1986;50:65–73.
263. Allessie MA, Schalij MJ, Kirchhof CJ, Boersma L, Huybers M, Hollen J. Experimental electrophysiology and arrhythmogenicity. Anisotropy and ventricular tachycardia. *Eur Heart J* 1989;10(Suppl. E):2–8.
264. El-Sherif N, Smith RA, Evans K. Canine ventricular arrhythmias in the late myocardial infarction period. 8. Epicardial mapping of reentrant circuits. *Circ Res* 1981;49:255–265.
265. El-Sherif N, Mehra R, Gough WB, Zeiler RH. Ventricular activation pattern of spontaneous and induced ventricular rhythms in canine one-day-old myocardial infarction. Evidence for focal and reentrant mechanisms. *Circ Res* 1982;51:152–166.
266. Mehra R, Zeiler RH, Gough WB, El-Sherif N. Reentrant ventricular arrhythmias in the late myocardial infarction period. 9. Electrophysiologic-anatomic correlation of reentrant circuits. *Circulation* 1983;67:11–24.
267. El-Sherif N, Mehra R, Gough WB, Zeiler RH. Reentrant ventricular arrhythmias in the late myocardial infarction period. Interruption of reentrant circuits by cyrothermal techniques. *Circulation* 1983;68:644–656.
268. Wit AL, Allessie MA, Bonke FIM, Lammers WJEP, Smeets JL, Fenoglio JJ. Electrophysiological mapping to determine the mechanisms of experimental ventricular tachycardia initiated by premature impulses. Experimental approach and initial results demonstrating reentrant excitation. *Am J Cardiol* 1982;49:166–185.
269. Dillon SM, Allessie MA, Ursell PC, Wit AL. Influences of anisotropic tissue structure on reentrant circuits in the epicardial border zone of subacute canine infarcts. *Circ Res* 1988;63:182–206.
270. Clerc L. Directional differences of impulse spread in trabecular muscle from mammalian heart. *J Physiol (Lond)* 1976;255:335–346.
271. Harumi K, Burgess MJ, Abildskov JA. A theoretic model of the T wave. *Circulation* 1966;34:657–668.
272. Spach MS, Kootsey JM, Sloan JD. Active modulation of electrical coupling between cardiac cells of the dog. A mechanism for transient and steady state variations in conduction velocity. *Circ Res* 1982;51:347–362.

273. El-Sherif N. The figure 8 model of reentrant excitation in the canine post-infarction heart. In: Zipes DP, Jalife J, Eds. *Cardiac Electrophysiology and Arrhythmias*. New York: Grune & Stratton, 1985:363–378.
274. Lin SF, Roth BJ, Wikswo JP Jr. Quatrefoil reentry in myocardium: An optical imaging study of the induction mechanism. *J Cardiovasc Electrophysiol* 1999;10:574–586.
275. Weiner N, Rosenblueth A. The mathematical formulation of the problem of conduction of impulses in a network of connected excitable elements, specifically in cardiac muscle. *Arch Inst Cardiol Mex* 1946;16:205–265.
276. Davidenko JM, Kent PF, Chialvo DR, Michaels DC, Jalife J. Sustained vortex-like waves in normal isolated ventricular muscle. *Proc Natl Acad Sci USA* 1990;87:8785–8789.
277. Pertsov AM, Davidenko JM, Salomonsz R, Baxter WT, Jalife J. Spiral waves of excitation underlie reentrant activity in isolated cardiac muscle. *Circ Res* 1993;72:631–650.
278. Winfree AT. How does ventricular tachycardia decay into ventricular fibrillation. In: Shenasa M, Borggrefe M, Breithardt G, Eds. *Cardiac Mapping*. Mount Kisco, NY: Futura Publishing Co., 1993: 655–680.
279. Lechleiter J, Girard S, Peralta E, Clapham D. Spiral calcium wave propagation and annihilation in Xenopus laevis oocytes. *Science* 1991;252:123–126.
280. Jalife J, Davidenko JM, Michaels DC. A new perspective on the mechanisms of arrhythmias and sudden cardiac death: Spiral wave of excitation in heart muscle. *J Cardiovasc Electrophysiol* 1991;2: S133–S152.
281. Athill CA, Ikeda T, Kim YH, Wu TJ, Fishbein MC, Karagueuzian HS, Chen PS. Transmembrane potential properties at the core of functional reentrant wave fronts in isolated canine right atria. *Circulation* 1998;98:1556–1567.
282. Jalife J, Delmar M, Davidenko JM, Anumonwo JMB. *Basic Cardiac Electrophysiology for the Clinician*. Armonk, NY: Futura Publishing, 1999.
283. Pertsov AM, Jalife J. Three-dimensional vortex-like reentry. In: Zipes DP, Jalife J, Eds. *Cardiac Electrophysiology: From Cell to Bedside*, 2nd ed. Philadelphia: W.B. Saunders, 1995:403–410.
284. Davidenko JM. Spiral wave activity: A possible common mechanism for polymorphic and monomorphic ventricular tachycardias. *J Cardiovasc Electrophysiol* 1993;4:730–746.
285. Garfinkel A, Qu Z. Nonlinear dynamics of excitation and propagation in cardiac muscle. In: Zipes DP, Jalife J, Eds. *Cardiac Electrophysiology: From Cell to Bedside*, 3rd ed. Philadelphia: W.B. Saunders, 1999:315–320.
286. De Bakker JMT, Van Capelle FJL, Janse MJ, *et al.* Reentry as a cause of ventricular tachycardia in patients with chronic ischemic disease: Electrophysiologic and anatomic correlation. *Circulation* 1988;77:589–606.
287. Stevenson WG, Nademanee K, Weiss JN, Weiner I, Baron K, Yeatman LA, Sherman CT. Programmed electrical stimulation at potential ventricular reentry circuit sites. Comparison of observations in humans with predictions from computer simulations. *Circulation* 1989;80:793–806.
288. Berenfeld O, Jalife J. Purkinje-muscle reentry as a mechanism of polymorphic ventricular arrhythmias in a 3-dimensional model of the ventricles. *Circ Res* 1998;82:1063–1077.
289. Comtois P, Kneller J, Nattel S. Of circles and spirals: Bridging the gap between the leading circle and spiral wave concepts of cardiac reentry. *Europace* 2005;7(Suppl. 2):10–20.
290. Wit AL, Janse MJ. *The Ventricular Arrhythmias of Ischemia and Infarction. Electrophysiological Mechanisms*. Mount Kisco, NY: Futura, 1993.
291. Moe GK, Rheinboldt WC, Abildskov JA. A computer model of atrial fibrillation. *Am Heart J* 1964; 67:200–220.
292. Scherf D, Romano FJ, Terranova R. Experimental studies on auricular flutter and auricular fibrillation. *Am Heart J* 1948;36:241–251.
293. Jalife J. Ventricular fibrillation: Mechanisms of initiation and maintenance. *Annu Rev Physiol* 2000;62:25–50.
294. Chen J, Mandapati R, Berenfeld O, Skanes AC, Jalife J. High-frequency periodic sources underlie ventricular fibrillation in the isolated rabbit heart. *Circ Res* 2000;86:86–93.
295. Schuessler RB, Grayson TM, Bromberg BI, Cox JL, Boineau JP. Cholinergically mediated tachyarrhythmias induced by a single extrastimulus in the isolated canine right atrium. *Circ Res* 1992;71: 1254–1267.
296. Zaitsev AV, Berenfeld O, Mironov SF, Jalife J, Pertsov AM. Distribution of excitation frequencies on the epicardial and endocardial surfaces of fibrillating ventricular wall of the sheep heart. *Circ Res* 2000;86:408–417.
297. Samie FH, Berenfeld O, Anumonwo J, Mironov SF, Udassi S, Beaumont J, Taffet S, Pertsov AM, Jalife J. Rectification of the background potassium current: A determinant of rotor dynamics in ventricular fibrillation. *Circ Res* 2001;89:1216–1223.

298. Zhou S, Chang CM, Wu TJ, Miyauchi Y, Okuyama Y, Park AM, Hamabe A, Omichi C, Hayashi H, Brodsky LA, Mandel WJ, Ting CT, Fishbein MC, Karagueuzian HS, Chen PS. Nonreentrant focal activations in pulmonary veins in canine model of sustained atrial fibrillation. *Am J Physiol* 2002;283: H1244–H1252.
299. Everett TH, Wilson EE, Foreman S, Olgin JE. Mechanisms of ventricular fibrillation in canine models of congestive heart failure and ischemia assessed by in vivo noncontact mapping. *Circulation* 2005;112:1532–1541.
300. Cabo C, Pertsov AM, Davidenko JM, Baxter WT, Gray RA, Jalife J. Vortex shedding as a precursor of turbulent electrical activity in cardiac muscle. *Biophys J* 1996;70:1105–1111.
301. Valderrabano M, Chen PS, Lin SF. Spatial distribution of phase singularities in ventricular fibrillation. *Circulation* 2003;108:354–359.
302. Ideker RE, Huang J. Our search for the porcine mother rotor. *Ann Noninvasive Electrocardiol* 2005;10:7–15.
303. Weiss JN, Qu Z, Chen PS, Lin SF, Karagueuzian HS, Hayashi H, Garfinkel A, Karma A. The dynamics of cardiac fibrillation. *Circulation* 2005;112: 1232–1240.
304. Qin H, Huang J, Rogers JM, Walcott GP, Rollins DL, Smith WM, Ideker RE. Mechanisms for the maintenance of ventricular fibrillation: The nonuniform dispersion of refractoriness, restitution properties, or anatomic heterogeneities? *J Cardiovasc Electrophysiol* 2005;16:888–897.
305. Wu TJ, Yashima M, Xie F, Athill CA, Kim YH, Fishbein MC, Qu Z, Garfinkel A, Weiss JN, Karagueuzian HS, Chen PS. Role of pectinate muscle bundles in the generation and maintenance of intra-atrial reentry: Potential implications for the mechanism of conversion between atrial fibrillation and atrial flutter. *Circ Res* 1998;83:448–462.
306. Hamabe A, Okuyama Y, Miyauchi Y, Zhou S, Pak HN, Karagueuzian HS, Fishbein MC, Chen PS. Correlation between anatomy and electrical activation in canine pulmonary veins. *Circulation* 2003;107:1550–1555.
307. Weiss JN, Chen PS, Qu Z, Karagueuzian HS, Lin SF, Garfinkel A. Electrical restitution and cardiac fibrillation. *J Cardiovasc Electrophysiol* 2002;13: 292–295.
308. Wu TJ, Lin SF, Weiss JN, Ting CT, Chen PS. Two types of ventricular fibrillation in isolated rabbit hearts: Importance of excitability and action potential duration restitution. *Circulation* 2002; 106:1859–1866.
309. Omichi C, Lamp ST, Lin SF, Yang J, Baher A, Zhou S, Attin M, Lee MH, Karagueuzian HS, Kogan B, Qu Z, Garfinkel A, Chen PS, Weiss JN. Intracellular Ca dynamics in ventricular fibrillation. *Am J Physiol* 2004;286:H1836–H1844.
310. Attuel P, Childers R, Cauchemez B, Poveda J, Mugica J, Coumel P. Failure in the rate adaptation of the atrial refractory period: Its relationship to vulnerability. *Int J Cardiol* 1982;2:179–197.
311. Wijffels MC, Kirchhof CJ, Dorland R, Allessie MA. Atrial fibrillation begets atrial fibrillation. A study in awake chronically instrumented goats. *Circulation* 1995;92:1954–1968.
312. Burashnikov A, Antzelevitch C. Role of repolarization restitution in the development of coarse and fine atrial fibrillation in the isolated canine right atria. *J Cardiovasc Electrophysiol* 2005;16:639–645.
313. Gray RA, Jalife J, Panfilov AV, Baxter WT, Cabo C, Davidenko JM, Pertsov AM. Mechanisms of cardiac fibrillation. *Science* 1995;270:1222–1223.
314. Janse MJ, Wilms-Schopman FJG, Coronel R. Ventricular fibrillation is not always due to multiple wavelet reentry. *J Cardiovasc Electrophysiol* 1995; 6:512–521.
315. Antzelevitch C. Ion channels and ventricular arrhythmias: Cellular and ionic mechanisms underlying the Brugada syndrome. *Curr Opin Cardiol* 1999;14:274–279.
316. Janse MJ, Van Capelle FJL, Morsink H, Kleber AG, Wilms-Schopman FJG, Cardinal R, Naumann D'Alnoncourt C, Durrer D. Flow of "injury" current and patterns of excitation during early ventricular arrhythmias in acute regional myocardial ischemia in isolated porcine and canine hearts. Evidence for two different arrhythmogenic mechanisms. *Circ Res* 1980;47:151–167.
317. Pogwizd SM, Corr PB. Mechanisms underlying the development of ventricular fibrillation during early myocardial ischemia. *Circ Res* 1990;66:672–695.
318. Riccio ML, Koller ML, Gilmour RF Jr. Electrical restitution and spatiotemporal organization during ventricular fibrillation. *Circ Res* 1999;84:955–963.
319. Rogers JC, Huang JL, Smith WM, Ideker RE. Incidence, evolution, and spatial distribution of functional reentry during ventricular fibrillation in pigs. *Circ Res* 1999;84:945–954.
320. Weiss JN, Garfinkel A, Karagueuzian HS, Qu Z, Chen PS. Chaos and the transition to ventricular fibrillation: A new approach to antiarrhythmic drug evaluation. *Circulation* 1999;99:2819–2826.

321. Choi BR, Liu T, Salama G. The distribution of refractory periods influences the dynamics of ventricular fibrillation. *Circ Res* 2001;88:E49–E58.
322. Chen PS, Wu TJ, Ting CT, Karagueuzian HS, Garfinkel A, Lin SF, Weiss JN. A tale of two fibrillations. *Circulation* 2003;108:2298–2303.
323. Li D, Zhang L, Kneller J, Nattel S. Potential ionic mechanism for repolarization differences between canine right and left atrium. *Circ Res* 2001;88:1168–1175.
324. Sarmast F, Kolli A, Zaitsev A, Parisian K, Dhamoon AS, Guha PK, Warren M, Anumonwo JM, Taffet SM, Berenfeld O, Jalife J. Cholinergic atrial fibrillation: I(K,ACh) gradients determine unequal left/right atrial frequencies and rotor dynamics. *Cardiovasc Res* 2003;59:863–873.
325. Antzelevitch C, Moe GK. Electrotonically-mediated delayed conduction and reentry in relation to "slow responses" in mammalian ventricular conducting tissue. *Circ Res* 1981;49:1129–1139.
326. Rozanski GJ, Jalife J, Moe GK. Reflected reentry in nonhomogeneous ventricular muscle as a mechanism of cardiac arrhythmias. *Circulation* 1984;69: 163–173.
327. Lukas A, Antzelevitch C. Reflected reentry, delayed conduction, and electrotonic inhibition in segmentally depressed atrial tissues. *Can J Physiol Pharmacol* 1989;67:757–764.
328. Davidenko JM, Antzelevitch C. The effects of milrinone on action potential characteristics, conduction, automaticity, and reflected reentry in isolated myocardial fibers. *J Cardiovasc Pharmacol* 1985;7:341–349.
329. Rosenthal JE, Ferrier GR. Contribution of variable entrance and exit block in protected foci to arrhythmogenesis in isolated ventricular tissues. *Circulation* 1983;67:1–8.
330. Antzelevitch C, Lukas A. Reflection and reentry in isolated ventricular tissue. In: Dangman KH, Miura DS, Eds. *Basic and Clinical Electrophysiology of the Heart.* New York: Marcel Dekker, 1991: 251–275.
331. Antzelevitch C, Moe GK. Electrotonic inhibition and summation of impulse conduction in mammalian Purkinje fibers. *Am J Physiol* 1983;245: H42–H53.
332. Jalife J, Moe GK. Excitation, conduction, and reflection of impulses in isolated bovine and canine cardiac Purkinje fibers. *Circ Res* 1981;49: 233–247.
333. Davidenko JM, Antzelevitch C. Electrophysiological mechanisms underlying rate-dependent changes of refractoriness in normal and segmentally depressed canine Purkinje fibers. The characteristics of post-repolarization refractoriness. *Circ Res* 1986;58:257–268.
334. Davidenko JM, Antzelevitch C. The effects of milrinone on conduction, reflection, and automaticity in canine Purkinje fibers. *Circulation* 984;69: 1026–1035.
335. Winkle RA. The relationship between ventricular ectopic beat frequency and heart rate. *Circulation* 1982;66:439–446.
336. Nau GJ, Aldariz AE, Acunzo RS, *et al.* Clinical studies on the mechanism of ventricular arrhythmias. In: Rosenbaum MB, Elizari MV, Eds. *Frontier of Cardiac Electrophysiology.* Amsterdam: Martinus Nijhoff, 1983:239–273.
337. Rosenthal JE. Reflected reentry in depolarized foci with variable conduction impairment in 1 day old infarcted canine cardiac tissue. *J Am Coll Cardiol* 1988;12:404–411.
338. Van Hemel NM, Swenne CA, De Bakker JMT, Defauw JAM, Guiraudon GM. Epicardial reflection as a cause of incessant ventricular bigeminy. *Pacing Clin Electrophysiol* 1988;11:1036–1044.
339. Litovsky SH, Antzelevitch C. Transient outward current prominent in canine ventricular epicardium but not endocardium. *Circ Res* 1988;62: 116–126.
340. Liu DW, Gintant GA, Antzelevitch C. Ionic bases for electrophysiological distinctions among epicardial, midmyocardial, and endocardial myocytes from the free wall of the canine left ventricle. *Circ Res* 1993;72:671–687.
341. Furukawa T, Myerburg RJ, Furukawa N, Bassett AL, Kimura S. Differences in transient outward currents of feline endocardial and epicardial myocytes. *Circ Res* 1990;67:1287–1291.
342. Fedida D, Giles WR. Regional variations in action potentials and transient outward current in myocytes isolated from rabbit left ventricle. *J Physiol (Lond)* 1991;442:191–209.
343. Clark RB, Bouchard RA, Salinas-Stefanon E, Sanchez-Chapula J, Giles WR. Heterogeneity of action potential waveforms and potassium currents in rat ventricle. *Cardiovasc Res* 1993;27: 1795–1799.
344. Wettwer E, Amos GJ, Posival H, Ravens U. Transient outward current in human ventricular myocytes of subepicardial and subendocardial origin. *Circ Res* 1994;75:473–482.
345. Nabauer M, Beuckelmann DJ, Uberfuhr P, Steinbeck G. Regional differences in current density and rate-dependent properties of the transient outward current in subepicardial and subendocardial myocytes of human left ventricle. *Circulation* 1996;93:168–177.

346. Di Diego JM, Sun ZQ, Antzelevitch C. I_{to} and action potential notch are smaller in left vs. right canine ventricular epicardium. *Am J Physiol* 1996;271: H548–H561.
347. Volders PG, Sipido KR, Carmeliet E, Spatjens RL, Wellens HJ, Vos MA. Repolarizing K+ currents ITO1 and IKs are larger in right than left canine ventricular midmyocardium. *Circulation* 1999;99: 206–210.
348. Takano M, Noma A. Distribution of the isoprenaline-induced chloride current in rabbit heart. *Pflugers Arch* 1992;420:223–226.
349. Zygmunt AC. Intracellular calcium activates chloride current in canine ventricular myocytes. *Am J Physiol* 1994;267:H1984–H1995.
350. Cordeiro JM, Greene L, Heilmann C, Antzelevitch D, Antzelevitch C. Transmural heterogeneity of calcium activity and mechanical function in the canine left ventricle. *Am J Physiol* 2004;286:H1471–H1479.
351. Banyasz T, Fulop L, Magyar J, Szentandrassy N, Varro A, Nanasi PP. Endocardial versus epicardial differences in L-type calcium current in canine ventricular myocytes studied by action potential voltage clamp. *Cardiovasc Res* 2003;58:66–75.
352. Wang HS, Cohen IS. Calcium channel heterogeneity in canine left ventricular myocytes. *J Physiol* 2003;547:825–833.
353. Sicouri S, Antzelevitch C. A subpopulation of cells with unique electrophysiological properties in the deep subepicardium of the canine ventricle. The M cell. *Circ Res* 1991;68:1729–1741.
354. Anyukhovsky EP, Sosunov EA, Rosen MR. Regional differences in electrophysiologic properties of epicardium, midmyocardium and endocardium: *In vitro* and *in vivo* correlations. *Circulation* 1996;94:1981–1988.
355. Zygmunt AC, Goodrow RJ, Antzelevitch C. I(NaCa) contributes to electrical heterogeneity within the canine ventricle. *Am J Physiol* 2000;278:H1671–H1678.
356. Brahmajothi MV, Morales MJ, Reimer KA, Strauss HC. Regional localization of ERG, the channel protein responsible for the rapid component of the delayed rectifier, K^+ current in the ferret heart. *Circ Res* 1997;81:128–135.
357. Antzelevitch C, Dumaine R. Electrical heterogeneity in the heart: Physiological, pharmacological and clinical implications. In: Page E, Fozzard HA, Solaro RJ, Eds. *Handbook of Physiology. Section 2 The Cardiovascular System.* New York: Oxford University Press, 2001:654–692.
358. Burashnikov A, Antzelevitch C. Differences in the electrophysiologic response of four canine ventricular cell types to α_1-adrenergic agonists. *Cardiovasc Res* 1999;43:901–908.
359. Yan GX, Shimizu W, Antzelevitch C. Characteristics and distribution of M cells in arterially-perfused canine left ventricular wedge preparations. *Circulation* 1998;98:1921–1927.
360. Antzelevitch C, Shimizu W, Yan GX, Sicouri S, Weissenburger J, Nesterenko VV, Burashnikov A, Di Diego JM, Saffitz J, Thomas GP. The M cell: Its contribution to the ECG and to normal and abnormal electrical function of the heart. *J Cardiovasc Electrophysiol* 1999;10:1124–1152.
361. Sicouri S, Antzelevitch C. Electrophysiologic characteristics of M cells in the canine left ventricular free wall. *J Cardiovasc Electrophysiol* 1995;6:591–603.
362. Sicouri S, Fish J, Antzelevitch C. Distribution of M cells in the canine ventricle. *J Cardiovasc Electrophysiol* 1994;5:824–837.
363. Stankovicova T, Szilard M, De Scheerder I, Sipido KR. M cells and transmural heterogeneity of action potential configuration in myocytes from the left ventricular wall of the pig heart. *Cardiovasc Res* 2000;45:952–960.
364. Drouin E, Charpentier F, Gauthier C, Laurent K, Le Marec H. Electrophysiological characteristics of cells spanning the left ventricular wall of human heart: Evidence for the presence of M cells. *J Am Coll Cardiol* 1995;26:185–192.
365. Weissenburger J, Nesterenko VV, Antzelevitch C. Transmural heterogeneity of ventricular repolarization under baseline and long QT conditions in the canine heart *in vivo*: Torsades de pointes develops with halothane but not pentobarbital anesthesia. *J Cardiovasc Electrophysiol* 2000;11: 290–304.
366. Sicouri S, Quist M, Antzelevitch C. Evidence for the presence of M cells in the guinea pig ventricle. *J Cardiovasc Electrophysiol* 1996;7:503–511.
367. Li GR, Feng J, Yue L, Carrier M. Transmural heterogeneity of action potentials and Ito1 in myocytes isolated from the human right ventricle. *Am J Physiol* 1998;275:H369–H377.
368. Rodriguez-Sinovas A, Cinca J, Tapias A, Armadans L, Tresanchez M, Soler-Soler J. Lack of evidence of M-cells in porcine left ventricular myocardium. *Cardiovasc Res* 1997;33:307–313.
369. Shimizu W, Antzelevitch C. Sodium channel block with mexiletine is effective in reducing dispersion of repolarization and preventing torsade de pointes in LQT2 and LQT3 models of the long-QT syndrome. *Circulation* 1997;96:2038–2047.
370. Weirich J, Bernhardt R, Loewen N, Wenzel W, Antoni H. Regional- and species-dependent effects

of K+-channel blocking agents on subendocardium and mid-wall slices of human, rabbit, and guinea pig myocardium. *Pflugers Arch* 1996;431:R 130 (abstract).

371. Shimizu W, McMahon B, Antzelevitch C. Sodium pentobarbital reduces transmural dispersion of repolarization and prevents torsade de pointes in models of acquired and congenital long QT syndrome. *J Cardiovasc Electrophysiol* 1999;10:156–164.
372. Shimizu W, Antzelevitch C. Cellular basis for the ECG features of the LQT1 form of the long QT syndrome: Effects of β-adrenergic agonists and antagonists and sodium channel blockers on transmural dispersion of repolarization and torsade de pointes. *Circulation* 1998;98:2314–2322.
373. Shimizu W, Antzelevitch C. Cellular and ionic basis for T-wave alternans under long QT conditions. *Circulation* 1999;99:1499–1507.
374. Yan GX, Antzelevitch C. Cellular basis for the normal T wave and the electrocardiographic manifestations of the long QT syndrome. *Circulation* 1998;98:1928–1936.
375. Balati B, Varro A, Papp JG. Comparison of the cellular electrophysiological characteristics of canine left ventricular epicardium, M cells, endocardium and Purkinje fibres. *Acta Physiol Scand* 1998;164:181–190.
376. McIntosh MA, Cobbe SM, Smith GL. Heterogeneous changes in action potential and intracellular Ca2+ in left ventricular myocyte sub-types from rabbits with heart failure. *Cardiovasc Res* 2000;45:397–409.
377. Viskin S, Lesh MD, Eldar M, Fish R, Setbon I, Laniado S, Belhassen B. Mode of onset of malignant ventricular arrhythmias in idiopathic ventricular fibrillation. *J Cardiovasc Electrophysiol* 1997;8:1115–1120.
378. Brugada P, Brugada J. Right bundle branch block, persistent ST segment elevation and sudden cardiac death: A distinct clinical and electrocardiographic syndrome: A multicenter report. *J Am Coll Cardiol* 1992;20:1391–1396.
379. Krishnan SC, Antzelevitch C. Sodium channel block produces opposite electrophysiological effects in canine ventricular epicardium and endocardium. *Circ Res* 1991;69:277–291.
380. Krishnan SC, Antzelevitch C. Flecainide-induced arrhythmia in canine ventricular epicardium. Phase 2 reentry? *Circulation* 1993;87:562–572.
381. Antzelevitch C, Fish JM. Therapy for the Brugada syndrome. In: Kass R, Clancy CE, Eds. *Handbook of Experimental Pharmacology*. New York: Springer-Verlag, 2006:305–330.
382. Antzelevitch C, Brugada P, Brugada J, Brugada R. *The Brugada Syndrome: From Bench to Bedside.* Oxford, UK: Blackwell Futura, 2005.
383. Antzelevitch C, Brugada P, Brugada J, Brugada R. The Brugada syndrome. From cell to bedside. *Curr Probl Cardiol* 2005;30:9–54.
384. Shimizu W. Does an overlap syndrome really exist between Brugada syndrome and progressive cardiac conduction defect (lenegre syndrome)? *J Cardiovasc Electrophysiol* 2006;17:276–278.
385. Roberts R. Genomics and cardiac arrhythmias. *J Am Coll Cardiol* 2006;47:9–21.
386. Brugada R, Brugada J, Antzelevitch C, Kirsch GE, Potenza D, Towbin JA, Brugada P. Sodium channel blockers identify risk for sudden death in patients with ST-segment elevation and right bundle branch block but structurally normal hearts. *Circulation* 2000;101:510–515.
387. Antzelevitch C, Brugada P, Brugada J, Brugada R, Nademanee K, Towbin JA. *Clinical Approaches to Tachyarrhythmias. The Brugada Syndrome.* Armonk, NY: Futura Publishing Company, Inc., 1999.
388. Yan GX, Antzelevitch C. Cellular basis for the Brugada syndrome and other mechanisms of arrhythmogenesis associated with ST segment elevation. *Circulation* 1999;100:1660–1666.
389. Dumaine R, Towbin JA, Brugada P, Vatta M, Nesterenko DV, Nesterenko VV, Brugada J, Brugada R, Antzelevitch C. Ionic mechanisms responsible for the electrocardiographic phenotype of the Brugada syndrome are temperature dependent. *Circ Res* 1999;85:803–809.
390. Chen Q, Kirsch GE, Zhang D, Brugada R, Brugada J, Brugada P, Potenza D, Moya A, Borggrefe M, Breithardt G, Ortiz-Lopez R, Wang Z, Antzelevitch C, O'Brien RE, Schultze-Bahr E, Keating MT, Towbin JA, Wang Q. Genetic basis and molecular mechanisms for idiopathic ventricular fibrillation. *Nature* 1998;392:293–296.
391. Rook MB, Alshinawi CB, Groenewegen WA, van Gelder IC, Van Ginneken AC, Jongsma HJ, Mannens MM, Wilde AA. Human SCN5A gene mutations alter cardiac sodium channel kinetics and are associated with the Brugada syndrome. *Cardiovasc Res* 1999;44:507–517.
392. Deschenes I, Baroudi G, Berthet M, Barde I, Chalvidan T, Denjoy I, Guicheney P, Chahine M. Electrophysiological characterization of SCN5A mutations causing long QT (E1784K) and Brugada (R1512W and R1432G) syndromes. *Cardiovasc Res* 2000;46:55–65.
393. Priori SG, Napolitano C, Glordano U, Collisani G, Memmi M. Brugada syndrome and sudden cardiac death in children. *Lancet* 2000;355:808–809 .

394. Bezzina C, Veldkamp MW, van Den Berg MP, Postma AV, Rook MB, Viersma JW, Van Langen IM, Tan-Sindhunata G, Bink-Boelkens MT, Der Hout AH, Mannens MM, Wilde AA. A single Na(+) channel mutation causing both long-QT and Brugada syndromes. *Circ Res* 1999;85:1206–1213.
395. Antzelevitch C, Brugada R. Fever and the Brugada syndrome. *Pacing Clin Electrophysiol* 2002;25:1537–1539.
396. Aramaki K, Okumura H, Shimizu M. Chest pain and ST elevation associated with fever in patients with asymptomatic Brugada syndrome: Fever and chest pain in Brugada syndrome. *Int J Cardiol* 2005;103:338–339.
397. Dinckal MH, Davutoglu V, Akdemir I, Soydinc S, Kirilmaz A, Aksoy M. Incessant monomorphic ventricular tachycardia during febrile illness in a patient with Brugada syndrome: Fatal electrical storm. *Europace* 2003;5:257–261.
398. Dulu A, Pastores SM, McAleer E, Voigt L, Halpern NA. Brugada electrocardiographic pattern in a postoperative patient. *Crit Care Med* 2005;33:1634–1637.
399. Keller DI, Huang H, Zhao J, Frank R, Suarez V, Delacretaz E, Brink M, Osswald S, Schwick N, Chahine M. A novel SCN5A mutation, F1344S, identified in a patient with Brugada syndrome and fever-induced ventricular fibrillation. *Cardiovasc Res* 2006;70:521–529.
400. Mok NS, Priori SG, Napolitano C, Chan NY, Chahine M, Baroudi G. A newly characterized SCN5A mutation underlying Brugada syndrome unmasked by hyperthermia. *J Cardiovasc Electrophysiol* 2003;14:407–411.
401. Ortega-Carnicer J, Benezet J, Ceres F. Fever-induced ST-segment elevation and T-wave alternans in a patient with Brugada syndrome. *Resuscitation* 2003;57:315–317.
402. Patruno N, Pontillo D, Achilli A, Ruggeri G, Critelli G. Electrocardiographic pattern of Brugada syndrome disclosed by a febrile illness: Clinical and therapeutic implications. *Europace* 2003;5:251–255.
403. Peng J, Cui YK, Yuan FH, Yi SD, Chen ZM, Meng SR. [Fever and Brugada syndrome: Report of 21 cases.]. *Di Yi Jun Yi Da Xue Xue Bao* 2005;25:432–434.
404. Porres JM, Brugada J, Urbistondo V, Garcia F, Reviejo K, Marco P. Fever unmasking the Brugada syndrome. *Pacing Clin Electrophysiol* 2002;25:1646–1648.
405. Saura D, Garcia-Alberola A, Carrillo P, Pascual D, Martinez-Sanchez J, Valdes M. Brugada-like electrocardiographic pattern induced by fever. *Pacing Clin Electrophysiol* 2002;25:856–859.
406. Weiss R, Barmada MM, Nguyen T, Seibel JS, Cavlovich D, Kornblit CA, Angelilli A, Villanueva F, McNamara DM, London B. Clinical and molecular heterogeneity in the Brugada syndrome. A novel gene locus on chromosome 3. *Circulation* 2002;105:707–713.
407. London B, Sanyal S, Michalec M, Pfahnl AE, Shang LL, Kerchner BS, Lagana S, Aleong RG, Mehdi H, Gutmann R, Weiss R, Dudley SC. AB16-1: A mutation in the glycerol-3-phosphate dehydrogenase 1-like gene (GPD1L) causes Brugada syndrome. *Heart Rhythm* 2006;3:S32 (abstract).
408. Yan GX, Antzelevitch C. Cellular basis for the electrocardiographic J wave. *Circulation* 1996;93:372–379.
409. Gussak I, Antzelevitch C, Bjerregaard P, Towbin JA, Chaitman BR. The Brugada syndrome: Clinical, electrophysiologic and genetic aspects. *J Am Coll Cardiol* 1999;33:5–15.
410. Miyazaki T, Mitamura H, Miyoshi S, Soejima K, Aizawa Y, Ogawa S. Autonomic and antiarrhythmic drug modulation of ST segment elevation in patients with Brugada syndrome. *J Am Coll Cardiol* 1996;27:1061–1070.
411. Tarin N, Farre J, Rubio JM, Tunon J, Castro-Dorticos J. Brugada-like electrocardiographic pattern in a patient with a mediastinal tumor. *Pacing Clin Electrophysiol* 1999;22:1264–1266.
412. Carlsson J, Erdogan A, Schulte B, Neuzner J, Pitschner HF. Possible role of left ventricular programmed stimulation in Brugada syndrome. *Pacing Clin Electrophysiol* 2001;24:247–249.
413. Litovsky SH, Antzelevitch C. Differences in the electrophysiological response of canine ventricular subendocardium and subepicardium to acetylcholine and isoproterenol. A direct effect of acetylcholine in ventricular myocardium. *Circ Res* 1990;67:615–627.
414. Matsuo K, Shimizu W, Kurita T, Suyama K, Aihara N, Kamakura S, Shimomura K. Increased dispersion of repolarization time determined by monophasic action potentials in two patients with familial idiopathic ventricular fibrillation. *J Cardiovasc Electrophysiol* 1998;9:74–83.
415. Schwartz PJ, Periti M, Malliani A. The long QT syndrome. *Am Heart J* 1975;89:378–390.
416. Moss AJ, Schwartz PJ, Crampton RS, Locati EH, Carleen E. The long QT syndrome: A prospective international study. *Circulation* 1985;71:17–21.
417. Zipes DP. The long QT interval syndrome: A Rosetta stone for sympathetic related ventricular tachyarrhythmias. *Circulation* 1991;84:1414–1419.
418. Shimizu W, Ohe T, Kurita T, Kawade M, Arakaki Y, Aihara N, Kamakura S, Kamiya T, Shimomura K. Effects of verapamil and propranolol on early

afterdepolarizations and ventricular arrhythmias induced by epinephrine in congenital long QT syndrome. *J Am Coll Cardiol* 1995;26:1299–1309.
419. Schwartz PJ. The idiopathic long QT syndrome: Progress and questions. *Am Heart J* 1985;109:399–411.
420. Moss AJ, Schwartz PJ, Crampton RS, Tzivoni D, Locati EH, MacCluer JW, Hall WJ, Weitkamp LR, Vincent GM, Garson A, Robinson JL, Benhorin J, Choi S. The long QT syndrome: Prospective longitudinal study of 328 families. *Circulation* 1991;84:1136–1144.
421. Wang Q, Shen J, Splawski I, Atkinson DL, Li ZZ, Robinson JL, Moss AJ, Towbin JA, Keating MT. *SCN5A* mutations associated with an inherited cardiac arrhythmia, long QT syndrome. *Cell* 1995;80:805–811.
422. Mohler PJ, Schott JJ, Gramolini AO, Dilly KW, Guatimosim S, duBell WH, Song LS, Haurogne K, Kyndt F, Ali ME, Rogers TB, Lederer WJ, Escande D, Le Marec H, Bennett V. Ankyrin-B mutation causes type 4 long-QT cardiac arrhythmia and sudden cardiac death. *Nature* 2003;421:634–639.
423. Plaster NM, Tawil R, Tristani-Firouzi M, Canun S, Bendahhou S, Tsunoda A, Donaldson MR, Iannaccone ST, Brunt E, Barohn R, Clark J, Deymeer F, George AL Jr, Fish FA, Hahn A, Nitu A, Ozdemir C, Serdaroglu P, Subramony SH, Wolfe G, Fu YH, Ptacek LJ. Mutations in Kir2.1 cause the developmental and episodic electrical phenotypes of Andersen's syndrome. *Cell* 2001;105:511–519.
424. Curran ME, Splawski I, Timothy KW, Vincent GM, Green ED, Keating MT. A molecular basis for cardiac arrhythmia: *HERG* mutations cause long QT syndrome. *Cell* 1995;80:795–803.
425. Wang Q, Curran ME, Splawski I, Burn TC, Millholland JM, Van Raay TJ, Shen J, Timothy KW, Vincent GM, De Jager T, Schwartz PJ, Towbin JA, Moss AJ, Atkinson DL, Landes GM, Connors TD, Keating MT. Positional cloning of a novel potassium channel gene: *KVLQT1* mutations cause cardiac arrhythmias. *Nat Genet* 1996;12:17–23.
426. Splawski I, Tristani-Firouzi M, Lehmann MH, Sanguinetti MC, Keating MT. Mutations in the hminK gene cause long QT syndrome and suppress I_{Ks} function. *Nat Genet* 1997;17:338–340.
427. Ye B, Tester DJ, Vatta M, Makielski JC, Ackerman MJ. AB1-1: Molecular and functional characterization of novel cav3-encoded caveolin-3 mutations in congenital long QT syndrome. *Heart Rhythm* 2006;3:S1 (abstract).
428. Domingo AM, Kaku T, Tester DJ, Torres PI, Itty A, Ye B, Valdivia CR, Makielski JC, Quintero SC, Luna TT, Ackerman MJ. AB16-6: Sodium channel ß4 subunit mutation causes congenital long QT syndrome. *Heart Rhythm* 2006;3:S34 (abstract).
429. Splawski I, Timothy KW, Sharpe LM, Decher N, Kumar P, Bloise R, Napolitano C, Schwartz PJ, Joseph RM, Condouris K, Tager-Flusberg H, Priori SG, Sanguinetti MC, Keating MT. Ca(V)1.2 calcium channel dysfunction causes a multisystem disorder including arrhythmia and autism. *Cell* 2004;119:19–31.
430. Schwartz PJ, Priori SG, Napolitano C. The long QT syndrome. In: Zipes DP, Jalife J, Eds. *Cardiac Electrophysiology: From Cell to Bedside*, 3rd ed. Philadelphia: W.B. Saunders, 2000:597–615.
431. Moss AJ, Zareba W, Hall WJ, Schwartz PJ, Crampton RS, Benhorin J, Vincent GM, Locati EH, Priori SG, Napolitano C, Medina A, Zhang L, Robinson JL, Timothy K, Towbin JA, Andrews ML. Effectiveness and limitations of beta-blocker therapy in congenital long-QT syndrome. *Circulation* 2000;101:616–623.
432. Schwartz PJ, Priori SG, Cerrone M, Spazzolini C, Odero A, Napolitano C, Bloise R, De Ferrari GM, Klersy C, Moss AJ, Zareba W, Robinson JL, Hall WJ, Brink PA, Toivonen L, Epstein AE, Li C, Hu D. Left cardiac sympathetic denervation in the management of high-risk patients affected by the long-QT syndrome. *Circulation* 2004;1826–1833.
433. Bednar MM, Harrigan EP, Anziano RJ, Camm AJ, Ruskin JN. The QT interval. *Prog Cardiovasc Dis* 2001;43:1–45.
434. Tomaselli GF, Marban E. Electrophysiological remodeling in hypertrophy and heart failure. *Cardiovasc Res* 1999;42:270–283.
435. Sipido KR, Volders PG, De Groot SH, Verdonck F, Van de WF, Wellens HJ, Vos MA. Enhanced Ca(2+) release and Na/Ca exchange activity in hypertrophied canine ventricular myocytes: Potential link between contractile adaptation and arrhythmogenesis. *Circulation* 2000;102:2137–2144.
436. Volders PG, Sipido KR, Vos MA, Spatjens RL, Leunissen JD, Carmeliet E, Wellens HJ. Downregulation of delayed rectifier K(+) currents in dogs with chronic complete atrioventricular block and acquired torsades de pointes. *Circulation* 1999;100:2455–2461.
437. Undrovinas AI, Maltsev VA, Sabbah HN. Repolarization abnormalities in cardiomyocytes of dogs with chronic heart failure: Role of sustained inward current. *Cell Mol Life Sci* 1999;55:494–505.
438. Antzelevitch C, Shimizu W. Cellular mechanisms underlying the long QT syndrome. *Curr Opin Cardiol* 2002;17:43–51.

439. Shimizu W, Antzelevitch C. Effects of a K(+) channel opener to reduce transmural dispersion of repolarization and prevent torsade de pointes in LQT1, LQT2, and LQT3 models of the long-QT syndrome. *Circulation* 2000;102:706–712.
440. Antzelevitch C. Heterogeneity of cellular repolarization in LQTS: The role of M cells. *Eur Heart J* 2001;(Suppl. 3):K-2–K-16.
441. Anyukhovsky EP, Sosunov EA, Gainullin RZ, Rosen MR. The controversial M cell. *J Cardiovasc Electrophysiol* 1999;10:244–260.
442. Crampton RS. Preeminence of the left stellate ganglion in the long Q-T syndrome. *Circulation* 1979;59:769–778.
443. Ali RH, Zareba W, Moss A, Schwartz PJ, Benhorin J, Vincent GM, Locati EH, Priori SG, Napolitano C, Towbin JA, Hall WJ, Robinson JL, Andrews ML, Zhang L, Timothy K, Medina A. Clinical and genetic variables associated with acute arousal and nonarousal-related cardiac events among subjects with long QT syndrome. *Am J Cardiol* 2000;85:457–461.
444. Noda T, Takaki H, Kurita T, Suyama K, Nagaya N, Taguchi A, Aihara N, Kamakura S, Sunagawa K, Nakamura S, Ohe T, Horie M, Napolitano C, Towbin JA, Priori SG, Shimizu W. Gene-specific response of dynamic ventricular repolarization to sympathetic stimulation in LQT1, LQT2 and LQT3 forms of congenital long QT syndrome. *Eur Heart J* 2002;23:975–983.
445. Schwartz PJ, Priori SG, Spazzolini C, Moss AJ, Vincent GM, Napolitano C, Denjoy I, Guicheney P, Breithardt G, Keating MT, Towbin JA, Beggs AH, Brink P, Wilde AA, Toivonen L, Zareba W, Robinson JL, Timothy KW, Corfield V, Wattanasirichaigoon D, Corbett C, Haverkamp W, Schulze-Bahr E, Lehmann MH, Schwartz K, Coumel P, Bloise R. Genotype-phenotype correlation in the long-QT syndrome: Gene-specific triggers for life-threatening arrhythmias. *Circulation* 2001;103: 89–95.
446. Windle JR, Geletka RC, Moss AJ, Zareba W, Atkins DL. Normalization of ventricular repolarization with flecainide in long QT syndrome patients with SCN5A:DeltaKPQ mutation. *Ann Noninvasive Electrocardiol* 2001;6:153–158.
447. Roden DM. Pharmacogenetics and drug-induced arrhythmias. *Cardiovasc Res* 2001;50:224–231.
448. Di Diego JM, Belardinelli L, Antzelevitch C. Cisapride-induced transmural dispersion of repolarization and torsade de pointes in the canine left ventricular wedge preparation during epicardial stimulation. *Circulation* 2003;108:1027–1033.
449. Antzelevitch C. Drug-induced Channelopathies. In: Zipes DP, Jalife J, Eds. *Cardiac Electrophysiology. From Cell to Bedside*, 4th ed. New York: W.B. Saunders, 2004:151–157.
450. Fenichel RR, Malik M, Antzelevitch C, Sanguinetti MC, Roden DM, Priori SG, Ruskin JN, Lipicky RJ, Cantilena LR. Drug-induced torsade de pointes and implications for drug development. *J Cardiovasc Electrophysiol* 2004;15:475–495.
451. Lubinski A, Lewicka-Nowak E, Kempa M, Baczynska AM, Romanowska I, Swiatecka G. New insight into repolarization abnormalities in patients with congenital long QT syndrome: The increased transmural dispersion of repolarization. *Pacing Clin Electrophysiol* 1998;21:172–175.
452. Wolk R, Stec S, Kulakowski P. Extrasystolic beats affect transmural electrical dispersion during programmed electrical stimulation. *Eur J Clinical Invest* 2001;31:293–301.
453. Tanabe Y, Inagaki M, Kurita T, Nagaya N, Taguchi A, Suyama K, Aihara N, Kamakura S, Sunagawa K, Nakamura K, Ohe T, Towbin JA, Priori SG, Shimizu W. Sympathetic stimulation produces a greater increase in both transmural and spatial dispersion of repolarization in LQT1 than LQT2 forms of congenital long QT syndrome. *J Am Coll Cardiol* 2001;37:911–919.
454. Frederiks J, Swenne CA, Kors JA, van Herpen G, Maan AC, Levert JV, Schalij MJ, Bruschke AV. Within-subject electrocardiographic differences at equal heart rates: Role of the autonomic nervous system. *Pflugers Arch* 2001;441:717–724.
455. Shimizu M, Ino H, Okeie K, Yamaguchi M, Nagata M, Hayashi K, Itoh H, Iwaki T, Oe K, Konno T, Mabuchi H. T-peak to T-end interval may be a better predictor of high-risk patients with hypertrophic cardiomyopathy associated with a cardiac troponin I mutation than QT dispersion. *Clin Cardiol* 2002;25:335–339.
456. Takenaka K, Ai T, Shimizu W, Kobori A, Ninomiya T, Otani H, Kubota T, Takaki H, Kamakura S, Horie M. Exercise stress test amplifies genotype-phenotype correlation in the LQT1 and LQT2 forms of the long-QT syndrome. *Circulation* 2003;107:838–844.
457. Watanabe N, Kobayashi Y, Tanno K, Miyoshi F, Asano T, Kawamura M, Mikami Y, Adachi T, Ryu S, Miyata A, Katagiri T. Transmural dispersion of repolarization and ventricular tachyarrhythmias. *J Electrocardiol* 2004;37:191–200.
458. Yamaguchi M, Shimizu M, Ino H, Terai H, Uchiyama K, Oe K, Mabuchi T, Konno T, Kaneda T, Mabuchi H. T wave peak-to-end interval and QT dispersion in acquired long QT syndrome: A

new index for arrhythmogenicity. *Clin Sci (Lond)* 2003;105:671–676.
459. Sicouri S, Moro S, Litovsky SH, Elizari MV, Antzelevitch C. Chronic amiodarone reduces transmural dispersion of repolarization in the canine heart. *J Cardiovasc Electrophysiol* 1997;8:1269–1279.
460. van Opstal JM, Schoenmakers M, Verduyn SC, De Groot SH, Leunissen JD, Der Hulst FF, Molenschot MM, Wellens HJ, Vos MA. Chronic amiodarone evokes no torsade de pointes arrhythmias despite QT lengthening in an animal model of acquired long-QT syndrome. *Circulation* 2001;104:2722–2727.
461. Gussak I, Brugada P, Brugada J, Wright RS, Kopecky SL, Chaitman BR, Bjerregaard P. Idiopathic short QT interval: A new clinical syndrome? *Cardiology* 2000;94:99–102.
462. Gussak I, Brugada P, Brugada J, Antzelevitch C, Osbakken M, Bjerregaard P. ECG phenomenon of idiopathic and paradoxical short QT intervals. *Cardiac Electrophysiol Rev* 2002;6:49–53.
463. Gaita F, Giustetto C, Bianchi F, Wolpert C, Schimpf R, Riccardi R, Grossi S, Richiardi E, Borggrefe M. Short QT syndrome: A familial cause of sudden death. *Circulation* 2003;108:965–970.
464. Brugada R, Hong K, Dumaine R, Cordeiro JM, Gaita F, Borggrefe M, Menendez TM, Brugada J, Pollevick GD, Wolpert C, Burashnikov E, Matsuo K, Wu YS, Guerchicoff A, Bianchi F, Giustetto C., Schimpf R, Brugada P, Antzelevitch C. Sudden death associated with short QT-syndrome linked to mutations in HERG. *Circulation* 2003;109: 30–35.
465. Bellocq C, Van Ginneken AC, Bezzina CR, Alders M, Escande D, Mannens MM, Baro I, Wilde AA. Mutation in the KCNQ1 gene leading to the short QT-interval syndrome. *Circulation* 2004;109:2394–2397.
466. Extramiana F, Antzelevitch C. Amplified transmural dispersion of repolarization as the basis for arrhythmogenesis in a canine ventricular-wedge model of short-QT syndrome. *Circulation* 2004; 110:3661–3666.
467. Janse MJ, Wit AL. Electrophysiological mechanisms of ventricular arrhythmias resulting from myocardial ischemia and infarction. *Physiol Rev* 1989;69:1049–1169.
468. Lukas A, Antzelevitch C. Differences in the electrophysiological response of canine ventricular epicardium and endocardium to ischemia: Role of the transient outward current. *Circulation* 1993; 88:2903–2915.
469. Di Diego JM, Antzelevitch C. Pinacidil-induced electrical heterogeneity and extrasystolic activity in canine ventricular tissues. Does activation of ATP-regulated potassium current promote phase 2 reentry? *Circulation* 1993;88:1177–1189.
470. Gilmour RF Jr, Zipes DP. Different electrophysiological responses of canine endocardium and epicardium to combined hyperkalemia, hypoxia, and acidosis. *Circ Res* 1980;46:814–825.
471. Kimura S, Bassett AL, Kohya T, Kozlovskis PL, Myerburg RJ. Simultaneous recording of action potentials from endocardium and epicardium during ischemia in the isolated cat ventricle: Relation of temporal electrophysiologic heterogeneities to arrhythmias. *Circulation* 1986;74:401–409.
472. Kimura S, Bassett AL, Furukawa T, Furukawa N, Myerburg RJ. Differences in the effect of metabolic inhibition on action potentials and calcium currents in endocardial and epicardial cells. *Circulation* 1991;84:768–777.
473. Guerchicoff A, Pollevick GD, Cordeiro JM, Dumaine R, Mazza M, Antzelevitch C, Di Diego JM. Transmural differences in expression of SCN5A may contribute to the greater sensitivity of ventricular epicardium to electrical depression. *Heart Rhythm* 2006;3:s302 (abstract).
474. Miller WT, Geselowitz DB. Simulation studies of the electrogram. 2. Ischemia and infarction. *Circ Res* 1978;43:315–323.
475. Miller WT, Geselowitz DB. Simulation studies of the electrocardiogram. 1. The normal heart. *Circ Res* 1978;43:301–315.
476. Mandel WJ, Burgess MJ, Neville J, Abildskov JA. Analysis of T-wave abnormalities associated with myocardial infarction using a theoretical model. *Circulation* 1968;38:178–188.
477. Haws CW, Lux RL. Correlation between *in vivo* transmembrane action potential durations and action-recovery intervals from electrograms. Effects of interventions that alter repolarization time. *Circulation* 1990;81:281–288.
478. Downar E, Janse MJ, Durrer D. The effect of acute coronary artery occlusion on subepicardial transmembrane potentials in the intact porcine heart. *Circulation* 1977;56:217–224.
479. Ejima J, Martin D, Engle CL, Gettes LS, Kunimoto S, Gettes LS. Ability of activation recovery intervals to assess action potential duration during acute no-flow ischemia in the in situ porcine heart. *J Cardiovasc Electrophysiol* 1998;9:832–844.
480. Madias JE. The earliest electrocardiographic signs of acute transmural myocardial infarction. *J Electrocardiol* 1977;10:193–196.

481. Di Diego JM, Antzelevitch C. Cellular basis for ST-segment changes observed during ischemia. *J Electrocardiol* 2003;36(Suppl.):1–5.
482. Olgin JE, Kalman JM, Lesh MD. Conduction barriers in human atrial flutter: Correlation of electrophysiology and anatomy. *J Cardiovasc Electrophysiol* 1996;7:1112–1126.
483. Cheung DW. Electrical activity of the pulmonary vein and its interaction with the right atrium in the guinea-pig. *J Physiol* 1981;314:445–456.
484. Wang TM, Chiang CE, Sheu JR, Tsou CH, Chang HM, Luk HN. Homogenous distribution of fast response action potentials in canine pulmonary vein sleeves: A contradictory report. *Int J Cardiol* 2003;89:187–195.
485. Zipes DP, Mihalick MJ, Robbins GT. Effects of selective vagal and stellate ganglion stimulation of atrial refractoriness. *Cardiovasc Res* 1974;8:647–655.
486. Liu L, Nattel S. Differing sympathetic and vagal effects on atrial fibrillation in dogs: Role of refractoriness heterogeneity. *Am J Physiol* 1997;273:H805–H816.
487. Burashnikov A, Antzelevitch C. Beta-adrenergic stimulation is highly arrhythmogenic following ischemia/reperfusion injury in the isolated canine right atrium. *Heart Rhythm* 2005;2:S179 (abstract).
488. Jais P, Hocini M, Macle L, Choi KJ, Deisenhofer I, Weerasooriya R, Shah DC, Garrigue S, Raybaud F, Scavee C, Le Metayer P, Clementy J, Haissaguerre M. Distinctive electrophysiological properties of pulmonary veins in patients with atrial fibrillation. *Circulation* 2002;106:2479–2485.
489. Arora R, Verheule S, Scott L, Navarrete A, Katari V, Wilson E, Vaz D, Olgin JE. Arrhythmogenic substrate of the pulmonary veins assessed by high-resolution optical mapping. *Circulation* 2003;107:1816–1821.
490. Wu S, Weiss JN, Chou CC, Attin M, Hayashi H, Lin SF. Dissociation of membrane potential and intracellular calcium during ventricular fibrillation. *J Cardiovasc Electrophysiol* 2005;16:186–192.
491. Burashnikov A, Di Diego JM, Belardinelli L, Antzelevitch C. Ranolazine suppresses artial fibrillation by exerting a marked use-dependent block of sodium channel current in canine atrium but not ventricle. *Heart Rhythm* 2006;3:s304 (abstract).
492. Wijffels MC, Crijns HJ. Recent advances in drug therapy for atrial fibrillation. *J Cardiovasc Electrophysiol* 2003;14:S40–S47.
493. Ferrier GR, Rosenthal JE. Automaticity and entrance block induced by focal depolarization of mammalian ventricular tissues. *Circ Res* 1980;47:238–248.
494. Wennemark JR, Ruesta VJ, Brody DA. Microelectrode study of delayed conduction in the canine right bundle branch. *Circ Res* 1968;23:753–769.
495. Downar E, Waxman MB. Depressed conduction and unidirectional block in Purkinje fibers. In: Wellens HJ, Lie KI, Janse MJ, Eds. *The Conduction System of the Heart.* Philadelphia: Lea & Febiger, 1976:393–409.
496. Antzelevitch C, Spach MS. Impulse conduction. Continuous and discontinuous. In: Spooner PM, Rosen MR, Eds. *Foundations of Cardiac Arrhythmias. Basic Concepts and Clinical Approaches.* New York: Marcel Dekker, Inc., 2000:205–241.
497. Spach MS, Miller WT, Geselowitz DB, Barr RC, Kootsey JM, Johnson EA. The discontinuous nature of propagation in normal canine cardiac muscle. Evidence for recurrent discontinuities of intracellular resistance that affect the membrane currents. *Circ Res* 1981;48:39–54.
498. Antzelevitch C, Jalife J, Moe GK. Frequency-dependent alternations of conduction in Purkinje fibers. A model of phase-4 facilitation and block. In: Rosenbaum MB, Elizari MV, Eds. *Frontiers of Cardiac Electrophysiology.* Amsterdam: Martinus Nijhoff, 1983:397–415.
499. Gilmour RF Jr, Salata JJ, Zipes DP. Rate-related suppression and facilitation of conduction in isolated canine cardiac Purkinje fibers. *Circ Res* 1985;57:35–45.
500. Gilmour RF Jr, Heger JJ, Prystowsky EN, Zipes DP. Cellular electrophysiologic abnormalities of diseased human ventricular myocardium. *Am J Cardiol* 1983;51:137–144.
501. Gilmour RF Jr, Zipes DP. Cellular basis for cardiac arrhythmias. *Cardiol Clin* 1983;1:3–11.
502. Antzelevitch C, Shimizu W, Yan GX. Electrical heterogeneity and the development of arrhythmias. In: Olsson SB, Yuan S, Amlie JP, Eds. *Dispersion of Ventricular Repolarization: State of the Art.* Armonk, NY: Futura Publishing Company, Inc., 2000:3–21.
503. Gilmour RF Jr. Phase resetting of circus movement reentry in cardiac tissue. In: Zipes DP, Jalife J, Eds. *Cardiac Electrophysiology, From Cell to Bedside.* New York: W.B. Saunders, 1989.
504. Matsuda K, Kamiyama A, Hoshi T. Configuration of the transmembrane action potential at the Purkinje-ventricular fiber junction and its analysis. In: Sano T, Mizuhira V, Matsuda K, Eds. *Electrophysiology and Ultrastructure of the Heart.* New York: Grune & Stratton, 1967:177–187.

505. Overholt ED, Joyner RW, Veenstra RD, Rawling DA, Wiedman R. Unidirectional block between Purkinje and ventricular layers of papillary muscles. *Am J Physiol* 1984;247:H-584–H-595.
506. Antzelevitch C. Electrotonus and reflection. In: Rosen MR, Janse MJ, Wit AL, Eds. *Cardiac Electrophysiology: A Textbook.* Mount Kisco, NY: Futura Publishing Company, Inc., 1990:491–516.
507. Antzelevitch C. The Brugada syndrome: Diagnostic criteria and cellular mechanisms. *Eur Heart J* 2001;22:356–363.

6
Mechanisms of Action of Antiarrhythmic Drugs

Shingo Murakami and Yoshihisa Kurachi

Introduction

Antiarrhythmic drugs have been used as an effective measure to treat or prevent tachyarrhythmias including ventricular tachycardia and fibrillation in clinics for a long time. Arrhythmias refer to changes from the normal sequence of electrical impulses and conduction, causing abnormal heart rhythms. They can be classified into two categories: bradyarrhythmias and tachyarrhythmias. Both can make the heart pump less effectively and, more seriously, cause sudden death. Possible treatments include electrical defibrillation, radio frequency ablation, implantable cardioverter defibrillators, artificial pacemakers, and medication. All these are used to prevent or terminate arrhythmias. Among them, arrhythmia medication is a nonsurgical and effective treatment and its major target has been tachyarrhythmias, mainly in the ventricle, including ventricular tachycardia and fibrillation. Of course, recently treatment of atrial tachyarrhythmias such as atrial fibrillation is also one of the major interests. However, its application may cause serious adverse effects.[1] Since usage of antiarrhythmic drugs tended to rely on clinicians' experience and to be based on clinical practice, the effects of antiarrhythmic drugs had been understood empirically. Accumulated studies on the mechanism of antiarrhythmic agents, however, have provided much basic understanding of drug action, especially on the electrophysiological properties of cardiac excitation. This will not only help clinicians to select proper antiarrhythmic drugs, but will also help in the development of new antiarrhythmic drugs.

Most antiarrhythmic drugs act on ion channels and alter the electrical properties of cardiac tissues, including excitation and conduction, which is beneficial in preventing or treating cardiac arrhythmias, though some of the effects are sometimes proarrhythmic. Therefore, it is necessary to understand the effects of various antiarrhythmic agents on cardiac ion channels and thus on excitation and conduction. Ion channels are generally specific for ion species (e.g., Na^+, K^+, Ca^{2+}), and movement of ions through ion channels generates current across the membrane and forms the action potential (AP). The cardiac AP (typically the ventricular AP) consists of four phases: shape depolarization from the resting potential due to Na^+ ions entering the myocyte through the Na^+ channel, phase 0; rapid initial repolarization due to a K^+ channel current and Cl^- channel current, phase 1; depolarization was maintained for 100 msec because of the Ca^{2+} channel current, phase 2; repolarization due to K^+ channel currents, phase 3; and the resting potential, phase 4 (Figure 6–1a). Different types of ion channels contribute to each phase of AP and mediate the transduction from membrane depolarization to the contraction of the cell, a process called excitation–contraction (EC) coupling (Figure 6–1a).

A number of classification systems of antiarrhythmic drugs based on their interaction with ion channels and receptors have been proposed including that by Vaughan-Williams.[2] Vaughan-Williams first proposed a scheme based on electrophysiological mechanisms of drug action to classify antiarrhythmic drug action.[3]

Although knowledge of the electrophysiological bases of arrhythmias and drug action at that time was limited, this classification is still commonly used. The Vaughan-Williams classification divides antiarrhythmic drugs into four major groups (Class I–IV) according to whether their major effect is to block the Na^+ channel (Class I drug), the β-adrenergic receptor (Class II drug), the K^+ channel (Class III drug), or the Ca^{2+} channel (Class IV drug) (Table 6–1). In general, by blocking the Na^+ channel, Class I drugs reduce the maximum rate of rise in phase 0 of the action potential without changing the resting potential, but have different effects on action potential duration (APD). The Class I drugs are further divided into three subgroups (Class Ia, Ib, Ic) according to their different effects on APD: Class Ia drugs prolong APD, Class Ib drugs shorten APD, and Class Ic drugs do not have significant effects on APD (Figure 6–1b). Class II drugs block β-adrenergic receptors. Class III drugs block K^+ channels of delayed-rectifier type and prolong APD. Class IV

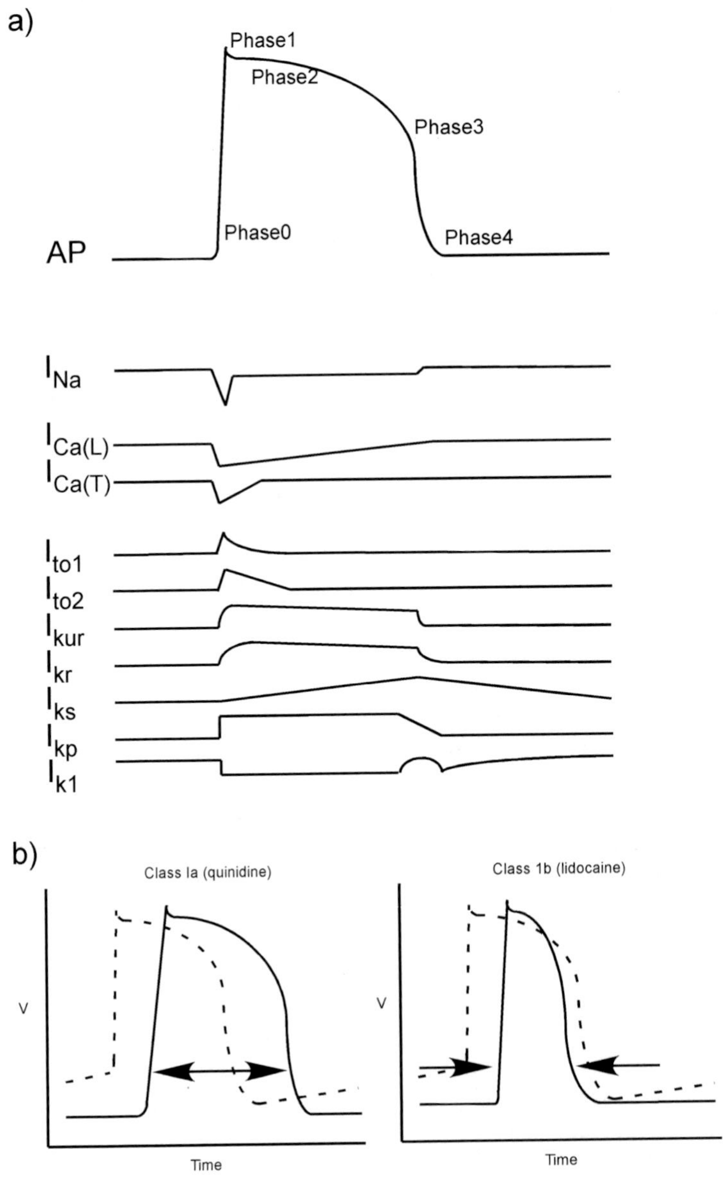

FIGURE 6–1. (a) Phases of a cardiac action potential and ion channel currents. (b) Blocking effects of lidocaine and quinidine on action potential duration.

TABLE 6–1. Vaughan-Williams classification of antiarrhythmic drug actions.

I	Na^+ channel block	Ia	Prolong action potential duration (APD)	Quinidine Procainamide Ajmaline Disopyramide Cibenzoline Pirmenol
		Ib	Shorten APD	Lidocaine Mexiletine Tocainide Aprindine (no effect on APD)
		Ic	No effect on APD	Flecainide Pilsicainide Propafenone
II	β-Adrenergic receptor block			Propranolol Metoprolol Atenolol
III	K^+ channel block		APD prolongation	Amiodarone Bretylium Sotalol Dofetilide E-4031
IV	Ca^{2+} channel block			Nifedipine Verapamil Diltiazem Bepridil

drugs block Ca^{2+} channels. The Vaughan-Williams classification has the virtue of simplicity. However, many antiarrhythmic drugs may block more than one type of ion channel. This classification cannot account for such complex phenomena and, moreover, some antiarrhythmic agents including digitalis and adenosine cannot be covered by the four groups. One important classification among others proposed to deal with these problems is the Sicilian Gambit.[4] The working group of the European Society of Cardiology met in Taormina, Sicily to consider the classification of antiarrhythmic drugs.[4] They criticized the Vaughan-Williams classification because of the following reasons. (1) The classification is a hybrid. A single class effect can be produced by multiple mechanisms and some drugs have several classes of actions. (2) Activation of channels or receptors is not considered. (3) The classification is incomplete. For example, α-adrenergic blockers, cholinergic agonists, digitalis, and adenosine are not included. The Sicilian Gambit group proposed that the Vaughan-Williams classification be replaced with a new classification. In the new classification, the vulnerable parameters associated with specific arrhythmic mechanisms are identified and the effects of each drug on each parameter are listed to characterize the profile of each drug in the termination or suppression of the arrhythmia depending on its underlying mechanisms. Thus, a most effective drug action with minimal possible adverse effects would be expected. This system can account for multiple drug actions and provides more flexibility for classifying antiarrhythmic drugs. However, this multidimensional classification system is significantly more complex than the standard Vaughan-Williams classification and may not be suitable for a basic understanding of antiarrhythmic drug actions. Because of its simplicity, the Vaughan-Williams classification will be used in this chapter to explain the mechanisms of antiarrhythmic drug action.

General Arrhythmia Suppression Mechanisms

Antiarrhythmic drugs can block cardiac arrhythmias by suppressing underlying mechanisms, such as abnormal automaticity, delayed afterdepolarization (DAD), early afterdepolarization (EAD), and reentry (Figure 6–2). Typically, the abnormal automaticity is caused by decrease of resting membrane conductance and/or enhancement of inward currents such as Ca^{2+} channel. The DAD is due to the overload of intracellular calcium ions (Figure 6–2b) and EAD is caused by the excessive prolongation of APD (Figure 6–2a). Establishment of microreentry requires the unidirectional conduction block and slow conduction of AP (Figure 6–2c). Abnormal automaticity can be altered by either changing the diastolic phase 4 slope, the threshold potential for rapid initial upstroke in phase 0, or APD. Generally speaking, Na^+ channel blockers and Ca^{2+} channel blockers elevate the threshold potential for action potential initiation, K^+ channel blockers prolong the APD, adenosine hyperpolarizes the cell membrane potential and shortens the APD, and β-adrenergic receptor blockers decrease phase 4 slope. Similarly, Na^+ channel blockers and Ca^{2+} channel blockers may suppress DAD by interfering with its upstroke. The EAD can be inhibited by shortening the APD. Reentry may be terminated by prolonging the refractory period, i.e., by blocking delayed rectifier K^+ channels or slowing recovery of Na^+ channels from inactivation. The main purpose of this chapter is to describe the basic mechanisms by which each class of drug affects cardiac ion channel activity.

Na^+ Channel Blocker (Class I Drugs)

Class I drugs in the Vaughan-Williams classification are primary Na^+ channel blockers and, historically, the blockers' effect on the Na^+ channel was first investigated to elucidate the mechanisms of antiarrhythmic drugs, before other antiarrhythmic drugs. Na^+ channels in many excitable cells generate a rapid regenerative upstroke of action potential and the Na^+ channel current is tetrodotoxin (TTX) sensitive and/or μ-conotoxin sensitive. Two independent gating mechanisms of the Na^+ channel (activation and inactivation) give rise to the fast onset and decay of the Na^+ channel current after the depolarizing pulse (Figure 6–3). The Na^+ channel in the atrium and ventricle accounts for the initial rapid depolarization (phase 0), which is responsible for the fast conduction of

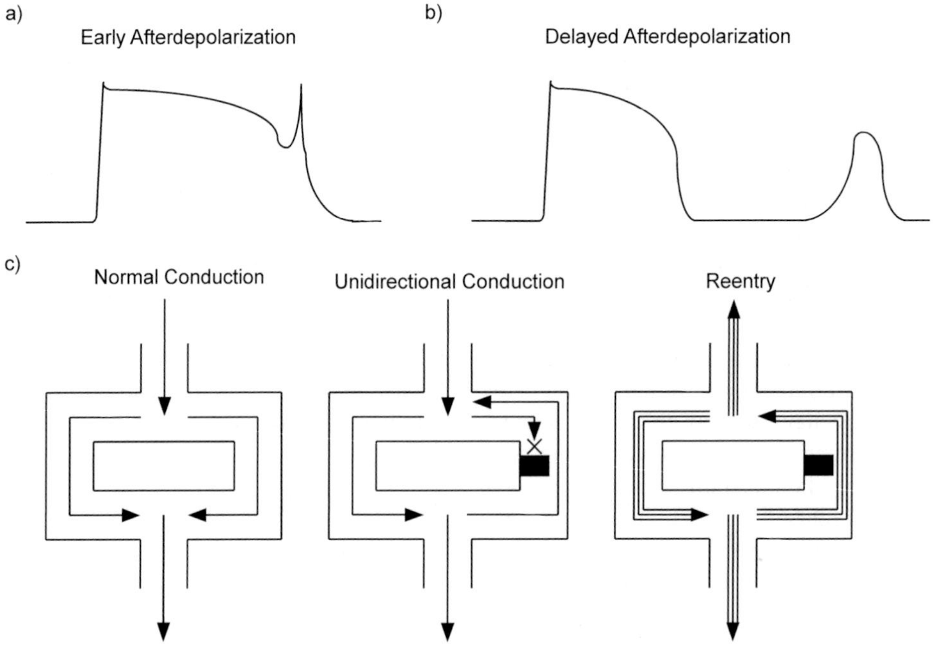

FIGURE 6–2. (a) Early afterdepolarization. (b) Delayed afterdepolarization. (c) Normal conduction, unidirectional conduction, and reentry.

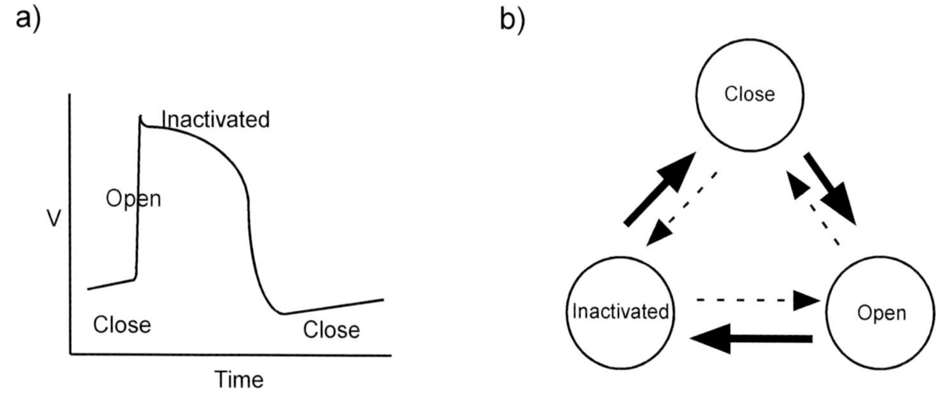

FIGURE 6–3. (a) States of the Na^+ channel during a cardiac action potential. (b) State diagram of the Na^+ channel.

excitation in cardiac tissues. Its maximum upstroke slope (dV/dt_{max}) is approximately proportional to the Na^+ channel current amplitude. And thus it has been used as the parameter to evaluate the effect of Class I drugs on the Na^+ channel. Therefore, the primary effect of Class I drugs is to slow the upstroke of cardiac AP. Class I drugs are further divided into three subgroups (Ia, Ib, Ic), according to their electrophysiological effects on APD. For example, Class Ia drugs such as quinidine slow the maximum upstroke slope and in addition prolong APD (Figure 6–1b). Because of its APD prolongation effect, quinidine is also known to cause so-called quinidine shock, i.e., a quinidine-related torsades de pointes type of polymorphic ventricular tachycardia. On the other hand, Class Ib drugs, such as lidocaine, also make the maximum upstroke slope gentle but shorten the APD (Figure 6–1b). Class Ic drugs slow the maximum upstroke slope but do not have a significant effect on APD. These differences among the Class I subtype drugs can be accounted for either by the kinetic properties of the drug action on Na^+ channels and/or by the action on other ion channels such as K^+ channels.

Drug Pathway to the Na Channel Binding Site and Modulated Receptor Hypothesis

The action of Class I drugs (Na^+ channel blockers) should be understood in two different ways: one is the pathway by which the drugs reach their binding site in the Na^+ channel to be blocked, and the other is how drugs in the channel interact with the binding site. The most important theory for this is the modulated receptor hypothesis. Differences in the drug action among antiarrhythmic drugs, such as state-dependent block, can be explained by the modulated receptor hypothesis. To understand the mechanism of antiarrhythmic drugs on the cardiac Na^+ channel, and that of local anesthesia on the nerve Na^+ channel, the modulated receptor hypothesis has been proposed.[5,6] This hypothesis features the following: (1) Na^+ channel block by drugs is caused by a binding between a drug molecule and a receptor in the channel pore or nearby; and (2) the affinity between a receptor and a drug depends on the channel state, such as resting, open, and inactivated (Figure 6–4). This hypothesis was developed by comparing a Class Ib open channel blocker, lidocaine, and a state-dependent blocker, QX-314. QX-314, a quaternary derivative of lidocaine, is a charged molecular and cannot go through the membrane. Application of QX-314 from extracellular space does not block the Na^+ channel at the resting potential. When applied from the inside site, the drug blocks the channel. However, the drug requires the channel to open for its action. Blockers with this kind of state-dependent block are generally called open channel blockers. In the application of open channel blockers, the magnitude of the Na^+ channel current at the first pulse is almost the same as that in the control, but it decreases gradually with additional pulses to a certain steady level. Independent of stimulus frequency, the drug effect accumulates at each AP

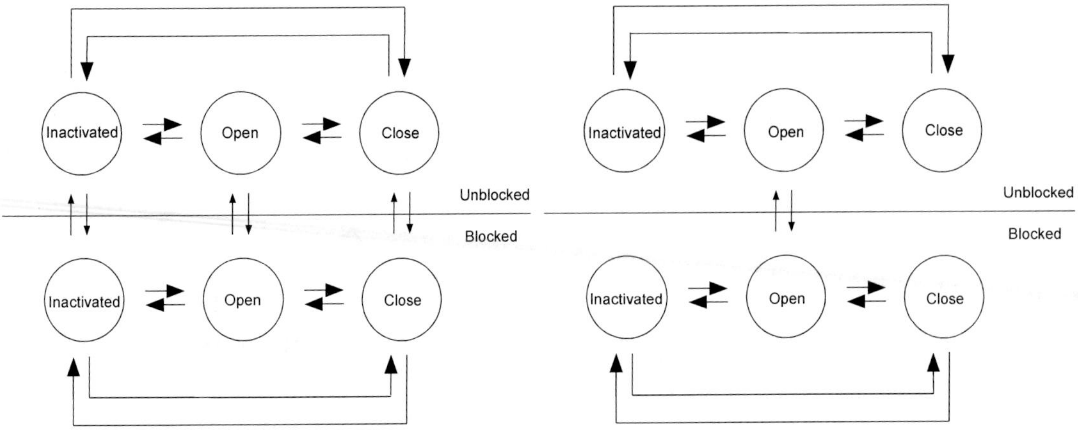

FIGURE 6–4. State-dependent ion channel block.

and reaches a certain steady state. The unblocking of QX-314 also requires the opening of the Na^+ channel. As long as the Na^+ channel is closed, the drug stays in the channel pore. When the Na^+ channel is open, the drug may leave the channel pore. This is because QX-314 can only go through a hydrophilic pathway (i.e., ion channel pores) (Figure 6–5). Thus, the action of QX-314 on the Na^+ channel is use dependent but frequency independent. However, the block by lidocaine, a neutral molecule, can either develop or recover even when the Na^+ channel is closed or inactivated. This is because lidocaine can go through not only the hydrophilic pathway (i.e., ion channel pores) but also the hydrophobic pathway (i.e., lipid bilayer) (Figure 6–5). Thus, the action of lidocaine is frequency dependent due to the balance between the onset and recovery of action. These properties of the drug pathway are important to characterize the state dependency of each drug.

In addition to the drug pathway, the voltage-dependent properties of the interaction between the drug and the binding site in the channel

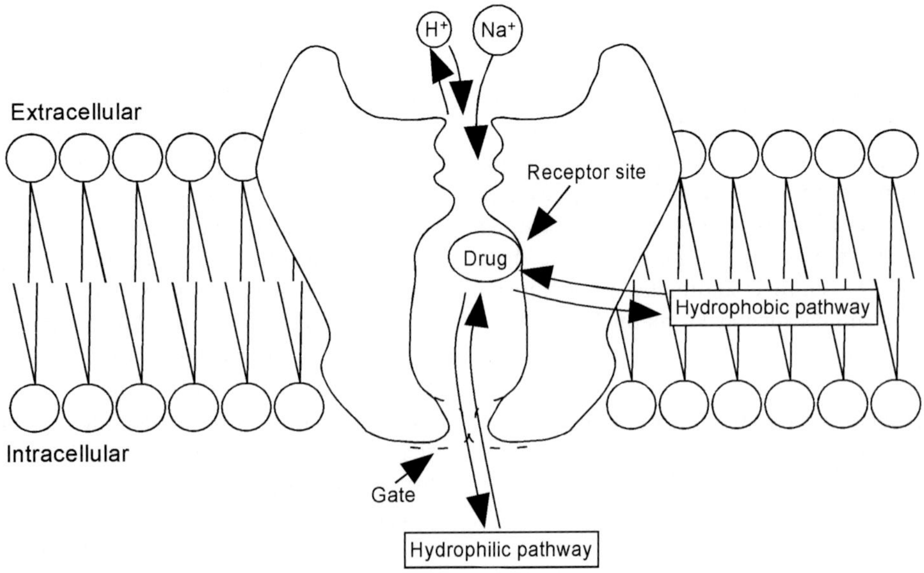

FIGURE 6–5. Binding site of Na^+ channel blockers and hydrophobic and hydrophilic pathways.

determine the net action of drugs on the Na^+ channel. Even if the drug goes through the channel pore and can bind to a receptor, the actual occurrence of the binding depends on the transmembrane potential. QX-314 strongly suppresses the Na^+ channel current at the depolarized potential and weakly at the hyperpolarized potential. In the same way, state-dependent unblocking can be accounted for by a similar explanation.

The analysis also suggests that the Na^+ channels blocked by Na^+ channel blockers have three states (the open state, inactivated state, and recovery from block) and each drug has a different preference for each channel state (Figure 6–4). These are determined by the properties of the drug in the access pathway and the interaction with the binding site. For example, quinidine shows open state block but not significant inactivated state block. Lidocaine shows both open state block and inactivated state block. These are probably due to the differences of these drugs in the access pathway to the binding site. Recovery from block with lidocaine is much faster than with quinidine, therefore, lidocaine induces use-dependent block and exhibits stronger block at a higher stimulus frequency, but quinidine does so even at a relatively low frequency (Figure 6–6). Since the open state block is dominant in quinidine and its recovery is slow (~5–7 sec), quinidine is effective in both the atrium where APD is short and in the ventricle where APD is long. In the case of lidocaine, open state block and inactivated state block work more or less in the same order. But the recovery of block is fast at a speed of ~100–200 msec. Therefore, lidocaine is also effective in the ventricle where APD is long, but is not so effective in the atrium where APD is so short that accumulation of block is not likely to happen.

This different behavior between charged and neutral drug molecules also underlies the effect of extracellular pH on drug action. Charged drug molecules, such as quinidine, have relatively stable properties as an open channel blocker at wide pH. Therefore, the effect on the inactivated state channel is weak and recovery is slow. In contrast, although lidocaine at neutral pH has the property of a neutral molecule and the effect on inactivated state channels is strong and recovery is fast, lidocaine at low pH becomes charged. Thus, at low pH it works as an open channel blocker and the effect on inactivated state channels becomes weak and recovery becomes slow. The effects of the extracellular acidification on the drugs are related to the phenomenon that the drugs inhibit excitability and conductance effectively in ischemic cardiac myocyte.

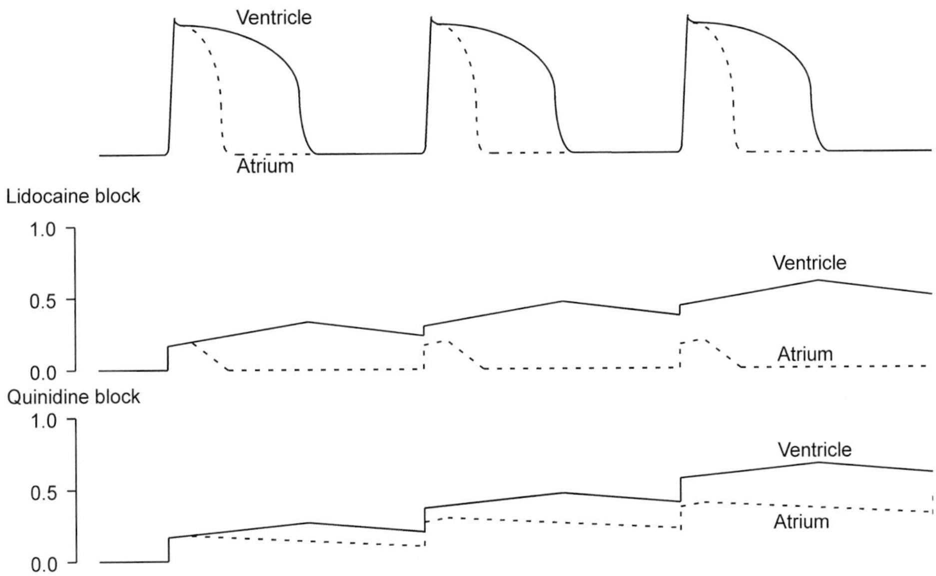

FIGURE 6–6. Accumulation of block effects of lidocaine and quinidine in the atria and ventricle action potentials.

Class I drugs may have other actions than Na^+ channel block. For example, Class Ia drugs such as quinidine and disopyramide can work as K^+ blockers and prolong APD. Because of this, quinidine is well known for starting drug-induced torsades de pointes. In addition, many Class I drugs, such as quinidine and disopyramide, have anticholinergic effects. Anticholinergic effects are due either to drug-induced inhibition of acetylcholine secretion from the nervous system or to inhibition of the effect of acetylcholine in the heart. The latter can be achieved by inhibition of the M_2-muscarinic receptor and/or inhibition of the muscarinic K^+ channel expressed in the sinoatrial and atrioventricular nodes and atrium. Therefore, Class Ia drugs may speed up the conduction in the atrioventricular node and could cause a serious adverse effect in atrial flutter. One reason why digitalis is given to patients with atrial flutter is to slow down the conduction in the atria before fibrillation treatment.

β-Adrenergic Blocker (Class II Drugs)

Stimulus of the β-adrenergic receptor enhances the Ca^{2+} channel current, repolarizing the K^+ and Cl^- channel currents, and may induce DAD- and EAD-related arrhythmias. Therefore, β-adrenergic receptor antagonists, such as propranolol, metoprolol, and atenolol, may work as antiarrhythmic drugs by decreasing sympathetic activity on the heart, and are classified as Class II drugs. β-Adrenergic blockers prolong atrioventricular nodal conduction time and refractoriness, and are useful in preventing or terminating reentrant arrhythmias involving the atrioventricular node in the reentrant pathways.

K Channel Blocker (Class III Drugs)

Reentry, one of the causes of arrhythmia, could be suppressed by removing the heterogeneity of the refractory period. For example, amiodarone is the best established antiarrhythmic drug for the treatment of ventricular arrhythmia in ischemic heart diseases. Amiodarone has multiple drug actions: it has β-block action and Ca^{2+} channel block action on the sinoatrial and atrioventricular nodes, acts on the Na^+ and K^+ channel to increase the refractory period, and acts on the Na^+ channel to slow down intracardiac conduction of the cardiac AP. But which action is mainly responsible for its antiarrhythmic effect has not yet been fully determined. However, amiodarone is generally classified as a Class III drug and APD prolongation is thought to be one of its major effects for effective antiarrhythmic action. As a result of this, a number of Class III drugs have been developed for prolonging APD and thus the refractory period for treatment of cardiac arrhythmia.

Most of the existing class III drugs such as dofetilide (which has recently been utilized to treat atrial fibrillation) and E-4031, and nifekalant, target the rapid delayed rectifier current (I_{kr}), which is one of the most important components of phase 3 repolarization. I_{kr} is a fast component of delayed rectifier K^+ currents and is presumably due to current flowing through the channel pore whose subunit is encoded by the human ether-à-go-go-related gene (hERG). The I_{kr} block effects of many class III drugs were studied as possible antiarrhythmic drugs and I_{kr} block-related adverse effects, such as torsades de pointes, were found in many Class III drugs specifically blocking I_{kr} (Table 6–2).[7] These I_{kr} blockers generally have a tendency to prolong APD as the stimulus frequency is decreased. More prominent prolongation of APD at lower stimulus frequency may cause excessive prolongation of QT at bradycardia, which results in ventricular tachycardia such as torsades de pointes. This reverse frequency-dependent nature of APD propagation by I_{Kr} blockers is known to be one of the underlying mechanisms that induce the life-threatening arrhythmias, torsades de pointes. Candidates for clinically effective I_{kr} blockers without this adverse effect include those that do not cause the reverse-frequency-dependent prolongation of APD.

Two factors may be involved in the reverse-frequency-dependent prolongation of APD upon I_{Kr} blockade. The first factor is the relative contribution of I_{Kr} to the total current for repolarization of the cardiac AP (phase 3) at various stimulus frequencies. The membrane current for AP repolarization is mainly composed of I_{Kr} and I_{Ks} (a slow component of the delayed rectifier K^+ current).[8] I_{Ks} is composed of KvLQT1and minK. Activation of I_{kr} is relatively fast (in the order of

TABLE 6–2. Cardiac and noncardiac drugs reported to block I_{Kr}.[a]

Drug	Blocks I_{Kr}	Prolongs QT interval	TdP reported	Induces EADs	Increases dispersion of repolarization
Antiarrhythmics					
Almokalant	+	+	+	+	+
Amiodarone	+	+	+	−	±
Azimilide	+	+	+	+	+
Dofetilide	+	+	+	+	+
Ibutilide	+	+	+	+	+
Quinidine	+	+	+	+	+
D-Sotalol	+	+	+	+	+
Antihistamines					
Astemizole	+	+	+	+	+
Terfenadine	+	+	+	+	+
Antibiotics					
Erythromycin	+	+	+	+	+
Clarithromycin	+	+	+	+	+
Ca^{2+} channel blockers					
Diltiazem	+	±	−	−	−
Verapamil	+	±	−	−	−
Mibefradil	+	+	+	+	−
Bepridil	+	+	+	+	+
Psychotherapeutics					
Sertindole	+	+	+	+	+
Droperidol	+	+	+	+	?
Fluoxetine	+	±	+	−	?
Miscellaneous					
Cisapride	+	+	+	+	+
Sodium pentobarbital	+	+	−	−	−
Ketanserin	+	+	+	+	+

Source: Modified from Belardinelli *et al.*[7]

[a]These cause torsades de pointes (TdP), induce early afterdepolarizations (EADs), and increase dispersion of ventricular repolarization.

10s of milliseconds) and can be fully activated even with low stimulus frequency. Since deactivation is also fast, I_{Kr} can recover fully before the next stimulus. On the other hand, the activation of I_{ks} is relatively slow, and I_{ks} cannot be fully activated during AP with low stimulus frequency. However, once it is activated, due to the slow deactivation, I_{Ks} cannot be fully deactivated during resting at high stimulus frequency and some of its fraction still remains to be activated at the next stimulus. Therefore, if the stimulus frequency is increased, I_{Ks} will accumulate. And thus the relative contribution of I_{Ks} to the total repolarization current (I_{Ks} plus I_{Kr}) will be increased. That is, when the stimulus frequency is low, the dominant repolarization current is I_{Kr}, and when stimulus frequency is high, it is I_{Ks}. If a Class III drug blocks only I_{Kr}, and blocks it completely, APD will be more prolonged as the frequency of stimulus becomes lower.

The second factor is that the speed of the recovery of open channel blockers of I_{Kr} may affect the reverse frequent dependence. Open channel blockers with slow recovery, such as E-4031 and dofetilide, have a stimulus frequency-independent effect after their blocks reach steady states. However, I_{Kr} blockers with fast recovery, such as vesnarione, exhibit clear use-dependent block at high stimulus frequency while they exhibit only limited use-dependent block at low stimulus frequency. Therefore, the fast recovery and consequent counterreverse frequency dependence work toward the cancellation of the reverse frequency dependence and these types of I_{Kr} blocks are expected to prolong APD without reverse frequency dependence.

In addition to the reverse frequency dependence of APD prolongation by the I_{Kr} blockers, the heterogeneity of depolarization in tissue caused by them is thought to be another underlying mechanism that causes torsades de points. In fact, it is known that amiodarone does not cause heterogeneity of excitation in tissue despite prominent prolongation of APD (Table 6–2).

Ca Channel Blocker (Class IV Drugs)

Cardiac Ca^{2+} channels activate at more depolarized potential than Na^{+} channels and their activation and inactivation are slower than Na^{+} channels. Together with outward K channel currents, inward currents through the activated Ca^{2+} channel shape the action potential plateau in phase 2. Because of these characteristics of Ca^{2+} channel current, its blockade leads to the reduction of amplitude and length of phase 2. The first generation of Ca^{2+} antagonists specifically inhibits L-type Ca^{2+} channels, and is categorized as class IV drugs in the Vaughan-Williams classification. These Ca^{2+} channel antagonists are divided into three subclasses: the benzothiazepine class (e.g., diltiazem), papaverine derivatives (e.g., verapamil), and dihydropyridines (e.g., nifedipine). These three first generation Ca^{2+} blockers also have a prominent effect on blood vessel smooth muscle and have been used as antihypertensive drugs. The second generation Ca^{2+} blockers, such as dilitiazem SR, verapamil SR, nifedipine SR, and istradipine, have extended-release mechanisms.[9] The third generation Ca^{2+} blockers, such as amlodipine, lacidipine, and lercanidipine, have slow onset and long acting hemodynamic effects-over days. Some of them have effects other than L-type Ca^{2+} channel blockade: nicardipine and amlodipine inhibit the N-type Ca^{2+} channel.

Binding Site of Ca Channel Blockers

After Numa and colleagues revealed the structure of the α_1 subunit of the L-type Ca^{2+} channel from skeletal muscle, Ca^{2+} channels from various tissues including cardiac myocytes were cloned. With these results, binding positions of Ca^{2+} blockers were elucidated. The three different blockers are known to bind to three different sites of the α_1 subunit: the 1,4-dihydropyridine (DHP) site, the phenylalkylamine site, and the benzothiazepine site. What makes the Ca^{2+} channel blocker different from the Na^{+} channel blocker is that the combined application of these Ca^{2+} channels can enhance or weaken the block effect. The multiple binding sites for the Ca^{2+} channel blocker account for this phenomenon.

Use Dependence

Each of the three different first-generation Ca^{2+} blockers shows different use dependence. Verapamil does not exhibit resting block and opening of the channel accumulates the block effect. Diltiazem has mild resting block and use-dependent block, which is stepwisely strengthened with the depolarizing pulse. Nifedipine shows distinct resting block and virtually no use-dependent block. The underlying mechanisms of these Ca^{2+} channel blockers can also be understood by the modulated receptor hypothesis. Verapamil may be a charged molecule, nifedipine may be a neutral molecule, and diltiazem may be between a charged and neutral molecule.

And as with the case of Na^{+} channel blockers, both hydrophilic and hydrophobic pathways exist for Ca^{2+} channel blockers. For example, the block effect of verapamil is obviously use dependent and verapamil can enter and exit from intracellular space through pores only when the channels are open. Therefore, the block effect of verapamil lasts a long time. Because verapamil and diltiazem enhance their use dependence under high-frequency stimulus, they presumably have a high affinity with activated state channels. Some dihydropyridine derivatives enhance L-type Ca^{2+} channel current, which cannot be explained by simple blockade of the channel pore, and have allosteric mechanisms with the concept of mode. Antagonists of dihydropyridines (nifedipine) move Ca^{2+} channel mode I to mode 0, and agonists of dihydropyridines (e.g., BAY K8644) move Ca^{2+} channel mode I to mode II.

Digitalis

The primary action of digitalis, such as digoxin, is to inhibit Na^+-K^+-ATPase, which results in an inotropic action on heart tissues and also an increase of vagal tone. As for the treatment of cardiac arrhythmia, digitalis is used to decrease the conduction of atrioventricular conduction. Thus, digitalis is used to (1) decrease the conduction of atrial excitation to the ventricle in tachyatrial fibrillation and (2) prevent paroxysmal supraventricular tachycardia (PSVT) with a Ca^{2+} channel blocker, verapamil.

Adenosine

Adenosine is a metabolite of ATP and is not included in the list of the Vaughan-Williams classification. This substance is able to stop the paroxysmal supraventricular tachycardia, which includes the atrioventricular node in its circuit and some of adrenaline (or excise)-induced ventricular tachycardia. Adenosine binds to the A_1-purinergic receptor of cardiac myocytes. The A_1-purinergic receptor couples to either adenylyl cyclase (AC) or inwardly rectifying muscarinic K^+ channels via trimeric pertussis toxin-sensitive $G_{i/o}$ proteins. Thus adenosine exhibits two actions: (1) an increase of K^+ conductance in sinoatrial and atrioventricular nodes and atria but not in the ventricle, and (2) inhibition of AC to reduce intracellular cyclic AMP in all types of cardiac myocytes including nodal, atrial, and ventricular myocytes (Figure 6–7).

Adenosine (5~10 mg) should be applied intravenously with a one-shot bolus injection, because the substance will be rapidly absorbed into cells via a cell membrane transporter. Thus, the time of action is transient and very short (less than several tenths of seconds). Dipyridamole prolongs the action of adenosine by disturbing the action of the transporter. The A_1-receptor antagonists, such as theophylline and aminophylline, abolish the action. ATP can also be used for the same purposes, because this substance will be metabolized to adenosine quickly in the blood. However, ATP may also binds to P_2-purinergic ATP receptors prior to being metabolized to adenosine. P_2 receptors either form ligand-gated nonselective cation channels (P2X) or couple to G_q proteins and the Ca^{2+} mobilization signal (P2Y). Thus, ATP causes abnormal excitation of cardiac tissues, such as premature ventricular excitation, in addition to the actions of adenosine-mediated A_1-receptor actions.

Cessation of PSVT: Adenosine injected intravenously transiently increases a K^+ conductance and causes bradycardia and various degrees of atrioventricular conduction block. Therefore, the tachyarrhythmia due to the macrocircuit reentrant involving the atrioventricular node can be transiently stopped because of the atrioventricular conduction block. A Ca^{2+} channel blocker, verapamil, is also often used for the same purpose because this drug prolongs atrioventricular conduction. However, it is necessary to be careful to use this Ca^{2+} channel blocker for this purpose, because verapamil possesses a prominent negative inotropic action by blocking the sarcolemmal

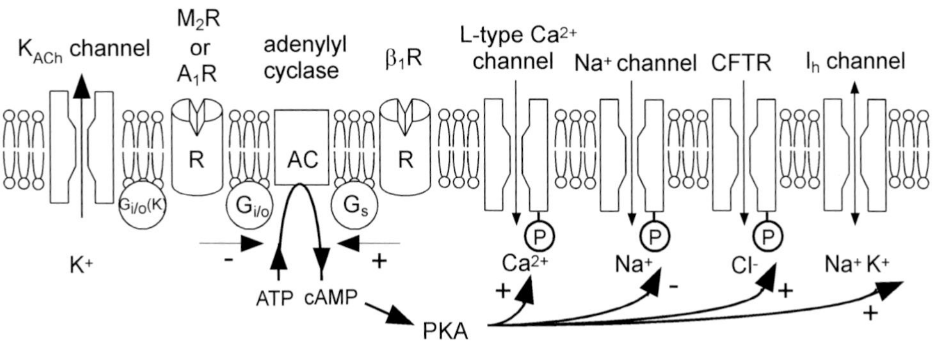

FIGURE 6–7. Intracellular signal transduction controlling cardiac ion channels.

Ca^{2+} channel and the washout of action takes a very long time (3–7 h).

Cessation of exercise-induced ventricular tachycardia: Exercise-induced or adrenaline-induced ventricular tachycardia is caused by an increase of intracellular cAMP due to β-adrenergic stimulation.[10] β_1-Adrenergic receptors in cardiac myocytes stimulate AC via G_s proteins. Stimulation of AC by G_s proteins is antagonized with $G_{i/o}$ proteins (dual control of AC by G proteins). Because the adenosine A_1-receptor couples to $G_{i/o}$ proteins, adenosine applied intravenously can decrease cAMP enhanced by β-adrenergic stimulation and thus stop the ventricular tachycardia.

References

1. Echt DS, Liebson PR, Mitchell LB, Peters RW, Obias-Manno D, Barker AH, Arensberg D, Baker A, Friedman L, Greene HL, *et al.* Mortality and morbidity in patients receiving encainide, flecainide, or placebo. The Cardiac Arrhythmia Suppression Trial. *N Engl J Med* 1991;324:781–788.
2. Vaughan Williams EM. A classification of antiarrhythmic actions reassessed after a decade of new drugs. *J Clin Pharmacol* 1984;24:129–147.
3. Vaughan Williams EM. Classification of antiarrhythmic drugs. In: Sandoe E, Flensted-Jensen E, Olsen EH, Eds. *Symposium on Cardiac Arrhythmias.* Sodertalje, Sweden: AB Astra, 1970:449–501.
4. Task Force of the Working Group on Arrhythmias of the European Society of Cardiology. The Sicilian Gambit: A new approach to the classification of antiarrhythmic drugs based on their actions on arrhythmogenic mechanisms. *Circulation* 1991;84: 1831–1851.
5. Hondeghem LM, Katzung BG. Time- and voltage-dependent interactions of antiarrhythmic drugs with cardiac sodium channels. *Biochim Biophys Acta* 1977;472:373–398.
6. Hille B. Local anesthetics: Hydrophilic and hydrophobic pathways for the drug-receptor reaction. *J Gen Physiol* 1977;69:497–515.
7. Belardinelli L, Antzelevitch C, Vos MA. Assessing predictors of drug-induced torsade de pointes. *Trends Pharmacol Sci* 2003;2412:619–625.
8. Zeng J, Laurita KR, Rosenbaum DS, Rudy Y. Two components of the delayed rectifier K+ current in ventricular myocytes of the guinea pig type. Theoretical formulation and their role in repolarization. *Circ Res* 1995;77:140–152.
9. Luscher TF, Cosentino F. The classification of calcium antagonists and their selection in the treatment of hypertension: a reappraisal. *Drugs* 1998;55: 509–517.
10. Lerman BB, Belardinelli L, West GA, Berne RM, DiMarco JP. Adenosine-sensitive ventricular tachycardia: Evidence suggesting cyclic AMP-mediated triggered activity. *Circulation* 1986;74:270–280.

7 Mechanoelectrical Interactions and Their Role in Electrical Function of the Heart

John Jeremy Rice and Peter Kohl

Integrated Cardiac Electromechanics

Introduction

The heart is an electrically controlled and chemically powered mechanical pump. There are complex interactions between cardiac electrophysiology, metabolism, and mechanics, with a multitude of interdigitating regulatory loops. This chapter will focus on the *cross-talk* between electrical and mechanical activity of the heart, and in particular its relevance for heart rhythm.

The cross-talk between cardiac electrics and mechanics can be viewed conceptually as a regulatory loop (Figure 7–1). In this loop, electrical control of cardiac contraction is afforded by excitation–contraction coupling (ECC)* while, in turn, the mechanical environment affects cardiac electrical activity via mechanoelectric feedback (MEF). This regulatory loop manifests itself at every level of structural integration, from whole heart to single cell. It supports the maintenance of steady-state cardiac performance, ensures adaptation to changing circulatory demands (even in the transplanted heart), and can contribute to both causation and termination of heart rhythm disturbances.[1]

Spatiotemporal Considerations

The heart is a spatially heterogeneous organ, both in terms of structure (e.g., variations in regional tissue architecture, cell distribution, coupling, innervation, blood supply) and function (active and passive tissue electromechanical properties). In addition, there are temporal gradients in key electromechanical behavior (e.g., activation, repolarization, shortening). Nonetheless, under physiological conditions the heart functions as a highly coordinated unit. This "externally homogeneous" mechanical performance at the organ level arises from, and necessarily requires, structural and functional heterogeneity at the (sub)cellular and tissue levels.[2]

While this appreciation has guided our thinking on structural and functional adaptation of the heart to (patho)physiological developments, it leaves the question as to how an individual cardiomyocyte inside this complex organization "knows" when and how to respond to beat-by-beat changes in electromechanical activity. The *when* is largely a function of the coordinated spread of electrical excitation (see Chapter 4 for details on the cardiac conduction system). The *how* requires subcellular regulatory pathways that match local mechanical performance to global mechanical demand; underlying processes are discussed next.

---

*Abbreviations: AP, action potential; ATP, adenosine triphosphate; $[Ca]_I$, free cytosolic Ca concentration; ECC, excitation–contraction coupling; ILCOR, International Liaison Committee on Resuscitation; LCC, L-type Ca channel; MEF, mechanoelectric feedback; NCX, Na/Ca exchanger; PT, precordial thump; RyR, ryanodine receptor; SAC, SAC_{NS}, SAC_K, stretch-activated channels of various ion selectivity; SERCA, sarcoplamsic/endoplasmic reticulum Ca^{2+}-ATPase; SL, sarcomere length; SR, sarcoplasmic reticulum; TnC, TnI, TnT, troponin C, troponin I, troponin T; VT,ventricular tachycardia; VF, ventricular fibrillation.

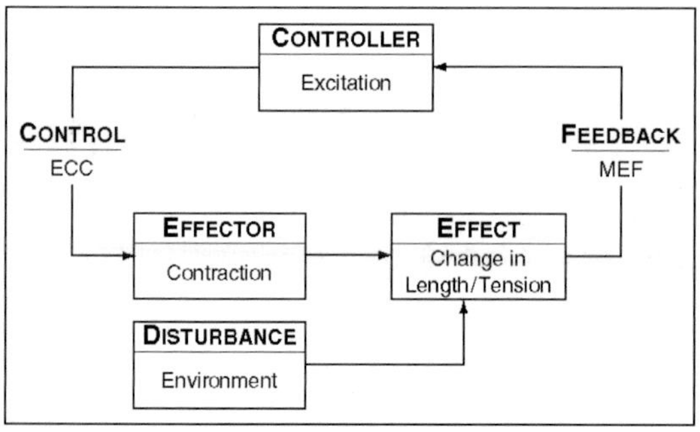

FIGURE 7–1. Conceptual scheme of cardiac electromechanical regulation. Electrical control of cardiac contraction is via excitation–contraction coupling (ECC), while the mechanical environment affects cardiac electrical behavior via mechanoelectric feedback (MEF). (From Kohl *et al.*,[1] with permission.)

Excitation–Contraction Coupling

Introduction

The process of ECC involves a transient rise in free cytosolic calcium concentration ($[Ca]_i$), as the intermediate signal between electrical depolarization of the cell membrane and activation of contractile myofilaments. The sequence is initiated by calcium (Ca) influx across the sarcolemma, which produces a secondary release of Ca from the sarcoplasmic reticulum (SR, a specialized Ca storage compartment in mammalian cardiac myocytes). The SR can rapidly release Ca in response to sarcolemmal Ca influx, a process termed "Ca-induced Ca release." The released Ca then binds to several intracellular Ca-binding proteins, including troponin, which in turn activates the myofilaments. The majority of Ca is resequestered back into the SR during each heartbeat, while the remainder (in steady state this is an amount equivalent to the initial transsarcolemmal influx) is extruded across the membrane.

In reality, the events involved in ECC are intimately connected and cannot be decomposed into discrete sets of spatially or temporally defined events. For example, SR Ca release occurs simultaneously with reuptake, with the net effect depending on the relative balance of the competing processes at any given time. Also, SR Ca storage involves "memory" mechanisms that render the amount of Ca stored in, and released from, the SR strongly dependent on stimulation history. Thus, the system shows complex behavior within single beats and between multiple beats. The following sections outline separate steps in the activation and relaxation sequence of cardiac muscle. However, care must be taken to remember that this decomposition into discrete steps is highly artificial and underestimates the complex dynamics of ECC.[3,4]

From Action Potential to Calcium Release

Figure 7–2 shows a conceptual model of Ca handling during a typical heartbeat. The trigger events (Figure 7–2A) involve sarcolemmal influx of Ca through L-type Ca channels (LCC; thick downward arrow), which produces a secondary and larger release of Ca from the SR (upward thick arrow), released via ryanodine receptors (RyR) into the diadic space (dotted box labeled DS). An important negative feedback pathway exists in that the released Ca, as well as LCC influx itself, causes Ca-induced inactivation of LCC, which reduces further influx (upward thin arrow with a "minus" sign). From the diadic space, Ca diffuses into the myoplasm (thick rightward arrow) to increase $[Ca]_i$ from approximately 0.1 μM to 1 μM (represented by the schematic Ca transient). The majority of this released Ca binds to intracellular buffers, including troponin and calmodulin (not shown). Ca can also enter the cell during the action potential (AP) upstroke and "notch" (rapid partial repolarization to plateau levels) via the Na/Ca exchanger (NCX), although this pathway is considered less important for ECC than Ca influx via LCC.

L-Type Ca Channel Influx

The LCC is the major influx pathway for Ca during each heartbeat. This current has multiple roles in producing the Ca transient, both by directly increasing $[Ca]_i$ and by triggering a larger secondary Ca release from the SR. Moreover this current contributes to AP morphology, especially in sustaining the AP plateau in spite of repolarizing K currents (see Chapters 13 and 14). LCC are activated by voltage and inactivated by both voltage and Ca.[5]

The Ca-induced inactivation is thought to play a primary role in determining the amplitude and

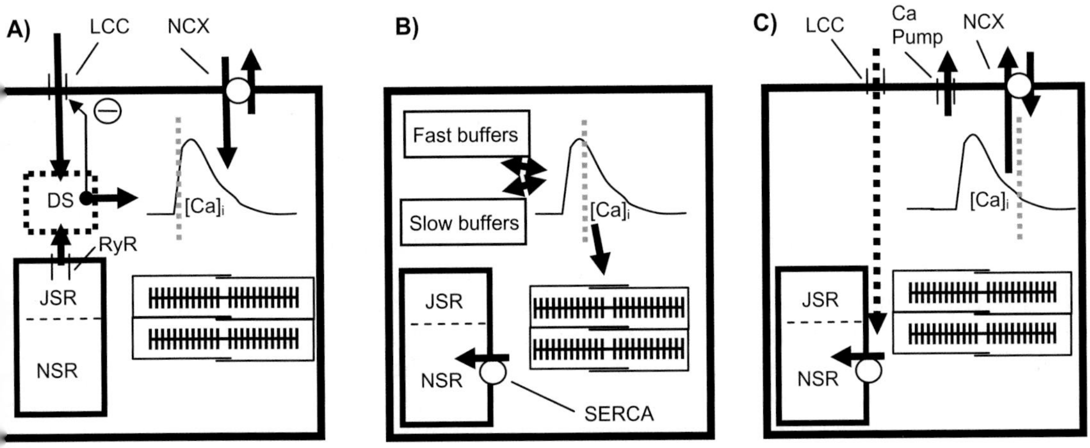

FIGURE 7–2. Schematic diagram of a cardiac cell, showing three conceptual steps in excitation–contraction coupling (ECC), with pseudorepresentative timing relative to cytosolic free Ca concentration ($[Ca]_i$) dynamics indicated by gray dotted lines. (A) Ca-induced Ca release; (B) cytosolic Ca buffering and contraction changes; (C) Ca reuptake and extrusion (for detail see text). DS, dyadic space; JSR, junctional sarcoplasmic reticulum; LCC, L-type Ca channel; NCX, Na/Ca exchanger; NSR, network sarcoplasmic reticulum; RyR, ryanodine receptor; SERCA, sarcoplasmic/endoplasmatic reticulum Ca-ATPase.

time course of LCC currents.[5,6] One potential role of this negative feedback (Figure 7–2A, thin arrow) is to limit Ca influx after triggering Ca-induced Ca release. However, longer-term roles in Ca homeostasis of both intracellular and SR Ca levels are also proposed.[4] Interestingly, LLC are generally assumed to sense diadic space Ca levels, determined largely by SR Ca release; this has a shorter latency, higher amplitude, and smaller overall duration than the cytosolic $[Ca]_i$ transient.[7] In contrast, Ca-induced LCC inactivation is generally seen to be prolonged, lasting as long as the AP.[5] These complex spatiotemporal dynamics may result from complicated molecular interactions with calmodulin, whose genetic manipulation to remove the negative feedback has surprisingly large side effects on AP duration (lengthening it by four or five times).[6] Thus, key electrophysiological parameters can be significantly more sensitive to Ca handling than customarily assumed.

Sarcoplasmic Reticulum Ca Release via Ryanodine Receptor Channels

Ca release from the SR via RyR has been shown to be roughly proportional to the trigger influx of Ca via LCC, although some variation exists, depending on how Ca flux is determined.[7] The system shows high gain, in that a small number of LLC will trigger release from a nearby cluster of RyR channels that open synchronously (see Chapter 15). As the discrete opening of LCC can modulate the number of activated RyR clusters, the large total Ca release tracks roughly linearly with total LCC Ca influx.

Another property of SR Ca release is that it appears to be a nonlinear function of SR Ca load. Essentially no SR release occurs below a threshold, after which SR release is usually a steeply increasing function of SR load.[7,8] Interestingly, there are indications that more than 100% of the original SR Ca content is released, suggesting that Ca is recycled back into SR during the release process, and rereleased again.[7] For a typical beat, though, the Ca release fraction is estimated at 60–80%.[8] Lastly, there appears to be a set maximum SR Ca load beyond which spontaneous RyR Ca release occurs, with potential for arrhythmogenesis (see Chapter 15). In addition, spontaneous RyR Ca release appears to also play critical roles in determining resting $[Ca]_i$.

From Calcium Release to Contraction

The translation of $[Ca]_i$ to force generation occurs at the level of the sarcomere, i.e., the basic subcellular unit of the contractile apparatus (Figure 7–3). The sarcomere is composed primarily of interdigitated thick myosin filaments that interact, when activated, with thinner actin filaments.[9,10]

While the basic interactions in the sarcomere are known, the underlying basis of several complex behavioral properties is still debated. For example, the myofilament system shows a high level of Ca sensitivity, as characterized by steep force–Ca relationships with a Hill coefficient equal to 7 or more (Figure 7–3B). Because each troponin binds a single Ca ion on the regulatory site of troponin C (TnC), a Hill coefficient of 1 is predicted; hence, the high Ca sensitivity is assumed to result from one or more cooperative mechanisms.[11]

Briefly, three types of cooperative interactions are most widely accepted. Attached crossbridges have been shown to increase the Ca affinity of TnC.[12–14] A second type of cooperativity among the regulatory proteins is thought to arise from nearest-neighbor interactions, produced by the overlap of adjacent tropomyosin units along the thin filament (Figure 7–3A).[9,10] A third proposed mechanism is that the binding of one myosin head increases the binding rate of neighboring heads by holding the regulatory proteins in a more permissive conformation.[15] Alternatively, the binding

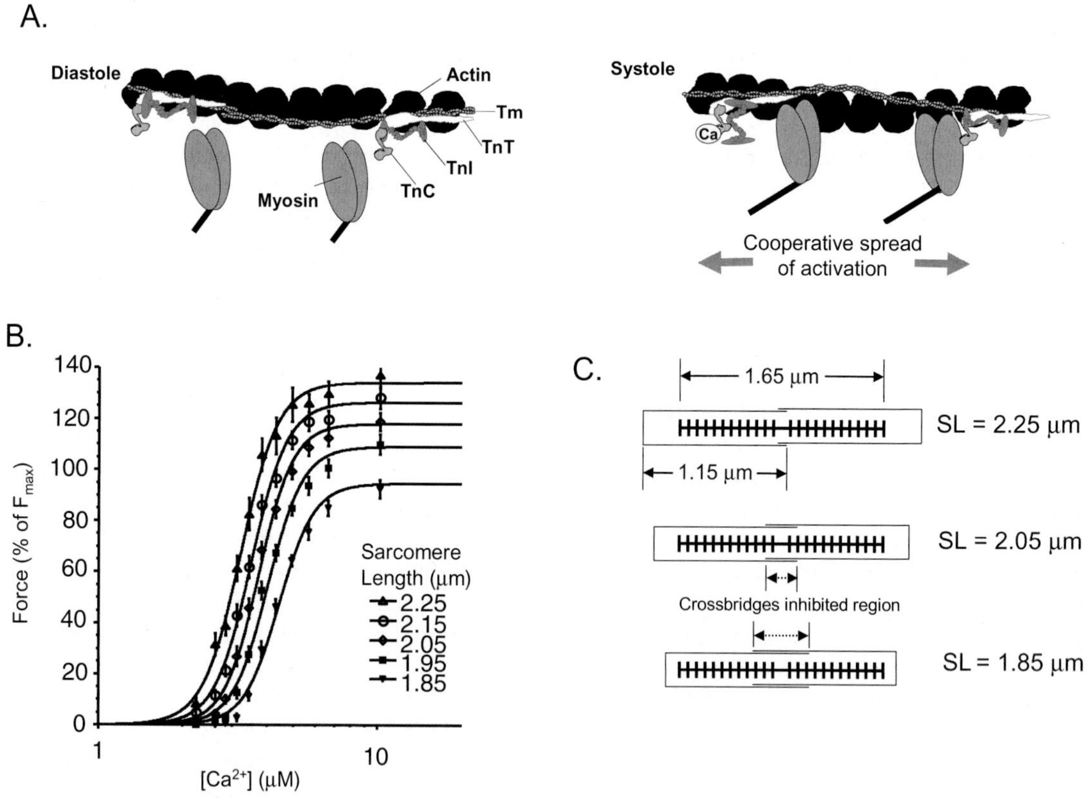

FIGURE 7–3. Contractile filaments and calcium. (A) Interrelation of a thin actin filament with nearby myosin heads. During diastole (left), tropomyosin (Tm) and troponin subunits (TnC, TnT, and TnI) sterically block crossbridge formation. During systole, elevated $[Ca]_i$ shifts the locations of tropomyosin/troponin to allow myosin head attachment and force generation. Note that cooperative activation can spread along the thin filament (see text for details). (From Bers,[3] with permission.) (B) Average force–Ca^{2+} relationships (pooled data, skinned rat cardiac trabeculae, $n = 10$) at five sarcomere lengths (SL); data are fitted to a Hill relationship. The level of cooperativity, assessed by the Hill coefficient, is not affected by SL. (From Dobesh *et al.*,[17] with permission.) (C) Diagram showing expected sarcomere geometry for three of the SL shown. Binding of crossbridges is assumed to be inhibited in the central region in which the thin filaments overlap.

of one crossbridge may pull binding sites on a compliant thin filament into register with myosin heads that have an inherently different characteristic distance in their repeating structure.[16]

Another complex phenomenon is the length dependence of force–Ca functions. Length-dependent effects can be separated into two main categories: changes in plateau force and changes in Ca sensitivity. As SL decreases, changes in plateau force may arise from overlap of thin filaments, which reduce the recruitable pool of crossbridges (Figure 7–3C; note that the lengths of the thick and thin filaments differ from the accepted values for skeletal muscle[11]). In support of this scheme, the developed force and ATPase rate of maximally activated cardiac muscle are linear functions of SL.[18] The second category is a decrease in myofilament Ca sensitivity, as shown by the rightward shift in force–Ca curves as SL shortens (Figure 7–3B). These length-dependent changes in Ca sensitivity are generally assumed to be the cellular basis of the Frank–Starling effect, although the biophysical mechanism is still under debate. One hypothesis suggests that SL changes the lattice spacing of the thick and thin filaments, with subsequent changes in crossbridge attachment.[19] Titin, a large protein that links myosin and actin lattices, could modify interfilament spacing[20] or act by additional mechanisms. However, other studies suggest that physiological changes in lattice spacing are insufficient to account for the observed changes in Ca sensitivity.[21,22] The changes in Ca sensitivity could result from cross-interactions of cooperative mechanisms and length-dependent changes in crossbridge recruitment as illustrated in Figure 7-3C.[11]

In addition to the immediate stretch-induced increase in cardiac force development, there is a secondary and more slowly occurring increase in force, which eventually reaches a plateau.[23] In contrast to the fast response, the slow force response involves an increase in Ca transient amplitude (Figure 7–4).[24] At the level of the myofilaments, there are no slow time-dependent changes in Ca sensitivity. In fact, length changes during the diastolic period alone are sufficient to generate a slow force response,[24,25,26] suggesting mechanisms that are independent of the ones discussed above. A full review of slow changes in force, and possible effects on membrane currents, is available elsewhere.[27] One obvious source of increased Ca is mechanically modulated ion channels (discussed below), which either directly conduct Ca ions or allow Na entry, which secondarily increases intracellular Ca, for example, via NCX. An alternative mechanism suggests Na influx via the Na/H exchanger, activated by a stretch-induced increase in angiotensin II and endothelin-1.[28,29]

Effects on the Ca Transient

While the exact mechanisms of length-dependent changes in Ca sensitivity are controversial, they may not be that important in understanding mechanical feedback on Ca transients. The amount of Ca bound to the myofilaments is generally assumed to be affected by the number of attached crossbridges (instead of length itself).[12–14] Hence, any feature that affects developed force can have secondary effects on Ca binding to troponin and on the Ca transient.

For example, increasing muscle length by 10% (see time points 3 and 4 in Figure 7–4) has a dramatic effect on developed force (see force in Figure 7–4B). This increase in developed force leads to greater Ca binding to TnC, initially lowering cytosolic $[Ca]_i$. Later, during the Ca transient, $[Ca]_i$ is slightly higher, as more Ca is slowly coming off TnC (compared with the low force case). Similar effects on the Ca transient have been seen elsewhere,[12,24,25,30,31] although details depend on the nature of mechanical perturbations and Ca monitoring agents used. Taken together, these results suggest that changes in force-dependent Ca binding to troponin have a noticeable, but not dramatic, effect on $[Ca]_i$ levels, which may restrict the role of this phase in mediating MEF effects.

Finally, a few more general comments should be made about Ca buffering. The cytosol of the cardiomyocyte is heavily buffered, and the vast majority of Ca ions are bound to several important buffers. For example, at diastolic $[Ca]_i$ of 0.1 μM, only ~2.5% of Ca ions are "free" in solution; this fraction increases to ~4.5% when systolic $[Ca]_i$ rises to 1 μM.[3] As shown in Figure 7–3B, fast and slow buffering systems exist in addition to troponin and the SR. Several fast buffers have dissociation constants near the operating range of

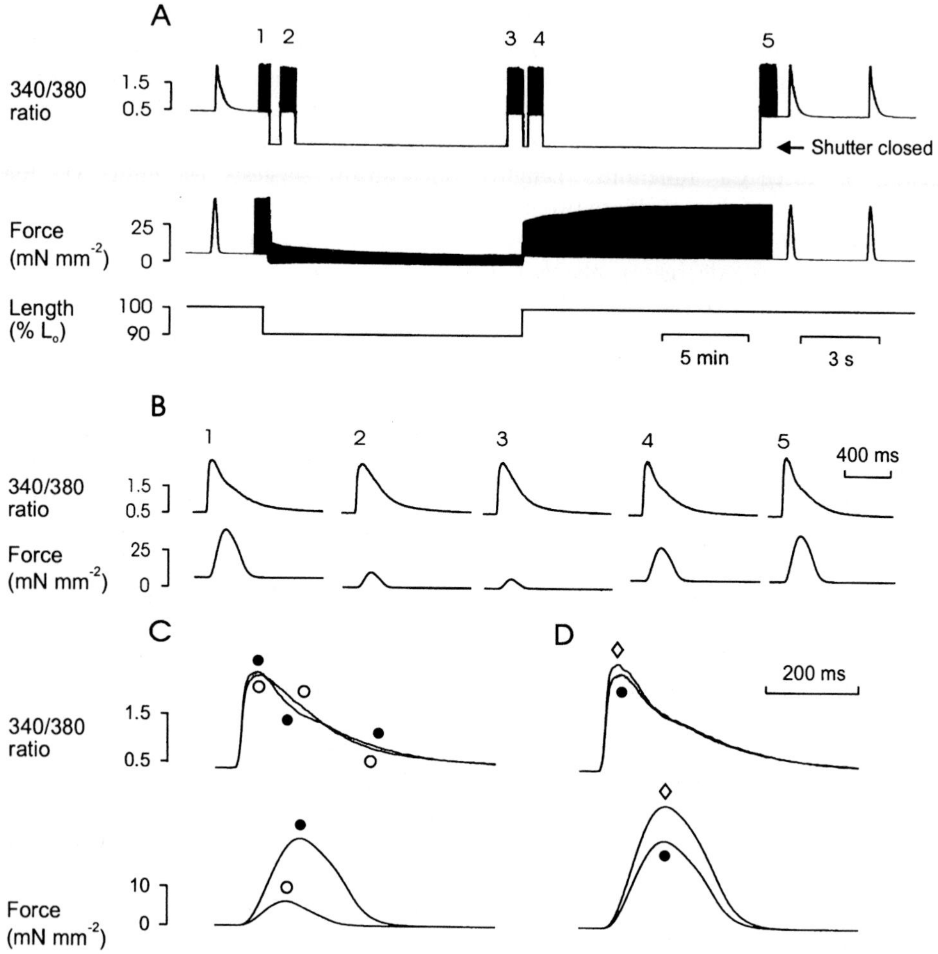

FIGURE 7–4. Illustration of immediate and slow changes in force after length changes. Records of the changes in fura2 fluorescence ratio and force produced by shortening a rat trabecula by 10% for 15 min. (A) Records of 340 nm/380 nm fluorescence ratio and force, with a representation of the length change from the initial length (L_0). A shutter in the excitation light pathway was opened only for discrete 48-sec recording periods (labeled 1–5) in order to avoid photobleaching of fura2. Note the slow changes in twitch force after the changes in muscle length. (B) Mean records (from 16 twitches) of fluorescence ratio and force measured during periods 1–5 in (A). (C) Overlaid traces of the fluorescence ratio and force averaged during periods 3 (○) and 4 (●) to illustrate the rapid effects of the length increase. Resting forces have been subtracted from these traces. (D) similar overlaid traces averaged during periods 4 (●) and 5 (◇) to illustrate the delayed effects of length increase. 24°C, 1 mM external Ca^{2+}, 0.33 Hz stimulation rate. (From Kentish *et al.*,[24] with permission.)

the Ca transient (0.1–1 μM), and these bind and release Ca on each heart beat. This group includes calmodulin, adenosine triphosphate (ATP), creatine phosphate, and the phospholipids of the sarcolemma. Slow buffers have dissociation constants that are much lower than the operating range of $[Ca]_i$, and hence Ca remains largely bound to these buffers throughout the heartbeat. Slow buffers include myosin and two high-affinity, nonregulatory sites on TnC. In addition, the mitochondria comprise roughly 35% of cytosolic volume and can potentially contain large amounts of Ca. Their large volume, coupled with close proximity to myofilaments and RyR, suggests a potentially significant active role for mitochondria in ECC.[3] However, most findings suggest little net Ca transit between mitochondria and cytosol on a beat-by-beat basis. In fact, mitochondrial Ca exchange may be an epiphenomenon of mechanisms that match ATP production to cellular demand, using intracellular Ca as a proxy for the energetic demand of a cell.

From Contraction to Relaxation

While "contraction" tends to be at the focus of attention, the process of relaxation is just as important for cardiac performance, yet is less well understood.[32] As diastolic filling occurs under low pressure, any residual force from incomplete relaxation can severely affect cardiac function. Relaxation is more than just elastic recoil of tissue, and complexities arise from the interplay of Ca release from the myofilaments, Ca reuptake into the SR, and crossbridge detachment (Figure 7–2C).

Besides serving as a trigger, LCC Ca influx also serves to load the SR (Figure 7–2C, dotted down arrow). This influx of Ca is thought mainly to influence the amount of Ca releasable by the SR on the subsequent beat (rather than the current beat). In steady-sate conditions, net loading is zero, as the amount of Ca extruded by NCX (and sarcolemmal Ca pumps) matches that of LCC influx.

The majority of $[Ca]_i$ (60–80%, depending on species) is recycled back into SR via the sarcoplasmic/endoplasmic reticulum Ca-ATPase (SERCA). Factors such as heart rate, inotrophic stimulation, or pathologies affect reuptake rates (heart failure can decrease SR uptake by 50%).[3,33] The major sarcolemmal efflux pathway is the NCX, extruding ~20–40% of Ca during the transient, whereas the sarcolemmal Ca-ATPase and mitochondrial uptake are generally thought to contribute less.[34]

With the decline of $[Ca]_i$, Ca ions unbind from TnC, starting the relaxation process. If TnC were a simple buffer, the process could be easily described. However, complexities arise from the presence of activated thin filaments and attached crossbridges, which increase TnC affinity for Ca (as described previously). Moreover, a small number of attached crossbridges are thought to be able to hold the thin filament in an activated state, even if Ca has dissociated from neighboring binding sites (Figure 7–3A). Thus, attached crossbridges can slow relaxation both by increasing Ca affinity of TnC and by holding the thin filament activated after Ca has dissociated from a fraction of TnC.

Because of these features, contractions involving high levels of developed force (and many attached crossbridges) are slower to relax than those with lower force development. This affects especially final relaxation, past 50% of maximum force.[35,36] Thus, a larger force transient as observed after application of stretch (see Figure 7–4C, lower panel) is noticeably slower to relax than a low force transient (note that for the two runs shown in Figure 7–4C, the activating Ca transients are very similar). Interestingly, increased force due to larger peak Ca transients also produces a slowed final relaxation, suggesting that the effect results from slow unbinding kinetics of crossbridges, not upstream Ca activation events.[32,36]

Finally, and as noted previously, complete relaxation is important for competent diastolic filling. Here, the steep Ca sensitivity of the myofilaments contributes to keeping the developed force minimal at diastolic $[Ca]_i$. Other features that may promote relaxation include the ability of myosin to detach under isometric or lengthening conditions (by quickly reversing the steps of attachment and head rotation) in a manner that retains most of the energy of ATP hydrolysis.[11,32] In contrast, the typical forward cycling scheme requires ADP dissociation and new ATP binding for a crossbridge to detach (if this slower detachment mechanism dominated, the relaxation rate would be greatly slowed). In fact, recent characterizations of isolated myofibrils suggest that relaxation is a nonuniform biphasic process,[32] and while isolated myofibril behavior may differ from intact muscle, the point is clear that relaxation is complex and is not just the reverse of activation.

Mechanoelectric Feedback

Diastolic Stretch Effects

As shown above, the heart is an exquisitely mechanosensitive organ. This also applies to mechanoelectrical transduction, as will be obvious

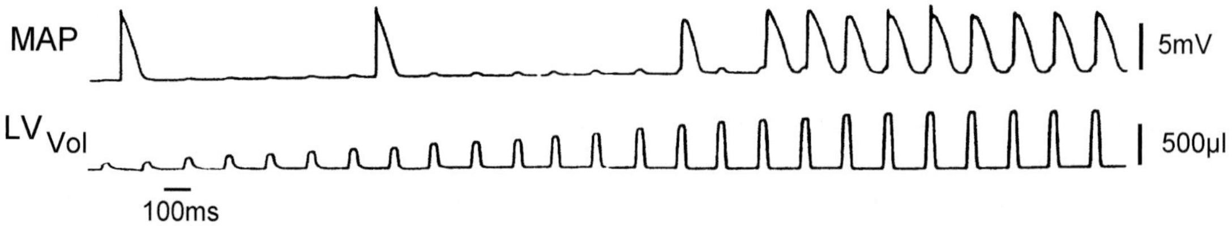

FIGURE 7–5. Diastolic stretch causes membrane depolarization. Monophasic action potential recordings (MAP) from an isolated rabbit heart (AV node disrupted) shows that injection of increasing amounts of fluid into a left ventricular balloon (LV_{Vol}) causes matching diastolic depolarizations that, once threshold is reached, will mechanically pace the preparation (note: the first two action potentials are spontaneous escape beats not related to mechanical stimulation). (From Franz *et al.*,[37] with permission.)

to anyone whose training involved the use of Langendorff-style heart preparations that can be stopped or started "by the flick of a finger." Mechanisms underlying these acute electrical responses to mechanical stimulation include stretch-activated ion channels (SAC), mechanical modulation of Ca handling, and effects mediated via communication with other cells.

As a rule, mechanical stimulation of resting cardiac tissue (during "electrical diastole") causes membrane depolarization (Figure 7–5).[37] This behavior can be observed across the whole range of structural integration, from whole organ to single cell, and it is understood to be largely mediated by depolarizing transmembrane currents through SAC.[38,39]

The SAC were discovered in mammalian cardiomyocytes about two decades ago,[40] and a number of channels with varying ion selectivity and gating properties have subsequently been described. Despite two decades of research, a uniform SAC classification has yet to emerge.

Meanwhile, SAC can be distinguished based on ion selectivity. The first group is composed of SAC that show little selectivity for the various cations normally present in physiological solutions (SAC_{NS}; for nonselective). The second group preferentially conducts potassium (SAC_K). A third group of chloride-selective channels[41] has been described in settings that involve centrifugal membrane deformation (most commonly in the context of pathophysiologically increased cell volumes). These channels show significant lag times between mechanical stimulus and increased channel open probability (1 min or more), rendering them less likely to underlie acute mechanical effects on heart rate and rhythm.[†]

The SAC_{NS} usually have reversal potentials between 0 and −20 mV. This is more positive than the membrane potential of resting cardiomyocytes, so that diastolic activation of SAC_{NS} will tend to depolarize cardiac cells. In working cardiomyocytes, SAC_{NS} activation may cause ectopic AP generation,[38] while in pacemaker cells a positive chronotropic response may be observed.[42]

The SAC_K will tend to shift the membrane potential toward the potassium equilibrium potential (negative to −90 mV), so their activation will oppose depolarization.

Given that diastolic stretch tends to depolarize myocardium, SAC_{NS} are generally assumed to be the leading contributors to acute electrophysiological responses of cardiac cells to stretch. In support of this idea, block of SAC_{NS} prevents mechanically induced extrasystoles.[43] In contrast, SAC_K appear to play secondary roles, at least under physiological conditions.

Systolic Stretch Effects

The AP upstroke, whether triggered by mechanical or electrical stimulation, is firmly governed by the fast sodium current. Any additional stimuli, including mechanical, have little appreciable effect.

[†]Mechanosensitive chloride channels are likely to affect electrophysiology predominantly in settings such as ischemia, reperfusion, or hypertrophy (where they are constitutently activated); for further detail see Baumgarten and Clemo.[41]

During the subsequent AP plateau, cardiomyocyte membranes are more positive than the reversal potentials of either SAC_{NS} or SAC_K, and stretch tends to have a repolarizing effect, which often leads to an overall reduction in AP duration.[44] However, AP lengthening[45] and crossover of repolarization[46] have also been observed. In particular, stretch applied during late repolarization often prolongs the AP, potentially giving rise to early or delayed afterdepolarization-like behavior. These afterdepolarizations may trigger extra beats, such as seen in patients during balloon valvuloplasty.[47]

Even when the immediate outcome of mechanically induced effects on systolic electrophysiology is less prominent, MEF can still affect electrical load, excitability, and refractoriness of cardiac tissue. This has implications for heart rhythm maintenance, as illustrated below.

Mechanisms

Most acute electrophysiological responses to mechanical stimulation, observed in cardiac cells, can be reconciled with SAC activation. That said, mechanically induced changes in Ca handling[27] and second messengers such as nitric oxide[48] are also likely to directly or indirectly contribute.

With respect to Ca handling, large changes in developed force or length produce generally small changes in the cytosolic Ca transient under normal conditions (see discussion of Figure 7–4). As such, mechanical perturbations alone are unlikely to produce large enough cell-wide perturbations in intracellular Ca concentration to be proarrhythmic by activating Ca-dependent inward currents (e.g., NCX), similar to that proposed in heart failure.[49] However, *in vitro* evidence suggests that stretch of locally weakened muscle regions can produce release of Ca from SR near the boundary of strong and weak cells.[50] Mechanically inhomogeneous myocardium (whether locally weakened, or stiffened, say by scarring or fibrosis) may give rise to proarrhythmic Ca release.

Finally, mechanosensitivity is not restricted to cardiomyocytes. Various mechanosensitive cell populations affect cardiac electrical responses to mechanical stimulation, either by paracrine pathways (e.g., neurons, endothelial cells, connective tissue),[51] or through direct electrotonic interaction via connexin-based coupling (fibroblasts).[52] Furthermore, several connexins have been found to exhibit mechanically modulated opening[53] that, if applicable to the heart, would have implications for signal propagation.

This dynamic area of research will benefit from the recent identification of a highly selective peptide blocker of SAC,[54] so that significant new insight into mechanisms of cardiac MEF can reasonably be expected in the next few years.[55]

Relevance for Electrical Function of the Heart

Mechanosensitivity of the Normal Heart

Manifestations of both the Frank–Starling effect (mechanically induced positive inotropy)[56] and the Bainbridge effect (stretch-induced positive chronotropy)[57] can be observed in human heart, even after denervation (e.g., recently transplanted heart). While the Frank–Starling effect is a well-established and efficient means of matching cardiac output to venous return, manifestations of the Bainbridge effect in humans are less evident. This is related to the fact that most interventions that temporarily raise venous return (e.g., tilt-table or orthostatic challenges) are associated with corresponding changes in arterial pressure. These, via reflex pathways, slow down (rather than accelerate) pacemaking. However, studies using autotransfusion (passive elevation of the legs) found that an isolated increase in venous return does indeed raise the heart rate in humans.[58] This response is believed to underlie the nonneural component of respiratory sinus arrhythmia (inspiration increases venous return, which raises beating rate), or the sometimes observed phase-inverted sinus arrhythmia during positive pressure ventilation (when forced inspiration impedes venous return, which reduces beating rate).

Mechanical Pacing in Asystole and Bradycardia

Precordial percussion of the asystolic heart was among the first documented mechanical interventions for heart rhythm management. As reported in 1920, Stokes–Adams syndrome patients could

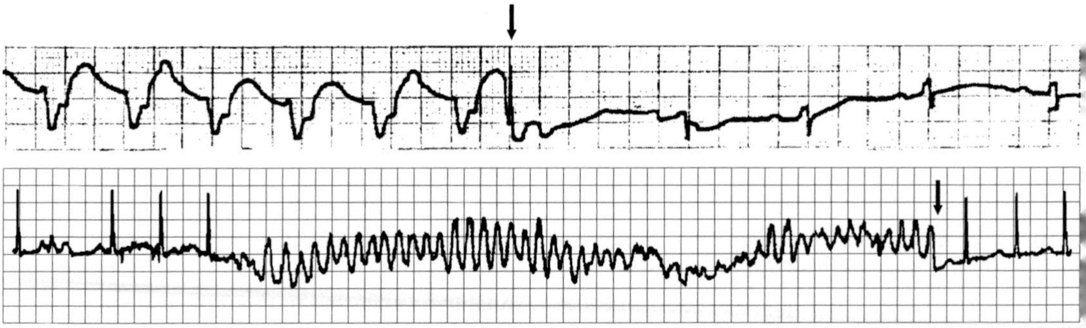

FIGURE 7–6. Tachyarrhythmia termination by precordial thump in humans. Case reports showing termination of ventricular tachycardia (top) and early ventricular fibrillation (bottom) by application of a fist thump to the precordium (arrows). (From Pennington *et al.*[66] and Barrett,[69] with permission.)

be kept conscious during periods of ventricular standstill by pacing the heart using fist impacts to the chest.[59]

Further applications include precordial thumps (PT) for the management of severe bradycardia, such as in the context of spinal anesthesia, or direct epicardial stimulation by "finger tap," which is regularly employed by surgeons to reinstate rhythmic activity in hearts that are weaned from cardiac bypass. The majority of case studies, conducted mainly in the 1970/1980s,[60,61] concluded that the fist is a suitable mechanical pacemaker, in particular in emergency situations where no alternative treatment modalities are available.[62] Of note, the impact energies required to trigger premature ventricular beats in humans are low,[‡] ranging from 0.04 to 1.5 J.[63] Underlying mechanisms of mechanically induced cardiac contractions are believed to be similar to those seen in isolated heart or tissue experiments, where diastolic stretch causes cardiomyocyte membrane depolarization that, if large enough, triggers AP generation (Figure 7–5) and subsequent ECC.

Of note, PT-induced ventricular contractions have significantly greater hemodynamic value than chest compressions, where blood is passively squeezed out of the heart (rather than actively ejected by the heart itself). In fact, the hemodynamic efficacy of mechanically induced beats matches that achieved with electrical pacing in patients.[64] Since adverse side effects are uncommon in this setting, the 2005 International Liaison Committee on Resuscitation (ILCOR) guidelines recommend fist pacing (at a rate of 50–70 bpm) for hemodynamically unstable bradyarrhythmias, until more enduring solutions (e.g., electrical pacemakers) can be employed.[65]

Mechanical Cardioversion in Tachycardia and Fibrillation

Single PT have been employed successfully as emergency resuscitation measures to terminate ventricular tachycardia and fibrillation (VT and VF, respectively; see Figure 7–6).[66,67] They are applied as a sharp impact to the lower half of the sternum, delivered from a height of 20–30 cm, using the ulnar edge of the tightly clinched fist, followed by active retraction after full impact (to emphasize the impulse-like nature of the stimulus).[68]

To date, no prospective study has evaluated the clinical utility of PT.[§] Case reports suggest that PT can be efficient in terminating witnessed cardiac arrest in about one-third of cases, and that VT is more amenable to mechanical cardioversion than VF.[67,68] However, severe preexisting hypoxia may render PT less efficient (which has implications for out-of-hospital PT success rates).[70]

Mechanisms underlying successful PT are believed to involve SAC_{NS}, which, via depolariza-

[‡]For comparison: 1 J of impact energy is released by dropping a standard can of soda from a 30 cm height.

[§]An out-of-hospital evaluation of PT for unwitnessed cardiac arrest is currently underway in the Pordenone region of Italy; results are expected in 2007.

tion of excitable gaps, may terminate reentry. The reduced efficacy of mechanical interventions in severely hypoxic hearts has been linked to the fact that reduced ATP levels preactivate at least some SAC_K.[71] This changes the overall electrophysiological response to mechanical stimulation, making it less efficient in depolarizing the excitable gap. In addition, more pronounced AP shortening may potentially render PT arrhythmogenic in severely ischaemic tissue.

Energy levels involved in PT termination of tachyarrhythmia range from 2 to 8 J.[68] This can be sustained by the conscious patient, in contrast to external electrical defibrillation involving more than one order of magnitude higher energy levels.

As PT is usually the fastest possible resuscitatory intervention "at hand,"[72] current ILCOR recommendations suggest considering it after monitored cardiac arrest, if no electrical defibrillator is immediately available.[73]

Mechanical Induction of Arrhythmia

Both acute and sustained stretch have been linked to atrial and ventricular arrhythmogenesis.[74,75]

The specific contribution of *sustained stretch* to cardiac arrhythmogenesis is difficult to clearly isolate, as pathologies that give rise to pressure and/or volume overload often carry an increased risk of heart rhythm disturbances via other mechanisms.

An interesting insight has been obtained, though, from the reverse conceptual approach, where volume overload was temporarily eliminated by conducting the Valsalva maneuver. This caused a reduction in venous return and cardiac dimensions, with subsequent temporary (while cardiac dimensions were reduced) termination of ventricular and supraventricular tachyarrhythmias,[75] even in heart transplant recipients,[76] suggesting that maintained stretch is proarrhythmogenic.

Underlying mechanisms are likely to involve SAC, whose pharmacological block prevents overload-mediated atrial fibrillation in isolated heart.[77] Similarly, activation of SAC has been implied to contribute to reduced defibrillation efficacy during volume overload.[78,79]

Acute mechanical stimulation of the heart can cause a range of electrophysiological responses, from single ectopic beats, to conduction abnormalities, runs of VT, and VF.[80] In the context of nonpenetrating extracorporeal impacts without cardiac structural damage, this is referred to as *Commotio cordis*.[81] Determinants of *C. cordis* outcome include impact type, location and energy,[82] as well as timing.[83]

The vulnerable window for mechanical induction of VF coincides, in a domestic pig model, with a 20-msec period prior to the peak of the ECG T-wave.[83] This vulnerable window is narrower than for electrical stimulation, and may explain why *C. cordis* is relatively rare.

Underlying mechanisms are likely to involve SAC activation, although the exact nature and individual contribution of subpopulations remain unresolved.[84,85] At the cellular level, mechanical stimulation during the T-wave affects cardiomyocytes differently, depending on their actual state of AP repolarization at the given point in time (Figure 7–7A–C). This may provide both trigger (ectopic AP) and sustaining mechanisms (heterogeneity of repolarization) for arrhythmogenesis.

The need to avoid both sustained overload (hemodynamic unloading, active and passive cardiac assist) and untoward acute mechanical stimulation of the heart (chest protectors) identifies important targets for prevention of arrhythmia.

Outlook

Cardiac mechanics is not merely an endpoint of heart rhythm management, but it is a rhythm moderator in its own right. Mechanical interventions affect the pace and force of cardiac contractions, and they may contribute to the induction, sustenance, and termination of arrhythmias.

Many of the links between electromechanical cross-talk, tissue and organ structure, and temporal organization of cardiac function are still poorly understood. This ranges from basic science questions, for example, regarding the modalities and mechanisms underlying mechanosensing, to clinical issues, such as the effects of various pathological factors (e.g., inhomogeneities, fibrosis) and treatment regimes (drugs, exercise) on mechanical arrhythmogenesis.

A better understanding of the cardiac electromechanical riddle will lead to more intelligent treatment strategies. This includes pharmacological leads,[77] as well as device development/

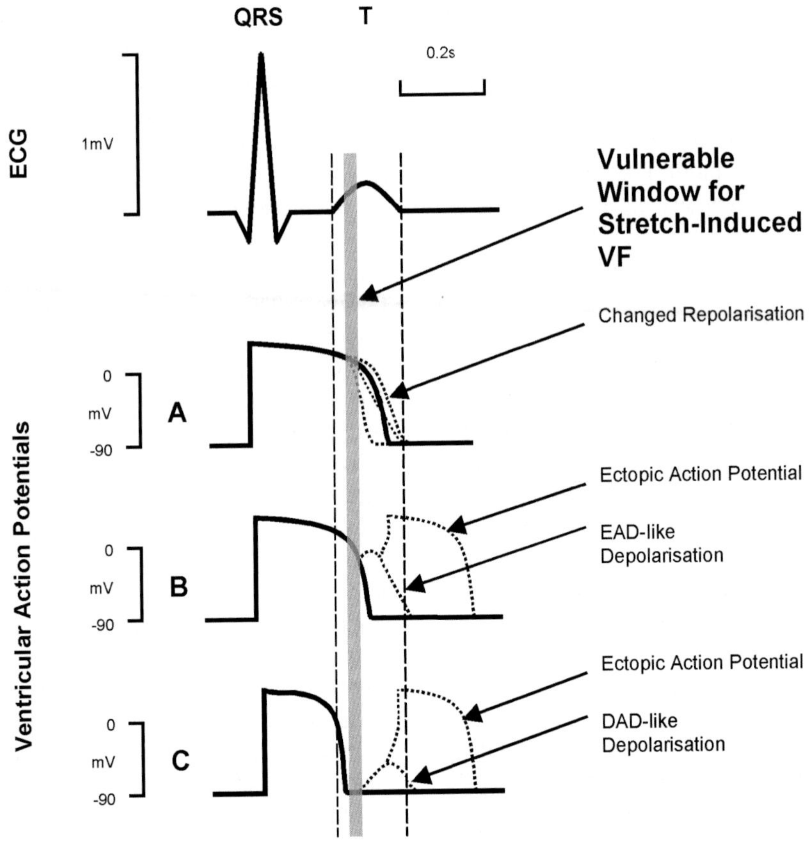

FIGURE 7–7. Schematic representation of cellular correlates of mechanical impacts during early repolarization (upstroke of the T-wave, see the gray band). Effects depend on the actual membrane potential of cardiomyocytes in different regions of the heart (A–C) and include (A) changes in action potential duration (shortening, prolongation, crossover of repolarization); (B) early afterdepolarization (EAD)-like behavior; or (C) delayed afterdepolarization (DAD)-like events, both of which may trigger extra beats. (From Kohl *et al.*,[85] with permission.)

improvement opportunities ranging from the use of ultrasound for cardiac pacing,[86] over active and passive cardiac assist technologies,[87] biventricular pacing/resynchronization,[88] and cardiac contractility modulating electrical stimulation,[89] to application of electrical defibrillation during peak chest compression and mechanical cardioversion, to name but a few.

References

1. Kohl P, Hunter P, Noble D. Stretch-induced changes in heart rate and rhythm: Clinical observations, experiments and mathematical models. *Prog Biophys Mol Biol* 1999;71(1):91–138.
2. Katz AM, Katz PB. Homogeneity out of heterogeneity. *Circulation* 1989;79:712–717.
3. Bers DM. *Excitation-Contraction Coupling and Cardiac Contractile Force*, 2nd ed. Boston: Kluwer Academic Publishers, 2001.
4. Eisner DA, Diaz ME, Li Y, O'Neill SC, Trafford AW. Stability and instability of regulation of intracellular calcium. *Exp Physiol* 2005;90(1):3–12.
5. Linz KW, Meyer R. Control of L-type calcium current during the action potential of guinea-pig ventricular myocytes. *J Physiol* 1998;513(Pt. 2): 425–442.
6. Alseikhan BA, DeMaria CD, Colecraft HM, Yue DT. Engineered calmodulins reveal the unexpected eminence of Ca2+ channel inactivation in controlling heart excitation. *Proc Natl Acad Sci USA* 2002; 99(26):17185–17190.
7. Shannon TR, Ginsburg KS, Bers DM. Potentiation of fractional sarcoplasmic reticulum calcium release by total and free intra-sarcoplasmic retic-

ulum calcium concentration. *Biophys J* 2000;78(1):334–343.
8. Trafford AW, Diaz ME, Eisner DA. A novel, rapid and reversible method to measure Ca buffering and time-course of total sarcoplasmic reticulum Ca content in cardiac ventricular myocytes. *Pflugers Arch* 1999;437(3):501–503.
9. Gordon AM, Regnier M, Homsher E. Skeletal and cardiac muscle contractile activation: Tropomyosin "rocks and rolls". *News Physiol Sci* 2001;16:49–55.
10. Solaro RJ, Rarick HM. Troponin and tropomyosin: Proteins that switch on and tune in the activity of cardiac myofilaments. *Circ Res* 1998;83(5):471–480.
11. Rice JJ, de Tombe PP. Approaches to modeling crossbridges and calcium-dependent activation in cardiac muscle. *Prog Biophys Mol Biol* 2004;85(2–3):179–195.
12. Allen DG, Kurihara S. The effects of muscle length on intracellular calcium transients in mammalian cardiac muscle. *J Physiol* 1982;327:79–94.
13. Bremel RD, Weber A. Cooperation within actin filament in vertebrate skeletal muscle. *Nat New Biol* 1972;238(82):97–101.
14. Hofmann PA, Fuchs F. Effect of length and cross-bridge attachment on Ca^{2+} binding to cardiac troponin C. Am *J Physiol Cell Physiol* 1987;253(1Pt. 1):C90–96.
15. Kad NM, Kim S, Warshaw DM, VanBuren P, Baker JE. Single-myosin crossbridge interactions with actin filaments regulated by troponin-tropomyosin. *Proc Natl Acad Sci USA* 2005;102(47):16990–16995.
16. Daniel TL, Trimble AC, Chase PB. Compliant realignment of binding sites in muscle: Transient behavior and mechanical tuning. *Biophys J* 1998;74(4):1611–1621.
17. Dobesh DP, Konhilas JP, de Tombe PP. Cooperative activation in cardiac muscle: Impact of sarcomere length. Am *J Physiol Heart Circ Physiol* 2002;282(3):H1055–1062.
18. Wannenburg T, Heijne GH, Geerdink JH, Van Den Dool HW, Janssen PM, De Tombe PP. Cross-bridge kinetics in rat myocardium: Effect of sarcomere length and calcium activation. Am *J Physiol Heart Circ Physiol* 2000;279(2):H779–790.
19. McDonald KS, Moss RL. Osmotic compression of single cardiac myocytes eliminates the reduction in Ca^{2+} sensitivity of tension at short sarcomere length. *Circ Res* 1995;77(1):199–205.
20. Cazorla O, Vassort G, Garnier D, Le Guennec JY. Length modulation of active force in rat cardiac myocytes: Is titin the sensor? *J Mol Cell Cardiol* 1999;31(6):1215–1227.
21. Konhilas JP, Irving TC, de Tombe PP. Length-dependent activation in three striated muscle types of the rat. *J Physiol* 2002;544(Pt. 1):225–236.
22. Konhilas JP, Irving TC, de Tombe PP. Frank-Starling law of the heart and the cellular mechanisms of length-dependent activation. *Pflugers Arch* 2002;445(3):305–310.
23. Parmley WW, Chuck L. Length-dependent changes in myocardial contractile state. *Am J Physiol* 1973;224:1195–1199.
24. Kentish JC, Wrzosek A. Changes in force and cytosolic Ca^{2+} concentration after length changes in isolated rat ventricular trabeculae. *J Physiol* 1998;506(Pt. 2):431–444.
25. Allen DG, Nichols CG, Smith GL. The effects of changes in muscle length during diastole on the calcium transient in ferret ventricular muscle. *J Physiol* 1988;406:359–370.
26. Nichols CG. The influence of "diastolic" length on the contractility of isolated cat papillary muscle. *J Physiol* 1985;361:269—279.
27. Calaghan SC, Belus A, White E. Do stretch-induced changes in intracellular calcium modify the electrical activity of cardiac muscle? *Prog Biophys Mol Biol* 2003;82(1–3):81–95.
28. Cingolani HE, Alvarez BV, Ennis IL, Camilion de Hurtado MC. Stretch-induced alkalinization of feline papillary muscle: An autocrine-paracrine system. *Circ Res* 1998;83(8):775–780.
29. Alvarez BV, Perez NG, Ennis IL, Camilion de Hurtado MC, Cingolani HE. Mechanisms underlying the increase in force and Ca(2+) transient that follow stretch of cardiac muscle: A possible explanation of the Anrep effect. *Circ Res* 1999;85(8):716–722.
30. Tavi P, Han C, Weckstrom M. Mechanisms of stretch-induced changes in [Ca2+]i in rat atrial myocytes: Role of increased troponin C affinity and stretch-activated ion channels. *Circ Res* 1998;83(11):1165–1177.
31. Janssen PM, de Tombe PP. Uncontrolled sarcomere shortening increases intracellular Ca2+ transient in rat cardiac trabeculae. *Am J Physiol Heart Circ Physiol* 1997;272(4Pt. 12):H1892–1897.
32. Poggesi C, Tesi C, Stehle R. Sarcomeric determinants of striated muscle relaxation kinetics. *Pflugers Arch* 2005;449(6):505–517.
33. Bassani JW, Yuan W, Bers DM. Fractional SR Ca release is regulated by trigger Ca and SR Ca content in cardiac myocytes. *Am J Physiol Cell Physiol* 1995;268(5Pt. 1):C1313–1319.
34. Puglisi JL, Bassani RA, Bassani JW, Amin JN, Bers DM. Temperature and relative contributions of Ca transport systems in cardiac myocyte relaxation.

Am J Physiol Heart Circ Physiol 1996;270(5Pt. 2): H1772–1888.
35. Janssen PM, Stull LB, Marban E. Myofilament properties comprise the rate-limiting step for cardiac relaxation at body temperature in the rat. Am J *Physiol Heart Circ Physiol* 2002;282(2):H499–507.
36. Janssen PM, Hunter WC. Force, not sarcomere length, correlates with prolongation of isosarcometric contraction. *Am J Physiol Heart Circ Physiol* 1995;269(2Pt. 2):H676–685.
37. Franz MR, Cima R, Wang D, Profitt D, Kurz R. Electrophysiological effects of myocardial stretch and mechanical determinants of stretch-activated arrhythmias. *Circulation* 1992;86:968–978.
38. Craelius W. Stretch-activation of rat cardiac myocytes. *Exp Physiol* 1993;78:411–423.
39. Kohl P, Bollensdorff C, Garny A. Mechano-sensitive ion channels in the heart: Experimental and theoretical models. *Exp Physiol* 2006;91:307–321.
40. Craelius W, Chen V, El-Sherif N. Stretch activated ion channels in ventricular myocytes. *BioSci Rep* 1988;8:407–414.
41. Baumgarten CM, Clemo HF. Swelling-activated chloride channels in cardiac physiology and pathophysiology. *Prog Biophys Mol Biol* 2003;82(1–3): 25–42.
42. Cooper PJ, Lei M, Cheng LX, Kohl P. Axial stretch increases spontaneous pacemaker activity in rabbit isolated sino-atrial node cells. *J Appl Physiol* 2000; 89:2099–2104.
43. Hansen DE, Borganelli M, Stacy GPJ, Taylor LK. Dose-dependent inhibition of stretch-induced arrhythmias by gadolinium in isolated canine ventricles. Evidence for a unique mode of antiarrhythmic action. *Circ Res* 1991;69:820–831.
44. White E, Le Guennec J-Y, Nigretto JM, Gannier F, Argibay JA, Garnier D. The effects of increasing cell length on auxotonic contractions; membrane potential and intracellular calcium transients in single guinea-pig ventricular myocytes. *Exp Physiol* 1993;78:65–78.
45. Zeng T, Bett GCL, Sachs F. Stretch-activated whole cell currents in adult rat cardiac myocytes. *Am J Physiol Heart Circ Physiol* 2000;278:H548–H557.
46. Zabel M, Coller B, Franz MR. Amplitude and polarity of stretch-induced systolic and diastolic voltage changes depend on the timing of stretch: A means to characterize stretch-activated channels in the intact heart. *Pacing Clin Electrophysiol* 1993;16: 886.
47. Levine JH, Guarnieri T, Kadish AH, White RI, Calkins H, Kan JS. Changes in myocardial repolarization in patients undergoing balloon valvuloplasty for congenital pulmonary stenosis: Evidence for contraction-excitation feedback in humans. *Circulation* 1988;77:70–77.
48. Vila-Petroff MG, Kim SH, Pepe S, Dessy C, Marbán E, Balligand J-L, Sollott SJ. Endogenous nitric oxide mechanisms mediate the stretch dependence of Ca^{2+} release in cardiomyocytes. *Nat Cell Biol* 2001; 3:867–873.
49. Pogwizd SM, Bers DM. Cellular basis of triggered arrhythmias in heart failure. *Trends Cardiovasc Med* 2004;14(2):61–66.
50. Ter Keurs HE, Wakayama Y, Miura M, Stuyvers BD, Boyden PA, Landesberg A. Spatial nonuniformity of contraction causes arrhythmogenic Ca2+ waves in rat cardiac muscle. *Ann NY Acad Sci* 2005;1047:345–365.
51. Giordano FJ, Gerber H-P, Williams S-P, *et al.* A cardiac myocyte vascular endothelial growth factor paracrine pathway is required to maintain cardiac function. *Proc Natl Acad Sci USA* 2001;98:5780–5785.
52. Camelliti P, Green CR, LeGrice I, Kohl P. Fibroblast network in rabbit sino-atrial node: Structural and functional identification of homo- and heterologous cell coupling. *Circ Res* 2004;94:828–835.
53. Bao L, Sachs F, Dahl G. Connexins are mechanosensitive. *Am J Physiol Cell Physiol* 2004;278: C1389–C1395.
54. Suchyna TM, Johnson JH, Hamer K, Leykam JF, Gage DA, Clemo HF, Baumgarten CM, Sachs F. Identification of a peptide toxin from Grammostola spatulata spider venom that blocks cation-selective stretch-activated channels. *J Gen Physiol* 2000;115: 583–598.
55. Kohl P, Sachs F, Franz MR. *Cardiac Mechano-Electric Feedback and Arrhythmias: From Pipette to Patient.* Philadelphia: Elsevier (Saunders), 2005.
56. Holubarsch C, Ruf T, Goldstein DJ, *et al.* Existence of the Frank-Starling mechanism in the failing human heart: Investigations on the organ, tissue, and sarcomere levels. *Circulation* 1996;94:683–689.
57. Slovut DP, Wenstrom JC, Moeckel RB, Wilson RF, Osborn JW, Abrams JH. Respiratory sinus dysrhythmia persists in transplanted human hearts following autonomic blockade. *Clin Exp Pharmacol Physiol* 1998;25:322–330.
58. Donald DE, Shepherd JT. Reflexes from the heart and lungs: Physiological curiosities or important regulatory mechanisms. *Cardiovasc Res* 1978;12:449–469.
59. Schott E. Über Ventrikelstillstand (Adams-Stokes'sche Anfälle) nebst Bemerkungen über andersartige Arhythmien passagerer Natur. *Deutsches Archiv Klinische Medizin* 1920;131:211–229.

60. Klumbies A, Paliege R, Volkmann H. Mechanical energy stimulation in asystole and extreme bradycardia [in German]. *Z Gesamte Exp Medizin* 1988; 43:348–352.
61. Zeh E, Rahner E. Die manuelle extrathorakale Stimulation des Herzens: zur Technik und Wirkung des "Prekordialschlages". *Z Kardiol* 1978;67:299–304.
62. Wild JB, Grover JD. The fist as a mechanical pacemaker. *Lancet* 1970;2:436–437.
63. Zoll PM, Belgard AH, Weintraub MJ, Frank HA. External mechanical cardiac stimulation. *N Engl J Med* 1976;294(23):1274–1275.
64. Chan L, Reid C, Taylor B. Effect of three emergency pacing modalities on cardiac output in cardiac arrest due to ventricular asystole. *Resuscitation* 2002;52(1):117–119.
65. International Liaison Committee on Resuscitation. 2005 International Consensus on Cardiopulmonary Resuscitation and Emergency Cardiovascular Care Science with Treatment Recommendations. Part 4: Advanced Life Support. *Resuscitation* 2005;67:213–247.
66. Pennington JE, Taylor J, Lown B. Chest thump for reverting ventricular tachycardia. *N Engl J Med* 1970;283:1192–1195.
67. Befeler B. Mechanical stimulation of the heart: Its therapeutic value in tachyarrhythmias. *Chest* 1978; 73(6):832–838.
68. Kohl P, King AM, Boulin C. Antiarrhythmic effects of acute mechanical stimulation. In: Kohl P, Sachs F, Franz MR, Eds. *Cardiac Mechano-Electric Feedback and Arrhythmias: From Pipette to Patient.* Philadelphia: Elsevier (Saunders), 2005:304–314.
69. Barrett JS. Chest thumps and the heart beat. *N Engl J Med* 1971;284(7):393.
70. Kohl P, Bollensdorff C, Garny A. Effects of mechanosensitive ion channels on ventricular electrophysiology: Experimental and theoretical models. *Exp Physiol* 2006;91:307–321.
71. van Wagoner DR, Lamorgese M. Ischemia potentiates the mechanosensitive modulation of atrial ATP-sensitive potassium channels. *Ann NY Acad Sci* 1994;723:392–395.
72. Caldwell G, Millar G, Quinn E, Vincent R, Chamberlain DA. Simple mechanical methods for cardioversion: Defence of the precordial thump and cough version. *Br Med J* 1985;291:627–630.
73. International Liaison Committee on Resuscitation. 2005 International Consensus on Cardiopulmonary Resuscitation and Emergency Cardiovascular Care Science with Treatment Recommendations. Part 3: Defibrillation. *Resuscitation* 2005;67:203–211.
74. Schotten U, Neuberger H-R, Allessie MA. The role of atrial dilatation in the domestication of atrial fibrillation. *Prog Biophys Mol Biol* 2003;82(1–3): 151–162.
75. Waxman MB, Wald RW, Finley JP, Bonet JF, Downar E, Sharma AD. Valsalva termination of ventricular tachycardia. *Circulation* 1980;62:843–851.
76. Ambrosi P, Habib G, Kreitmann B, Faugère G, Métras D. Valsalva manoeuvre for supraventricular tachycardia in transplanted heart recipient. *Lancet* 1995;346:713.
77. Bode F, Sachs F, Franz MR. Tarantula peptide inhibits atrial fibrillation. *Nature* 2001;409:35–36.
78. Strobel JS, Kay GN, Walcott GP, Smith WM, Ideker RE. Defibrillation efficacy with endocardial electrodes is influenced by reductions in cardiac preload. *J Intervent Cardiac Electrophysiol* 1997; 1(2):95–102.
79. Trayanova N, Li W, Eason J, Kohl P. The effect of stretch-activated channels on defibrillation efficacy: A simulation study. *Heart Rhythm* 2004;1: 67–77.
80. Maron BJ, Link MS, Wang PJ, Estes III NAM. Clinical profile of Commotio cordis: An under appreciated cause of sudden death in the young during sports and other activities. *J Cardiovasc Electrophysiol* 1999;10:114–120.
81. Riedinger F. Über Brusterschütterung. In: *Festschrift zur dritten Saecularfeier der Alma Julia Maximiliana Leipzig.* Leipzig: Verlag von F.C.W. Vogel, 1882:221–234.
82. Schlomka G. Commotio cordis und ihre Folgen. Die Einwirkung stumpfer Brustwandtraumen auf das Herz. *Ergebnisse inneren Med Kinderheilkunde* 1934;47:1–91.
83. Link MS, Wang PJ, Pandian NG, *et al.* An experimental model of sudden cardiac death due to low-energy chest-wall impact (Commotio cordis). *N Engl J Med* 1998;338:1805–1811.
84. Link MS, Wang PJ, VanderBrink BA, Avelar E, Pandian NG, Maron BJ, Estees III M. Selective activation of the K^{+}_{ATP} channel is a mechanism by which sudden death is produced by low-energy chest-wall impact (Commotio cordis). *Circulation* 1999;100:413–418.
85. Kohl P, Nesbitt AD, Cooper PJ, Lei M. Sudden cardiac death by *Commotio cordis*: Role of mechano-electric feedback. *Cardiovasc Res* 2001;50(2):280–289.
86. Towe BC, Rho R. Ultrasonic cardiac pacing in the porcine model. *IEEE Trans Biomed Eng* 2006;53: 1446–1448.
87. Cheng A, Nguyen TC, Malinowski M, Langer F, Liang D, Daughters GT, Ingels NB Jr, Miller DC. Passive ventricular constraint prevents transmural

shear strain progression in left ventricle remodeling. *Circulation* 2006;114:I79–I86.
88. Boriani G, Gasparini M, Lunati M, *et al.* Characteristics of ventricular tachyarrhythmias occurring in ischemic versus nonischemic patients implanted with a biventricular cardioverter-defibrillator for primary or secondary prevention of sudden death. *Am Heart J* 2006;152:527–536.
89. Sabbah HN, Gupta RC, Rastogi S, Mishra S, Mika Y, Burkhoff D. Treating heart failure with cardiac contractility modulation electrical signals. *Curr Heart Fail Rep* 2006;3:21–24.

8
The Role of Cellular Sodium and Calcium Loading in Cardiac Energetics and Arrhythmogenesis: Contribution of the Late Sodium Current

John C. Shryock, Luiz Belardinelli, and Sridharan Rajamani

Introduction

An imbalance between myocardial oxygen supply and demand, as occurs during ischemia, leads to increases of cellular concentrations of sodium and calcium (Figure 8–1).[1] Reperfusion of the ischemic heart may further exacerbate an ischemia-induced loss of ionic homeostasis. Ischemia and ischemic metabolites can increase the influx of sodium into myocytes.[2–7] Concurrent reduction of sodium efflux during ischemia, as a consequence of reductions of cellular ATP and activity of the cell membrane Na^+–K^+-ATPase, allows the intracellular sodium concentration to rise. By virtue of the coupled exchange of sodium and calcium facilitated by the cell membrane Na^+–Ca^{2+} exchanger (NCX), an elevation of the intracellular sodium concentration leads to an increased influx of calcium. An excessive or prolonged increase of the intracellular sodium concentration leads to intracellular calcium ($[Ca^{2+}]_i$) overload. The mechanisms and consequences of sodium and calcium overload are the subject of this review. Evidence supporting a role for the late sodium current (late I_{Na}) as a mechanism of calcium overloading and cardiac dysfunction is emphasized.

Causes of Sodium Overload

The influx of sodium ions through sodium channels is responsible for the upstroke (phase 0) of the cardiac action potential. The magnitude of peak sodium current during phase 0 of an action potential is thus correlated with cardiac excitability and the speed of impulse propagation. Reduction of peak I_{Na} (as in Brugada syndrome) may cause inexcitability and conduction block. However, for every sodium ion that enters a cardiac cell, one must be extruded. Cellular ATP is consumed in this process. Ideally, therefore, I_{Na} should be of large magnitude, but brief. Rapid inactivation of I_{Na} is important for curtailing the influx of sodium into the cell during an action potential, and thus for avoiding sodium overload. An increase of the frequency of excitation of myocytes increases sodium influx and the intracellular concentration of sodium.[8]

The concentration of intracellular sodium is elevated in cardiac myocytes or myocardium exposed to hypoxia, ischemic metabolites, reactive oxygen species, and selected toxins and drugs.[2–7,9–11] It is also increased in myocardium and myocytes isolated from failing hearts[12–14] and from postinfarction remodeled myocardium.[15] Increases of both sodium/hydrogen exchange (NHE) and late I_{Na} [3,5,6,10,16–18] appear to contribute to the rise of the intracellular sodium concentration that is observed during hypoxia, ischemia or simulated ischemia/reperfusion, and heart failure. Inhibitions of either NHE[2,10,11,16,19–21] or late I_{Na}[2,6,16,17,19] in these conditions attenuate the rise in intracellular sodium and are cardioprotective. The sea anemone toxin ATX-II,[22–24] many other natural toxins,[22,25] and agents such as DPI 201–106[26] that increase late I_{Na} by direct actions to interfere with sodium channel inactivation also cause sodium overload that can lead to calcium overload and myocardial electrical and mechanical dysfunction.

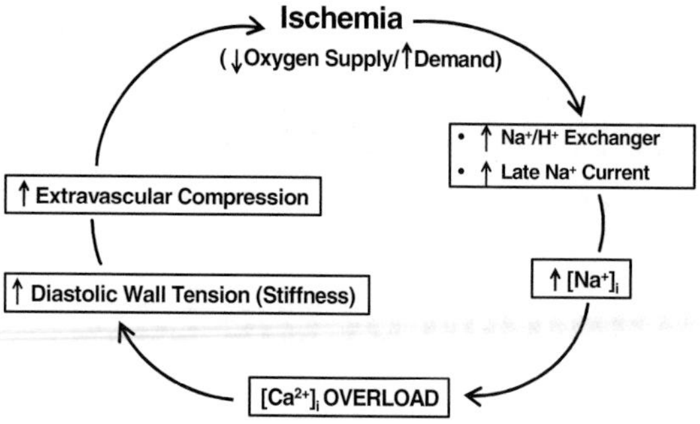

FIGURE 8–1. Positive feedback during ischemia increases the imbalance between myocardial oxygen supply and demand. In this deleterious positive feedback cycle, the $[Na^+]_i$-dependent calcium overload caused by the imbalance between O_2 supply and demand results in a further decrease in O_2 supply and increase in O_2 demand (see text for details).

An increase of sodium influx through sodium channels, NHE, or other membrane transporters must be matched by an equal increase of sodium extrusion via the Na^+–K^+-ATPase (Na pump). Sodium extrusion rises as the intracellular sodium concentration rises, and equilibrium of influx and efflux is reached at a higher intracellular sodium concentration. Activity of the Na pump is reduced when the cellular content of ATP falls. The fall of cellular ATP content during ischemia/reperfusion is thus associated with a large increase of intracellular sodium, at a time when late I_{Na} and NHE are increased. It is not clear, however, that the activity of the Na^+ pump is reduced or limited in other conditions wherein late I_{Na} is increased. Sodium pump activity was found to be increased in myocytes from failing rabbit hearts.[12] On the other hand, expression of the sodium–potassium ATPase in human myocardium appears to be reduced in heart failure.[27] Regardless, the sodium concentration in myocytes from failing hearts is elevated.[13]

The Late Sodium Current

Late I_{Na} is sodium channel current that persists from 10 to hundreds of milliseconds after the large, brief "spike" of peak I_{Na} that is elicited by depolarization. It may persist throughout the duration of the action potential plateau. Late I_{Na} has no recognized physiological role in the heart, although the relatively large magnitude of this current in Purkinje and M cells may explain the long durations of action potentials in these cells.[28] Random brief openings and long bursts of multiple openings of single sodium channels are responsible for late I_{Na}.[29,30] These openings are normally rare, and late I_{Na} is typically a small current (≈0.1% of peak I_{Na}) in ventricular myocytes. Evidence indicates that channels conducting late and peak I_{Na} are similar; for example, both peak and late I_{Na} are blocked by tetrodotoxin. Late I_{Na} can be distinguished from the sodium "window current"[31] by its presence at voltages outside the range at which window current is observed (which is roughly −40 to −60 mV with a peak at approximately −52 mV);[5] however, when present, the sodium window current contributes to late I_{Na}.[13]

Although late I_{Na} is known to be increased during exposure of myocardial cells to hypoxia and ischemic metabolites,[2,3,5,7,15,32,33] and is increased in myocytes from failing hearts,[14,34] the nature of the modification(s) of the sodium channel that leads to an increase in late I_{Na} during these circumstances is unknown. Reactive oxygen species may be important. Formation of reactive oxygen species is increased during ischemia and greatly increased upon reperfusion of the ischemic myocardium.[5,35,36] Oxidants appear to act either directly on the sodium channel or on a closely associated protein to alter channel inactivation and increase late I_{Na}.[9,36] The ischemic metabolites palmitoylcarnitine,[7] lysophosphatidylcholine,[33] and hydrogen peroxide[37,38] increase late I_{Na} and appear to interfere with sodium channel inactivation. Calcium/calmodulin-dependent kinase II is implicated as a cause of increased late I_{Na}[39] and sodium channel activity can also be modulated by protein kinase A-dependent phosphorylation.[40] In long QT syndrome type 3, an increase of late I_{Na} is caused by sodium channel mutations (most commonly these are single amino acid substitutions in the gene *SCN5A*) that increase the probability that a channel will fail to inactivate properly or will more readily reopen from a closed state.[41–45] Modeling studies suggest that persistent late openings of a relatively small number of sodium channels in LQT3 can significantly increase sodium influx during the cardiac ventricular action potential, and action potential duration.[46]

Consequences of an Increase of Late I_{Na}

Although late I_{Na} is small relative to peak I_{Na}, it persists for the duration of an action potential. It may contribute more to sodium influx than the much larger but briefer peak I_{Na}.[47] Furthermore, late I_{Na} is a depolarizing current during the action potential plateau when total membrane current is relatively small. Thus, small increases of late I_{Na} during the action potential plateau can markedly increase its duration and exacerbate both temporal and spatial dispersions of action potential duration across the ventricular wall.[48] The increases of sodium influx and of action potential duration may be expected to increase the activity of the Na pump and reverse mode NCX, and calcium entry through the L-type calcium channel, respectively. These direct and indirect consequences of late I_{Na} may themselves lead to electrical dysfunction [i.e., increased dispersion of repolarization, early afterdepolarizations (EADs), arrhythmias] and calcium overloading.[49]

Much experimental data suggest that late I_{Na} can contribute to myocardial pathology. Sodium influx via late I_{Na} appears to be a major contributor to the rise of intracellular sodium that is observed during ischemia[19] and hypoxia.[3] Myocardial ischemia is known to cause increases of lysophosphatidylcholine, palmitoyl-L-carnitine, and reactive oxygen species (e.g., hydrogen peroxide), and these substances are themselves reported to cause increases of late I_{Na}.[7,33,37,38] Sodium channel blockers (e.g., tetrodotoxin, lidocaine) have been shown to reduce the rise of sodium in rat ventricular myocytes and isolated hearts during hypoxia and ischemia, respectively.[3,5,6,10,11,16,17] This action of sodium channel blockers is associated with an improvement of contractile function and with reduction of the hypoxia/ischemia-induced increase in intracellular calcium concentration.[2,5,6,17,32,50] An increase of late I_{Na} is also arrhythmogenic[14,34,48,51–53] and is the cause of the long QT3 (LQT3) syndrome.[41–45,54] Drug-induced reduction of late I_{Na} is protective against arrhythmias caused by human ether-à-go-go-related gene (hERG) channel blockers[18,51–53,55] and sodium channel mutations that cause LQT3 syndrome.[54,56]

Recent evidence suggests that an increase of the intracellular sodium concentration leads to a decrease of the calcium concentration in the mitochondrion, and a reduction of mitochondrial NADH production.[57] An increase of intracellular sodium accelerates calcium efflux from the mitochondrion via the mitochondrial NCX. It was hypothesized that this may reduce the ability of mitochondria to increase ATP production in response to an increase of ATP consumption, as when heart rate and/or preload are increased, and a relative energy starvation.[57] When isolated guinea pig myocytes were stimulated at 4 Hz in the presence of isoproterenol, mitochondrial calcium concentration and NADH decreased when the intracellular sodium concentration was elevated from 5 to 15 mM.[57]

Sodium-Calcium Exchange

An increase of the intracellular sodium concentration reduces the chemical potential for coupled sodium entry/calcium extrusion via NCX. In a ventricular myocyte, forward exchange (net sodium entry/calcium extrusion) normally exists for all but a few milliseconds following the upstroke of the action potential.[58,59] During this early period of the action potential plateau, both the positive membrane voltage and the elevated subsarcolemmal sodium concentration favor reverse exchange (net sodium extrusion/calcium entry), and the reversal potential of the exchanger is thus positive relative to the membrane potential. If, however, the subsarcolemmal concentration of sodium and/or the membrane voltage during the action potential plateau is abnormally elevated, reverse NCX may persist for a longer time during the action potential plateau. During this time cellular calcium entry via NCX is increased and efflux is decreased. These conditions are expected to increase calcium uptake and loading of the sarcoplasmic reticulum, and thus to increase the magnitude and/or duration of the calcium transient during the next systolic contraction. An elevation of calcium content in the sarcoplasmic reticulum may also trigger calcium release either during repolarization of the action potential or during diastole. This untimely calcium release may cause EADs and delayed afterdepolarizations (DADs) and aftercontractions.[49,60]

A rise in the intracellular concentration of sodium will lead to an increased exchange of intracellular sodium for extracellular calcium via the "reverse" mode of NCX. There is in general agreement with the fact that the cellular calcium overload that occurs during ischemia and reperfusion is a result of a combination of decreased efflux of calcium ions via the forward mode of NCX and increased influx of calcium ions via the reverse mode of NCX.[1,61–68] A relative increase of activity of NCX in the reverse mode (sodium efflux and calcium influx) is a predictable outcome of both a rise in the intracellular sodium concentration and an increase in duration of the action potential. As noted above, an increase of late I_{Na} causes both an increase of the intracellular sodium concentration and a prolongation of action potential duration, and thus increased activity of NCX in the reverse mode, and calcium influx. Direct evidence in support of the critical role of the reverse mode of NCX in intracellular calcium overload during reperfusion or reoxygenation after ischemia is derived from the observations that inhibitors of NCX,[63,66,67] antisense inhibition of NCX,[62] and knockout of NCX[65] markedly decrease either contractile dysfunction or the rise in intracellular calcium in myocardial cells.

Consequences of an Increase of Intracellular Calcium

An increase of the cytosolic concentration of Ca^{2+} is expected to increase the uptake and loading of calcium into the sarcoplasmic reticulum, cell calcium efflux and sodium influx via NCX (forward mode), and calcium binding by and kinase activity of calmodulin, and to enhance I_{Ks},[69] reduce I_{K1},[70] and decrease the chemical potential gradient for calcium influx through the L-type calcium channel.

Mechanical effects of an increase of the cytosolic concentration of Ca^{2+} become apparent during both systole and diastole. Cytosolic calcium overload causes an increased actin/myosin filament interaction and an increase in left ventricular diastolic tension (i.e., "stiffness," a failure to relax normally). As a result, both myocardial contractile work and oxygen consumption, and compression of the vascular space, become abnormally elevated. The result is a reduction of myocardial blood flow during diastole. Consequently, oxygen supply is reduced (especially in the subendocardial region of the left ventricle) while the demand for oxygen to support contraction is further increased. This pattern of cause and effect has the characteristics of a deleterious positive feedback system wherein ischemia leads to further ischemia (Figure 8–1).

Physiological adjustment of calcium uptake and filling of the sarcoplasmic reticulum is a mechanism for rapid regulation of cardiac contractile force in response to changes in heart rate and adrenergic tone.[60] Phosphorylation of phospholamban by cAMP-dependent protein kinase A removes inhibition of Ca^{2+} release channels (ryanodine receptors) and facilitates rapid release of Ca^{2+} in response to calcium influx (i.e., calcium-induced calcium release) after excitation of the myocyte. However, an increase in calcium loading of the sarcoplasmic reticulum also increases the probability of spontaneous calcium release during diastole. An increase of the cytoplasmic concentration of calcium may also trigger spontaneous calcium release from the sarcoplasmic reticulum.[60,71,72] Calcium release during diastole causes an aftercontraction and a transient depolarization of the cell membrane. Some of the released calcium exits the cell via NCX in exchange for extracellular sodium. This coupled exchange of three Na^+ for one Ca^{2+} is electrogenic, and the transient inward current thus produced causes a DAD that may initiate an action potential.[60,73] Thus, DADs may serve as a trigger of arrhythmic activity.[74,75] The spontaneous "unloading" of calcium from the sarcoplasmic reticulum during diastole also causes a relative depletion of the calcium store available for the following systolic contraction, thus reducing contractility.

An increase of the intracellular calcium concentration may cause increased activation of Ca^{2+}/calmodulin-dependent kinase II. Calcium-mediated activation of Ca^{2+}/calmodulin-dependent kinase II is followed by increased phosphorylation of phospholamban, L-type calcium channels, and nitric oxide synthase. The results of increased phosphorylation of these proteins include reduced inhibition by phospholamban of SERCA-mediated uptake of calcium by the sarcoplasmic reticulum (thus speeding relaxation of contraction), increased I_{Ca}, and increased formation of nitric oxide (NO), respectively. Increased formation of NO may be involved in the induction of late I_{Na}[9] and may mediate enhancement of I_{Ks} by increased intracellular calcium[69] and activation of NCX.[76] Activity of Ca^{2+}/calmodulin-dependent kinase may increase late I_{Na},[39] and inhibition of the enzyme was shown to suppress the NCX-mediated transient inward current.[77]

The Therapeutic Potential of Decreasing Late I_{Na}

Inhibitors of late I_{Na} are reported to reduce the effects of hypoxia or simulated ischemia on isolated, *in vitro* cardiac preparations and the effects of ischemia on animal hearts *in vivo*. Although current inhibitors of late I_{Na} (lidocaine, amiodarone, flecainide, mexiletine, ranolazine, RSD1235, R56865, KC12291, tetrodotoxin, saxitoxin, and n-3 polyunsaturated fatty acids) are only relatively selective inhibitors of this current (versus peak I_{Na} or I_{Kr}, for example), there is substantial evidence that inhibition of late I_{Na} by these compounds is cardioprotective. Inhibitors of late I_{Na} have been shown to attenuate ionic, metabolic, electrical, and mechanical dysfunction in preclinical models of hypoxia, ischemia, heart failure, or sodium overload.[2,5,6,10,16,17,32,50,51,78–82]

In ventricular myocytes from dogs and humans with chronic heart failure, wherein late I_{Na} is augmented,[14] the duration of the action potential (APD) is prolonged[34,82] and EADs are common.[83] The sodium channel blockers tetrodotoxin, saxitoxin, and lidocaine were shown to shorten the APD and suppress EADs in ventricular myocytes from failing hearts.[34,84] Ranolazine is reported to inhibit late I_{Na} in ventricular myocytes from dogs with chronic heart failure with a potency of 6.4 μM and to shorten APD and suppress EADs in these myocytes at concentrations of 5 and 10 μM.[85]

Dispersion of ventricular repolarization and beat-to-beat variability of APD (also referred to as instability of APD) are frequently observed in myocytes from failing dog hearts, in ischemic preparations, and in myocardial tissue exposed to either ATX-II or drugs and ionic conditions that prolong the QT interval. An increased dispersion of repolarization is associated with electrical (T-wave) and mechanical alternans and proarrhythmia,[86] and is predictive of torsades de pointes ventricular tachyarrhythmia.[87] The role of late I_{Na} in increasing beat-to-beat variability of APD and the suppression of this variability by tetrodotoxin, saxitoxin, and lidocaine have been reported.[34,84,88] Ranolazine (5 and 10 μM) reduces the variability of APD in single ventricular myocytes from dogs with heart failure[85] and in myocytes exposed to ATX-II.[52] Thus, inhibition of late I_{Na} with sodium channel blockers suppresses arrhythmogenic abnormalities of ventricular repolarization (i.e., EADs and increased dispersion of ventricular repolarization) that are associated with abnormal intracellular sodium and calcium homeostasis and with the occurrence of ventricular tachycardias.[53,79,89,90]

Selective inhibitors of late I_{Na} have therapeutic potential in the treatment of cardiac disease. Inhibitors of cardiac late I_{Na} are expected to be safe and effective because late I_{Na} is both significant and common in pathological settings such as ischemic heart failure, but not in healthy myocardium where its inhibition is presumably without consequence. Ranolazine was recently approved for the treatment of chronic stable angina[91] with the rationale that reduction of late I_{Na} should reduce Na-induced calcium overload, improve diastolic relaxation, and reduce ischemia (see Figure 8–1). Ranolazine appears to be the most selective inhibitor of the late sodium current in current clinical practice.[81] It binds to the local anesthetic binding site of the sodium channel and selectively reduces late relative to peak sodium current.[92] It does not reduce heart rate, cardiac output, or blood pressure, and is not a vasodilator. Ranolazine does not appear to be arrhythmogenic.[53,90,93] However, ranolazine and other inhibitors of late I_{Na} may decrease arrhythmic activity caused by blockers of I_{Kr}.[18,52,53,55,90,94] Further studies are needed to investigate the antiarrhythmic effects of blockers of the late sodium current.[48,94]

In summary, sodium and sodium-induced calcium overloading are characteristic of ischemia and contribute to electrical and mechanical dysfunction. An increase of the late sodium current is proposed as a mechanism causing sodium overloading during hypoxia/reperfusion and heart failure, and in patients with gain-of-function *SCN5A* mutations and possibly in other cardiac diseases. Evidence suggests that late I_{Na} is increased by ischemia, hypoxia, and reperfusion of ischemic myocardium. It appears that the timing of the increase of late I_{Na} precedes electrical and mechanical dysfunction, but more experiments are needed to determine the timing of ionic and functional events in ischemia. Enhancers of late I_{Na}, such as ATX-II, H_2O_2, and ischemic metabolites, and *SCN5A* mutations cause functional effects that mimic many but not all (e.g., ischemia-induced activation of $I_{K,ATP}$ and shortening of APD are not a result of increased late I_{Na}) of the effects of ischemia/reperfusion and hypoxia. Blockers of late I_{Na} reduce mechanical and electrical dysfunction caused by ischemia/reperfusion and hypoxia. Selective inhibition of late I_{Na} has not been demonstrated to be detrimental to normal cardiac function, but further studies of late I_{Na} in noncardiac tissues are needed to identify the physiological and/or pathological roles of late I_{Na} in these tissues. The therapeutic potential of selective inhibitors of late I_{Na} is under investigation.

References

1. Silverman HS, Stern MD. Ionic basis of ischaemic cardiac injury: Insights from cellular studies. *Cardiovasc Res* 1994;28:581–597.
2. Eng S, Maddaford TG, Kardami E, Pierce GN. Protection against myocardial ischemic/reperfusion injury by inhibitors of two separate pathways of Na+ entry. *J Mol Cell Cardiol* 1998;30:829–835.
3. Ju YK, Saint DA, Gage PW. Hypoxia increases persistent sodium current in rat ventricular myocytes. *J Physiol* 1996;497:337–347.
4. Pike MM, Kitakaze M, Marban E. 23Na-NMR measurements of intracellular sodium in intact perfused ferret hearts during ischemia and reperfusion. *Am J Physiol* 1990;259:H1767–H1773.
5. Saint DA. The role of the persistent Na(+) current during cardiac ischemia and hypoxia. *J Cardiovasc Electrophysiol* 2006;17(Suppl. 1):S96–S103.
6. van Emous JG, Nederhoff MG, Ruigrok TJ, van Echteld CJ. The role of the Na+ channel in the accumulation of intracellular Na+ during myocardial ischemia: Consequences for post-ischemic recovery. *J Mol Cell Cardiol* 1997;29:85–96.
7. Wu J, Corr PB. Palmitoylcarnitine increases [Na+]i and initiates transient inward current in adult ventricular myocytes. *Am J Physiol* 1995;268:H2405–H2417.
8. Cohen CJ, Fozzard HA, Sheu SS. Increase in intracellular sodium ion activity during stimulation in mammalian cardiac muscle. *Circ Res* 1982;50:651–662.
9. Ahern GP, Hsu SF, Klyachko VA, Jackson MB. Induction of persistent sodium current by exogenous and endogenous nitric oxide. *J Biol Chem* 2000;275:28810–28815.
10. Eigel BN, Hadley RW. Contribution of the Na(+) channel and Na(+)/H(+) exchanger to the anoxic rise of [Na(+)] in ventricular myocytes. *Am J Physiol* 1999;277:H1817–H1822.
11. Xiao XH, Allen DG. Role of Na(+)/H(+) exchanger during ischemia and preconditioning in the isolated rat heart. *Circ Res* 1999;85:723–730.
12. Despa S, Islam MA, Weber CR, Pogwizd SM, Bers DM. Intracellular Na(+) concentration is elevated in heart failure but Na/K pump function is unchanged. *Circulation* 2002;105:2543–2548.
13. Pieske B, Houser SR. [Na+]i handling in the failing human heart. *Cardiovasc Res* 2003;57:874–886.
14. Valdivia CR, Chu WW, Pu J, Foell JD, Haworth RA, Wolff MR, Kamp TJ, Makielski JC. Increased late sodium current in myocytes from a canine heart failure model and from failing human heart. *J Mol Cell Cardiol* 2005;38:475–483.
15. Huang B, El Sherif T, Gidh-Jain M, Qin D, El Sherif N. Alterations of sodium channel kinetics and gene expression in the postinfarction remodeled myocardium. *J Cardiovasc Electrophysiol* 2001;12:218–225.
16. Decking UK, Hartmann M, Rose H, Bruckner R, Meil J, Schrader J. Cardioprotective actions of KC 12291. I. Inhibition of voltage-gated Na+ channels in ischemia delays myocardial Na+ overload. *Naunyn Schmiedebergs Arch Pharmacol* 1998;358: 547–553.
17. Haigney MC, Lakatta EG, Stern MD, Silverman HS. Sodium channel blockade reduces hypoxic sodium loading and sodium-dependent calcium loading. *Circulation* 1994;90:391–399.
18. Hallman K, Carlsson L. Prevention of class III-induced proarrhythmias by flecainide in an animal model of the acquired long QT syndrome. *Pharmacol Toxicol* 1995;77:250–254.
19. Baetz D, Bernard M, Pinet C, Tamareille S, Chattou S, El Banani H, Coulombe A, Feuvray D. Different pathways for sodium entry in cardiac cells during ischemia and early reperfusion. *Mol Cell Biochem* 2003;242:115–120.
20. Hartmann M, Decking UK. Blocking Na(+)-H+ exchange by cariporide reduces Na(+)-overload in

ischemia and is cardioprotective. *J Mol Cell Cardiol* 1999;31:1985–1995.
21. Scholz W, Albus U, Counillon L, Gogelein H, Lang HJ, Linz W, Weichert A, Scholkens BA. Protective effects of HOE642, a selective sodium-hydrogen exchange subtype 1 inhibitor, on cardiac ischaemia and reperfusion. *Cardiovasc Res* 1995;29:260–268.
22. Benzinger GR, Kyle JW, Blumenthal KM, Hanck DA. A specific interaction between the cardiac sodium channel and site-3 toxin anthopleurin B. *J Biol Chem* 1998;273:80–84.
23. El Sherif N, Fozzard HA, Hanck DA. Dose-dependent modulation of the cardiac sodium channel by sea anemone toxin ATXII. *Circ Res* 1992;70:285–301.
24. Hoey A, Harrison SM, Boyett MR, Ravens U. Effects of the Anemonia sulcata toxin (ATX II) on intracellular sodium and contractility in rat and guinea-pig myocardium. *Pharmacol Toxicol* 1994;75:356–365.
25. Denac H, Mevissen M, Scholtysik G. Structure, function and pharmacology of voltage-gated sodium channels. *Naunyn Schmiedebergs Arch Pharmacol* 2000;362:453–479.
26. Kuhlkamp V, Mewis C, Bosch R, Seipel L. Delayed sodium channel inactivation mimics long QT syndrome 3. *J Cardiovasc Pharmacol* 2003;42:113–117.
27. Schwinger RH, Bundgaard H, Muller-Ehmsen J, Kjeldsen K. The Na, K-ATPase in the failing human heart. *Cardiovasc Res* 2003;57:913–920.
28. Zygmunt AC, Eddlestone GT, Thomas GP, Nesterenko VV, Antzelevitch C. Larger late sodium conductance in M cells contributes to electrical heterogeneity in canine ventricle. *Am J Physiol Heart Circ Physiol* 2001;281:H689–H697.
29. Kiyosue T, Arita M. Late sodium current and its contribution to action potential configuration in guinea pig ventricular myocytes. *Circ Res* 1989;64:389–397.
30. Li CZ, Wang XD, Wang HW, Bian YT, Liu YM. Four types of late Na channel current in isolated ventricular myocytes with reference to their contribution to the lastingness of action potential plateau. *Sheng Li Xue Bao* 1997;49:241–248.
31. Attwell D, Cohen I, Eisner D, Ohba M, Ojeda C. The steady state TTX-sensitive ("window") sodium current in cardiac Purkinje fibres. *Pflugers Arch* 1979;379:137–142.
32. Le Grand B, Vie B, Talmant JM, Coraboeuf E, John GW. Alleviation of contractile dysfunction in ischemic hearts by slowly inactivating Na+ current blockers. *Am J Physiol* 1995;269:H533–H540.
33. Undrovinas AI, Fleidervish IA, Makielski JC. Inward sodium current at resting potentials in single cardiac myocytes induced by the ischemic metabolite lysophosphatidylcholine. *Circ Res* 1992;71:1231–1241.
34. Undrovinas AI, Maltsev VA, Sabbah HN. Repolarization abnormalities in cardiomyocytes of dogs with chronic heart failure: Role of sustained inward current. *Cell Mol Life Sci* 1999;55:494–505.
35. Becker LB. New concepts in reactive oxygen species and cardiovascular reperfusion physiology. *Cardiovasc Res* 2004;61:461–470.
36. Hammarstrom AK, Gage PW. Hypoxia and persistent sodium current. *Eur Biophys J* 2002;31:323–330.
37. Ma JH, Luo AT, Zhang PH. Effect of hydrogen peroxide on persistent sodium current in guinea pig ventricular myocytes. *Acta Pharmacol Sin* 2005;26:828–834.
38. Ward CA, Giles WR. Ionic mechanism of the effects of hydrogen peroxide in rat ventricular myocytes. *J Physiol* 1997;500:631–642.
39. Maier LS, Hasenfuss G. Role of [Na+]i and the emerging involvement of the late sodium current in the pathophysiology of cardiovascular disease. *Eur Heart J* 2006;(Suppl. A):A6–A9.
40. Tateyama M, Rivolta I, Clancy CE, Kass RS. Modulation of cardiac sodium channel gating by protein kinase A can be altered by disease-linked mutation. *J Biol Chem* 2003;278:46718–46726.
41. Bennett PB, Yazawa K, Makita N, George AL Jr. Molecular mechanism for an inherited cardiac arrhythmia. *Nature* 1995;376:683–685.
42. Clancy CE, Rudy Y. Linking a genetic defect to its cellular phenotype in a cardiac arrhythmia. *Nature* 1999;400:566–569.
43. Clancy CE, Tateyama M, Liu H, Wehrens XH, Kass RS. Non-equilibrium gating in cardiac Na+ channels: An original mechanism of arrhythmia. *Circulation* 2003;107:2233–2237.
44. Splawski I, Timothy KW, Tateyama M, Clancy CE, Malhotra A, Beggs AH, Cappuccio FP, Sagnella GA, Kass RS, Keating MT. Variant of SCN5A sodium channel implicated in risk of cardiac arrhythmia. *Science* 2002;297:1333–1336.
45. Wang Q, Shen J, Splawski I, Atkinson D, Li Z, Robinson JL, Moss AJ, Towbin JA, Keating MT. SCN5A mutations associated with an inherited cardiac arrhythmia, long QT syndrome. *Cell* 1995;80:805–811.
46. Sakmann BF, Spindler AJ, Bryant SM, Linz KW, Noble D. Distribution of a persistent sodium current across the ventricular wall in guinea pigs. *Circ Res* 2000;87:910–914.
47. Makielski JC, Farley AL. Na(+) current in human ventricle: Implications for sodium loading and

homeostasis. *J Cardiovasc Electrophysiol* 2006;17(Suppl. 1):S15–S20.

48. Antzelevitch C, Belardinelli L. The role of sodium channel current in modulating transmural dispersion of repolarization and arrhythmogenesis. *J Cardiovasc Electrophysiol* 2006;17(Suppl. 1):S79–S85.
49. Volders PG, Vos MA, Szabo B, Sipido KR, de Groot SH, Gorgels AP, Wellens HJ, Lazzara R. Progress in the understanding of cardiac early afterdepolarizations and torsades de pointes: Time to revise current concepts. *Cardiovasc Res* 2000;46:376–392.
50. John GW, Letienne R, Le Grand B, Pignier C, Vacher B, Patoiseau JF, Colpaert FC, Coulombe A. KC 12291: An atypical sodium channel blocker with myocardial antiischemic properties. *Cardiovasc Drug Rev* 2004;22:17–26.
51. Orth PM, Hesketh JC, Mak CK, Yang Y, Lin S, Beatch GN, Ezrin AM, Fedida D. RSD1235 blocks late INa and suppresses early afterdepolarizations and torsades de pointes induced by class III agents. *Cardiovasc Res* 2006;70:486–496.
52. Song Y, Shryock JC, Wu L, Belardinelli L. Antagonism by ranolazine of the pro-arrhythmic effects of increasing late INa in guinea pig ventricular myocytes. *J Cardiovasc Pharmacol* 2004;44:192–199.
53. Wu L, Shryock JC, Song Y, Li Y, Antzelevitch C, Belardinelli L. Antiarrhythmic effects of ranolazine in a guinea pig in vitro model of long-QT syndrome. *J Pharmacol Exp Ther* 2004;310:599–605.
54. Tian XL, Yong SL, Wan X, Wu L, Chung MK, Tchou PJ, Rosenbaum DS, Van Wagoner DR, Kirsch GE, Wang Q. Mechanisms by which SCN5A mutation N1325S causes cardiac arrhythmias and sudden death in vivo. *Cardiovasc Res* 2004;61:256–267.
55. Abrahamsson C, Carlsson L, Duker G. Lidocaine and nisoldipine attenuate almokalant-induced dispersion of repolarization and early afterdepolarizations in vitro. *J Cardiovasc Electrophysiol* 1996;7:1074–1081.
56. Wang DW, Yazawa K, Makita N, George AL Jr, Bennett PB. Pharmacological targeting of long QT mutant sodium channels. *J Clin Invest* 1997;99:1714–1720.
57. Maack C, Cortassa S, Aon MA, Ganesan AN, Liu T, O'Rourke B. Elevated cytosolic Na+ decreases mitochondrial Ca2+ uptake during excitation-contraction coupling and impairs energetic adaptation in cardiac myocytes. *Circ Res* 2006;99:172–182.
58. Bers DM. Cardiac excitation-contraction coupling. *Nature* 2002;415:198–205.
59. Weber CR, Piacentino V, III, Ginsburg KS, Houser SR, Bers DM. Na(+)-Ca(2+) exchange current and submembrane [Ca(2+)] during the cardiac action potential. *Circ Res* 2002;90:182–189.
60. Bers DM. *Excitation-Contraction Coupling and Cardiac Contractile Force*. Dordrecht, The Netherlands: Kluwer Academic Publishers, 2001.
61. Bers DM, Barry WH, Despa S. Intracellular Na+ regulation in cardiac myocytes. *Cardiovasc Res* 2003;57:897–912.
62. Eigel BN, Hadley RW. Antisense inhibition of Na+/Ca2+ exchange during anoxia/reoxygenation in ventricular myocytes. *Am J Physiol Heart Circ Physiol* 2001;281:H2184–H2190.
63. Hagihara H, Yoshikawa Y, Ohga Y, Takenaka C, Murata KY, Taniguchi S, Takaki M. Na+/Ca2+ exchange inhibition protects the rat heart from ischemia-reperfusion injury by blocking energy-wasting processes. *Am J Physiol Heart Circ Physiol* 2005;288:H1699–H1707.
64. Haigney MC, Miyata H, Lakatta EG, Stern MD, Silverman HS. Dependence of hypoxic cellular calcium loading on Na(+)-Ca2+ exchange. *Circ Res* 1992;71:547–557.
65. Imahashi K, Pott C, Goldhaber JI, Steenbergen C, Philipson KD, Murphy E. Cardiac-specific ablation of the Na+-Ca2+ exchanger confers protection against ischemia/reperfusion injury. *Circ Res* 2005;97:916–921.
66. Schafer C, Ladilov Y, Inserte J, Schafer M, Haffner S, Garcia-Dorado D, Piper HM. Role of the reverse mode of the Na+/Ca2+ exchanger in reoxygenation-induced cardiomyocyte injury. *Cardiovasc Res* 2001;51:241–250.
67. Wagner S, Seidler T, Picht E, Maier LS, Kazanski V, Teucher N, Schillinger W, Pieske B, Isenberg G, Hasenfuss G, Kogler H. Na(+)-Ca(2+) exchanger overexpression predisposes to reactive oxygen species-induced injury. *Cardiovasc Res* 2003;60:404–412.
68. Zeitz O, Maass AE, Van Nguyen P, Hensmann G, Kogler H, Moller K, Hasenfuss G, Janssen PM. Hydroxyl radical-induced acute diastolic dysfunction is due to calcium overload via reverse-mode Na(+)-Ca(2+) exchange. *Circ Res* 2002;90:988–995.
69. Bai CX, Namekata I, Kurokawa J, Tanaka H, Shigenobu K, Furukawa T. Role of nitric oxide in Ca2+ sensitivity of the slowly activating delayed rectifier K+ current in cardiac myocytes. *Circ Res* 2005;96:64–72.
70. Fauconnier J, Lacampagne A, Rauzier JM, Vassort G, Richard S. Ca2+-dependent reduction of IK1 in rat ventricular cells: A novel paradigm for arrhythmia in heart failure? *Cardiovasc Res* 2005;68:204–212.
71. Fabiato A, Fabiato F. Contractions induced by a calcium-triggered release of calcium from the sarcoplasmic reticulum of single skinned cardiac cells. *J Physiol* 1975;249:469–495.

72. Katra RP, Laurita KR. Cellular mechanism of calcium-mediated triggered activity in the heart. *Circ Res* 2005;96:535–542.
73. Lederer WJ, Tsien RW. Transient inward current underlying arrhythmogenic effects of cardiotonic steroids in Purkinje fibres. *J Physiol* 1976;263:73–100.
74. Pogwizd SM, Schlotthauer K, Li L, Yuan W, Bers DM. Arrhythmogenesis and contractile dysfunction in heart failure: Roles of sodium-calcium exchange, inward rectifier potassium current, and residual beta-adrenergic responsiveness. *Circ Res* 2001;88:1159–1167.
75. Wit AL, Rosen MR. Afterdepolarizations and triggered activity: Distinction from automaticity as an arrhythmogenic mechanism. In: Fozzard HA, Habert E, Jennings RB, Katz AM, Morgan HE, Eds. *Heart and Cardiovascular System: Scientific Foundations.* New York: Raven Press, 1992:2113–2163.
76. Eigel BN, Gursahani H, Hadley RW. ROS are required for rapid reactivation of Na+/Ca2+ exchanger in hypoxic reoxygenated guinea pig ventricular myocytes. *Am J Physiol Heart Circ Physiol* 2004;286:H955–H963.
77. Wu Y, Roden DM, Anderson ME. Calmodulin kinase inhibition prevents development of the arrhythmogenic transient inward current. *Circ Res* 1999;84:906–912.
78. Belardinelli L, Shryock JC, Fraser H. Inhibition of the late sodium current as a potential cardioprotective principle: Effects of the late sodium current inhibitor ranolazine. *Heart* 2006;92(Suppl. 4): iv6–iv14.
79. Fedida D, Orth PM, Hesketh JC, Ezrin AM. The role of late I and antiarrhythmic drugs in EAD formation and termination in Purkinje fibers. *J Cardiovasc Electrophysiol* 2006;17(Suppl. 1):S71–S78.
80. Pu J, Balser JR, Boyden PA. Lidocaine action on Na+ currents in ventricular myocytes from the epicardial border zone of the infarcted heart. *Circ Res* 1998;83:431–440.
81. Undrovinas AI, Belardinelli L, Undrovinas NA, Sabbah HN. Ranolazine improves abnormal repolarization and contraction in left ventricular myocytes of dogs with heart failure by inhibiting late sodium current. *J Cardiovasc Electrophysiol* 2006; 17(Suppl. 1):S169–S177.
82. Ver Donck L, Borgers M, Verdonck F. Inhibition of sodium and calcium overload pathology in the myocardium: A new cytoprotective principle. *Cardiovasc Res* 1993;27:349–357.
83. Li GR, Lau CP, Ducharme A, Tardif JC, Nattel S. Transmural action potential and ionic current remodeling in ventricles of failing canine hearts. *Am J Physiol Heart Circ Physiol* 2002;283:H1031–H1041.
84. Maltsev VA, Sabbah HN, Higgins RS, Silverman N, Lesch M, Undrovinas AI. Novel, ultraslow inactivating sodium current in human ventricular cardiomyocytes. *Circulation* 1998;98:2545–2552.
85. CV Therapeutics. Ranexa (ranolazine) review documents NDA. CV Therapeutics, Ed. 2003:21-526.
86. Shimizu W, Antzelevitch C. Cellular and ionic basis for T-wave alternans under long-QT conditions. *Circulation* 1999;99:1499–1507.
87. Belardinelli L, Antzelevitch C, Vos MA. Assessing predictors of drug-induced torsade de pointes. *Trends Pharmacol Sci* 2003;24:619–625.
88. Zaniboni M, Pollard AE, Yang L, Spitzer KW. Beat-to-beat repolarization variability in ventricular myocytes and its suppression by electrical coupling. *Am J Physiol Heart Circ Physiol* 2000;278: H677–H687.
89. Antzelevitch C, Belardinelli L, Wu L, Fraser H, Zygmunt AC, Burashnikov A, Diego JM, Fish JM, Cordeiro JM, Goodrow RJ Jr, Scornik F, Perez G. Electrophysiologic properties and antiarrhythmic actions of a novel antianginal agent. *J Cardiovasc Pharmacol Ther* 2004;9(Suppl. 1):S65–S83.
90. Wu L, Shryock JC, Song Y, Belardinelli L. An increase in late sodium current potentiates the proarrhythmic activities of low-risk QT-prolonging drugs in female rabbit hearts. *J Pharmacol Exp Ther* 2006;316:718–726.
91. Chaitman BR. Ranolazine for the treatment of chronic angina and potential use in other cardiovascular conditions. *Circulation* 2006;113:2462–2472.
92. Fredj S, Sampson KJ, Liu H, Kass RS. Molecular basis of ranolazine block of LQT-3 mutant sodium channels: Evidence for site of action. *Br J Pharmacol* 2006;148:16–24.
93. Antzelevitch C, Belardinelli L, Zygmunt AC, Burashnikov A, Di Diego JM, Fish JM, Cordeiro JM, Thomas G. Electrophysiological effects of ranolazine, a novel antianginal agent with antiarrhythmic properties. *Circulation* 2004;10:904–910.
94. Makielski JC, Valdivia CR. Ranolazine and late cardiac sodium current–a therapeutic target for angina, arrhythmia and more? *Br J Pharmacol* 2006;48:4–6.

9
Sodium Ion Channelopathies

Simona Casini, Arthur A.M. Wilde, and Hanno L. Tan

Introduction

Voltage-gated Sodium (Na^+) channels are sarcolemmal proteins that are responsible for the rapid upstroke of the cardiac action potential (AP), and for rapid impulse conduction through cardiac tissue. Therefore, Na^+ channel function plays a major role in initiation, propagation, and maintenance of the normal cardiac rhythm. Mutations in SCN5A, the gene encoding for the α-subunit of the cardiac Na^+ channel, the so-called "inherited sodium channelopathies," are known to evoke multiple life-threatening disorders of cardiac rhythm that can vary from tachyarrhythmias to bradyarrhythmias and may require implantation of pacemakers or implantable cardioverter/defibrillators (ICDs). However, recent studies have also linked Na^+ current (I_{Na}) dysfunction to structural cardiac defects, notably cardiac fibrosis, dilated cardiomyopathy, and, possibly, arrhythmogenic right ventricular cardiomyopathy. These structural changes may also be conducive to (reentrant) arrhythmias.

The identification of mutant Na^+ channels in inherited arrhythmia syndromes and the studies of their functional properties have significantly enhanced our knowledge of Na^+ channel function and our understanding of how Na^+ channel dysfunction may act as a major pathophysiological mechanism in various diseases, including common acquired disease (Table 9–1). Clearly, these observations highlight the cardiac Na^+ channel as an interesting target for novel therapy strategies. Accordingly, this chapter aims to provide an overview of presently identified disease entities with involvement of SCN5A variants, and concepts regarding arrhythmia susceptibility derived from studies of these conditions.

Na Channel Structure and Function

The cardiac Na^+ channel is a molecular complex consisting of various subunits: a main pore-forming subunit (α), encoded by SCN5A, and smaller accessory proteins, known as β-subunits.

The α-subunit consists of four homologous domains (DI–DIV), each composed of six membrane-spanning segments (S1–S6) linked by intracellular and extracellular loops (Figure 9–1). The linkers between S5 and S6 control ion selectivity and permeation[1] of the channel, while the positively charged segments S4 act as a voltage sensor.[2] Na^+ channels are dynamic molecules that undergo rapid structure rearrangements in response to changes in the electric field across the sarcolemma, a process known as "gating." Upon membrane depolarization, all four S4 segments move in a concerted way in an outward direction allowing the opening of the channel (activation).[2,3] This increase in Na^+ permeability causes the sudden membrane depolarization that characterizes the rapid upstroke of the AP. Activation of the channel lasts a few milliseconds and is followed by fast inactivation, a nonconducting state from which the channel cannot reopen. Finally, membrane repolarization is necessary to allow Na^+

TABLE 9–1. Sodium ion channelopathies.

Inherited primary electrical disease	**Reported changes in I_{Na}**
Brugada syndrome	↓
SUDS	↓
LQT3 syndrome	↑
SIDS	↑↓
Conduction disease	↓
Atrial standstill	↓
Sick sinus syndrome	↓
Structural disease	
Fibrosis	↓
Arrythmogenic right ventricular cardiomyopathy*	↓
Dilated cardiomyopathy	↓
Acquired disease	
Acquired Brugada syndrome	↓
Acquired long QT syndrome	↑
Congestive heart failure	↑↓
Ischemic heart disease	↑↓

↑ increased net I_{Na}; ↓ reduced net I_{Na}.
*Not fully resolved.

channels to recover from inactivation to the resting state (closed state).

Fast inactivation is primarily mediated by the intracellular linker between domains III and IV that acts as a lid, occluding the inner vestibule of the pore.[2,4] It was recently demonstrated that interactions between the C-terminus and the intracellular III–IV linker are required to stabilize channel inactivation. This interaction plays a critical role in the heart by preventing a small persistent inward Na^+ current (also called late I_{Na}) that would prolong the AP and render the heart susceptible to arrhythmias that are initiated by secondary depolarizations occurring before the

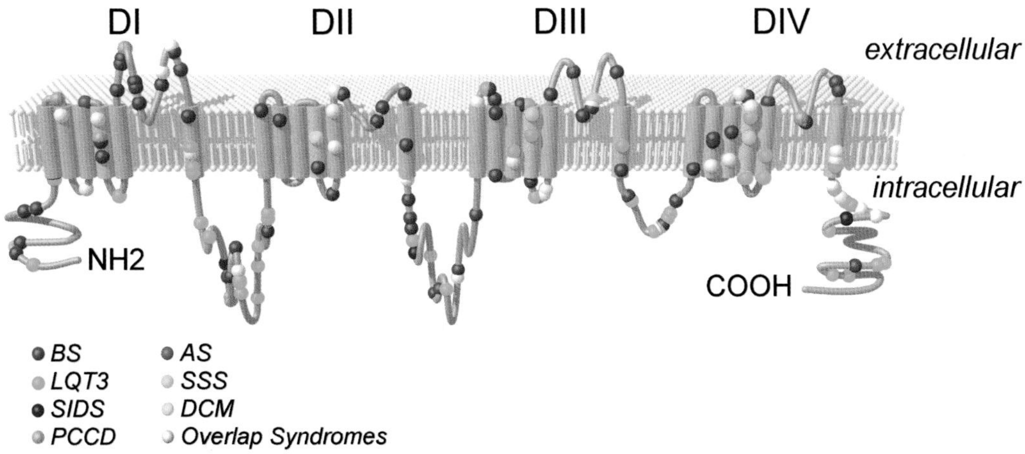

FIGURE 9–1. Schematic representation of the voltage-gated Na^+ channel α-subunit. The protein consists of four domains (D1–D4), each composed of six membrane-spanning segments (S1–S6) linked by intracellular and extracellular loops. The linkers between S5 and S6 control ion selectivity and permeation of the channel, while the positively charged segments S4 (in pink) act as a voltage sensor. Differently colored circles display the location of mutations associated with Brugada syndrome (BS), long QT syndrome 3 (LQT3), sudden infant death syndrome (SIDS), conduction disease (PCCD), atrial standstill (AS), sick sinus syndrome (SSS), dilated cardiomyopathy (DCM), and overlap syndromes.

cell has fully repolarized, called early afterdepolarizations (EADs).[5,6]

Beside this fast inactivation process (time frame: a few milliseconds), Na^+ channels can undergo a slower inactivation process (intermediate inactivation) when the membrane remains depolarized for a longer time. That more stable, nonconducting conformational state develops in cardiac Na^+ channels in about 50–100 msec and requires a prolonged period of hyperpolarization from which to recover.[7,8] Intermediate inactivation involves residues located in the outer pore and the C-terminus.[9,10] Finally, closed-state inactivation (inactivation from the closed-state without prior activation) may also occur[11] and can be clinically relevant.[12] The regions involved in closed-state inactivation await identification.

This spatial organization of gating functions suggests that single amino acid substitutions or deletions within the SCN5A coding region can evoke a broad spectrum of cardiac rhythm derangements by modulating this gating process. At the same time, common sequence variants (polymorphisms) in the Na^+ channel have also been implicated as risk factors in cardiac disease[13,14] and determinants of drug sensitivity.[15]

The α subunit interacts with smaller accessory proteins known as β-subunits. β-Subunits are glycoproteins with a single sarcolemma-spanning segment, a large immunoglobulin-like extracellular domain, and a small intracellular portion.[16] So far, four β-subunit isoforms (β_1–β_4) were identified and all are present in the heart.[17–19] Moreover, alternative RNA splicing has also been described for the β_1 subunit (β_{1A} and β_{1B}).[20,21] β_1 and β_3 share significant homology and are both not covalently associated with the α-subunit. On the other hand, β_2 and β_4 are similar and are linked to the α-subunit via disulfide bonds. β-subunits modulate the kinetic properties and the expression levels of the α subunit, and can play a role in cell adhesion.[22]

Inherited Primary Electrical Disease

Brugada Syndrome

Brugada syndrome (BS) is a cardiac disorder characterized by sudden death (especially at night and rest) due to ventricular tachyarrhythmias in the absence of structural heart disease as can be detected by routine cardiac examination. The electrocardiogram (ECG) of BS patients is characterized by ST-segment elevation in the right precordial leads (V1–V3), often in conjunction with signs of conduction slowing[23,24] (Figure 9–2). The ECG signs of the syndrome are dynamic and often concealed, but can be unmasked by Na^+ channel blockers, or during a febrile state.[25,26] Although the syndrome typically manifests during adulthood, with a peak around 40 years, arrhythmic events may occur at all ages. In western countries, the prevalence is estimated at 5–50 cases per 10,000 inhabitants.[27,28] In Southeast Asia, the disease is the leading cause of death in males under the age of 40, second only to car accidents.

Brugada syndrome exhibits an autosomal dominant pattern of inheritance, with incomplete penetrance and male predominance. Most drugs are not effective as a treatment in this syndrome

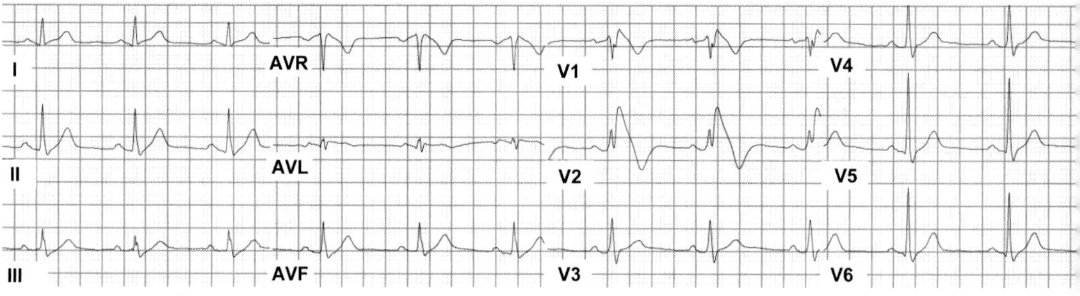

FIGURE 9–2. Representative electrocardiogram of Brugada syndrome. Note ST-segment elevation with high take-off (J point), and negative T waves, typically seen in right precordial leads V^1-V^2.

TABLE 9–2. Reported biophysical mechanisms of increase in net sodium current (gain-of-function) and reduction in net sodium current (loss-of-function).

Gain of function
Persistent current (disruption of fast inactivation)
Changes in voltage dependence of activation (hyperpolarizing shift) and inactivation (depolarizing shift)
Faster recovery from inactivation
Slower inactivation
Loss of function
Reduction in current density
Reduced number of functional sodium channels in sarcolemma
Truncated protein due to premature stop codon
Retention in endoplasmic reticulum (trafficking defect)
Mutation located in ion-conducting pore
Gating changes
Changes in voltage dependence of activation (depolarizing shift) and inactivation (hyperpolarizing shift)
Slower recovery from inactivation
Accelerated inactivation
Enhanced intermediate inactivation
Enhanced closed-state inactivation

and ICDs are the only recommended form of therapy to prevent sudden death.[29]

To date, a significant number of SCN5A gene mutations have been reported to contribute to BS. Functional analysis employing expression systems showed that all produce Na[4] channel loss of function. However, various mechanisms of I_{Na} reduction have been described (Table 9–2): (1) failure to express in the sarcolemma; (2) changes in the voltage and time dependence of activation, inactivation, and recovery from inactivation; (3) enhanced intermediate inactivation; (4) accelerated inactivation; and (5) trafficking defect. Of note, SCN5A mutations account for only 18–30% of BS cases, suggesting that other genes might be involved.[30] In 2002, a second locus on chromosome 3, close to but apart from the SCN5A locus, was linked to BS.[31] Here, an A280V mutation in the glycerol-3-phosphate dehydrogenase 1-like gene (GPD1L) was identified. This mutant, when transiently transfected into a HEK293 cell line that stably expressed SCN5A, resulted in reduction in I_{Na} when compared to wild type. Thus, GPD1L is a novel Na^+ channel modulator in the heart.[32] Another study showed a modulatory effect on the BS phenotype of the delayed rectifier potassium current encoded by KCNH2.[33]

How I_{Na} reduction causes the characteristic features of BS is unresolved. One hypothesis (repolarization disorder hypothesis) proposes that reduced I_{Na} may exacerbate the effects of the intrinsic difference in density of the transient outward current, I_{to}, between epicardial (high I_{to} density) and endocardial (low I_{to} density) layers.[34] According to this hypothesis, this strong repolarizing current renders epicardial cells more sensitive than endocardial cells to reductions in Na^+ current. An alternative hypothesis revolves around slowing of impulse propagation in the right ventricle, particularly the right ventricular outflow tract (depolarization disorder hypothesis).[35,36] Both hypotheses are supported by clinical and experimental data, rendering it likely that BS is not fully explained by one single mechanism. Yet evidence of conduction abnormalities in patients with BS is accumulating. Widening of P-wave and QRS duration and prolongation of the PQ and HV intervals, all of which represent conduction abnormalities, are often observed in BS patients. Smits *et al.* showed that greater prolongation of PQ and HV intervals at baseline and excessive QRS interval prolongation after Na^+ channel blockade are more likely to be found in BS patients who carry a SCN5A mutation than in those who do not.[37] Moreover, in a study of 78 individuals carrying a SCN5A mutation associated with BS, resting ECGs showed a spontaneous BS ECG pattern in 28 of 78 (36%) gene carriers, while 59 of 78 (76%) exhibited conduction defects. Moreover, the conduction defects worsened with age in mutation carriers, leading in five cases to pacemaker implantation.[38] This study showed that the most common phenotype of gene carriers of a BS-type SCN5A mutation is a progressive cardiac conduction defect similar to the Lenègre disease phenotype (see the section on "Conduction Disease" below).

Finally, recent studies highlight the role of other pathophysiological derangements, e.g., fibrosis[39,40] (see the section on "Cardiac Fibrosis" below), thereby contributing to the emerging notion that BS is not a monofactorial disease.

Sudden Unexplained Death Syndrome

Sudden unexplained death syndrome (SUDS) is characterized by sudden death, typically during sleep, in young- and middle-aged males in South East Asian countries. The syndrome is the leading natural cause of death in young Thai men.[41] The patients, almost exclusively men, have structurally normal hearts and ECG patterns similar to BS. SCN5A mutations were identified in SUDS patients, which resulted in "loss-of-function" alterations such as in BS. These data suggest that SUDS and BS are phenotypically, genetically, and functionally the same disorder.[42]

Long QT Syndrome

The congenital long QT syndrome (LQTS) is an inherited disorder estimated to affect 1/5000 individuals, with the onset of symptoms typically occurring within the first two decades of life. The syndrome is mostly transmitted in an autosomal dominant fashion (Romano–Ward syndrome) and rarely as an autosomal recessive disease associated with congenital deafness (Jervell and Lange–Nielsen syndrome). The syndrome derives its name from the characteristic prolongation of the QT interval on the surface ECG (Figure 9–3), which is coupled at the cellular level to prolonged AP duration and delay in myocardial repolarization. AP prolongation can lead to EADs, which may initiate a life-threatening form of polymorphic ventricular tachycardia called torsade de pointes (TdP).[43] LQTS is a heterogeneous disorder with different genotypes and corresponding phenotypes. So far, mutations in eight different genes were associated with LQTS. Mutations in SCN5A characterize LQT3. LQT3 accounts for 8% of LQTS patients.[44]

In general, Na^+ channel mutations linked to LQT3 are associated with disrupted inactivation, as was originally identified in the ΔKPQ mutation,[45] a three amino acid deletion in the DIII–DIV linker. This intracellular segment is critically involved in Na^+ channel fast inactivation. Accordingly, this mutation results in a noninactivating persistent Na^+ current (gain-of-function) during the AP plateau that prolongs the AP duration and may account for the development of arrhythmogenic triggered activity, such as EADs. Although most of the mutations associated with LQT3 show a persistent inward current, some mutations exhibited other gating disorders that also led to the prolongation of the QT interval. These include faster recovery from inactivation, shift in voltage dependence of activation and inactivation, and a slower inactivation[46–49] (Table 9–2). Because a very delicate balance of inward and outward currents maintains the AP plateau, these subtle current alterations during repolarization may provoke QT prolongation and TdP.

Genotype–phenotype studies have shown that the risk of cardiac events differs among the different LQTS genotypes. In the case of LQT3, symptoms occur especially at rest or during sleep, when sympathetic nerve activity is expected to be low. These differences must be taken into account during diagnosis and treatment.

β-Adrenergic blockers remain the cornerstone of therapy in LQTS, although this treatment may be less efficacious in SCN5A mutation carriers.[5] Clinical and *in vitro* evidence suggests that mexiletine may reduce persistent Na^+ current and shorten the QT interval in SCN5A mutation

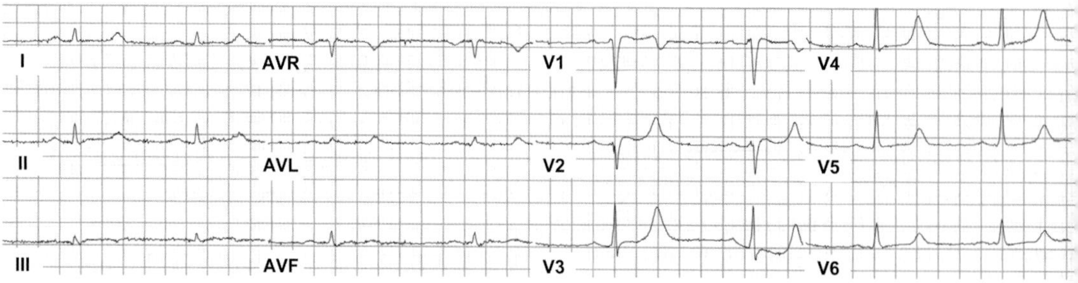

FIGURE 9–3. Representative electrocardiogram of long QT syndrome type 3. Note the marked QT interval prolongation with late peaked T waves.

carriers, although there are no data to indicate a reduction in mortality.[51,52] Flecainide has also been observed to shorten QT intervals,[53,54] but some have argued over the safety of this therapy.[55]

Sudden Infant Death Syndrome

Sudden infant death syndrome (SIDS) continues to be the most common cause of postneonatal infant death, accounting for about 25% of all deaths between 1 month and 1 year of age. It is a complex, multifactorial disorder, the cause of which is still not fully understood. However, much is now known about environmental risk factors, some of which are modifiable. These include maternal and antenatal risk factors, such as smoking during pregnancy, the use of alcohol and drugs, and infant-related risk factors, such as nonsupine sleeping position and soft bedding. Emerging evidence also shows an increased number of genetic risk factors responsible for SIDS. Overall, it is estimated that 5–10% of SIDS are associated with a defective cardiac ion channel and, therefore, an increased potential for lethal arrhythmias.[56]

Schwartz *et al.* provided the first molecular proof that LQTS may be involved in SIDS by studying an infant who experienced cardiac arrest from ventricular fibrillation (VF). Genetic analysis demonstrated a sporadic *de novo* SCN5A mutation (S941N).[57] Subsequent studies reported other mutations linked to LQT3.[49,58] Other studies demonstrated that BS can also be considered as a cause of sudden death in children.[59,60] In conclusion, complex interactions between genetic and environmental risk factors have to be taken into account to determine the risk of SIDS in individual infants.

Conduction Disease

Progressive cardiac conduction defect (PCCD), also known as Lenègre disease, is characterized by progressive slowing of conduction velocity through the His–Purkinje system with right or left bundle branch block, manifesting on the surface ECG as PR interval prolongation and QRS widening, usually in older individuals (Figure 9–4). Complete atrioventricular (AV) block can occur, resulting in syncope or sudden death. Implantation of a pacemaker is the treatment of choice. The disorder has been linked to mutations in SCN5A and in another chromosomal locus (19q13.2–q13.3)[61,62] at which the involved gene is yet unknown. The first description of a SCN5A mutation was in a large French family. In this family, P-wave width, PR, and QRS intervals prolonged with age.[63] However, in a Dutch family, where the disease was caused by another SCN5A mutation, the proband was a child.[63] This suggests that the resulting phenotype may be progressive or immediate. The first study on the biophysical properties of a PCCD-associated SCN5A mutation (G514C) showed reduced I_{Na}.[12] Patch-clamp studies revealed opposing gating changes that resulted in attenuated I_{Na} reduction. As confirmed by modeling studies, this decrease in Na^+ current was sufficient to cause conduction disease, but insufficient to cause BS. Although

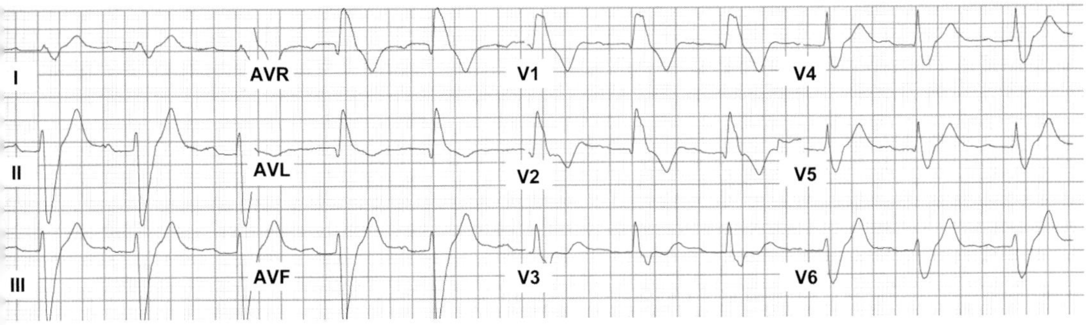

FIGURE 9–4. Representative electrocardiogram of conduction disease. Note the marked QRS widening, PQ interval prolongation, and left QRS axis deviation.

through different mechanisms, all subsequent SCN5A mutants studied were characterized by a loss of Na^+ channel function.[14,64–67] The decreased I_{Na} would result in a reduction of the AP upstroke velocity, thereby slowing the conduction velocity. Recently, in a large Finnich family, the loss-of-function mutation D1275N was identified. The affected individuals showed cardiac conduction defects and atrial arrhythmias.[68] Of note, the same mutation was found in families with atrial standstill[69] and with dilated cadiomyopathy.[70,71]

Atrial Standstill

Atrial standstill (AS) is a rare arrhythmia that consists of loss in electrical and mechanical activity of the atria. It is characterized by bradycardia, absence of P-waves, and junctional escape rhythm.[72] Whereas in most reports, AS is secondary to other diseases, familial AS without underlying cardiac disorder is extremely rare and identification of genetic factors for AS is hampered by the small number of affected individuals in each family. The first mutation associated with AS was found in SCN5A (D1275N) and resulted in a loss-of-function Na^+ channel. Of interest, the affected individuals carried the mutation and were homozygous for two linked polymorphisms in Cx40, the gene encoding the atrium-specific gap junction protein connexin 40.[69] These Cx40 polymorphisms were localized in the promoter region and resulted in reduced Cx40 expression. This was predicted to hamper cell-to-cell electrical coupling in the atrium, thereby reducing atrial excitability. At the same time, the requirement of this Cx40 variant was used to explain why the phenotype in this family was restricted to the atrium. Recently, another SCN5A mutation (L212P) linked to AS was identified.[73] When expressed in a heterologous system, this mutation showed opposing gating changes, resulting in a net loss-of-function of I_{Na}. Further screening for genetic variations revealed that the affected individual carried the same Cx40 polymorphisms as described previously[69] but was heterozygous for them. Taken together, these studies indicate that genetic defects in SCN5A most likely underlie AS, but that additional genetic factors that modulate atrial electrical coupling are relevant to the clinical manifestation of this inherited arrhythmia.

Sick Sinus Syndrome

Idiopathic sick sinus syndrome (SSS) is characterized by sinus bradycardia and sinus arrest in the absence of any structural heart disease. In three independent studies, mutations in HCN4, the gene encoding the α-subunit of the pacemaker current, I_f, were identified.[74–76] These HCN4 mutations resulted in loss-of-function of I_f. Although the role of I_{Na} in sinoatrial node depolarization is less clear, SCN5A mutations were also identified in 5 of 10 children (three families) with sinus node disease.[77] Compound heterozygosity was, however, necessary, as members of the studied families who carried mutations in only one allele were clinically unaffected. The SCN5A mutations resulted in loss-of-function of I_{Na}. The phenotype in these individuals included bradycardia that progressed to atrial inexcitability. Thus, there may be substantial overlap with the atrial standstill phenotype. The available data suggest, similar to other channelopathies, that idiopathic SSS is genetically heterogeneous.

Variant Na^+ Channels in Structural Defects

Cardiac Fibrosis

The first association between reduced I_{Na} and structural defects was derived from a study of two infants of asymptomatic parents who exhibited prolonged conduction intervals (PR, QRS) associated with episodes of wide complex tachycardia.[64] Genetic analysis revealed compound heterozygosity for two SCN5A mutations that both caused I_{Na} reduction (due to a truncated protein resulting from a premature stop codon in W156X, in conjunction with severely reduced I_{Na} density of R225W channels). The postmortem examination of the heart of one of the children who died from severe reduction in cardiac excitability and ventricular tachyarrhythmias showed fibrosis and necrosis in the left and right ventricle, and fibrosis of the AV node and specialized conduction system, providing the first evidence that a monogenic channel defect can progressively lead to myocardial structural abnormalities in humans.

Similarly, studies of the explanted heart of a BS patient with a loss-of-function SCN5A mutation

(G1935S) revealed severe fibrosis in the right ventricular midmyocardial free wall.[39] Of note, this region was critically involved in tachyarrhythmias elicited by programmed electrical stimulation. Finally, in a study of 18 unrelated patients with the clinical phenotype of BS and normal cardiac structure and function on noninvasive examinations, endomyocardial biopsies revealed structural derangements in all. Mutations in SCN5A were identified in 4 of 18 patients.[40] All mutations resulted in loss-of-function I_{Na}, characteristic of BS. One mutation carrier showed fibrofatty myocardial replacement, suggestive of arrhythmogenic right ventricular cardiomyopathy (ARVC). Of note, in the BS patients with SCN5A mutations, myocyte apoptosis in both the left and the right ventricle was significantly higher than in control.

The association between reduced I_{Na} and structural defects is supported by experimental studies. In a SCN5A knockout mouse model, mice that were homozygous for the null allele died before birth, with profound derangements in cardiac development. Heterozygous mice survived, and exhibited severe conduction abnormalities, resembling the PCCD phenotype, along with a 50% reduction in I_{Na}, as found in patch-clamp studies.[78] In a follow-up study, it was found that old (but not young) heterozygous mice had prominent cardiac fibrosis in the left and right ventricular free walls and the interventricular septum. In addition to fibrosis, altered expression of connexin was also identified.[79] Finally, in aged heterozygous mice, reduced I_{Na} in combination with interstitial fibrosis and disarrangement of gap junctions resulted in severe conduction impairment.[80]

Arrhythmogenic Right Ventricular Cardiomyopathy

Arrhythmogenic right ventricular cardiomyopathy (ARVC) is an inherited heart muscle disease characterized pathologically by specific derangements of the right ventricle (RV) (fibrosis, fibrofatty replacement of myocardium) and clinically by ventricular tachycardia that may culminate in ventricular fibrillation and sudden death. Of interest, the clinical features of ARVC may exihibit significant overlap with those of BS.[81–83] Most notably, the hallmark ST elevations of BS have also been reported in ARVC, and may be provoked by Na^+ channel blockers, similar to BS.[84] Conversely, autopsy studies of BS patients revealed fatty tissue deposition in the RV.[85,86] Moreover, in biopsies from the RV, fatty tissue infiltration mimicking ARVC was observed in 8 of 22 BS cases (36%).[86] Most recently, in a study of 18 unrelated patients with the clinical phenotype of BS, endomyocardial biopsies revealed structural derangements in all, with histopathological findings suggestive of ARVC in a patient who carried a SCN5A mutation.[40] Although overlap may exist between ARVC and BS, at present, ARVC has been linked to genes that are different from those responsible for BS. Only the ARVC5 locus has been mapped to a region on the same chromosome that contains SCN5A and GPD1L, the two genes associated with BS, but the gene has not been identified yet.[87] These data not only substantiate an overlap between ARVC and BS[88] but may also exemplify the potential of SCN5A mutations to be causally involved in structural cardiac defects.

Dilated Cardiomyopathy

Dilated cardiomyopathy (DCM) is an idiopathic, genetically heterogeneous disorder characterized by heart failure and an enhanced incidence of arrhythmias. The majority of the identified genes encode structural proteins of the contractile apparatus and cytoskeleton. In 1996, a locus for DCM was identified on chromosome 3 (3p22–p25), which contains SCN5A.[89] Subsequent screening of SCN5A revealed the missense mutation D1275N, as reported in studies by McNair *et al.*[70] and Olson *et al.*[71] In these studies, affected members had dilated cardiomyopathy and signs of conduction disease, along with atrial fibrillation. Of interest, this phenotype is distinct from a previous study by Groenewegen *et al.*, in which the D1275N mutation caused familial AS, when combined with a rare Cx40 polymorphism (in the study of McNair *et al.*, DCM did not correlate with the presence of Cx40 polymorphisms).[69] A more recent study by Laitinen-Forsblom *et al.* also linked the D1275N mutation with cardiac conduction defects and atrial arrhythmias, while no contractile dysfunction was observed.[68] Why the D1275N mutation caused DCM in the family reported by Olson *et al.* and McNair *et al.*, but not in the families reported by Groenewegen *et al.* and Laitinen-Forsblom *et al.*, remains a matter of debate.[90] It was proposed that contractile dysfunction and DCM may be secondary to chronically increased heart rates from atrial fibrillation. Still, the possible role of SCN5A mutations in causing DCM was supported by the presentation by Olson *et al.* of loss-of-function SCN5A mutations in four other DCM families (T220I, R814W, D1595H, and the basepair insertion 2550–2551insTG, leading to a stop codon), with histopathological derangements in two of four mutation carriers (in the T220I and R814W families).[71] In conclusion, while this study[71] supports the proposed link between reduced I_{Na} and structural derangements, it is unclear how identical loss-of function mutations in SCN5A may lead to different phenotypes.

Overlap Syndromes and Modulating Factors

Several SCN5A mutations have been identified, which resulted in overlapping phenotypes characterized by a combination of various features of the above described disorders. The 1795insD mutant was the first to be reported. Carriers of this mutation exhibited features of LQT3 and BS[7]. Patch-clamp studies revealed that these opposing phenotypes (gain of function in LQT3, and loss-of-function in BS) may be explained by distinct gating changes. Thus, enhanced persistent I_{Na} accounted for AP prolongation and LQT3, while, concurrently, enhanced intermediate inactivation resulted in reduced I_{Na} availability and ST elevation at fast heart rates. A subsequent study revealed that this SCN5A variant is also associated with sinus rate slowing, and that this phenomenon may equally be explained by altered biophysical properties, notably prolongation of the sinus node AP by persistent I_{Na}.[91] Additionally, mutation of the same residue to a histidine (Y1795H) or cysteine (Y1795C) resulted in BS and LQTS, respectively.[92] Kyndt *et al.*[93] described a large French family with a missense mutation (G1406R) in which mutation carriers exhibited either BS or PCCD phenotypes, suggesting that modifier gene(s) may influence the phenotypic consequence of this SCN5A mutation. Similarly, the deletion of a lysine (ΔK1500) was associated with BS, LQTS, and PCCD.[94] Later studies have also reported combinations of others phenotypes, e.g. SSS in conjunction with conduction disease and BS.[95] Probably the most consistent link is that between BS and PCCD. In a study of 78 individuals carrying a SCN5A mutation associated with BS, the spontaneous (i.e., in the absence of pharmacological challenge) BS phenotypes were present only in 36%, while 76% exhibited conduction defects. Moreover, the conduction defects worsened with age in mutation carriers.[38]

How a single mutation can result in a different and sometimes opposing phenotype, is not fully resolved. In addition to specific gating changes (as described for the 1795insD mutation[7]), other explanations have been proposed. For instance, the intrinsic heterogeneity of the myocardial substrate with which the mutant Na^+ channel interacts may be relevant. Epicardial myocytes have a characteristic spike-and-dome AP morphology due to a large I_{to}, while endocardial cells do not. Mutations that act to reduce I_{Na}, in the presence of a large repolarizing current, may result in premature AP repolarization, loss of AP dome, and BS-type ST elevation on the ECG (repolarization disorder hypothesis). Conversely, in endocardial cells, persistent I_{Na}, in the presence of smaller repolarizing currents, may prolong AP duration (LQT3 phenotype).[96] Still, this theory does not explain why a single mutation may cause different phenotypes in various members of the same family. Other studies have revealed the role of gender. In a single family, the G1406R mutant caused BS only in male carriers (four of six), while PCCD was found in six of six female and two of six male carriers.[93] This is consistent with the observation that while SCN5A variants are equally transmitted between both sexes, the BS phenotype is more prevalent in males. The male predominance might be partially due to the intrinsic differences in ventricular AP between males and females.[97] I_{to} density is higher in males, rendering them more susceptible to the effect of I_{Na} reduction. In men, this may result more readily in excessive repolarization as proposed in the repolarization disorder hypothesis.[98] Conversely, females may be protected, because $I_{Ca\text{-}L}$ is more strongly expressed in their epicardium.[99] Moreover, other studies suggested that the male hormone testosterone may be accountable for the gender differences in BS.[100]

Of note, the modulating role of genetic factors in determining the clinical phenotype is now emerging from recent studies. For instance, the D1275N mutation caused atrial standstill in the presence of homozygous loss-of-function Cx40 promoter polymorphisms,[69] but DCM and conduction defects in their absence.[68,70] Similarly, the common polymorphism H558R in SCN5A produced no appreciable I_{Na} gating changes in isolation, but it attenuated the gating defects caused by a SCN5A mutation identified in a child with conduction disease.[14] Another study also reported a modulatory role of this polymorphism on a LQT3-linked SCN5A mutant.[101] The presence of such polymorphisms and differences in their prevalence among various ethnic groups may underlie clinically relevant differences among ethnic groups. For instance, the S1102Y polymorphism in SCN5A is mainly present in subjects of African descent[15] (it was also found in a single white family, but there, it was deemed a disease-causing mutation responsible for LQT3[102]). S1102Y was found in a patient of African descent who sustained QT prolongation and TdP on amiodarone (with associated hypokalemia and dilated cardiomyopathy as confounders for QT prolongation).[15] Similarly, Bezzina *et al.*[13] recently identified a haplotype variant in the promoter region of SCN5A that occurred with an allele frequency of 22% in Asian subjects, but was absent in whites and blacks. This haplotype resulted in reduced SCN5A transcription and was associated with slower cardiac conduction. It was suggested that this variability in SCN5A transcription may contribute to differences in phenotype as a function of ethnicity.[13]

Acquired Cardiac Arrhythmias

Whereas the inherited arrhythmias described above are explained by disturbed properties of mutant Na^+ channels, "acquired arrhythmias" are precipitated by environmental factors that act on the electrical activity of the heart.

It is increasingly recognized that acquired arrhythmias may involve subclinical genetic variations (polymorphisms) that can alter the structure or the electrophysiological properties of the myocardial substrate, thereby contributing to unique drug responses in carriers of these gene variants. Similarly, some of the knowledge obtained in the study of rare inherited SCN5A-related disorders can be now extended to common acquired diseases. Na^+ channel gating derangements caused by these conditions may have relevance both in the presence of Na^+ channel polymorphisms and in their absence.

Drug-Induced Brugada Syndrome

Given the role of I_{Na} reduction in BS, various conditions and drugs that reduce I_{Na} may cause/mimic BS. Class IC Na^+ channel blockers are the most frequent causes of acquired BS, but many other drugs (not necessarily drugs aimed primarily at cardiac disease) are able to induce ST-segment elevations. Moreover, a BS-like phenotype may be evoked by environmental factors, including electrolyte abnormalities, hyperthermia, hypothermia, elevated insulin level, acute ischemia, and mechanical compression of the right ventricular outflow tract (RVOT).[103] It is likely that polymorphisms can enhance individual susceptibility to the BS phenotype in the presence of drugs or other triggers, although up to now no cases were reported.

Drug-Induced Long QT Syndrome

A SCN5A polymorphism (S1102Y) was found in a patient of African descent who sustained QT prolongation and TdP on amiodarone (with associated hypokalemia and dilated cardiomyopathy as confounders for QT prolongation).[15] This polymorphism appeared to be ethnicity related, being commonly present in subjects of African descent. Subsequent biophysical analysis revealed mild Na^+ channel gain-of-function, primarily caused by enhanced persistent I_{Na} and increased I_{Na} density. The biophysical effects of S1102Y are so subtle that it is anticipated that most individuals who carry it do not develop arrhythmias, unless additional acquired risk factors are present, such as drug use, hypokalemia, or structural heart disease.

A SCN5A mutation (L1825P) was isolated in a woman who showed drug-induced LQTS after cisapride treatment.[104] In isolation, this mutation was subclinical, and exerted clinical effects only when uncovered by the use of cisapride. The mutant channel exhibited both gain-of-function Na^+ channel features (persistent I_{Na}, slowed decay of inactivation), characteristic of LQT3, and loss-of-function features (decreased peak current, negative shift of inactivation, positive shift of activation, enhanced closed-state inactivation) typical of BS. It was suggested that the superimposition of the subclinical features of L1825P channels at baseline, and the proarrhythmic effects of cisapride, may have been the cause of the LQTS phenotype in the patient.

Congestive Heart Failure

AP and QT prolongation are well-known features of congestive heart failure (HF) that contribute to enhanced risk of arrhythmias and sudden death in this disease. An increased persistent I_{Na}, which can contribute to AP prolongation, was shown in two different dog models of HF[105,106] and in failing human ventricular myocytes.[106] Accordingly, experimental block of persistent I_{Na} by saxitoxin or lidocaine shortened AP duration and abolished EADs in myocytes of failing hearts.[105] In contrast, down-regulation of I_{Na} was found in two different canine HF models,[106–108] and in human ventricular cells.[106] A decrease in I_{Na} density may reduce excitability, thereby slowing myocardial conduction and contributing to reentrant arrhythmias. However, Wiegerinck *et al.*[109] did not observe any differences in peak current between HF and CTR in a volume/pressure overload HF rabbit model, in line with another study that did not reveal changes in I_{Na} in dogs with pacing-induced HF.[110] The contrasting results of these studies may be due to species/model differences.

While these studies did not address the possible presence of Na^+ channel polymorphisms, these observations may point to a novel target for a reduction in risk of arrhythmia in congestive heart failure.

Ischemic Heart Disease

Although several studies have revealed ischemia-related functional changes in various cardiac ion channels and transporters,[111] it is likely that Na^+ channel dysfunction plays an important role in reentrant arrhythmias under ischemic conditions.[112] Ischemia-induced arrhythmias can evolve from a site of slowed conduction near the ischemic border zone,[113] consistent with a loss of Na^+ channel function.

Supporting these findings, in an experimental dog model of chronic ischemia, myocytes obtained from the ischemic zone exhibited reduced I_{Na} and altered inactivation gating properties (negative shift of inactivation, slowed recovery from inactivation, enhanced closed-state inactivation) when compared to myocytes of nonischemic regions.[114] These results are consistent with previous findings in which maximal AP upstroke velocity (V_{max}), a measure of I_{Na}, was found to be significantly reduced in myocytes of infarction border zones.[115,116] The reduced I_{Na} can contribute to conduction slowing, thereby facilitating reentrant arrhythmias.

Consistent with a higher affinity for the inactivated channel conformation(s), lidocaine is able to produce an enhanced use-dependent I_{Na} block in border zone cells, suggesting that changes in Na^+ channel inactivation gating in ischemic border zones may provoke a proarrhythmic pharmacological effect.[117] This could be a molecular mechanism for the enhanced risk of life-threatening proarrhythmia conferred by potent Na^+ channel blockers in patients who experienced cardiac ischemia in the CAST trial.[118]

These data suggest that gating changes may contribute to electrophysiological heterogeneity during ischemia, which predispose to reentrant arrhythmias. Accordingly, in rats with 3- to 4-week-old experimentally induced myocardial infarctions, an increased persistent Na^+ was found when compared to controls.[119]

Other experiments revealed that Na^+ influx carried by the persistent Na^+ current appeared to be a major contributor to the rise of intracellular Na^+ observed during ischemia[120] and hypoxia.[121] Moreover, exposure of the heart to ischemia is known to increase lysophosphatidylcholine, palmitoyl-L-carnitine, and reactive oxygen species (e.g., hydrogen peroxide), and these substances are themselves reported to increase persistent I_{Na}.[122–124] Persistent I_{Na} can trigger arrhythmias either by prolonging AP duration with subsequent EADs or by increasing intracellular Na^+ loading, leading to calcium overload, and, consequently, to delayed afterdepolarizations (DADs).[125] In both mechanisms, persistent I_{Na} represents an attractive target for therapeutic intervention. A selective blocker of this current without significant action on peak Na^+ current may be a promising development.[126,127]

Summary

While the spectrum of diseases associated with SCN5A mutations is still expanding, it is becoming increasingly clear that even subtle changes in Na^+ channel gating can dramatically affect cardiac rhythm, especially if exacerbated by environmental factors that act on the electrical activity of the heart. Biophysical studies have revealed Na^+ channel gating defects that, in many cases, can explain the phenotype associated with the rhythm disorder. However, recent studies have shown significant overlap between aberrant rhythm phenotypes, and single mutations have been found to evoke different rhythm disorders. It is now evident that the correlation between mutation and the clinical phenotype is not always straightforward. Many factors, such as the presence of polymorphisms, humoral regulation, auxiliary subunits, and transcriptional regulation may play a role. Moreover, it is becoming clear that Na^+ channel-related diseases involve not only derangements in cardiac excitability, but also structural cardiac derangements, that may not be detectable using current clinical imaging modalities, but that nevertheless may act in concert with reductions in cardiac excitability to facilitate reentrant arrhythmias. With the discovery of novel disease entities associated with SCN5A variants, and the elucidation of the biophysical ways in which these variants impact on I_{Na}, we are now beginning to obtain the insights needed to apply the concepts derived from studies of rare inherited SCN5A-associated diseases to common acquired disease.

Acknowledgments. The authors thank Dr. Andre Linnenbank for providing Figure 9–1 and Dr. Connie Bezzina for valuable discussions. Dr. Tan was supported by the Royal Netherlands Academy of Arts and Sciences (KNAW), the Netherlands Heart Foundation (NHS2002B191), and the Bekales Foundation.

References

1. Heinemann SH, Terlau H, Stuhmer W, *et al.* Calcium channel characteristics conferred on the sodium channel by single mutations. *Nature* 1992;356:441–443.
2. Stuhmer W, Conti F, Suzuki H, *et al.* Structural parts involved in activation and inactivation of the sodium channel. *Nature* 1989;339:597–603.
3. Kontis KJ, Rounaghi A, Goldin AL. Sodium channel activation gating is affected by substitutions of voltage sensor positive charges in all four domains. *J Gen Physiol* 1997;110:391–401.
4. West JW, Patton DE, Scheuer T, *et al.* A cluster of hydrophobic amino acid residues required for fast Na(+)-channel inactivation. *Proc Natl Acad Sci USA* 1992;89:10910–10914.
5. Kass RS. Sodium channel inactivation in heart: A novel role of the carboxy-terminal domain. *J Cardiovasc Electrophysiol* 2006;17(Suppl. 1):S21–S5.
6. Motoike HK, Liu H, Glaaser IW, *et al.* The Na+ channel inactivation gate is a molecular complex: A novel role of the COOH-terminal domain. *J Gen Physiol* 2004;123:155–165.
7. Veldkamp MW, Viswanathan PC, Bezzina C, *et al.* Two distinct congenital arrhythmias evoked by a multidysfunctional Na(+) channel. *Circ Res* 2000;86:E91–97.
8. Wang DW, Makita N, Kitabatake A, *et al.* Enhanced Na(+) channel intermediate inactivation in Brugada syndrome. *Circ Res* 2000;87:E37–43.
9. Balser JR. The cardiac sodium channel: Gating function and molecular pharmacology. *J Mol Cell Cardiol* 2001;33:599–613.
10. Tan HL, Kupershmidt S, Zhang R, *et al.* A calcium sensor in the sodium channel modulates cardiac excitability. *Nature* 2002;415:442–447.
11. Horn R, Patlak J, Stevens CF. Sodium channels need not open before they inactivate. *Nature* 1981;291:426–427.
12. Tan HL, Bink-Boelkens MT, Bezzina CR, *et al.* A sodium-channel mutation causes isolated cardiac conduction disease. *Nature* 2001;409:1043–1047.
13. Bezzina CR, Shimizu W, Yang P, *et al.* Common sodium channel promoter haplotype in asian subjects underlies variability in cardiac conduction. *Circulation* 2006;113:338–344.
14. Viswanathan PC, Benson DW, Balser JR. A common SCN5A polymorphism modulates the biophysical effects of an SCN5A mutation. *J Clin Invest* 2003;111:341–346.
15. Splawski I, Timothy KW, Tateyama M, *et al.* Variant of SCN5A sodium channel implicated in risk of cardiac arrhythmia. *Science* 2002;297:1333–1336.

16. Isom LL, Catterall WA. Na+ channel subunits and Ig domains. *Nature* 1996;383:307–308.
17. Makita N, Sloan-Brown K, Weghuis DO, *et al.* Genomic organization and chromosomal assignment of the human voltage-gated Na+ channel beta 1 subunit gene (SCN1B). *Genomics* 1994;23: 628–634.
18. Morgan K, Stevens EB, Shah B, *et al.* beta 3: An additional auxiliary subunit of the voltage-sensitive sodium channel that modulates channel gating with distinct kinetics. *Proc Natl Acad Sci USA* 2000;97:2308–2313.
19. Yu FH, Westenbroek RE, Silos-Santiago I, *et al.* Sodium channel beta4, a new disulfide-linked auxiliary subunit with similarity to beta2. *J Neurosci* 2003;23:7577–7585.
20. Kazen-Gillespie KA, Ragsdale DS, D'Andrea MR, *et al.* Cloning, localization, and functional expression of sodium channel beta1A subunits. *J Biol Chem* 2000;275:1079–1088.
21. Qin N, D'Andrea MR, Lubin ML, *et al.* Molecular cloning and functional expression of the human sodium channel beta1B subunit, a novel splicing variant of the beta1 subunit. *Eur J Biochem* 2003;270:4762–4770.
22. Isom LL. Sodium channel beta subunits: Anything but auxiliary. *Neuroscientist* 2001;7:42–54.
23. Brugada P, Brugada J. Right bundle branch block, persistent ST segment elevation and sudden cardiac death: A distinct clinical and electrocardiographic syndrome. A multicenter report. *J Am Coll Cardiol* 1992;20:1391–1396.
24. Brugada J, Brugada R, Brugada P. Right bundle-branch block and ST-segment elevation in leads V1 through V3: A marker for sudden death in patients without demonstrable structural heart disease. *Circulation* 1998;97:457–460.
25. Antzelevitch C, Brugada R. Fever and Brugada syndrome. *Pacing Clin Electrophysiol* 2002;25: 1537–1539.
26. Brugada R, Brugada J, Antzelevitch C, *et al.* Sodium channel blockers identify risk for sudden death in patients with ST-segment elevation and right bundle branch block but structurally normal hearts. *Circulation* 2000;101:510–515.
27. Alings M, Wilde A. "Brugada" syndrome: Clinical data and suggested pathophysiological mechanism. *Circulation* 1999;99:666–673.
28. Sreeram N, Simmers T, Brockmeier K. The Brugada syndrome. Its relevance to paediatric practice. *Z Kardiol* 2004;93:784–790.
29. Antzelevitch C, Brugada P, Borggrefe M, *et al.* Brugada syndrome: Report of the second consensus conference: Endorsed by the *Heart Rhythm* Society and the European *Heart Rhythm* Association. *Circulation* 2005;111:659–670.
30. Shimizu W. The Brugada syndrome–an update *Intern Med* 2005;44:1224–1231.
31. Weiss R, Barmada MM, Nguyen T, *et al.* Clinical and molecular heterogeneity in the Brugada syndrome: A novel gene locus on chromosome 3. *Circulation* 2002;105:707–713.
32. London B, Sanyal S, Michalec M, *et al.* A mutation in the glycerol-3-phosphate dehydrogenase 1-like gene (GPD1L) causes Brugada syndrome. *Heart Rhythm* 2006;3(Suppl.):S32.
33. Verkerk AO, Wilders R, Schulze-Bahr E, *et al.* Role of sequence variations in the human ether-a-go-go-related gene (HERG, KCNH2) in the Brugada syndrome. *Cardiovasc Res* 2005;68:441–453.
34. Yan GX, Antzelevitch C. Cellular basis for the Brugada syndrome and other mechanisms of arrhythmogenesis associated with ST-segment elevation. *Circulation* 1999;100:1660–1666.
35. Meregalli PG, Wilde AA, Tan HL. Pathophysiological mechanisms of Brugada syndrome: Depolarization disorder, repolarization disorder, or more? *Cardiovasc Res* 2005;67:367–378.
36. Tukkie R, Sogaard P, Vleugels J, *et al.* Delay in right ventricular activation contributes to Brugada syndrome. *Circulation* 2004;109:1272–1277.
37. Smits JP, Eckardt L, Probst V, *et al.* Genotype-phenotype relationship in Brugada syndrome: Electrocardiographic features differentiate SCN5A-related patients from non-SCN5A-related patients. *J Am Coll Cardiol* 2002;40:350–356.
38. Probst V, Allouis M, Sacher F, *et al.* Progressive cardiac conduction defect is the prevailing phenotype in carriers of a Brugada syndrome SCN5A mutation. *J Cardiovasc Electrophysiol* 2006;17: 270–275.
39. Coronel R, Casini S, Koopmann TT, *et al.* Right ventricular fibrosis and conduction delay in a patient with clinical signs of Brugada syndrome: A combined electrophysiological, genetic, histopathologic, and computational study. *Circulation* 2005;112:2769–2777.
40. Frustaci A, Priori SG, Pieroni M, *et al.* Cardiac histological substrate in patients with clinical phenotype of Brugada syndrome. *Circulation* 2005;112:3680–3687.
41. Nademanee K, Veerakul G, Nimmannit S, *et al.* Arrhythmogenic marker for the sudden unexplained death syndrome in Thai men. *Circulation* 1997;96:2595–2600.
42. Vatta M, Dumaine R, Varghese G, *et al.* Genetic and biophysical basis of sudden unexplained nocturnal death syndrome (SUNDS), a disease allelic

to Brugada syndrome. *Hum Mol Genet* 2002;11: 337–345.
43. Tan HL, Hou CJ, Lauer MR, *et al.* Electrophysiologic mechanisms of the long QT interval syndromes and torsade de pointes. *Ann Intern Med* 1995;122:701–714.
44. Splawski I, Shen J, Timothy KW, *et al.* Spectrum of mutations in long-QT syndrome genes. KVLQT1, HERG, SCN5A, KCNE1, and KCNE2. *Circulation* 2000;102:1178–1185.
45. Bennett PB, Yazawa K, Makita N, *et al.* Molecular mechanism for an inherited cardiac arrhythmia. *Nature* 1995;376:683–685.
46. Abriel H, Cabo C, Wehrens XH, *et al.* Novel arrhythmogenic mechanism revealed by a long-QT syndrome mutation in the cardiac Na(+) channel. *Circ Res* 2001;88:740–745.
47. Kambouris NG, Nuss HB, Johns DC, *et al.* Phenotypic characterization of a novel long-QT syndrome mutation (R1623Q) in the cardiac sodium channel. *Circulation* 1998;97:640–644.
48. Rivolta I, Clancy CE, Tateyama M, *et al.* A novel SCN5A mutation associated with long QT-3: Altered inactivation kinetics and channel dysfunction. *Physiol Genomics* 2002;10:191–197.
49. Wedekind H, Smits JP, Schulze-Bahr E, *et al.* De novo mutation in the SCN5A gene associated with early onset of sudden infant death. *Circulation* 2001;104:1158–1164.
50. Priori SG, Napolitano C, Schwartz PJ, *et al.* Association of long QT syndrome loci and cardiac events among patients treated with beta-blockers. *JAMA* 2004;292:1341–1344.
51. Schwartz PJ, Priori SG, Locati EH, *et al.* Long QT syndrome patients with mutations of the SCN5A and HERG genes have differential responses to Na+ channel blockade and to increases in heart rate. Implications for gene-specific therapy. *Circulation* 1995;92:3381–3386.
52. Wang DW, Yazawa K, Makita N, *et al.* Pharmacological targeting of long QT mutant sodium channels. *J Clin Invest* 1997;99:1714–1720.
53. Abriel H, Wehrens XH, Benhorin J, *et al.* Molecular pharmacology of the sodium channel mutation D1790G linked to the long-QT syndrome. *Circulation* 2000;102:921–925.
54. Windle JR, Geletka RC, Moss AJ, *et al.* Normalization of ventricular repolarization with flecainide in long QT syndrome patients with SCN5A:DeltaKPQ mutation. *Ann Noninvasive Electrocardiol* 2001;6:153–158.
55. Priori SG, Napolitano C, Schwartz PJ, *et al.* The elusive link between LQT3 and Brugada syndrome: The role of flecainide challenge. *Circulation* 2000; 102:945–947.
56. Hunt CE, Hauck FR. Sudden infant death syndrome. *Can Med Assoc J* 2006;174:1861–1869.
57. Schwartz PJ, Priori SG, Dumaine R, *et al.* A molecular link between the sudden infant death syndrome and the long-QT syndrome. *N Engl J Med* 2000;343:262–267.
58. Ackerman MJ, Siu BL, Sturner WQ, *et al.* Postmortem molecular analysis of SCN5A defects in sudden infant death syndrome. *JAMA* 2001;286: 2264–2269.
59. Priori SG, Napolitano C, Giordano U, *et al.* Brugada syndrome and sudden cardiac death in children. Lancet 2000;355:808–809.
60. Skinner JR, Chung SK, Montgomery D, *et al.* Near-miss SIDS due to Brugada syndrome. Arch Dis Child 2005;90:528–529.
61. Brink PA, Ferreira A, Moolman JC, *et al.* Gene for progressive familial heart block type I maps to chromosome 19q13. *Circulation* 1995;91:1633–1640.
62. de Meeus A, Stephan E, Debrus S, *et al.* An isolated cardiac conduction disease maps to chromosome 19q. *Circ Res* 1995;77:735–740.
63. Schott JJ, Alshinawi C, Kyndt F, *et al.* Cardiac conduction defects associate with mutations in SCN5A. *Nat Genet* 1999;23:20–21.
64. Bezzina CR, Rook MB, Groenewegen WA, *et al.* Compound heterozygosity for mutations (W156X and R225W) in SCN5A associated with severe cardiac conduction disturbances and degenerative changes in the conduction system. *Circ Res* 2003;92:159–168.
65. Herfst LJ, Potet F, Bezzina CR, *et al.* Na+ channel mutation leading to loss of function and non-progressive cardiac conduction defects. *J Mol Cell Cardiol* 2003;35:549–557.
66. Probst V, Kyndt F, Potet F, *et al.* Haploinsufficiency in combination with aging causes SCN5A-linked hereditary Lenegre disease. *J Am Coll Cardiol* 2003;41:643–652.
67. Wang DW, Viswanathan PC, Balser JR, *et al.* Clinical, genetic, and biophysical characterization of SCN5A mutations associated with atrioventricular conduction block. *Circulation* 2002;105:341–346.
68. Laitinen-Forsblom PJ, Makynen P, Makynen H, *et al.* SCN5A mutation associated with cardiac conduction defect and atrial arrhythmias. *J Cardiovasc Electrophysiol* 2006;17:480–485.
69. Groenewegen WA, Firouzi M, Bezzina CR, *et al.* A cardiac sodium channel mutation cosegregates with a rare connexin40 genotype in familial atrial standstill. *Circ Res* 2003;92:14–22.

70. McNair WP, Ku L, Taylor MR, *et al.* SCN5A mutation associated with dilated cardiomyopathy, conduction disorder, and arrhythmia. *Circulation* 2004;110:2163–2167.
71. Olson TM, Michels VV, Ballew JD, *et al.* Sodium channel mutations and susceptibility to heart failure and atrial fibrillation. *JAMA* 2005;293:447–454.
72. Nakazato Y, Nakata Y, Hisaoka T, *et al.* Clinical and electrophysiological characteristics of atrial standstill. *Pacing Clin Electrophysiol* 1995;18:1244–1254.
73. Makita N, Sasaki K, Groenewegen WA, *et al.* Congenital atrial standstill associated with coinheritance of a novel SCN5A mutation and connexin 40 polymorphisms. *Heart Rhythm* 2005;2:1128–1134.
74. Ueda K, Nakamura K, Hayashi T, *et al.* Functional characterization of a trafficking-defective HCN4 mutation, D553N, associated with cardiac arrhythmia. *J Biol Chem* 2004;279:27194–27198.
75. Schulze-Bahr E, Neu A, Friederich P, *et al.* Pacemaker channel dysfunction in a patient with sinus node disease. *J Clin Invest* 2003;111:1537–1545.
76. Milanesi R, Baruscotti M, Gnecchi-Ruscone T, *et al.* Familial sinus bradycardia associated with a mutation in the cardiac pacemaker channel. *N Engl J Med* 2006;354:151–157.
77. Benson DW, Wang DW, Dyment M, *et al.* Congenital sick sinus syndrome caused by recessive mutations in the cardiac sodium channel gene (SCN5A). *J Clin Invest* 2003;112:1019–1028.
78. Papadatos GA, Wallerstein PM, Head CE, *et al.* Slowed conduction and ventricular tachycardia after targeted disruption of the cardiac sodium channel gene Scn5a. *Proc Natl Acad Sci USA* 2002;99:6210–6215.
79. Royer A, van Veen TA, Le Bouter S, *et al.* Mouse model of SCN5A-linked hereditary Lenegre's disease: Age-related conduction slowing and myocardial fibrosis. *Circulation* 2005;111:1738–1746.
80. van Veen TA, Stein M, Royer A, *et al.* Impaired impulse propagation in Scn5a-knockout mice: Combined contribution of excitability, connexin expression, and tissue architecture in relation to aging. *Circulation* 2005;112:1927–1935.
81. Martini B, Nava A, Thiene G, *et al.* Ventricular fibrillation without apparent heart disease: Description of six cases. *Am Heart J* 1989;118:1203–1209.
82. Corrado D, Nava A, Buja G, *et al.* Familial cardiomyopathy underlies syndrome of right bundle branch block, ST segment elevation and sudden death. *J Am Coll Cardiol* 1996;27:443–448.
83. Corrado D, Basso C, Buja G, *et al.* Right bundle branch block, right precordial ST-segment elevation, and sudden death in young people. *Circulation* 2001;103:710–717.
84. Peters S, Trummel M, Denecke S, *et al.* Results of ajmaline testing in patients with arrhythmogenic right ventricular dysplasia-cardiomyopathy. *Int J Cardiol* 2004;95:207–210.
85. Morimoto S, Uemura A, Hishida H. An autopsy case of Brugada syndrome with significant lesions in the sinus node. *J Cardiovasc Electrophysiol* 2005;16:345–347.
86. Morimoto S, Uemura A, Watanabe E, *et al.* A multicentre histological study of autopsied and biopsied speciments in Brugada syndrome. *Eur Heart J* 2003;24(Suppl.):147.
87. Ahmad F, Li D, Karibe A, *et al.* Localization of a gene responsible for arrhythmogenic right ventricular dysplasia to chromosome 3p23. *Circulation* 1998;98:2791–2795.
88. Perez Riera AR, Antzelevitch C, Schapacknik E, *et al.* Is there an overlap between Brugada syndrome and arrhythmogenic right ventricular cardiomyopathy/dysplasia? *J Electrocardiol* 2005;38:260–263.
89. Olson TM, Keating MT. Mapping a cardiomyopathy locus to chromosome 3p22–p25. *J Clin Invest* 1996;97:528–532.
90. Groenewegen WA, Wilde AA. Letter regarding article by McNair et al, "SCN5A mutation associated with dilated cardiomyopathy, conduction disorder, and arrhythmia". *Circulation* 2005;112:e9; author reply e10.
91. Veldkamp MW, Wilders R, Baartscheer A, *et al.* Contribution of sodium channel mutations to bradycardia and sinus node dysfunction in LQT3 families. *Circ Res* 2003;92:976–983.
92. Rivolta I, Abriel H, Tateyama M, *et al.* Inherited Brugada and long QT-3 syndrome mutations of a single residue of the cardiac sodium channel confer distinct channel and clinical phenotypes. *J Biol Chem* 2001;276:30623–30630.
93. Kyndt F, Probst V, Potet F, *et al.* Novel SCN5A mutation leading either to isolated cardiac conduction defect or Brugada syndrome in a large French family. *Circulation* 2001;104:3081–3086.
94. Grant AO, Carboni MP, Neplioueva V, *et al.* Long QT syndrome, Brugada syndrome, and conduction system disease are linked to a single sodium channel mutation. *J Clin Invest* 2002;110:1201–1209.
95. Smits JP, Koopmann TT, Wilders R, *et al.* A mutation in the human cardiac sodium channel (E161K) contributes to sick sinus syndrome, conduction

disease and Brugada syndrome in two families. *J Mol Cell Cardiol* 2005;38:969–981.
96. Sarkozy A, Brugada P. Sudden cardiac death and inherited arrhythmia syndromes. *J Cardiovasc Electrophysiol* 2005;16(Suppl. 1):S8–20.
97. Di Diego JM, Cordeiro JM, Goodrow RJ, *et al.* Ionic and cellular basis for the predominance of the Brugada syndrome phenotype in males. *Circulation* 2002;106:2004–2011.
98. Verkerk AO, Wilders R, de Geringel W, *et al.* Cellular basis of sex disparities in human cardiac electrophysiology. *Acta Physiol* 2006;187:459–477.
99. Pham TV, Robinson RB, Danilo P Jr, *et al.* Effects of gonadal steroids on gender-related differences in transmural dispersion of L-type calcium current. *Cardiovasc Res* 2002;53:752–762.
100. Matsuo K, Akahoshi M, Seto S, *et al.* Disappearance of the Brugada-type electrocardiogram after surgical castration: A role for testosterone and an explanation for the male preponderance. *Pacing Clin Electrophysiol* 2003;26:1551–1553.
101. Ye B, Valdivia CR, Ackerman MJ, *et al.* A common human SCN5A polymorphism modifies expression of an arrhythmia causing mutation. *Physiol Genomics* 2003;12:187–193.
102. Chen S, Chung MK, Martin D, *et al.* SNP S1103Y in the cardiac sodium channel gene SCN5A is associated with cardiac arrhythmias and sudden death in a white family. *J Med Genet* 2002;39:913–915.
103. Shimizu W. Acquired forms of the Brugada syndrome. *J Electrocardiol* 2005;38:22–25.
104. Makita N, Horie M, Nakamura T, *et al.* Drug-induced long-QT syndrome associated with a subclinical SCN5A mutation. *Circulation* 2002;106:1269–1274.
105. Undrovinas AI, Maltsev VA, Sabbah HN. Repolarization abnormalities in cardiomyocytes of dogs with chronic heart failure: Role of sustained inward current. *Cell Mol Life Sci* 1999;55:494–505.
106. Valdivia CR, Chu WW, Pu J, *et al.* Increased late sodium current in myocytes from a canine heart failure model and from failing human heart. *J Mol Cell Cardiol* 2005;38:475–483.
107. Maltsev VA, Sabbab HN, Undrovinas AI. Down-regulation of sodium current in chronic heart failure: Effect of long-term therapy with carvedilol. *Cell Mol Life Sci* 2002;59:1561–1568.
108. Zicha S, Maltsev VA, Nattel S, *et al.* Post-transcriptional alterations in the expression of cardiac Na+ channel subunits in chronic heart failure. *J Mol Cell Cardiol* 2004;37:91–100.
109. Wiegerinck RF, Verkerk AO, Belterman CN, *et al.* Larger cell size in rabbits with heart failure increases myocardial conduction velocity and QRS duration. *Circulation* 2006;113:806–813.
110. Kaab S, Nuss HB, Chiamvimonvat N, *et al.* Ionic mechanism of action potential prolongation in ventricular myocytes from dogs with pacing-induced heart failure. *Circ Res* 1996;78:262–273.
111. Carmeliet E. Cardiac ionic currents and acute ischemia: From channels to arrhythmias. *Physiol Rev* 1999;79:917–1017.
112. Kimura S, Bassett AL, Furukawa T, *et al.* Electrophysiological properties and responses to simulated ischemia in cat ventricular myocytes of endocardial and epicardial origin. *Circ Res* 1990;66:469–477.
113. Pogwizd SM, Corr PB. Reentrant and nonreentrant mechanisms contribute to arrhythmogenesis during early myocardial ischemia: Results using three-dimensional mapping. *Circ Res* 1987;61:352–371.
114. Pu J, Boyden PA. Alterations of Na+ currents in myocytes from epicardial border zone of the infarcted heart. A possible ionic mechanism for reduced excitability and postrepolarization refractoriness. *Circ Res* 1997;81:110–119.
115. Lue WM, Boyden PA. Abnormal electrical properties of myocytes from chronically infarcted canine heart. Alterations in Vmax and the transient outward current. *Circulation* 1992;85:1175–1188.
116. Patterson E, Scherlag BJ, Lazzara R. Rapid inward current in ischemically-injured subepicardial myocytes bordering myocardial infarction. *J Cardiovasc Electrophysiol* 1993;4:9–22.
117. Pu J, Balser JR, Boyden PA. Lidocaine action on Na+ currents in ventricular myocytes from the epicardial border zone of the infarcted heart. *Circ Res* 1998;83:431–440.
118. Echt DS, Liebson PR, Mitchell LB, *et al.* Mortality and morbidity in patients receiving encainide, flecainide, or placebo. The Cardiac Arrhythmia Suppression Trial. *N Engl J Med* 1991;324:781–788.
119. Huang B, El-Sherif T, Gidh-Jain M, *et al.* Alterations of sodium channel kinetics and gene expression in the postinfarction remodeled myocardium. *J Cardiovasc Electrophysiol* 2001;12:218–225.
120. Baetz D, Bernard M, Pinet C, *et al.* Different pathways for sodium entry in cardiac cells during ischemia and early reperfusion. *Mol Cell Biochem* 2003;242:115–120.

121. Ju YK, Saint DA, Gage PW. Hypoxia increases persistent sodium current in rat ventricular myocytes. *J Physiol* 1996;497(Pt. 2):337–347.
122. Wu J, Corr PB. Palmitoyl carnitine modifies sodium currents and induces transient inward current in ventricular myocytes. *Am J Physiol* 1994;266:H1034–1046.
123. Undrovinas AI, Fleidervish IA, Makielski JC. Inward sodium current at resting potentials in single cardiac myocytes induced by the ischemic metabolite lysophosphatidylcholine. *Circ Res* 1992;71:1231–1241.
124. Ward CA, Giles WR. Ionic mechanism of the effects of hydrogen peroxide in rat ventricular myocytes. *J Physiol* 1997;500(Pt. 3):631–642.
125. Pogwizd SM, Bers DM. Cellular basis of triggered arrhythmias in heart failure. *Trends Cardiovasc Med* 2004;14:61–66.
126. Belardinelli L, Shryock JC, Fraser H. Inhibition of the late sodium current as a potential cardioprotective principle: Effects of the late sodium current inhibitor ranolazine. *Heart* 2006;92:6–14.
127. Undrovinas AI, Belardinelli L, Undrovinas NA, *et al.* Ranolazine improves abnormal repolarization and contraction in left ventricular myocytes of dogs with heart failure by inhibiting late sodium current. *J Cardiovasc Electrophysiol* 2006;17(Suppl. 1):S169–S177.

10
L-Type Calcium Channel Disease

Yanfei Ruan, Raffaella Bloise, Carlo Napolitano, and Silvia G. Priori

Introduction

In recent years, the progress of molecular genetics of inherited arrhythmogenic diseases portrays an unexpected complexity of clinical phenotypes associated with mutations in several genes that control cardiac excitability. Among the most recent findings, the voltage-gated L-type cardiac calcium channel (Cav1.2) has been involved in the pathogenesis of Timothy syndrome (TS). TS is a variant of the long QT syndrome (also LQT8) and it is a rare and severe genetic disorder characterized by a spectrum of complex phenotypes including QT interval prolongation, congenital heart defects, syndactyly, and distinctive dysmorphic features. So far TS is the only inherited arrhythmogenic disorder linked to cardiac calcium channel mutations. In this chapter, we will briefly review the structure, physiology, and pathophysiology of the cardiac Cav1.2 encoded by the *CACNA1c* gene.

L-Type Calcium Channel

Structure of the Cardiac Cav1.2 Channel

Cav1.2 constitutes the pore-forming protein (α_1 subunit) responsible for the voltage-dependent L-type Ca^{2+} channel in the heart. However, the channel may be considered as a macromolecular complex, made up of α_1, α_2/δ, and β subunits. The α_1 subunit is a protein of about 2000 amino acidic residues and consists of four homologous domains (I–IV), each one formed by transmembrane spanning segments (S1–S6), and a membrane-associated loop between S5 and S6[1] (Figure 10–1). The α_1 subunit forms the ion-selective pore, the voltage sensor, the gating machinery, and the binding sites for channel-modulating drugs. The positively charged S4 of each domain serves as the voltage sensors for channel activation. It is thought that the S4 moves outward and rotates under the influence of the electric field so as to induce a conformational change that opens the pore.[2] The pore-conducting calcium ions are composed of S5 and S6 and the loop between them. The pore is asymmetric: the outside pore is constructed by the pore loop, which contains highly conserved glutamate residues (EEEE) for calcium ion selectivity.[3] The inside pore is composed of the S6 segments, which include the receptor sites for L-type Ca^{2+} channel antagonist drugs.[1]

The β, α_2, and δ subunits appear to have a regulatory effect. Interestingly, the α_2 and δ subunits are encoded by a single gene that is translated as a precursor polypeptide and is posttranslationally cleaved into the two subunits. The transmembrane δ subunit anchors the α_2 protein to the membrane via a single putative transmembrane segment. This association is mediated by disulfide bridges. A range of functional effects has been identified for the associated subunits, especially the β subunit, including ligand binding, increasing peak currents, and modulation of activation and inactivation (increasing the rate of both voltage and Ca^{2+}-dependent inactivation) rates.[4,5]

Calcium Channel Function

Cav1.2 is the major calcium channel expressed in the ventricular myocytes. It produces a voltage-dependent inward Ca^{2+} current (I_{Ca}) that activates

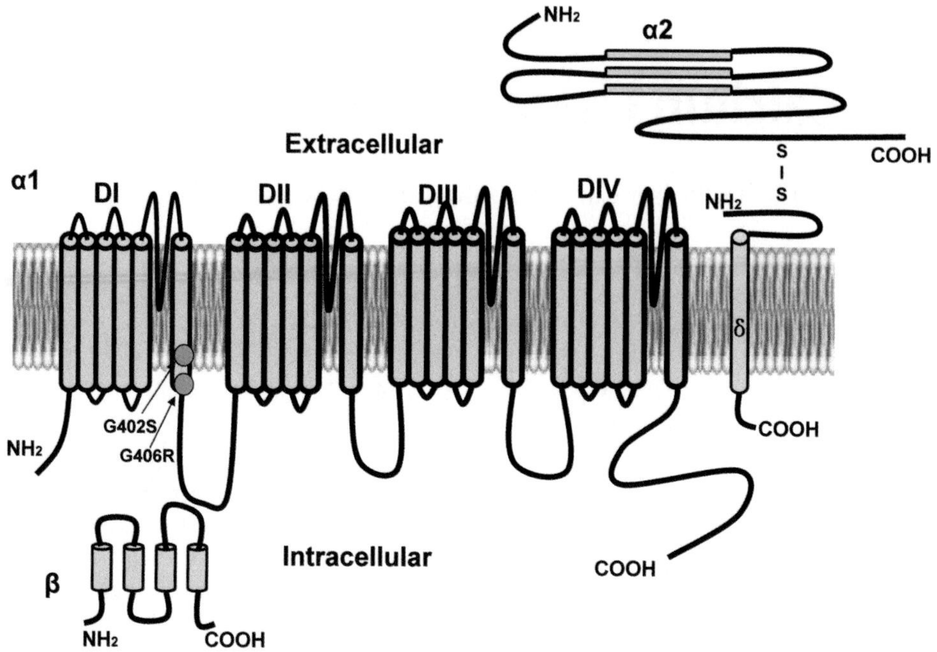

FIGURE 10–1. Predicted topology of Cav1.2, showing the location of the mutations. (From Splawski *et al.*[15])

upon depolarization and it is a crucial player in the maintenance of the plateau of the cardiac action potential; thus I_{Ca} modulation can greatly affect the action potential duration. Furthermore, Ca^{2+} ions play an important role in excitation–contraction coupling, since I_{Ca} triggers the release of the calcium ion from the sarcoplasmic reticulum and thereby elevates cytoplasmic Ca^{2+} to initiate contraction. Overall, any perturbation of this channel has a great potential of inducing an arrhythmogenic substrate.

Regulation and Tissue Distribution of the Cardiac Cav1.2 Channel

Besides voltage, many factors are important for regulation of cardiac Cav1.2 channel. Protein kinase A (PKA), protein kinase C (PKC), and Ca^{2+}-binding protein calmodulin constitute a key mechanism for controlling Ca^{2+} influx.[6–9] Furthermore, Cav1.2 channel activity is also enhanced by calcium, catecholamine[10] and Ca^{2+}-calmodulin-dependent protein kinase II (CaMKII).[11,12] This latter interaction appears to have an important role for Timothy syndrome pathogenesis (see below).

Cav1.2 protein is expressed in several tissues including heart, the peripheral and central nervous system, liver, testis, spleen, connective tissue, and bone marrow. (see details at: http://www.ncbi.nlm.nih.gov/UniGene/ESTProfileViewer.cgi?uglist=Hs.372570). On the basis of such widespread tissue distribution it is conceivable that mutations in this gene may perturb the function of several organs.

Furthermore, it must be emphasized that the *CACNA1c* gene (the gene encoding for Cav1.2) undergoes extensive alternative splicing, producing splice variants with distinct electrophysiological and pharmacological properties.[13] Cell-selective expression of Cav1.2 channels containing a specific alternatively spliced exon increases the functional variations for specific cellular activities in response to changing physiological signals.

Although the control pathways of such alternative splicing are unknown, this evidence highlights the complexity of regulation of the calcium current and it emphasizes the difficulty in predicting the clinical manifestation of mutants Cav1.2 proteins. This concept is well confirmed by the recent genetic findings linking Cav1.2 mutations to a severe inherited arrhythmogenic disease, the Timothy syndrome,[14,15] which will be described below.

Timothy Syndrome

Historical Notes

Until recently only anecdotal reports of QT interval prolongation, arrhythmias, and syndactyly were given in the literature. In 1992, Reichenbach reported and defined it as a novel clinical entity, a case of a male infant born at week 36 of gestation by cesarean section (because of intrauterine bradycardia) who died suddenly at age 5 months. Second degree atrioventricular (AV) block, QT interval prolongation and syndactyly were observed.[16] Subsequently Marks *et al.* reported additional three cases of long QT syndrome (LQTS) and syndactyly,[17] confirming the typical features of this disorder.

The first systematic description of the disease was jointly reported in a collaborative study by the group of Mark Keating and our group. In this study we described 13 cases of this distinctive form of LQTS, presenting with a complex disorder (Figure 10–2) (see below) with multiorgan involvement and defined the disease as Timothy syndrome (MIM:601005).[14]

Phenotype and Natural History of Timothy Syndrome

The initial clinical abnormalities of TS may manifest during gestation with bradycardia and 2:1 AV block, but diagnosis is often made within the first few days of life due to abnormal ventricular repolarization and soft tissue syndactyly of hands and toes. With few exceptions (possibly related to a different genetic substrate, see below), syndactyly has been observed in the majority of cases.

The QT interval is markedly prolonged in TS (mean value 600 msec); such extreme QT prolongation often causes 2:1 functional AV block. Remarkable abnormalities of T-wave morphology consisting of long and straight ST segment, negative T-wave, and macroscopic T-wave alternans are also evident.

The most frightful manifestations of the disease are represented by cardiac tachyarrhythmia [ventricular tachycardia (VT) or ventricular fibrillation (VF)], which occurs in 79% of patients and is the most frequent cause of mortality (Figure 10–3). Ten of the 17 patients described in the past decade died at a mean age of 2.5 years. In 12 of 17 patients life-threatening ventricular arrhythmias have been documented. The most severe variant of LQTS is probably TS.

Several additional pathological (cardiac and extracardiac) phenotypes contribute to the TS phenotype:

1. Congenital heart disease (patent ductus arteriosus, ventricular septal defect, patent foramen ovalis, Tetralogy of Fallot) (55% of cases).
2. Hypertrophic cardiomyopathy,[18] cardiomegaly, and ventricular systolic dysfunction (30% of cases).
3. Facial dysmorphisms (91% of cases).
4. Predisposition to sepsis (50% of cases).
5. Metabolic (severe hypoglycemia) and immunological (recurrent infections) disturbances (40% of cases).
6. Neuropsychiatric involvement (autism, seizures, psychological developmental delays) (83%).

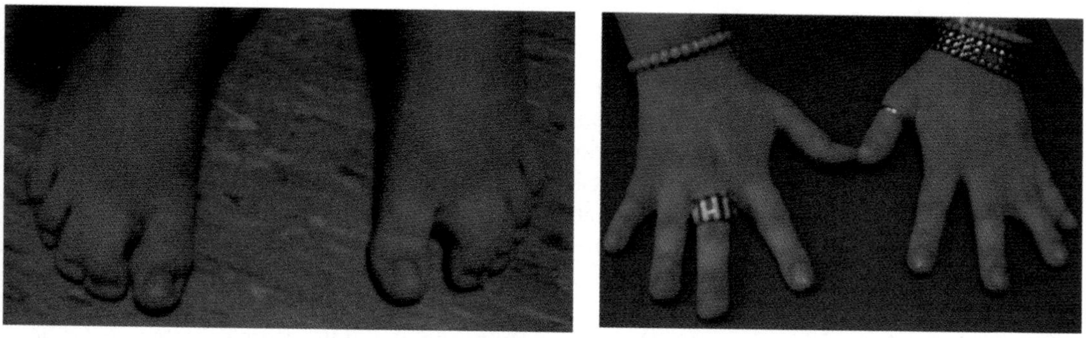

FIGURE 10–2. Syndactyly of feet (left panel) and hands (right panel) in patients with TS.

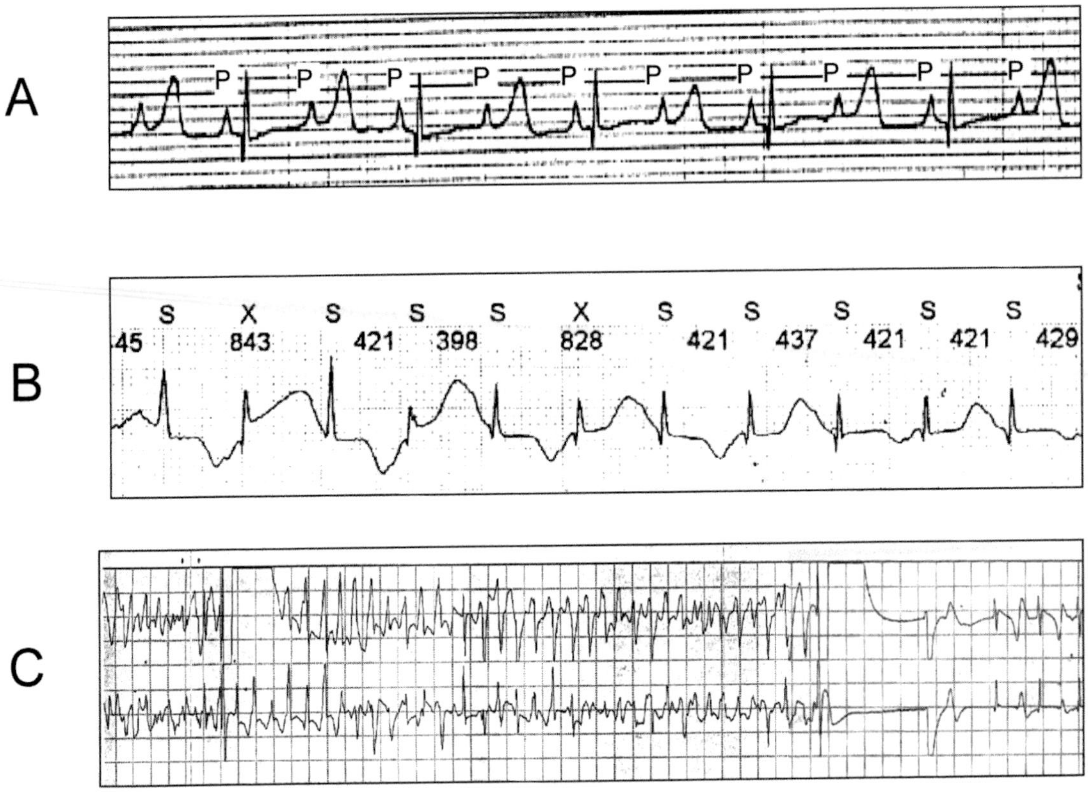

FIGURE 10–3. ECG recording in a TS patient. (A) Long QT and 2:1 atrioventricular block. (B) T-wave alternans. (C) Ventricular fibrillation.

Genetics of Timothy Syndrome

The ST-T wave morphology in TS patients resembles that of LQTS patients with sodium channel mutations (LQT3, see Chapter 11), suggesting the involvement of an inward current active during the plateau phase of the cardiac action potential. However, the screening of the *SCN5A* gene (as well as that of the other known LQTS genes) was negative. Thus the *CACNA1c* gene (encoding for Cav1.2) was considered a plausible candidate. In 2004, Splawski *et al.* identified the G1216A transition in exon 8A (an alternatively spliced exon), which caused the G406R amino acid transition in DI/S6 in TS patients.[14] Subsequently, Splawski *et al.* reported two individuals with a severe variant of TS but without syndactyly, which they named TS2.[15] Genetic analyses show G1216A and G1204A in exon 8, which caused a G406R and G402S amino acid transition, respectively (Figure 10–1).

By means of immunostaining experiments it was shown that exon 8A is expressed in the central nervous system, including hippocampus, cerebellum, and amygdala. Abnormalities of these brain regions have been implicated in autism, a typical feature of TS. Thus, TS may represent the first evidence for a genetic predisposition to behavioral disorders. Interestingly, the clinical relevance of transmembrane Ca^{2+} current alterations and behavioral abnormalities has been further supported by the association between allelic variants in the *CACNA1h* gene (Cav3.2, T-type calcium channel) in patients with autism spectrum disorder.[19] Although not directly related to TS pathogenesis these data strengthen the concept that Ca^{2+} dysfunction may be involved in severe neuropsychological disorders and indirectly the direct pathogenetic role of Cav1.2 in autism.

Exon 8A of *CACNA1c* is also expressed throughout the heart and the vascular system in developing digits and teeth. Thus, the expression pattern of exon 8A is consistent with the phenotypic abnormalities associated with TS.[14]

Exons 8 and 8A are mutually exclusive as they encode the same structural domain (DI/S6), but one of the two must be present to encode a functional channel. In the human heart it has been experimentally shown that 22.8% of Cav1.2 proteins contain exon 8A and 77.2% contain exon 8. In the brain, 23.2% contain exon 8A and 76.8% contain exon 8. Compared to exon 8A, exon 8 is very highly expressed in the heart and brain. Consistent with the expression, TS2 patients having a mutation in exon 8 appear to have a longer QTc than TS1, and a more severe pattern of arrhythmias. Interestingly, the TS2 patients reported so far do not show syndactyly, possibly because of the differential expression of exons 8 and 8A.[15]

Familial recurrence of the TS phenotype is rare. Indeed, the disease results from *de novo* mutation in most of the probands. Parent-to-offspring transmission of the phenotype has never been reported, probably because the high rate of malignancy associated with the disease prevents the majority of affected patients from reaching reproductive age. Familial recurrence in the offspring of normal parents has been reported in only three families and it was attributed to mosaicism. The evidence that a normal couple with no previous family history of TS may have children affected by this severe disease has a relevant impact for genetic counseling of TS patients/families.

Mechanism of Arrhythmogenesis

In the experiment of Splawski *et al.*,[14] the current–voltage (I/V) relationship and voltage dependence of activation were similar for wild-type (WT) and mutant channels. The difference between WT and G406R channels was the extent of inactivation. Inactivation of WT channel current was nearly complete in 300 msec, while G406R channels were only slightly inactivated during the same time frame. In the voltage dependence of inactivation curves, WT channel inactivation was complete at +20 mV. In contrast, inactivation was only 56% for the G406R channels (Figure 10–4). Thus, the likely mechanism of G406R mutation was assumed to be an increase of inward I_{Ca} due to loss of voltage-dependent inactivation.[14] The altered L-type calcium channel inactivation caused by the mutations was also simulated in a dynamic model of a human ventricular myocyte.[15] This model confirmed that the action potential is significantly prolonged as a consequence of this TS mutation and suggested that delayed afterdepolarizations and triggered activity are the final mechanisms for the onset of arrhythmias.

Recently Erxleben C *et al.* proposed a more complex model to explain the cellular phenotype

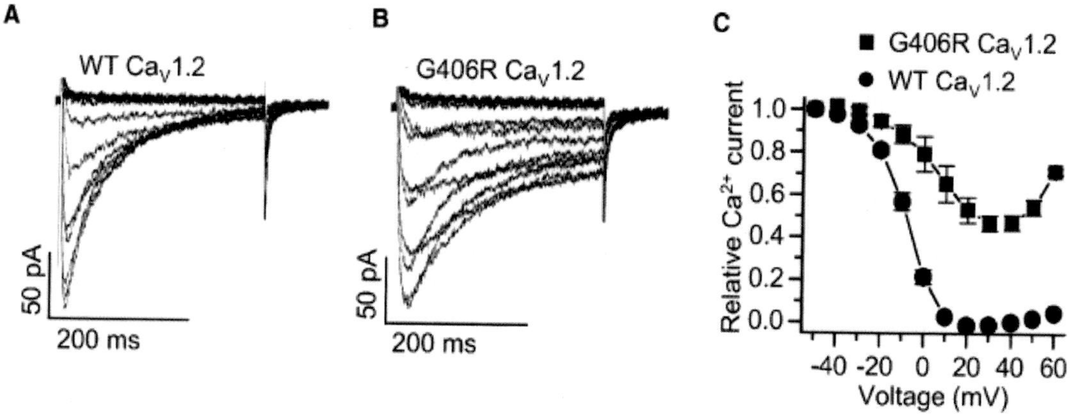

FIGURE 10–4. Wild-type (A) and G406R (B) Cav1.2 channel currents recorded from CHO cells in response to voltage pulses applied in 10 mV increments from −40 to +60 mV. (C) Voltage dependence of Ca^{2+} current inactivation for WT and G406R channels. (From Splawski *et al.*[14]).

caused by the G406R mutation.[20] By means of single channel recordings, they observed a decrease in unitary channel conductance and an increase in spontaneous "mode 2 gating" (which is characterized by increased open probability and longer channel activations). Such mode 2 gating could produce the apparent loss of macroscopic current inactivation at the whole cell level.

They further explored the role of G436R mutation (the rabbit homolog for human TS mutation G406R) on Cav1.2 channel phosphorylation. The presence of the TS mutation in rabbit Cav1.2 makes the protein much more sensitive to CaMKII (Ca^{2+}-calmodulin-dependent protein kinase II) and the channel is less easily dephosphorylated. Thus, the mutation is likely to be a kind of hyperphosphorylated state that in addition to the above-mentioned electrophysiological effect can also create a cytotoxic effect due to chronic intracellular calcium overload.

Therapy for Timothy Syndrome

As pointed out previously, ventricular tachyarrhythmias (VT or VF) are the leading cause of death in TS. At present, most TS patients have been treated with β-blockers, since it is considered a generally effective therapy in patients with congenital long QT syndromes. However, no data are available concerning the effectiveness of this approach in the TS subgroup. Additional pharmacological therapies (mexiletine, calcium channel blockers) have been proposed in an attempt to shorten ventricular repolarization, restore 1:1 conduction, and reduce the risk of arrhythmias, but their use still has to be considered in a experimental evaluation phase. Therefore an implantable cardioverter defibrillator (ICD) is the most important tool to prevent sudden cardiac death in TS patients. The implant should be considered in all patients with confirmed diagnosis as soon as body weight allows the procedure.

Although prevention of cardiac arrhythmia is the primary goal of therapy, it is very important to note that TS patient may die of other causes. (1) Severe infections, probably the consequence of altered immune responses, are frequent in TS patients, and deaths have been reported despite aggressive antibiotic therapy. (2) Intractable hypoglycemia has also been reported as a cause of death. A close monitoring of glucose levels, especially in patients treated with β-blockers, is required since these drugs may mask hypoglycemic symptoms.

Finally, it is important keep in mind that severe ventricular arrhythmias have been reported in TS patients during induction of anesthesia: whether the increased susceptibility to arrhythmias is a nonspecific response related to adrenergic activation or is the consequence of the specific pharmacological activity of the drugs used is currently unknown.

Conclusion

Timothy syndrome is a genetic channelopathy with a complex clinical presentation. Mutations in Cav1.2 cause LQTS associated with dysfunction in multiple organ systems, including congenital heart disease, syndactyly, immune deficiency, hypoglycemia, and autism. Impaired gating caused by mutation is supposed to be the underlying mechanism. An implantable cardioverter defibrillator and β-blockers are the recommended treatments.

References

1. Catterall WA. Structure and regulation of voltage-gated Ca^{2+} channels. *Annu Rev Cell Dev Biol* 2000;16: 521–555.
2. Bezanilla F. Voltage sensor movements. *J Gen Physiol* 2002;120:465–473.
3. Klockner U, Mikala G, Schwartz A, *et al.* Molecular studies of the asymmetric pore structure of the human cardiac voltage-dependent Ca^{2+} channel. Conserved residue, Glu-1086, regulates proton-dependent ion permeation. *J Biol Chem* 1996;271: 22293–22296.
4. Hanlon MR, Wallace BA. Structure and function of voltage-dependent ion channel regulatory β subunits. *Biochemistry* 2002;41:2886–2894.
5. Klugbauer N, Marais E, Hofmann F. Calcium channel a2d subunits: Differential expression, function, and drug binding. *J Bioenerg Biomembr* 2003;35: 639–647.
6. De Jongh KS, Murphy BJ, Colvin AA, *et al.* Specific phosphorylation of a site in the full-length form of the alpha 1 subunit of the cardiac L-type calcium

channel by adenosine 3',5'-cyclic monophosphate-dependent protein kinase. *Biochemistry* 1996;35: 10392–10402.
7. Lacerda AE, Rampe D, Brown AM. Effects of protein kinase C activators on cardiac Ca^{2+} channels. *Nature* 1988;335:249–251.
8. Qin N, Olcese R, Bransby M, *et al.* Ca^{2+}-induced inhibition of the cardiac Ca^{2+} channel depends on calmodulin. *Proc Natl Acad Sci USA* 1999;96:2435–2438.
9. Zuhlke RD, Pitt GS, Deisseroth K, *et al.* Calmodulin supports both inactivation and facilitation of L-type calcium channels. *Nature* 1999;399:159–162.
10. Van der Heyden MA, Wijnhoven TJ, Opthof T. Molecular aspects of adrenergic modulation of cardiac L-type Ca^{2+} channels. *Cardiovasc Res* 2005; 65:28–39.
11. Gurney AM, Charnet P, Pye JM, *et al.* Augmentation of cardiac calcium current by flash photolysis of intracellular caged-Ca^{2+} molecules. *Nature* 1989; 341:65–68.
12. Dzhura I, Wu Y, Colbran RJ, *et al.* Calmodulin kinase determines calcium-dependent facilitation of L-type calcium channels. *Nat Cell Biol* 2000;2: 173–177.
13. Liao P, Yong TF, Liang MC, *et al.* Splicing for alternative structures of Cav1.2 Ca^{2+} channels in cardiac and smooth muscles. *Cardiovasc Res* 2005;68:197–203.
14. Splawski I, Timothy KW, Sharpe LM, *et al.* Cav1.2 calcium channel dysfunction causes a multisystem disorder including arrhythmia and autism. *Cell* 2004;119:19–31.
15. Splawski I, Timothy KW, Decher N, *et al.* Severe arrhythmia disorder caused by cardiac L-type calcium channel mutations. *Proc Natl Acad Sci USA* 2005;102:8089–8096.
16. Reichenbach H, Meister EM, Theile H. The heart-hand syndrome. A new variant of disorders of heart conduction and syndactylia including osseous changes in hands and feet. *Kinderarztl Prax* 1992; 60:54–56.
17. Marks ML, Whisler SL, Clericuzio C, et al. A new form of long QT syndrome associated with syndactyly. *J Am Coll Cardiol* 1995;25:59–64.
18. Lo-A-Njoe SM, Wilde AA, van Erven L, *et al.* Syndactyly and long QT syndrome (Cav1.2 missense mutation G406R) is associated with hyperotrophic cardiomyopathy. *Heart Rhythm* 2005;2: 1365–1368.
19. Splawski I, Yoo DS, Stotz SC, *et al.* CACNA1H mutations in autism spectrum disorders. *J Biol Chem* 2006;281(31):22085–22091.
20. Erxleben C, Liao Y, Gentile S, *et al.* Cyclosporin and Timothy syndrome increase mode 2 gating of Cav1.2 calcium channels through aberrant phosphorylation of S6 helices. *Proc Natl Acad Sci USA* 2006;103:3932–3937.

11
K$^+$ Channelopathies (I_{Ks} and I_{Kr})

Nicolas Lindegger and Robert S. Kass

Ion Channels

Ion channels are pore-forming proteins that cross the lipid membrane of cells and selectively conduct ions across this hermetic wall. Ion channels are responsible for the generation of electrical signals in most tissues and thus are involved in every heart beat, every perception, every thought, etc. Opening of ion channels allows ions to move along their electrochemical gradient thus either depolarizing the membrane or repolarizing it and creating electrical patterns such as the action potential (see Chapter 9 and Figure 11–1).

Before 1982, the understanding of cellular excitation was limited to model systems and the work of Hodgkin, Huxley, and Cole, who first described the ionic basis of the electrical activity in the giant squid axon.[1–4] Similar electrical activity in mammalian heart cells was found, but its human physiology remained indirect.[5] The first cloning of the α subunit of the acetylcholine receptor in 1982 marked the beginning of a new era in which molecular tools allowed the discovery of many physiologically crucial channels.[6,7] In combination with the development of electrophysiology, detailed functional properties of channels were described, especially when these were expressed in cells with minimal electrical activity.[8,9]

The crystal structure of a bacterial potassium channel was solved in 1988, revealing at the atomic level the structural basis of the fundamental mechanism of this class of ion channels.[10] It rapidly became clear how channels open and close, how ion selectivity was based on the channel structure, and how changes in transmembrane voltage were sensed by proteins, thus controlling the open and closed conformational states.[11]

Channels + Pathology = Channelopathy

While the investigation of ion channel structures bridges the biophysical properties of channels, the link to human disease came from clinical investigations of congenital disorders and the discoveries that defects in gene coding for ion channels (α) or their regulatory subunits (β) cause diverse pathological states. The number of diseases linked to these mutations is so large that the term "channelopathy" has been introduced to define this class of diseases.

Acquired or Inherited

Channelopathies are commonly divided into two primary clinical categories: inherited and acquired. The inherited form involves the mutation of an ion channel and its transmission to the family descendants. The Romano–Ward syndrome, for example, is an autosomal-dominant form of the long QT syndrome (LQTS) that involves a large collection of ion channel mutants, including K$^+$ channels, which will be discussed bellow.[12] The acquired form of channelopathies, in addition to the mutation, generally results from pharmacological intervention, often for the purpose of treating unrelated disorders. Among others, antihistaminics, antipsychotics, antibiotics, and

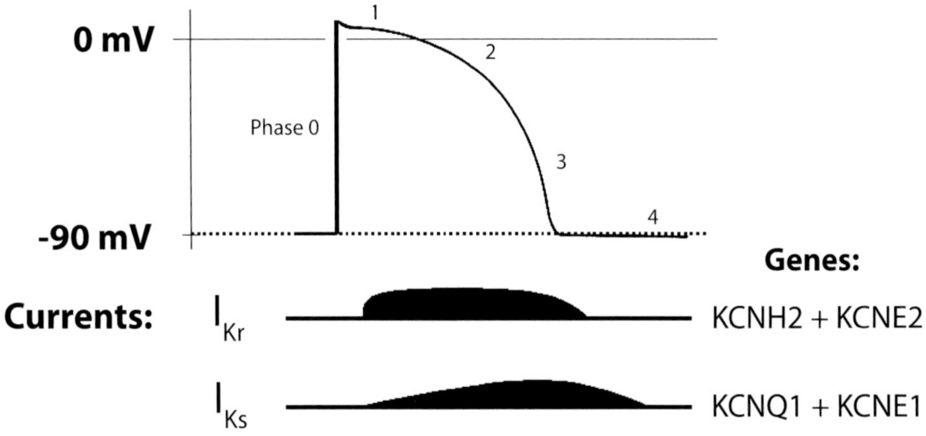

FIGURE 11–1. I_{Kr}, and I_{Ks}, their respective genes, and their role in the repolarization of the ventricular action potential (phases 2 to 4).

certain antiarrhythmics can predispose patients to lethal arrhythmias by blocking the rapidly activating component of the delayed rectifier K^+ current (I_{Kr}) (see bellow).[13]

K^+ Channelopathies

This chapter will now focus on two voltage-gated K^+ channels involved in the generation of the slowly and the rapidly activating component of the delayed rectifier K^+ current, I_{Ks} and I_{Kr}, respectively. Whether the pore subunit is affected or its accessory subunit, all mutations affecting the channel ion conductance lead to the generation of either prolonged or shortened action potentials, as the delicate balance of currents involved in its generation is affected (see Chapter 9 and Figure 11–1). Such alterations have been shown to trigger cardiac arrhythmias and even lead to unfortunate sudden death.

Historically, pathologies due to ion channel mutations were described many years before an actual understanding of the electrical issues involved was available. The Romano–Ward and the Jervell and Lange–Nielsen syndromes, both congenital LQTSs, were first described from a purely clinical point of view in 1964–1965 and 1957, respectively.[14,15] But it was only many years later that the link between K^+ channels and the failing action potential repolarization was made.[16,17] Due to these reports and in conjunction with the functional and structural knowledge of K^+ channels, people started to understand why certain drugs ironically used to prevent cardiac arrhythmia could induce similar disorders.[13,18] In a similar manner and very recently, the same K^+ channels were found to be involved in familial atrial fibrillation and the short QT syndrome.[19] Involvement of K^+ channels and their respective currents I_{Kr} and I_{Ks} in channelopathies such as LQTS or short QT syndrome (SQTS) could be done only with an understanding of normal channels. We will thus discuss bellow the normal structural and biophysical characteristics of the channels responsible for the generation of I_{Kr} and I_{Ks}.

Voltage-Gated K^+ Channels

The great functional diversity among voltage-gated K^+ channels can be classified in two broad classes. At least two types of transient outward currents ($I_{to,f}$ and $I_{to,s}$) and several delayed-rectifying current (I_{Kr}, I_{Ks}, and I_{Kur}) have been identified. Although functional diversity is so vast, isolated currents from voltage-gated K^+ channels (I_K) in different species and in different regions in the heart are very similar, suggesting that similar molecular entities contribute to each I_K in different species or cardiac regions. In addition, the expression heterogeneity accounts for the important action potential waveform regional differences, as seen between the epicardium and the endocardium ventricular walls.[20]

Molecular Determinants of Voltage-Gated K^+ Channels

Most of what is known about the biophysical basis of voltage-gated K^+ channel gating is derived from studies of Shaker (Kv1.1) channels. The crystal structures of bacterial and mammalian K^+ channels were solved by the group of Rod MacKinnon.[21] Voltage-gated K^+ channels are usually composed of two subunits: the α subunits are the pore-forming subunits that carry voltage-gated properties (see Figure 11–2A); and the β subunits are accessory subunits that affect the channel-gating properties. This was observed when α and β subunits were coexpressed in cultured human embryonic kidney cells (HEK 293), a heterologous expression system that has almost no background currents but the one investigated.

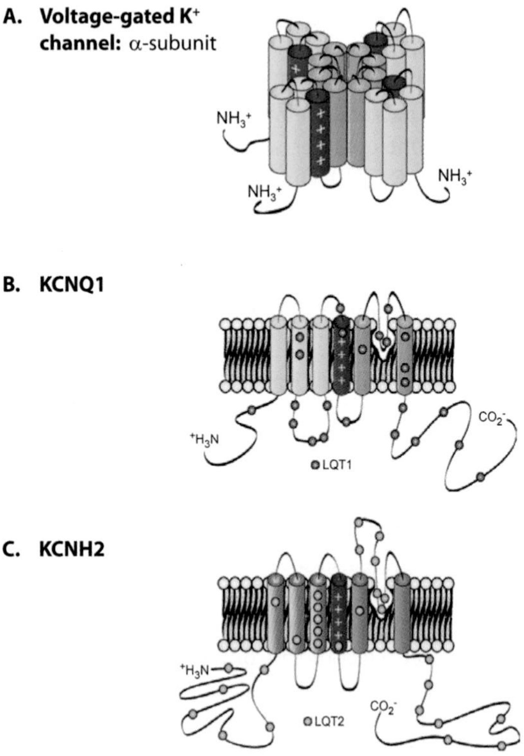

FIGURE 11–2. Molecular topologies of voltage-gated K^+ channels. (A) Functional homotetrameric α subunit complex. (B) KCNQ1 responsible for I_{Ks}. (C) KCNH2 responsible for I_{Kr}. Circles represent known mutations that cause either LQT1 or LQT2 (B and C).

The α subunits belong to the "S4" superfamily of voltage-gated channels.[22] They are composed of six transmembrane spans (S1–S6) and functional voltage-gated K^+ channels are composed of four α subunits with a central ion-conducting pore (see Figure 11–2B and C). Like all voltage-gated channels, the pore loop located between S5 and S6 in each domain is though to be involved in channel selectivity. Similarly, the S4 span has a highly conserved stretch where every third amino acid is positively charged and serves as the membrane potential sensor.[23,24] Nine subfamilies of α subunits have been identified, where Kv1–Kv4 reveal functional voltage-gated K^+ channels and Kv5–Kv9 are electrically silent. Nevertheless "silent" voltage-gated K^+ channel α subunits may affect functionality, since it was shown that functional diversity arises through alternate splicing of transcripts[25] as well as through formation of heteromultimers.[26,27] The voltage-gated K^+ channels accessory subunits protein sequence is not as conserved as it is for α subunits. There are small 130-amino-acid-long single transmembrane spans, as is the case for MinK and MiRP1, a 574-amino-acid-long KChAP with no transmembrane domains, Kvβ1, 2, and 3, which share similar COOH- and NH_2-terminal domains with specific enzymatic activity, and finally KChIP2, which belongs to the recoverin family of neuronal Ca^{2+}-sensing proteins.

Localization

Delayed-rectifying currents were first described in sheep Purkinje fibers,[28,29] and following characterization were made in atrial and ventricular cells as well as in pacemaker cells from various species.[20]

The two prominent components first described in atrial and ventricular guinea pig myocytes based on their differences in time- and voltage-dependent properties were I_{Ks} ($I_{K,slow}$) and I_{Kr} ($I_{K,rapid}$).[30–32] I_{Kr} is known to activate rapidly and inactivate even faster. In addition, I_{Kr} displays a marked inward rectification that is ion conduction favored inwardly. However, I_{Ks} does not display any inward rectification and activates slowly.[31,32] These currents can be found in human atrial and ventricular myocytes, in canine and rabbit ventricular cells, and in canine Purkinje fibers.[20] In rodent ventricles the current densities are very low or even undetectable.[33]

Other specific components of I_K were detected in various species such as in rats (I_K, I_{Klate}, I_{ss}) or in mice (I_{Kslow1}, I_{Kslow2}, and I_{ss} for steady state). In addition, a very rapidly activating and noninactivating outward I_K, referred to as I_{KUR} (for ultrarapid), was described in rat, canine, and human atrial myocytes, but not in human ventricular myocytes or in Purkinje fibers.[20,34]

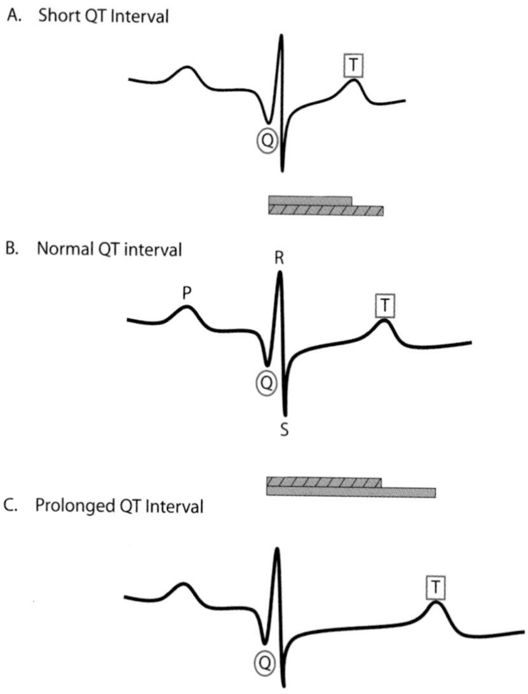

FIGURE 11–3. Schematic representations of normal (B), short (A), and long (C) QT interval durations.

Congenital Channelopathies

In the following section, we will focus on congenital K^+ channelopathies. Since the discovery that family-linked QT prolongation could be caused by mutation in the K^+ channel responsible for the rapidly and the slowly activating component of the delayed rectifier K^+ current (I_{Kr} and I_{Ks}, respectively), other congenital K^+ channelopathies were described, such as the SQTS (see chapter 35) or certain forms of atrial fibrillation (AF, see Chapter 41).

Long QT Syndrome

Long QT syndrome (LQTS) is a collection of cardiac disorders characterized by a prolongation of the QT interval on the ECG that affects an estimated 1 in 5000 to 10,000 people worldwide (see Figure 11–3C and Chapter 34).

The autosomal dominant inherited form of LQTS, called the Romano–Ward syndrome, is a collection of more than 300 mutations distributed over seven different genes responsible for seven different LQTS types, LQT1–LQT7.[35] Another much more rare inherited LQTS is autosomal recessive and is called the Jervell and Lange-Nielsen syndrome. In this pathology, the arrhythmic disorder is only part of the pathological picture since the severity of the cardiac symptoms vary from case to case and since it is associated with sensorineural deafness at birth.[36] Both congenital forms of LQTS result from mutations of ionic channels (α) and their accessory subunit (β), thus disrupting the delicate interplay between inward and outward currents generating the action potential. To date four genes, KCNQ1, KCNE1, KCNH2, and MiRP1, responsible for the slowly activating component of the delayed rectifier K^+ current (I_{Ks}) and the rapidly activating component of the delayed rectifier K^+ current (I_{Kr}), have been implicated in K^+-linked LQTS types 1, 5, 2, and 6, respectively (see Table 11–1).

I_{Ks}

I_{Ks} is a major contributor to cardiac action potential repolarization (phases 2 and 3, see Figure 11–1 and Chapter 9). KCNQ1 which shares a structure similar to other voltage-gated K^+ channels, is 676 amino acid long and is mapped to chromosome

TABLE 11–1. K^+ channel LQT-associated genes, proteins, and currents.

LQT type	1	2	5	6
Gene	KCNQ1	KCNH2	KCNE1	KCNE2
Protein	KCNQ1	hERG	KCNE1 or MinK	MiRP1
Function	α Subunit	α Subunit	β Subunit	β Subunit
Current	I_{Ks}	I_{Kr}	I_{Ks}	I_{Kr}

11 (see Figure 11–2B).[17] Expression of KCNQ1 alone in a heterologous system such as human embryonic kidney (HEK) cells, which have virtually no overlapping current to the one expressed, leads to rapidly activating and noninactivation outward K^+ currents (see Figure 11–4A1).[37,38] Similarly, KCNE1, a 130-amino-acid-long protein forming a single transmembrane spans, which is also called MinK, which stands for minimal K^+, and is now known to be the channel accessory subunit (β), was first shown to produce functional voltage-gated K^+ channels when expressed alone.[39,40] Because coexpression of KCNQ1 and KCNE1 produces slow activating noninactivating currents ressembling I_{Ks} (see Figure 11–4A2), it was deducted that I_{Ks} may result from the coassem-

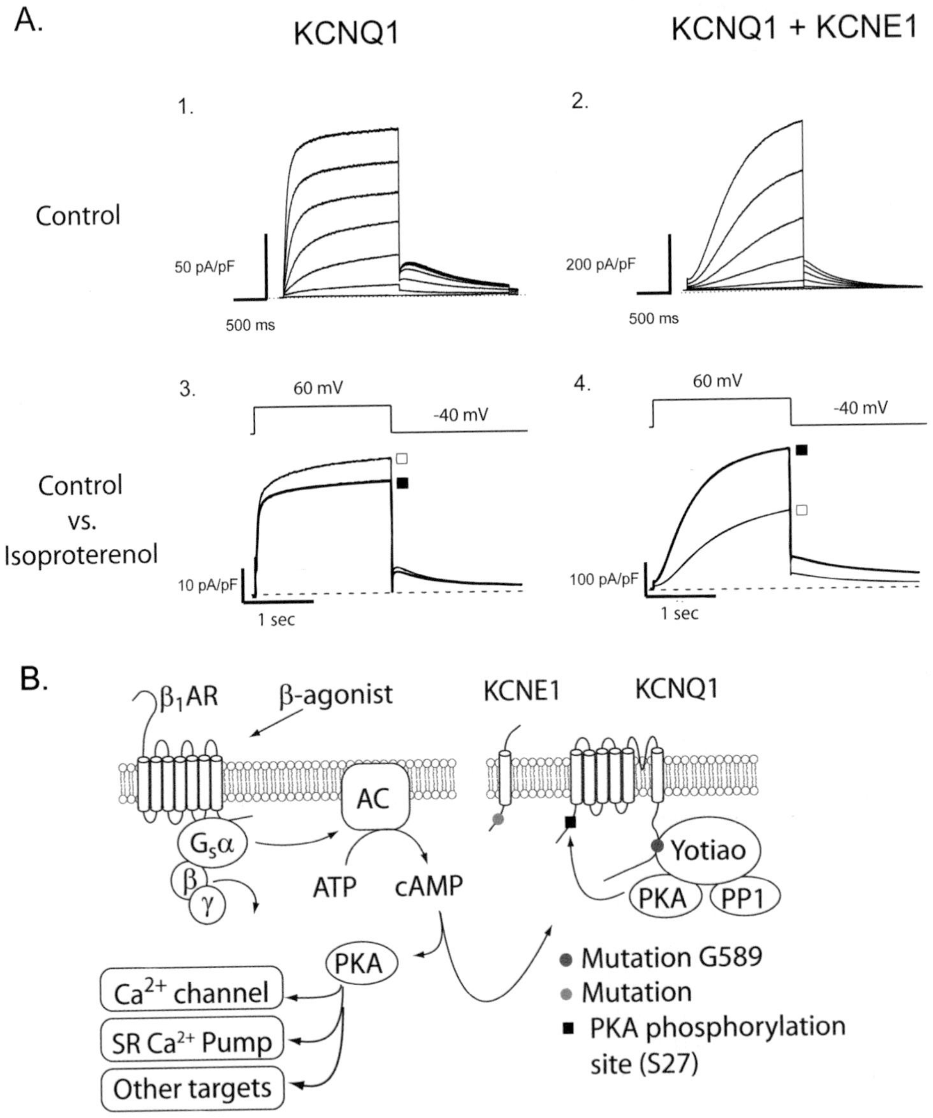

Figure 11–4. (A) Currents from KCNQ1 expressed alone (A1) and from KCNQ1 and KCNE1 coexpressed (A2) in heterologous expression sytems. The β-adrenergic stimulatory effect (■) requires coexpression of both subunits, KCNQ1 and KCNE1 (A4). If KCNQ1 is expressed alone, stimulation fails (A3). The β-adrenergic stimulation pathway, as depicted in (B), involves the synthesis of cAMP that stimulates protein kinase A (PKA), which in turn phosphorylates various targets, among which is KCNQ1 at serine 27 (S27).

bly of an α subunit, KCNQ1, and a β subunit, KCNE1.[37,38] At fast rates, that is during short diastolic recovery intervals preventing complete I_{Ks} deactivation, I_{Ks} sums and results in instantaneous repolarizing currents that underlie the rate-dependent shortening of the action potential.[12]

In heterologous expression systems I_{Ks} shows only activation and no inactivation. The kinetics are slow; the time course of the rise in current is sigmoidal, whereas the decay of the tails is monoexponential at voltages negative to −50 mV and biexponential at more positive potentials. Deactivation is also generally slow. The selectivity for K^+ is quite high, but not as high as other K^+ channels, thus shifting the reversal potential toward values more positive than what would be expected for K^+. Finally the fully activated current–voltage relation approaches linearity.[41]

Sympathetic Nervous Stimulation of I_{Ks}

Binding of epinephrin to β-adrenergic receptors that couple to stimulatory G_s proteins leads to activation of adenylyl cyclase. Adenylyl cyclase synthesizes cyclic adenosine monophosphate (cAMP) from adenosine trisphosphate (ATP), which eventually leads to an increased activity of the cAMP-dependent protein kinase A (PKA). PKA has many targets and I_{Ks} is one of these. I_{Ks} amplitude is directly modulated by β-adrenergic stimulation (see Figure 11–4b). Indeed, it was shown that the coassembly KCNQ1–KCNE1 was a functional macromolecuar complex physically coupling PKA to the channel. PKA-dependent phosphorylation of KCNQ1 significantly increases the rate of channel activation, resulting in a larger peak, and reducing the rate of channel deactivation (see Figure 11–4A3 and 4).[8] Such an increase in the repolarizing I_{Ks} coupled to its summation will reduce the duration of the action potential and its corresponding QT interval resulting in a rapid increase in heart rate.[42]

LQT1 and LQT

Mutations in KCNQ1 and KCNE1 both affect I_{Ks} amplitude, resulting in abnormal action potential durations and the development of cardiac arrhythmias (see Figure 11–3C). Mutations in the gene KCNQ1 have been linked to LQT1 syndrome (see Figure 11–2B).[43,44] It was suggested that the various LQT1-associated mutations in KCNQ1 were in general loss of function, resulting in a decreased functional I_{Ks}. This was confirmed by *in silico* experiments where a decreased I_{Ks} channel expression led to a significantly prolonged ventricular action potential duration.[20] To date 240 different mutations were isolated from LQT1 patients, all resulting in QT prolongation. The role of KCNE1 in the generation of cardiac K^+ current was clearly demonstrated by the identification of a mutation, S74L, associated with inherited LQT5.[35,45] Two other mutations in KCNE1, linked to LQT5, V47F, and W87R, later confirmed these observations.[46] Since then, 43 other mutations were described from LQT5 patients.

In these two types of LQTS (1 and 5), more time than usual is taken between repolarization of the ventricles and repolarization of the atria, especially during stimulation by the sympathetic nervous system, leading to subsequent syncope and arrhythmias and sudden death.[47] The point mutation G589D, where a glycine at position 589 is replaced by an aspartic acid, was also shown to reduce the response to sympathetic nervous stimulation disrupting the leucine zipper motif and preventing cAMP-dependent regulation of I_{Ks}.[8,48] Similarly, the two LQT5-linked point mutations D76N, originally described by Splawski *et al.*, and W87R were shown to disrupt the adrenergic answer, suggesting that KCNE1 is required for the adrenergic modulation of I_{Ks}.[45,49]

I_{Kr}

The importance of hERG, the human ether-à-go-go-related gene, in normal human cardiac electrical activity became obvious when inherited mutations in KCNH2 were found to cause LQTS type 2.[16,50] But before this discovery it was known that a similar long QT disorder could be induced by a high dose of some I_{Kr} blockers[13] (see Acquired Channelopathies bellow and Figure 11–5B). MiRP1 (KCNE2), an MinK-related peptide from the MiRP subfamily, has been shown to function as an accessory subunit of KCNH2 to generate cardiac I_{Kr}.[51] Its physiological implication became important when MiRP1 variants were associated with congenital and drug-induced LQT.[35,52,53] I_{Kr} activates rapidly, allowing outward diffusion of K^+ ions in accordance with its electrochemical driving

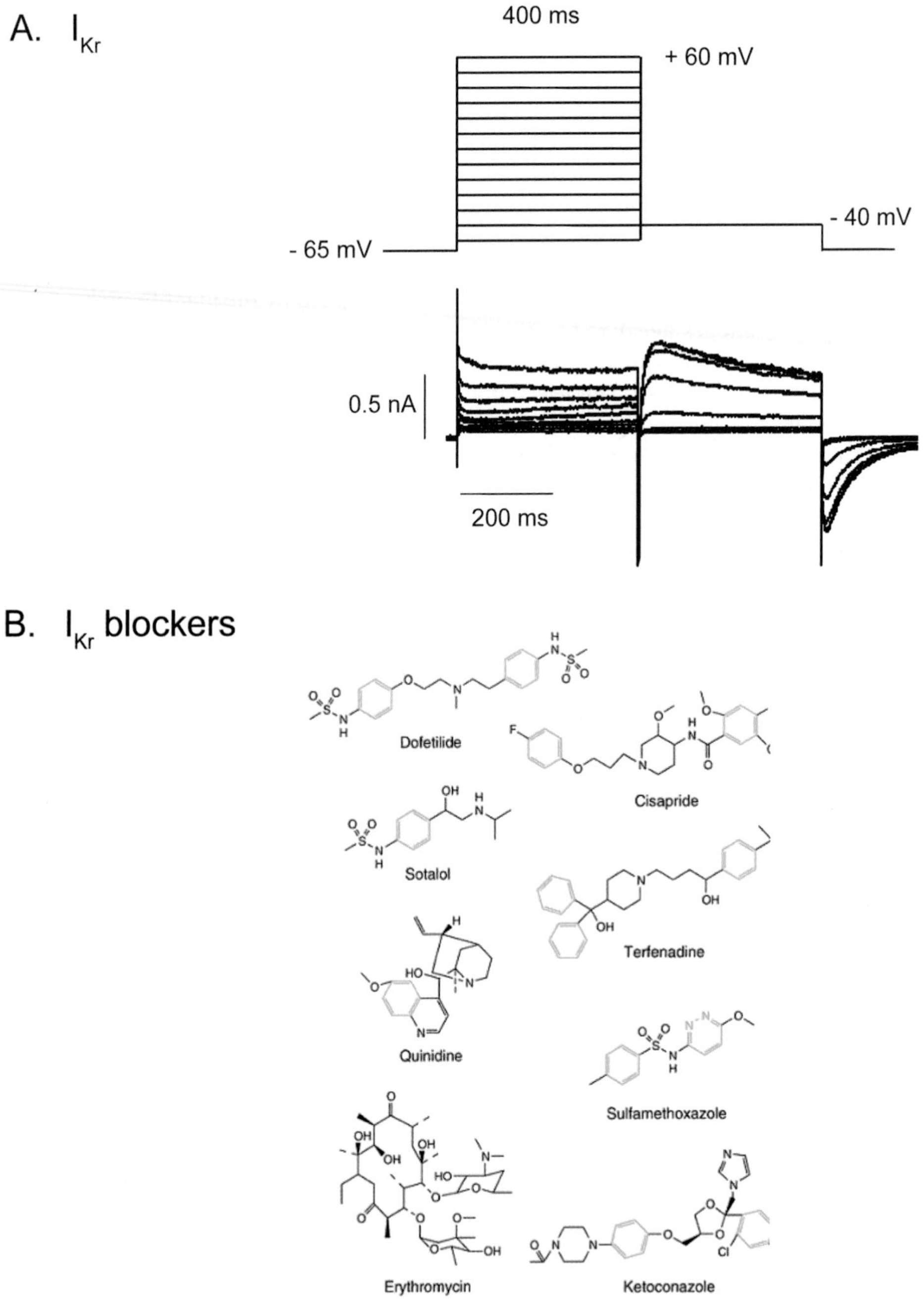

Figure 11–5. (A) The protocol used to record a current–voltage relationship of I_{Kr} (up) and the resultant currents as recorded in a heterologous expression system (down). Cells are first depolarized from a resting potential of −65 mV to different test potentials ranging from −60 mV to +60 mV for 400 msec and repolarized for the same amount of time to −40 mV to estimate the amount of channel deactivation prior to a complete repolarization to the imposed resting potential. Note the typical presence of a "hook" in the current recording upon repolarization to −40 mV (down). (B) The structures of known I_{Kr} blockers. Treating patients with such drugs may trigger fatal arrhythmias.

force (see Figure 11–5A). Time constants of activation vary among species and membrane potentials. For example, I_{Kr} generally activates faster in guinea pig than in rabbit ventricular cells.[54,55] Compared with I_{Ks}, these time constants are shorter, a finding on which the distinction between the two currents has been based. The time course of the macroscopic current recorded using the patch-clamp technique shows saturation with no indication of a secondary decrease. The "tail" currents during repolarization, however, are preceded by a "hook," and the current temporarily increases before it declines exponentially (see Figure 11–5A).[55,56] This observation was interpreted as being the result of the recovery from the inactivation state, which implies the existence of a steady-state inactivation, a nonconducting configuration, responsible for current rectification. As is the case for I_{Ks}, and although preferentially permeable to K^+, the channel's K^+ selectivity is less pronounced than that of other K^+ channels such as I_{K1}, especially at a lower external K^+ concentration ($[K^+]_o$). External bivalent and trivalent cations were shown to block the channel. I_{Kr} is especially sensitive to block by Co^{2+} and La^{3+}. The block by Ca^{2+} and Mg^{2+} is reduced by elevating $[K^+]_o$, but does not change the inward rectification.[41,57]

LQT2 and LQT6

Mutations in KCNH2 are found throughout the protein sequence (see Figure 11–2C). Single-strand conformation polymorphism and DNA sequence analyses revealed hERG mutations in six LQT families, including two intragenic deletions, one splice-donor mutation, three missense mutations, and one *de novo*.[16] All of these mutations resulted in a loss of function decreasing I_{Kr}, possibly through dominant-negative effects or alteration in channel processing and trafficking.[43,58,59] Several other mutations having a dominant-negative effect have been characterized. The substitution of a glycine for a serine at position 638 (G638S) caused a loss of function and altered the K^+ pore sequence. Similarly, the substitution of N470D resulted in currents that were smaller and that deactivated more slowly than expected.[60] To date 272 mutations affecting I_{Kr} gating have been described and it is very likely that new ones will be discovered in LQT2 patients. Similar to LQT5, 14 mutations in MiRP1 were described and linked to LQT6.

In conclusion, K^+-linked LQTS are most often caused by mutations in KCNQ1 or KCNH2 and less frequently by mutations in β accessory subunits (KCNE1 and KCNE2). While β-blocker therapy was shown to be effective in decreasing the incidence of syncope and sudden death in K^+-linked LQTS, LQT2/6 patients are still more prone to develop fatal cardiac arrhythmias.[61] Prophylactic and preventive therapy thus depends on the specific type of LQTS and includes β-blocker therapy, left cervicothoracic sympathetic ganglionectomy, pacemakers, implanted defibrillators, and gene-specific pharmacological therapy.[62]

Short QT Syndrome

Among inherited arrhythmogenic diseases, the most recently identified is the SQTS.[63] A short QT interval (see Figure 11–3A) was identified in three people from the same family, one of whom had several episodes of paroxysmal atrial fibrillation. Further characterization was made by Gaita *et al.*[64] in 2003, who showed that SQTS was linked to a familial history of ventricular fibrillation and sudden death.

SQTS was shown to be caused by gain-of-functions mutations. Gain-of-function mutations are mutations enhancing the normal function of the channel, as opposed to loss-of-function mutations similar to those described earlier for voltage-gated K^+ channel-linked LQTS (for example see Figure 11–6). These gain-of-function mutations were found in three different genes, thus characterizing three different types of SQTS. The first mutations described were found in the gene KCNH2, which encodes for hERG. Two different missense mutations were identified, resulting in the same amino acid change (N588K) in the S5-P loop region of the cardiac I_{Kr} channel. The mutations dramatically increase I_{Kr}, leading to heterogeneous abbreviation of action potential duration and refractoriness, and reduce the affinity of the channels to I_{Kr} blockers.[65] This is now described as the first form of SQTS (SQT1). A few months later another gain-of-function mutation was found in a patient suffering from idiopathic ventricular fibrillation. The substitution of a valine by an leucine occurred at position 307 (V307L) in the

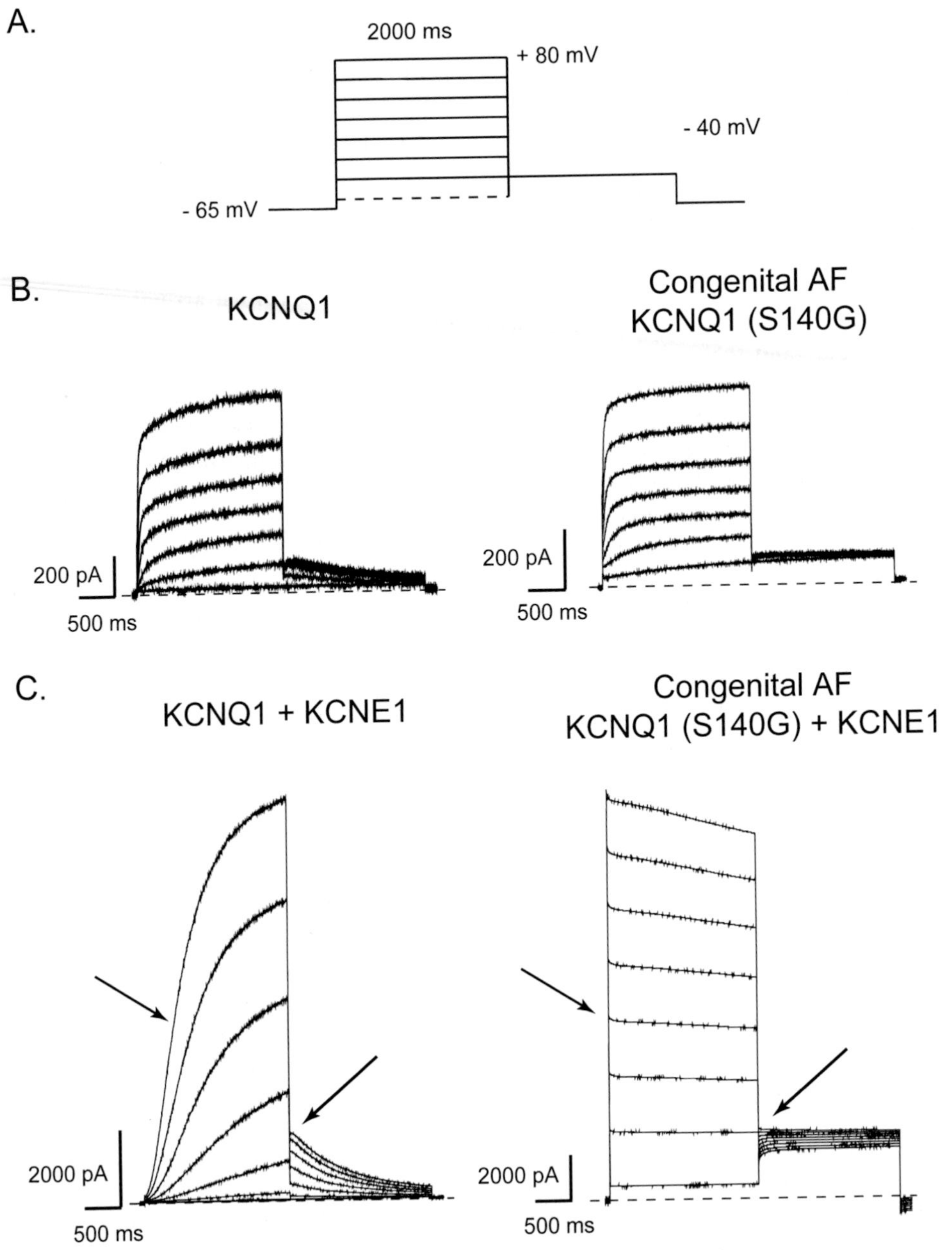

FIGURE 11–6. Current–voltage relationships were recorded according to the voltage-clamp protocol (A). Cells were depolarized from a resting potential of −65 mV to various test potentials, from −60 mV to +80 mV, for 2 sec. They were then repolarized to −40 mV for an additional 2 sec to measure the amount of channel deactivation before being brought back to the resting potential of −65 mV. (B) The typical currents triggered by such a protocol in normal (left) and AF-linked KCNQ1 mutant (S140G, right) expressed alone in heterologous systems. (C) The typical current–voltage relationship of I_{Ks}, as expected from the coexpression of KCNQ1 and KCNE1 (C, left), and the currents recorded from coexpressed S140G mutant KCNQ1 and normal KCNE1 (C, right). Mutant channels (C, right) were detected in the open state (left arrow) and very little deactivation was observed within seconds of return to negative potentials (right arrow).

gene KCNQ1, which now characterizes the second form of SQTS (SQT2).[66] Finally, a last and third type of SQTS (SQT3) was characterized by a gain-of-function mutation in the gene KCNJ2 (D172N) that encodes for a K^+ inward rectifier channel Kir2.1, which is thought to be the major channel involved in the generation of IK1. Interestingly loss-of-function mutations of KCNJ2 are known to cause the Andersen–Tawil syndrome (see Chapters 14 and 38).[67] All 5 mutations described to date dramatically shorten the action potential duration, thus shortening the excitatory refractory period and creating a substrate for ventricular and atrial fibrillations (see Chapters 41 and 42). Indeed, most patients suffering from any SQTS seem to have a high incidence of supraventricular arrhythmias, particularly atrial fibrillations.[64]

Atrial Fibrillation

Atrial fibrillation is the most common cardiac arrhythmia. It is estimated that 2.2 millions Americans have this rhythm disorder, which causes a 2-fold increase in mortality and a 2- to 6-fold increased risk for stroke. Despite its high prevalence and severe complications, a definitive treatment approach has not been established.[68] Atrial fibrillation is characterized by a rapid and irregular atrial activation. Whatever the initiating mechanism for AF is, whether this is the consequence of a channelopathy or any other AF-promoting factor, multiple wavelet reentry has been widely accepted to be the maintaining mechanism for AF.[69] For more details, see Chapter 41.

Interestingly, KCNQ1 and KCNE2 were both recently involved in familial AF. In January 2003 Chen *et al.*[19] reported for the first time a KCNQ1 mutation in a three generation family with AF in the absence of structural cardiac disease. In this particular case a missense mutation due to the substitution of a highly conserved serine by a glycine at position 140 (S140G) led to a gain-of-function effect correlated with a significant increase in I_{Ks}. Representative current–voltage relationships of normal and S140G mutant channels expressed in heterologous expression systems with or without KCNE1 are shown in Figure 11–6. When the S140G mutant was coexpressed with a normal KCNE1 β subunit (Figure 11–6B), channels were immediately detected in the open state upon depolarization (left arrow). Upon repolarization, very little evidence for deactivation was detected within seconds (right arrow).

Interestingly, some of these patients presented a prolonged QT interval, the phenotype of which contrasts with the phenotype observed *in vitro*. In November 2004 Yang *et al.*[68] reported the results of the molecular screening of 28 unrelated Chinese kindreds with AF. They analyzed eight genes from K^+ channels and reported an arginine-to-cysteine mutation at position 27 (R27C) in KCNE2 in all the affected patients. Interestingly, currents recorded from cotransfected cells with hERG/MiRP1 were not impaired. As a consequence, they looked at the cotransfected pair KCNQ1/MiRP1, known to produce a resting membrane potential stabilizing the background K^+ current.[70] Similar to the KCNQ1 mutation discussed above, the mutation had a gain-of-function effect. But compared to the people carrying the KCNQ1 S140G mutation, patients who had the KCNE2 R27C mutation had a less severe phenotype, with paroxysmal AF instead of a permanent type. In conclusion, although AF is usually known to be a complication of cardiac valvular disease or systemic hyperthyroidism, to mention just a few possibilities from the long list of causal factors, little is known about the familial forms of this disease.

Acquired Channelopathies

The acquired form of channelopathies linked to voltage-gated K^+ channels generally results from pharmacological intervention, often for the purpose of treating disorders unrelated to cardiac dysfunction. Among others antihistaminics, antipsychotics, antibiotics, and certain antiarrhythmics can predispose patients to lethal arrhythmias (see Figure 11–5B).[42]

hERG Drug Block

It has long been known that common medications could prolong the QT interval, leading to symptoms similar to those found in patients suffering from inherited LQTS (see Figure 11–5B). For example, drug-induced torsade de pointe by the antiarrhythmic drug quinidine is a relatively frequent side effect, affecting 2–9% of the treated patients.[13] Similarly, induction of arrhythmias by other than antiarrhythmic drugs is rare. Cisapride-induced torsade de pointe occurred in only one patient out of 1200. It is thus a high risk for patients being treated for gastrointestinal disorders and allergies. As a consequence, drugs such as cisapride, sertindole, grepafloxacin, terfenadine, and astemizole were removed from the market. The common property of all these drugs is that they affect hERG channel current by depressing its gating or interfering with its trafficking to the cell surface, thus causing a drug-induced QT prolongation and significantly increasing the risks for arrhythmias and sudden death.[13] Indeed, the hERG is unusually susceptible to blockage by drugs in comparison with other voltage-gated K^+ channels. Further investigations were carried out and a unique drug-binding site was found. Two residues located at the base of the pore and two others found in the S6 helix, when mutated to alanines, significantly decreased the affinity of potent hERG inhibitors.[71] While the two pore helix residues are highly conserved in voltage-gated K^+ channels and cannot easily explain the susceptibility of hERG blockade, the two aromatic S6 residues are not conserved, thus partially explaining the surprising chemical diversity of hERG blockers.[71]

Acknowledgment. The authors would like to acknowledge David Y. Chung for providing the material used in Figure 11-6.

References

1. Cole KS. Mostly membranes. *Annu Rev Physiol* 1979;41:1–24.
2. Hodgkin AL, Huxley AF. Propagation of electrical signals along giant nerve fibers. *Proc R Soc Lond B Biol Sci* 1952;140(899):177–183.
3. Hodgkin AL, Huxley AF. A quantitative description of membrane current and its application to conduction and excitation in nerve. *J Physiol* 1952; 117(4):500–544.
4. Hodgkin AL, Rushton WAH. The electrical constants of a crustacean nerve fiber. *Proc R Soc* 1946; B133:444–479.
5. Weidmann S. The electrical constants of Purkinje fibres. *J Physiol* 1952;118(3):348–360.
6. Giraudat J, Devillers-Thiery A, Auffray C, Rougeon F, Changeux JP. Identification of a cDNA clone coding for the acetylcholine binding subunit of Torpedo marmorata acetylcholine receptor. *EMBO J* 1982;1(6):713–717.
7. Noda M, Takahashi H, Tanabe T, *et al.* Primary structure of alpha-subunit precursor of Torpedo californica acetylcholine receptor deduced from cDNA sequence. *Nature* 1982;299(5886):793–797.
8. Marx SO, Kurokawa J, Reiken S, *et al.* Requirement of a macromolecular signaling complex for beta adrenergic receptor modulation of the KCNQ1-KCNE1 potassium channel. *Science* 2002;295(5554): 496–499.
9. Neher E, Sakmann B. Single-channel currents recorded from membrane of denervated frog muscle fibres. *Nature* 1976;260(5554):799–802.
10. Doyle DA, Morais Cabral J, Pfuetzner RA, *et al.* The structure of the potassium channel: Molecular basis of K+ conduction and selectivity. *Science* 1998;280(5360):69–77.
11. MacKinnon R. Potassium channels. *FEBS Lett* 2003;555(1):62–65.
12. Clancy CE, Kass RS. Inherited and acquired vulnerability to ventricular arrhythmias: Cardiac Na+ and K+ channels. *Physiol Rev* 2005;85(1):33–47.
13. Sanguinetti MC, Tristani-Firouzi M. hERG potassium channels and cardiac arrhythmia. *Nature* 2006;440(7083):463–469.
14. Jervell A, Lange-Nielsen F. Congenital deaf-mutism, functional heart disease with prolongation of the Q-T interval and sudden death. *Am Heart J* 1957; 54(1):59–68.
15. Ward OC. A new familial cardiac syndrome in children. *J Ir Med Assoc* 1964;54:103–106.
16. Curran ME, Splawski I, Timothy KW, Vincent GM, Green ED, Keating MT. A molecular basis for cardiac arrhythmia: HERG mutations cause long QT syndrome. *Cell* 1995;80(5):795–803.
17. Wang Q, Curran ME, Splawski I, *et al.* Positional cloning of a novel potassium channel gene: KVLQT1 mutations cause cardiac arrhythmias. *Nat Genet* 1996;12(1):17–23.
18. Haverkamp W, Breithardt G, Camm AJ, *et al.* The potential for QT prolongation and proarrhythmia by non-antiarrhythmic drugs: Clinical and regulatory implications. Report on a policy conference of the European Society of Cardiology. *Eur Heart J* 2000;21(15):1216–1231.
19. Chen YH, Xu SJ, Bendahhou S, *et al.* KCNQ1 gain-of-function mutation in familial atrial fibrillation. *Science* 2003;299(5604):251–254.
20. Nerbonne JM, Kass RS. Molecular physiology of cardiac repolarization. *Physiol Rev* 2005;85(4):1205–1253.

21. Long SB, Campbell EB, Mackinnon R. Crystal structure of a mammalian voltage-dependent Shaker family K+ channel. *Science* 2005;309(5736):897–903.
22. Pond AL, Scheve BK, Benedict AT, *et al.* Expression of distinct ERG proteins in rat, mouse, and human heart. Relation to functional I(Kr) channels. *J Biol Chem* 2000;275(8):5997–6006.
23. Mannuzzu LM, Moronne MM, Isacoff EY. Direct physical measure of conformational rearrangement underlying potassium channel gating. *Science* 1996; 271(5246):213–216.
24. Yang N, George AL Jr, Horn R. Molecular basis of charge movement in voltage-gated sodium channels. *Neuron* 1996;16(1):113–122.
25. Attali B, Lesage F, Ziliani P, *et al.* Multiple mRNA isoforms encoding the mouse cardiac Kv1-5 delayed rectifier K+ channel. *J Biol Chem* 1993; 268(32):24283–24289.
26. Covarrubias M, Wei AA, Salkoff L. Shaker, Shal, Shab, and Shaw express independent K+ current systems. *Neuron* 1991;7(5):763–773.
27. Guo W, Li H, Aimond F, *et al.* Role of heteromultimers in the generation of myocardial transient outward K+ currents. *Circ Res* 2002;90(5): 586–593.
28. Noble D, Tsien RW. Reconstruction of the repolarization process in cardiac Purkinje fibres based on voltage clamp measurements of membrane current. *J Physiol* 1969;200(1):233–254.
29. Noble D, Tsien RW. Outward membrane currents activated in the plateau range of potentials in cardiac Purkinje fibres. *J Physiol* 1969;200(1): 205–231.
30. Horie M, Hayashi S, Kawai C. Two types of delayed rectifying K+ channels in atrial cells of guinea pig heart. *Jpn J Physiol* 1990;40(4):479–490.
31. Sanguinetti MC, Jurkiewicz NK. Delayed rectifier outward K+ current is composed of two currents in guinea pig atrial cells. *Am J Physiol* 1991;260(2Pt. 2):H393–399.
32. Sanguinetti MC, Jurkiewicz NK. Role of external Ca2+ and K+ in gating of cardiac delayed rectifier K+ currents. *Pflugers Arch* 1992;420(2):180–186.
33. Xu H, Guo W, Nerbonne JM. Four kinetically distinct depolarization-activated K+ currents in adult mouse ventricular myocytes. *J Gen Physiol* 1999; 113(5):661–678.
34. Sanguinetti MC, Bennett PB. Antiarrhythmic drug target choices and screening. *Circ Res* 2003;93(6): 491–499.
35. Splawski I, Shen J, Timothy KW, *et al.* Spectrum of mutations in long-QT syndrome genes. KVLQT1, HERG, SCN5A, KCNE1, and KCNE2. *Circulation* 2000;102(10):1178–1185.
36. Chen Q, Zhang D, Gingell RL, *et al.* Homozygous deletion in KVLQT1 associated with Jervell and Lange-Nielsen syndrome. *Circulation* 1999;99(10): 1344–1347.
37. Barhanin J, Lesage F, Guillemare E, Fink M, Lazdunski M, Romey G. K(V)LQT1 and lsK (minK) proteins associate to form the I(Ks) cardiac potassium current. *Nature* 1996;384(6604):78–80.
38. Sanguinetti MC, Curran ME, Zou A, *et al.* Coassembly of K(V)LQT1 and minK (IsK) proteins to form cardiac I(Ks) potassium channel. *Nature* 1996;384 (6604):80–83.
39. Folander K, Smith JS, Antanavage J, Bennett C, Stein RB, Swanson R. Cloning and expression of the delayed-rectifier IsK channel from neonatal rat heart and diethylstilbestrol-primed rat uterus. *Proc Natl Acad Sci USA* 1990;87(8):2975–2979.
40. Murai T, Kakizuka A, Takumi T, Ohkubo H, Nakanishi S. Molecular cloning and sequence analysis of human genomic DNA encoding a novel membrane protein which exhibits a slowly activating potassium channel activity. *Biochem Biophys Res Commun* 1989;161(1):176–181.
41. Carmeliet E. Cardiac ionic currents and acute ischemia: From channels to arrhythmias. *Physiol Rev* 1999;79(3):917–1017.
42. Clancy CE, Kurokawa J, Tateyama M, Wehrens XH, Kass RS. K+ channel structure-activity relationships and mechanisms of drug-induced QT prolongation. *Annu Rev Pharmacol Toxicol* 2003;43: 441–461.
43. Keating MT, Sanguinetti MC. Molecular and cellular mechanisms of cardiac arrhythmias. *Cell* 2001; 104(4):569–580.
44. Maruoka ND, Steele DF, Au BP, *et al.* alpha-Actinin-2 couples to cardiac Kv1.5 channels, regulating current density and channel localization in HEK cells. *FEBS Lett* 2000;473(2):188–194.
45. Splawski I, Tristani-Firouzi M, Lehmann MH, Sanguinetti MC, Keating MT. Mutations in the hminK gene cause long QT syndrome and suppress IKs function. *Nat Genet* 1997;17(3):338–340.
46. Bianchi L, Shen Z, Dennis AT, *et al.* Cellular dysfunction of LQT5-minK mutants: Abnormalities of IKs, IKr and trafficking in long QT syndrome. *Hum Mol Genet* 1999;8(8):1499–1507.
47. Schwartz PJ, Priori SG, Spazzolini C, *et al.* Genotype-phenotype correlation in the long-QT syndrome: Gene-specific triggers for life-threatening arrhythmias. *Circulation* 2001;103(1):89–95.
48. Piippo K, Swan H, Pasternack M, *et al.* A founder mutation of the potassium channel KCNQ1 in long QT syndrome: Implications for estimation of disease prevalence and molecular diagnostics. *J Am Coll Cardiol* 2001;37(2):562–568.

49. Kurokawa J, Motoike HK, Rao J, Kass RS. Regulatory actions of the A-kinase anchoring protein Yotiao on a heart potassium channel downstream of PKA phosphorylation. *Proc Natl Acad Sci USA* 2004;101(46):16374–16378.
50. Warmke JW, Ganetzky B. A family of potassium channel genes related to eag in Drosophila and mammals. *Proc Natl Acad Sci USA* 1994;91(8):3438–3442.
51. Abbott GW, Goldstein SA. A superfamily of small potassium channel subunits: Form and function of the MinK-related peptides (MiRPs). *Q Rev Biophys* 1998;31(4):357–398.
52. Abbott GW, Sesti F, Splawski I, *et al.* MiRP1 forms IKr potassium channels with HERG and is associated with cardiac arrhythmia. *Cell* 1999;97(2):175–187.
53. Sesti F, Abbott GW, Wei J, *et al.* A common polymorphism associated with antibiotic-induced cardiac arrhythmia. *Proc Natl Acad Sci USA* 2000; 97(19):10613–10618.
54. Carmeliet E. Voltage- and time-dependent block of the delayed K+ current in cardiac myocytes by dofetilide. *J Pharmacol Exp Ther* 1992;262(2):809–817.
55. Sanguinetti MC, Jurkiewicz NK. Two components of cardiac delayed rectifier K+ current. Differential sensitivity to block by class III antiarrhythmic agents. *J Gen Physiol* 1990;96(1):195–215.
56. Shibasaki T. Conductance and kinetics of delayed rectifier potassium channels in nodal cells of the rabbit heart. *J Physiol* 1987;387:227–250.
57. Sanguinetti MC, Jurkiewicz NK. Lanthanum blocks a specific component of IK and screens membrane surface change in cardiac cells. *Am J Physiol* 1990; 259(6Pt. 2):H1881–1889.
58. Antzelevitch C. Molecular genetics of arrhythmias and cardiovascular conditions associated with arrhythmias.*JCardiovascElectrophysiol*2003;14(11): 1259–1272.
59. Delisle BP, Anson BD, Rajamani S, January CT. Biology of cardiac arrhythmias: Ion channel protein trafficking. *Circ Res* 2004;94(11):1418–1428.
60. Sanguinetti MC. Dysfunction of delayed rectifier potassium channels in an inherited cardiac arrhythmia. *Ann NY Acad Sci* 1999;868:406–413.
61. Priori SG, Napolitano C, Schwartz PJ, *et al.* Association of long QT syndrome loci and cardiac events among patients treated with beta-blockers. *JAMA* 2004;292(11):1341–1344.
62. Moss AJ, Kass RS. Long QT syndrome: From channels to cardiac arrhythmias. *J Clin Invest* 2005; 115(8):2018–2024.
63. Gussak I, Brugada P, Brugada J, *et al.* Idiopathic short QT interval: A new clinical syndrome? *Cardiology* 2000;94(2):99–102.
64. Gaita F, Giustetto C, Bianchi F, *et al.* Short QT Syndrome: A familial cause of sudden death. *Circulation* 2003;108(8):965–970.
65. Brugada R, Hong K, Dumaine R, *et al.* Sudden death associated with short-QT syndrome linked to mutations in HERG. *Circulation* 2004;109(1): 30–35.
66. Bellocq C, van Ginneken AC, Bezzina CR, *et al.* Mutation in the KCNQ1 gene leading to the short QT-interval syndrome. *Circulation* 2004;109(20): 2394–2397.
67. Priori SG, Pandit SV, Rivolta I, *et al.* A novel form of short QT syndrome (SQT3) is caused by a mutation in the KCNJ2 gene. *Circ Res* 2005;96(7):800–807.
68. Yang Y, Xia M, Jin Q, *et al.* Identification of a KCNE2 gain-of-function mutation in patients with familial atrial fibrillation. *Am J Hum Genet* 2004; 75(5):899–905.
69. Nattel S. New ideas about atrial fibrillation 50 years on. *Nature* 2002;415(6868):219–226.
70. Tinel N, Diochot S, Borsotto M, Lazdunski M, Barhanin J. KCNE2 confers background current characteristics to the cardiac KCNQ1 potassium channel. *EMBO J* 2000;19(23):6326–6330.
71. Sanguinetti MC, Mitcheson JS. Predicting drug-hERG channel interactions that cause acquired long QT syndrome. *Trends Pharmacol Sci* 2005; 26(3):119–124.

12 Channelopathies of Cardiac Inwardly Rectifying Potassium Channels

Andre Terzic, Michel Vivaudou, Christophe Moreau, Timothy M. Olson, Arshad Jahangir, Leonid V. Zingman, and Alexey E. Alekseev

Kir Channels and Channelopathies: An Overview

Diseases resulting from impaired ion channel function—channelopathies—are increasingly recognized pathologies in human cardiovascular medicine.[1] Understanding the molecular basis of an ion channel disease has provided new opportunities for screening, early diagnosis, and therapy of these commonly life-threatening conditions.[2,3] A case in point is the identification of molecular genetic defects in inwardly rectifying potassium (Kir, *KCNJ*) channels.

Inwardly rectifying potassium channels, also referred as Kir channels, are a distinct family of ion channels encoded by 15 genes, grouped into seven channel subfamilies (Figure 12–1).[4] Structurally and functionally unique, Kir channels are ubiquitously expressed and serve vital functions as diverse as regulation of resting membrane potential and excitability, maintenance of potassium homeostasis, control of heart rate, and hormone secretion.[4,5] Persistent hyperinsulinemic hypoglycemia of infancy, a disorder affecting the function of pancreatic β-cells, and Bartter's syndrome, characterized by hypokalemic alkalosis, hypercalciuria, increased serum aldosterone, and plasma renin activity, were the two human disease conditions initially linked to mutations in a Kir channel or associated protein.[6,7] Mutations in genes encoding myocardial ion channels,[8,9] including subunits of Kir channel complexes—namely the IK_1 (Kir2.1, *KCNJ2*) tetramer and the ATP-sensitive K^+ (K_{ATP}; Kir6.2/SUR2A, *KCNJ11/ABCC9*) heteromultimer—have also been more recently linked to human channelopathies and increased susceptibility to cardiac disease. Specifically, IK_1 channelopathies have been reported in three conditions: Andersen cardiodysrhythmic periodic paralysis syndrome,[10] short QT syndrome,[11] and atrial fibrillation.[12] Mutations in the regulatory subunit of the K_{ATP} channel complex have been demonstrated in patients with dilated cardiomyopathy and ventricular arrhythmia,[13] as well as in adrenergic atrial fibrillation.[14]

We here provide an overview of cardiac IK_1 (Kir2.1) and K_{ATP} (Kir6.2/SUR2A) channels and highlight progress made in the identification of molecular defects associated with human disease. IK_{Ach} (Kir3.1/Kir3.4), the third inwardly rectifying potassium channel functionally expressed in the myocardium (Figure 12–1), responsible for the negative chronotropic and inotropic effects of vagal stimulation, will not be discussed in detail as human disease has not yet been associated with malfunction in this channel. As Kir channels serve multiple roles in the heart (Figure 12–1), it is conceivable that molecular defects in members of this channel family will, in the near future, be linked to additional clinical conditions. Indeed, further genetic investigation and epidemiological studies, along with the full understanding of the consequences that a defect in an Kir channel or associated protein would have on disease prediction, progression, and management, are among the priorities in the emerging field of individualized molecular medicine.

A

Current	Major function	Effectors	Human disease	IUPHAR nomenclature	Alias	HUGO Gene nomenclature	Chromosomal location
IK_{ATP}	Adjusts membrane excitability to match cell energy status	ATP/ADP	Dilated cardiomyopathy & ventricular tachycardia; Atrial fibrillation	Kir6.2	-	*KCNJ11*	11p15.1
				-	SUR2A	*ABCC9*	12p12.1
IK_1	Sets resting membrane potential	-	Anderson's syndrome; Short QT syndrome; Atrial fibrillation	Kir2.1	IRK1	*KCNJ2*	17q23.1
IK_{Ach}	Regulates autonomic-modulated heart rate	Gβγ subunits	-	Kir3.1	GIRK1	*KCNJ3*	2q24.1
				Kir3.4	GIRK4	*KCNJ5*	11q24

B

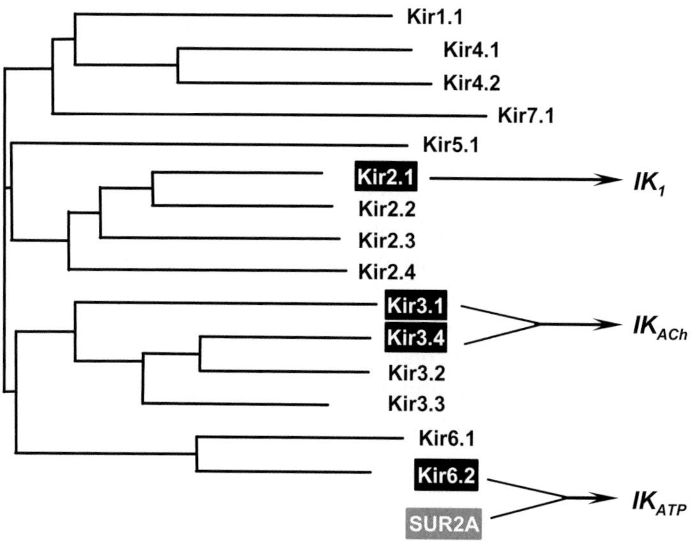

FIGURE 12–1. Molecular constituents of cardiac inwardly rectifying potassium currents. (A) Nomenclature and main features. (B) Phylogenetic tree based on the full amino acid sequences of all known human inward rectifier potassium channel proteins produced by ClustalX (Thompson JD, *et al.*, *Nucleic Acids Res* 1997;25:4876–4882) and drawn using Treeview (Page RD, *Comput Appl Biosci* 1996;12:357–358). Channel-forming proteins found in cardiomyocytes and linked to regulation of cell function are highlighted.

Inwardly Rectifying Potassium Channels in Health

Structure

While initially conceptualized over six decades ago,[15] the molecular identity of Kir channels has only recently been solved with the cloning of genes encoding individual Kir proteins (Figure 12–1).[16] These include *KCNJ2* (localized on human chromosome 17q23) and *KCNJ11* (localized on chromosome 11q15) that encode Kir2.1 and Kir6.2, respectively, as well as *KCNJ3*/*KCNJ5* encoding Kir3.1/Kir3.4 (localized on chromosomes 2q24/11q24), each expressed in the heart.[4,17–19] The Kir family of genes encodes ~360–500 amino acid proteins folded into canonical structures consisting of two membrane-spanning domains (M1 and M2) flanking a highly conserved pore (P) region that contains the H5 segment (Figure 12–2). In accordance with an early emergence in evolution, Kir channels have an apparently simpler structure than that of other ion channel families.[16] The H5 and M2 segments, in conjunction with the carboxyl terminus hydrophilic domain, are critical for potassium ion permeation.[20,21] Resolving the architecture of the pore has established the structural determinants underlying selective K^+ conduction.[22,23] Four channel subunits assemble to form functional Kir channels. A tetrameric channel complex can be formed by the physical association of identical ("homomers") or different ("heteromers") subunits. The amino acid sequences of various Kir channels diverge at the distal carboxy and amino termini, as well as in the extracellular loop linking the M1 and P regions. Further diversity is achieved through association of Kir subunits with additional, structurally unrelated protein(s) that play important roles in the expression, distribution, or regulation of channel activity.[16,20,21]

The biophysical fingerprint of Kir channels is inward rectification in the current–voltage relationship, which limits potassium efflux at potentials more positive than the reversal potassium potential (Figure 12–3).[20] Rectification describes the fundamental property of certain ion channels to preferentially allow currents to flow in one direction, or equivalently to limit currents from flowing in the other direction. In the case of Kir channels, rectification has come to designate the latter phenomenon. The term "inward rectification" refers, perhaps somewhat confusingly, to a reduction in outward current. It is now recognized that rectification in Kir channels is not solely an intrinsic property of the channel protein, as it is in certain voltage-dependent channel counterparts,[24] but is mediated by interaction with cytosolic multivalent cations, such as Mg^{2+} and polyamines.[25,26] These cations bind within the channel and impede outward K^+ movement at depolarized voltages, but are displaced by incoming K^+ ions at hyperpolarized voltages.[25,26] High-affinity binding and strong voltage dependence of these blocking molecules are made possible by an ion conduction pore that extends toward the cytosol (Figure 12–2).[27] How effectively these blockers bind, and how strong rectification is, is determined by the nature of several residues lining the cytoplasmic access pathway of the channel. These include a negatively charged amino acid residue, termed the "rectification controller" in the region of the M2 helix that delineates the proximal entrance of the channel,[20,25] as well as

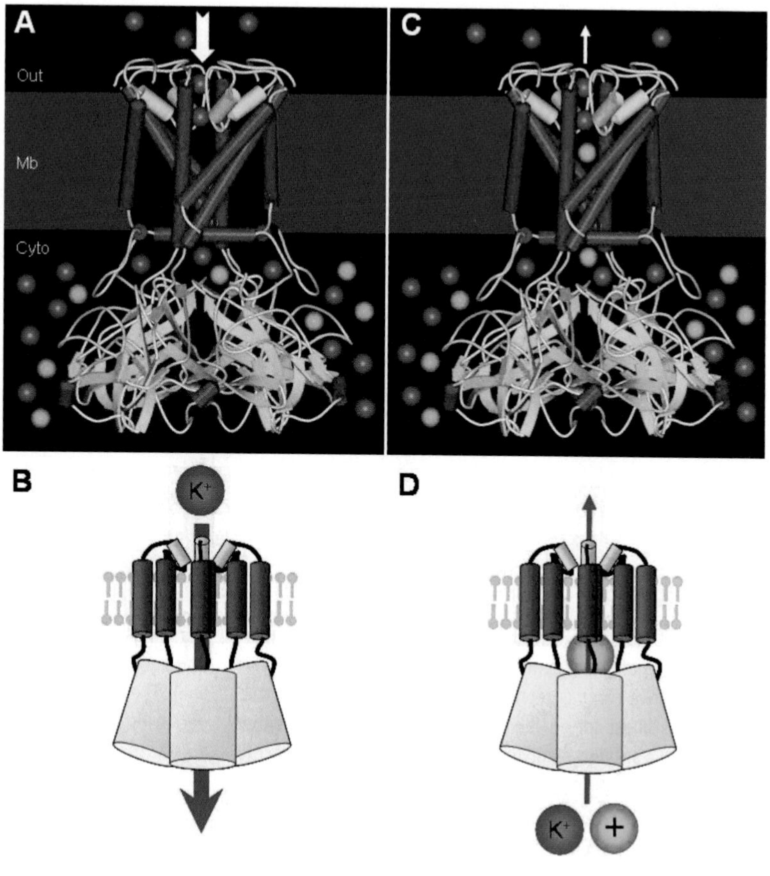

FIGURE 12–2. Molecular architecture of inwardly rectifying K^+ channels. Four Kir proteins assemble to form a pore (A–D). The core transmembrane structure of the pore consists of a rigid K^+ selectivity filter (yellow) and a cytoplasm-facing vestibule delimited by flexible helices involved in channel gating (red), and is rather conserved among K^+ channels. Inwardly rectifying channels possess a large cytoplasmic domain (blue) that forms a pore extension important for inward rectification. At hyperpolarized potentials, K^+ ions can move freely from the extracellular to the intracellular milieu (A and B). At depolarized potentials, the electrochemical gradient drives cations into the pore, K^+ ions (purple) but also polyamines and Mg^{2+} (green) that dock tightly to negative charges within the cytoplasmic extension and the inner vestibule, and impede outward K^+ flux. (A and B) The predicted molecular structure of Kir6.2 constructed by homology modeling from the crystallographic structure of the bacterial KirBac1.1 channel. (From Kuo *et al.*[23])

several acidic and hydrophobic amino acids along the inner wall of the cytoplasmic pore that create a favorable docking environment for polyamines.[27] Rectification properties are considered static and are determined by the amino acid sequence of a given channel, although they may also be dynamically regulated by environmental conditions.[28]

A prototype of a weakly rectifying channel, Kir6.2, allows considerable outward current at depolarized potentials, whereas strongly rectifying channels, such as Kir2.1 and Kir3.x, significantly prevent ion permeation in the outward direction (Figure 12–3).[20,25] These observations correlate with the distinct identity of a few key rectification residues within the amino acid sequence of each of these proteins, implying that the permeation pathways of Kir channels conform to the same structural blueprint with minor evolutionary alterations.

Beyond this common architecture, divergences in channel function arise from structural differences in the large cytoplasmic domains of the Kir proteins, which harbor specific binding sites for cytosolic effectors, such as nucleotides for IK_{ATP} and G-proteins for IK_{ACh}. Divergences also stem from different multimeric assemblies. IK_1 channels are predominantly homotetramers of Kir2.1 proteins.[29] In the heart, the K_{ACh} channel is a Kir3.1/Kir3.4 heterotetramer,[30,31] while the K_{ATP} channel is typically built as a Kir6.2 homotetramer surrounded by four *ABCC9*-encoded SUR2A proteins that act as regulatory subunits (Figure 12–4).[32] In the case of Kir6.2/SUR2A, tetramers of Kir6.2 subunits comprise the pore of K_{ATP} channel complexes, but pore-forming Kir6.2 subunits cannot readily traffic to the plasma membrane, without the regulatory SUR module, due to a C-terminal RKR endoplasmic reticulum retention signal.[33–35]

Function

Kir2.1 = IK_1

Kir2.1 channels and associated IK_1 current are abundant in atria and ventricle, where they set the resting membrane potential and regulate cellular excitability.[35] Indeed, the principle underlying the functional role of any ion channel, including

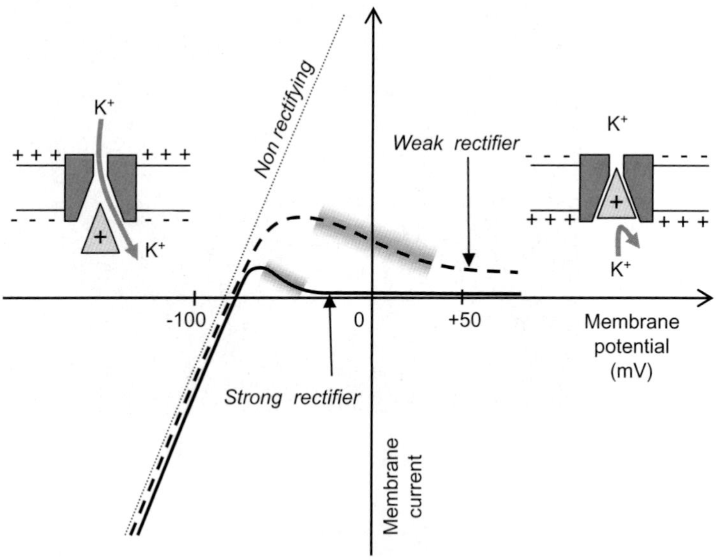

FIGURE 12–3. Idealized current–voltage relationships for channels displaying different degrees of inward rectification. By convention, positive currents represent ions moving out of the cell. The curve is linear for an ideal nonrectifying "ohmic" channel (dotted line). A strongly rectifying channel behaves like an electric diode, and allows little or no outward ion flux (solid line). A weakly rectifying channel has an intermediate behavior, allowing reduced but significant outward current at depolarized potentials (solid line). The "negative slope conductance" regions, where current decreases as potential becomes more positive, are shown as gray areas.

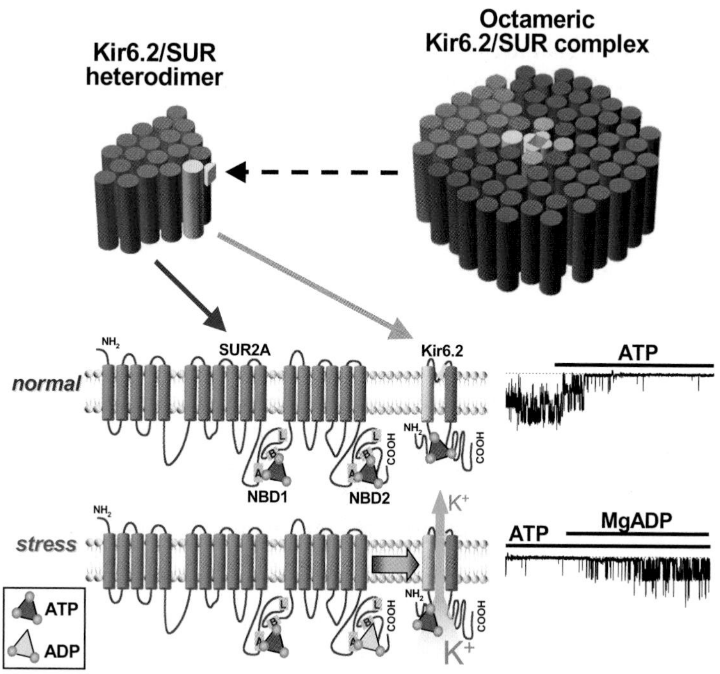

FIGURE 12–4. Cardiac K_{ATP} channels are heteromultimers composed of the *ABCC9*-encoded SUR2A subunit (containing nucleotide-binding domains NBD1/NBD2 with Walker A/B motifs and linker L region) and the *KCNJ11*-encoded Kir6.2 pore. Intracellular ATP normally keeps K_{ATP} channels closed. Stress-induced build-up of MgADP at NBD2 of SUR2A antagonizes ATP-induced channel inhibition, promoting K^+ efflux. Original patch-clamp recordings demonstrate nucleotide-dependent gating of K_{ATP} channels.

Kir2.1 channels, is their fundamental aptitude to bring and maintain the membrane potential to values that are close to the reversal potential for the conducting ion. In this way, Kir2.1 channel closure, due to time-independent inward rectification, allows nonpotassium channels to initiate membrane depolarization essential for cardiac excitation–contraction coupling. IK_1 current, with no significant K^+ outflow between −50 and 0 mV, allows membrane depolarization following sodium channel activation, and does not interfere with calcium channel activity during the action potential plateau. During the late phase of the action potential, a progressive increase in Kir2.1 conductance, as the membrane potential decreases and reaches the −30 to −80 mV negative slope conductance range (Figure 12–3), accelerates repolarization.[36,37] This mechanism explains the steep repolarization phase in ventricles, where IK_1 is particularly prominent, and the more shallow phase in atria, where IK_1 is less abundant.[38] While IK_1 mediates the outflow of K^+ during the terminal phase of atrial and ventricular action potential repolarization, this current is almost nonexistent in sinoatrial node cells, allowing for a relatively depolarized resting membrane potential compared to atrial or ventricular cardiomyocytes.[39] Studies of Kir2.1 knockout or overexpressing mice, antisense oligonucleotide targeting of Kir2.1, and plasmid transfection with a dominant-negative construct have collectively provided definitive evidence for the essential role of IK_1 in cardiac excitability. IK_1 is not detectable in myocytes isolated from neonatal Kir2.1 knockouts, and action potentials are significantly broader than those of wild-type mice.[29] Lack of IK_1 disrupts effective clamping of the resting membrane potential, precipitating spontaneous action potential activity in otherwise nonpacemaking cardiac cells. While overexpression of IK_1 hyperpolarizes, suppression of I_{K1} depolarizes the resting membrane potential. Accordingly, while greater IK_1 current shortens, suppression of IK_1 prolongs action potential duration at 90% of repolarization.[40] Indeed, overexpression of a dominant-negative Kir2.1 decreases IK_1, reducing the rate of change in membrane potential during the final phase of repolarization.[40] On electrocardiograms, overexpression of IK_1 results in a shorter QT interval, whereas suppression of IK_1 leads to a long QT phenotype.[37]

Kir6.2/SUR2A = K_{ATP}

Kir6.2, the K^+ conducting pore, and SUR2A, the regulatory ATP-binding cassette protein, form cardiac K_{ATP} channels gated by cellular energetic metabolism.[41] Under metabolic surplus, the cardiac K_{ATP} channel responds by closure, while metabolic challenge provokes channel opening with consequent K^+ efflux, action potential shortening, and limitation of potentially damaging intracellular Ca^{2+} loading.[42] The gating of the K_{ATP} channel reflects the balance at the channel site of inhibitory and stimulatory nucleotides, ATP and ADP, respectively (Figure 12–4). Kir6.2 is the principal site of ATP-induced channel inhibition, while SUR2A regulates K^+ flux through adenine nucleotide binding and catalysis.[32,43,44] Readout of the cellular metabolic state involves delivery of nucleotide signals to the K_{ATP} channel subunits and nucleotide interactions with specialized channel domains that secure signal translation into pore gating.[42] The cooperative interaction of nucleotide binding domains and the ATPase-driven conformations within SUR2A defines nucleotide-dependent K_{ATP} channel regulation.[45,46] Integration of K_{ATP} channels with the cellular energetic network, facilitated through phosphotransfer enzyme-mediated transmission of energetic signals, renders K_{ATP} channels high-fidelity metabolic sensors.[47–49] In this way, K_{ATP} channels mediate a homeostatic response to the metabolic insults of ischemia or hypoxia, contributing to a cardioprotective outcome.[50,51] Recent studies indicate an even broader function for cardiac K_{ATP} channels in providing tolerance to sympathetic surge and physical training, protecting against cellular injury and/or arrhythmia.[52–54] In fact, K_{ATP} channels have now been identified as critical endogenous elements for cardiac adaptation not only in the ischemic myocardium,[50] but also in the "flight-or-fight" response[52] and heart failure.[55,56] Mutations that disrupt K_{ATP} channel function[13] and/or defects in signaling pathways proximal to the channel site[57] are now established mechanisms for compromise of the channel's ability to optimally respond to metabolic challenge.

Inwardly Rectifying Potassium Channels in Human Disease

Andersen Cardiodysrhythmic Periodic Paralysis Syndrome

Andersen cardiodysrhythmic periodic paralysis syndrome, also known as Andersen syndrome, Andersen–Tawil syndrome, or long QT 7 syndrome (OMIM #170390, Online Mendelian Inheritance in Man database, National Center for Biotechnology Information), is an autosomal dominant genetic disorder characterized by a clinical triad of potassium-sensitive periodic paralysis, ventricular ectopy, and dysmorphic features.[58] The skeletal muscle phenotype involves abnormal muscle relaxation associated with weakness and tubular aggregates on histopathology. The cardiac arrhythmogenic phenotype manifests as variable prolongation of the QT interval, adrenergically mediated multifocal ventricular ectopy, ventricular bigeminy, and short runs of ventricular tachycardia. Developmental dysmorphology includes short stature, scoliosis, clinodactyly, hypertelorism, low-set small ears, micrognathia, and a broad forehead.

Significant genetic linkage of the disease locus for Andersen syndrome was found on the long arm of chromosome 17 that overlapped the *KCNJ2* gene locus (region 17q23.1–q24.2), encoding Kir2.1.[10] Mutations in *KCNJ2* have been identified in >50% of patients with Andersen syndrome, and allelic heterogeneity indicated by the discovery of >20 distinct missense mutations reported in the heterozygous state.[59,60] Heterologous expression of mutant Kir2.1 channel subunits has revealed a loss of channel function, with a dominant-negative effect of mutant subunits on wild-type protein resulting in a large reduction of IK_1 current or abnormal binding of phosphatidylinositol-4,5-bisphosphate (PIP_2) at the cytoplasmic C-terminus of Kir2.1 subunits, required for regular Kir2.1 channel activity.[10,61,62] *KCNJ2* loss-of-function mutations that reduce IK_1 current decelerate action potential repolarization, prolong action potential duration, and, by depolarizing and destabilizing the resting membrane potential, are proarrhythmogenic and cause myotonic skeletal muscle contractions. Moreover, the dysmorphic phenotypic spectrum of Andersen syndrome patients indicates that Kir2.1 dysfunction and IK_1 reduction also impair developmental signaling in nonmuscle tissues.[60]

Short QT Syndrome

Short QT syndrome is an inheritable primary electrical disease of the heart.[63] The disorder is characterized by an abnormally short QT interval (<300 msec) and a propensity for accelerated ventricular and/or atrial repolarization. Patients with short QT syndrome have a high risk for ventricular and/or atrial fibrillation and sudden death. Shortening of the effective refractory period combined with increased dispersion of repolarization is the likely substrate for reentry and life-threatening tachyarrhythmias predisposing to cardiovascular collapse.[63]

The short QT syndrome is genetically heterogeneous as its clinical and genetic counterpart, the long QT syndrome.[60] Both syndromes reflect the extremes of cardiac repolarization defects attributable to potassium channel mutations. The original forms of the short QT syndrome, SQT1 (OMIM #609620) and SQT2 (OMIM #609621), were linked to gain-of-function amino acid substitutions in noninwardly rectifying potassium channels, i.e., hERG (I_{Kr}) and KvLQT1 (I_{Ks}) encoded by *KCNH2* and *KCNQ1*, respectively.[64,65] The third subtype, SQT3 (OMIM #609622), which displays a unique electrocardiographic phenotype characterized by asymmetrical T waves, has been associated with a defect in the *KCNJ2* gene coding for Kir2.1.[11] The identified missense mutation in SQT3 replaces the key rectification residue at position 172, aspartic acid, with asparagine (D172N) attenuating rectification, widening the negative slope conductance range and increasing the outward current.[11] Overexpression of Kir2.1 by gene transfer generates significantly shorter action potential duration due to accelerated terminal repolarization, translating into abbreviated QT intervals that provide a substrate for the disease-associated SQT3 phenotype.[40] This is in contrast to loss of Kir2.1 channel function mutations that tend to induce a prolonged QT interval, as observed in Andersen syndrome. The most effective treatment of short QT syndrome is implantation of a cardioverter defibrillator for prevention of sudden cardiac death.[66]

Atrial Fibrillation

Atrial fibrillation is characterized by rapid and irregular electrical activation of the atrium, and is traditionally viewed as an acquired disorder attributable to structural heart disease in patients with comorbidities. However, recognition of familial aggregation has more recently implicated a heritable basis for atrial fibrillation.[67] A primary genetic defect is particularly likely in familial cases of early-onset lone atrial fibrillation. In this regard, gain-of-function mutations in the *KCNQ1* and *KCNE2* genes,[68,69] encoding subunits of the cardiac voltage-dependent channel I_{Ks}, were the first molecular defects identified as a cause for atrial fibrillation, based on action potential shortening and proarrhythmogenic reduction in the refractory period (OMIM #607554). More recently, identification of a loss-of-function mutation in *KCNA5*, encoding the voltage-dependent Kv1.5 channel, has provided an alternate mechanism for atrial fibrillation.[70] Kv1.5 channelopathy increased the propensity for prolongation of action potential duration, providing a substrate for triggered activity in the human atrium.[70]

With regard to the involvement of Kir channels in disease pathogenesis, a valine-to-isoleucine substitution at position 93 (V93I) of *KCNJ2*-encoded Kir2.1 was found in atrial fibrillation, and was proposed to a role in initiating and/or maintaining arrhythmia.[12] This residue and its flanking region are highly conserved, with functional analysis demonstrating gain-of-function in mutant Kir2.1 channels. This effect is similar to that observed in short QT syndrome and is opposite to the loss-of-function effect of previously reported *KCNJ2* mutations in Andersen's syndrome. The significance of Kir channels in atrial fibrillation is further underscored by the recent report of a K_{ATP} channel mutation conferring risk for adrenergic atrial fibrillation originating from the vein of Marshall.[14] The vein of Marshall, a remnant of the left superior vena cava rich in sympathetic fibers, is a recognized source for adrenergic atrial fibrillation. Genetic investigation uncovered a missense mutation (T1547I) in the *ABCC9* gene, encoding the regulatory subunit of cardiac K_{ATP} channels. Structural modeling of mutant K_{ATP} channels predicted, and patch-clamp electrophysiology demonstrated, compromised function with defective stress responsiveness. Targeted knockout of the K_{ATP} channel verified the pathogenic link between channel dysfunction and predisposition to adrenergic atrial fibrillation. In this first report of genetic susceptibility to the adrenergic vein of Marshall atrial fibrillation, radiofrequency ablation was curative, disrupting the gene–environment substrate for arrhythmia conferred by K_{ATP} channelopathy.[14]

Dilated Cardiomyopathy with Ventricular Tachycardia

Dilated cardiomyopathy is an idiopathic form of heart failure characterized by ventricular dilation and reduced contractile function. This phenotype may occur as an isolated trait or in association with rhythm disorder. It has been recognized that dilated cardiomyopathy is familial in >20% of cases, and over 20 distinct genes have so far been linked to the heritable form of the disease.[71] The ontological spectrum of dilated cardiomyopathy-associated mutant genes has traditionally included those encoding contractile (e.g., actin), cytoskeletal (e.g., dystrophin), or nuclear (e.g., lamin A/C) proteins, and was more recently expanded to the distinct class of proteins (e.g., phospholamban) that regulates ion homeostasis. This later group includes the K_{ATP} channel, as mutations in the *ABCC9*-encoded regulatory channel subunit SUR2A have been demonstrated in a subset of patients with dilated cardiomyopathy and ventricular arrhythmia.[13] The identified missense and frameshift mutations were mapped to domains bordering the catalytic ATPase pocket within SUR2A. Mutant SUR2A proteins reduced the intrinsic channel ATPase activity, altering reaction kinetics, and translating into dysfunctional channel phenotype with impaired metabolic signal decoding and processing capabilities. These data implicate a link between mutations in the cardioprotective K_{ATP} channel and susceptibility to myopathic disease and electrical instability.[13] Dilated cardiomyopathy with ventricular tachycardia due to *ABCC9* K_{ATP} channel mutations has been designated CMD10 (OMIM #608569) to distinguish this entity from other etiologies causing this heterogeneous condition.

Acknowledgments. This work was supported by grants from the National Institutes of Health, Marriott Heart Disease Research Program, Marriott Foundation, Ted Nash Long Life Foundation, and Ralph Wilson Medical Research Foundation.

References

1. Ashcroft FM. From molecule to malady. *Nature* 2006;440:440–447.
2. Ackerman MJ. Cardiac channelopathies: It's in the genes. *Nat Med* 2004;10:463–464.
3. Priori SG, Napolitano C. Role of genetic analyses in cardiology: Cardiac channelopathies. *Circulation* 2006;113:1130–1135.
4. Kubo Y, Adelman JP, Clapham DE, Jan LY, Karschin A, Kurachi Y, Lazdunski M, Nichols CG, Seino S, Vandenberg CA. Nomenclature and molecular relationships of inwardly rectifying potassium channels. *Pharmacol Rev* 2005;57:509–526.
5. Bichet D, Haass FA, Jan LY. Merging functional studies with structures of inward rectifier K^+ channels. *Nat Rev Neurosci* 2003;4:957–967.
6. Abraham MR, Jahangir A, Alekseev AE, Terzic A. Channelopathies of inwardly rectifying potassium channels. *FASEB J* 1999;13:1901–1910.
7. Ashcroft FM. ATP-sensitive potassium channelopathies: Focus on insulin secretion. *J Clin Invest* 2005; 115:2047–2058.
8. Marban E. Cardiac channelopathies. *Nature* 2002; 415:213–218.
9. Charpentier F, Demolombe S, Escande D. Cardiac channelopathies: From men to mice. *Ann Med* 2004;36:28–34.
10. Plaster N, Tawil R, Tristani-Firouzi M, Canun S, Bendahhou S, Tsunoda A, Donaldson M, Iannaccone S, Brunt E, Barohn R, Clark J, Deymeer F, George AL, Fish F, Hahn A, Nitu A, Ozdemir C, Serdaroglu P, Subramony S, Wolfe G, Fu Y, Ptacek L. Mutations in Kir2.1 cause the developmental and episodic electrical phenotypes of Andersen's syndrome. *Cell* 2001;105:511–519.
11. Priori SG, Pandit SV, Rivolta I, Berenfeld O, Ronchetti E, Dhamoon A, Napolitano C, Anumonwo J, Raffaele dB, Gudapakkam S, Bosi G, Stramba-Badiale M, Jalife J. A novel form of short QT syndrome (SQT3) is caused by a mutation in the *KCNJ2* gene. *Circ Res* 2005;96:800–807.
12. Xia M, Jin Q, Bendahhou S, He Y, Larroque MM, Chen Y, Zhou Q, Yang Y, Liu Y, Liu B, Zhu Q, Zhou Y, Lin J, Liang B, Li L, Dong X, Pan Z, Wang R, Wan H, Qiu W, Xu W, Eurlings P, Barhanin J, Chen Y. A Kir2.1 gain-of-function mutation underlies familial atrial fibrillation. *Biochem Biophys Res Commun* 2005;332:1012–1019.
13. Bienengraeber M, Olson TM, Selivanov VA, Kathmann EC, O'Cochlain F, Gao F, Karger AB, Ballew JD, Hodgson DM, Zingman LV, Pang YP, Alekseev AE, Terzic A. *ABCC9* mutations identified in human dilated cardiomyopathy disrupt catalytic K_{ATP} channel gating. *Nat Genet* 2004;36:382–387.
14. Olson TM, Alekseev AE, Moreau C, Liu XK, Zingman LV, Miki T, Seino S, Asirvatham SJ, Jahangir A, Terzic A. K_{ATP} channel mutation confers risk for adrenergic atrial fibrillation originating from the vein of Marshall. *Nat Clin Pract Cardiovasc Med* 2007;4:110–116.
15. Katz B. Les constantes electriques de la membrane du muscle. *Arch Sci Physiol* 1949;2:285–299.
16. Jan LY, Jan YN. Cloned potassium channels from eukaryotes and prokaryotes. *Annu Rev Neurosci* 1997;20:91–123.

17. Kubo Y, Baldwin TJ, Jan YN, Jan LY. Primary structure and functional expression of a mouse inward rectifier potassium channel. *Nature* 1993;362:127–133.
18. Kubo Y, Reuveny E, Slesinger P, Jan Y, Jan LY. Primary structure and functional expression of a rat G-protein-coupled muscarinic potassium channel. *Nature* 1993;364:802–806.
19. Inagaki N, Gonoi T, Clement JP, Namba N, Inazawa J, Gonzalez G, Aguilar-Bryan L, Seino S, Bryan J. Reconstitution of IK_{ATP}: An inward rectifier subunit plus the sulfonylurea receptor. *Science* 1995;270:1166–1170.
20. Nichols CG, Lopatin AN. Inward rectifier potassium channels. *Annu Rev Physiol* 1997;59:171–191.
21. Isomoto S, Kondo C, Kurachi Y. Inwardly rectifying potassium channels: Their molecular heterogeneity and function. *Jpn J Physiol* 1997;47:11–39.
22. Doyle DA, Morais CJ, Pfuetzner RA, Kuo A, Gulbis JM, Cohen SL, Chait BT, MacKinnon R. The structure of the potassium channel: Molecular basis of K^+ conduction and selectivity. *Science* 1998;280:69–77.
23. Kuo AL, Gulbis JM, Antcliff JF, Rahman T, Lowe ED, Zimmer J, Cuthbertson J, Ashcroft FM, Ezaki T, Doyle DA. Crystal structure of the potassium channel KirBac1.1 in the closed state. *Science* 2003;300:1922–1926.
24. Smith PL, Baukrowitz T, Yellen G. The inward rectification mechanism of the HERG cardiac potassium channel. *Nature* 1996;379:833–836.
25. Lu Z. Mechanism of rectification in inward rectifier K^+ channels. *Annu Rev Physiol* 2004;66:103–129.
26. Lopatin AN, Makhina EN, Nichols CG. Potassium channel block by cytoplasmic polyamines as the mechanism of intrinsic rectification. *Nature* 1994;372:366–369.
27. Nishida M, MacKinnon R. Structural basis of inward rectification: Cytoplasmic pore of the G protein-gated inward rectifier GIRK1 at 1.8 angstrom resolution. *Cell* 2002;111:957–965.
28. Baukrowitz T, Tucker S, Schulte U, Benndorf K, Ruppersberg JP, Fakler B. Inward rectification in K_{ATP} channels: A pH switch in the pore. *EMBO J* 1999;18:848–853.
29. Zaritsky JJ, Redell JB, Tempel BL, Schwarz TL. The consequences of disrupting cardiac inwardly rectifying K^+ current (IK_1) as revealed by the targeted deletion of the murine Kir2.1 and Kir2.2 genes. *J Physiol* 2001;533:697–710.
30. Krapivinsky G, Gordon EA, Wickman K, Velimirovic B, Krapivinsky L, Clapham DE. The G-protein-gated atrial K^+ channel IK_{ACh} is a heteromultimer of two inwardly rectifying K^+-channel proteins. *Nature* 1995;374:135–141.
31. Corey S, Krapivinsky G, Krapivinsky L, Clapham DE. Number and stoichiometry of subunits in the native atrial G-protein-gated K^+ channel, IK_{ACh}. *J Biol Chem* 1998;273:5271–5278.
32. Mikhailov MV, Campbell JD, de-Wet H, Shimomura K, Zadek B, Collins RF, Sansom MS, Ford RC, Ashcroft FM. 3-D structural and functional characterization of the purified K_{ATP} channel complex Kir6.2-SUR1. *EMBO J* 2005;24:4166–4175.
33. Inagaki N, Gonoi T, Clement JP, Wang CZ, Aguilar-Bryan L, Bryan J, Seino S. A family of sulfonylurea receptors determines the pharmacological properties of ATP-sensitive K^+ channels. *Neuron* 1996;16:1011–1017.
34. Aguilar-Bryan L, Clement JP IV, Gonzalez G, Kunjilwar K, Babenko A, Bryan J. Toward understanding the assembly and structure of K_{ATP} channels. *Physiol Rev* 1998;78:227–245.
35. Zerangue N, Schwappach B, Jan Y, Jan L. A new ER trafficking signal regulates the subunit stoichiometry of plasma membrane K_{ATP} channels. *Neuron* 1999;22;537–548.
36. Lopatin AN, Nichols CG. Inward rectifiers in the heart: An update on I_{K1}. J *Mol Cell Cardiol* 2001;33:625–638.
37. Dhamoon AS, Jalife J. The inward rectifier current IK_1 controls cardiac excitability and is involved in arrhythmogenesis. *Heart Rhythm* 2005;2:316–324.
38. Giles WR, Imaizumi Y. Comparison of potassium currents in rabbit atrial and ventricular cells. *J Physiol* 1988;405:123–145.
39. Schram G, Pourrier M, Melnyk P, Nattel S. Differential distribution of cardiac ion channel expression as a basis for regional specialization in electrical function. *Circ Res* 2002;90:939–950.
40. Miake J, Marban E, Nuss HB. Functional role of inward rectifier current in heart probed by Kir2.1 overexpression and dominant-negative suppression. *J Clin Invest* 2003;111:1529–1536.
41. Nichols CG. K_{ATP} channels as molecular sensors of cellular metabolism. *Nature* 2006;440:470–476.
42. Alekseev AE, Hodgson D, Karger A, Park S, Zingman LV, Terzic A. ATP-sensitive K^+ channel channel/enzyme multimer: Metabolic gating in the heart. *J Mol Cell Cardiol* 2005;38:895–905.
43. Tucker SJ, Gribble FM, Zhao C, Trapp S, Ashcroft FM. Truncation of Kir6.2 produces ATP-sensitive K^+ channels in the absence of the sulphonylurea receptor. *Nature* 1997;387:179–183.
44. Bienengraeber M, Alekseev AE, Abraham MR, Carrasco AJ, Moreau C, Vivaudou M, Dzeja PP, Terzic A. ATPase activity of the sulfonylurea

receptor: A catalytic function for the K_{ATP} channel complex. *FASEB J* 2000;14:1943–1952.
45. Zingman LV, Alekseev AE, Bienengraeber M, Hodgson D, Karger AB, Dzeja PP, Terzic A. Signaling in channel/enzyme multimers: ATPase transitions in SUR module gate ATP-sensitive K^+ conductance. *Neuron* 2001;31:233–245.
46. Zingman LV, Hodgson DM, Bienengraeber M, Karger AB, Kathmann EC, Alekseev AE, Terzic A. Tandem function of nucleotide binding domains confers competence to sulfonylurea receptor in gating ATP-sensitive K^+ channels. *J Biol Chem* 2002; 277:14206–14210.
47. Carrasco AJ, Dzeja PP, Alekseev AE, Pucar D, Zingman LV, Abraham MR, Hodgson D, Bienengraeber M, Puceat M, Janssen E, Wieringa B, Terzic A. Adenylate kinase phosphotransfer communicates cellular energetic signals to ATP-sensitive potassium channels. *Proc Natl Acad Sci USA* 2001; 98:7623–7628.
48. Abraham MR, Selivanov VA, Hodgson DM, Pucar D, Zingman LV, Wieringa B, Dzeja PP, Alekseev AE, Terzic A. Coupling of cell energetics with membrane metabolic sensing: Integrative signaling through creatine kinase phosphotransfer disrupted by M-CK gene knock-out. *J Biol Chem* 2002;277: 24427–24434.
49. Selivanov VA, Alekseev AE, Hodgson DM, Dzeja PP, Terzic A. Nucleotide-gated K_{ATP} channels integrated with creatine and adenylate kinases: Amplification, tuning and sensing of energetic signals in the compartmentalized cellular environment. *Mol Cell Biochem* 2004;256–257:243–256.
50. Gumina RJ, Pucar D, Bast P, Hodgson DM, Kurtz CE, Dzeja PP, Miki T, Seino S, Terzic A. Knockout of Kir6.2 negates ischemic preconditioning-induced protection of myocardial energetics. *Am J Physiol* 2003;284:H2106–2113.
51. Kane GC, Liu XK, Yamada S, Olson TM, Terzic A. Cardiac K_{ATP} channels in health and disease. *J Mol Cell Cardiol* 2005;38:937–943.
52. Zingman LV, Hodgson DM, Bast PH, Kane GC, Perez-Terzic C, Gumina RJ, Pucar D, Bienengraeber M, Dzeja PP, Miki T, Seino S, Alekseev AE, Terzic A. Kir6.2 is required for adaptation to stress. *Proc Natl Acad Sci USA* 2002;99:13278–13283.
53. Kane GC, Behfar A, Yamada S, Perez-Terzic C, O'Cochlain F, Reyes S, Dzeja PP, Miki T, Seino S, Terzic A. ATP-sensitive K^+ channel knockout compromises the metabolic benefit of exercise training, resulting in cardiac deficits. *Diabetes* 2004;53: S169–175.
54. Liu XK, Yamada S, Kane GC, Alekseev AE, Hodgson DM, O'Cochlain F, Jahangir A, Miki T, Seino S, Terzic A. Genetic disruption of Kir6.2 the pore-forming subunit of ATP-sensitive K^+ channel, predisposes to catecholamine-induced ventricular dysrhythmia. *Diabetes* 2004;53: S165–168.
55. Kane GC, Behfar A, Dyer RB, O'cochlain DF, Liu XK, Hodgson DM, Reyes S, Miki T, Seino S, Terzic A. *KCNJ11* gene knockout of the Kir6.2 K_{ATP} channel causes maladaptive remodeling and heart failure in hypertension. *Hum Mol Genet* 2006;15:2285–2297.
56. Yamada S, Kane GC, Behfar A, Liu X-K, Dyer RB, Faustino RS, Miki T, Seino S, Terzic A. Protection conferred by myocardial ATP-sensitive K^+ channels in pressure overload-induced congestive heart failure revealed in *KCNJ11* Kir6.2-null mutant. *J Physiol* 2006;577:1053–1065.
57. Hodgson DM, Zingman LV, Kane GC, Perez-Terzic C, Bienengraeber M, Ozcan C, Gumina RJ, Pucar D, O'Coclain F, Mann DL, Alekseev AE, Terzic A. Cellular remodeling in heart failure disrupts K_{ATP} channel-dependent stress tolerance. *EMBO J* 2003; 22:1732–1742.
58. Tawil R, Ptacek L J, Pavlakis SG, DeVivo DC, Penn AS, Ozdemir C, Griggs RC. Andersen's syndrome: Potassium-sensitive periodic paralysis, ventricular ectopy, and dysmorphic features. *Ann Neurol* 1994; 35:326–330.
59. Andelfinger G, Tapper AR, Welch RC, Vanoye CG, George AL Jr, Benson DW. KCNJ2 mutation results in Andersen syndrome with sex-specific cardiac and skeletal muscle phenotypes. *Am J Hum Genet* 2002;71:663–668.
60. Schulze-Bahr E. Short QT syndrome or Andersen syndrome: Yin and Yang of Kir2.1 channel dysfunction. *Circ Res* 2005;96:703–704.
61. Tristani-Firouzi M, Jensen JL, Donaldson MR, Sansone V, Meola G, Hahn A, Bendahhou S, Kwiecinski H, Fidzianska A, Plaster N, Fu Y-H, Ptacek LJ, Tawil R. Functional and clinical characterization of KCNJ2 mutations associated with LQT7 (Andersen syndrome). *J Clin Invest* 2002;110:381–388.
62. Lopes CMB, Zhang H, Rohacs T, Jin T, Yang J, Logothetis DE. Alterations in conserved Kir channel-PIP_2 interactions underlie channelopathies. *Neuron* 2002;34:933–944.
63. Bjerregaard P, Gussak I. Short QT syndrome: Mechanisms, diagnosis and treatment. *Nat Clin Pract Cardiovasc Med* 2005;2:84–87.
64. Brugada R, Hong K, Dumaine R, Cordeiro J, Gaita F, Borggrefe M, Menendez TM, Brugada J, Pollevick GD, Wolpert C, Burashnikov E, Matsuo K, Wu YS, Guerchicoff A, Bianchi F, Giustetto C, Schimpf R, Brugada P, Antzelevitch C. Sudden death associ-

ated with short-QT syndrome linked to mutations in HERG. *Circulation* 2004;109:30–35.
65. Bellocq C, van Ginneken AC, Bezzina CR, Alders M, Escande D, Mannens MM, Baro I, Wilde AA. Mutation in the KCNQ1 gene leading to the short QT-interval syndrome. *Circulation* 2004;109:2394–2397.
66. Bjerregaard P, Jahangir A, Gussak I. Targeted therapy for short QT syndrome. *Expert Opin Ther Targets* 2006;10:393–400.
67. Darbar D, Herron KJ, Ballew JD, Jahangir A, Gersh BJ, Shen WK, Hammill SC, Packer DL, Olson TM. Familial atrial fibrillation is a genetically heterogeneous disorder. *J Am Coll Cardiol* 2003;41:2185–2192.
68. Chen YH, Xu SJ, Bendahhou S, Wang XL, Wang Y, Xu WY, Jin HW, Sun H, Su XY, Zhuang QN, Yang YQ, Li YB, Liu Y, Xu HJ, Li XF, Ma N, Mou CP, Chen Z, Barhanin J, Huang W. KCNQ1 gain-of-function mutation in familial atrial fibrillation. *Science* 2003;299:251–254.
69. Yang Y, Xia M, Jin Q, Bendahhou S, Shi J, Chen Y, Liang B, Lin J, Liu Y, Liu B, Zhou Q, Zhang D, Wang R, Ma N, Su X, Niu K, Pei Y, Xu W, Chen Z, Wan H, Cui J, Barhanin J, Chen Y. Identification of a KCNE2 gain-of-function mutation in patients with familial atrial fibrillation. *Am J Hum Genet* 2004;75:899–905.
70. Olson TM, Alekseev AE, Liu XK, Park S, Zingman LV, Bienengraeber M, Sattiraju S, Ballew JD, Jahangir A, Terzic A. Kv1.5 channelopathy due to KCNA5 loss-of-function mutation causes human atrial fibrillation. *Hum Mol Genet* 2006;15:2185–2191.
71. Ahmad F, Seidman JG, Seidman CE. The genetic basis for cardiac remodeling. *Annu Rev Genomics Hum Genet* 2005;6:185–216.

13
Calcium Release Channels (Ryanodine Receptors) and Arrhythmogenesis

Subeena Sood and Xander H.T. Wehrens

Introduction

Intracellular calcium release channels (ryanodine receptors, RyR) are present on the sarcoplasmic reticulum (SR) in cardiomyocytes and are required for excitation–contraction (EC) coupling in cardiac muscle. Each RyR channel consists of four pore-forming subunits that contain large cytoplasmic domains, which serve as scaffolds for proteins that regulate the activity of the channel. An important regulatory protein is calstabin2 (FKBP12.6), a subunit that stabilizes the closed state of the channel to prevent aberrant calcium (Ca^{2+}) leak from the SR.[1] Direct targeting of several protein kinases and phosphatases to the type 2 cardiac RyR channel (RyR2) allows for rapid and localized modulation of SR Ca^{2+} release in response to extracellular signals.[2]

Recent studies have provided new mechanistic insight into the role of diastolic SR Ca^{2+} leak through RyR2 as a trigger of cardiac arrhythmias. Inherited mutations in the RyR2 gene have been linked to cardiac arrhythmia syndromes including catecholaminergic polymorphic ventricular tachycardia (CPVT, see also Chapter 37) and arrhythmogenic right ventricular cardiomyopathy (ARVD).[3–5] Moreover, defective regulation of RyRs may contribute to arrhythmogenesis in heart failure.[6,7] These findings have initiated the development of a new class of drugs called "calcium channel stabilizers" that specifically target these molecular defects, improve cardiac function, and prevent arrhythmias in relevant animal models.[8–11]

Excitation–Contraction Coupling in the Heart

The process of EC coupling involves a sequence of events that translates electrical membrane depolarization into contraction of the cardiomyocyte.[12] During cardiac muscle contraction (systole), Ca^{2+} is released from a network of intracellular Ca^{2+} stores referred to as the sarcoplasmic reticulum (Figure 13–1). When the heart subsequently relaxes to fill with blood (diastole), the cytoplasmic Ca^{2+} is actively pumped back into the SR. Cyclic release of Ca^{2+} from the SR Ca^{2+} store and Ca^{2+} uptake from the cytosol are thus critical for continuous performance of the heart.[13]

Depolarization of the cardiomyocyte membrane leads to activation of voltage-gated L-type Ca^{2+} channels (LTCC) located in plasma membrane invaginations called transverse or T-tubules (Figure 13–1). Entry of Ca^{2+} through LTCCs triggers a much greater release of Ca^{2+} from the SR via the RyR2 intracellular Ca^{2+} release channels, which is known as Ca^{2+}-induced Ca^{2+} release (CICR).[14] For relaxation to occur during diastole, Ca^{2+} is extruded from the cytoplasm via a specialized Ca^{2+} pump known as the SR Ca^{2+}-ATPase (SERCA2a). SERCA2a activity is regulated by phospholamban, which inhibits SR Ca^{2+} uptake in its nonphosphorylated form. Finally, cytosolic Ca^{2+} is also extruded from the cardiomyocyte via the electrogenic plasma membrane Na^+–Ca^{2+} exchanger (NCX).[13,15]

Advanced imaging techniques have revealed that cytosolic Ca^{2+} transients in cardiomyocytes represent the summation of 10^4 to 10^6 localized

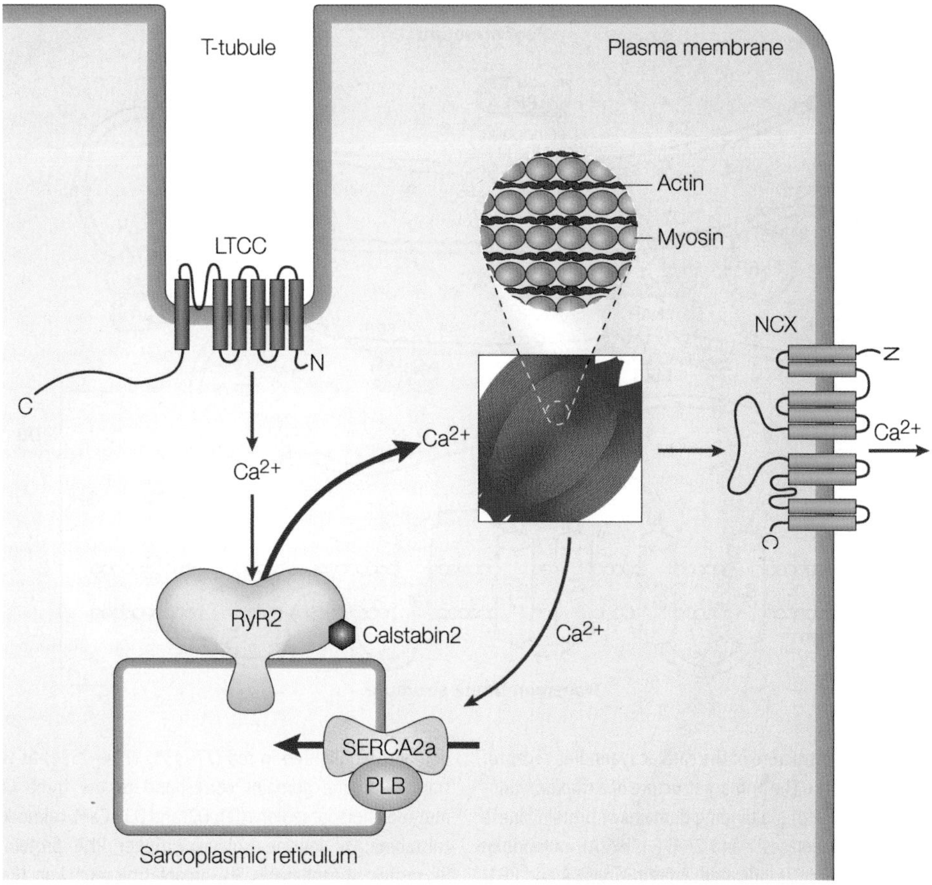

IGURE 13–1. Excitation–contraction coupling in the heart. xcitation–contraction coupling in cardiomyocytes involves epolarization of the transverse (T) tubule, which activates oltage-gated L-type Ca^{2+} channels (LTCC). The small influx of a^{2+} through LTCC triggers a much larger Ca^{2+} release from the arcoplasmic reticulum (SR) through ryanodine receptors (RyR2). The increase in cytoplasmic Ca^{2+} concentration induces muscle contraction. To enable relaxation, intracellular Ca^{2+} is returned into the SR via SR Ca^{2+}-ATPase (SERCA2a), which is regulated by phospholamban (PLB), or extruded from the cell via the Na^{+}–Ca^{2+} exchanger (NCX). (Reproduced with permission from Wehrens *et al.*[84])

ubcellular Ca^{2+} release events called Ca^{2+} sparks.[16] he CICR process amplifies and scales the intraclular Ca^{2+} signal via summation of functionally ndependent Ca^{2+} sparks.[17] Moreover, Ca^{2+} sparks re characterized by local refractoriness, suggestng that local SR Ca^{2+} release is independent of the uration of the LTCC-mediated Ca^{2+} influx.[18] It is stimated that about 100 or more RyR2 channels nay become functionally coupled in a Ca^{2+} release nit in order to open and close simultaneously by he process of coupled gating.[19] However, Ca^{2+} elease from the SR also results in local Ca^{2+} depleion in subcompartments of the SR Ca^{2+} stores.[20] herefore, the intrinsic (e.g., channel composition) and extrinsic (e.g., regulation by extracellular signals) properties of RyR2 channel gating are important determinants of the net Ca^{2+} concentration in the cytosol and the SR at any given time point during the cardiac contraction–relaxation cycle.

Cardiac Ryanodine Receptors

Ryanodine receptors are composed of four 560-kDa pore-forming subunits that form tetrameric ion channels located on the SR membranes.[21] RyR2 is the predominant isoform in the heart and

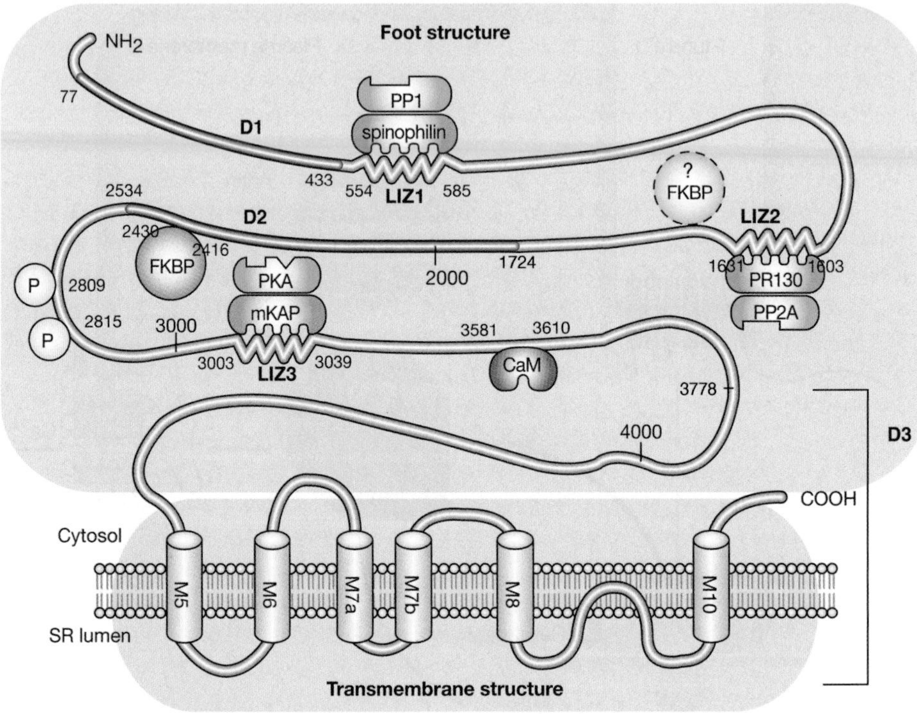

FIGURE 13–2. Primary structure of the cardiac ryanodine receptor macromolecular complex. The primary structure of a cardiac ryanodine receptor subunit, with the binding domains of protein kinase A (PKA), protein phosphatases 1 and 2A (PP1, PP2A), calmodulin and calstabin2 (FKBP12.6), is indicated. Protein kinase A and PP1/PP2A are bound to RyR2 via their specific adaptor proteins. The domains highlighted in red (77–433, 1724–2534) as well as th transmembrane domains correspond to the three CPVT/ARVD mutation hotspot regions (D1, D2, and D3). CaM, calmodulin; FKBP calstabin2; LIZ, leucine–isoleucine zipper; PKA, protein kinase A PP, protein phosphatases; SR, sarcoplasmic reticulum. (Reproduce with permission from Yano *et al.*,[87] Macmillan Publishers, Ltd.)

functions as the principal intracellular Ca^{2+} release channel during EC coupling.[22] Apart from a relatively small C-terminal pore-forming domain, approximately 90% of the RyR2 N-terminal sequence forms the electron-dense cytosolic foot structure in the junctional space between the T-tubule and the SR. This cytoplasmic RyR2 domain (Figure 13–2) functions as a scaffold for modulating proteins, which regulate gating of the transmembrane Ca^{2+}-conducting pore (for a more extensive review, see also Wehrens *et al.*[15]).

The Ryanodine Receptor Macromolecular Complex

A major regulatory subunit interacting with RyR2 calcium release channels is calstabin2, also known as the 12.6-kDa cytosolic FK506-binding protein (FKBP12.6).[23,24] Calstabin2, a peptidyl-prolyl *cis-trans* isomerase that tightly associates with RyR2 monomers, stabilizes the closed conformational state of RyR2, enabling the channel to close completely during diastolic.[25,26] Therefore in the heart an important physiological role of calstabin2 appears to be inhibiting the RyR2 channel at low intracellular Ca^{2+} concentrations to ensure muscle relaxation and preventing detrimental effects of intracellular Ca^{2+} leak during diastole.[11,26] In addition, calstabin2 plays a role in the orchestration of simultaneous RyR2 gating in Ca^{2+} release units composed of functionally linked RyR2.[19,27]

Other modulators associated with the large cytosolic RyR2 domain include calmodulin (CaM),[28] sorcin,[29] the protein kinases A (PKA) and Ca^{2+}/CaM-dependent kinase II (CaMKII),[30,3 and the phosphatases PP1 and PPA2A.[2] These kinases and phosphatases are targeted to RyR2 by the anchoring proteins mAKAP, spinophilin, and PR130 (Figure 13–2). Conserved leucine/isoleucine zipper (LIZ) motifs in the targeting proteins correspond to complementary LIZ domains in RyR2, allowing for highly localized RyR2 regulation.

Ryanodine receptors also associate with proteins at the luminal surface within the SR membrane. Junctin and triadin are most likely involved in anchoring RyR2 to the SR membrane.[32,33] Calsequestrin (CSQ) is the major Ca^{2+}-binding protein in the SR and provides a high capacity intra-SR Ca^{2+} buffer.[34] Recent studies suggest that Ca^{2+}-dependent conformational changes in CSQ modulate RyR2 channel activity, and that dysfunctional luminal regulation of RyR2 may lead to cardiac arrhythmias (see below).[35]

Phosphorylation-Dependent Regulation of RyR2 in the Heart

The maximal cardiac force development during systole (inotropy) can be enhanced by increasing the amplitude of the intracellular Ca^{2+} transient, which is dependent on the amount of intracellular Ca^{2+} released via RyR2.[36] Sustained upregulation of SR Ca^{2+} cycling is achieved by phosphorylation of proteins involved in SR Ca^{2+} release and Ca^{2+} uptake pathways by cAMP-dependent PKA,[6] CaMKII,[31] and protein kinase C (PKC).[37] The most potent mechanism to rapidly increase cardiac contractility is mediated by stress-mediated activation of β-adrenergic receptors by catecholamines resulting in increased intracellular cAMP synthesis and activation of PKA.[38] Protein kinase A phosphorylates both RyR2 to increase SR Ca^{2+} release,[2] as well as phospholamban to enhance activity of SERCA2a.[39] The net effect of β-adrenergic receptor activation is amplification of the EC coupling gain such that for any given LTCC Ca^{2+} current more SR Ca^{2+} release is triggered.[40]

Phosphorylation by PKA increases RyR2 channel open probability by increasing the sensitivity to Ca^{2+}-dependent activation.[6,26,41,42] PKA phosphorylates serine 2808 on RyR2, which results in transient dissociation of the channel-stabilizing protein calstabin2 and an increase in the sensitivity to Ca^{2+}-dependent activation.[6,43] Although some studies suggest PKA might phosphorylate an additional residue on RyR2 *in vitro*,[44] PKA phosphorylation of RyR2 is completely prevented in RyR2–S2808A knockin mice, in which serine 2808 is replaced by an alanine.[45] RyR2 channels can also be modulated by CaMKII, which phosphorylates a distinct site (serine 2814) on RyR2 and does not decrease the binding affinity of calstabin2.[31] CaMKII phosphorylation of RyR2 increases channel open probability, which is believed to increase cardiac output at higher heart rates (i.e., the staircase phenomenon).[31]

The transient nature of RyR2 activation by PKA phosphorylation in cells suggests powerful negative feedback mechanisms that prevent uncontrolled intracellular Ca^{2+} release. Indeed, RyR2 phosphorylation is locally regulated by protein phosphatases, which are targeted to the channel complex.[2,46] Moreover, we have found that the phosphodiesterase PDE4D3 associates with RyR2, limiting excessive phosphorylation of the channel, which has been shown to detrimentally affect cardiac function in disease states of the heart.[47]

Mutations in RyR2 Linked to Cardiac Arrhythmias

In humans, two distinct clinical syndromes causing exercise-induced sudden cardiac death, catecholaminergic polymorphic ventricular tachycardia type 1 (CPVT-1) and arrhythmogenic right ventricular cardiomyopathy/dysplasia type 2 (ARVD-2), have been linked to mutations in the human *RyR2* gene (see Table 13–1).[3–5] Unlike ARVD, which is associated with progressive degeneration of the right ventricular myocardium, CPVT is not characterized by structural heart degeneration. The *RyR2* mutations linked to CPVT-1 and ARVD-2 cluster in three domains of the channel, corresponding to similar mutation domains in the type 1 ryanodine receptor (RyR1) linked to malignant hyperthermia and central core disease (Figure 13–2).

Catecholaminergic Polymorphic Ventricular Tachycardia

Patients with CPVT characteristically develop arrhythmias during exercise or emotional stress (see also Chapter 37). Clinical electrophysiological

TABLE 13–1. Mutations in the cardiac ryanodine receptor (RyR2) gene associated with CPVT and ARVD-2.[a]

Amino acid	Nucleotide	Disease	Number of probands	Domain	Reference
A77V	230 C > T	ARVD-2/CPVT	1	D1	48, 49
R176Q	527 G > A	ARVD-2	1	D1	3
R414C	1361 T > C	CPVT	1	D1	50
R414L	1241 A > T	CPVT	1	D1	51
I419F	1255 A > T	CPVT	1	D1	51
R420W	1258 C > T	ARVD-2	3	D1	52, 53
L433P	1298 T > C	ARVD-2	1	D1	3
P466A	1396C > G	CPVT	1	D1	51
E1724K	N/A	CPVT	1	D2	54
S2246L	6737 C > T	CPVT	4	D2	4, 53, 55
A2254V	N/A	CPVT	1	D2	54
V2306I	6916 G > A	CPVT	1	D2	56
E2311D	N/A	CPVT	1	D2	55
P2328S	6982 C > T	CPVT	1	D2	5
F2331S	7113 T > C	CPVT	1	D2	50
A2394G	N/A	CPVT	1	D2	54
N2386I	7157 A > T	ARVD-2	2	D2	3
A2387T	7158 G > A	CPVT	1	D2	51
A2387P	7159 G > C	CPVT	1	D2	57
Y2392C	7175 A > G	ARVD-2	1	D2	52
R2401H	7202 G > A	CPVT	1	D2	58
R2401L	7323 G > T	CPVT	1	D2	50
A2403T	7207 G > A	CPVT	1	D2	51
R2474S	7422 G > C	CPVT	1	D2	4
T2504M	7511 C > T	ARVD-2	1	D2	3
L2534V	N/A	CPVT	1	D2	59
L3778F	11332 C > T	CPVT	1	D3	55
C3800F	11399 G > T	CPVT	1	D3	51
G3946S	11836 G > A	CPVT	2	D3	55
F4020L	N/A	CPVT	1	D3	54
E4076K	N/A	CPVT	2	D3	54
N4097S	12290 A > G	CPVT	1	D3	53
N4104K	12312 C > G	CPVT	1	D3	4
N4104I	N/A	CPVT	1	D3	54
H4108N	N/A	CPVT	1	D3	54
H4108Q	N/A	CPVT	1	D3	54
S4124T	12371 G > C	CPVT	1	D3	51
E4146K	12436 G > A	CPVT	1	D3	53
T4158P	12472 A > C	CPVT	1	D3	53
Q4201R	12601 C > A	CPVT	1	D3	5
R4497C	13610 C > T	CPVT	2	D3	4, 53
F4499C	13496 T > G	CPVT	1	D3	51
M4504I	13512 G > A	CPVT	1	D3	57
A4510T	13528 G > A	CPVT	1	D3	51
A4556T	13666 G > A	CPVT	1	D3	51
A4607P	13819 G > C	CPVT	1	D3	57
V4653F	13957 A > G	CPVT	1	D3	5
Ins (EY4657–4658)	Dupl 13967–13972	CPVT	1	D3	51
G4662S	N/A	CPVT	1	D3	54
G4671R	14010 G > C	CPVT	1	D3	51
H4762P	N/A	CPVT	2	D3	54
V4771I	14311 G > A	CPVT	1	D3	54, 55
I4848V	14542 A > G	CPVT	2	D3	51
A4860G	14579 C > G	CPVT	1	D3	55
I4867M	14601 T > G	CPVT	1	D3	55
V4880A	14639 T > C	CPVT	1	D3	57
N4895D	N/A	CPVT	1	D3	55
P4902L	14705 C > T	CPVT	1	D3	56
P4902S	N/A	CPVT	1	D3	54
E4950K	14848 G > A	CPVT	1	D3	55
R4959Q	14876 G > A	CPVT	4	D3	51, 56, 60

[a]CPVT, catecholaminergic polymorphic ventricular tachycardia; ARVD-2, arrhythmogenic right ventricular cardiomyopathy/dysplasia type 2.

studies of patients with *RyR2* mutations have revealed that CPVT can be induced by catecholamine infusion, but typically not by programmed electrical stimulation.[55,61] These clinical findings strongly suggest that catecholamine-sensitive automaticity functions as a cellular mechanism of CPVT.

Cerrone *et al.*[62] developed a knockin mouse model of the RyR2–R4496C mutation, the mouse equivalent of the R4497C mutation identified in CPVT families. Following exercise stress testing and epinephrine administration, RyR2–R4496C knockin mice developed bidirectional ventricular tachycardia (Figure 13–3). Interestingly, pretreatment with β-adrenergic receptor blockers did not prevent the occurrence of these arrhythmias in this mouse model of CPVT, which is consistent with the observation in CPVT patients that β-blockers provide incomplete protection against arrhythmias and sudden cardiac death.[55] Additional evidence for a causal role of *RyR2* mutations in CPVT was provided by the observation that mutation R176Q, linked to exercise-induced arrhythmias in patients, also caused ventricular arrhythmias and sudden cardiac death in RyR2–R176Q heterozygous knockin mice.[63] These genetic mouse models have provided strong experimental evidence for a causal link between abnormalities in RyR2 and triggers for cardiac arrhythmias.

Planar lipid bilayer studies of single RyR2 channels with CPVT-associated mutations show features consistent with the clinical phenotype.[26] Mutant RyR2 channels show gain-of-function defects in response to PKA phosphorylation[26,64] or caffeine-induced channel activation,[65] suggesting that mutant RyR2 channels fail to completely close during diastole resulting in diastolic SR Ca^{2+} leak during stress or exercise (Figure 13–3). Consistent with these studies, intracellular Ca^{2+} leak was observed after β-adrenergic stimulation in HL-1 atrial tumor cells expressing the same CPVT mutant RyR2 channels.[66] The findings that RyR2 missense mutations result in SR Ca^{2+} leak only after activation of the β-adrenergic signaling cascade[26,64] are in agreement with the fact that affected mutation carriers develop arrhythmias only during stress or exercise.[55,67]

Wehrens *et al.*[26] reported that CPVT mutant RyR2 channels have a decreased binding affinity for the channel-stabilizing subunit calstabin2 (FKBP12.6), although this was not observed by George *et al.*[66] under different experimental conditions. However, calstabin2 haploinsufficient mice show a phenotype similar to that observed in RyR2–R4496C knockin mice (i.e., bidirectional ventricular tachycardia), suggesting that calstabin2 deficiency in the RyR2 channel complex is an important pathogenic mechanism in CPVT.[68] Since CPVT mutations in RyR2 decrease the

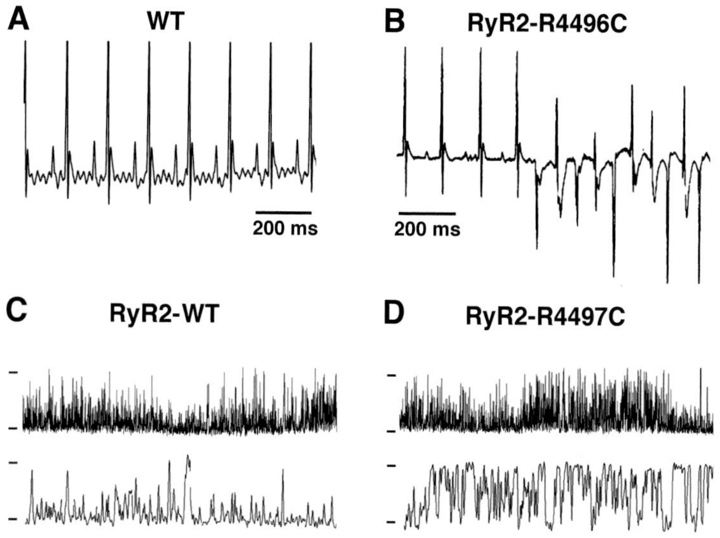

FIGURE 13–3. The CPVT mutations cause ventricular tachycardia and leaky RyR2 channels. (A) The ECG recordings show sinus rhythm in wild-type (WT) mouse and (B) bidirectional ventricular tachycardia in a CPVT knockin mouse heterozygous for RyR2 mutation R4496C. (Reproduced with permission from Cerrone *et al.*[62]) Planar lipid bilayer recordings of (C) a single human RyR2–WT channel showing low open probability at low cytosolic Ca^{2+} concentrations (150 nM), and (D) an RyR2–R4497C channel (equates to R4496C in the mouse) showing higher channel activity indicative of diastolic Ca^{2+} leakage. (Reprinted from Wehrens *et al.*, with permission from Elsevier.[26])

binding affinity of calstabin2, excessive dissociation of calstabin2 might be expected following PKA phosphorylation during stress or exercise, leading to incomplete channel closure and diastolic SR Ca^{2+} leak in patients with CPVT.[8,26]

Additional mechanisms might contribute to diastolic SR Ca^{2+} leak through CPVT mutant RyR2. Jiang *et al.*[69] expressed wild-type and mutant RyR2 in HEK293 cells and found altered luminal Ca^{2+} activation in cells expressing mutant RyR2. They proposed that a reduced threshold for store overload-induced Ca^{2+} release (SOICR) in CPVT-linked RyR2 mutations triggers arrhythmias.[35,69] However, it should be noted that these studies were conducted in HEK293 cells that are nonmuscular in origin and lack junctional SR, which is crucial for proper Ca^{2+} handling in cardiomyocytes. Moreover, they reported that CPVT mutant channels are defective under baseline conditions, which is at odds with the clinical disease phenotype (i.e., exercise-induced cardiac arrest). Nevertheless, most functional characterizations of RyR2 mutants performed so far agree on the presence of a diastolic SR Ca^{2+} leak upon β-adrenergic stimulation and on a lower threshold for Ca^{2+} spilling from the SR. These dysfunctions are likely to promote the development of delayed afterdepolarizations (DADs) and triggered arrhythmias in CPVT.

Finally, a less common type of CPVT (CPVT-2) is caused by mutations in the cardiac calsequestrin gene (*CASQ2*). Although the pathogenetic mechanisms of CPVT-2 are beyond the scope of this chapter, it is thought that mutations in CASQ2 may lead to destabilization of the Ca^{2+}-induced Ca^{2+} release mechanism by reducing effective Ca^{2+} buffering inside the SR,[34] by or causing altered interactions with the RyR2 channel complex leading to impaired RyR2 regulation by luminal Ca^{2+}.[70]

Arrhythmogenic Right Ventricular Dysplasia

Arrhythmogenic right ventricular dysplasia is one of the leading causes of sudden cardiac death in young children and athletes. Missense mutations in *RyR2* have also been linked to arrhythmogenic right ventricular cardiomyopathy/dysplasia type 2 (ARVD-2),[3] in which exercise-induced arrhythmias as well as structural abnormalities of the right ventricle were reported. The report that one variant of ARVD might be caused by mutations in a calcium release channel has raised substantial interest and scientific debate, as ARVD was generally believed to be a disease of adhesion molecules.[71] After several years of discussion among cardiogenetic research groups, it is currently believed that the presence of some minor structural abnormalities of the ventricle may be part of the CPVT phenotype that nonetheless remains a condition that is clinically and physiologically distinct from ARVD.[72] Consistent with this hypothesis is the finding that knockin mice with the ARVD2-associated RyR2–R176Q mutation develop mild right ventricular contractile defects in addition to stress-induced ventricular tachycardia, although right ventricular dysplesia was not observed.[63]

Triggered Arrhythmias in CPVT

Patients with CPVT often develop a rare and unusual arrhythmia, known as bidirectional ventricular tachycardia.[4,5] This type of arrhythmia, better known for its association with digoxin toxicity,[73] is characterized by broad complex tachycardia with alternating QRS complex polarity. Delayed afterdepolarizations are believed to be the underlying cause of these arrhythmias observed in CPVT. The cellular basis for DADs is Ca^{2+} aftertransients resulting from spontaneous SR Ca^{2+} release followed by activation of a transient inward current (I_{ti}) under conditions that favor accumulation of intracellular Ca^{2+}.[74] If the amplitude of the inward current exceeds the threshold membrane potential, depolarization will occur.[75] Propagation of the triggered impulse may subsequently deteriorate into a ventricular arrhythmia.

Factors that increase the likelihood that the threshold depolarization will be reached include a faster heart rate and intracellular Ca^{2+} overload.[76] The association with faster heart rates may explain why arrhythmias in CPVT almost exclusively occur during exercise or stress.[55] Intracellular Ca^{2+} loading is enhanced by cardiac glycoside toxicity and might explain triggered activity in patients with digoxin toxicity. However, hypercalcemia alone does not appear to cause bidirectional ventricular tachycardia, presumably because the increased Ca^{2+} entry into the cytoplasm is sufficiently buffered or balanced by Ca^{2+} efflux. Aberrant diastolic release of SR Ca^{2+} through leaky CPVT-associated RyR2 mutations, however, may trigger arrhythmias due to temporal–spatial proximity and function coupling of RyR2 Ca^{2+} leak with depolarizing membrane transport mechanisms (i.e., Na^+–Ca^{2+} exchanger).[68]

Ryanodine Receptor Defects in Heart Failure

Alterations in intracellular Ca^{2+} handling play an important role in depressing intracellular Ca^{2+} transients and cardiac contractility in heart failure.[15,77] Increased SR Ca^{2+} leak via RyR2 has been proposed to be an important contributor to a reduction in SR Ca^{2+} load and, thus, to a reduced intracellular Ca^{2+} transient.[6,77] Chronic activation of the β-adrenergic pathways in heart failure results in maladaptive changes in the heart, including downregulation and uncoupling of β-adrenergic receptors.[78] Therefore, the finding that RyR2 is PKA hyperphosphorylated in heart failure may have seemed counterintuitive at first.[6,79] However, subsequent studies have demonstrated that changes in the RyR2 macromolecular signaling complex are responsible for chronically increased PKA hyperphosphorylation of RyR2. Reduced levels of PP1 and PP2A contribute to the maintenance of long-term hyperphosphorylation of RyR2 by PKA.[6,80] In addition, we recently demonstrated a downregulation of the phosphodiesterase PDE4D3 in the RyR2 complex in failing hearts.[47] Since PDEs regulate local concentrations of 3′,5′-cyclic adenosine monophosphate (cAMP), decreased activity of PDE4D3 in the RyR2 complex leads to increased activity of cAMP-dependent PKA. Indeed, PDE4D knockout mice develop defective RyR2 channel function associated with heart failure.[47] Furthermore, PDE4D deficiency in the RyR2 channel complex and PKA hyperphosphorylation increase the susceptibility to cardiac arrhythmias in PDE4D-deficient mice. These findings suggest that PDE4 inhibitors might increase the risk for cardiac arrhythmias due to "leaky" RyR2 channels in patients with heart failure and genetic forms of sudden cardiac death linked to mutations in RyR2.[26,64]

Ryanodine Receptors as a Therapeutic Target

Clinical studies support the concept that systemic β-adrenergic receptor blockers can prevent, at least in part, cardiac arrhythmias in patients with CPVT.[55,81] These findings are consistent with cellular studies showing that PKA phosphorylation results in SR Ca^{2+} leak by gain-of-function defects in mutant RyR2 channels.[26,35] However, the fact that patients with CPVT still develop sudden cardiac death despite treatment with β-blockers warrants the development of more effective treatments for these lethal arrhythmias.[61,67,82]

The identification of calstabin2 deficiency in the RyR2 channel complex as a source of diastolic SR Ca^{2+} leak has led to the hypothesis that increasing calstabin2 binding to RyR2 could constitute a new molecular target for the treatment of exercise-induced arrhythmias.[6,26] In proof-of-principle experiments, we demonstrated that a genetically modified calstabin2 protein is capable of binding to PKA-phosphorylated CPVT-mutant RyR2 channels.[26] The association of mutant calstabin2 to RyR2 restored defective single-channel gating of CPVT mutant or PKA-hyperphosphorylated channels.[26,83] These studies suggested that enhancing calstabin2 binding to RyR2 might provide a very effective and specific therapy for the prevention of triggered arrhythmias in CPVT.

In 2003, Yano *et al.*[8] showed that the compound JTV519, a 1,4-benzothiazepine derivative, slows the progression of canine heart failure by inhibiting RyR2 hyperactivity and intracellular Ca^{2+} leak. Using a genetic mouse model of calstabin2 deficiency, we demonstrated that ventricular arrhythmias induced by an exercise-stress test protocol in haploinsufficient calstabin2 mice could be effectively prevented by treatment with JTV519.[8] Treatment with JTV519 increases calstabin2 binding to RyR2, which inhibits diastolic Ca^{2+} leak from the SR and prevents cardiac arrhythmias (Figure 13–4).[8,84] In agreement with these findings are cellular studies by Venetucci *et al.*,[85] which teach that reducing RyR2 open probability in Ca^{2+} overloaded myocytes suppresses arrhythmogenic spontaneous Ca^{2+} release while maintaining Ca^{2+} homeostasis.

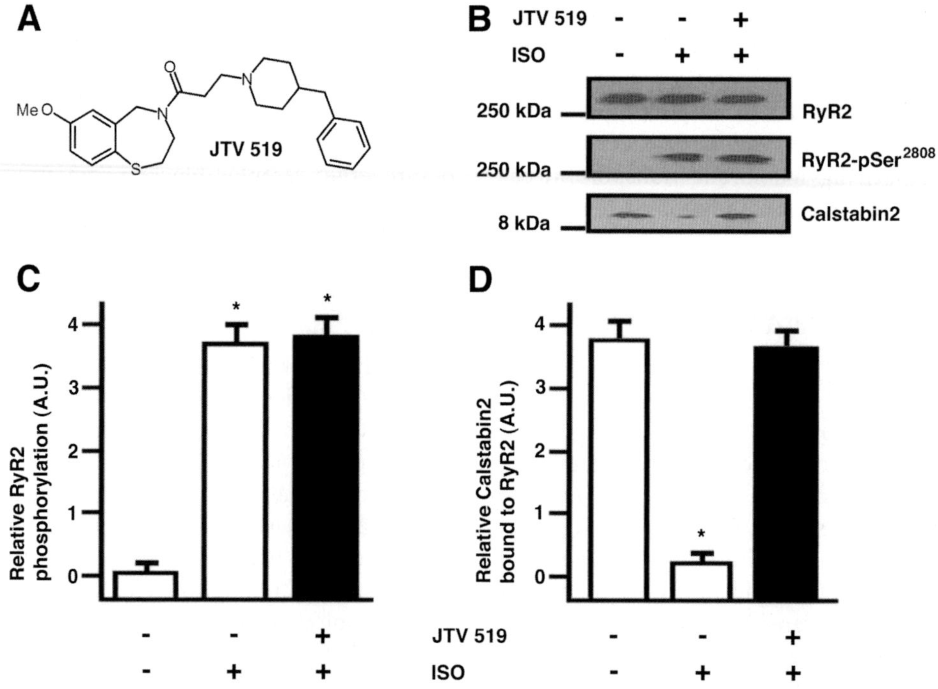

Figure 13–4. The compound JTV519 prevents cardiac arrhythmias by preventing RyR2 Ca^{2+} leak. (A) Chemical structure of the 1,4-benzothiazepine JTV519. (B) RyR2 immunoprecipitation from calstabin2 plus or minus cardiomyocyte lysate demonstrating increased PKA phosphorylation of RyR2 and calstabin2 dissociation after a 30-min exposure to 100 nM isoproterenol. Pretreatment with JTV519 prevented calstabin2 release from RyR2 despite PKA hyperphosphorylation of serine 2808. (C and D) Bar graphs summarizing results from three myocyte isolations each measured in triplicate. (Reproduced with permission from Lehnart *et al.*,[68] copyright 2006, National Academy of Sciences USA.)

The effectiveness of JTV519 in preventing SR Ca^{2+} leak is not limited to CPVT, as this drug also exerts therapeutic effects in the failing heart.[8,11] This finding is of particular interest considering that ~50% of patients with heart failure (HF) die suddenly due to cardiac arrhythmias.[86] In a genetic mouse model of ischemic heart failure, we were able to demonstrate that JTV519 can prevent SR Ca^{2+} leak by increasing the binding affinity of calstabin2 for PKA-hyperphosphorylated RyR2.[11] Increased binding of calstabin2 resulted in improved cardiac function and normalized single channel gating properties of PKA-hyperphosphorylated RyR2.[11] Thus, JTV519-based therapies may provide the unique advantage of treating both contractile dysfunction as well as cardiac arrhythmias in patients with heart failure.[11] These new compounds, referred to as "calcium channel stabilizers," could potentially be developed into highly specific therapeutics for cardiac arrhythmias and heart failure.

Summary and Conclusions

Ryanodine receptor intracellular calcium release channels on the SR are required for excitation–contraction coupling in cardiac muscle. RyRs are macromolecular channel complexes associated with regulatory proteins that modulate RyR2 function in response to extracellular signals. Cardiac arrhythmia is an important cause of death in patients with HF and inherited arrhythmia syndromes, such as CPVT. Alterations in RyR2 function in CPVT cause diastolic calcium leak from the SR, which may lead to DADs and triggered cardiac arrhythmias (Figure 13–5). Novel therapeutic approaches, based on recent advances in

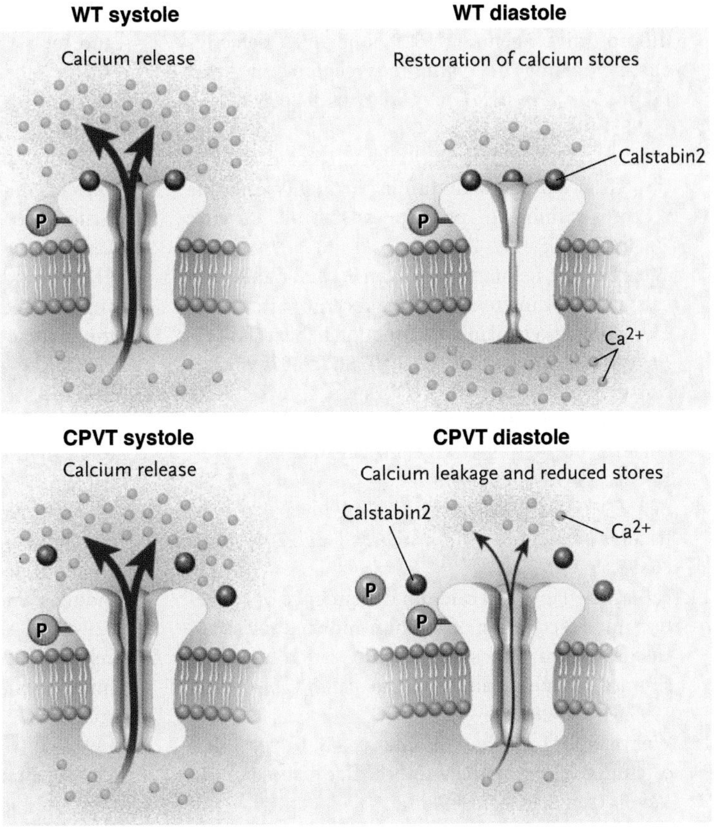

FIGURE 13–5. The CPVT-associated mutations in RyR2 cause intracellular Ca^{2+} leak and arrhythmias. In the normal heart, cyclic AMP-mediated activation of protein kinase A in response to adrenergic stimuli causes phosphorylation (P) of the cardiac ryanodine recetor (RyR2) and dissociation of calstabin2. The result is the release of stored calcium from the sarcoplasmic reticulum (SR) through the RyR2 complex into the cytoplasm, where Ca^{2+} initiates actin–myosin cross-bridging and myocyte contraction during systole. In CPVT, mutant RyR2 (x) are not fully bound by calstabin2, resulting in channels that remain partially open during diastole with consequent calcium leakage and cardiac arrhythmias. (Reproduced with permission from Farr *et al.*[88])

the understanding of the cellular mechanisms underlying arrhythmias in heart failure and CPVT, are currently being evaluated to specifically correct defects in RyR2 Ca^{2+} release in these lethal syndromes.

References

1. Jayaraman T, Brillantes AM, Timerman AP, *et al.* FK506 binding protein associated with the calcium release channel (ryanodine receptor). *J Biol Chem* 1992;267:9474–9477.
2. Marx SO, Reiken S, Hisamatsu Y, *et al.* Phosphorylation-dependent regulation of ryanodine receptors. A novel role for leucine/isoleucine zippers. *J Cell Biol* 2001;153(4):699–708.
3. Tiso N, Stephan DA, Nava A, *et al.* Identification of mutations in the cardiac ryanodine receptor gene in families affected with arrhythmogenic right ventricular cardiomyopathy type 2 (ARVD2). *Hum Mol Genet* 2001;10(3):189–194.
4. Priori SG, Napolitano C, Tiso N, *et al.* Mutations in the cardiac ryanodine receptor gene (hRyR2) underlie catecholaminergic polymorphic ventricular tachycardia. *Circulation* 2001;103(2):196–200.
5. Laitinen PJ, Brown KM, Piippo K, *et al.* Mutations of the cardiac ryanodine receptor (RyR2) gene in familial polymorphic ventricular tachycardia. *Circulation* 2001;103(4):485–490.
6. Marx SO, Reiken S, Hisamatsu Y, *et al.* PKA phosphorylation dissociates FKBP12.6 from the calcium release channel (ryanodine receptor): Defective regulation in failing hearts. *Cell* 2000;101:365–376.
7. Yano M, Ono K, Ohkusa T, *et al.* Altered stoichiometry of FKBP12.6 versus ryanodine receptor as a cause of abnormal Ca^{2+} leak through ryanodine receptor in heart failure. *Circulation* 2000;102(17):2131–2136.
8. Yano M, Kobayashi S, Kohno M, *et al.* FKBP12.6-mediated stabilization of calcium-release channel (ryanodine receptor) as a novel therapeutic strategy against heart failure. *Circulation* 2003;107(3):477–484.

9. Kohno M, Yano M, Kobayashi S, *et al.* A new cardioprotective agent, JTV519, improves defective channel gating of ryanodine receptor in heart failure. *Am J Physiol Heart Circ Physiol* 2003;284(3): H1035–1042.
10. Wehrens XH, Lehnart SE, Reiken SR, *et al.* Protection from cardiac arrhythmia through ryanodine receptor-stabilizing protein calstabin2. *Science* 2004;304(5668):292–296.
11. Wehrens XH, Lehnart SE, Reiken S, *et al.* Enhancing calstabin binding to ryanodine receptors improves cardiac and skeletal muscle function in heart failure. *Proc Natl Acad Sci USA* 2005;102(27):9607–9612.
12. Nabauer M, Callewart G, Cleeman L, Morad M. Regulation of calcium release is gated by calcium current, not gating charge, in cardiac, myocytes. *Science* 1989;244:800–803.
13. Bers DM, Guo T. Calcium signaling in cardiac ventricular myocytes. *Ann NY Acad Sci* 2005;1047: 86–98.
14. Fabiato A. Time and calcium dependence of activation and inactivation of calcium-induced release of calcium from the sarcoplasmic reticulum of a skinned canine cardiac Purkinje cell. *J Gen Physiol* 1985;85:247–289.
15. Wehrens XHT, Lehnart SE, Marks AR. Intracellular calcium release channels and cardiac disease. *Annu Rev Physiol* 2005;67:69–98.
16. Cheng H, Lederer WJ, Cannell MB. Calcium sparks: Elementary events underlying excitation-contraction coupling in heart muscle. *Science* 1993; 262(5134):740–744.
17. Lindegger N, Niggli E. Paradoxical SR Ca^{2+} release in guinea-pig cardiac myocytes after β-adrenergic stimulation revealed by two-photon photolysis of caged Ca^{2+}. *J Physiol* 2005;565(3):801–813.
18. Cannell MB, Cheng H, Lederer WJ. The control of calcium release in heart muscle. *Science* 1995; 268(5213):1045–1049.
19. Marx SO, Gaburjakova J, Gaburjakova M, Henrikson C, Ondrias K, Marks AR. Coupled gating between cardiac calcium release channels (ryanodine receptors). *Circ Res* 2001;88(11):1151–1158.
20. Brochet DX, Yang D, Di Maio A, Lederer WJ, Franzini-Armstrong C, Cheng H. Ca2+ blinks: Rapid nanoscopic store calcium signaling. *Proc Natl Acad Sci USA* 2005;102(8):3099–3104.
21. Otsu K, Willard HF, Khanna VK, Zorzato F, Green NM, MacLennan DH. Molecular cloning of cDNA encoding the Ca^{2+} release channel (ryanodine receptor) of rabbit cardiac muscle sarcoplasmic reticulum. *J Biol Chem* 1990;265:13472–13483.
22. Tunwell RE, Wickenden C, Bertrand BM, *et al.* The human cardiac muscle ryanodine receptor-calcium release channel: Identification, primary structure and topological analysis. *Biochem J* 1996;318:477–487.
23. Marks AR, Tempst P, Hwang KS, *et al.* Molecular cloning and characterization of the ryanodine receptor/junctional channel complex cDNA from skeletal muscle sarcoplasmic reticulum. *Proc Natl Acad Sci USA* 1989;86:8683–8687.
24. Lam E, Martin MM, Timerman AP, *et al.* A novel FK506 binding protein can mediate the immunosuppressive effects of FK506 and is associated with the cardiac ryanodine receptor. *J Biol Chem* 1995; 270:26511–26522.
25. Brillantes AB, Ondrias K, Scott A, *et al.* Stabilization of calcium release channel (ryanodine receptor) function by FK506-binding protein. *Cell* 1994; 77(4):513–523.
26. Wehrens XH, Lehnart SE, Huang F, *et al.* FKBP12.6 deficiency and defective calcium release channel (ryanodine receptor) function linked to exercise-induced sudden cardiac death. *Cell* 2003;113(7): 829–840.
27. Lehnart SE, Huang F, Marx SO, Marks AR. Immunophilins and coupled gating of ryanodine receptors. *Curr Top Med Chem* 2003;3(12):1383–1391.
28. Chu A, Sumbilla C, Inesi G, Jay SD, Campbell KP. Specific association of calmodulin-dependent protein kinase and related substrates with the junctional sarcoplasmic reticulum of skeletal muscle. *Biochemistry* 1990;29(25):5899–5905.
29. Meyers MB, Pickel VM, Sheu SS, Sharma VK, Scotto KW, Fishman GI. Association of sorcin with the cardiac ryanodine receptor. *J Biol Chem* 1995; 270(44):26411–26418.
30. Currie S, Loughrey CM, Craig MA, Smith GL. Calcium/calmodulin-dependent protein kinase IIdelta associates with the ryanodine receptor complex and regulates channel function in rabbit heart. *Biochem J* 2004;377(Pt. 2):357–366.
31. Wehrens XH, Lehnart SE, Reiken SR, Marks AR. Ca^{2+}/calmodulin-dependent protein kinase II phosphorylation regulates the cardiac ryanodine receptor. *Circ Res* 2004;94(6):e61–70.
32. Zhang L, Kelley J, Schmeisser G, Kobayashi YM, Jones LR. Complex formation between junctin, triadin, calsequestrin, and the ryanodine receptor. Proteins of the cardiac junctional sarcoplasmic reticulum membrane. *J Biol Chem* 1997;272(37): 23389–23397.
33. Gyorke I, Hester N, Jones LR, Gyorke S. The role of calsequestrin, triadin, and junctin in conferring cardiac ryanodine receptor responsiveness to luminal calcium. *Biophys J* 2004;86:2121–2128.

34. Terentyev D, Viatchenko-Karpinski S, Gyorke I, Volpe P, Williams SC, Gyorke S. Calsequestrin determines the functional size and stability of cardiac intracellular calcium stores: Mechanism for hereditary arrhythmia. *Proc Natl Acad Sci USA* 2003;100(20):11759–11764.
35. Jiang D, Wang R, Xiao B, *et al.* Enhanced store overload-induced Ca2+ release and channel sensitivity to luminal Ca2+ activation are common defects of RyR2 mutations linked to ventricular tachycardia and sudden death. *Circ Res* 2005; 97(11):1173–1181.
36. Stull LB, Leppo MK, Marban E, Janssen PM. Physiological determinants of contractile force generation and calcium handling in mouse myocardium. *J Mol Cell Cardiol* 2002;34(10):1367–1376.
37. Braz JC, Gregory K, Pathak A, *et al.* PKC-alpha regulates cardiac contractility and propensity toward heart failure. *Nat Med* 2004;10(3):248–254.
38. Lefkowitz RJ, Rockman HA, Koch WJ. Catecholamines, cardiac beta-adrenergic receptors, and heart failure. *Circulation* 2000;101(14):1634–1637.
39. Jones LR, Simmerman HK, Wilson WW, Gurd FR, Wegener AD. Purification and characterization of phospholamban from canine cardiac sarcoplasmic reticulum. *J Biol Chem* 1985;260(12):7721–7730.
40. Gomez AM, Valdivia HH, Cheng H, *et al.* Defective excitation-contraction coupling in experimental cardiac hypertrophy and heart failure. *Science* 1997; 276(5313):800–806.
41. Hain J, Onoue H, Mayrleitner M, Fleischer S, Schindler H. Phosphorylation modulates the function of the calcium release channel of sarcoplasmic reticulum from cardiac muscle. *J Biol Chem* 1995;270(5): 2074–2081.
42. Valdivia HH, Kaplan JH, Ellis-Davies GC, Lederer WJ. Rapid adaptation of cardiac ryanodine receptors: Modulation by Mg^{2+} and phosphorylation. *Science* 1995;267(5206):1997–2000.
43. Wehrens XH, Marks AR. *Ryanodine Receptors. Structure, Function and Dysfunction in Clinical Disease.* New York: Springer, 2004.
44. Xiao B, Jiang MT, Zhao M, *et al.* Characterization of a novel PKA phosphorylation site, serine-2030, reveals no PKA hyperphosphorylation of the cardiac ryanodine receptor in canine heart failure. *Circ Res* 2005;96(8):847–855.
45. Wehrens XH, Lehnart SE, Reiken S, Vest JA, Wronska A, Marks AR. Ryanodine receptor/calcium release channel PKA phosphorylation: A critical mediator of heart failure progression. *Proc Natl Acad Sci USA* 2006;103(3):511–518.
46. Lokuta AJ, Rogers TB, Lederer WJ, Valdivia HH. Modulation of cardiac ryanodine receptors of swine and rabbit by a phosphorylation-dephosphorylation mechanism. *J Phys* 1995;487(Pt. 3):609–622.
47. Lehnart SE, Wehrens XH, Reiken S, *et al.* Phosphodiesterase 4D deficiency in the ryanodine-receptor complex promotes heart failure and arrhythmias. *Cell* 2005;123(1):25–35.
48. d'Amati G, Bagattin A, Bauce B, *et al.* Juvenile sudden death in a family with polymorphic ventricular arrhythmias caused by a novel RyR2 gene mutation: Evidence of specific morphological substrates. *Hum Pathol* 2005;36(7):761–767.
49. Tiziana di Gioia CR, Autore C, Romeo DM, *et al.* Sudden cardiac death in younger adults: Autopsy diagnosis as a tool for preventive medicine. *Hum Pathol* 2006;37(7):794–801.
50. Creighton W, Virmani R, Kutys R, Burke A. Identification of novel missense mutations of cardiac ryanodine receptor gene in exercise-induced sudden death at autopsy. *J Mol Diagn* 2006;8(1):62–67.
51. Tester DJ, Kopplin LJ, Will ML, Ackerman MJ. Spectrum and prevalence of cardiac ryanodine receptor (RyR2) mutations in a cohort of unrelated patients referred explicitly for long QT syndrome genetic testing. *Heart Rhythm* 2005;2(10):1099–1105.
52. Bauce B, Rampazzo A, Basso C, *et al.* Screening for ryanodine receptor type 2 mutations in families with effort-induced polymorphic ventricular arrhythmias and sudden death: Early diagnosis of asymptomatic carriers. *J Am Coll Cardiol* 2002; 40(2):341–349.
53. Tester DJ, Spoon DB, Valdivia HH, Makielski JC, Ackerman MJ. Targeted mutational analysis of the cardiac ryanodine receptor (RyR2) in sudden unexplained death: A molecular autopsy of 51 medical examiner/coroner's cases. *Mayo Clin Proc* 2004; 79(11):1380–1384.
54. Postma AV, Denjoy I, Kamblock J, *et al.* Catecholaminergic polymorphic ventricular tachycardia: RYR2 mutations, bradycardia, and follow up of the patients. *J Med Genet* 2005;42(11):863–870.
55. Priori SG, Napolitano C, Memmi M, *et al.* Clinical and molecular characterization of patients with catecholaminergic polymorphic ventricular tachycardia. *Circulation* 2002;106(1):69–74.
56. Laitinen PJ, Swan H, Kontula K. Molecular genetics of exercise-induced polymorphic ventricular tachycardia: Identification of three novel cardiac ryanodine receptor mutations and two common calsequestrin 2 amino-acid polymorphisms. *Eur J Hum Genet* 2003;11(11):888–891.
57. Bagattin A, Veronese C, Bauce B, *et al.* Denaturing HPLC-based approach for detecting RYR2 mutations involved in malignant arrhythmias. *Clin Chem* 2004;50(7):1148–1155.

58. Aizawa Y, Ueda K, Komura S, *et al.* A novel mutation in FKBP12.6 binding region of the human cardiac ryanodine receptor gene (R2401H) in a Japanese patient with catecholaminergic polymorphic ventricular tachycardia. *Int J Cardiol* 2005; 99(2):343–345.
59. Hasdemir C, Priori SG, Overholt E, Lazzara R. Catecholaminergic polymorphic ventricular tachycardia, recurrent syncope, and implantable loop recorder. *J Cardiovasc Electrophysiol* 2004;15(6): 729.
60. Allouis M, Probst V, Jaafar P, Schott JJ, Le Marec H. Unusual clinical presentation in a family with catecholaminergic polymorphic ventricular tachycardia due to a G14876A ryanodine receptor gene mutation. *Am J Cardiol* 2005;95(5):700–702.
61. Sumitomo N, Harada K, Nagashima M, *et al.* Catecholaminergic polymorphic ventricular tachycardia: Electrocardiographic characteristics and optimal therapeutic strategies to prevent sudden death. *Heart* 2003;89(1):66–70.
62. Cerrone M, Colombi B, Santoro M, *et al.* Bidirectional ventricular tachycardia and fibrillation elicited in a knock-in mouse model carrier of a mutation in the cardiac ryanodine receptor. *Circ Res* 2005;96(10):e77–82.
63. Kannankeril P, Mitchell B, Goonasekera S, *et al.* Mice with the R176Q cardiac ryanodine receptor mutation exhibit catecholamine-induced ventricular tachycardia and mild cardiomyopathy. *Proc Natl Acad Sci USA* 2006;103(32):12179–12184.
64. Lehnart SE, Wehrens XHT, Laitinen PJ, *et al.* Sudden death in familial polymorphic ventricular tachycardia associated with calcium release channel (ryanodine receptor) leak. *Circulation* 2004(109): r113–119.
65. George CH, Jundi H, Walters N, Thomas NL, West RR, Lai FA. Arrhythmogenic mutation-linked defects in ryanodine receptor autoregulation reveal a novel mechanism of Ca2+ release channel dysfunction. *Circ Res* 2006;98(1):88–97.
66. George CH, Higgs GV, Lai FA. Ryanodine receptor mutations associated with stress-induced ventricular tachycardia mediate increased calcium release in stimulated cardiomyocytes. *Circ Res* 2003;93(6): 531–540.
67. Swan H, Piippo K, Viitasalo M, *et al.* Arrhythmic disorder mapped to chromosome 1q42-q43 causes malignant polymorphic ventricular tachycardia in structurally normal hearts. *J Am Coll Cardiol* 1999; 34(7):2035–2042.
68. Lehnart SE, Terrenoire C, Reiken S, *et al.* Stabilization of cardiac ryanodine receptor prevents intracellular calcium leak and arrhythmias. *Proc Natl Acad Sci USA* 2006;103(20):7906–7910.
69. Jiang D, Xiao B, Yang D, *et al.* RyR2 mutations linked to ventricular tachycardia and sudden death reduce the threshold for store-overload-induced Ca2+ release (SOICR). *Proc Natl Acad Sci USA* 2004;101(35):13062–13067.
70. Terentyev D, Nori A, Santoro M, *et al.* Abnormal interactions of calsequestrin with the ryanodine receptor calcium release channel complex linked to exercise-induced sudden cardiac death. *Circ Res* 2006;98(9):1151–1158.
71. Corrado D, Thiene G. Arrhythmogenic right ventricular cardiomyopathy/dysplasia: Clinical impact of molecular genetic studies. *Circulation* 2006; 113(13):1634–1637.
72. Priori SG, Napolitano C. Intracellular calcium handling dysfunction and arrhythmogenesis: A new challenge for the electrophysiologist. *Circ Res* 2005;97(11):1077–1079.
73. Ma G, Brady WJ, Pollack M, Chan TC. Electrocardiographic manifestations: Digitalis toxicity. *J Emerg Med* 2001;20(2):145–152.
74. Scoote M, Williams AJ. The cardiac ryanodine receptor (calcium release channel): Emerging role in heart failure and arrhythmia pathogenesis. *Cardiovasc Res* 2002;56(3):359–372.
75. Wehrens XH, Lehnart SE, Marks AR. Ryanodine receptor-targeted anti-arrhythmic therapy. *Ann NY Acad Sci* 2005;1047:366–375.
76. Santana LF, Cheng H, Gomez AM, Cannell MB, Lederer WJ. Relation between the sarcolemmal Ca^{2+} current and Ca^{2+} sparks and local control theories for cardiac excitation-contraction coupling. *Circ Res* 1996;78(1):166–171.
77. Bers DM, Eisner DA, Valdivia HH. Sarcoplasmic reticulum Ca2+ and heart failure: Roles of diastolic leak and Ca2+ transport. *Circ Res* 2003;93(6):487–490.
78. Daaka Y, Luttrell LM, Lefkowitz RJ. Switching of the coupling of the beta2-adrenergic receptor to different G proteins by protein kinase A. *Nature* 1997;390(6655):88–91.
79. Marks AR. Ryanodine receptors/calcium release channels in heart failure and sudden cardiac death. *J Mol Cell Cardiol* 2001;33(4):615–624.
80. Reiken S, Wehrens XH, Vest JA, *et al.* Beta-blockers restore calcium release channel function and improve cardiac muscle performance in human heart failure. *Circulation* 2003;107(19):2459–2466.
81. De Rosa G, Delogu AB, Piastra M, Chiaretti A, Bloise R, Priori SG. Catecholaminergic polymorphic ventricular tachycardia: Successful emergency treatment with intravenous propranolol. *Pediatr Emerg Care* 2004;20(3):175–177.
82. Fisher JD, Krikler D, Hallidie-Smith KA. Familial polymorphic ventricular arrhythmias: A quarter

century of successful medical treatment based on serial exercise-pharmacologic testing. *J Am Coll Cardiol* 1999;34(7):2015–2022.

83. Huang F, Shan J, Reiken S, Wehrens XH, Marks AR. Analysis of calstabin2 (FKBP12.6)-ryanodine receptor interactions: Rescue of heart failure by calstabin2 in mice. *Proc Natl Acad Sci USA* 2006; 103(9):3456–3461.

84. Wehrens XH, Marks AR. Novel therapeutic approaches for heart failure by normalising calcium cycling. *Nat Rev Drug Discov* 2004;3:565–573.

85. Venetucci LA, Trafford AW, Diaz ME, O'Neill SC, Eisner DA. Reducing ryanodine receptor open probability as a means to abolish spontaneous Ca2+ release and increase Ca2+ transient amplitude in adult ventricular myocytes. *Circ Res* 2006; 98(10):1299–1305.

86. Pratt NG. Pathophysiology of heart failure: Neuroendocrine response. *Crit Care Nurs Q* 1995;18(1): 22–31.

87. Yano M, Yamamoto T, Ikeda Y, Matsuzaki M. Mechanisms of disease: Ryanodine receptor defects in heart failure and fatal arrhythmia. *Nat Clin Pract Cardiovasc Med* 2006;3(1):43–52.

88. Farr MA, Basson CT. Sparking the failing heart. *N Engl J Med* 2004;351(2):185–187.

14
Caveolae and Arrhythmogenesis

Matteo Vatta

Introduction

The plasma membrane is a semipermeable barrier composed of a lipid bilayer, which defines the boundaries between the intracellular and extracellular space. However, unlike the historical model of the "fluid mosaic" for the plasma membrane, in which integral membrane proteins are evenly distributed and free to diffuse, current knowledge suggests a more heterogeneous view of the plasma membrane in which proteins and lipids are clustered within specialized vesicular microdomains termed lipid rafts. This novel scenario for the cell surface has dramatic implications in cardiomyocytes, where the plasma membrane contributes to the correct exchange of electrolytes and ions essential for membrane depolarization and excitation–contraction coupling (ECC), which are at the basis for normal cardiac function. All major ion channels implicated in the regulation of the cardiac action potential mainly localize at the cell surface and the cellular membrane provides these specialized proteins with a formidable interface capable of regulating the cellular response and the modulation of ion channel function upon various stimuli from the extracellular and intracellular environment. The structural support, protein turnover, and functional regulation of ion channels on the plasma membrane occur through self renewal and molecular adaptation, which represent the molecular plasticity of the plasmalemma and its ability to maintain an adequate composition to ensure an adequate cellular performance and response.

Cell trafficking through the endoplasmic reticulum (ER) and the Golgi apparatus, which represent a source of bilipid vesicles and posttranslationally modified proteins, is the mechanism that modifies the cell surface arrangement and intertalks with the main subcellular compartments.

Caveolae (little caves in Latin) are plasmalemmal organelles, deeply involved in vesicular transport from the ER and Golgi compartments to the cell surface. They are characterized by a peculiar "flask-like" shape and are virtually ubiquitous, but are particularly abundant in cells of the cardiovascular system, including endothelial cells, smooth muscle cells, macrophages, cardiomyocytes, and fibroblasts. In addition, many channels, instrumental for ion homeostasis and regulation of the cardiac action potential, have been colocalized within caveolae, suggesting an increasingly important role of these plasmalemmal organelles in trafficking and regulation of ion channel function.

In this chapter, we will discuss the overall function of caveolae and the relationship between caveolae and ion channel function as the base of their involvement in arrhythmogenesis. Caveolae and their major component caveolins may represent a novel molecular machinery implicated in ion channels function.

Caveolae: Discovery

The tale of caveolae started in 1953, when at the dawn of the biological application of electron microscopy (EM) to investigate the cellular ultrastructure, George Palade observed large numbers of narrow-necked small plasma membrane invaginations in endothelial cells of the heart.[1] Palade named these invaginations "plasmalemmal vesicles." Two years later, in 1955, Yamada confirmed Palade's observation, identifying 50- to 100-nm "flask-shaped" invaginations of the plasma membrane in the gallbladder.[2] Yamada proposed the name caveolae, which in Latin means "little caves," to describe this morphological structure.[2] Since that initial finding, further EM studies have identified caveolae in most cell types, especially endothelial cells and adipocytes, but not in red blood cells, platelets, lymphocytes, some neuronal tissues, and CaCo-2 human fibroblasts.[3–5] All these ultrastructural investigations achieved a detailed morphological definition of caveolae.

In fact, caveolae have been defined as flask-shaped invaginations of the plasma membrane that are regular in shape and size but are distinct from the larger electron-dense clathrin-coated vesicles involved in various phenomena of endocytosis.

Caveolae: Tissue Distribution

Caveolae have been identified in most tissues and cell types, although at a different surface density. In particular, caveolae are intensely abundant in endothelial cells, adipocytes, and type I pneumocytes, which are the major constituents of lung alveoli.[6] However, a distinction can occur within the same cellular type, as has been observed in continuous endothelium, with a higher density of caveolae in contrast to the fenestrated endothelium with a more modest number of caveolae.[7] Although the absolute number of caveolae measured in the aforementioned endothelial cells has been challenged by studies using different tissue preparations, the ratio of caveolae in the two endothelial cell types appears to be conserved.[8–10]

Ultrastructural analysis has demonstrated that adipose tissue is the prevalent source of caveolae with up to 20% of the adipocyte plasma membrane occupied by caveolae.[11] Endothelial and pneumocyte cells of the lung are the second major source of lipid raft vesicles, with a relatively high abundance of these plasma membrane microdomains.[6] Thus caveolae can greatly increase the surface area of numerous cell types, an observation that lends credence to the original speculation that caveolae are involved in macromolecular transport and mechanotransduction events.

In addition, caveolae are also abundant in the skeletal muscle and in the cardiovascular system. In particular, caveolae are particularly abundant in the endothelial and smooth muscle cells of the vasculature as well as in the myocardium.[12]

Caveolae: Structure and Composition

The caveolae are smooth uncoated plasma membrane microdomains of 50–100 nm in diameter that are easily distinguishable from clathrin-coated vesicles. Caveolae can be isolated or can occur in clusters with a peculiar rosette formation deriving from the fusion of individual caveolae. In muscle cells, caveolae usually occur individually, although clusters have been reported.[13,14] In particular, EM analysis of myocardial and skeletal muscle caveolae demonstrated that when they cluster, caveolae occur in ordered linear arrays, suggesting a possible association with the cytoskeletal structure.[15–20] This observation was confirmed by studying caveolae in cell migration. In fact, caveolae are preferentially distributed to the retracting edge of the migrating cell.[21–23] Although extensive investigations revealed the various morphological subsets of caveolae, it is still unclear what the overall function of the archetypal caveolae organelle is, and, in particular, if each different subset of caveolae represents a specialized function.

The first clue to understanding what caveolae are and what their biological significance is comes from biochemical studies of caveolae composition.

Caveolae can be distinguished from the plasma membrane due to their peculiar composition; they are extremely rich in proteins and lipids such as cholesterol, ceramide, and diacylglycerol (DAG), sphingomyelin, and *cis*-unsaturated phospholipids such as phosphatidylserine, phosphatidylethanolamine, phosphatidylinositol, and phosphatidylinositol biphosphate.[24] Due to their high content in specific lipids, caveolae have also been defined as lipids rafts. Caveolae are formed

TABLE 14–1. Principal lipids and protein component of caveolae.

Lipids		
	Cholesterol	
	Ceramide	
	Sphingomyelin	
	Diacylglycerol (DAG)	
	cis-Unsaturated phospholipids	
		Phosphatidylserine
		Phosphatidylethanolamine
		Phosphatidylinositol
		Phosphatidylinositol biphosphate (PIP_2)
Protein		
	Caveolins (-1, -2, and -3)	
	G proteins	
		G-α, G-β
	Adrenergic receptor (AR)	
		β_1, β_2, β_3?
	Cytokine receptors	
		Epidermal growth factor receptor (EGFR)
		Platelet-derived growth factor receptor (PDGFR)
		Insulin receptor
		Bradykinin receptor
		Endothelin receptor
		GRB-2—growth factor receptor bound protein 2
		SOS—son of sevenless
	Signal transduction	
		Protein kinase C (PKC) α subunit
		Phosphatidylinositol 3-kinase (PI3K)
		Mitogen-activated protein kinase (MAPK)
		eNOS, nNOS
		Calmodulin
	Cytoskeletal	
		Actin
		Myosin
		Ezrin

by the aggregation of glycosphingolipids and sphingomyelin in the Golgi apparatus, which are transported to the plasma membrane as concentrated units.[6] There are multiple types of rafts categories depending on the presence of specific marker proteins, ultrastructure data, and varying lipid compositions.[25] Caveolae are considered one subpopulation of lipid rafts because of their lipid constituents and biochemical characteristics (Table 14–1). However, their specific morphology and the presence of a scaffolding protein such as caveolin, the principal marker of the caveolae, distinguish them from other raft types.[26]

Caveolins: Markers for Caveolae

Caveolins not only are the main elements of caveolae, but they are the "cornerstone" of these lipid rafts.

Caveolins were identified quite fortuitously at the end of the 1980s, when investigators studying chicken embryonic fibroblasts transformed with Rous sarcoma virus (RSV) purified several phosphotyrosine-containing proteins, one of these being resistant to nonionic detergent extraction.[27] This 22-kDa protein, later identified in caveolae by EM analysis and thus termed caveolin, showed an immunohistochemical pattern consistent with parallel arrays of individual vesicles along the actin stress fibers, and with altered localization after cellular transformation.[28] The latter observation supported the hypothesis that the phosphorylation of caveolin occurred upon transformation with v-Src, suggesting a possible role of caveolin and caveolae in oncogenesis.[28]

In 1992, studies on cellular trafficking determined that caveolin (also called VIP21) localized to the Golgi apparatus, the plasma membrane, and membrane-bound vesicles.[29]

Caveolin Genes and Their Products

Caveolin-1 and -2

Caveolin is the general term used to define the three members of the three caveolin (*CAV1–3*) gene families identified so far, each encoded by a separate gene (Figure 14–1). The gene coding for caveolin-1 (*CAV1*) is the first gene to be identified, and is composed of three exons that are highly conserved in sequence and structure across species, while the gene coding for caveolin-2 (*CAV2*) was discovered by protein microsequencing of purified adipocyte caveolae membrane domains in which the polypeptide revealed a remarkable similarity to caveolin-1, but differed in some key conserved caveolin-1 residues.[30]

Finally, using the sequence of *CAV1* as a probe, Lisanti's group cloned the gene coding for caveolin-3 (*CAV3*), and characterized its expression to be mainly, if not exclusively, muscle specific.[31]

The *CAV1* and *CAV2* genes are expressed almost ubiquitously, and, in particular, they are coexpressed in most differentiated cells types, especially in adipocytes, endothelial cells, fibroblasts, and type I pneumocytes, but they are absent in striated muscle.[32]

Unfortunately, the caveolin family became more complex with the discovery of multiple isoforms for both caveolin-1 and -2. Caveolin-1

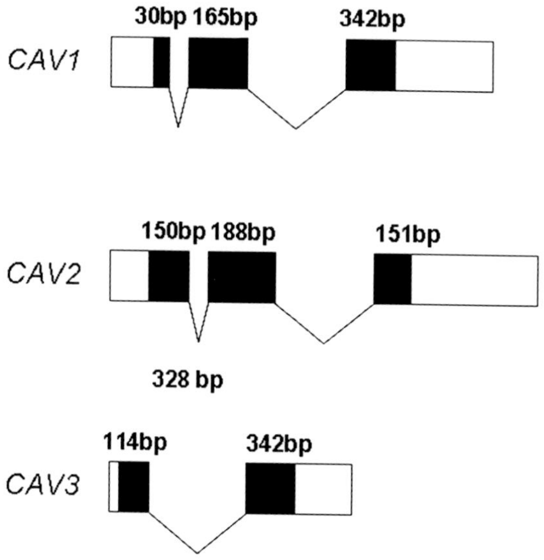

FIGURE 14–1. Schematic depiction of the caveolin gene family. Black boxes indicate the exon coding sequence for each caveolin family member. The numbers indicate the number of coding sequence nucleotides in each exon.

presents with two isoforms, termed α and β; caveolin-1α consists of residues 1–178, while caveolin-1β, originating from an alternate translation initiation site occurring at a methionine in position 32, contains residues 32–178, resulting in a protein ~3 kDa smaller in size.[32] Although shorter than caveolin-1α, caveolin-1β represents a functional isoform able to drive caveolae formation similar to caveolin-1α in *Drosophila melanogaster* Sf21 cells, which lack endogenous caveolae.[33]

The functional significance of these distinct caveolin-1 isoforms remains uncertain, although caveolin-1α appears to be localized primarily to deeply invaginated caveolae and more efficiently drive the formation of caveolae than caveolin-1β.[34,20]

Three isoforms have been identified for caveolin-2, the full-length caveolin-2α and two alternate splice variants, called caveolin-2β and caveolin-2γ (see Figure 14–3 later), which show a subcellular distribution distinct from caveolin-2α, although their functional significance is largely unknown.[6]

Caveolin-3

The tissue distribution of CAV3 has been intensely studied in mouse, in which CAV3 expression appears to be restricted to differentiated skeletal components and cardiomyocytes, while it is absent in nonproliferating C2C12 skeletal murine myoblasts compared to the proliferating precursor myoblasts, which express both caveolin-1 and -2.[35] In addition, caveolin-3 levels are intimately associated with muscle development, and experiments on the differentiation of C2C12 skeletal myoblasts in culture showed CAV3 upregulation,[36] while treatment with a *CAV3* antisense prevented myotube fusion *in vitro*.[37]

Caveolin-3 has been shown to function in a manner similar to caveolin-1, with which it shares high protein homology. In fact, caveolin-3 is connected to the sarcolemma and modulates the function of the dystrophin glycoprotein complex (DGC), the major protein ensemble linking the contractile apparatus to the plasma membrane in striated muscle, and is associated with a variety of muscular dystrophies with cardiac involvement and primary heart diseases all presenting with frequent arrhythmias.[38–40] Dystrophin, as well as several members of the DGC including α-sarcoglycan and β-dystroglycan, cofractionate with caveolin-3 in cultured mouse C2C12 myocytes.[36] In addition, coimmunoprecipitation (Co-IP) experiments demonstrated that dystrophin forms a stable complex with caveolin-3 and that dystrophin and caveolin-3 colocalize.[41] In addition, since the WW-like domain of caveolin-3 binds the C-terminus of β-dystroglycan, a region containing a PPXY motif, it is possible that caveolin-3 competes with dystrophin for the binding to β-dystroglycan; this will inhibit dystrophin binding with subsequent reduced dystrophin presentation to the sarcolemma.[41] In fact, in muscle biopsies from patients suffering from Duchenne muscular dystrophy (DMD) with progressive muscle weakness, respiratory failure and the development of dilated cardiomyopathy (DCM) associated with arrhythmias, caveolin-3 is shown to be upregulated along with an increased number and size of caveolae on the plasma membrane.[42,43] Similarly, caveolin-3 overexpression and increased caveolae number and size also occur in dystrophin-deficient *mdx* mice.[43,44]

Caveolins and Animal Models

One of the first experimental approaches to study the unknown role of a known protein is to generate an animal model in which the target gene has been ablated. Knockout mice have been generated for all known caveolins, but only the $CAV1^{-/-}$ and $CAV3^{-/-}$ mice have been particularly interesting in studying caveolin function in the biology of the myocardium.

It is interesting to note that all the caveolin-deficient mouse models generated ($CAV1^{-/-}$, $CAV2^{-/-}$, $CAV3^{-/-}$, $CAV1/3^{-/-}$ double knockout mice) are viable and fertile, despite the tissue distribution and the involvement in a variety of biological processes observed for caveolins.

$CAV1^{-/-}$ Mice

Two independent groups generated *CAV1* null mice. Drab *et al.*, in 2001, showed that upon targeted disruption of *CAV1*, the animals showed an absence of caveolae in all tissues usually expressing caveolin-1; this led to impaired nitric oxide and calcium signaling in the cardiovascular system, causing aberrations in endothelium-dependent relaxation, contractility, and maintenance of muscular tone.[45] In addition, the lungs of $CAV1^{-/-}$ mice exhibited alveolar thickening due to unrestrained endothelial cell proliferation and fibrosis.[45]

In the same year, Razani and colleagues generated viable and fertile caveolin-1 null mice demonstrating the same caveolar aberration previously affirmed and showing that absence of caveolin-1 could not prevent the formation of normal caveolae in tissues expressing caveolin-3, such as skeletal and cardiac muscles.[46] In addition, the $CAV1^{-/-}$ mouse demonstrated an almost complete loss of caveolin-2, confirming the role of caveolin-1 in heterooligomerization with caveolin-2, and the ability of caveolin-1 to recruit caveolin-2 from the Golgi to the plasma membrane.[45,46]

Although *CAV1* expression cannot be detectable in cardiomyocytes, it is surprising that $CAV1^{-/-}$ animals also demonstrate cardiovascular abnormalities including DCM, which was shown by transthoracic echocardiographic (TEE) analysis of 5-month-old $CAV1^{-/-}$ mice.[47] Similarly, another group analyzed $CAV1^{-/-}$ mice at age 2, 4, and 12 months by cardiac- gated magnetic resonance imagining (MRI) and TEE, revealing progressive concentric left ventricular hypertrophy, severe right ventricular dilation, and sudden cardiac death (SCD).[48] The SCD phenotype in $CAV1^{-/-}$ mice has been associated with the occurrence of hypertrophic cardiomyopathy (HCM) which is classically associated with arrhythmias and premature sudden death secondary to the progressive disorganization of cardiac tissue.[49,50]

$CAV3^{-/-}$ Mice

The caveolin-3 null mouse demonstrates the absence of muscular caveolae, while expression of caveolin-1 and -2 was normal in nonmuscle cells.[51,52] The animals developed a muscular dystrophy phenotype similar to limb girdle muscular dystrophy (LGMD) observed in patients with LGMD-1C. In addition, $CAV3^{-/-}$ demonstrates a cardiomyopathy phenotype similar to that described above in $CAV1^{-/-}$ animals.

Using cardiac-gated MRI and TEE, Woodman *et al.* found that at 4 months of age, $CAV3^{-/-}$ showed significant cardiac hypertrophy and reduced fractional shortening.[53]

Cardiac histological analysis revealed perivascular fibrosis, myocyte hypertrophy, and cellular infiltration, derived from the exclusion of the DGC from lipid rafts and hyperactivation of the Ras-p42/44 mitogen-activated protein (MAP) kinase cascade in *CAV3* null cardiac tissue.[53] These changes are consistent with the known role of p42/44 MAP kinase activation in cardiac hypertrophy and the role of caveolin-3 as a negative regulator of the Ras-p42/44 MAP kinase cascade, similar to that of caveolin-1.[53]

Interestingly, the caveolin-3 T63S mutation has been recently identified in patients with HCM and DCM, although the exact pathological mechanism is unknown.[54]

$CAV1/3^{-/-}$ Mice

The generation of truly caveolae-deficient animals was accomplished by interbreeding Cav-1 and Cav-3 null mice, to produce caveolin-1/3 double knockout mice (Cav-1/3 dKO). Surprisingly, Cav-1/3 dKO mice are viable and fertile, despite a complete absence of morphologically identifiable caveolae in muscle and nonmuscle cells.[55] Additionally, these mice are deficient in the expression of all three caveolin family members, as caveolin-2 is unstable and degraded in the absence of caveolin-1.

The dKO mice present with a severe cardiomyopathy phenotype, already evident at 2 months of age, with more pronounced left ventricular wall thickness and ventricular septum thickness, accompanied by dramatic cardiac hypertrophic, interstitial inflammation, perivascular fibrosis, and myocyte necrosis.[55] Thus the combined ablation of both caveolin-1 and -3 profoundly alters cardiac structure and function leading to a remarkable risk of SCD.

Caveolins: Biochemistry

Caveolin Protein Domains

Regardless of isoform variability, all three caveolin proteins contain some protein motifs highly conserved throughout evolution such as the eight amino acid FEDVIAEP, which constitutes the "caveolin signature sequence" and is localized proximal to the N-terminus of the protein.[6]

Another characteristic protein domain present in caveolins is the "scaffolding domain," a motif proximal to the hydrophobic transmembrane domain, which interacts with different signal transduction molecules (Figure 14–2).[56,57] Although researchers recognize the importance of each protein domain present in caveolins, it appears that proper caveolin function, such as lipid raft association, extrusion from the Golgi apparatus, and caveolae targeting, greatly if not solely depends on the overall protein folding and tertiary structure.[58]

Despite the high amino acid sequence similarity among the different caveolins, human caveolin-1 and -3 share the highest protein homology with ~65% identity and ~85% similarity, while caveolin-2 shares only ~38% identity and ~58% similarity to human caveolin-1. This remarkable resemblance between caveolin-1 and -3 and their divergence from caveolin-2 may explain why both caveolin-1 and -3, but not caveolin-2, can form caveolae alone or in association with other caveolins in cells lacking caveolae structures such as Madin–Darby canine kidney (MDCK) and epithelial Caco-2 cells.[59] In addition, caveolin-1 and -3, but not caveolin-2, undergo an irreversible posttranslational modification inserting a palmitoyl acid molecule on a cysteine residue at their C-terminus.[60] It is believed that palmitoylation of caveolin-1 and -3 stabilizes the caveolin oligomers and increases the association with the membrane through hydrophobic domains.[61,62] The expression of both caveolin-1 and -3 is also necessary to stabilize caveolin-1/-2 and caveolin-3/-2 heterodimers and to ensure the correct membrane localization of caveolin-2.[63]

Caveolin Protein Topology

Both the N- and the C-termini of the prototypical caveolin are localized to the cytoplasm, while the central hydrophobic domains are "embedded" in the plasma membrane, and no extracellular segments were detected (Figure 14–3).[64] This spatial conformation allows the N-terminal phosphorylation of caveolin-1 by the α subunit of protein kinase C (PKCα) and, as previously mentioned, the palmitoylation at the C-terminus of both caveolin-1 and -3.[33,60] The ultimate protein structure and topology of caveolins originate in the ER, where caveolins are believed to be introduced in the plasma membrane and form a hairpin loop configuration through a transmembrane domain containing 32 hydrophobic amino acids (residues 102–134), which prevents caveolins from completely extending across the plasma membrane.[65]

In addition, the scaffolding domain (residues 82–101) proximal to the N-terminus and the segment 135–150 proximal to the C-terminus are tightly connected to the membranes.[6] Caveolin-1 constructs containing residues 1–101 are

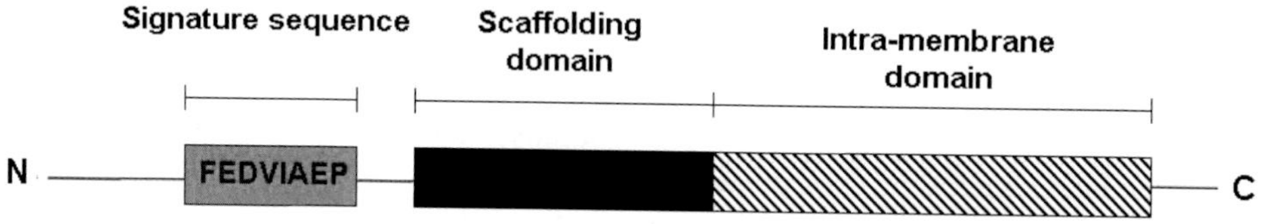

FIGURE 14–2. Prototypic caveolin structure and critical protein motifs.

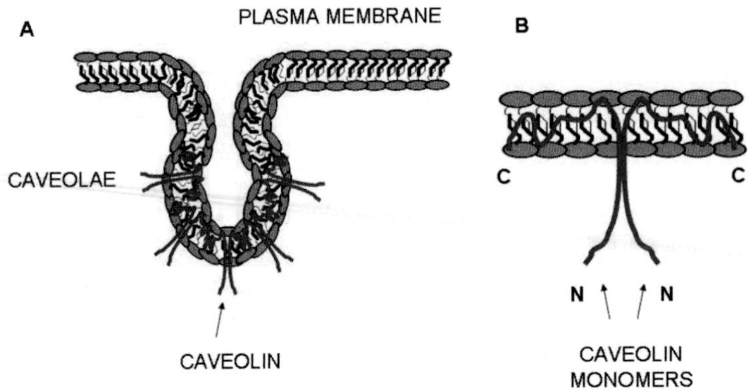

FIGURE 14–3. Caveolae and caveolin topology. (A) Caveolae form plasma membrane invaginations that differ from the clathrin coated endocytic vesicles. (B) Caveolins exhibit both N- and C-terminus ends into the cytoplasm, although their central portion is tightly embedded into the plasma membrane, where most of the interactions with ion channels are hypothesized to occur. Caveolin topology dramatically determines the role of these proteins in lipid raft internalization and functional modulation of its binding partners.

sufficient for membrane localization, while segment 1–82 remained in the cytoplasm.[66] It has been established that the (KYWFYR) motif was sufficient to confer membrane localization to a green fluorescent protein (GFP) fusion protein.[67] In addition, residues 135–150 include a unique Golgi-targeting sequence, and a construct including only this segment of caveolin shows a prevalent Golgi localization.[68,69]

Caveolin-1 contains an oligomerization domain (residues 61–101), which promotes the homooligomerization of up to 16 individual caveolin-1 molecules,[56] while a second stage of oligomerization occurs during transport from the *trans*-Golgi to the plasma membrane, thus forming a large network of caveolin.[70] In contrast, caveolin-2 is unable to generate large homooligomeric complexes and so develop caveolae by itself,[30] while it can form heterooligomers with caveolin-1 in the ER to stabilize caveolin-2 against proteasomal degradation and consent to its transport from the Golgi apparatus to the plasma membrane.[46,71–73]

Similar to caveolin-1, caveolin-3 forms large homooligomeric complexes in striated muscle, and Co-IP and membrane cofractionation studies in rat neonatal cardiomyocytes demonstrated that caveolin-3 associates with caveolin-2 in heterooligomers as occurs for caveolin-1/-2.[74,75]

Caveolae: Function

Caveolae and Lipid Regulation

Due to their high lipid content, it is not surprising that caveolae are involved in lipid metabolism, in particular in the regulation of cholesterol.

Studies employing cholesterol-binding agents such as filipin and nystatin resulted in the disruption of caveolae, suggesting the importance of cellular cholesterol balance on caveolar structure.[2] In addition, an increase in cholesterol levels upregulates caveolin-1 expression through specific binding to two steroid regulatory elements (SRE) on the caveolin-1 promoter, while decreased cholesterol levels result in *CAV1* downregulation.[76,77] Moreover, oxidation of cholesterol into cholesterone by cholesterol oxidase alters the cellular cholesterol balance and results in caveolin-1 internalization from the plasma membrane to the ER and the Golgi apparatus.[78]

Caveolin-1 transports newly synthesized cholesterol from the ER to membrane caveolae, and than to plasma high-density lipoproteins (HDL), while extracellular cholesterol primarily enters cells via clathrin-mediated endocytosis of low-density lipoproteins (LDL).[79] Therefore, caveolae may represent the principal location for cholesterol exchanged between HDL and the cell membrane.

Caveolae and Endocytosis

Caveolae are believed to play a role in endocytosis, oncogenesis, and internalization of pathogenic bacteria.[80]

Caveolae represent a clathrin-independent mechanism of endocytosis for the turnover of adhesive complexes, and since their discovery, they were believed to play a role in endocytosis because they protrude from the plasma membrane into the cytoplasm. However, there is conflicting evidence involving caveolae in constitutive endocytic trafficking. Caveolin-1 cloned as N- and

C-terminus GFP fusion protein and expressed in HeLa, A431, and MDCK cells demonstrated that caveolae require both cholesterol and an intact actin cytoskeleton to maintain their integrity.[81] This may support the hypothesis that caveolae are intimately connected to the actin network. Conversely, Pelkmans and colleagues demonstrated that caveolae play an instrumental role in the internalization of SV40 viral particles, and that this internalization was triggered by molecular signals from the virus, able to activate the caveolae otherwise "dormant" in the stable state previously described.[82]

Caveolae and Signal Transduction

Caveolae play an essential role in signal transduction since biochemically purified caveolae contain multiple signaling molecules, including heterotrimeric G proteins, which in the myocardium are involved in sympathetic tone response though β-adrenergic receptors (β-AR).[83,84] In addition, other signaling factors such as H-Ras, Src-family kinases, and endothelial nitric oxide synthase (eNOS) have been isolated from caveolae.[6]

Other pathways important in cardiac remodeling have been associated with caveolae. For instance, it has been shown that key components of the Ras-p42/44 MAP kinase cascade (MEK and ERK), involved in cardiac hypertrophy, reside within caveolae and are negatively regulated by a direct interaction with caveolin.[36,85–89]

Transient transfection of caveolin dramatically inhibits Raf-1/MEK/ERK and p42/44 MAP kinase signaling, while *in vitro* expression of the caveolin scaffolding domain inhibits the kinase activity of MEK-1 and ERK-2.[83,85] The finding of such a concentration of signaling molecules in caveolae suggests that caveolins act as scaffolding proteins, through the amino acid 82–101 motif, to concentrate and localize these elements for a rapid and specific cell response.[83]

Caveolae and Ion Channels

Being highly expressed in excitable cells of the nervous system, skeletal muscle, and myocardium, a variety of ion channels are localizing to caveolae (Table 14–2). However, it took more than a decade to obtain evidence that these plasmalemmal vesicles not only cluster and scaffold a plethora of cell membrane proteins including signaling molecules, but also anchor, distribute, transport, and possibly modify ion channels on the cell surface.

TABLE 14–2. Ion channels localizing to cardiac caveolae.

Cardiac ion channels
Cardiac sodium channel (Nav1.5)[94]
L-type Ca^{2+} (Cav1.2a)[123,124]
Voltage-gated Kv1.5[91]
Pacemaker channel HCN4[125]
Na^{+}–Ca^{2+} exchanger (NCX)[126]

In 2000, Martens and colleagues identified the relationship of Shaker-like K^{+} channels (Kv2.1) to noncaveolar lipid rafts[90]; the role of these vesicles in Kv2.1 function regulation was elucidated a year later by the same laboratory, showing that cyclodextrin treatment not only led to cholesterol depletion, but also caused a significant shift in steady-state inactivation of the Kv2.1 channel.[91] This first evidence that ion channels localize to lipid rafts suggested that other ion channels may be present in caveolae and that caveolins may regulate ion channel function.

In fact, in 2001 Martens and colleagues localized the voltage-gated potassium channel Kv1.5 to caveolae in transfected fibroblasts.[91] It is interesting to note that Kv1.5 binds the major protein of the Z-line, α-actinin-2,[92] which is connected to the actin network, supporting the concept that caveolae interact with the cytoskeleton (Figure 14–4).

The Kv1.5 channels are expressed in the intercalated disk of human cardiomyocytes and are associated with connexin 43 and N-cadherin.[93] Cytoskeletal alteration using cytochalasin D, which disrupts the filament actin (F-actin), leads to a massive increase in I_{K+}, while the phenomenon was totally abolished when the cells were preincubated with phalloidin, an F-actin-stabilizing agent.[92]

Probably the most intriguing discovery concerning the relationship between cardiac ion channels and caveolae was that the *SCN5A*-coded voltage-gated Na^{+} channels (Nav1.5) have been reported to localize to "caveolin-rich membranes" in cardiac myocytes.[94] In addition, the α subunit of the L-type Ca^{2+} channel (Cav1.2) was originally found in caveolin-enriched membranes in smooth muscle.[95]

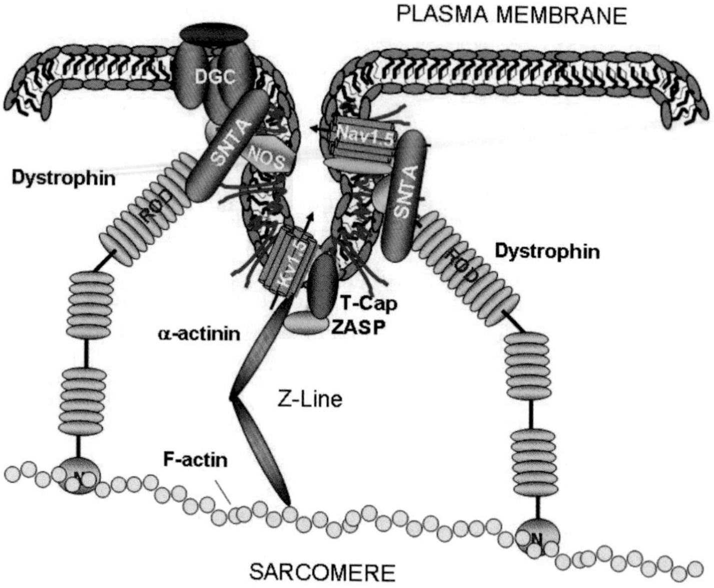

FIGURE 14–4. Cytoskeleton, caveolae, and caveolins. Caveolae are intimately associated with the cytoskeleton of the cardiomyocytes, and are ultimately linked to the contractile apparatus of the myocardial cells. DGC, dystrophin glycoprotein complex; SNTA, α_1-syntrophin.

It is interesting to note that mutations in both Nav1.5 and Cav1.2 have been associated with a primary arrhythmogenic disorder such as the long QT syndrome (LQTS) in human subjects.[96–98]

Similarly, skeletal muscle caveolae have also been found to contain the 1,4-dihydropyridine receptor (DHPR or RyR) in the subsarcolemmal region of the myofibers.[99] In addition, caveolin expression induces Cl_2 channel function.[100]

It is hypothesized that ion channels, which localize to caveolae probably through the scaffolding domain of caveolin-3, reach these lipid rafts after posttranslational modifications such as palmitoylation and myristoylation, or by glycophosphatidylinositol (GPI) membrane anchors, mostly occurring in the Golgi apparatus.[101]

It is still unclear whether caveolin, which can independently drive caveolae formation, can organize membrane lipids and stabilize transient membrane rafts, so that channel proteins might perform as a focal point in raft development.

Alternatively, the association between ion channels and caveolae may not occur through protein/lipid interactions but rather through protein/protein interactions with the direct involvement of caveolins such as caveolin-3, or the direct binding of other caveolin-associated proteins such as the PDZ motif containing protein PSD95 (postsynaptic density protein 95), which has been reported to associate with low-density lipid rafts in mammalian cells.[102] However, the PDZ protein domain may be only one player in the localization of ion channels to raft domains. In fact, Kv2.1 channels do not contain standard PDZ binding sequences,[103] and removal of the PDZ binding motif from the Kv1.5 channel does not prevent its lipid raft association.[91]

Caveolae: Cytoskeleton and Ion Channels

It is interesting to note that many key structural elements, such as the Z-band alternatively spliced PDZ motif protein (ZASP), signaling molecules such as eNOS, and an Nav1.5 modulator, such as α_1-syntrophin (SNTA), contain a PDZ domain, and both eNOS and SNTA also localize to caveolae and directly bind caveolin-3.[104–107] In addition, all the aforementioned proteins localize or are associated with the sarcolemma via direct or indirect interaction with the large protein dystrophin and the DGC, thus modulating ion channel regulation.[38–40]

Caveolin-3; Cytoskeleton and Ion Channels

Syntrophins are known to contain two pleckstrin homology (PH) domains, a PDZ domain, and a syntrophin-unique (SU) at its C-terminus. Syntrophins directly bind dystrophin through their PH domain distal to the N-terminus and the highly conserved SU domain.[108,109] The PH domain proximal to the N-terminus and the PDZ domain interact with other membrane components such as phosphatidylinositol-4,5-bisphosphate (PIP_2),[110] neuronal NOS (nNOS),[111] aquaporin-4,[112] stress-activated protein kinase-3,[113] and Nav1.5,[114] thereby linking all these molecules to the dystrophin complex (Figure 14–4).[115]

In addition, syntrophins bind the C-terminus of Nav1.5 through its PDZ domain, regulating the gating properties of the sodium channel.[116]

Remarkably, caveolae not only cluster syntrophins, but caveolin-3 directly binds syntrophin[107] as well as other important factors such as the Na^+–Ca^{2+} exchanger,[117] the L-type Ca^{2+} channel,[107] eNOS and nNOS, and the DGC (Figure 14–4).[104–106] Therefore, the association of caveolin-3 with α_1-syntrophin, through its binding to F-actin, nNOS, and Nav1.5, appears to be involved in regulating structural and electrical functions as well as signal transduction in heart failure.[107]

Caveolae and Ion Channel Regulation

As previously discussed, due to their physical localization into caveolae and their direct binding to caveolins, it should not be surprising that ion channels might be functionally regulated by lipid rafts such as caveolae. However, the precise mechanism by which caveolins modulate ion channel function, either via direct protein/lipid or protein/protein interactions, as well as through indirect signaling mechanisms, remains unknown.

It is known that caveolin-3 is associated with G protein-coupled receptors (GPCR), which upon stimulation of sympathetic adrenergic receptors triggers G protein-mediated activation of both cAMP-dependent protein kinase A (PKA) and phospholipase C (PLC)-activated protein kinase C (PKC). Both PKA and PKC are known to directly phosphorylate Nav1.5 and modulate its function.[118]

In addition, Kv channels can be phosphorylated by tyrosine kinase such as c-Src, present particularly in caveolae leading to a reduced I_{K+}.[24,119] The two proteins interact through the N-terminal proline-rich sequence of the Kv1.5 channel and the Src homology region 3 (SH3) of Src.[24]

It is also known that CAV3 binds calmodulin (CaM), which in response to a regional increase of Ca^{2+} concentration binds SCN5A increasing its slow-inactivation kinetics.[118] Moreover, SNTA binds Nav1.5 through its PDZ domain at the C-terminus of the sodium channel, altering its gating properties, markedly shifting its activation kinetics, and reducing Na^+-current availability. Therefore, it is possible that mutated CAV3 could modulate ion channel activity directly or via altered structural support on the plasma membrane resulting in uncoupling of ion channels from the cytoskeleton.

Also altered membrane cholesterol can directly modulate ion channel function.[120–122]

All this evidence points toward an increasingly important role of caveolae and caveolin-3 in particular in the regulation of gating, activation/inactivation kinetics, as well as conductance of cardiac ion channels.

Conclusions and Future Directions

Caveolae are peculiar plasma membrane vesicles with an important biological function and role in various cellular processes. The discovery of their main constituents, the caveolins, suggested that caveolae and caveolins are implicated in a variety of important cellular activity, including vesicular trafficking, cholesterol homeostasis, signal transduction, and ion channel regulation.

Since caveolins act as oligomeric scaffolding elements responsible for the clustering and localization of numerous proteins, it was not surprising to discover that caveolin aberration is associated with human diseases.

The ultrastructural, genetic, and molecular analysis of caveolae and caveolins both *in vitro* and *in vivo* provided increasing evidence that these components were instrumental in a range of pathological processes such as muscular dystrophy, cardiac dysfunction, and probably arrhythmias.

The generation of caveolin-deficient mice, and in particular the *CAV3*$^{-/-}$, provides further evidence that although caveolins are not indispensable for life, caveolin alterations are significant in the pathogenesis of human striated muscle abnormalities such as muscular dystrophies and cardiomyopathies, often associated with arrhythmogenesis. Only recently have investigators accumulated increasing evidence of the important role of caveolins in arrhythmogenesis.

There is still a need for further investigation of caveolin-3 abnormalities in patients with primary arrhythmogenic syndromes such as LQTS and Brugada syndrome (BrS). This may help in understanding pivotal protein domains for ion channel function regulation and in designing novel therapeutic approaches to prevent lethal arrhythmic events such as sudden cardiac death.

References

1. Palade GE. An electron microscope study of the mitochondrial structure. *J Histochem Cytochem* 1953;1(4):188–211.
2. Yamada E. The fine structure of the gall bladder epithelium of the mouse. *J Biophys Biochem Cytol* 1955;1(5):445–458.
3. Fra AM, Williamson E, Simons K, Parton RG. De novo formation of caveolae in lymphocytes by expression of VIP21-caveolin. *Proc Natl Acad Sci USA* 1995;92(19):8655–8659.
4. Gorodinsky A, Harris DA. Glycolipid-anchored proteins in neuroblastoma cells form detergent-resistant complexes without caveolin. *J Cell Biol* 1995;129(3):619–627.
5. Mirre C, Monlauzeur L, Garcia M, Delgrossi MH, Le Bivic A. Detergent-resistant membrane microdomains from Caco-2 cells do not contain caveolin. *Am J Physiol* 1996;271(3Pt. 1):C887–894.
6. Cohen AW, Hnasko R, Schubert W, Lisanti MP. Role of caveolae and caveolins in health and disease. *Physiol Rev* 2004;84(4):1341–1379.
7. Simionescu M, Simionescu N, Palade GE. Morphometric data on the endothelium of blood capillaries. *J Cell Biol* 1974;60(1):128–152.
8. McGuire PG, Twietmeyer TA. Morphology of rapidly frozen aortic endothelial cells. Glutaraldehyde fixation increases the number of caveolae. *Circ Res* 1983;53(3):424–429.
9. Noguchi Y, Shibata Y, Yamamoto T. Endothelial vesicular system in rapid-frozen muscle capillaries revealed by serial sectioning and deep etching. *Anat Rec* 1987;217(4):355–360.
10. Wood MR, Wagner RC, Andrews SB, Greener DA, Williams SK. Rapidly-frozen, cultured, human endothelial cells: An ultrastructural and morphometric comparison between freshly-frozen and glutaraldehyde prefixed cells. *Microcirc Endothelium Lymphatics* 1986;3(5–6):323–358.
11. Fan JY, Carpentier JL, van Obberghen E, Grunfel C, Gorden P, Orci L. Morphological changes of th 3T3-L1 fibroblast plasma membrane upon differ entiation to the adipocyte form. *J Cell Sci* 1983;6 219–230.
12. Gratton JP, Bernatchez P, Sessa WC. Caveolae an caveolins in the cardiovascular system. *Circ Re* 2004;94(11):1408–1417.
13. Ishikawa H. Formation of elaborate networks o T-system tubules in cultured skeletal muscle wit special reference to the T-system formation. *J Ce Biol* 1968;38(1):51–66.
14. Parton RG, Way M, Zorzi N, Stang E. Caveolin- associates with developing T-tubules during muscl differentiation. *J Cell Biol* 1997;136(1):137–154.
15. Gabella G, Blundell D. Effect of stretch and con traction on caveolae of smooth muscle cells. *Cel Tissue Res* 1978;190(2):255–271.
16. Sawada H, Ishikawa H, Yamada E. High resolutio scanning electron microscopy of frog sartoriu muscle. *Tissue Cell* 1978;10(1):179–190.
17. Frank JS, Beydler S, Kreman M, Rau EE. Structur of the freeze-fractured sarcolemma in the norma and anoxic rabbit myocardium. *Circ Res* 1980;47(1) 131–143.
18. Severs NJ. Plasma membrane cholesterol i myocardial muscle and capillary endothelial cells Distribution of filipin-induced deformations i freeze-fracture. *Eur J Cell Biol* 1981;25(2):289–299.
19. Izumi T, Shibata Y, Yamamoto T. Striped struc tures on the cytoplasmic surface membranes o the endothelial vesicles of the rat aorta reveale by quick-freeze, deep-etching replicas. *Anat Re* 1988;220(3):225–232.
20. Fujimoto T. Cell biology of caveolae and its impli cation for clinical medicine. Nagoya *J Med Sc* 2000;63(1–2):9–18.
21. Isshiki M, Ando J, Korenaga R, *et al.* Endothelia Ca2+ waves preferentially originate at specific loci in caveolin-rich cell edges. *Proc Natl Acad Sci USA* 1998;95(9):5009–5014.
22. Isshiki M, Ando J, Yamamoto K, Fujita T, Ying Y, Anderson RG. Sites of Ca(2+) wave initiation move with caveolae to the trailing edge of migrating cells. *J Cell Sci* 2002;115(Pt. 3):475–484.
23. Parat MO, Anand-Apte B, Fox PL. Differential caveolin-1 polarization in endothelial cells during migration in two and three dimensions. *Mol Biol Cell* 2003;14(8):3156–3168.
24. Anderson RG. The caveolae membrane system. *Annu Rev Biochem* 1998;67:199–225.
25. Edidin M. The state of lipid rafts: From model membranes to cells. *Annu Rev Biophys Biomol Struct* 2003;32:257–283.

26. Rothberg KG, Heuser JE, Donzell WC, Ying YS, Glenney JR, Anderson RG. Caveolin, a protein component of caveolae membrane coats. *Cell* 1992;68(4):673–682.
27. Glenney JR Jr, Kindy MS, Zokas L. Isolation of a new member of the S100 protein family: Amino acid sequence, tissue, and subcellular distribution. *J Cell Biol* 1989;108(2):569–578.
28. Glenney JR Jr. Tyrosine phosphorylation of a 22-kDa protein is correlated with transformation by Rous sarcoma virus. *J Biol Chem* 1989;264(34): 20163–20166.
29. Kurzchalia TV, Dupree P, Parton RG, *et al.* VIP21, a 21-kD membrane protein is an integral component of trans-Golgi-network-derived transport vesicles. *J Cell Biol* 1992;118(5):1003–1014.
30. Scherer PE, Okamoto T, Chun M, Nishimoto I, Lodish HF, Lisanti MP. Identification, sequence, and expression of caveolin-2 defines a caveolin gene family. *Proc Natl Acad Sci USA* 1996;93(1): 131–135.
31. Tang Z, Scherer PE, Okamoto T, *et al.* Molecular cloning of caveolin-3, a novel member of the caveolin gene family expressed predominantly in muscle. *J Biol Chem* 1996;271(4):2255–2261.
32. Stan RV. Structure of caveolae. *Biochim Biophys Acta* 2005;1746(3):334–348.
33. Li S, Song KS, Koh SS, Kikuchi A, Lisanti MP. Baculovirus-based expression of mammalian caveolin in Sf21 insect cells. A model system for the biochemical and morphological study of caveolae biogenesis. *J Biol Chem* 1996;271(45):28647–28654.
34. Scherer PE, Tang Z, Chun M, Sargiacomo M, Lodish HF, Lisanti MP. Caveolin isoforms differ in their N-terminal protein sequence and subcellular distribution. Identification and epitope mapping of an isoform-specific monoclonal antibody probe. *J Biol Chem* 1995;270(27):16395–16401.
35. Way M, Parton RG. M-caveolin, a muscle-specific caveolin-related protein. *FEBS Lett* 1995;376(1–2): 108–112.
36. Song KS, Scherer PE, Tang Z, *et al.* Expression of caveolin-3 in skeletal, cardiac, and smooth muscle cells. Caveolin-3 is a component of the sarcolemma and co-fractionates with dystrophin and dystrophin-associated glycoproteins. *J Biol Chem* 1996;271(25):15160–15165.
37. Galbiati F, Volonte D, Engelman JA, Scherer PE, Lisanti MP. Targeted down-regulation of caveolin-3 is sufficient to inhibit myotube formation in differentiating C2C12 myoblasts. Transient activation of p38 mitogen-activated protein kinase is required for induction of caveolin-3 expression and subsequent myotube formation. *J Biol Chem* 1999;274(42):30315–30321.
38. Ahn AH, Yoshida M, Anderson MS, *et al.* Cloning of human basic A1, a distinct 59-kDa dystrophin-associated protein encoded on chromosome 8q23–24. *Proc Natl Acad Sci USA* 1994;91(10): 4446–4450.
39. Adams ME, Dwyer TM, Dowler LL, White RA, Froehner SC. Mouse alpha 1- and beta 2-syntrophin gene structure, chromosome localization, and homology with a discs large domain. *J Biol Chem* 1995;270(43):25859–25865.
40. Piluso G, Mirabella M, Ricci E, *et al.* Gamma1- and gamma2-syntrophins, two novel dystrophin-binding proteins localized in neuronal cells. *J Biol Chem* 2000;275(21):15851–15860.
41. Sotgia F, Lee JK, Das K, *et al.* Caveolin-3 directly interacts with the C-terminal tail of beta-dystroglycan. Identification of a central WW-like domain within caveolin family members. *J Biol Chem* 2000;275(48):38048–38058.
42. Bonilla E, Fischbeck K, Schotland DL. Freeze-fracture studies of muscle caveolae in human muscular dystrophy. *Am J Pathol* 1981;104(2):167–173.
43. Repetto S, Bado M, Broda P, *et al.* Increased number of caveolae and caveolin-3 overexpression in Duchenne muscular dystrophy. *Biochem Biophys Res Commun* 1999;261(3):547–550.
44. Vaghy PL, Fang J, Wu W, Vaghy LP. Increased caveolin-3 levels in mdx mouse muscles. *FEBS Lett* 1998;431(1):125–127.
45. Drab M, Verkade P, Elger M, *et al.* Loss of caveolae, vascular dysfunction, and pulmonary defects in caveolin-1 gene-disrupted mice. *Science* 2001; 293(5539):2449–2452.
46. Razani B, Engelman JA, Wang XB, *et al.* Caveolin-1 null mice are viable but show evidence of hyperproliferative and vascular abnormalities. *J Biol Chem* 2001;276(41):38121–38138.
47. Zhao YY, Liu Y, Stan RV, *et al.* Defects in caveolin-1 cause dilated cardiomyopathy and pulmonary hypertension in knockout mice. *Proc Natl Acad Sci USA* 2002;99(17):11375–11380.
48. Park DS, Cohen AW, Frank PG, *et al.* Caveolin-1 null (–/–) mice show dramatic reductions in life span. *Biochemistry* 2003;42(51):15124–15131.
49. Maron BJ. Cardiology patient pages. Hypertrophic cardiomyopathy. *Circulation* 2002;106(19):2419–2421.
50. Tin LL, Beevers DG, Lip GY. Hypertension, left ventricular hypertrophy, and sudden death. *Curr Cardiol Rep* 2002;4(6):449–457.
51. Galbiati F, Engelman JA, Volonte D, *et al.* Caveolin-3 null mice show a loss of caveolae, changes in

the microdomain distribution of the dystrophin-glycoprotein complex, and T-tubule abnormalities. *J Biol Chem* 2001;276(24):21425–21433.
52. Hagiwara Y, Sasaoka T, Araishi K, *et al.* Caveolin-3 deficiency causes muscle degeneration in mice. *Hum Mol Genet* 2000;9(20):3047–3054.
53. Woodman SE, Park DS, Cohen AW, *et al.* Caveolin-3 knock-out mice develop a progressive cardiomyopathy and show hyperactivation of the p42/44 MAPK cascade. *J Biol Chem* 2002;277(41): 38988–38997.
54. Hayashi T, Arimura T, Ueda K, *et al.* Identification and functional analysis of a caveolin-3 mutation associated with familial hypertrophic cardiomyopathy. *Biochem Biophys Res Commun* 2004; 313(1):178–184.
55. Park DS, Woodman SE, Schubert W, *et al.* Caveolin-1/3 double-knockout mice are viable, but lack both muscle and non-muscle caveolae, and develop a severe cardiomyopathic phenotype. *Am J Pathol* 2002;160(6):2207–2217.
56. Sargiacomo M, Scherer PE, Tang Z, *et al.* Oligomeric structure of caveolin: Implications for caveolae membrane organization. *Proc Natl Acad Sci USA* 1995;92(20):9407–9411.
57. Schlegel A, Arvan P, Lisanti MP. Caveolin-1 binding to endoplasmic reticulum membranes and entry into the regulated secretory pathway are regulated by serine phosphorylation. Protein sorting at the level of the endoplasmic reticulum. *J Biol Chem* 2001;276(6):4398–4408.
58. Ren X, Ostermeyer AG, Ramcharan LT, Zeng Y, Lublin DM, Brown DA. Conformational defects slow Golgi exit, block oligomerization, and reduce raft affinity of caveolin-1 mutant proteins. *Mol Biol Cell* 2004;15(10):4556–4567.
59. Vogel U, Sandvig K, van Deurs B. Expression of caveolin-1 and polarized formation of invaginated caveolae in Caco-2 and MDCK II cells. *J Cell Sci* 1998;111(Pt. 6):825–832.
60. Dietzen DJ, Hastings WR, Lublin DM. Caveolin is palmitoylated on multiple cysteine residues. Palmitoylation is not necessary for localization of caveolin to caveolae. *J Biol Chem* 1995;270(12): 6838–6842.
61. Monier S, Dietzen DJ, Hastings WR, Lublin DM, Kurzchalia TV. Oligomerization of VIP21-caveolin in vitro is stabilized by long chain fatty acylation or cholesterol. *FEBS Lett* 1996;388(2–3):143–149.
62. Parat MO, Fox PL. Palmitoylation of caveolin-1 in endothelial cells is post-translational but irreversible. *J Biol Chem* 2001;276(19):15776–15782.
63. Razani B, Woodman SE, Lisanti MP. Caveolae: From cell biology to animal physiology. *Pharmacol Rev* 2002;54(3):431–467.
64. Dupree P, Parton RG, Raposo G, Kurzchalia TV Simons K. Caveolae and sorting in the trans-Golg network of epithelial cells. *EMBO J* 1993;12(4) 1597–1605.
65. Monier S, Parton RG, Vogel F, Behlke J, Henske A Kurzchalia TV. VIP21-caveolin, a membrane protein constituent of the caveolar coat, oligomerizes in vivo and in vitro. *Mol Biol Cell* 1995;6(7) 911–927.
66. Schlegel A, Schwab RB, Scherer PE, Lisanti MP. A role for the caveolin scaffolding domain in mediating the membrane attachment of caveolin-1. The caveolin scaffolding domain is both necessary and sufficient for membrane binding in vitro. *J Biol Chem* 1999;274(32):22660–22667.
67. Woodman SE, Schlegel A, Cohen AW, Lisanti MP. Mutational analysis identifies a short atypical membrane attachment sequence (KYWFYR) within caveolin-1. *Biochemistry* 2002;41(11):3790–3795.
68. Luetterforst R, Stang E, Zorzi N, Carozzi A, Way M, Parton RG. Molecular characterization of caveolin association with the Golgi complex: Identification of a cis-Golgi targeting domain in the caveolin molecule. *J Cell Biol* 1999;145(7):1443–1459.
69. Schlegel A, Pestell RG, Lisanti MP. Caveolins in cholesterol trafficking and signal transduction: Implications for human disease. *Front Biosci* 2000;5:D929–937.
70. Song KS, Tang Z, Li S, Lisanti MP. Mutational analysis of the properties of caveolin-1. A novel role for the C-terminal domain in mediating homo-typic caveolin-caveolin interactions. *J Biol Chem* 1997;272(7):4398–4403.
71. Mora R, Bonilha VL, Marmorstein A, *et al.* Caveolin-2 localizes to the Golgi complex but redistributes to plasma membrane, caveolae, and rafts when co-expressed with caveolin-1. *J Biol Chem* 1999;274(36):25708–25717.
72. Parolini I, Sargiacomo M, Galbiati F, *et al.* Expression of caveolin-1 is required for the transport of caveolin-2 to the plasma membrane. Retention of caveolin-2 at the level of the golgi complex. *J Biol Chem* 1999;274(36):25718–25725.
73. Scherer PE, Lewis RY, Volonte D, *et al.* Cell-type and tissue-specific expression of caveolin-2. Caveolins 1 and 2 co-localize and form a stable hetero-oligomeric complex in vivo. *J Biol Chem* 1997; 272(46):29337–29346.
74. Rybin VO, Grabham PW, Elouardighi H, Steinberg SF. Caveolae-associated proteins in cardiomyocytes: Caveolin-2 expression and interactions with caveolin-3. *Am J Physiol Heart Circ Physiol* 2003;285(1):H325–332.

75. Woodman SE, Sotgia F, Galbiati F, Minetti C, Lisanti MP. Caveolinopathies: Mutations in caveolin-3 cause four distinct autosomal dominant muscle diseases. *Neurology* 2004;62(4):538–543.
76. Bist A, Fielding PE, Fielding CJ. Two sterol regulatory element-like sequences mediate up-regulation of caveolin gene transcription in response to low density lipoprotein free cholesterol. *Proc Natl Acad Sci USA* 1997;94(20):10693–10698.
77. Fielding CJ, Bist A, Fielding PE. Caveolin mRNA levels are up-regulated by free cholesterol and down-regulated by oxysterols in fibroblast monolayers. *Proc Natl Acad Sci USA* 1997;94(8):3753–3758.
78. Smart EJ, Ying YS, Conrad PA, Anderson RG. Caveolin moves from caveolae to the Golgi apparatus in response to cholesterol oxidation. *J Cell Biol* 1994;127(5):1185–1197.
79. Graf GA, Matveev SV, Smart EJ. Class B scavenger receptors, caveolae and cholesterol homeostasis. *Trends Cardiovasc Med* 1999;9(8):221–225.
80. Frank PG, Lisanti MP. Caveolin-1 and caveolae in atherosclerosis: Differential roles in fatty streak formation and neointimal hyperplasia. *Curr Opin Lipidol* 2004;15(5):523–529.
81. Thomsen P, Roepstorff K, Stahlhut M, van Deurs B. Caveolae are highly immobile plasma membrane microdomains, which are not involved in constitutive endocytic trafficking. *Mol Biol Cell* 2002;13(1):238–250.
82. Pelkmans L, Helenius A. Endocytosis via caveolae. *Traffic* 2002;3(5):311–320.
83. Lisanti MP, Scherer PE, Tang Z, Sargiacomo M. Caveolae, caveolin and caveolin-rich membrane domains: A signalling hypothesis. *Trends Cell Biol* 1994;4(7):231–235.
84. Sargiacomo M, Sudol M, Tang Z, Lisanti MP. Signal transducing molecules and glycosyl-phosphatidylinositol-linked proteins form a caveolin-rich insoluble complex in MDCK cells. *J Cell Biol* 1993;122(4):789–807.
85. Engelman JA, Chu C, Lin A, *et al.* Caveolin-mediated regulation of signaling along the p42/44 MAP kinase cascade in vivo. A role for the caveolin-scaffolding domain. *FEBS Lett* 1998;428(3):205–211.
86. Galbiati F, Volonte D, Engelman JA, *et al.* Targeted downregulation of caveolin-1 is sufficient to drive cell transformation and hyperactivate the p42/44 MAP kinase cascade. *EMBO J* 1998;17(22):6633–6648.
87. Liu P, Ying Y, Ko YG, Anderson RG. Localization of platelet-derived growth factor-stimulated phosphorylation cascade to caveolae. *J Biol Chem* 1996;271(17):10299–10303.
88. Liu P, Ying Y, Anderson RG. Platelet-derived growth factor activates mitogen-activated protein kinase in isolated caveolae. *Proc Natl Acad Sci USA* 1997;94(25):13666–13670.
89. Smart EJ, Ying YS, Anderson RG. Hormonal regulation of caveolae internalization. *J Cell Biol* 1995;131(4):929–938.
90. Martens JR, Navarro-Polanco R, Coppock EA, *et al.* Differential targeting of Shaker-like potassium channels to lipid rafts. *J Biol Chem* 2000;275(11):7443–7446.
91. Martens JR, Sakamoto N, Sullivan SA, Grobaski TD, Tamkun MM. Isoform-specific localization of voltage-gated K+ channels to distinct lipid raft populations. Targeting of Kv1.5 to caveolae. *J Biol Chem* 2001;276(11):8409–8414.
92. Maruoka ND, Steele DF, Au BP, *et al.* Alpha-actinin-2 couples to cardiac Kv1.5 channels, regulating current density and channel localization in HEK cells. *FEBS Lett* 2000;473(2):188–194.
93. Mays DJ, Foose JM, Philipson LH, Tamkun MM. Localization of the Kv1.5 K+ channel protein in explanted cardiac tissue. *J Clin Invest* 1995;96(1):282–292.
94. Yarbrough TL, Lu T, Lee HC, Shibata EF. Localization of cardiac sodium channels in caveolin-rich membrane domains: Regulation of sodium current amplitude. *Circ Res* 2002;90(4):443–449.
95. Darby PJ, Kwan CY, Daniel EE. Caveolae from canine airway smooth muscle contain the necessary components for a role in Ca(2+) handling. *Am J Physiol Lung Cell Mol Physiol* 2000;279(6):L1226–1235.
96. Jiang C, Atkinson D, Towbin JA, *et al.* Two long QT syndrome loci map to chromosomes 3 and 7 with evidence for further heterogeneity. *Nat Genet* 1994;8(2):141–147.
97. Splawski I, Timothy KW, Sharpe LM, *et al.* Ca(V)1.2 calcium channel dysfunction causes a multisystem disorder including arrhythmia and autism. *Cell* 2004;119(1):19–31.
98. Splawski I, Timothy KW, Decher N, *et al.* Severe arrhythmia disorder caused by cardiac L-type calcium channel mutations. *Proc Natl Acad Sci USA* 2005;102(23):8089–8096; discussion 8086–8088.
99. Jorgensen AO, Shen AC, Arnold W, Leung AT, Campbell KP. Subcellular distribution of the 1,4-dihydropyridine receptor in rabbit skeletal muscle in situ: An immunofluorescence and immunocolloidal gold-labeling study. *J Cell Biol* 1989;109(1):135–147.
100. Okada Y. A scaffolding for regulation of volume-sensitive Cl^- channels. *J Physiol* 1999;520(Pt. 1):2.

101. Melkonian KA, Ostermeyer AG, Chen JZ, Roth MG, Brown DA. Role of lipid modifications in targeting proteins to detergent-resistant membrane rafts. Many raft proteins are acylated, while few are prenylated. *J Biol Chem* 1999;274(6):3910–3917.
102. Perez AS, Bredt DS. The N-terminal PDZ-containing region of postsynaptic density-95 mediates association with caveolar-like lipid domains. *Neurosci Lett* 1998;258(2):121–123.
103. Scannevin RH, Murakoshi H, Rhodes KJ, Trimmer JS. Identification of a cytoplasmic domain important in the polarized expression and clustering of the Kv2.1 K+ channel. *J Cell Biol* 1996;135(6 Pt. 1):1619–1632.
104. Venema VJ, Ju H, Zou R, Venema RC. Interaction of neuronal nitric-oxide synthase with caveolin-3 in skeletal muscle. Identification of a novel caveolin scaffolding/inhibitory domain. *J Biol Chem* 1997;272(45):28187–28190.
105. Campbell KP, Kahl SD. Association of dystrophin and an integral membrane glycoprotein. *Nature* 1989;338(6212):259–262.
106. Durbeej M, Campbell KP. Muscular dystrophies involving the dystrophin-glycoprotein complex: An overview of current mouse models. *Curr Opin Genet Dev* 2002;12(3):349–361.
107. Feron O, Kelly RA. Gaining respectability: Membrane-delimited, caveolar-restricted activation of ion channels. *Circ Res* 2002;90(4):369–370.
108. Ahn AH, Kunkel LM. Syntrophin binds to an alternatively spliced exon of dystrophin. *J Cell Biol* 1995;128(3):363–371.
109. Kachinsky AM, Froehner SC, Milgram SL. A PDZ-containing scaffold related to the dystrophin complex at the basolateral membrane of epithelial cells. *J Cell Biol* 1999;145(2):391–402.
110. Chockalingam PS, Gee SH, Jarrett HW. Pleckstrin homology domain 1 of mouse alpha 1-syntrophin binds phosphatidylinositol 4,5-bisphosphate. *Biochemistry* 1999;38(17):5596–5602.
111. Brenman JE, Chao DS, Gee SH, *et al.* Interaction of nitric oxide synthase with the postsynaptic density protein PSD-95 and alpha1-syntrophin mediated by PDZ domains. *Cell* 1996;84(5):757–767.
112. Frigeri A, Nicchia GP, Verbavatz JM, Valenti G, Svelto M. Expression of aquaporin-4 in fast-twitch fibers of mammalian skeletal muscle. *J Clin Invest* 1998;102(4.):695–703.
113. Hasegawa M, Cuenda A, Spillantini MG, *et al.* Stress-activated protein kinase-3 interacts with the PDZ domain of alpha1-syntrophin. A mechanism for specific substrate recognition. *J Biol Chem* 1999;274(18):12626–12631.
114. Gee SH, Madhavan R, Levinson SR, Caldwell JH, Sealock R, Froehner SC. Interaction of muscle and brain sodium channels with multiple members c the syntrophin family of dystrophin-associate proteins. *J Neurosci* 1998;18(1):128–137.
115. Adams ME, Mueller HA, Froehner SC. In viv requirement of the alpha-syntrophin PDZ domai for the sarcolemmal localization of nNOS an aquaporin-4. *J Cell Biol* 2001;155(1):113–122.
116. Ou Y, Strege P, Miller SM, *et al.* Syntrophin gamm 2 regulates SCN5A gating by a PDZ domain mediated interaction. *J Biol Chem* 2003;278(3): 1915–1923.
117. Bossuyt J, Taylor BE, James-Kracke M, Hale CC Evidence for cardiac sodium-calcium exchange association with caveolin-3. *FEBS Lett* 2002 511(1–3):113–117.
118. Abriel H, Kass RS. Regulation of the voltage-gate cardiac sodium channel Nav1.5 by interactin proteins. *Trends Cardiovasc Med* 2005;15(1) 35–40.
119. Holmes TC, Fadool DA, Ren R, Levitan IB. Association of Src tyrosine kinase with a human potassium channel mediated by SH3 domain. *Scienc* 1996;274(5295):2089–2091.
120. Romanenko VG, Rothblat GH, Levitan I. Modulation of endothelial inward-rectifier K+ current b optical isomers of cholesterol. *Biophys J* 2002;83(6) 3211–3222.
121. Hajdu P, Varga Z, Pieri C, Panyi G, Gaspar R Jr Cholesterol modifies the gating of Kv1.3 in huma T lymphocytes. *Pflugers Arch* 2003;445(6):674-682.
122. Barrantes FJ. Lipid matters: nicotinic acetylcholine receptor-lipid interactions (Review). *Mo Membr Biol* 2002;19(4):277–284.
123. Galbiat F, Engelman JA, Volonte D, Zhang XL Minetti C, Li M, et al., Caveolin-3 null mice shov a loss of caveolae, changes in the microdomair distribution of the dystrophinglycoprotein complex, and t-tubule abnormalities. *J Biol Chem* 2001;276:21425–21433.
124. Balijepalli RC, Foell JD, Hall DD, Hell JW, Kamp TJ. Localization of cardiac L-type Ca(2+) channels to a caveolar macromolecular signaling complex is required for beta(2)-adrenergic regulation. *Proc Natl Acad Sci USA* 2006;103(19):7500–7505.
125. Barbuti A, Terragni B, Brioschi C, DiFrancesco D. Localization of f-channels to caveolae mediates specific beta2-adrenergic receptor modulation of rate in sinoatrial myocytes. *J Mol Cell Cardiol* 2007;42(1):71–78.
126. Teubl M, Groschner K, Kohlwein SD, Mayer B, Schmidt K. Na(+)/Ca(2+) exchange facilitates Ca(2+)-dependent activation of endothelial nitric-oxide synthase. *J Biol Chem* 1999;274(41);29529–29535.

15 Senescence and Arrhythmogenesis

Arshad Jahangir, Srinivasan Sattiraju, and Win-Kuang Shen

Introduction

Aging is associated with an increased incidence of cardiac arrhythmias that contributes significantly to the increased morbidity and mortality of old age.[1–3] The increased susceptibility to both ventricular and atrial arrhythmias in the senescent heart occurs despite the absence of apparent disease and is exaggerated in the presence of underlying comorbidities.[4,5] Cardiac dysrhythmias not only adversely affect the quality of life but also contribute to deterioration in myocardial function, increasing the susceptibility to heart failure, stroke, and sudden death.[5–7] With the rapid increase in the elderly population and the prevalence of cardiovascular diseases in the elderly, it is projected that the number of patients with cardiac arrhythmias and associated disability will more than double in 30 years, placing an enormous burden on health care resources.[8–10] Although progress is being made in understanding the pathogenesis of age-related cardiac diseases and therapies are being developed for these diseases, advanced age by itself poses significant dilemmas in therapy due to the lack of a full understanding of the molecular basis for the aging-associated increase in the susceptibility of the heart to arrhythmogenesis and the paucity of outcome studies in the very elderly.[6,11] This chapter summarizes the epidemiology, aging-associated changes in cardiac structure and function, basis for arrhythmogenesis, and evaluation and management of elderly patients with ventricular tachyarrhythmias causing sudden death.

Ventricular Arrhythmias and Sudden Cardiac Death

Unexpected death from cardiovascular causes, ranging from 300,000 to 350,000 deaths annually in the United States, is one of the most common modes of death in the elderly.[12] It accounts for 13% of all natural deaths and 50% of all deaths from cardiovascular causes.[4,13] Its incidence increases with advancing age in both those with structural heart disease, as well as those without recognizable risk factors for SCD.[4,14] In patients with coronary disease, sudden cardiac death (SCD) may occur as the first clinical event in 50% of the patients.[14] Despite advances in the management of cardiovascular diseases, the overall incidence of SCD in the general population (0.1–0.2% per year) has decreased only marginally and is expected to increase with the aging of the population and the increased prevalence of chronic heart disease.[15,16] Therefore, effective means to identify those at the highest risk of sudden death and development of strategies for the primary and secondary prevention of SCD in the elderly remain a priority.

Substrates for Sudden Cardiac Death in the Elderly

The substrate for SCD in the elderly varies depending on the underlying heart disease. The effect of aging alone on cardiac structure and function in humans is difficult to study because of difficulties in separating the effect of aging from the effect of diseases associated with aging. The majority of sudden deaths in the elderly occur in the setting of coronary artery disease caused by ventricular arrhythmias, often triggered by acute ischemia.[12,14,17] Approximately 80% of patients who die suddenly from cardiac causes have underlying coronary artery disease and in 50% sudden death may be the first manifestation of their disease.[14] Active coronary lesions or acute changes in plaque morphology, such as plaque disruption or thrombus, may be present in more than 50% of the victims of sudden death.[18–20] The risk for ventricular arrhythmias increases after a myocardial infarction due to the presence of scar and the reduction in left ventricular systolic function. Other substrates for ventricular arrhythmias and sudden death in the elderly include ventricular hypertrophy, nonischemic cardiomyopathy, valvular diseases, or inflammatory or infiltrative diseases.[4,21–25] Only a small percentage of SCDs in the elderly occur due to a primary defect in ion channels responsible for sudden death in younger patients with inherited arrhythmia syndromes, such as the congenital long QT syndrome, short QT syndrome, Brugada syndrome, or catecholaminergic polymorphic ventricular tachycardia.[26–28] Familial clustering of cardiac events, however, does suggest a role of hereditary factors in the predisposition to sudden death,[29,30] which in the elderly appears to be due to genetic influences that increase the risk of a coronary event.[11,28,31–34] The presence of obesity, hypertension, and lipid abnormalities, and a history of smoking and diabetes increase the risk for sudden death.[35–37]

Mechanisms of Sudden Cardiac Death

Despite our understanding of risk factors and substrate for arrhythmogenesis, the exact mechanisms underlying initiation, propagation, maintenance, or prediction of timing for cardiac dysrhythmias causing SCD in the elderly are not fully understood. This is mainly due to the complex interactions between myocardial substrate and triggers that define the overall risk of susceptibility to arrhythmia.[38,39] Age-related changes in cardiac structure and function occur at macroscopic and microscopic levels in both the cellular and extracellular matrix.[1,40] This results in altered cellular excitability and cell-to cell coupling creating a proarrhythmic milieu that increases the predisposition to arrhythmogenesis due to abnormalities in impulse initiation and/or propagation. Failure of impulse initiation or conduction results in bradyarrhythmias, whereas enhanced impulse generation due to increased automaticity or triggered activity or slowed conduction resulting in reentry causes tachyarrhythmias.

Bradyarrhythmias, due to reduced normal automaticity and delayed conduction, are common in the very elderly, even in the absence of apparent heart diseases.[41,42] The intrinsic heart rate as measured following blockade of the parasympathetic and sympathetic nervous system and heart rate reserve decrease with aging.[43] This is related to aging-associated replacement of pacemaker cells within the sinoatrial node and atrioventricular conduction fibers with collagenous and elastic matrix[3] and impairment of signaling via cardiac G protein-coupled receptors, specifically β-adrenergic receptors contributing to diminished cardiac exercise reserve, spontaneous heart rate variability, and maximum heart rate achieved during stress resulting in a reduction in the aerobic work capacity in the elderly.[3,41,44] Myocyte hypertrophy and interstitial fibrosis also accompany aging, which alter cellular coupling and exaggerate directional differences in conduction (anisotropy); this increasing heterogeneity in conduction and refractoriness promotes the formation of zones of functional slowing or conduction block that stabilize reentry-enhancing susceptibility to arrhythmogenesis.[45,46] In addition, aging causes changes in expression, distribution, and/or functioning of ion channels, which alter action potential waveforms and propagation, further increasing vulnerability to dysrhythmias.[47–49] The action potential duration and repolarization are prolonged in the senescent heart,[50,51] in part due to the delay in the inactivation of the calcium current (I_{CaL})[52–54] and in part due to downregulation of potassium currents, including the transient outward (I_{to}) current, Ca^{2+}-activated potassium current, and ATP-sensitive potassium channel current that along with an increase in the sodium–calcium exchanger increase the predisposition to Ca^{2+} overload-mediated triggered activity and reentrant arrhythmias.[51,54–59] Advanced age is also associated with a reduction of expression of the sarcoplasmic reticulum Ca^{2+}-ATPase (SERCA-2)[60,61] and posttranslational modifications causing phosphorylation-dependent changes in the function of SERCA-2, phospholamban, and other Ca^{2+} transport proteins, including the ryanodine receptor, the sarcoplasmic reticulum Ca^{2+} release channel.[62,63] The contribution of age-related changes in cardiac microstructure, including mitochondria[64] and other intracellular organelles, cytoskeleton, sarcolemma, intercellular gap junctions, cellular geometry, and interstitium on regulation of cardiac excitability or arrhythmogenesis is not well defined and warrants further studies.

Ventricular arrhythmias are common in the elderly, being present in more than 70% of persons over the age of 60 years. The incidence, prevalence, and complexity of ventricular arrhythmias and their prognostic significance increase with advancing age[35] and the presence of heart disease.[4,65–67] In the absence of heart disease, asymptomatic premature ventricular complexes (PVC) observed at rest do not carry an adverse prognosis, but when elicited during exercise[68] or the postexercise recovery period[69] are associated with an increased risk of cardiovascular death. In those with structural heart disease, PVCs do indicate an increased mortality risk, especially if ventricular function is reduced.[35,70–76] The mechanisms underlying ventricular arrhythmias vary depending on the underlying substrate. During the acute phase of myocardial infarction or with acute ischemia, ventricular fibrillation may result from functional reentry, whereas in patients with healed myocardial infarction, a reentry circuit can form around scarred tissue causing ventricular tachycardia that can then degenerate into fibrillation, even in the absence of active ischemia. In the peri-infarction period, the senescent heart is more vulnerable to arrhythmogenesis, with a greater likelihood of in-hospital cardiac arrest in those 75 years and older compared to younger patients.[77] Although ventricular tachyarrhythmias occurring within 48 h of the acute coronary syndrome is associated with an increase in hospital mortality, long-term mortality is not affected unless significant ventricular dysfunction persists.[78] The incidence of scar-related reentrant ventricular arrhythmias, however, increases following myocardial infarction, increasing exponentially as the left ventricular ejection fraction falls below 30%.[12,17]

The exact electrophysiological basis for SCD in the elderly is difficult to determine and results from multiple factors depending on the underlying cardiac substrate with which dynamic transient factors (such as ischemia, hypoxia, catecholamine, pH and electrolyte changes, stretch, or inflammation) interact to precipitate arrhythmias.[12] In addition, an arrhythmia may be initiated by one mechanism, perpetuated by another, and then degenerate into a different mechanism. At the time of cardiac arrest, ventricular fibrillation is, however, the most commonly recorded rhythm observed in 75–80% of patients compared to advanced atrioventricular block or asystole documented in 15–20% of the cases.[79,80] The true incidence of bradyarrhythmias causing sudden death in the elderly is not known because by the time the first rhythm is recorded, an arrhythmia beginning as ventricular tachyarrhythmia may degenerate into or appear as asystole.

Evaluation of Elderly Patients at Risk for Sudden Cardiac Death

Several risk stratification protocols have been developed for the identification of patients at risk for ventricular arrhythmias who may benefit from interventions to reduce the risk of sudden death. These include noninvasive tests, such as a standard 12 lead electrocardiogram (ECG), exercise tests or parameters to determine the severity of left ventricular systolic dysfunction, the presence of late potentials on signal-average electrocardiography (SAECG), the severity of ventricular arrhythmias determined by ambulatory cardiac monitoring, the detection of repolarization instability by measurement of QT interval, QT dispersion, and microvolt T-wave alternans, and autonomic balance by heart rate variability or baroreflex sensitivity, or invasive tests to determine inducibility of sustained ventricular arrhythmias by programmed electrical stimulation.[4]

A standard 12-lead ECG allows identification of underlying structural disease, such as conduction system abnormalities with heart block, bundle-branch block, intraventricular conduction delay, ventricular hypertrophy, or prior infarction, as well as primary electrical disorders, such as the long QT syndrome, short QT syndrome, Brugada syndrome, or arrhythmogenic right ventricular cardiomyopathy. A prolonged QRS duration >120 msec in patients with a severely depressed ventricular function or a prolonged QTc interval in the elderly predict a higher risk of SCD.[2,81] The absence of a slowly conducting zone, the electrophysiological substrate for reentrant ventricular arrhythmias that is otherwise detected as late potentials on SAECG, may be useful with its high negative predictive value to exclude a wide-complex tachycardia as a cause of unexplained syncope in the elderly patient with coronary artery disease.[82,83] An exercise ECG may also provide useful diagnostic and prognostic information in the evaluation of patients with known or suspected coronary artery disease, cardiomyopathies, or frequent premature ventricular complexes. The appearance of exercise-induced complex ventricular ectopy or ventricular tachycardia in the elderly may predict an increased risk of mortality compared to patients with simple ectopy observed at rest only.[68,69,84] T-wave alternans detected as microvolt fluctuation in the amplitude or morphology of the T-wave during exercise testing or atrial pacing is also a useful tool for identifying high-risk patients after myocardial infarction or with cardiomyopathy and carries a high negative predictive accuracy.[85,86]

Assessment of left ventricular systolic function and other structural and functional information about myocardial dimensions, wall thickness, and valvular and congenital heart disorders with imaging techniques, such as echocardiogram, is an essential part of risk stratification of patients with ventricular arrhythmias at risk for SCD.[87] Cardiac magnetic resonance imaging (MRI) or computed tomography (CT) scan is helpful in patients with suspected arrhythmogenic right ventricular cardiomyopathy.[88] Myocardial perfusion single-photon emission computed tomography (SPECT) using exercise or pharmacological agents is useful for the detection of ischemia in those suspected of having ventricular arrhythmias triggered by ischemia.[89] Coronary angiography is useful in the assessment of obstructive coronary artery disease in patients with ventricular arrhythmias or aborted sudden death,

The utility of electrophysiology (EP) testing with intracardiac recording and electrical stimulation in the elderly varies with the type and severity of heart disease.[90–92] It is useful for the assessment of arrhythmia and risk stratification for SCD in elderly patients with ischemic heart disease and left ventricular dysfunction or syncope, but plays only a minor role in the evaluation of patients with dilated cardiomyopathy (DCM) or inherited arrhythmia syndromes, such as the long or short QT syndrome.[90–94] Its utility in patients with Brugada syndrome or hypertrophic cardiomyopathy is controversial.[95–97] In patients with coronary artery disease, nonsustained ventricular tachycardia, and left ventricular ejection fraction (EF) less than 40%, the inducibility of sustained ventricular tachycardia identifies patients at high risk for ventricular arrhythmias and predicts a worse prognosis.[98] However, in those with severe ventricular dysfunction (EF <30%), noninducibility of ventricular tachycardia with program electrical stimulation does not indicate a good prognosis[99] and is not helpful in risk stratification.

Management of Elderly Patients at Risk for Sudden Cardiac Death

Antiarrhythmic Drugs

The essential goals of antiarrhythmic therapy in the elderly are acute termination of an ongoing arrhythmia and/or prevention of the recurrence of arrhythmia. Although antiarrhythmic agents, except for the β-blockers, have not been shown to reduce mortality in randomized trials,[100–103] they continue to play an important role for symptom relief by suppression of recurrences of arrhythmia in elderly patients. However, these agents should be used with caution as they can also cause arrhythmia in susceptible individuals.[104] Selection of an effective yet safe medication in the elderly is challenging due to variability in the pathophysiological substrate, mechanisms of arrhythmia, clinical presentation, and prognostic implications of the arrhythmia.[105] In addition, the presence of comorbidities, concomitant drug use, and variability in drug disposition, and/or responses due to aging-associated physiological changes that alter the pharmacokinetics and pharmacodynamics of a drug, require careful adjustment of drug regimens and frequent monitoring for efficacy and side effects.[106] The empiric use of antiarrhythmic drugs regardless of the prognostic significance of an arrhythmia or choosing antiarrhythmic drugs by trial and error is not acceptable due to deleterious effects, including the risk of proarrhythmia,[107,108] which may be increased in the elderly due to impaired renal clearance and the potential for drug interactions.[106] There is no evidence that suppression of asymptomatic nonsustained ventricular tachycardia prolongs life, and the only indication to treat these arrhythmias is for symptom control due to frequent recurrences of rapid tachycardia compromising hemodynamics. These could be managed with antiarrhythmic therapy, preferably with β-blockers, sotalol, or amiodarone, or with catheter ablation. In the presence of structural heart disease or myocardial ischemia, class I antiarrhythmic agents should be avoided as clinical trials, such as the Cardiac Arrhythmia Suppression Trial, have demonstrated increased mortality or incessant arrhythmias in patients treated with antiarrhythmic agents compared to placebo.[107] Patients with atrial fibrillation treated with a class I antiarrhythmic agent may become symptomatic with a rapid 1:1 atrioventricular response as the atrial rhythm becomes more organized and if used these agents should be given with drugs that slows atrioventricular node conduction. In addition, use of class I antiarrhythmic agents in patients with a pacemaker or implantable cardioverter defribillator (ICD) may result in an increase in pacing threshold or defibrillation energy requirement[109,110] necessitating reprogramming of pacing or ICD systems.

Overall, class I or III antiarrhythmic drugs should not be used as primary therapy in the management of ventricular arrhythmias or the prevention of SCD in the elderly. Its use as a hybrid treatment with ICD implantation, however, can be considered for symptom control and improvement in quality of life by suppression of recurrences of arrhythmia and frequency of ICD discharges.[111,112] Amiodarone, a complex drug with multiple electrophysiological effects, is useful for the termination and suppression of ventricular arrhythmias, especially when used with β-blockers. However, the long-term survival benefit from amiodarone alone was not shown in most of the randomized, placebo-controlled studies, demonstrating no significant benefit over standard of care in high-risk patients with heart failure or coronary artery disease.[113–115] Similarly, use of sotalol, despite its effectiveness in suppressing ventricular arrhythmias, has not been shown to improve survival.[116] Use of amiodarone (with a β-blocker) or sotalol is recommended in patients who do not meet the criteria for ICD implantation, or in those who have an ICD with the therapeutic goal of reducing the recurrence of ventricular arrhythmias and the frequency of ICD shocks.[111,112]

Drugs that are relatively safe and have been shown to be effective in improving survival in high-risk elderly patients include β-blockers, angiotensin converting enzyme inhibitors, angiotensin receptor antagonists, and statins; these do not possess classic antiarrhythmic properties and should be considered in high-risk patients after myocardial infarction or with heart failure.[117,118] The combination of β-blockers and amiodarone appears to be more effective in reducing overall mortality and sudden death than amiodarone alone.[119,120]

Implantable Cardioverter Devices

Patients who had cardiac arrest due to ventricular fibrillation or sustained ventricular tachycardia in the absence of a removable cause or those with persistent severe left ventricular dysfunction (EF <35%) due to nonischemic or ischemic cardiomyopathy 40 days after acute myocardial infarction are at increased risk of SCD and should be considered for ICD implantation.[4,121,122] Randomized, prospective trials comparing antiarrhythmic drug therapy to ICD have demonstrated the efficacy of ICDs in primary and secondary prevention of sudden death in those at high risk of SCD or in those resuscitated after cardiac arrest.[100–102,123–125] However, none of these trials has focused specifically on the efficacy of ICD in the elderly. The survival benefit of ICD in those 65 years or older appears to be similar to those <65 years of age,[126–128] with the benefit of ICD therapy apparently greater in those in whom an ICD is implanted for primary prophylaxis of SCD than in those for secondary prevention after a life-threatening arrhythmic event or in those with advanced heart failure and a higher risk of nonarrhythmic cardiac or noncardiac death.[129,130] Because of the limited availability of data, the efficacy of ICD therapy in the older elderly with limited life expectancy is not clear, as only a very small number of elderly above 80 years of age have been included in these trials; these trials may also suffer from selection bias for the use of more expensive devices in "healthier" elderly patients with a lower risk of noncardiac or cardiac death.[131] Pooled analysis of the secondary prevention trials does indicate that the very elderly may derive less benefit from an ICD than younger patients, due to an increased number of nonarrhythmic cardiac and noncardiac deaths.[132] Similarly, cohort studies reporting an equivalent survival benefit in the elderly and younger patients may not reflect the true benefit of ICD therapy in the overall elderly population as selection bias may be present, with use of more expensive device implantation considered in only "healthier elderly" free of serious comorbidities with a better functional capacity.[131,133–135] In the absence of symptomatic arrhythmias in those with preserved ventricular function (EF >40%), the risk for SCD is relatively low, and at this time ICD therapy is not indicated.[4] In addition, in the very elderly patient who has multiple comorbidities with a limited life expectancy from nonarrhythmic causes, ICD may not prolong survival and could have an adverse impact on quality of life, and therefore should be avoided. Patients with ICD with compromised ventricular function who require pacing may have exacerbation of heart failure when paced from the right ventricular (RV) apex.[136] In these patients RV pacing should be minimized by selecting a low minimum rate, programming a long AV interval, selecting an ICD with algorithms utilizing automatic mode selection that favors atrial over ventricular pacing, or using ICDs with biventricular pacing capabilities.[137]

Radiofrequency Ablation

Ablation therapy should be considered in the elderly as adjunctive therapy for recurrent ventricular tachycardia in those with recurrent ICD shocks not manageable by reprogramming of ICD or antiarrhythmic therapy or who do not wish long-term drug therapy.[4,138–141] Ablation as primary therapy is indicated only in those who are otherwise at low risk for SCD and have symptomatic predominantly monomorphic ventricular arrhythmias that are drug resistant, or in patients who are drug intolerant or do not wish long-term drug therapy.[4,142] Ablation of the tachycardia circuit involving the bundle branches in bundle branch ventricular tachycardia may be curative, but these patients typically have severe ventricular dysfunction with an underlying substrate that increases the risk for other arrhythmias and therefore may need ICD. Ventricular arrhythmias arising from the right and less commonly the left ventricular outflow tract are usually seen in healthy young individuals, but may present in the elderly. They are associated with a good prognosis[143] and often respond to treatment with β-blockers and calcium channel blockers or class IC antiarrhythmic drugs. In those who remain symptomatic or do not respond to drug therapy, catheter ablation should be considered.[4]

Other Interventions

Ablation of the tachycardia circuit using surgery to resect or modify the arrhythmia substrate is an alternative therapy that may be suitable for patients in whom catheter ablation is unsuccessful and who are otherwise fit to undergo cardiac surgery. Coronary revascularization with percutaneous coronary intervention or bypass surgery reduces myocardial ischemia and SCD during long-term follow-up,[144] but controlled trials evaluating the effect of myocardial revascularization on ventricular arrhythmias in the elderly have not been conducted. If ventricular arrhythmias are triggered by acute ischemia, coronary revascularization helps reduce the frequency and complexity of the arrhythmias. However, sustained monomorphic ventricular tachycardia in patients with scarred myocardium from a previous infarction is not affected by revascularization[145]; neither is the risk of recurrent cardiac arrest in patients with markedly reduced ventricular function eliminated with revascularization even if the original arrhythmia appeared to result from transient ischemia.[146]

With the continuing rise in medical costs and the rapid increase in the elderly population and in the prevalence of cardiovascular diseases and associated disability, urgency exists to better integrate our efforts in basic science and clinical practice to enhance our understanding of arrhythmogenesis and its effect on outcomes in the elderly, so as to advance both therapeutic and preventive strategies to improve health and longevity of elderly patients.

References

1. Lakatta EG, Sollott SJ. Perspectives on mammalian cardiovascular aging: Humans to molecules. *Comp Biochem Physiol A Mol Integr Physiol* 2002; 132:699–721.
2. Chugh SS, Jui J, Gunson K, Stecker EC, John BT, Thompson B, Ilias N, Vickers C, Dogra V, Daya M, Kron J, Zheng ZJ, Mensah G, McAnulty J. Current burden of sudden cardiac death: Multiple source surveillance versus retrospective death certificate-based review in a large U.S. community. *J Am Coll Cardiol* 2004;44:1268–1275.
3. Lakatta EG. Cardiovascular regulatory mechanisms in advanced age. *Physiol Rev* 1993;73:413–467.
4. Zipes DP, Camm AJ, Borggrefe M, Buxton AE, Chaitman B, Fromer M, Gregoratos G, Klein G, Moss AJ, Myerburg RJ, Priori SG, Quinones MA, Roden DM, Silka MJ, Tracy C. ACC/AHA/ESC 2006 guidelines for management of patients with ventricular arrhythmias and the prevention of sudden cardiac death: A report of the American College of Cardiology/American Heart Association Task Force and the European Society of Cardiology Committee for Practice Guidelines (Writing Committee to Develop Guidelines for Management of Patients with Ventricular Arrhythmias and the Prevention of Sudden Cardiac Death). *J Am Coll Cardiol* 2006;48:e247–e346.
5. Fuster V, Ryden LE, Cannom DS, Crijns HJ, Curtis AB, Ellenbogen KA, Halperin JL, Le Heuzey J-Y, Kay GN, Lowe JE, Olsson SB, Prystowsky EN, Tamargo JL, Wann S, Smith SC Jr, Jacobs AK, Adams CD, Anderson JL, Antman EM, Hunt SA, Nishimura R, Ornato JP, Page RL, Riegel B, Priori SG, Blanc J-J, Budaj A, Camm AJ, Dean V, Deckers JW, Despres C, Dickstein K, Lekakis J, McGregor K, Metra M, Morais J, Osterspey A, Zamorano JL. ACC/AHA/ESC 2006 guidelines for the management of patients with atrial fibrillation-executive summary: A report of the American College of Cardiology/American Heart Association Task Force on Practice Guidelines and the European Society of Cardiology Committee for Practice Guidelines (Writing Committee to Revise the 2001 Guidelines for the Management of Patients with Atrial Fibrillation). *Circulation* 2006;114:700–752.
6. Aronow WS. Heart disease and aging. *Med Clin North Am* 2006;90:849–862.
7. Thom T, Haase N, Rosamond W, Howard VJ, Rumsfeld J, Manolio T, Zheng Z-J, Flegal K, O'Donnell C, Kittner S, Lloyd-Jones D, Goff DC Jr, Hong Y, Members of the Statistics Committee and Stroke Statistics Subcommittee, Adams R, Friday G, Furie K, Gorelick P, Kissela B, Marler J, Meigs J, Roger V, Sidney S, Sorlie P, Steinberger J, Wasserthiel-Smoller S, Wilson M, Wolf P. Heart Disease and Stroke Statistics—2006 Update: A Report from the American Heart Association Statistics Committee and Stroke Statistics Subcommittee. *Circulation* 2006;113:e85–151.
8. Go AS, Hylek EM, Phillips KA, Chang Y, Henault LE, Selby JV, Singer DE. Prevalence of diagnosed atrial fibrillation in adults: National implications for rhythm management and stroke prevention: The Anticoagulation and Risk Factors in Atrial Fibrillation (ATRIA) Study. *JAMA* 2001;285:2370–2375.
9. Jahangir A, Shen WK. Pacing in elderly patients. *Am Heart J* 2003;146:750–753.
10. Miyasaka Y, Barnes ME, Gersh BJ, Cha SS, Bailey KR, Abhayaratna WP, Seward JB, Tsang TSM. Secular trends in incidence of atrial fibrillation in Olmsted County, Minnesota, 1980 to 2000, and implications on the projections for future prevalence. *Circulation* 2006;114:119–125.
11. Myerburg RJ. Scientific gaps in the prediction and prevention of sudden cardiac death. *J Cardiovasc Electrophysiol* 2002;13:709–723.
12. Myerburg RJ, Castellanos A. Emerging paradigms of the epidemiology and demographics of sudden cardiac arrest. *Heart Rhythm* 2006;3:235–239.
13. Gillum RF. Geographic variation in sudden coronary death. *Am Heart J* 1990;119:380–389.
14. Myerburg RJ. Sudden cardiac death: Exploring the limits of our knowledge. *J Cardiovasc Electrophysiol* 2001;12:369–381.
15. Braunwald E. Shattuck lecture cardiovascular medicine at the turn of the millennium: Triumphs, concerns, and opportunities. *N Engl J Med* 1997; 337:1360–1369.
16. Schatzkin A, Cupples LA, Heeren T, *et al.* Sudden death in the Framingham Heart Study.

Differences in incidence and risk factors by sex and coronary disease status. *Am J Epidemiol* 1984;120:888–899.
17. Huikuri HV, Castellanos A, Myerburg RJ. Medical progress: Sudden death due to cardiac arrhythmias. *N Engl J Med* 2001;345:1473–1482.
18. Theroux P, Fuster V. Acute coronary syndromes: Unstable angina and non-Q-wave myocardial infarction. *Circulation* 1998;97:1195–1206.
19. Naghavi M, Falk E, Hecht HS, Jamieson MJ, Kaul S, Berman D, Fayad Z, Budoff MJ, Rumberger J, Naqvi TZ, Shaw LJ, Faergeman O, Cohn J, Bahr R, Koenig W, Demirovic J, Arking D, Herrera VL, Badimon J, Goldstein JA, Rudy Y, Airaksinen J, Schwartz RS, Riley WA, Mendes RA, Douglas P, Shah PK; SHAPE Task Force. From vulnerable plaque to vulnerable patient—Part III: Executive summary of the Screening for Heart Attack Prevention and Education (SHAPE) Task Force report. *Am J Cardiol* 2006;17:2H–15H.
20. Farb A, Tang AL, Burke AP, Sessums L, Liang Y, Virmani R. Sudden coronary death: Frequency of active coronary lesions, inactive coronary lesions, and myocardial infarction. *Circulation* 1995;92: 1701–1709.
21. Hulot JS, Jouven X, Empana JP, Frank R, Fontaine G. Natural history and risk stratification of arrhythmogenic right ventricular dysplasia/cardiomyopathy. *Circulation* 2004;110:1879–1884.
22. Klein GJ, Krahn AD, Skanes AC, Yee R, Gula LJ. Primary prophylaxis of sudden death in hypertrophic cardiomyopathy, arrhythmogenic right ventricular cardiomyopathy, and dilated cardiomyopathy. *J Cardiovasc Electrophysiol* 2005;16: S28–34.
23. Maron BJ, McKenna WJ, Danielson GK, Kappenberger LJ, Kuhn HJ, Seidman CE, Shah PM, Spencer I, William H., Spirito P. American College of Cardiology/European Society of Cardiology Clinical Expert Consensus Document on Hypertrophic Cardiomyopathy: A report of the American College of Cardiology Foundation Task Force on Clinical Expert Consensus Documents and the European Society of Cardiology Committee for Practice Guidelines. *J Am Coll Cardiol* 2003;42: 1687–1713.
24. Maron BJ, Estes NA III, Maron MS, Almquist AK, Link MS, Udelson JE. Primary prevention of sudden death as a novel treatment strategy in hypertrophic cardiomyopathy. *Circulation* 2003; 107:2872–2875.
25. More D, O'Brien K, Shaw J. Arrhythmogenic right ventricular dysplasia in the elderly. *Pacing Clin Electrophysiol* 2002;25:1266–1269.
26. Locati EH, Zareba W, Moss AJ, Schwartz PJ, Vincent GM, Lehmann MH, Towbin JA, Priori SG, Napolitano C, Robinson JL, Andrews M, Timothy K, Hall WJ. Age- and sex-related differences in clinical manifestations in patients with congenital long-QT syndrome: Findings from the international LQTS registry. *Circulation* 1998;97:2237–2244.
27. Bjerregaard P, Jahangir A, Gussak I. Targeted therapy for short QT syndrome. *Expert Opin Ther Targets* 2006;10:393–400.
28. Spooner PM, Albert C, Benjamin EJ, Boineau R, Elston RC, George AL Jr, Jouven X, Kuller LH, MacCluer JW, Marban E, Muller JE, Schwartz PJ, Siscovick DS, Tracy RP, Zareba W, Zipes DP. Sudden cardiac death, genes, and arrhythmogenesis: Consideration of new population and mechanistic approaches from a National Heart, Lung, and Blood Institute workshop, part I. *Circulation* 2001;103:2361–2364.
29. Friedlander Y, Siscovick DS, Weinmann S, Austin MA, Psaty BM, Lemaitre RN, Arbogast P, Raghunathan TE, Cobb LA. Family history as a risk factor for primary cardiac arrest. *Circulation* 1998; 97:155–160.
30. Jouven X, Desnos M, Guerot C, Ducimetiere P. Predicting sudden death in the population. The Paris prospective study I. *Circulation* 1999;99: 1978–1983.
31. Boerwinkle E, Ellsworth DL, Hallman DM, Biddinger A. Genetic analysis of atherosclerosis: A research paradigm for the common chronic diseases. *Human Mol Genet* 1996;5:1405–1410.
32. Faber BCG, Cleutjens KB, Niessen RL, Aarts PL, Boon W, Greenberg AS, Kitslaar PJ, Tordoir JH, Daemen MJ. Identification of genes potentially involved in rupture of human atherosclerotic plaques. *Circ Res* 2001;89:547–554.
33. Topol EJ, McCarthy J, Gabriel S, Moliterno DJ, Rogers WJ, Newby LK, Freedman M, Metivier J, Cannata R, O'Donnell CJ, Kottke-Marchant K, Murugesan G, Plow EF, Stenina O, Daley GQ. Single nucleotide polymorphisms in multiple novel thrombospondin genes may be associated with familial premature myocardial infarction. *Circulation* 2001;104:2641–2644.
34. Splawski I, Timothy KW, Tateyama M, Clancy CE, Malhotra A, Beggs AH, Cappuccio FP, Sagnella GA, Kass RS, Keating MT. Variant of SCN5A sodium channel implicated in risk of cardiac arrhythmia. *Science* 2002;297:1333–1336.
35. Kannel WB, Cupples LA, D'Agostino RB. Sudden death risk in overt coronary heart disease: The Framingham Study. *Am Heart J* 1987;113:799–804.

36. Alpert MA. Obesity cardiomyopathy: Pathophysiology and evolution of the clinical syndrome. *Am J Med Sci* 2001;321:225–236.
37. Luscher TF, Creager MA, Beckman JA, Cosentino F. Diabetes and vascular disease: Pathophysiology, clinical consequences, and medical therapy: Part II. *Circulation* 2003;108:1655–1661.
38. Myerburg RJ, Kessler KM, Castellanos A. Sudden cardiac death: Epidemiology, transient risk, and intervention assessment. *Ann Intern Med* 1993; 119:1187–1197.
39. Adamson P, Barr RC, Callans DJ, Chen PS, Lathrop DA, Makielski JC, Nerbonne JM, Nuss HB, Olgin JE, Przywara DA, Rosen MR, Rozanski GJ, Spach MS, Yamada KA. The perplexing complexity of cardiac arrhythmias: Beyond electrical remodeling. *Heart Rhythm* 2005;2:650–659.
40. Juhaszova M, Rabuel C, Zorov DB, Lakatta EG, Sollott SJ. Protection in the aged heart: Preventing the heart-break of old age? *Cardiovasc Res* 2005; 66:233–244.
41. Gregoratos G, Abrams J, Epstein AE, Freedman RA, Hayes DL, Hlatky MA, Kerber RE, Naccarelli GV, Schoenfeld MH, Silka MJ, Winters SL. 2. ACC/AHA/NASPE 2002 guideline update for implantation of cardiac pacemakers and antiarrhythmia devices: A report of the American College of Cardiology/American Heart Association Task Force on Practice Guidelines (ACC/AHA/NASPE Committee on Pacemaker Implantation). Available at www.acc.org/clinical/guidelines/pacemaker/pacemaker.pdf, 2002.
42. Vlietstra RE, Jahangir A, Shen WK. Choice of pacemakers in patients aged 75 years and older: Ventricular pacing mode vs. dual-chamber pacing mode. *Am J Geriatr Cardiol* 2005;14:35–38.
43. Jose A. Effect of combined sympathetic and parasympathetic blockade on heart rate and cardiac function in man. *Am J Cardiol* 1966;18: 476–478.
44. Fleg JL, O'Connor F, Gerstenblith G, Becker LC, Clulow J, Schulman SP, Lakatta EG. Impact of age on the cardiovascular response to dynamic upright exercise in healthy men and women. *J Appl Physiol* 1995;78:890–900.
45. Koura T, Hara M, Takeuchi S, Ota K, Okada Y, Miyoshi S,Watanabe A, Shiraiwa K, Mitamura H, Kodama I, Ogawa S. Anisotropic conduction properties in canine atria analyzed by high-resolution optical mapping: Preferential direction of conduction block changes from longitudinal to transverse with increasing age. *Circulation* 2002; 105:2092–2098.
46. de Bakker JM, van Rijen HM. Continuous and discontinuous propagation in heart muscle. *J Cardiovasc Electrophysiol* 2006;17:567–573.
47. Schram G, Pourrier M, Melnyk P, Nattel S. Differential distribution of cardiac ion channel expression as a basis for regional specialization in electrical function. *Circ Res* 2002;90:939–950.
48. Nerbonne JM, Kass RS. Physiology and molecular biology of ion channels contributing to ventricular repolarization. In: Gussak I, Antzelevitch C, Hammill SC, Shen WK, Bjerregaard P, Eds. *Cardiac Repolarization: Bridging Basic and Clinical Science (Contemporary Cardiology)*. Totowa, NJ: Humana Press, 2003:25–62.
49. Kléber AG, Rudy Y. Basic mechanisms of cardiac impulse propagation and associated arrhythmias. *Physiol Rev* 2004;84:431–488.
50. Josephson IR, Guia A, Stern MD, Lakatta EG. Alterations in properties of L-type Ca channels in aging rat heart. *J Mol Cell Cardiol* 2002;34:297–308.
51. Jahangir A, Cabrera Aguilera CC, Oberlin AS, Ashfaque N, Alexei A, Terzic A. Molecular basis for the increased vulnerability of the aging heart to injury. *Eur Heart J* 2006;27:875.
52. Janczewski AM, Spurgeon HA, Lakatta EG. Action potential prolongation in cardiac myocytes of old rats is an adaptation to sustain youthful intracellular Ca2+ regulation. *J Mol Cell Cardiol* 2002;34: 641–648.
53. Walker KE, Lakatta EG, Houser SR. Alterations in properties of L-type Ca channels in aging rat heart. *J Mol Cell Cardiol* 2002;34:297–308.
54. Walker KE, Lakatta EG, Houser SR. Age associated changes in membrane currents in rat ventricular myocytes. *Cardiovasc Res* 1993;27: 1968–1977.
55. Jahangir A, Terzic A. KATP channel therapeutics at the bedside. *J Mol Cell Cardiol* 2005;39:99–112.
56. Toro L, Marijic J, Nishimaru K, Tanaka Y, Song M, Stefani E. Aging, ion channel expression, and vascular function. *Vasc Pharmacol* 2002;38:73–80.
57. Zhou YY, Lakatta EG, Xiao RP. Age-associated alterations in calcium current and its modulation in cardiac myocytes. *Drugs Aging* 1998;13:159–171.
58. Xiao R-P, Tomhave ED, Wang D-J, Ji X, Boluyt MO, Cheng H, Lakatta EG, Koch WJ. Age-associated reductions in cardiac beta 1- and beta 2-adrenergic responses without changes in inhibitory G proteins or receptor kinases. *J Clin Invest* 1998; 101:1273–1282.
59. Xiao R-P, Zhu W, Zheng M, Cao C, Zhang Y, Lakatta EG, Han Q. Subtype-specific [alpha]1- and

[beta]-adrenoceptor signaling in the heart. *Trends Pharmacol Sci China* 2006;27:330–337.

60. Lompre AM, Lambert F, Lakatta EG, Schwartz K. Expression of sarcoplasmic reticulum Ca2.-ATPase and calsequestrin genes in rat heart during ontogenic development and aging. *Circ Res* 1991; 69:1380–1388.
61. Taffet GE, Tate CA. ATPase content is lower in cardiac sarcoplasmic reticulum isolated from old rats. *Am J Physiol* 1993;264:H1609–H1614.
62. Koban MU, Moorman AF, Holtz J, Yacoub MH, Boheler KR. Expressional analysis of the cardiac Na-Ca exchanger in rat development and senescence. *Cardiovasc Res* 1998;37:405–423.
63. Xu A, Narayanan N. Effects of aging on sarcoplasmic reticulum Ca2.-cycling proteins and their phosphorylation in rat myocardium. *Am J Physiol* 1998;275:H2087–H2094.
64. Jahangir A, Ozcan C, Holmuhamedov EL, Terzic A. Increased calcium vulnerability of senescent cardiac mitochondria: Protective role for a mitochondrial potassium channel opener. *Mech Ageing Dev* 2001;122:1073–1086.
65. Fleg JL, Kennedy HL. Cardiac arrhythmias in a healthy elderly population: Detection by 24-hour ambulatory electrocardiography. *Chest* 1982;81: 302–307.
66. Kennedy HL, Whitlock JA, Sprague MK, Kennedy LJ, Buckingham TA, Goldberg RJ. Long-term follow-up of asymptomatic healthy subjects with frequent and complex ventricular ectopy. *N Engl J Med* 1985;312:193–197.
67. Hinkle LEJ, Carver ST, Stevens M. The frequency of asymptomatic disturbances of cardiac rhythm and conduction in middle-aged men. *Am J Cardiol* 1969;24:629–650.
68. Jouven X, Zureik M, Desnos M, Courbon D, Ducimetiere P. Long-term outcome in asymptomatic men with exercise-induced premature ventricular depolarizations. *N Engl J Med* 2000;343: 826–833.
69. Frolkis JP, Pothier CE, Blackstone EH, Lauer MS. Frequent ventricular ectopy after exercise as a predictor of death. *N Engl J Med* 2003;348:781–790.
70. Messerli FH, Ventura HO, Elizardi DJ, Dunn FG, Frohlich ED. Hypertension and sudden death: Increased ventricular ectopic activity in left ventricular hypertrophy. *Am J Med* 1984;77:18–22.
71. Bigger JT Jr, Fleiss JL, Kleiger R, *et al.* The relationships among ventricular arrhythmias, left ventricular dysfunction, and mortality in the 2 years after myocardial infarction. *Circulation* 1984;69:250–258.
72. Huikuri HV, Makikallio TH, Raatikainen MJP, Perkiomaki J, Castellanos A, Myerburg RJ. Prediction of sudden cardiac death: Appraisal of the studies and methods assessing the risk of sudden arrhythmic death. *Circulation* 2003;108: 110–115.
73. Stevenson WG, Stevenson LW, Middlekauff HR, Saxon LA. Sudden death prevention in patients with advanced ventricular dysfunction. *Circulation* 1993;88:2953–2961.
74. Aronow WS, Ahn C, Mercando AD, Epstein S, Kronzon I. Prevalence and association of ventricular tachycardia and complex ventricular arrhythmias with new coronary events in older men and women with and without cardiovascular disease. *J Gerontol Ser A Biol Sci Med Sci* 2002;57:M178–M180.
75. Volpi A, Cavalli A, Turato R, Barlera S, Santoro E, Negri E. Incidence and short-term prognosis of late sustained ventricular tachycardia after myocardial infarction: Results of the Gruppo Italiano per lo Studio della Sopravvivenza nell'Infarto Miocardico (GISSI-3) Data Base. *Am Heart J* 2001;142:87–92.
76. Trusty JM, Beinborn DS, Jahangir A. Dysrhythmias and the athlete. *AACN Clin Issues* 2004;15: 432–448.
77. Ornato JP, Peberdy MA, Tadler SC, Strobos NC. Factors associated with the occurrence of cardiac arrest during hospitalization for acute myocardial infarction in the second national registry of myocardial infarction in the US. *Resuscitation* 2001; 48:117–123.
78. Behar S, Goldbourt U, Reicher-Reiss H, Kaplinsky E, The Principal Investigators of the SPRINT Study. Prognosis of acute myocardial infarction complicated by primary ventricular fibrillation. *Am J Cardiol* 1990;66:1208–1211.
79. Luu M, Stevenson WG, Stevenson LW, Baron K, Walden J. Diverse mechanisms of unexpected cardiac arrest in advanced heart failure. *Circulation* 1989;80:1675–1680.
80. Bayes de Luna A, Coumel P, Leclercq JF. Ambulatory sudden cardiac death: Mechanisms of production of fatal arrhythmia on the basis of data from 157 cases. *Am Heart J* 1989;117:151–159.
81. Schouten EG, Dekker JM, Meppelink P, Kok FJ, Vandenbroucke JP, Pool J. QT interval prolongation predicts cardiovascular mortality in an apparently healthy population. *Circulation* 1991;84: 1516–1523.
82. Steinberg JS, Berbari EJ. The signal-averaged electrocardiogram: Update on clinical applications. *J Cardiovasc Electrophysiol* 1996;7:972–988.

83. Cook JR, Flack JE, Gregory CA, Deaton DW, Rousou JA, Engelman RM, The CABG Patch Trial. Influence of the preoperative signal-averaged electrocardiogram on left ventricular function after coronary artery bypass graft surgery in patients with left ventricular dysfunction. *Am J Cardiol* 1998;82:285–289.
84. Podrid PJ, Graboys TB. Exercise stress testing in the management of cardiac rhythm disorders. *Med Clin North Am* 1984;68:1139–1152.
85. Bloomfield DM, Bigger JT, Steinman RC, Namerow PB, Parides MK, Curtis AB, Kaufman ES, Davidenko JM, Shinn TS, Fontaine JM. Microvolt T-wave alternans and the risk of death or sustained ventricular arrhythmias in patients with left ventricular dysfunction. *J Am Coll Cardiol* 2006;47:456–463.
86. Chow T, Kereiakes DJ, Bartone C, Booth T, Schloss EJ, Waller T, Chung ES, Menon S, Nallamothu BK, Chan PS. Prognostic utility of microvolt T-wave alternans in risk stratification of patients with ischemic cardiomyopathy. *J Am Coll Cardiol* 2006; 47:1820–1827.
87. Cheitlin MD, Armstrong WF, Aurigemma GP, Beller GA, Bierman FZ, Davis JL, Douglas PS, Faxon DP, Gillam LD, Kimball TR. ACC/AHA/ASE 2003 guideline update for the clinical application of echocardiography: Summary article: A report of the American College of Cardiology/American Heart Association Task Force on Practice Guidelines (ACC/AHA/ASE Committee to Update the 1997 Guidelines for the Clinical Application of Echocardiography). *J Am Coll Cardiol* 2003;42:954–970.
88. Kies P, Bootsma M, Bax J, Schalij MJ, van der Wall EE. Arrhythmogenic right ventricular dysplasia/cardiomyopathy: Screening, diagnosis, and treatment. *Heart Rhythm* 2006;3:225–234.
89. Klocke FJ, Baird MG, Lorell BH, Bateman TM, Messer JV, Berman DS, O'Gara PT, Carabello BA. ACC/AHA/ASNC Guidelines for the Clinical Use of Cardiac Radionuclide Imaging—Executive Summary: A Report of the American College of Cardiology/American Heart Association Task Force on Practice Guidelines (ACC/AHA/ASNC Committee to Revise the 1995 Guidelines for the Clinical Use of Cardiac Radionuclide Imaging). *J Am Coll Cardiol* 2003;42:1318–1333.
90. Wilber DJ, Garan H, Finkelstein D, Kelly E, Newell J, McGovern B, Ruskin JN. Out-of-hospital cardiac arrest. Use of electrophysiologic testing in the prediction of long-term outcome. *N Engl J Med* 1988;318:19–24.
91. Bachinsky WB, Linzer M, Weld L, Estes I, Mark NA. Usefulness of clinical characteristics in predicting the outcome of electrophysiologic studies in unexplained syncope. *Am J Cardiol* 1992;69: 1044–1049.
92. Chen LY, Jahangir A, Decker WW, Smars PA, Wieling W, Hodge DO, Gersh BJ, Hammill SC, Shen WK. Score indices for predicting electrophysiologic outcomes in patients with unexplained syncope. *J Interv Card Electrophysiol* 2005;14:99–105.
93. Brignole M, Alboni P, Benditt DG, Bergfeldt L, Blanc J-J, Thomsen PEB, Gert van Dijk J, Fitzpatrick A, Hohnloser S, Janousek, *et al.* Guidelines on management (diagnosis and treatment) of syncope-update 2004. Executive Summary. *Eur Heart J* 2004;25:2054–2072.
94. Priori SG, Schwartz PJ, Napolitano C, Bloise R, Ronchetti E, Grillo M, Vicentini A, Spazzolini C, Nastoli J, Bottelli G, Folli R, Cappelletti D. Risk stratification in the long-QT syndrome. *N Engl J Med* 2003;348:1866–1874.
95. Priori SG, Napolitano C, Gasparini M, Pappone C, Della Bella P, Giordano U, Bloise R, Giustetto C, De Nardis R, Grillo M, Ronchetti E, Faggiano G, Nastoli J. Natural history of Brugada syndrome: Insights for risk stratification and management. *Circulation* 2002;105:1342–1347.
96. Brugada J, Brugada R, Brugada P. Determinants of sudden cardiac death in individuals with the electrocardiographic pattern of Brugada syndrome and no previous cardiac arrest. *Circulation* 2003; 108:3092–3096.
97. Nienaber CA, Hiller S, Spielmann RP, Geiger M, Kuck KH. Syncope in hypertrophic cardiomyopathy: Multivariate analysis of prognostic determinants. *J Am Coll Cardiol* 1990;15:948–955.
98. Schmitt C, Barthel P, Ndrepepa G, Schreieck J, Plewan A, Schomig A, Schmidt G. Value of programmed ventricular stimulation for prophylactic internal cardioverter-defibrillator implantation in postinfarction patients preselected by noninvasive risk stratifiers. *J Am Coll Cardiol* 2001;37: 1901–1907.
99. Buxton AE, Lee KL, Hafley GE, Wyse DG, Fisher JD, Lehmann MH, Pires LA, Gold MR, Packer DL, Josephson ME, Prystowsky EN, Talajic MR. Relation of ejection fraction and inducible ventricular tachycardia to mode of death in patients with coronary artery disease: An analysis of patients enrolled in the multicenter unsustained tachycardia trial. *Circulation* 2002;106:2466–2472.
100. Buxton AE, Lee KL, Fisher JD, Josephson ME, Prystowsky EU, Hafley G. A randomized study of

the prevention of sudden death in patients with coronary artery disease. *N Engl J Med* 1999;341: 1882–1890.

101. Moss AJ, Hall WJ, Cannom DS, Daubert JP, Higgins SL, Klein H, Levine JH, Saksena S, Waldo AL, Wilber D, Brown MW, Heo M. Improved survival with an implanted defibrillator in patients with coronary disease at high risk for ventricular arrhythmia. *N Engl J Med* 1996;335:1933–1940.
102. Moss AJ, Zareba W, Hall WJ, Klein H, Wilber DJ, Cannom DS, Daubert JP, Higgins SL, Brown MW, Andrews ML. Prophylactic implantation of a defibrillator in patients with myocardial infarction and reduced ejection fraction. *N Engl J Med* 2002; 346:877–883.
103. Connolly SJ, Hallstrom AP, Cappato R, Schron EB, Kuck KH, Zipes DP, Greene HL, Boczor S, Domanski M, Follmann, *et al.* Meta-analysis of the implantable cardioverter defibrillator secondary prevention trials. AVID, CASH and CIDS studies. Antiarrhythmics vs implantable defibrillator study. Cardiac Arrest Study Hamburg. Canadian Implantable Defibrillator Study. *Eur Heart J* 2000; 21:2071–2078.
104. Roden DM. Drug-induced prolongation of the QT interval. *N Engl J Med* 2004;350:1013–1022.
105. Jahangir A, Terzic A, Shen WK. Antiarrhythmic drugs and future direction In: Gussak I, Antzelevitch C, Hammill SC, Shen WK, Bjerregaard P, Eds. *Cardiac Repolarization: Bridging Basic and Clinical Science (Contemporary Cardiology)*. Totowa, NJ: Humana Press, 2003:387–404.
106. Williams BR. Cardiovascular drug therapy in the elderly: Theoretical and practical considerations. *Drugs Aging* 2003;20:445–463.
107. The Cardiac Arrhythmia Suppression Trial (CAST) Investigators. Preliminary report effect of encainide and flecainide on mortality in a randomized trial of arrhythmia suppression after myocardial infarction. *N Engl J Med* 1989;321: 406–412.
108. Waldo AL, Camm AJ, deRuyter H, Friedman PL, MacNeil DJ, Pauls JF, Pitt B, Pratt CM, Schwartz PJ, Veltri EP. Effect of d-sotalol on mortality in patients with left ventricular dysfunction after recent and remote myocardial infarction. *Lancet* 1996;348:7–12.
109. Hellestrand KJ, Burnett PJ, Milne JR, *et al.* Effect of the antiarrhythmic agent flecainide acetate on acute and chronic pacing thresholds. *Pacing Clin Electrophysiol* 1983;6:892–899.
110. Echt DS, Black JN, Barbey JT, Coxe DR, Cato E. Evaluation of antiarrhythmic drugs on defibrillation energy requirements in dogs. Sodium channel block and action potential prolongation. *Circulation* 1989;79:1106–1117.
111. Connolly SJ, Dorian P, Roberts RS, Gent M, Bailin S, Fain ES, Thorpe K, Champagne J, Talajic M, Coutu B, Gronefeld GC, Hohnloser SH. Comparison of [beta]-blockers, amiodarone plus [beta]-blockers, or sotalol for prevention of shocks from implantable cardioverter defibrillators—The OPTIC study: A randomized trial. *JAMA* 2006;295:165–171.
112. Pacifico A, Hohnloser SH, Williams JH, Tao B, Saksena S, Henry PD, Prystowsky EN. Prevention of implantable-defibrillator shocks by treatment with sotalol. *N Engl J Med* 1999;340:1855–1862.
113. Connolly SJ. Meta-analysis of antiarrhythmic drug trials. *Am J Cardiol* 1999;84:90R-93R.
114. Farre J, Romero J, Rubio JM, Ayala R, Castro-Dorticos J. Amiodarone and "primary" prevention of sudden death: Critical review of a decade of clinical trials. *Am J Cardiol* 1999;83:55D-63D.
115. Steinberg JS, Martins J, Sadanandan S, Goldner B, Menchavez E, Domanski M, Russo A, Tullo N, Hallstrom A. Antiarrhythmic drug use in the implantable defibrillator arm of the antiarrhythmics versus implantable defibrillators (AVID) study. *Am Heart J* 2001;142:520–529.
116. Kuhlkamp V, Mewis C, Mermi J, Bosch RF, Seipel L. Suppression of sustained ventricular tachyarrhythmias: A comparison of d,l-sotalol with no antiarrhythmic drug treatment. *J Am Coll Cardiol* 1999;33:46–52.
117. Alberte C, Zipes DP. Use of nonantiarrhythmic drugs for prevention of sudden cardiac death. *J Cardiovasc Electrophysiol* 2003;14:S87–S95.
118. Woods KL, Ketley D, Lowy A, Agusti A, Hagn C, Kala R, Karatzas NB, Leizorowicz A, Reikvam A, Schilling J, Seabra-Gomes R, Vasiliauskas D, Wilhelmsen L. Beta-blockers and antithrombotic treatment for secondary prevention after acute myocardial infarction. Towards an understanding of factors influencing clinical practice. *Eur Heart J* 1998;19:74–79.
119. Cairns JA, Connolly SJ, Roberts R, Gent M. Randomised trial of outcome after myocardial infarction in patients with frequent or repetitive ventricular premature depolarisations: CAMIAT. *Lancet* 1997;349:675–682.
120. Julian D, Camm A, Frangin G, Janse M, Munoz A, Schwartz P, Simon P. Randomised trial of effect of amiodarone on mortality in patients with left-ventricular dysfunction after recent myocardial infarction: EMIAT. *Lancet* 1997;349:667–674.
121. Wilber DJ, Zareba W, Hall WJ, Brown MW, Lin AC, Andrews ML, Burke M, Moss AJ. Time dependence of mortality risk and defibrillator benefit

after myocardial infarction. *Circulation* 2004;109:1082–1084.

122. Hohnloser SH, Kuck KH, Dorian P, Roberts RS, Hampton JR, Hatala R, Fain E, Gent M, Connolly SJ. Prophylactic use of an implantable cardioverter-defibrillator after acute myocardial infarction. *N Engl J Med* 2004;351:2481–2488.
123. Connolly SJ, Gent M, Roberts RS, Dorian P, Roy D, Sheldon RS, Mitchell LB, Green MS, Klein GJ, O'Brien B. Canadian implantable defibrillator study (CIDS): A randomized trial of the implantable cardioverter defibrillator against amiodarone. *Circulation* 2000;101:1297–1302.
124. Lee KL, Hafley G, Fisher JD, Gold MR, Prystowsky EN, Talajic M, Josephson ME, Packer DL, Buxton AE, for the Multicenter Unsustained Tachycardia Trial Investigators. Effect of implantable defibrillators on arrhythmic events and mortality in the Multicenter Unsustained Tachycardia Trial. *Circulation* 2002;106:233–238.
125. Kuck K-H, Cappato R, Siebels J, Ruppel R. Randomized comparison of antiarrhythmic drug therapy with implantable defibrillators in patients resuscitated from cardiac arrest: The Cardiac Arrest Study Hamburg (CASH). *Circulation* 2000;102:748–754.
126. Trappe H-J, Pfitzner P, Achtelik M, Fieguth H-G. Age dependent efficacy of implantable cardioverter-defibrillator treatment: Observations in 450 patients over an 11 year period. *Heart* 1997;78:364–370.
127. Duray G, Richter S, Manegold J, Israel CW, Granefeld G, Hohnloser SH. Efficacy and safety of ICD therapy in a population of elderly patients treated with optimal background medication. *J Interv Cardiac Electrophysiol* 2005;14:169–173.
128. Daubert J, Sesselberg H, Huang D. Implantable cardioverter-defibrillators for primary prevention: How do the data pertain to the aged? *Am J Geriatr Cardiol* 2006;15:88–92.
129. Bardy GH, Lee KL, Mark DB, *et al.* Amiodarone or an implantable cardioverter-defibrillator for congestive heart failure. *N Engl J Med* 2005;352:225–237.
130. Cleland JGF, Daubert J-C, Erdmann E, Freemantle N, Gras D, Kappenberger L, Tavazzi L. The effect of cardiac resynchronization on morbidity and mortality in heart failure. *N Engl J Med* 2005;352:1539–1549.
131. Jahangir A, Shen WK, Neubauer SA, Ballard DJ, Hammill SC, Hodge DO, Lohse CM, Gersh BJ, Hayes DL. Relation between mode of pacing and long-term survival in the very elderly. *J Am Coll Cardiol* 1999;33:1208–1216.
132. Krahn AD, Connolly SJ, Roberts RS, Gent M. Diminishing proportional risk of sudden death with advancing age: Implications for prevention of sudden death. *Am Heart J* 2004;147:837–840.
133. Geelen P, Lorga Filho A, Primo J, Wellens F, Brugada P. Experience with implantable cardioverter defibrillator therapy in elderly patients. *Eur Heart J* 1997;18:1339–1342.
134. Panotopoulos PT, Axtell K, Anderson AJ, Sra J, Blanck Z, Deshpande S, Biehl M, Keelan ET, Jazayeri MR, Akhtar M, Dhala A. Efficacy of the implantable cardioverter-defibrillator in the elderly. *J Am Coll Cardiol* 1997;29:556–560.
135. Saksena S, Mathew P, Giorgberidze I, Krol RB, Kaushik R. Implantable defibrillator therapy for the elderly. *Am J Geriatr Cardiol* 1998;7:11–13.
136. Wilkoff BL, *et al.* Dual-chamber pacing or ventricular backup pacing in patients with an implantable defibrillator: The Dual Chamber and VVI Implantable Defibrillator (DAVID) Trial. *JAMA* 2002;288:3115–3123.
137. Kocovic DZ. Cardiac resynchronization therapy and other new approaches for the treatment of heart failure in the elderly. *Am J Geriatr Cardiol* 2006;15:108–113.
138. Silva RM, Mont L, Nava S, Rojel U, Matas M, Brugada J. Radiofrequency catheter ablation for arrhythmic storm in patients with an implantable cardioverter defibrillator. *Pacing Clin Electrophysiol* 2004;27:971–975.
139. Scheinman MM. NASPE survey on catheter ablation. *Pacing Clin Electrophysiol* 1995;18:1474–1478.
140. Tchou P, Jazayeri M, Denker S, Dongas J, Caceres J, Akhtar M. Transcatheter electrical ablation of right bundle branch. A method of treating macroreentrant ventricular tachycardia attributed to bundle branch reentry. *Circulation* 1988;78:246–257.
141. Stevenson WG, Khan H, Sager P, Saxon LA, Middlekauff HR, Natterson PD, Wiener I. Identification of reentry circuit sites during catheter mapping and radiofrequency ablation of ventricular tachycardia late after myocardial infarction. *Circulation* 1993;88:1647–1670.
142. Gurevitz OT, Glikson M, Asirvatham S, Kester TA, Grice SK, Munger TM, Rea RF, Shen WK, Jahangir A, Packer DL, Hammill SC, Friedman PA. Use of advanced mapping systems to guide ablation in complex cases: Experience with noncontact mapping and electroanatomic mapping systems. *Pacing Clin Electrophysiol* 2005;28:316–323.
143. Joshi S, Wilber DJ. Ablation of idiopathic right ventricular outflow tract tachycardia: Current

perspectives *J Cardiovasc Electrophysiol* 2005;16: S52–S58.

144. Kelly P, Ruskin JN, Vlahakes GJ, Buckley MJJ, Freeman CS, Garan H. Surgical coronary revascularization in survivors of prehospital cardiac arrest: Its effect on inducible ventricular arrhythmias and long-term survival. *J Am Coll Cardiol* 1990;15:267–273.
145. Brugada J, Aguinaga L, Mont L, Betriu A, Mulet J, Sanz G. Coronary artery revascularization in patients with sustained ventricular arrhythmias in the chronic phase of a myocardial infarction: Effects on the electrophysiologic substrate and outcome. *J Am Coll Cardiol* 2001;37:529–533.
146. Natale A, Sra J, Axtell K, Maglio C, Dhala A, Blanck Z, Deshpande S, Jazayeri M, Akhtar M. Ventricular fibrillation and polymorphic ventricular tachycardia with critical coronary artery stenosis: Does bypass surgery suffice? *J Cardiovasc Electrophysiol* 1994;5:988–994.

16
Comparisons of Substrates Responsible for Atrial Versus Ventricular Fibrillation

Brett Burstein, Philippe Comtois, and Stanley Nattel

Introduction

The fundamental mechanisms underlying fibrillation have long been debated (Figure 16–1). The classical notion of multiple circuit reentry (Figure 16–1C) has been challenged by recent ideas suggesting that in some cases a single high-frequency rotor (Figure 16–1B)[1] or even a rapidly firing focus (Figure 16–1A)[2] can underlie fibrillation. In the latter two cases, although the primary source may be firing regularly, the inability of tissues to follow 1:1 causes wave breakup and fibrillation. Ironically, these recent ideas echo notions first put forward in the early twentieth century.[3]

There is increasing awareness that arrhythmias do not usually begin in perfectly normal tissue, but require changes in tissue structure or function that constitute the arrhythmic substrate. The principal mechanisms underlying ectopic complex formation and reentry are illustrated in Figure 16–2, along with the determinants of their substrates. Abnormal automaticity results from enhanced spontaneous phase 4 depolarization and causes premature beats that can trigger reentry in a vulnerable substrate. Early afterdepolarizations (EADs) are caused by failure of normal repolarization, prolonging the action potential (AP) plateau and allowing L-type Ca^{2+} channel reactivation to produce abnormal depolarization before repolarization can occur. Delayed afterdepolarizations (DADs) are due to spontaneous Ca^{2+} leak from sarcoplasmic reticulum (SR) Ca^{2+} stores. The released Ca^{2+} is exchanged for extracellular Na^+ by the Na^+-Ca^{2+} exchanger (NCX) in a fashion that generates a depolarizing current and a DAD. Early afterdepolarizations and DADs can cause extrasystoles that trigger reentrant ventricular fibrillation (VF), but when repetitive can also cause sustained tachyarrhythmias that degenerate to VF. This chapter examines critically the substrates that underlie atrial fibrillation (AF) and VF, to inform the reader about their properties and to evaluate their similarities and differences.

Biophysical Substrate

In biophysical terms, fibrillation represents self-sustaining rapid and irregular electrical activity. Fibrillation can be sustained by either a single rotor, a so-called "mother wave," or by multiple smaller wavelets.[4] Mathematical modeling of AF shows that it can be sustained by either mechanism under different spatial distributions of acetylcholine,[5] thus relating the mechanism to the degree of dispersion of refractoriness and regional ion channel expression. Ectopic complexes arising by automatic, DAD or EAD mechanisms contribute to the fibrillation substrate by providing the critical premature activation that initiates reentrant activity.

Figure 16–3A and B compares the features of the classical leading-circle reentry concept to those of the spiral-wave formalism, which is the presently accepted biophysical representation of functional reentrant activity in cardiac tissue.[6] The transition between tachycardia and

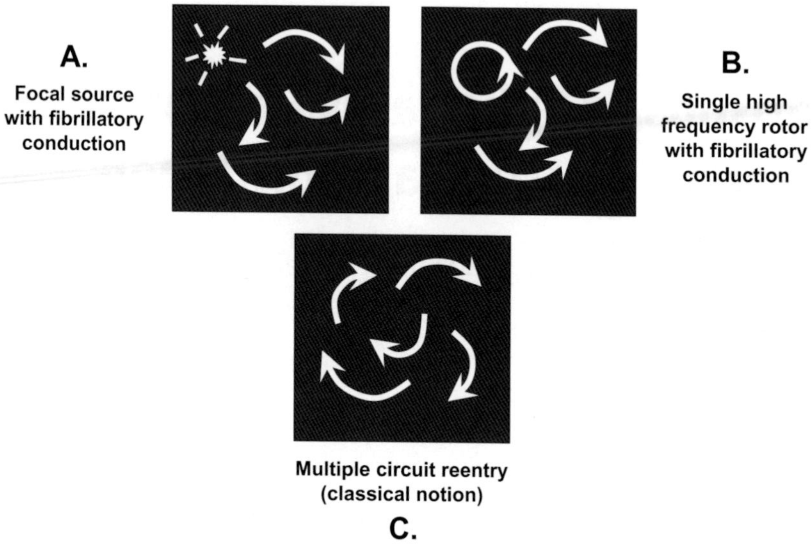

Figure 16–1. Potential mechanisms of fibrillation. Fibrillation may be initiated by a rapidly discharging, spontaneously active, ectopic focus (A), by a single high-frequency rotor (B), or by multiple functional reentrant circuits (C).

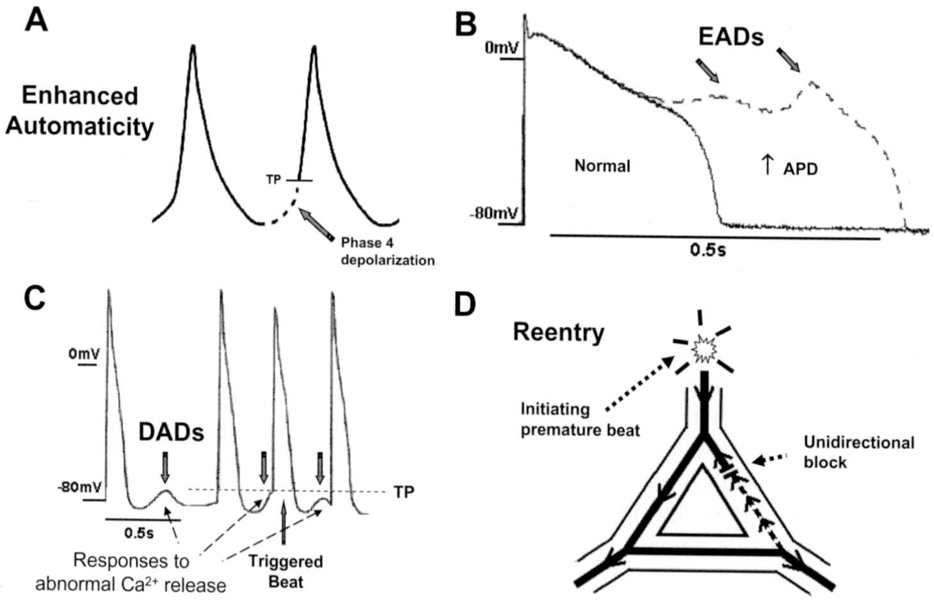

Figure 16–2. Mechanisms of arrhythmia generation. (A) Enhanced automaticity: abnormal impulse formation can result from a region of cardiac tissue prematurely brought to threshold potential (TP) by an increased slope of spontaneous phase 4 diastolic depolarization. (B) Early afterdepolarizations (EADs): reductions in repolarizing currents and/or increases in depolarizing plateau currents can delay repolarization, prolonging action potential duration (APD). This can cause abnormal depolarizations (EADs, arrows) by reactivation of L-type Ca^{2+} channels. (C) Delayed afterdepolarizations (DADs): under pathological conditions (e.g., Ca^{2+} overload, ryanodine receptor dysfunction) Ca^{2+} is released from SR stores in diastole. This Ca^{2+} is exchanged by the Na^+–Ca^{2+} exchanger for three times as many extracellular Na^+ ions, producing an inward current. The inward current depolarizes the cell, producing delayed afterdepolarizations (DADs, downward arrows). If DADs are large enough to reach threshold potential (TP), they can trigger beats (upward arrow). (D) Reentry: reentry may result from a premature initiating beat that fails to conduct in a region that is still refractory (unidirectional block), while conducting through an alternative connecting pathway that is no longer refractory. The impulse can then return backward (retrogradely, dashed line) in the previously blocked pathway, and if enough time has elapsed for recovery of excitability, reenter through that pathway. Reentry requires a crucial balance between conduction and refractoriness to be maintained. It is favored by brief refractory periods and slow conduction. Because variable refractoriness is needed to initiate reentry, spatial variability in refractoriness is an important predisposing condition.

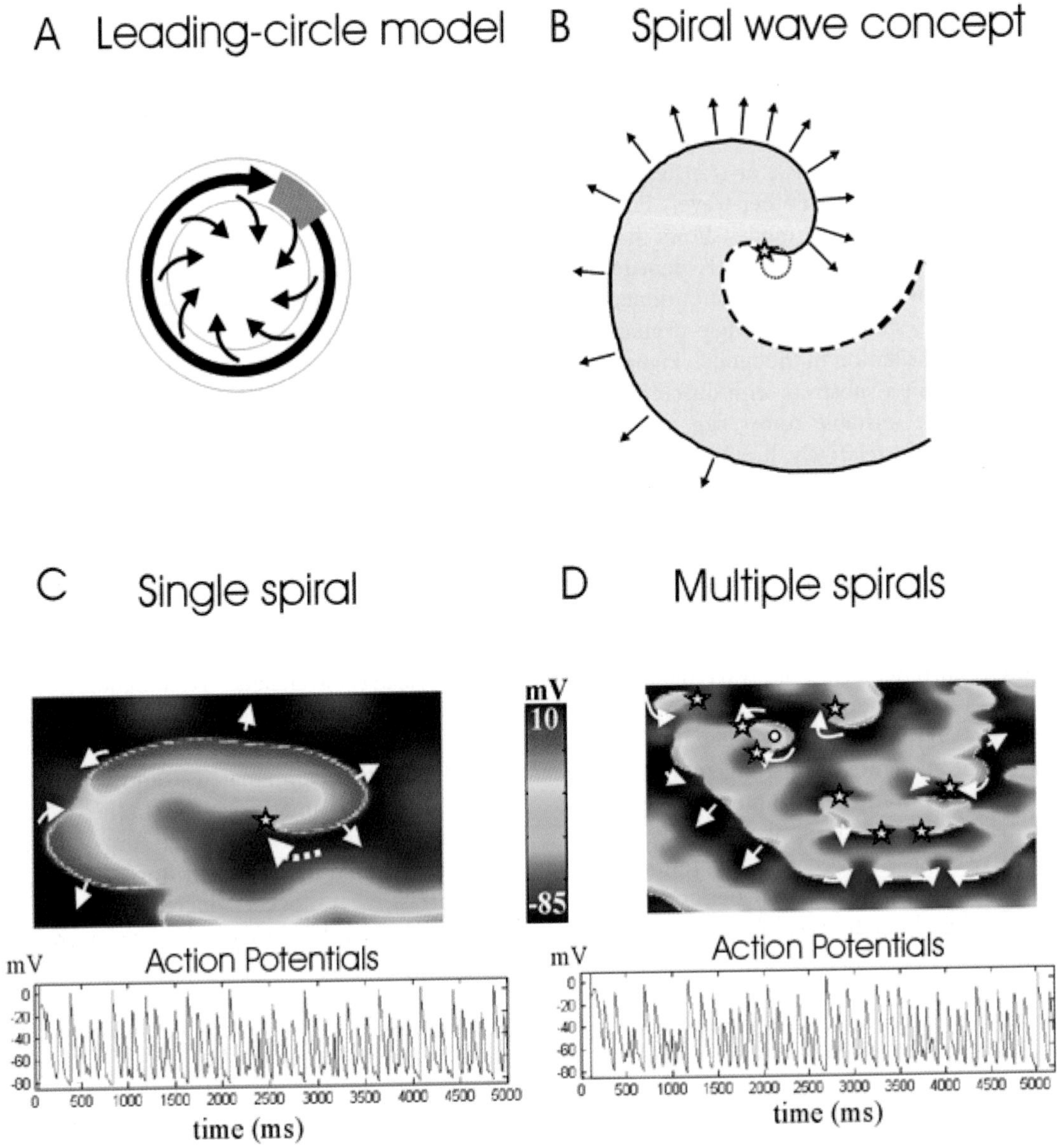

FIGURE 16–3. (A) The leading circle model: schematic diagram of a leading circle reentry wave (shown here as a large black arrow). Activity establishes itself in the smallest pathway that can support reentry, given by the distance traveled by electrical activity in one refractory period (refractory period × conduction velocity). The length of this pathway is also called the wavelength for reentry. Inside the leading circle, centripetal wavelets (small arrows) emanating from the leading circle wavefront constantly maintain the central core in a refractory state. The wave tip and tail are separated by a region (shown in gray) that must be excitable, called the "excitable gap." (B) Spiral wave concept: schematic diagram of a spiral wave with the activation front shown by a continuous line and the repolarization front by a dashed line. The point at which the continuous and dashed curves meet (shown with a star) has an undefined voltage state, and is usually called the phase singularity point. There is no unexcitable core in the spiral wave model. (C) Example of fibrillation sustained by a single spiral wave. Top panel: snapshot of a transmembrane potential (color coded: red = fully depolarized tissue, blue = resting tissue, yellow and green correspond to the AP plateau) during AF. The phase singularity of the single spiral is indicated by the star, and the dashed arrow shows the direction of rotation. The smaller arrows indicate the directions of electrical propagation. Bottom panel: action potentials over 5 sec, showing the nonperiodic fibrillatory activity in a cell near the rotor core. (D) Example of fibrillation sustained by multiple spiral wave rotors. Top panel: snapshot of a transmembrane potential during AF. Generator rotors existing for between 100 msec and 1 sec are indicated by stars. In this case, longer-lasting rotors that maintained AF were always multiple and none of them lasted for long periods. However, they have generated daughter waves, some of which avoided annihilation and were able to maintain generator function when the initial generator extinguished. Bottom panel: action potentials over 5 sec, showing fibrillatory activity at the position pinpointed by the white circle in the top panel. (For more detailed information and access to illustrative videos, see Zou *et al.*[7] Reproduced with permission of the American Physiological Society Inc.)

fibrillation proceeds through partial electrical wave breakup and the formation of secondary reentrant spiral waves that can either be sustained (consistent with the "multiple-wavelet hypothesis," Figure 16–1C) or transient (fibrillatory response to the "mother-wave," Figure 16–1B). An AP-based atrial model shows that either form of activity can underlie AF, depending on functional properties and tissue dimensions.[7] Figure 16–3C shows how a single primary rotor maintains fibrillation in the model. Figure 16–3D shows how, in a substrate with different properties, multiple unstable rotors can coexist, each continuing for relatively brief periods of time (up to 1–2 sec) but spawning sufficient daughter rotors before extinction to perpetuate AF. For further details and access to on-line movies, the interested reader is referred to the original paper.[7]

The first stage in the formation of a spiral wave is the occurrence of partial wave block, equivalent to "unidirectional block" in classical reentry theory. Wave block occurs when the electrical wavefront encounters still-refractory tissue, creating a free wavetip that reenters through excitable tissue. Sustained spiral waves necessitate a sensitive balance between the time for the wavetip to reenter and the refractory period,[6] analogous to the conduction velocity-refractory period requirements for classical reentry. For a more detailed discussion of the relationship between classical reentry theory and the spiral wave formulation, see Comtois *et al.*[8]

Two different substrate characteristics play a role in initiating and sustaining fibrillation. Refractoriness (static) heterogeneity can provide the conditions for reentrant fibrillatory activity. Alternatively, dynamic spatial dispersion related to beat-to-beat variation in AP duration (APD) may be involved.[9] The APD restitution relation (relation between APD and recovery time) and conduction-velocity restitution relation are crucial determinants of this dynamic instability.

Atrial Fibrillation Substrate

Primarily nondynamic mechanisms involving heterogeneity of ERP are thought to initiate breakup within atrial tissue.[10] Variations in neural innervation can also increase ERP heterogeneity. For example, remodeling of atrial electrical characteristics and innervation following left ventricular infarction, causing increased slope of the APD restitution curve, may promote AF via dynamic mechanisms.[11] Atrial shape details, including a range of complicated anatomical factors like pectinate muscles, pulmonary veins, and limited interatrial connections, are likely important in AF, although the transmural electrical complexity of the ventricles is absent. Only recently have computational AF models been developed that consider the anatomical complexity of the atria.[12]

The efficacy of Na^+ channel blockade in terminating AF may be a unique feature of the atrial biophysical substrate. I_{Na} blockers terminate AF[13] via mechanisms demonstrated in AP-based computational models.[14] Na^+ channel blockade slows AF and underlying rotors without increasing wavelength. Termination occurs because of the increased size and meandering of the primary generator rotor, which becomes more likely to be annihilated against a boundary, as well as a dramatic decrease in the number of daughter wavelets that could provide new generators should the primary rotor extinguish.[14] In contrast, I_{Na} blockers increase VF-related mortality in post-MI patients,[15] suggesting a VF-promoting action. In ventricular computational models, behaviors qualitatively similar to those in AF are seen with VF, but spiral wave stabilization occurs rather than termination.[16] Possible explanations of the failure of VF (in contrast to AF) to terminate with Na^+ channel blockade are (1) spiral wave stabilization by anchoring to structures like the papillary muscles[17] instead of terminating on boundary conditions, and (2) limited atrial tissue mass that lacks the three-dimensional transmural complexities of the ventricle and favors spiral wave termination at boundaries.

Ventricular Fibrillation Substrate

Wave breakup occurs in VF mainly via a dynamic mechanism, often first preceded by APD alternans, in particular discordant alternans. Although the importance of APD restitution has been emphasized, recent work points to Ca^{2+} handling properties as the prime culprit.[18,19] Tissue thickness and intramural reentry play a key role in VF.[20] Transmural heterogeneity and repolarization gradients[21] favor wave breakup and reentrant wave formation. Because of its tridimensionality, VF is based on scroll waves rotating around filaments, counterparts to spiral waves/core tips in AF. Mathematical modeling shows that transmural changes in ventricular fiber orientation (rotational anisotropy) can induce filament destabilization,[22,23] with filament twisting leading to wave breakup.[24] Large twisting causes a transition to a turbulent regime characterized by a high density of moving filaments and secondary three-dimensional spiral sources.

Summary of Biophysical Determinants

Similar general biophysical principles apply to AF and VF (Figure 16–4). Important differences result primarily from discrepant structural characteristics of atria versus ventricles. The much greater thickness and transmural properties of the ventricles add an additional level of complexity to VF that may account for the discrepant responses to Na^+ channel blockers, which terminate AF but increase the likelihood of VF.

Ischemic Substrates

Ventricular tachyarrhythmias are the commonest cause of death, usually sudden, in the early phase of acute myocardial infarction (MI).[25] Prior MI is a primary risk factor for VF.[26] Atrial fibrillation also complicates acute MI quite regularly.[27] Acute ischemia promotes ion-channel dysfunction and tissue electrical dyssynchrony in relation to impairments in cell-to-cell coupling, intracellular acidosis, and accumulating extracellular K^+. Coronary artery disease (CAD) is one of the conditions most commonly associated with AF.[28] The association could be due to secondary factors like congestive heart failure (CHF) caused by CAD, but could also be due to ischemia-induced AF.

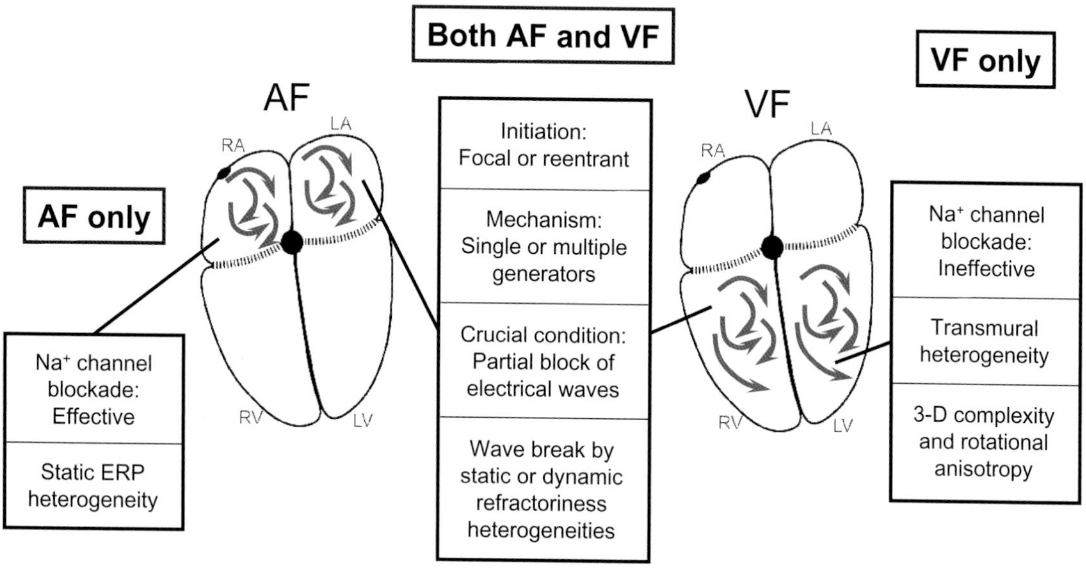

FIGURE 16–4. A comparison of the biophysical properties of AF and VF substrates. The most important differences relate to the transmural complexities of the ventricle and the differential response to Na^+ channel blockers.

Atrial Fibrillation Substrate

Atrial ischemia in itself promotes AF by impairing conduction, thus stabilizing atrial reentry that underlies AF and allowing AF to be much more readily sustained.[29] In contrast to ventricular MI,[30] almost nothing is known about the effects of healed atrial MI. Studies of AF in small-animal MI models have described changes that more likely reflect the effects of post-MI hypertrophy and/or CHF than ischemia per se. Atrial fibrosis provides a substrate for AF in MI rats with CHF.[31] Chronic ventricular MI with no atrial involvement causes heterogeneous alteration of atrial electrical restitution related to atrial sympathetic hyperinnervation, a form of neural remodeling that provides a substrate for increased AF vulnerability.[11]

Ventricular Fibrillation Substrate

The presence of a zone of slow propagation and propagation block is an important common feature shared by the AF and VF substrates caused by acute myocardial ischemia/infarction. With subacute and healed ventricular infarction, a complex set of electrophysiological changes occurs that creates a substrate for ventricular tachycardia (VT) and VF.[32] Surviving cardiomyocytes in the MI border have reduced AP amplitude and phase 0 upstroke velocity (dV/dt_{max})[33] and increased the phase 4 depolarization slope, in addition to prolonged APD.[34] Most K^+ currents are downregulated in post-MI border-zone cells.[35] These conditions are associated with enhanced automaticity and EADs.[36]

Ca^{2+} handling is altered in border-zone and Purkinje cells post-MI, with I_{CaL} diminished in several large animal models,[37,38] showing slower recovery[37] and hyperpolarizing shifts in inactivation voltage dependence.[38] Cardiac contraction is based on Ca^{2+} released into the cytoplasm from SR Ca^{2+} stores in response to Ca^{2+} entry through L-type Ca^{2+} channels during the AP. The SR has specialized channels, called Ca^{2+} release channels or ryanodine receptors (RyRs, co-called because they were first isolated based on high affinity to the blocker ryanodine), that are responsible for releasing Ca^{2+} with the appropriate stimulus and then remaining closed until the next AP. Altered RyR function is importantly altered post-MI,[39,40] whereas NCX function appears unaltered.[41] These MI-induced disturbances in SR Ca^{2+} handling favor the occurrence of arrhythmogenic DADs.

Abnormalities of activation cause slow and often discontinuous conduction within and around the MI region.[42,43] Marked changes in border-zone I_{Na}, including reduced current density, accelerated inactivation, and slowed reactivation,[44] impair conduction and excitability, promoting unidirectional block and reentry. Electrical conduction is also hindered by altered cell-to-cell coupling caused by gap junction dysfunction.[43] Gap junctions are smaller and less numerous in the peri-MI region.[45] Decreased side-to-side connections favor conduction block perpendicular to fiber orientation, producing a substrate for anisotropic reentry that underlies inducible VT/VF.[46,47] Connexin proteins form the cell-to-cell connections in gap junctions that maintain low-resistance intercellular coupling. Altered expression of the principal ventricular connexin, connexin43, is a primary factor in post-MI gap junction dysfunction and the substrate for VT/VF.[46]

Summary of the Role of Myocardial Ischemia

Figure 16–5 summarizes the mechanisms demonstrated to provide substrates for AF and VF in relation to myocardial ischemia and infarction. A favorable VF substrate is present at various phases of the acute ventricular ischemic process: immediately after acute MI, during the subacute phase, and during the chronic healed phase. Important contributors include abnormalities in impulse propagation, heterogeneity in electrical properties, impairments in myocardial repolarization, and disturbances in Ca^{2+} handling. Much less is known about the role of ischemia in the AF substrate. It is clear that severe acute atrial ischemia/infarction can produce a substrate for AF. There are presently no data regarding the role of healed atrial infarctions or less severe atrial ischemia in AF, but it is likely that the types of disturbances seen with a prior ventricular MI can also occur in the atria and promote AF.

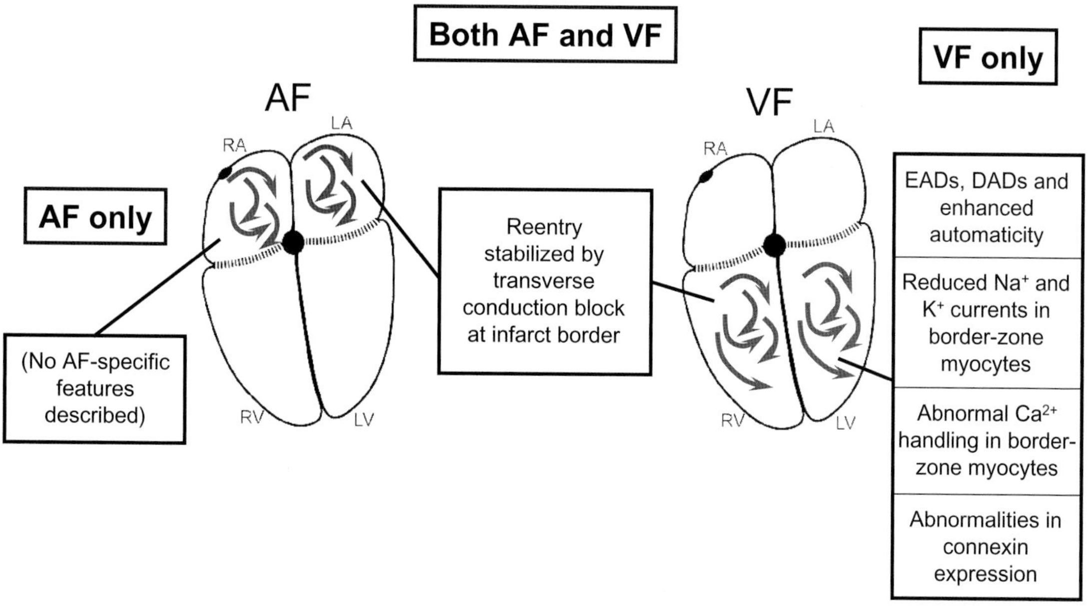

FIGURE 16–5. Promotion of AF and VF by myocardial ischemia and infarction. Acute ischemia seems to affect the atria and ventricles similarly. There is nothing known about longer-term effects of previous ischemia/infarction on the atria. Vastly more work has been done on the ventricles.

Congestive Heart Failure

In the CHF population, sudden cardiac death, largely due to VF, is responsible for up to 50% of CHF-associated mortality.[48] CHF is also one of the most common clinical causes of AF.[49]

Atrial Fibrillation Substrate

Sinoatrial (SA) node function is abnormal in CHF.[50] Bradycardia enhances refractoriness heterogeneity and thereby facilitates reentry,[51] and can also promote the emergence of ectopic foci.[52] Atrial APD is unchanged or increased in CHF.[53] The only study available of atrial ionic-current changes in CHF showed decreased transient-outward current (I_{to}) and slow delayed-rectifier current (I_{Ks}), along with increased NCX current.[53] NCX carries a depolarizing diastolic current because it exchanges one intracellular Ca^{2+} ion (total charge +2) for three extracellular Na^+ ions (total charge +3), carrying net inward current, when Ca^{2+} is extruded. This depolarizing current generates DADs, which can reach threshold and result in triggered activity, particularly in a setting of Ca^{2+} overload. There is evidence for DAD-induced focal atrial tachyarrhythmias in experimental CHF.[54,55] These tachyarrhythmias may be very rapid and mimic AF. In addition, mapping studies have provided evidence for rapidly discharging focal sources with fibrillatory conduction during AF in CHF dogs,[56] as in Figure 16–1A, suggesting that DAD-induced sustained triggered activity may be able to maintain AF.

Structural remodeling and fibrosis appear to be significant factors in the CHF-induced AF substrate.[57] Localized regions of conduction slowing occur and manifest as increased conduction heterogeneity that favors AF.[58] In some cases, this has been shown to result in single macroreentry circuits underlying AF,[59] consistent with the mechanism shown in Figure 16–1B.

Ventricular Fibrillation Substrate

As in the atria, ventricular K^+ currents, including both I_{to} and I_{Ks}, are downregulated by CHF.[60,61] Additionally, many studies show reduced I_{K1}.[60] One study showed reduced I_{Kr},[62] but most found I_{Kr} to be unchanged.[60,61] Downregulation of K^+

currents increases APD (APD prolongation is a consistent feature in CHF[63]) and can lead to EAD-related tachyarrhythmias.

Significant Ca^{2+} handling changes occur in CHF ventricles. Both NCX expression and activity are enhanced.[64,65] Congestive heart failure also causes SR Ca^{2+} leak due to abnormal RyR function.[66] Hyperphosphorylated RyRs, whether by protein kinase A or Ca^{2+} calmodulin-dependent protein kinase II (CaMKII), are prone to abnormal spontaneous diastolic Ca^{2+} release.[66] CaMKII-induced RyR hyperphosphorylation produces important SR diastolic Ca^{2+} leaks despite the decreased SR Ca load in CHF.[66] Ca^{2+} leaked from hyperphosphorylated RyRs is exchanged for extracellular Na^+ by the NCX, producing DADs. These DADs can cause extrasystoles that may initiate reentry in a vulnerable VF substrate or directly lead to triggered-activity tachyarrhythmias that degenerate to VF.[67] In addition, spontaneous SR Ca^{2+} release promotes abnormal automaticity in latent pacemaker cells.[68] Ca^{2+} release-induced DADs are enhanced by two other factors[64]: (1) increased NCX activity, which increases the amount of current generated for any level of Ca^{2+} release, and (2) downregulation of I_{K1}, which increases membrane resistance, resulting in a larger depolarization for a given inward current.

Extensive ventricular structural remodeling occurs with end-stage CHF in humans[69] and experimental models.[46] Areas of interstitial fibrosis cause ventricular conduction slowing and promote reentry. However, CHF-related fibrosis is much more extensive in atria than in ventricles,[7] suggesting a more important role in AF than VF. Connexin43 expression is downregulated in human and experimental CHF.[71–74] Moreover, gap junctional distribution and regulation are altered, with connexins redistributed to the cardiomyocyte lateral borders and dephosphorylated.[72] Along with tissue fibrosis, the changes in connexin43 expression and phosphorylation lead to conduction slowing[71,72] and APD heterogeneity[74] in the failing heart, predisposing to reentry.

Summary of the Role of CHF

CHF creates a substrate for both AF and VF. Table 16–1 compares the underlying changes in the two tissues and Figure 16–6 summarizes the known

TABLE 16–1. Substrate: congestive heart failure.[a]

Feature	AF	VF
Potassium currents		
I_{to}	↓	↓
I_{K1}	↔	↓
I_{Kr}	↔	↔ (↓)
I_{Ks}	↓	↓
Sodium currents		
I_{Na}	?	↓
Calcium handling		
I_{CaL}	↓	↓, ↔
NCX	↑	↑
SERCA	?	↓
CaRC	?	DS, Ph ↑
Structural changes		
Fibrosis	↑↑↑	↑
Connexins	?	↓, lateralization
APD	↔ (↑)	↑
CV	↓	↓
EADs	?	+
DADs	+	+
Reentry	+	+

[a]↑, increased; ↓, decreased; ↔, unaffected; +, present; Ph, phosphorylation; DS, dyssynchronous release; AF, atrial fibrillation; VF, ventricular fibrillation; NCX, Na^+–Ca^{2+} exchanger; CaRC, calcium release channel; APD, action potential duration; CV, cardiac volume; EADs, early afterdepolarization; DADs, delayed afterdepolarization; ( ), effect reported less frequently than the primary effect shown; ?, unknown.

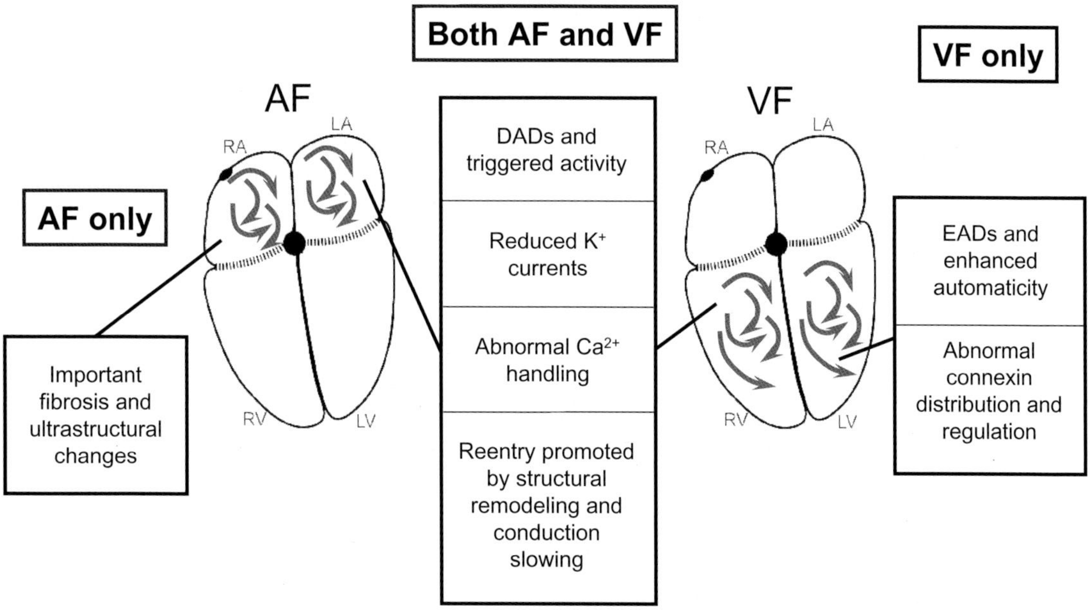

FIGURE 16–6. The CHF-related changes underlying AF and VF substrates. Many similar changes occur with CHF in both atria and ventricles. The roles of EADs and connexin changes are more clearly established in the ventricles.

contributors to AF and VF substrates in CHF. Many similar alterations occur in each, and form substrates for EAD, DAD, and reentry-based arrhythmic activity. The main differences appear to be more prominent and functionally important fibrosis at the atrial level and a clearer role for connexin alterations and EADs at the ventricular level.

Genetic Factors

Recent advances in genetics have pinpointed a wide range of primary fibrillation-inducing mutations,[75] which provide novel insights into molecular mechanisms. Two important fibrillation-promoting disorders of repolarization are the short QT syndromes (SQTSs) and long QT syndromes (LQTSs). The SQTS causes early-onset paroxysmal AF[76] and VF.[77] The prolonged APD in LQTS patients often leads to the EAD-associated polymorphic ventricular tachyarrhythmia torsades de pointes (TdP), which can degenerate to VF.[78] Arrhythmic mutations can also affect conduction properties, like the loss-of-function mutations in cardiac Na^+ channels that cause the arrhythmic Brugada syndrome[79] and probably also AF.[80] Inherited arrhythmia predilections can also affect Ca^{2+} handling and connexin function.

Atrial Fibrillation Substrate

While SQTS most strikingly causes VF-related sudden death, SQTS clearly also predisposes to AF.[76,77,81,82] The AF substrate is presumably based on accelerated repolarization, which makes the atria highly vulnerable to reentry, as seen with many acquired arrhythmia paradigms.[83] Atrial and ventricular ERPs are very short and both AF and VF are readily inducible in SQTS.[76] A *KCNQ1* mutation causes familial AF by increasing I_{Ks} and giving it a time-independent behavior.[84] A mutation in *KCNE2*, a β subunit of uncertain function, has been described in a familial AF kindred.[85] Mutated subunits produce gain-of-function in a time-independent I_{Ks} component upon coexpression with *KCNQ1*. It is not clear why these two gain-of-function I_{Ks} mutations do not cause SQTS and ventricular tachyarrhythmias. There is some evidence suggesting that LQTS can lead to AF,[86] but this remains controversial. Recently, other paradigms of AF apparently associated with delayed repolarization have been described.[87,88] Prolonged atrial APs could lead to AF either by

EAD-mediated mechanisms in susceptible patients or by favoring wavefront breakup at critical rates.[87]

Slow conduction favors reentry by leaving more time for recovery of excitability in potential reentrant pathways (Figure 16–2). Conduction can be slowed by altering the Na^+ current that provides the energy for electrical conduction or by affecting cell-to-cell coupling. Several mutations in *SCN5A*, which encodes the cardiac Na^+ channel, lead to a variety of phenotypes including AF.[80] A single-nucleotide polymorphism (SNP) in the connexin40 promoter that reduces Cx40 transcription is associated with AF vulnerability.[89,90] Gollob *et al.* have recently reported the intriguing observation that several patients with idiopathic, early-onset AF have somatic mutations in Cx40.[91]

Ventricular Fibrillation Substrate

Short QT syndrome produces transmurally heterogeneous APD abbreviation by preferentially abbreviating repolarization in M-cells, promoting reentry.[92] A variety of loss-of-function K^+ channel mutations or gain-of-function Na^+ and Ca^{2+} channel mutations can lead to impaired repolarization, LQTS, TdP, and VF precipitation.[93]

The Brugada syndrome is characterized by ST segment elevation in right precordial leads, right bundle branch block, and susceptibility to VF.[79] Loss-of-function *SCN5A* genes are causal in ~25% of Brugada syndrome patients.[94] Loss of *SCN5A* function can promote reentry by slowing conduction. However, a major component of the pathophysiology in the Brugada syndrome appears to be loss of the action potential plateau in the epicardium, where large I_{to} can cause very early repolarization in the absence of countervailing I_{Na}, with current spread from normal AP plateaus in the endocardium causing "phase 2 reentry" (for detailed review, see Antzelevitch *et al.*[95]).

A variety of genetic syndromes promote VF by impairing Ca^{2+} handling. Catecholaminergic polymorphic ventricular tachycardia (CPVT) mutations affect Ca^{2+} handling and buffering. Missense mutations in the *CASQ2* gene, encoding the principal SR Ca^{2+} buffer calsequestrin, are associated with autosomal-recessive CPVT.[96] Mutations in the gene encoding RyRs are the most common cause of CPVT.[97] Alterations in these CPVT-related gene products cause abnormal diastolic SR Ca^{2+} release, producing DADs. Catecholamine-induced β-adrenergic receptor stimulation promotes VT/VF in CPVT patients by increasing Ca^{2+}

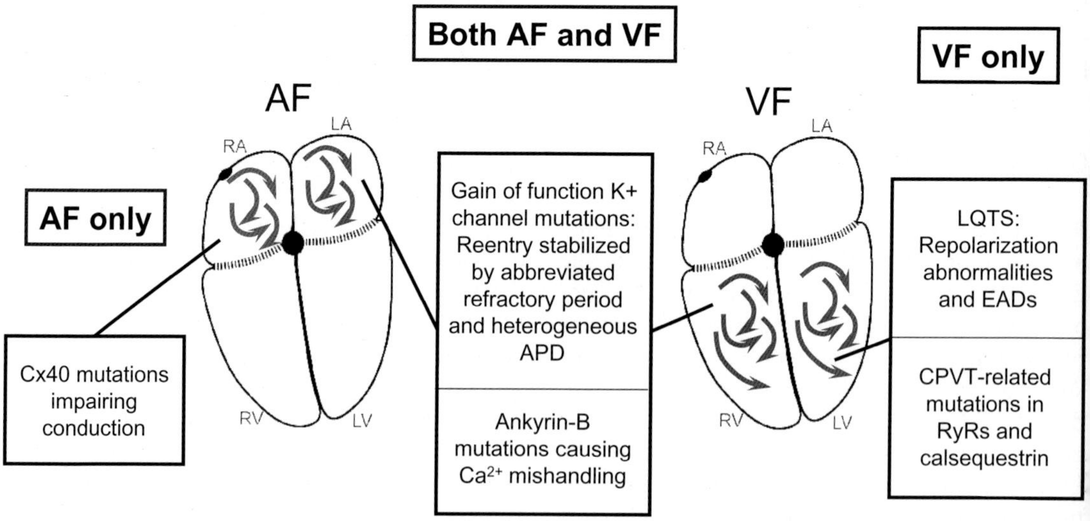

FIGURE 16–7. Genetically determined AF and VF substrates. The role of connexin40 abnormalities in AF is clear, as is the role of SQTS, LQTS, and CPVT mutations in VF. In addition, gain-of-function K^+ channel mutations have been described that appear to cause AF but not VF, for presently unclear reasons. Ankyrin-B mutations cause both AF and VF. Recently, repolarization-delaying genetic alterations have been described as associated with AF, but the precise mechanisms remain unclear.

entry through L-type Ca^{2+} channels, increasing Ca^{2+} loading, and enhancing spontaneous diastolic Ca^{2+} release and DADs. Ankyrin-B mutations disrupt the cellular localization of a variety of proteins, including Na^{+}-K^{+}-ATPase and NCX, and ankyrin-B deficiency produces defects in Ca^{2+} handling and afterdepolarizations that may be responsible for fibrillation-induced cardiac death, as well as AF.[98,99]

Summary of the Role of Genetic Determinants

There is considerable overlap in genetic AF and VF determinants (Figure 16–7), but the unique role of connexin40 in the atrium is reflected in the lack of ventricular arrhythmias with connexin40 gene abnormalities. Repolarization abnormalities predispose much more clearly to VF than AF, presumably because of the much longer AP durations in Purkinje and M-cells than the atrium, predisposing to EADs and repolarization heterogeneity. CPVT-related mutations also seem to be much more likely to lead to VF than AF.

Neuroregulatory Factors

It has long been recognized that the autonomic nervous system (ANS) plays a potentially important role in AF and VF.[100,101] The spatial heterogeneity of ANS actions increases refractoriness dispersion,[102] favoring fibrillation. This is particularly important in vagal AF, a well-recognized clinical entity.[103] Alterations in neurohormonal function can also play a critical modulating role for fibrillation substrates. For example, adrenergic stimulation is a well-recognized precipitator of ventricular tachyarrhythmias in LQTS and CPVT. β-Adrenergic stimulation is also an important contributor to ischemic VF, since β-adrenoceptor blockers are among the only drugs known to prevent VF post-MI in patients with CAD.[104]

Atrial Fibrillation Substrate

Vagal stimulation produces high vulnerability to sustained AF.[105] Spatially heterogeneous refractoriness abbreviation appears particularly important in the pathogenesis of vagal AF.[106] The local (intrinsic) cardiac nervous system is affected by pathology associated with AF.[107] Atrial arrhythmias can be induced by stimulating mediastinal nerve branches of the thoracic vagosympathetic complex[108] or mediastinal nerves associated with pulmonary veins.[109,110]

Significant nerve sprouting and spatially heterogeneous sympathetic hyperinnervation occur in a canine model of sustained AF produced by prolonged right atrial pacing.[111] Heterogeneous sympathetic denervation in a canine model also facilitates AF.[112] Sympathetic hyperinnervation may also increase AF vulnerability in a canine post-MI model.[11]

Ventricular Fibrillation Substrate

In contrast to AF, vagal influences do not appear to play a major role in VF substrates. Ventricular nerve sprouting is related to ventricular tachyarrhythmia-associated sudden death,[11,113] apparently by effects on repolarization.[114,115] Mice with MIs show sympathetic nerve sprouting with upregulation of nerve growth factor peri-MI and, to a lesser extent, in remote areas.[116] The ability of β-adrenergic stimulation to increase I_{CaL} accounts for its well-recognized role as a promoting effect on EAD-related arrhythmias associated with the LQTS and DAD-related arrhythmias in CPVT. The contribution of β-adrenergic stimulation to the VF substrate in acute MI and CHF may be related to the promotion of EADs and DADs, but also to other factors such as an enhancement in metabolic needs, stimulation of hypertrophic/remodeling pathways, and increased ischemia.

Summary of the Role of Neuroregulatory Determinants

Figure 16–8 summarizes the contribution of neural regulation to AF and VF substrates. Vagal factors play a prominent role in the AF substrate. Adrenergic stimulation contributes particularly to EAD and DAD mechanisms, and potentially plays a role in reentrant substrates by enhancing refractoriness heterogeneity.

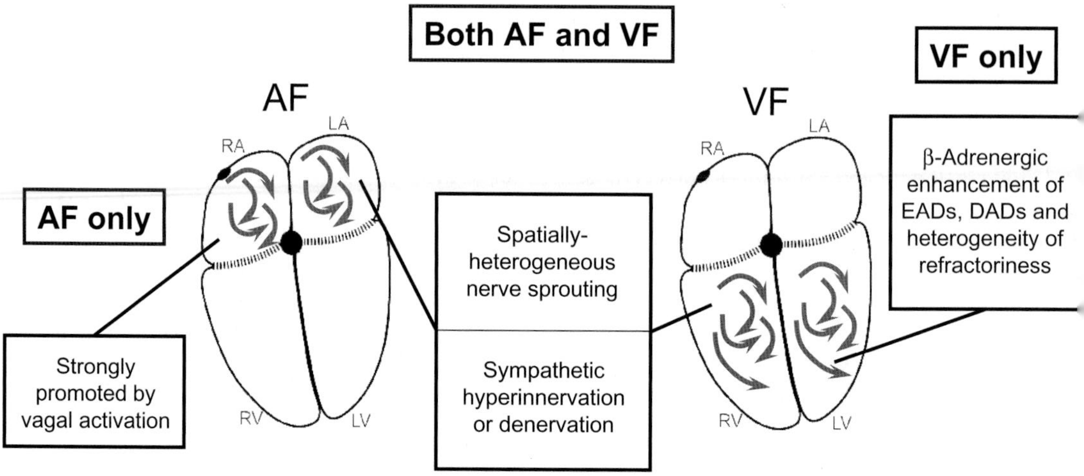

Figure 16–8. Neuroregulatory contributions to AF and VF substrates. Vagal effects are particularly important in AF and much less so in VF. Sympathetic enhancement of EAD- and DAD-related arrhythmia syndromes is well established in the ventricles but has not been shown in the atria.

Arrhythmic Remodeling

Accumulating evidence indicates that cardiac rhythm disturbances may cause persistent changes in cardiac electrophysiology. The clearest example is AF itself, which by virtue of the rapid atrial rate causes atrial changes that promote AF occurrence ("AF begets AF"),[117,118] a process sometimes called "atrial tachycardia remodeling" (ATR). Atrial fibrillation-induced remodeling has most clearly been demonstrated in humans by the reversal of remodeling changes in atrial refractoriness and conduction after AF cardioversion.[119] Remodeling is believed to underlie the tendency of paroxysmal AF to become permanent, of longer-lasting AF to be refractory to drug therapy, and of AF recurrence to be most likely within the first few days postcardioversion.[117] Ventricular arrhythmic remodeling is most clearly manifested by electrical changes caused by abnormal activation sequences, as occurs with ectopic beats, so-called "T-wave memory."[120] The implications of T-wave memory for VF are poorly defined.

Atrial Fibrillation Substrate

A consistent feature of ATR is a reduction in APD and consequently ERP.[117,118,121] Atrial tachycardia remodeling-induced refractoriness shortening is maximal within 2 days, whereas AF promotion occurs over several weeks.[117,118] Action potential duration abbreviation results from reduced I_{CaL},[122] along with increased I_{K1}[123] and acetylcholine-regulated K^+ current.[124] I_{Kr} and I_{Ks} are unchanged, but I_{to} is reduced.[122] There is evidence for ATR-induced I_{Na} reductions in dogs,[125] which could contribute to conduction slowing and AF promotion, but these have not been seen in atrial cardiomyocytes from AF patients.[126]

Atrial tachycardia remodeling alters Ca^{2+} handling, reducing cellular Ca^{2+} transients.[127] There is evidence for defective RyR function related to hyperphosphorylation in ATR/AF,[128] as well as for spontaneous, potentially DAD-promoting, SR Ca^{2+} release.[129]

A variety of changes in connexin expression and distribution have been described in ATR and AF. The most consistent findings are connexin lateralization[130,131] and increased hemichannel subunit heterogeneity[130] with spatially variable loss of connexin40.[132] The connexin alterations may promote AF by causing spatially heterogeneous conduction disturbances.

Ventricular Fibrillation Substrate

Sustained ventricular tachyarrhythmias[133] and even frequent ventricular ectopy[134] can produce ventricular cardiomyopathy and CHF; however, most associated electrical remodeling changes are

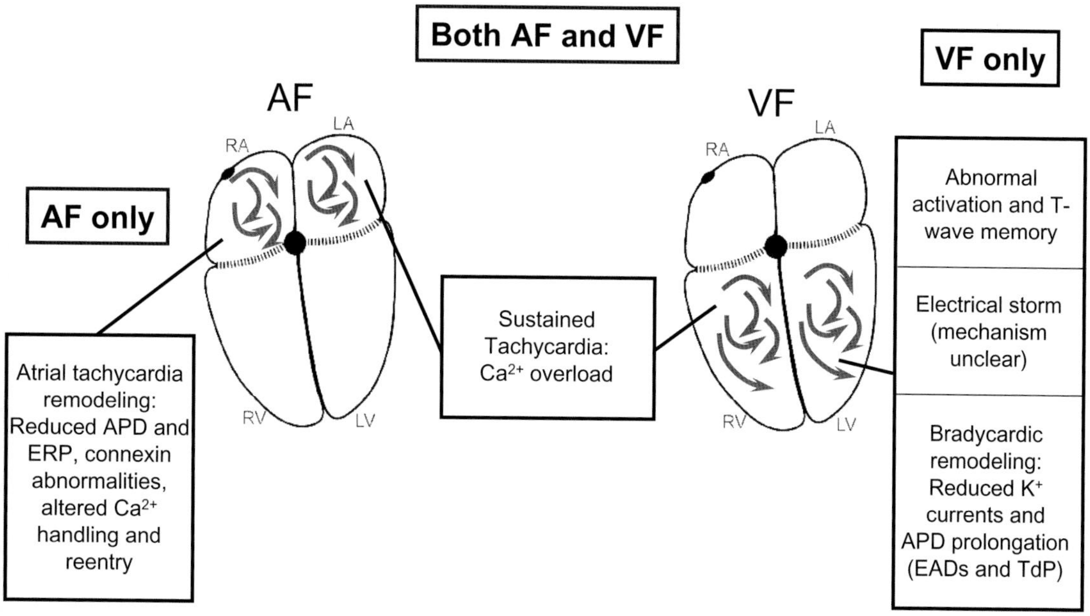

FIGURE 16–9. Contribution of arrhythmic remodeling to fibrillation substrates. Arrhythmia itself can cause electrical and structural changes that promote the initiation and maintenance of fibrillation. The classical example of such arrhythmic remodeling is atrial tachycardia remodeling (ATR, or so called "AF begets AF"). Atrial tachycardia remodeling results in alterations of ionic currents and Ca^{2+} handling that lead to refractoriness shortening, conduction disturbances, and triggered activity. The purely rate-dependent mechanisms underlying ventricular tachycardia-induced remodeling cannot be dissociated from the major changes caused by the accompanying CHF, and so are unknown. The mechanisms underlying refractory VT/VF episodes of electrical storm have yet to be defined. Bradycardic states produce a substrate for VF by causing K^+ current downregulation, repolarization delays, and a potential for TdP.

likely due to associated CHF. Electrical storm is characterized by a clustering of intractable VT or VF episodes,[135] suggesting a positive-feedback system caused by ventricular tachyarrhythmias. The pathophysiology of electrical storm is poorly understood. Ca^{2+} overload likely plays a pivotal role by reducing myofilament responsiveness and promoting postdefibrillation reinitiation of VF.[136–138]

Bradycardic states are also associated with ventricular electrical remodeling, predisposing to lethal ventricular tachyarrhythmias.[139,140] Sustained bradycardia decreases I_{Kr} and I_{Ks},[61,141,142] causing QT interval prolongation and prominent repolarization delays leading to spontaneous TdP. I_{Kr} alterations with simultaneous I_{Ks} downregulation (reduced repolarization reserve) appear to be particularly important in the resulting long QT phenotype, which may explain the association of AV block and clinical TdP syndromes.[143]

Summary of the Role of Arrhythmic Remodeling

Arrhythmic remodeling contributions to fibrillation substrates are shown in Figure 16–9. Atrial tachycardia remodeling promotes AF by abbreviating refractoriness and possibly by causing abnormal SR Ca^{2+} handling and connexin remodeling. Bradycardic remodeling produces a substrate for VF due to repolarization abnormalities caused by K^+ current downregulation, and electrical storm may be an extreme form of ventricular tachyarrhythmia-induced VF promotion.

Conclusions

The AF and VF substrates have many features in common but also a number of important specific differences. Consideration of these mechanistic features will lead to improved understanding of the pathophysiology of AF and VF, and possibly to newer, arrhythmia-specific therapeutic approaches.

Acknowledgments. Supported by the Canadian Institutes of Health Research, the Quebec Heart and Stroke Foundation, and the Mathematics of Information Technology and Complex Systems Network of Centers of Excellence.

References

1. Jalife J, Anumonwo JM, Berenfeld O. Toward an understanding of the molecular mechanisms of ventricular fibrillation. *J Interv Card Electrophysiol* 2003;9:119–129.
2. Oral H. Mechanisms of atrial fibrillation: Lessons from studies in patients. *Prog Cardiovasc Dis* 2005; 48:29–40.
3. Nattel S. New ideas about atrial fibrillation 50 years on. *Nature* 2002;415:219–226.
4. Jalife J, Berenfeld O, Mansour M. Mother rotors and fibrillatory conduction: A mechanism of atrial fibrillation. *Cardiovasc Res* 2002;54:204–216.
5. Kneller J, Zou R, Vigmond EJ, Wang Z, Leon LJ, Nattel S. Cholinergic atrial fibrillation in a computer model of a two-dimensional sheet of canine atrial cells with realistic ionic properties. *Circ Res* 2002;90:73–87.
6. Winfree AT. Electrical instability in cardiac muscle: Phase singularities and rotors. *J Theor Biol* 1989;138:353–405.
7. Zou R, Kneller J, Leon LJ, Nattel S. Substrate size as a determinant of fibrillatory activity maintenance in a mathematical model of canine atrium. *Am J Physiol Heart Circ Physiol* 2005;289:H1002–H1012.
8. Comtois P, Kneller J, Nattel S. Of circles and spirals: Bridging the gap between the leading circle and spiral wave concepts of cardiac reentry. *Europace* 2005;7(Suppl. 2):10–20.
9. Karma A. Spiral breakup in model equations of action potential propagation in cardiac tissue. *Phys Rev Lett* 1993;71:1103–1106.
10. Fareh S, Villemaire C, Nattel S. Importance of refractoriness heterogeneity in the enhanced vulnerability to atrial fibrillation induction caused by tachycardia-induced atrial electrical remodeling. *Circulation* 1998;98:2202–2209.
11. Miyauchi Y, Zhou S, Okuyama Y, Miyauchi M, Hayashi H, Hamabe A, Fishbein MC, Mandel WJ, Chen LS, Chen PS, Karagueuzian HS Altered atrial electrical restitution and heterogeneous sympathetic hyperinnervation in hearts with chronic left ventricular myocardial infarction: Implications for atrial fibrillation. *Circulation* 2003;108:360–366.
12. Vigmond EJ, Tsoi V, Kuo S, Arevalo H, Kneller J, Nattel S, Trayanova N. The effect of vagally induced dispersion of action potential duration on atrial arrhythmogenesis. *Heart Rhythm* 2004;1:334–344.
13. Wijffels MC, Dorland R, Mast F, Allessie MA. Widening of the excitable gap during pharmacological cardioversion of atrial fibrillation in the goat: Effects of cibenzoline, hydroquinidine, flecainide, and d-sotalol. *Circulation* 2000;102:260–267.
14. Kneller J, Kalifa J, Zou R, Zaitsev AV, Warren M, Berenfeld O, Vigmond EJ, Leon LJ, Nattel S, Jalife J. Mechanisms of atrial fibrillation termination by pure sodium channel blockade in an ionically-realistic mathematical model. *Circ Res* 2005;96: 35–47.
15. Preliminary report: Effect of encainide and flecainide on mortality in a randomized trial of arrhythmia suppression after myocardial infarction. The Cardiac Arrhythmia Suppression Trial (CAST) Investigators. *N Engl J Med* 1989;321:406–412.
16. Qu Z, Weiss JN. Effects of Na(+) and K(+) channel blockade on vulnerability to and termination of fibrillation in simulated normal cardiac tissue. *Am J Physiol Heart Circ Physiol* 2005;289:1692–1701.
17. Kim YH, Xie F, Yashima M, Wu TJ, Valderrabano M, Lee MH, Ohara T, Voroshilovsky O, Doshi RN, Fishbein MC, Qu Z, Garfinkel A, Weiss JN, Karagueuzian HS, Chen PS. Role of papillary muscle in the generation and maintenance of reentry during ventricular tachycardia and fibrillation in isolated swine right ventricle. *Circulation* 1999;100:1450–1459.
18. Pruvot EJ, Katra RP, Rosenbaum DS, Laurita KR. Role of calcium cycling versus restitution in the mechanism of repolarization alternans. *Circ Res* 2004;94:1083–1090.
19. Weiss JN, Karma A, Shiferaw Y, Chen PS, Garfinkel A, Qu Z. From pulsus to pulseless: The saga of cardiac alternans. *Circ Res* 2006;98:1244–1253.
20. Zaitsev AV, Berenfeld O, Mironov SF, Jalife J, Pertsov AM. Distribution of excitation frequencies on the epicardial and endocardial surfaces of fibrillating ventricular wall of the sheep heart. *Circ Res* 2000;86:408–417.
21. Janse MJ, Sosunov EA, Coronel R, Opthof T, Anyukhovsky EP, de Bakker JM, Plotnikov AN, Shlapakova IN, Danilo P Jr, Tijssen JG, Rosen MR.

Repolarization gradients in the canine left ventricle before and after induction of short-term cardiac memory. *Circulation* 2005;112:1711–1718.
22. Fenton F, Karma A. Fiber-rotation-induced vortex turbulence in thick myocardium. *Phys Rev Lett* 1998;81:481–484.
23. Panfilov AV, Keener JP. Reentry in 3-dimensional Fitzhugh-Nagumo medium with rotational anisotropy. *Physica D* 1995;84:545–552.
24. Qu Z, Kil J, Xie F, Garfinkel A, Weiss JN. Scroll wave dynamics in a three-dimensional cardiac tissue model: Roles of restitution, thickness, and fiber rotation. *Biophys J* 2000;78:2761–2775.
25. Hurwitz JL, Josephson ME. Sudden cardiac death in patients with chronic coronary heart disease. *Circulation* 1992;85:I43–I49.
26. Henkel DM, Witt BJ, Gersh BJ, Jacobsen SJ, Weston SA, Meverden RA, Roger VL. Ventricular arrhythmias after acute myocardial infarction: A 20-year community study. *Am Heart J* 2006;151:806–812.
27. Wong CK, White HD, Wilcox RG, Criger DA, Califf RM, Topol EJ, Ohman EM. Significance of atrial fibrillation during acute myocardial infarction, and its current management: Insights from the GUSTO-3 trial. *Card Electrophysiol Rev* 2003; 7:201–207.
28. Allessie MA, Boyden PA, Camm AJ, Kleber AG, Lab MJ, Legato MJ, Rosen MR, Schwartz PJ, Spooner PM, Van Wagoner DR, Waldo AL. Pathophysiology and prevention of atrial fibrillation. *Circulation* 2001;103:769–777.
29. Sinno H, Derakhchan K, Libersan D, Merhi Y, Leung TK, Nattel S. Atrial ischemia promotes atrial fibrillation in dogs. *Circulation* 2003;107:1930–1936.
30. Janse MJ, Wit AL. Electrophysiological mechanisms of ventricular arrhythmias resulting from myocardial ischemia and infarction. *Physiol Rev* 1989;69:1049–1169.
31. Boixel C, Fontaine V, Rucker-Martin C, Milliez P, Louedec L, Michel JB, Jacob MP, Hatem SN. Fibrosis of the left atria during progression of heart failure is associated with increased matrix metalloproteinases in the rat. *J Am Coll Cardiol* 2003; 42:336–344.
32. Wit AL, Janse MJ. Experimental models of ventricular tachycardia and fibrillation caused by ischemia and infarction. *Circulation* 1992;85:I32–I42.
33. Lue WM, Boyden PA. Abnormal electrical properties of myocytes from chronically infarcted canine heart. Alterations in Vmax and the transient outward current. *Circulation* 1992;85:1175–1188.
34. Cabo C, Boyden PA. Electrical remodeling of the epicardial border zone in the canine infarcted heart: A computational analysis. *Am J Physiol Heart Circ Physiol* 2003;284:H372–H384.
35. Dun W, Boyden PA. Diverse phenotypes of outward currents in cells that have survived in the 5-day-infarcted heart. *Am J Physiol Heart Circ Physiol* 2005;289:H667–H673.
36. Gough WB, Hu D, el Sherif N. Effects of clofilium on ischemic subendocardial Purkinje fibers 1 day postinfarction. *J Am Coll Cardiol* 1988;11:431–437.
37. Dun W, Baba S, Yagi T, Boyden PA. Dynamic remodeling of K^+ and Ca^{2+} currents in cells that survived in the epicardial border zone of canine healed infarcted heart. *Am J Physiol Heart Circ Physiol* 2004;287:H1046–H1054.
38. Pinto JM, Yuan F, Wasserlauf BJ, Bassett AL, Myerburg RJ. Regional gradation of L-type calcium currents in the feline heart with a healed myocardial infarct. *J Cardiovasc Electrophysiol* 1997;8: 548–560.
39. Litwin SE, Zhang D, Bridge JH. Dyssynchronous Ca(2+) sparks in myocytes from infarcted hearts. *Circ Res* 2000;87:1040–1047.
40. Boyden PA, Dun W, Barbhaiya C, ter Keurs HE. 2APB- and JTV519(K201)-sensitive micro Ca^{2+} waves in arrhythmogenic Purkinje cells that survive in infarcted canine heart. *Heart Rhythm* 2004; 1:218–226.
41. Pu J, Robinson RB, Boyden PA. Abnormalities in Ca(i) handling in myocytes that survive in the infarcted heart are not just due to alterations in repolarization. *J Mol Cell Cardiol* 2000;32:1509–1523.
42. de Bakker JM, van Capelle FJ, Janse MJ, Wilde AA, Coronel R, Becker AE, Dingemans KP, van Hemel NM, Hauer RN. Reentry as a cause of ventricular tachycardia in patients with chronic ischemic heart disease: Electrophysiologic and anatomic correlation. *Circulation* 1988;77:589–606.
43. Spear JF, Michelson EL, Moore EN. Reduced space constant in slowly conducting regions of chronically infarcted canine myocardium. *Circ Res* 1983; 53:176–185.
44. Pu J, Boyden PA. Alterations of Na+ currents in myocytes from epicardial border zone of the infarcted heart. A possible ionic mechanism for reduced excitability and postrepolarization refractoriness. *Circ Res* 1997;81:110–119.
45. Peters NS. Myocardial gap junction organization in ischemia and infarction. *Microsc Res Tech* 1995;31:375–386.
46. Peters NS, Coromilas J, Severs NJ, Wit AL. Disturbed connexin43 gap junction distribution correlates with the location of reentrant circuits in the

epicardial border zone of healing canine infarcts that cause ventricular tachycardia. *Circulation* 1997;95:988–996.
47. Yao JA, Hussain W, Patel P, Peters NS, Boyden PA, Wit AL. Remodeling of gap junctional channel function in epicardial border zone of healing canine infarcts. *Circ Res* 2003;92:437–443.
48. Kjekshus J. Arrhythmias and mortality in congestive heart failure. *Am J Cardiol* 1990;65:42I-48I.
49. Ehrlich JR, Nattel S, Hohnloser SH. Atrial fibrillation and congestive heart failure: Specific considerations at the intersection of two common and important cardiac disease sets. *J Cardiovasc Electrophysiol* 2002;13:399–405.
50. Zicha S, Fernandez-Velasco M, Lonardo G, L'Heureux N, Nattel S. Sinus node dysfunction and hyperpolarization-activated (HCN) channel subunit remodeling in a canine heart failure model. *Cardiovasc Res* 2005;66:472–481.
51. Han J, Millet D, Chizzonitti B, Moe GK. Temporal dispersion of recovery of excitability in atrium and ventricle as a function of heart rate. *Am Heart J* 1966;71:481–487.
52. Goel BG, Han J. Atrial ectopic activity associated with sinus bradycardia. *Circulation* 1970;42:853–858.
53. Li D, Melnyk P, Feng J, Wang Z, Petrecca K, Shrier A, Nattel S. Effects of experimental heart failure on atrial cellular and ionic electrophysiology. *Circulation* 2000;101:2631–2638.
54. Fenelon G, Shepard RK, Stambler BS. Focal origin of atrial tachycardia in dogs with rapid ventricular pacing-induced heart failure. *J Cardiovasc Electrophysiol* 2003;14:1093–1102.
55. Stambler BS, Fenelon G, Shepard RK, Clemo HF, Guiraudon CM. Characterization of sustained atrial tachycardia in dogs with rapid ventricular pacing-induced heart failure. *J Cardiovasc Electrophysiol* 2003;14:499–507.
56. Ryu K, Shroff SC, Sahadevan J, Martovitz NL, Khrestian CM, Stambler BS. Mapping of atrial activation during sustained atrial fibrillation in dogs with rapid ventricular pacing induced heart failure: Evidence for a role of driver regions. *J Cardiovasc Electrophysiol* 2005;16:1348–1358.
57. Shinagawa K, Shi YF, Tardif JC, Leung TK, Nattel S. Dynamic nature of atrial fibrillation substrate during development and reversal of heart failure in dogs. *Circulation* 2002;105:2672–2678.
58. Li D, Fareh S, Leung TK, Nattel S. Promotion of atrial fibrillation by heart failure in dogs: Atrial remodeling of a different sort. *Circulation* 1999;100:87–95.
59. Derakhchan K, Li D, Courtemanche M, Smith B, Brouillette J, Page PL, Nattel S. Method for simultaneous epicardial and endocardial mapping of in vivo canine heart: Application to atrial conduction properties and arrhythmia mechanisms. *J Cardiovasc Electrophysiol* 2001;12:548–555.
60. Li GR, Lau CP, Leung TK, Nattel S. Ionic current abnormalities associated with prolonged action potentials in cardiomyocytes from diseased human right ventricles. *Heart Rhythm* 2004;1:460–468.
61. Tsuji Y, Zicha S, Qi XY, Kodama I, Nattel S. Potassium channel subunit remodeling in rabbits exposed to long-term bradycardia or tachycardia: Discrete arrhythmogenic consequences related to differential delayed-rectifier changes. *Circulation* 2006;113:345–355.
62. Tsuji Y, Opthof T, Kamiya K, Yasui K, Liu W, Lu Z, Kodama I. Pacing-induced heart failure causes a reduction of delayed rectifier potassium currents along with decreases in calcium and transient outward currents in rabbit ventricle. *Cardiovasc Res* 2000;48:300–309.
63. Nuss HB, Kaab S, Kass DA, Tomaselli GF, Marban E. Cellular basis of ventricular arrhythmias and abnormal automaticity in heart failure. *Am J Physiol* 1999;277:H80–H91.
64. Pogwizd SM, Schlotthauer K, Li L, Yuan W, Bers DM. Arrhythmogenesis and contractile dysfunction in heart failure. Roles of sodium-calcium exchange, inward rectifier potassium current, and residual beta-adrenergic responsiveness. *Circ Res* 2001;88:1159–1167.
65. Xiong W, Tian Y, DiSilvestre D, Tomaselli GF. Transmural heterogeneity of Na^+-Ca^{2+} exchange: Evidence for differential expression in normal and failing hearts. *Circ Res* 2005;97:207–209.
66. Ai X, Curran JW, Shannon TR, Bers DM, Pogwizd SM. $Ca2^+$/calmodulin-dependent protein kinase modulates cardiac ryanodine receptor phosphorylation and sarcoplasmic reticulum Ca^{2+} leak in heart failure. *Circ Res* 2005;97:1314–1322.
67. Schlotthauer K, Bers DM. Sarcoplasmic reticulum Ca(2+) release causes myocyte depolarization. Underlying mechanism and threshold for triggered action potentials. *Circ Res* 2000;87:774–780.
68. Huser J, Blatter LA, Lipsius SL. Intracellular Ca^{2+} release contributes to automaticity in cat atrial pacemaker cells. *J Physiol* 2000;524(Pt. 2):415–422.
69. Kawara T, Derksen R, de Groot JR, Coronel R, Tasseron S, Linnenbank AC, Hauer RN, Kirkels H, Janse MJ, de Bakker JM. Activation delay after premature stimulation in chronically diseased human myocardium relates to the architecture of

interstitial fibrosis. *Circulation* 2001;104:3069–3075.

70. Hanna N, Cardin S, Leung TK, Nattel S. Differences in atrial versus ventricular remodeling in dogs with ventricular tachypacing-induced congestive heart failure. *Cardiovasc Res* 2004;63:236–244.
71. Ai X, Pogwizd SM. Connexin 43 downregulation and dephosphorylation in nonischemic heart failure is associated with enhanced colocalized protein phosphatase type 2A. *Circ Res* 2005;96:54–63.
72. Akar FG, Spragg DD, Tunin RS, Kass DA, Tomaselli GF. Mechanisms underlying conduction slowing and arrhythmogenesis in nonischemic dilated cardiomyopathy. *Circ Res* 2004;95:717–725.
73. Dupont E, Matsushita T, Kaba RA, Vozzi C, Coppen SR, Khan N, Kaprielian R, Yacoub MH, Severs NJ. Altered connexin expression in human congestive heart failure. *J Mol Cell Cardiol* 2001;33:359–371.
74. Poelzing S, Rosenbaum DS. Altered connexin43 expression produces arrhythmia substrate in heart failure. *Am J Physiol Heart Circ Physiol* 2004;287:H1762–H1770.
75. Roberts R. Genomics and cardiac arrhythmias. *J Am Coll Cardiol* 2006;47:9–21.
76. Hong K, Bjerregaard P, Gussak I, Brugada R. Short QT syndrome and atrial fibrillation caused by mutation in KCNH2. *J Cardiovasc Electrophysiol* 2005;16:394–396.
77. Gussak I, Brugada P, Brugada J, Wright RS, Kopecky SL, Chaitman BR, Bjerregaard P. Idiopathic short QT interval: A new clinical syndrome? *Cardiology* 2000;94:99–102.
78. Moss AJ, Schwartz PJ, Crampton RS, Tzivoni D, Locati EH, MacCluer J, Hall WJ, Weitkamp L, Vincent GM, Garson A, *et al.* The long QT syndrome. Prospective longitudinal study of 328 families. *Circulation* 1991;84:1136–1144.
79. Brugada P, Brugada J. Right bundle branch block, persistent ST segment elevation and sudden cardiac death: A distinct clinical and electrocardiographic syndrome. A multicenter report. *J Am Coll Cardiol* 1992;20:1391–1396.
80. Olson TM, Michels VV, Ballew JD, Reyna SP, Karst ML, Herron KJ, Horton SC, Rodeheffer RJ, Anderson JL. Sodium channel mutations and susceptibility to heart failure and atrial fibrillation. *JAMA* 2005;293:447–454.
81. Gaita F, Giustetto C, Bianchi F, Wolpert C, Schimpf R, Riccardi R, Grossi S, Richiardi E, Borggrefe M. Short QT Syndrome: A familial cause of sudden death. *Circulation* 2003;108:965–970.
82. Hong K, Piper DR, Diaz-Valdecantos A, Brugada J, Oliva A, Burashnikov E, Santos-de-Soto J, Grueso-Montero J, Diaz-Enfante E, Brugada P, Sachse F, Sanguinetti MC, Brugada R. De novo KCNQ1 mutation responsible for atrial fibrillation and short QT syndrome in utero. *Cardiovasc Res* 2005;68:433–440.
83. Nattel S, Shiroshita-Takeshita A, Brundel BJ, Rivard L. Mechanisms of atrial fibrillation: Lessons from animal models. *Prog Cardiovasc Dis* 2005;48:9–28.
84. Chen YH, Xu SJ, Bendahhou S, Wang XL, Wang Y, Xu WY, Jin HW, Sun H, Su XY, Zhuang QN, Yang YQ, Li YB, Liu Y, Xu HJ, Li XF, Ma N, Mou CP, Chen Z, Barhanin J, Huang W. KCNQ1 gain-of-function mutation in familial atrial fibrillation. *Science* 2003;299:251–254.
85. Yang Y, Xia M, Jin Q, Bendahhou S, Shi J, Chen Y, Liang B, Lin J, Liu Y, Liu B, Zhou Q, Zhang D, Wang R, Ma N, Su X, Niu K, Pei Y, Xu W, Chen Z, Wan H, Cui J, Barhanin J, Chen Y. Identification of a KCNE2 gain-of-function mutation in patients with familial atrial fibrillation. *Am J Hum Genet* 2004;75:899–905.
86. Kirchhof P, Eckardt L, Franz MR, Monnig G, Loh P, Wedekind H, Schulze-Bahr E, Breithardt G, Haverkamp W. Prolonged atrial action potential durations and polymorphic atrial tachyarrhythmias in patients with long QT syndrome. *J Cardiovasc Electrophysiol* 2003;14:1027–1033.
87. Ehrlich JR, Zicha S, Coutu P, Hebert TE, Nattel S. Atrial fibrillation-associated minK38G/S polymorphism modulates delayed rectifier current and membrane localization. *Cardiovasc Res* 2005;67:520–528.
88. Olson TM, Alekseev AE, Liu XK, Park S, Zingman LV, Bienengraeber M, Sattiraju S, Ballew JD, Jahangir A, Terzic A. Kv1.5 channelopathy due to KCNA5 loss-of-function mutation causes human atrial fibrillation. *Hum Mol Genet* 2006;15:2185–2191.
89. Firouzi M, Ramanna H, Kok B, Jongsma HJ, Koeleman BP, Doevendans PA, Groenewegen WA, Hauer RN. Association of human connexin40 gene polymorphisms with atrial vulnerability as a risk factor for idiopathic atrial fibrillation. *Circ Res* 2004;95:e29–e33.
90. Juang JM, Chern YR, Tsai CT, Chiang FT, Lin JL, Hwang JJ, Hsu KL, Tseng CD, Tseng YZ, Lai LP. The association of human connexin 40 genetic polymorphisms with atrial fibrillation. *Int J Cardiol* 2006;116(1):107–112.

91. Gollob MH, Jones DL, Krahn AD, Danis L, Gong XQ, Shao Q, Liu X, Veinot JP, Tang AS, Stewart AF, Tesson F, Klein GJ, Yee R, Skanes AC, Guiraudon GM, Ebihara L, Bai D. Somatic mutations in the connexin 40 gene (GJA5) in atrial fibrillation. *N Engl J Med* 2006;354:2677–2688.
92. Extramiana F, Antzelevitch C. Amplified transmural dispersion of repolarization as the basis for arrhythmogenesis in a canine ventricular-wedge model of short-QT syndrome. *Circulation* 2004; 110:3661–3666.
93. Modell SM, Lehmann MH. The long QT syndrome family of cardiac ion channelopathies: A HuGE review. *Genet Med* 2006;8:143–155.
94. Priori SG, Napolitano C, Gasparini M, Pappone C, Della Bella P, Giordano U, Bloise R, Giustetto C, De Nardis R, Grillo M, Ronchetti E, Faggiano G, Nastoli J. Natural history of Brugada syndrome: Insights for risk stratification and management. *Circulation* 2002;105:1342–1347.
95. Antzelevitch C, Brugada P, Brugada J, Brugada R. Brugada syndrome: From cell to bedside. *Curr Probl Cardiol* 2005;30:9–54.
96. Eldar M, Pras E, Lahat H. A missense mutation in the CASQ2 gene is associated with autosomal-recessive catecholamine-induced polymorphic ventricular tachycardia. *Trends Cardiovasc Med* 2003;13:148–151.
97. Priori SG, Napolitano C, Memmi M, Colombi B, Drago F, Gasparini M, DeSimone L, Coltorti F, Bloise R, Keegan R, Cruz Filho FE, Vignati G, Benatar A, DeLogu A. Clinical and molecular characterization of patients with catecholaminergic polymorphic ventricular tachycardia. *Circulation* 2002;106:69–74.
98. Mohler PJ, Schott JJ, Gramolini AO, Dilly KW, Guatimosim S, duBell WH, Song LS, Haurogne K, Kyndt F, Ali ME, Rogers TB, Lederer WJ, Escande D, Le Marec H, Bennett V. Ankyrin-B mutation causes type 4 long-QT cardiac arrhythmia and sudden cardiac death. *Nature* 2003;421:634–639.
99. Mohler PJ, Splawski I, Napolitano C, Bottelli G, Sharpe L, Timothy K, Priori SG, Keating MT, Bennett V. A cardiac arrhythmia syndrome caused by loss of ankyrin-B function. *Proc Natl Acad Sci USA* 2004;101:9137–9142.
100. Garrey WE. Auricular fibrillation. *Physiol Rev* 1924;4:215–250.
101. Zipes DP, Barber MJ, Takahashi N, Gilmour RF Jr. Influence of the autonomic nervous system on the genesis of cardiac arrhythmias. *Pacing Clin Electrophysiol* 1983;6:1210–1220.
102. Alessi R, Nusynowitz M, Abildskov JA, Moe GK. Nonuniform distribution of vagal effects on the atrial refractory period. *Am J Physiol* 1958;194 406–410.
103. Coumel P. Paroxysmal atrial fibrillation: A disorder of autonomic tone? *Eur Heart J* 1994;15(Suppl A):9–16.
104. Hohnloser SH. Ventricular arrhythmias: Antiadrenergic therapy for the patient with coronary artery disease. *J Cardiovasc Pharmacol Ther* 2005 10(Suppl. 1):S23–S31.
105. Nattel S, Bourne G, Talajic M. Insights into mechanisms of antiarrhythmic drug action from experimental models of atrial fibrillation. *J Cardiovasc Electrophysiol* 1997;8:469–480.
106. Liu L, Nattel S. Differing sympathetic and vagal effects on atrial fibrillation in dogs: Role of refractoriness heterogeneity. *Am J Physiol* 1997;273:H805-H816.
107. Arora RC, Cardinal R, Smith FM, Ardell JL Dell'Italia LJ, Armour JA. Intrinsic cardiac nervous system in tachycardia induced heart failure. *Am J Physiol Regul Integr Comp Physiol* 2003;285:1212-1223.
108. Armour JA, Hageman GR, Randall WC. Arrhythmias induced by local cardiac nerve stimulation. *Am J Physiol* 1972;223:1068–1075.
109. Schauerte P, Scherlag BJ, Patterson E, Scherlag MA, Matsudaria K, Nakagawa H, Lazzara R Jackman WM. Focal atrial fibrillation: Experimental evidence for a pathophysiologic role of the autonomic nervous system. *J Cardiovasc Electrophysiol* 2001;12:592–599.
110. Scherlag BJ, Yamanashi WS, Schauerte P, Scherlag M, Sun YX, Hou Y, Jackman WM, Lazzara R Endovascular stimulation within the left pulmonary artery to induce slowing of heart rate and paroxysmal atrial fibrillation. *Cardiovasc Res* 2002;54:470–475.
111. Chang CM, Wu TJ, Zhou S, Doshi RN, Lee MH Ohara T, Fishbein MC, Karagueuzian HS, Chen PS, Chen LS. Nerve sprouting and sympathetic hyperinnervation in a canine model of atrial fibrillation produced by prolonged right atrial pacing. *Circulation* 2001;103:22–25.
112. Olgin JE, Sih HJ, Hanish S, Jayachandran JV, Wu J, Zheng QH, Winkle W, Mulholland GK, Zipes DP, Hutchins G. Heterogeneous atrial denervation creates substrate for sustained atrial fibrillation *Circulation* 1998;98:2608–2614.
113. Swissa M, Zhou S, Gonzalez-Gomez I, Chang CM Lai AC, Cates AW, Fishbein MC, Karagueuzian HS, Chen PS, Chen LS. Long-term subthreshold electrical stimulation of the left stellate ganglion and a canine model of sudden cardiac death. *J Am Coll Cardiol* 2004;43:858–864.

114. Cao JM, Fishbein MC, Han JB, Lai WW, Lai AC, Wu TJ, Czer L, Wolf PL, Denton TA, Shintaku IP, Chen PS, Chen LS. Relationship between regional cardiac hyperinnervation and ventricular arrhythmia. *Circulation* 2000;101:1960–1969.
115. Zhou S, Cao JM, Tebb ZD, Ohara T, Huang HL, Omichi C, Lee MH, KenKnight BH, Chen LS, Fishbein MC, Karagueuzian HS, Chen PS. Modulation of QT interval by cardiac sympathetic nerve sprouting and the mechanisms of ventricular arrhythmia in a canine model of sudden cardiac death. *J Cardiovasc Electrophysiol* 2001;12:1068–1073.
116. Oh YS, Jong AY, Kim DT, Li H, Wang C, Zemljic-Harpf A, Ross RS, Fishbein MC, Chen PS, Chen LS. Spatial distribution of nerve sprouting after myocardial infarction in mice. *Heart Rhythm* 2006;3:728–736.
117. Nattel S. Atrial electrophysiological remodeling caused by rapid atrial activation: Underlying mechanisms and clinical relevance to atrial fibrillation. *Cardiovasc Res* 1999;42:298–308.
118. Wijffels MC, Kirchhof CJ, Dorland R, Allessie MA. Atrial fibrillation begets atrial fibrillation. A study in awake chronically instrumented goats. *Circulation* 1995;92:1954–1968.
119. Raitt MH, Kusumoto W, Giraud G, McAnulty JH. Reversal of electrical remodeling after cardioversion of persistent atrial fibrillation. *J Cardiovasc Electrophysiol* 2004;15:507–512.
120. Patberg KW, Shvilkin A, Plotnikov AN, Chandra P, Josephson ME, Rosen MR. Cardiac memory: Mechanisms and clinical implications. *Heart Rhythm* 2005;2:1376–1382.
121. Morillo CA, Klein GJ, Jones DL, Guiraudon CM. Chronic rapid atrial pacing. Structural, functional, and electrophysiological characteristics of a new model of sustained atrial fibrillation. *Circulation* 1995;91:1588–1595.
122. Yue L, Feng J, Gaspo R, Li GR, Wang Z, Nattel S. Ionic remodeling underlying action potential changes in a canine model of atrial fibrillation. *Circ Res* 1997;81:512–525.
123. Van Wagoner DR, Pond AL, McCarthy PM, Trimmer JS, Nerbonne JM. Outward K+ current densities and Kv1.5 expression are reduced in chronic human atrial fibrillation. *Circ Res* 1997;80:772–781.
124. Cha TJ, Ehrlich JR, Zhang L, Nattel S. Atrial ionic remodeling induced by atrial tachycardia in the presence of congestive heart failure. *Circulation* 2004;110:1520–1526.
125. Gaspo R, Bosch RF, Bou-Abboud E, Nattel S. Tachycardia-induced changes in Na+ current in a chronic dog model of atrial fibrillation. *Circ Res* 1997;81:1045–1052.
126. Bosch RF, Zeng X, Grammer JB, Popovic K, Mewis C, Kuhlkamp V. Ionic mechanisms of electrical remodeling in human atrial fibrillation. *Cardiovasc Res* 1999;44:121–131.
127. Sun H, Gaspo R, Leblanc N, Nattel S. Cellular mechanisms of atrial contractile dysfunction caused by sustained atrial tachycardia. *Circulation* 1998;98:719–727.
128. Vest JA, Wehrens XH, Reiken SR, Lehnart SE, Dobrev D, Chandra P, Danilo P, Ravens U, Rosen MR, Marks AR. Defective cardiac ryanodine receptor regulation during atrial fibrillation. *Circulation* 2005;111:2025–2032.
129. Hove-Madsen L, Llach A, Bayes-Genis A, Roura S, Rodriguez FE, Aris A, Cinca J. Atrial fibrillation is associated with increased spontaneous calcium release from the sarcoplasmic reticulum in human atrial myocytes. *Circulation* 2004;110:1358–1363.
130. Kostin S, Klein G, Szalay Z, Hein S, Bauer EP, Schaper J. Structural correlate of atrial fibrillation in human patients. *Cardiovasc Res* 2002;54:361–379.
131. Polontchouk L, Haefliger JA, Ebelt B, Schaefer T, Stuhlmann D, Mehlhorn U, Kuhn-Regnier F, De Vivie ER, Dhein S. Effects of chronic atrial fibrillation on gap junction distribution in human and rat atria. *J Am Coll Cardiol* 2001;38:883–891.
132. van der Velden HM, Ausma J, Rook MB, Hellemons AJ, van Veen TA, Allessie MA, Jongsma HJ. Gap junctional remodeling in relation to stabilization of atrial fibrillation in the goat. *Cardiovasc Res* 2000;46:476–486.
133. Rakovec P, Lajovic J, Dolenc M. Reversible congestive cardiomyopathy due to chronic ventricular tachycardia. *Pacing Clin Electrophysiol* 1989;12:542–545.
134. Chugh SS, Shen WK, Luria DM, Smith HC. First evidence of premature ventricular complex-induced cardiomyopathy: A potentially reversible cause of heart failure. *J Cardiovasc Electrophysiol* 2000;11:328–329.
135. Verma A, Kilicaslan F, Marrouche NF, Minor S, Khan M, Wazni O, Burkhardt JD, Belden WA, Cummings JE, Abdul-Karim A, Saliba W, Schweikert RA, Tchou PJ, Martin DO, Natale A. Prevalence, predictors, and mortality significance of the causative arrhythmia in patients with electrical storm. *J Cardiovasc Electrophysiol* 2004;15:1265–1270.
136. Merillat JC, Lakatta EG, Hano O, Guarnieri T. Role of calcium and the calcium channel in the initiation and maintenance of ventricular fibrillation. *Circ Res* 1990;67:1115–1123.

137. Zaugg CE, Wu ST, Barbosa V, Buser PT, Wikman-Coffelt J, Parmley WW, Lee RJ. Ventricular fibrillation-induced intracellular Ca2+ overload causes failed electrical defibrillation and post-shock reinitiation of fibrillation. *J Mol Cell Cardiol* 1998; 30:2183–2192.

138. Zaugg CE, Ziegler A, Lee RJ, Barbosa V, Buser PT. Postresuscitation stunning: Postfibrillatory myocardial dysfunction caused by reduced myofilament Ca2+ responsiveness after ventricular fibrillation-induced myocyte Ca2+ overload. *J Cardiovasc Electrophysiol* 2002;13:1017–1024.

139. Tsuji Y, Opthof T, Yasui K, Inden Y, Takemura H, Niwa N, Lu Z, Lee JK, Honjo H, Kamiya K, Kodama I. Ionic mechanisms of acquired QT prolongation and torsades de pointes in rabbits with chronic complete atrioventricular block. *Circulation* 2002; 106:2012–2018.

140. Vos MA, de Groot SH, Verduyn SC, van der ZJ, Leunissen HD, Cleutjens JP, van Bilsen M, Daemen MJ, Schreuder JJ, Allessie MA, Wellens H Enhanced susceptibility for acquired torsade d pointes arrhythmias in the dog with chronic, com plete AV block is related to cardiac hypertroph and electrical remodeling. *Circulation* 1998;98 1125–1135.

141. Suto F, Zhu W, Cahill SA, Greenwald I, Navarr AL, Gross GJ. Ventricular rate determines earl bradycardic electrical remodeling. *Heart Rhythm* 2005;2:293–300.

142. Volders PG, Sipido KR, Vos MA, Spatjens RI Leunissen JD, Carmeliet E, Wellens HJ. Down regulation of delayed rectifier K(+) currents in dogs with chronic complete atrioventricular block and acquired torsades de pointes. *Circulation* 1999;100:2455–2461.

143. Maor N, Weiss D, Lorber A. Torsade de pointe complicating atrioventricular block: Report o two cases. *Int J Cardiol* 1987;14:235–238.

17

ingle Nucleotide Polymorphisms n Health and Cardiac Disease

ric Schulze-Bahr

ntroduction

he prevalence of many complex human diseases uch as asthma, cardiovascular disease, and diaetes has risen greatly over the past two decades n developed countries. In addition, the genetic auses of monogenic diseases have been identied, leading to a better understanding of their athogenesis and to the development of preventive strategies, diagnostic tools, and treatment. onsiderable effort has been made to detect enetic loci contributing to quantitative phenoypes and complex arrhythmogenic diseases. enetic association and linkage studies comprise he two dominant strategies: association studies im to find disease-predisposing alleles [from ingle nucleotide polymorphisms (SNPs) or nicrosatellite markers] at the population level, vhereas linkage studies focus on familial segregaion. Predisposition to arrhythmia, e.g., acquired T prolongation or torsade de pointes (TdP) luring treatment with cardiac and noncardiac lrugs, is still a major challenge for physicians. ecent advances in the knowledge of the genomic nd physiological regulation of myocardial repoarization suggest that common alterations of ardiac (ion channel) genes are associated with light electrophysiological changes and an ncreased susceptibility for ventricular arrhythnia. The extent to which common genetic factors lay a role is under current investigation and emains to be determined. The availability of xtensive catalogues of SNPs in cardiac and nonardiac genes across the human genome is appliable for further genetic and functional studies to address the issue of genetically determined arrhythmogenesis.

Human Genome and Single Nucleotide Polymorphisms: A Revival in Genomic Medicine

The annotated draft sequence of approximately three billion base pairs (bp) of the human genome has been completed much sooner than expected.[1,2] This was a major scientific and technological development for researchers with an interest in the molecular bases of rare and common disorders, since awareness of the genomic diversity and molecular differences is expected to help in understanding the role of genetic contributions between individuals and disease. The variations at the nucleotide level are implemented to determine the physiological differences and individual phenotypic variance, including major biological functions at the cellular and body level. Single nucleotide polymorphisms (SNPs) were the first type of genetic markers that were used to make chromosomal genetic maps.[3] However, due to a lower degree of heterozygosity and less genetic information when compared to polymorphic length (repeat) markers, SNPs became temporarily less attractive, until the completion of the human genome was done. In general, SNPs are single nucleotide base substitutions at a certain gene or genomic position and represent the major part of interindividual variability that accounts for only 0.1% of genome sequences between individuals in health and disease. These small differences in the genetic code can be linked to unique personal features (e.g., eye color, height) and alterations of regular physiological function, varied response to environmental conditions, and predisposition for certain diseases. Of the approximately 10^6 million SNPs in the human genome, only a fraction has been directly associated with functional significance and related to complex traits so far. Thus, the complexity of the entire human genome map is undermined by distinct effects of SNPs that depend on the nucleotide subtype, their genomic location and effect on protein structure/function, their abundance (allele frequency), and their contribution to subchromosomal compartments of SNPs in linkage disequilibrium (haplotypes). The SNPs differ in their location within the genomic sequence (coding vs. noncoding areas), in the type of nucleotide exchange and the consequences for the amino acid sequence, and in their frequency (relative occurrence) in the human genome (Table 17–1). Polymorphisms that potentially have the greatest impact of phenotypic disease are rare within the genome.[4] Current estimates of the degree of diversity range from 1:500 to 1:1000, resulting in millions of variants in the human genome. An understanding of the genetic diversity and of its contribution to variations in normal and abnormal physiology will have a potentially powerful effect on cardiovascular and genomic medicine.

Genetic association studies (or case–control studies) are an analysis of statistically significant relationships between SNP alleles and phenotypic differences. The power of a genetic association study is a direct function of the number and quality of the SNPs used to screen a population for phenotypic variability. Because SNPs and haplotypes can vary in their prevalence among different populations, an SNP associated with a particular phenotype or quantitative trait in one population may not have the same frequency or effect in another population, e.g., when the population is of different ethnicity, age, or gender. Large datasets of chromosomal SNPs have been published since 2000[2,5–8] along with improved methods to screen immense numbers of SNP candidates. Nearly three million variants have been reported and are catalogued in public databases (http://www.ncbi.nlm.nih.gov/SNP/) (http://www.ncbi.nlm.nih.gov/projects/SNP/). Newer techniques allow high-throughput genotyping to study simultaneously large numbers of SNP loc

TABLE 17–1. Types and sequence location of DNA variation.[a]

Polymorphism type	Sequence location	Predicted protein and potential functional effects	Occurrence in genome	Potential disease impact
Nonsense	Coding	Prematurely truncated, most likely loss of protein function	Very low	High
Missense, nonsynonymous	Coding, nonconserved	Altered amino acid chain, mostly similar protein properties	Low	Low (to high)
Missense, nonsynonymous	Coding, conserved	Altered amino acid chain, mostly different protein properties	Low	Medium to high
Rearrangements (insertion/deletion)	Coding	Altered amino acid chain, mostly different protein properties	Low	High
Sense, synonymous	Coding	Unchanged amino acid chain, rarely an effect on exon splicing	Medium	Low (to medium)
Promotor and regulatory sequences	Noncoding, Promotor/UTR	Unchanged amino acid chain, but may affect gene expression	Low to medium	Low to high, depending on site
Intronic nucleotide exchange (<40 bp)	Noncoding, Splice/Lariat sites	Altered amino acid chain, failed recognition of exonic structure	Low	Low to high, depending on site
Intronic nucleotide exchange (>40 bp)	Noncoding, between introns	Unchanged amino acid chain, rarely abnormal splicing or mRNA instability, site for gene rearrangements	Medium	Very low
Intergenic nucleotide exchange	Noncoding, between genes	Unchanged amino acid chain, may affect gene expression, site for gross rearrangements	High	Very low

Source: From Kääb and Schulze-Bahr.[4]

[a]UTR, untranslated region (5′ or 3′ region of a gene); bp, base pairs.

currently 500K per chip) and are based on matrix-assisted laser desorption ionization time-of-flight (MALDI-TOF; e.g., Sequenom MassARRAY), pyrosequencing, or hybridization. There are, however, some inherent limitations to SNP studies. The two major issues are *statistical power* and *replication* of genetic findings in another population. In association studies, the prevalence of genetic marker alleles in unrelated subjects with a certain phenotype and (unaffected) controls will be compared, with the aim of correlating differences in disease frequencies between groups (or in trait levels for continuously varying characters) and allele frequencies for an SNP. Thus, the frequencies of the two variant forms (alleles) of an SNP are of primary interest for the identification of genes affecting disease. The traditional case–control approach assumes that any noted difference in allele frequencies is related to the outcome measured and that there are no unobserved confounding effects. Unfortunately, allele frequencies are known to vary widely within and between populations, irrespective of disease status. For an appropriate study, an adequate sample size of the groups and a relatively high frequency of the minor SNP allele (to facilitate detection of allele frequency differences between the investigated populations) are needed. Studies with small sample sizes may result in *type II errors*, i.e., not declaring a statistically significant result when there may be a difference. These underpowered studies can be misleading because genes may be undetected, and reporting the odds ratio and 95% confidence interval is recommended.[9] The term β (beta) is defined as the chance of making a type II error. Values for β are typically 10–20%, meaning a power $(1 - \beta)$ between 80% and 90%. In contrast, a sample size that is much larger than required may indicate that small differences are statistically significant and thus commit *type I errors* (i.e., declaring a statistically significant difference when it may not be present). The term α (alpha) refers to the chance of making a *type I error*; usually, a level of 0.05 or less is chosen.

Proposed guidelines have been developed that should facilitate the quality of association studies,[10,11] including strategies to ascertain *heritability and exact phenotyping of a trait*, to perform *population stratification of cases and controls* (ethnicity, age, and gender distribution), *to select physiologically and genetically meaningful markers*, to address the *probability of association*, and to *replicate* initial results in independent studies. To date, only a few of the several thousand published association studies strictly meet the criteria to ascertain a ("true") genetic association. For arrhythmogenic disorders, first studies exist,[12–15] but the majority of data is still unreplicated by independent approaches. Differences in study outcome may be related to population stratification, study design, still inappropriate marker selection, and lack of statistical power.[4] Discovery of meaningful SNP markers, e.g., indicating an elevated risk of sudden cardiac death (SCD), is still far from being established. Common weaknesses of many association studies include a study design that fails to adequately identify true positives while eliminating false positives, poorly defined phenotypes and sampling from heterogeneous patient populations, inappropriately matched controls, small sample sizes relative to the magnitude of the genetic effects, failure to account for multiple testing, population and sample stratification, failure to replicate marginal findings, and overemphasizing the interpretation of the study results. In the past, the optimum study design for association studies has been discussed because, often, studies were prone to population stratification and biased or spurious results. Thus, replication of the findings from genetic association studies in other populations became a cornerstone for maintaining data quality, and, so far, only a few studies merit these criteria. A shift from case–control and cohort studies toward a family-based association designs has therefore been noted. These study designs have fewer problems with population stratification, but have greater genotyping and sampling requirements, and data can be difficult or impossible to gather.

Analysis of Single Nucleotide Polymorphisms in Arrhythmias: Toward Common Genetic Constellations for Arrhythmogenesis

Phenotypic variation in the development of arrhythmia is well known from families with inherited, arrhythmogenic disorders that have demonstrated an important phenotypic spectrum of the same mutation in affected family members.[16,17] These observations are also seen in patients with more polygenic disorders, such as myocardial infarction, for which not every patient develops ventricular fibrillation during acute ischemia.[18] In a case–control study in patients with a first ST elevation myocardial infarction (STEMI) and similar infarct sizes and locations, it was recently shown that (cumulative) ST segment elevation was significantly higher among cases and that familial sudden death occurred more frequently among cases than controls.[18] Thus, development of arrhythmia may have a common substrate modification in both, rare inherited and common, polygenic forms of various arrhythmias, and a positive family history can be noted in both. In addition, multiple factors—such as age, gender, and environmental conditions—play an important role in the modulation of the phenotype. Structural and electrical remodeling during acute ischemia, altered hemodynamic loads, or changes in neurohormonal signaling are recognized as key features that alter ion channel gene expression. Downregulation of major repolarizing potassium currents, I_{to}, I_{Kr}, I_{Ks}, and I_{K1}, has been described in several models of heart failure and resembles a condition of "acquired QT prolongation." Cellular abnormalities through disturbances in electrical cell–cell coupling and a local reduction of conduction velocity facilitate reentrant ventricular arrhythmias. These cellular abnormalities can be found in the structurally diseased heart. The extent of the genetically controlled variation is not clear to date, but it is of potential interest and has recently been investigated.

Population-based studies demonstrated an increased risk of SCD among patients with a parental history of cardiac arrest,[19,20] but a clearly defined genetic basis is not known.[21] In contrast to patients with cardiac dysfunction, in patients without intraventricular conduction defects or a normal cardiac function, QTc prolongation is a nonnegligible risk factor for sudden cardiac death independent of age, history of myocardial infarction, heart rate, and drug use. This has been shown in the Rotterdam Study, a prospective population-based cohort study, in which 125 patients died of sudden cardiac death (mean follow-up of 6.7 years) and patients had a 3-fold increased risk for a prolonged QTc interval.[21–2] Recently, a quantitative influence of ion channe gene variation on myocellular repolarization was described in twins[14] and in the general population.[12,13,24] Genomic studies are currently making progress in narrowing these candidate gene regions and in identifying these variants (SNPs or haplotype constellations) in coding and noncoding sequences. Also, patients with drug-induced QT prolongation have been investigated for the presence of (clinically inapparent) gene mutations in long QT syndrome (LQTS) genes. In 10-15% of patients such mutations can be found.[25–27] Recently, common protein variants (SNPs) in cardiac ion channels have been identified (Table 17–2), which also may have a potential impact on susceptibility to arrhythmia and pharmacogenetic strategies for circumvention of arrhythmia as well as for therapy. Yang *et al.* screened the coding regions of the three major LQT genes (LQT1-3) in 92 patients with drug-induced LQTS and additional controls.[28] The allele frequencies of three common, nonsynonymous polymorphisms (*SCN5A*-H558R, *SCN5A*-R34C, *HERG*-K897T) did not significantly differ between the two groups. Similar findings were reported by Paulussen *et al.*[29] and indicate no particular concomitant effect of the presence of an LQTS gene polymorphism and the occurrence of TdP.

These observations and more general considerations led to the concept that beyond the "rare disease paradigm" [meaning that rare gene mutations cause (rare) Mendelian disorders] a "common variant–common disease hypothesis" may be present. Here, common SNPs in ion channel genes may determine arrhythmogenesis. It is anticipated that not a single SNP, but several SNPs in one or more genes together exhibit a detectable, functional effect. For severe atrial conduction impairment, a heterozygous mutation (D1275N) in the cardiac sodium channel gene *SCN5A* has been reported that was probably aggravated by the presence of two SNPs within regulatory regions of gap junction protein connexin 40.[30,31] For patients with Brugada syndrome as well as control individuals, an *SCN5A* promoter haplotype (so-called HapB) was associated with longer PR and QRS interval durations and response to sodium channel blockers.[32] These examples of genomic interplay are assumed to

Table 17–2. Ion channel gene variants identified in patients with drug-induced QT prolongation or torsade de pointes occurrence.

Gene	Current	Amino acid alteration	Drug/setting	Functional assay	Minor allele	Reference
KCNE2	I_{Kr}	T8E	Trimethoprim (TMX)/sulfamethoxazole (SMX); quinidine; amiodarone	E8-MiRP1 weakly reduced I_{Kr} current peak density; Chinese hamster ovary (CHO) cells; SMX and TMX had almost no effecton on wild-type channels, but SMX was reported to inhibit more than 50% of A8-MiRP1 at −40 mV; mutant channels were four times more sensitive to SMX than wild type	1.6%	29, 45, 46
	I_{Kr}	Q9E	Clarithromycin, low K^+		Rare in whites, but not in Afro-Americans	33, 45
	I_{Kr}	M54T	Procainamide	T54-MiRP1 significantly reduced I_{Kr} current peak density (CHO cells); no influence on drug-related channel inhibition was seen	Rare	46
	I_{Kr}	M57T	Oxatomide	T57-MiRP1 significantly reduced I_{Kr} current peak density (CHO cells); no influence on drug-related channel inhibition was seen	Rare	46
	I_{Kr}	A116V	Quinidine	V116-MiRP1 significantly reduced I_{Kr} current peak density (CHO cells); no influence on drug-related channel inhibition was seen	Rare	46
KCNH2	I_{Kr}	M124T	Probucol	Coexpression of wild-type hERG and T124-hERG resulted in markedly smaller amplitudes of I_{Kr} (*Xenopus* oocytes); probucol decreased the amplitude of the hERG tail current, decelerated the rate of channel activation, accelerated the rate of channel deactivation, and shifted the reversal potential to a more positive value	Rare	47
	I_{Kr}	R328C	Not reported		Rare	48
	I_{Kr}	P347S	Cisapride/clarithromycin		Rare	29, 49
	I_{Kr}	R486H	Quinidine		Rare[a]	25
	I_{Kr}	A561P	Clobutinol	P561-hERG led to an intracellular trafficking defect; when coexpressed with wild-type hERG, voltage dependence was shifted toward more negative potentials (3–3.5 mV); clobutinol further blocked heteromeric channels	Rare[a]	50
						51
	I_{Kr}	R784W	Amiodarone	W784-hERG mediated a reduced I_{Kr} current (by ~75%) and a positive shift of voltage dependence of activation	Rare	28
KCNQ1	I_{Ks}	R243H	Halofantrine; hydrochinine		Rare[a,b]	25
	I_{Ks}	Y315C	Cisapride	*In vitro* expression of mutant KvLQT1 protein showed a severe loss of current with a dominant negative effect on the WT-KvLQT1 channel	Rare[a]	52
	I_{Ks}	R555C	Terfenadine		Rare	53, 54
	I_{Ks}	R583C	Dofetilide	C583-KvLQT1-mediated I_{Ks} was reduced by ~50% compared with wild type, and the voltage dependence of activation was shifted positively by 19.6 mV (CHO cells)	Rare	28
SCN5A	I_{Na}	G615E	Quinidine	E615-SCN5A was indistinguishable from wild-type mediated I_{Na} currents (tsa-201 cells)	Rare	28
	I_{Na}	L618F	Quinidine	F618-SCN5A was indistinguishable from wild-type mediated I_{Na} currents (tsa-201 cells)	Rare	28
	I_{Na}	S1103Y	Amiodarone	Y1103-SCN5A mediated an increased I_{Na} channel activation (HEK 293)	7–10% (Afro-Americans or West Africans/Caribbeans only)	28

TABLE 17–2. *Continued*

Gene	Current	Amino acid alteration	Drug/setting	Functional assay	Minor allele	Reference
	I_{Na}	F1250L	Sotalol	L1250-SCN5A was indistinguishable from wild-type mediated I_{Na} currents (tsa-201 cells)	Rare	28
	I_{Na}	P1825L	Cisapride	The C-terminal mutant L1825-SCN5A mediated I_{Na} current with slow decay and prominent TTX- insensitive, noninactivating component (gain of function), a reduced peak density (loss of function), shifted voltage dependence of activation (more positive potentials) and of inactivation (more negative potentials) (tsA-201 cells)		55
				L1825-SCN5A channels showed impairment of intracellular trafficking (CHO cells) and failed to generate QT prolongation; exposure with cisapride rescued cell surface expression of L1825-SCN5A and exaggerated the LQT3 phenotype		56

[a]Heterozygous mutation carriers may have a normal QT interval; for SCN5A, amino acid residues are numerated according to their position on the long splice variant.
[b]Reported from recessive forms of long QT syndrome.

alter the designation of a specific phenotype from mild to pronounced, even in carriers of the same mutation. Typically, more frequently occurring SNPs should be used, but large numbers of cases and controls would still be needed because of their low phenotypic impact. The following assumptions underlie these investigations:

1. An important fraction of susceptibility to a given disease may be explained by the relatively modest effects of a small number of relatively common variants.
2. Many of these common variants are either SNPs themselves or genomic markers in linkage disequilibrium with the functional variant, and arise at rates lower than the rate at which new SNPs appear.
3. Rates at which SNPs become common are low enough that many of the SNP carriers inherited this variant from a single ancestor.
4. Recombination rates at SNP loci are low; therefore carriers of a common disease-linked variant will have the same SNP (haplotype) pattern that appeared on the ancestral chromosomal locus near the causal variant.

Ethnicity-specific and population-specific differences in the frequency of an SNP allele in cardiac ion channel genes have to be considered, since they recently became evident.[33] The SNP *KCNH2*-K897T (rs1805123) has been investigated in different studies to address an effect on QT interval duration. So far, no convincing data were reported, because some,[12,35,35] but not all studies[28,36,37] suggested an effect on QTc interval duration. *SCN5A*-S1103Y (also *SCN5A*-S1102Y, referring to the shorter splice form of *SCN5A*) is another frequent LQT gene polymorphism that has been identified primarily in West Africans and Caribbeans (ca. 19%) and in Afro-Americans (ca. 13%), but is very rare in whites, Asians, and Hispanics.[38] Y1103 allele carriers (YY or SY) were reported to have a higher relative risk for ventricular arrhythmia, which was not linked to baseline repolarization parameters[38] and sudden cardiac death in infants (SIDS).[39,40,41]

The majority is related to sudden cardiac death in myocardial ischemia or during heart failure. The instability of membrane electrophysiological properties of myocardium and local conduction impairment led to lethal ventricular arrhythmias. Since ATP-sensitive potassium (KATP) channels are involved in membrane regulation during metabolic stress, studies focused on identifying variants in the *KCNJ11* gene associated with SCD after myocardial infarction.[42] These channels are composed of four pore-forming Kir6.2 (*KCNJ11*) subunits and four sulfonylurea receptor subunits (*SUR2A*); sarcolemmal KATP channels regulate membrane potential and action potential duration, whereas the mitochondrial KATP channels are involved in ischemic preconditioning. So far, two nonsynonymous polymorphisms (R371H, P266T) in two highly conserved pore regions are known that show altered modulation by intracellular ATP and protons and differences in channel density[43] and, thus, are potential candidates for genetically determined electrophysiological differences under ischemic conditions.

Future Directions

Recent advances in our knowledge of the genomic structure of ion channel genes and their physiological role in myocardial repolarization have shown that genetic alterations of these key molecular components are associated with slight *in vitro* effects and changes in finetuning normal repolarization. The extent to which minor genetic factors are associated with susceptibility to arrhythmias remains to be determined, but initial evidence for this is present. Following the concept of "repolarization reserve,"[44] it is likely that TdP as well as arrhythmia during acute myocardial infarction or drug response (as well as side effects) are also dependent on individual genetic backgrounds. The genetic factors involved in arrhythmogenesis switch from gene identification and single pathway understanding to genomic medicine by integrating complex gene and environmental information. Future research will

1. Identify all relevant genes and their genomic structure for repolarization.
2. Determine the extent of the variability of the QT interval and of the response to action potential prolongation that is genetically controlled.
3. Investigate the role of functionally relevant SNPs and haplotype constellations in LQTS and other gene loci for their quantitative contribution to repolarization.
4. Integrate identified genetic factors with other known factors for TdP risk, according to their relative importance, in a network algorithm for arrhythmogenesis.

These data should be available within the next few years and advances, along with additional technological improvements in DNA analysis and data management, will enable researchers to lower the costs of complex genotyping and to implement these data into a personalized, genomic-oriented medicine.

Acknowledgments. This work was supported by the Leducq Foundation, Paris, France, and by the German Research Foundation, Bonn, Germany (DFG Schu1082/3-1 and 3-2, DFG Ki653/13-1, and SFB 656-C1) and by the Interdisciplinary Center for Cardiovascular Research (IZKF) of the University of Münster, Germany.

References

1. Venter JC, Adams MD, Myers EW, *et al.* The sequence of the human genome. *Science* 2001; 291(5507):1304–1351.
2. Lander ES, Linton LM, Birren B, *et al.* Initial sequencing and analysis of the human genome. *Nature* 2001;409(6822):860–921.
3. Botstein D, White RL, Skolnick M, *et al.* Construction of a genetic linkage map in man using restriction fragment length polymorphisms. *Am J Hum Genet* 1980;32(3):314–331.
4. Kääb S, Schulze-Bahr E. Susceptibility genes and modifiers for cardiac arrhythmias. *Cardiovasc Res* 2005;67(3):397–413.
5. Altshuler D, Pollara VJ, Cowles CR, *et al.* An SNP map of the human genome generated by reduced representation shotgun sequencing. *Nature* 2000; 407(6803):513–516.
6. Lindblad-Toh K, Winchester E, Daly MJ, *et al.* Large-scale discovery and genotyping of single-nucleotide polymorphisms in the mouse. *Nat Genet* 2000;24(4):381–386.
7. Mullikin JC, Hunt SE, Cole CG, *et al.* An SNP map of human chromosome 22. *Nature* 2000;407(6803): 516–520.
8. Sachidanandam R, Weissman D, Schmidt SC, *et al.* A map of human genome sequence variation containing 1.42 million single nucleotide polymorphisms. *Nature* 2001;409(6822):928–933.
9. Au WW, Oh HY, Grady J, *et al.* Usefulness of genetic susceptibility and biomarkers for evaluation of environmental health risk. *Environ Mol Mutagen* 2001;37(3):215–225.
10. Editorial. Freely associating. *Nat Genet* 1999;22: 1–2.

11. Cooper DN, Nussbaum RL, Krawczak M. Proposed guidelines for papers describing DNA polymorphism-disease associations. *Hum Genet* 2002;110(3):207–208.
12. Pfeufer A, Jalilzadeh S, Perz S, *et al.* Common variants in myocardial ion channel genes modify the QT interval in the general population: Results from the KORA study. *Circ Res* 2005;96(6):693–701.
13. Arking DE, Pfeufer A, Post W, *et al.* A common genetic variant in the NOS1 regulator NOS1AP modulates cardiac repolarization. *Nat Genet* 2006; 38(6):644–651.
14. Busjahn A, Knoblauch H, Faulhaber HD, *et al.* QT interval is linked to 2 long-QT syndrome loci in normal subjects. *Circulation* 1999;99(24):3161–3164.
15. Newton-Cheh C, Larson MG, Corey DC, *et al.* QT interval is a heritable quantitative trait with evidence of linkage to chromosome 3 in a genome-wide linkage analysis: The Framingham Heart Study. *Heart Rhythm* 2005;2(3):277–284.
16. Kaufman ES, Priori SG, Napolitano C, *et al.* Electrocardiographic prediction of abnormal genotype in congenital long QT syndrome: Experience in 101 related family members. *J Cardiovasc Electrophysiol* 2001;12(4):455–461.
17. Zareba W, Moss AJ, Sheu G, *et al.* Location of mutation in the KCNQ1 and phenotypic presentation of long QT syndrome. *J Cardiovasc Electrophysiol* 2003;14(11):1149–1153.
18. Dekker LR, Bezzina CR, Henriques JP, *et al.* Familial sudden death is an important risk factor for primary ventricular fibrillation: A case-control study in acute myocardial infarction patients. *Circulation* 2006;114(11):1140–1145.
19. Spooner PM, Albert C, Benjamin EJ, *et al.* Sudden cardiac death, genes, and arrhythmogenesis: Consideration of new population and mechanistic approaches from a national heart, lung, and blood institute workshop, part I. *Circulation* 2001;103(19): 2361–2364.
20. Jouven X, Desnos M, Guerot C, *et al.* Predicting sudden death in the population: The Paris Prospective Study I. *Circulation* 1999;99(15):1978–1983.
21. de Bruyne MC, Hoes AW, Kors JA, *et al.* Prolonged QT interval predicts cardiac and all-cause mortality in the elderly. The Rotterdam Study. *Eur Heart J* 1999;20(4):278–284.
22. Algra A, Tijssen JG, Roelandt JR, *et al.* QTc prolongation measured by standard 12-lead electrocardiography is an independent risk factor for sudden death due to cardiac arrest. *Circulation* 1991;83(6):1888–1894.
23. Straus SM, Kors JA, De Bruin ML, *et al.* Prolonged QTc interval and risk of sudden cardiac death in a population of older adults. *J Am Coll Cardiol* 2006; 47(2):362–367.
24. Newton-Cheh C, Larson MG, Corey DC, *et al.* QT interval is a heritable quantitative trait with evidence of linkage to chromosome 3 in a genome-wide linkage analysis: The Framingham Heart Study. *Heart Rhythm* 2005;2(3):277–284.
25. Schulze-Bahr E, Haverkamp W, Hördt M, *et al.* Do mutations in cardiac ion channel genes predispose to drug-induced (acquired) long-QT syndrome? *Circulation* 1997;96(8):I–210(Suppl.).
26. Roden DM, Viswanathan PC. Genetics of acquired long QT syndrome. *J Clin Invest* 2005;115(8):2025–2032.
27. Roden DM. Long QT syndrome: Reduced repolarization reserve and the genetic link. *J Intern Med* 2006;259(1):59–69.
28. Yang P, Kanki H, Drolet B, *et al.* Allelic variants in long-QT disease genes in patients with drug-associated torsades de pointes. *Circulation* 2002; 105(16):1943–1948.
29. Paulussen ADC, Gilissen RAHJ, Armstrong M, *et al.* Genetic variations of KCNQ1, KCNH2, SCN5A, KCNE1, and KCNE2 in drug-induced long QT syndrome patients. *J Mol Med* 2004;82(3):182–188.
30. Groenewegen WA, Firouzi M, Bezzina CR, *et al.* A cardiac sodium channel mutation cosegregates with a rare connexin40 genotype in familial atrial standstill. *Circ Res* 2003;92(1):14–22.
31. Makita N, Sasaki K, Groenewegen WA, *et al.* Congenital atrial standstill associated with coinheritance of a novel SCN5A mutation and connexin 40 polymorphisms. *Heart Rhythm* 2005;2(10):1128–1134.
32. Bezzina CR, Shimizu W, Yang P, *et al.* Common sodium channel promoter haplotype in asian subjects underlies variability in cardiac conduction. *Circulation* 2006;113(3):338–344.
33. Ackerman MJ, Tester DJ, Jones GS, *et al.* Ethnic differences in cardiac potassium channel variants: Implications for genetic susceptibility to sudden cardiac death and genetic testing for congenital long QT syndrome. *Mayo Clinic Proc* 2003;78(12): 1479–1487.
34. Bezzina CR, Verkerk AO, Busjahn A, *et al.* A common polymorphism in KCNH2 (HERG) hastens cardiac repolarization. *Cardiovasc Res* 2003;59(1): 27–36.
35. Gouas L, Nicaud V, Berthet M, *et al.* Association of KCNQ1, KCNE1, KCNH2 and SCN5A polymorphisms with QTc interval length in a healthy

population. *Eur J Hum Genet* 2005;13(11):1213–1222.
36. Paavonen KJ, Chapman H, Laitinen PJ, *et al.* Functional characterization of the common amino acid 897 polymorphism of the cardiac potassium channel KCNH2 (HERG). *Cardiovasc Res* 2003; 59(3):603–611.
37. Pietila E, Fodstad H, Niskasaari E, *et al.* Association between HERG K897T polymorphism and QT interval in middle-aged Finnish women. *J Am Coll Cardiol* 2002;40(3):511–514.
38. Splawski I, Timothy KW, Tateyama M, *et al.* Variant of SCN5A sodium channel implicated in risk of cardiac arrhythmia. *Science* 2002;297(5585):1333–1336.
39. Burke A, Creighton W, Mont E, Li L, Hogan S, Kutys R, *et al.* Role of SCN5A Y1102 polymorphism in sudden cardiac death in blacks. *Circulation* 2005;112(6):798–802.
40. Plant LD, Bowers PN, Liu Q, Morgan T, Zhang T, State MW, *et al.* A common cardiac sodium channel variant associated with sudden infant death in African Americans, SCN5A S1103Y. *J Clin Invest* 2006;116(2):430–435.
41. Etzrodt D, Schulze-Bahr E. Letter regarding article by Burke *et al.*, "role of SCN5A Y1102 polymorphism in sudden cardiac death in blacks." *Circulation* 2006;113(15):e709.
42. Jeron A, Hengstenberg C, Holmer S, *et al.* KCNJ11 polymorphisms and sudden cardiac death in patients with acute myocardial infarction. *J Mol Cell Cardiol* 2004;36(2):287–293.
43. Cui N, Li L, Wang X, *et al.* Elimination of allosteric modulation of myocardial KATP channels by ATP and protons in two Kir6.2 polymorphisms found in sudden cardiac death. *Physiol Genomics* 2006;25(1):105–115.
44. Roden DM. Taking the "idio" out of "idiosyncratic": Predicting torsades de pointes. *Pacing Clin Electrophysiol* 1998;21(5):1029–1034.
45. Abbott GW, Sesti F, Splawski I, *et al.* MiRP1 forms IKr potassium channels with HERG and is associated with cardiac arrhythmia. *Cell* 1999;97(2):175–187.
46. Sesti F, Abbott GW, Wei J, *et al.* A common polymorphism associated with antibiotic-induced cardiac arrhythmia. *Proc Natl Acad Sci USA* 2000; 97(19):10613–10618.
47. Hayashi K, Shimizu M, Ino H, *et al.* Probucol aggravates long QT syndrome associated with a novel missense mutation M124T in the N-terminus of HERG. *Clin Sci (Lond)* 2004;107(2):175–182.
48. Splawski I, Shen J, Timothy KW, *et al.* Genomic structure of three long QT syndrome genes: KVLQT1, HERG, and KCNE1. *Genomics* 1998;51(1):86–97.
49. Piquette RK. Torsade de pointes induced by cisapride/clarithromycin interaction. *Ann Pharmacother* 1999;33(1):22–26.
50. Bellocq C, Wilders R, Schott JJ, *et al.* A common antitussive drug, clobutinol, precipitates the long QT syndrome 2. *Mol Pharmacol* 2004;66(5):1093–1102.
51. Chevalier P, Rodriguez C, Bontemps L, *et al.* Noninvasive testing of acquired long QT syndrome: Evidence for multiple arrhythmogenic substrates. *Cardiovasc Res* 2001;50(2):386–398.
52. Napolitano C, Schwartz PJ, Brown AM, *et al.* Evidence for a cardiac ion channel mutation underlying drug-induced QT prolongation and life-threatening arrhythmias. *J Cardiovasc Electrophysiol* 2000;11(6):691–696.
53. Berthet M, Denjoy I, Donger C, *et al.* C-terminal HERG mutations: The role of hypokalemia and a KCNQ1-associated mutation in cardiac event occurrence. *Circulation* 1999;99(11):1464–1470.
54. Donger C, Denjoy I, Berthet M, *et al.* KVLQT1 C-terminal missense mutation causes a forme fruste long-QT syndrome. *Circulation* 1997;96(9):2778–2781.
55. Makita N, Horie M, Nakamura T, *et al.* Drug-induced long-QT syndrome associated with a subclinical SCN5A mutation. *Circulation* 2002;106(10):1269–1274.
56. Liu J, Laurita KR. The mechanism of pause-induced torsade de pointes in long QT syndrome. *J Cardiovasc Electrophysiol* 2005;16(9):981–987.

18
Electrophysiological Remodeling in Dilated Cardiomyopathy and Heart Failure

Fadi G. Akar and Gordon F. Tomaselli

Introduction

Cardiac remodeling commonly refers to a persistent change in the properties of the myocardium in response to external stress. Cardiac remodeling occurs prominently in the setting of structural heart disease such as myocardial infarction, hypertrophy, and heart failure (HF), but may also occur in the absence of mechanical dysfunction, as is the case during abrupt changes in heart rate and/or activation sequence. As such, remodeling is a prominent feature of atrial fibrillation, flutter, complete heart block, ventricular pacing, and tachycardia. Remodeling is induced by changes in gene expression, which, in turn, alter the expression of key regulatory proteins, the distribution and function of subcellular organelles, the size and morphology of individual cells, the properties of the extracellular matrix, and ultimately those of the entire organ.

Remodeling, whether electrical or structural, is an important adaptive mechanism that allows the heart to maintain its primary blood pumping function in the face of external stress. However, remodeling also imposes maladaptive consequences that contribute significantly to mortality and morbidity in patients with heart disease, particularly those with congestive HF. Despite remarkable improvements in medical therapy, the prognosis of patients with myocardial failure remains very poor,[1] with over 15% of patients dying within 1 year of initial diagnosis and 80% within 6 years.[2] Interestingly, of the deaths in patients with HF, up to 50% are sudden and unexpected, and presumably the consequence of lethal ventricular tachyarrhythmias,[3] secondary to electrical and structural remodeling. Therefore, a better understanding of the mechanisms that underlie the maladaptive electrophysiological remodeling processes in HF will aid in the design of both pharmacological and nonpharmacological treatment strategies for patients.

In HF, the myocardium undergoes a complex series of changes in both myocyte and nonmyocyte elements. In an attempt to compensate for reduced cardiac function, the sympathetic nervous system (SNS), the rennin–angiotensin–aldosterone system (RAAS), and other neurohumoral mechanisms are activated, initiating fundamental changes in gene expression that result in myocyte hypertrophy. Ultimately, these changes become maladaptive, predisposing to myocyte loss, interstitial hyperplasia, and chamber remodeling.

Both intrinsic (i.e., cardiac) as well as peripheral responses to myocardial failure adversely alter the electrophysiology of the heart, predisposing patients to an increased risk for arrhythmic events. With progression of HF, the frequency and complexity of ventricular ectopy are enhanced.[4] Although total mortality in HF patients correlates well with left ventricular (LV) function and the presence of complex ventricular ectopy,[5] there is no clear correlation between sudden cardiac death (SCD) and LV function. In fact, data from VheFT-I (Veteran's Administration Heart Failure Trial) and other trials suggest that the percentage of SCD is greater in more modest compared to severe ventricular dysfunction.[6] A major caveat is that the mechanism of SCD is highly heterogeneous, even when exclusively considering those patients whose death was arrhythmic. Here we provide an overview of the electrophysiological remodeling that accompanies HF and that occurs at the molecular, cellular, and tissue network levels.

Cellular Electrophysiology of the Failing Ventricle

An elementary and distinctive signature of any excitable tissue is its action potential profile. In myocardial cells, which possess a characteristically long action potential, an initial rapid upstroke is followed by a plateau phase of maintained depolarization, and a subsequent gradual return to rest (Figure 18–1). Therefore, the duration of the action potential is primarily responsible for the time course of cardiac repolarization. Consequently, prolongation of the action potential produces significant repolarization delays, which often predispose to malignant arrhythmias by mechanisms involving either triggered activity (secondary to early afterdepolarizations) or reentry (secondary to unidirectional conduction block).

Prolongation of the action potential is a hallmark of cells and tissues isolated from failing hearts independent of etiology. These include pressure and/or volume overload,[7–14] genetic,[15] metabolic, and ischemia/infarction,[16] and chronic pacing tachycardia models.[17–19] The pathophysiological significance of action potential prolongation in cells isolated from hypertrophied and failing hearts has been challenged on several grounds. First, most action potential recordings have been performed at unphysiologically slow rates, and indeed differences in action potential duration between cells of failing and normal hearts are expected to converge at high stimulation frequencies (Figure 18–2). However, since slow heart rates and pauses following premature ventricular contractions are common in HF, pause-dependent prolongation of the action potential duration may be highly relevant. Moreover, cell-to-cell electrotonic coupling in the intact heart is expected to appreciably modulate repolarization in a manner that reduces the effective spatial dispersion of refractoriness. However, qualitatively similar action potential prolongation was recently demonstrated in intact muscle preparations from failing hearts using optical dye recordings.[20] Finally, the duration of the action potential is quite sensitive to mechanical load, which may shorten action potential duration and refractoriness disproportionately in failing versus normal hearts.[21] These effects are likely to be heterogeneous, resulting in further enhancement of repolarization heterogeneity in the failing heart.

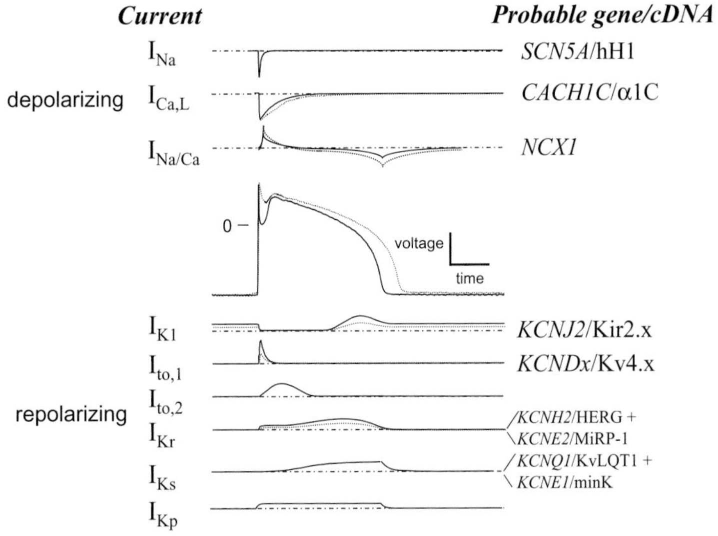

FIGURE 18–1. Schematic of inward and outward ionic currents, pumps, and exchangers, which underlie ventricular action potentials in the mammalian heart. Control (bold line) and failing action potential profiles are shown on the top. Each phase of the action potential is also labeled. A schematic of the time course of each current is shown, and the gene product that underlies the current is indicated.

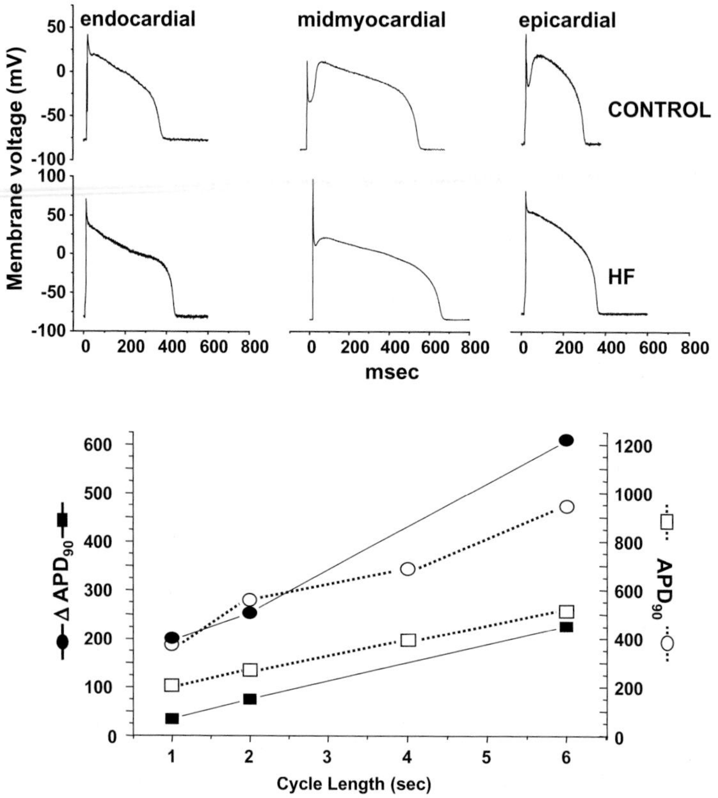

FIGURE 18–2. (Top) Action potential (APs) recorded from cells isolated from dif ferent transmural layers of the normal an failing canine ventricle. The APs are pro longed in each layer and exhibit significan changes in morphology. (Bottom) Plots o the dispersion in APD_{90} (ΔAPD_{90}, solid line and solid symbols) and APD_{90} (dotted line and open symbols) of myocytes from th midmyocardial layer tend to converge a more rapid pacing rates.

An important question is the effect of HF on regional differences in action potential duration. Even in normal hearts, intrinsic variations in action potential durations are considerable across the myocardial wall[22–25] and in different regions. Furthermore, data from experimental animal models of hypertrophy and failure demonstrate regional heterogeneity in action potential prolongation,[10,12] predisposing to intramural conduction block and reentrant excitation underlying polymorphic ventricular tachycardia resembling torsade de pointes.[26]

The morphology and duration of the action potential are sculpted by a delicate balance between multiple inward and outward currents. In the mammalian heart, repolarization is achieved primarily by the activity of potassium selective ionic currents. Ventricular myocytes contain several distinct classes of voltage-gated K channels. Although the relative densities and exact molecular compositions of these currents vary considerably across species, they can be categorized as follows. (1) The inward rectifier K curren (I_{K1}) sets the resting membrane potential and contributes to the terminal phase of repolarization (2) The calcium-independent transient outwar current (I_{to}), which is expressed in a species- an cell type-specific fashion, plays a critical role i the early phase of repolarization, and may contribute to phase 2 reentry, underlying arrhythmogenesis in the Brugada syndrome.[27] (3) Th delayed rectifier K current (I_K), composed o molecularly distinct rapidly (I_{Kr}) and slowly (I_{Ks} activating components, is dominant during phas 3 of repolarization. Importantly, I_{to} and I_K densities vary regionally and transmurally,[28,29] underlying the spatial heterogeneity in the AP profile an duration (Figure 18–2). I_{Kr} is the target of severa antiarrhythmic drugs with Vaughan-William class III action. Genetic mutations or pharmacological interventions that reduce the activity o these currents cause the congenital and acquire forms of the long QT syndrome (LQTS) respectively.

Transient Outward Potassium Current

Downregulation of I_{to} is arguably the most consistent ionic change in cardiac hypertrophy and failure. Several notable exceptions are studies of compensated pressure overload hypertrophy in which either no change[9] or an increase[30] in I_{to} density was observed. Downregulation of I_{to}, without a significant change in its voltage dependence or kinetics, has also been observed in cells isolated from terminally failing human hearts.[31–33] Since I_{to} is a transient current, its density may not directly affect the action potential duration, particularly in larger mammals such as dogs and humans that have relatively long action potentials. However, it was recently shown that I_{to} profoundly influences the depth of the phase 1 notch and the takeoff potential at the plateau onset, thereby affecting all ensuing currents.[18,19] In fact, a reduction in I_{to} results in a paradoxical shortening of the action potential by reducing the availability of $I_{Ca\text{-}L}$ in canine and rabbit myocytes.

Mechanisms underlying regional and transmural heterogeneities of I_{to} remain unclear. Some data suggest that there are differences in the level of expression of the main K channel gene (Kv4.x) thought encodes I_{to} in humans and large animals. Alternatively, distinct gene products may underlie I_{to} in different regions of the heart and at various stages of cardiac development.[34,35] For example, Kv1.4 plays a prominent role in endocardial I_{to} in some species, while Kv4.3 underlies mid-myocardial and epicardial I_{to}.[32] Interestingly, these two K channels exhibit distinct kinetic behaviors when heterologously expressed. Since Kv1.4 has significantly slower inactivation recovery kinetics than Kv4.x,[36,37] its preferential expression in the endocardium may underlie the differential behavior of I_{to} in that myocardial layer.[32,33] Whether this indeed is the case in humans and dogs remains a matter of debate, since recently we demonstrated that I_{to} in both canine and human myocytes is not modulated by Kv1.4 expression.[38] Moreover, there is further evidence challenging the role of Kv1.4 in the mammalian heart by demonstrating that I_{to} in Purkinje cells of subendocardial origin is not encoded by Kv1.4.[39]

The molecular mechanism of I_{to} downregulation in HF is likely to be multifactorial. For example, I_{to} is regulated by neurohumoral mechanisms, including α-adrenergic stimulation, which reduces the current size. In animal models[40] and human HF,[41] a reduction in the steady-state level of Kv4 mRNA was associated with functional downregulation of I_{to}. In the rat, reduction in mRNA was associated with a commensurate decrease in the level of Kv4 immunoreactive protein.[40] Reduced Kv4 mRNA levels result from a change in the balance between transcription and mRNA degradation, the precise molecular mechanism of which remains elusive. It is also noteworthy that regulated expression of I_{to} and Kv4 mRNA and protein occurs during development[34] and exposure to thyroid hormone.[35]

Inward Rectifier Potassium Current

Changes in other K currents in HF have also been reported, but not with the consistency of I_{to} downregulation. The inward rectifier K current (Kir2 family of genes) maintains the resting membrane potential and contributes to the terminal phase of repolarization in the ventricular myocyte. The important component of I_{K1} for action potential repolarization is the outward current present at voltages positive to the equilibrium potential for K^+. In mild ventricular hypertrophy increased, decreased,[9] and unchanged[10,13] I_{K1} densities have been reported. Even in the same experimental model of HF (i.e., pacing tachycardia), similar inconsistencies have been observed: Reduced I_{K1} density was demonstrated in dog,[19] and both reduced and unchanged current densities were found in rabbit.[18] In human HF, significantly reduced I_{K1} is observed at negative voltages. The underlying basis of I_{K1} downregulation in human HF is uncertain, but Kääb *et al.* reported no change in the steady-state level of Kir2.1 mRNA in failing compared to normal hearts.[41] Interestingly, a differential reduction in I_{K1} was noted between cells isolated from failing hearts with dilated versus ischemic cardiomyopathy, with the former group exhibiting a lower whole-cell slope conductance at the reversal potential for K^+ than the latter.[42] Also, cells isolated from hearts with dilated cardiomyopathy displayed longer action potentials and slower terminal (phase 3) repolarization than those from the ischemic group.[42]

While ventricular myocytes isolated from normal hearts and hearts with ischemic cardiomyopathy exhibited clear voltage dependence of I_{K1} open probability, those from hearts with dilated cardiomyopathy lacked such dependence, further highlighting the importance of disease etiology in the details of electrical remodeling.

Delayed Rectifier Potassium Currents

Delayed rectifier K currents do not significantly contribute to repolarization in the adult rodent heart and studies of these currents in failing hearts are more limited than other potassium currents. However, reduced I_K density, slower activation, and faster deactivation kinetics were shown in feline hypertrophied ventricles.[43] Also, Tsuji *et al.* reported downregulation of both I_{Kr} and I_{Ks} in a rabbit model of tachycardia pacing HF.[44] This reduction in the outward current over the plateau voltage range may predispose the animal to the development of potentially arrhythmogenic early afterdepolarizations (EADs).[43] In contrast, studies of cells isolated from pressure-overload guinea pigs[14] or spontaneously hypertensive rats[9] demonstrate no change in I_K. To date, there are no studies comparing I_K in control and failing human hearts. Although downregulation of I_{Ks} has been observed in cells isolated from explanted human right ventricles exhibiting abnormal histological findings compared with cells isolated from right ventricles with relatively normal histology.[45] We measured the mRNA of hERG, the protein encoding I_{Kr}, in normal and failing canine hearts and found no statistical difference.[41]

ATP-Sensitive Potassium Current

The ATP-sensitive potassium current ($I_{K\text{-}ATP}$) is the principal mediator of ischemia-induced action potential shortening. Therefore, differences in the behavior of $I_{K\text{-}ATP}$ in hypertrophied or failing hearts may have profound implications for susceptibility to arrhythmia in the setting of myocardial ischemia. Human ventricular $I_{K\text{-}ATP}$ in cells isolated from failing ventricles is less sensitive to ATP inhibition than that from normal hearts.[46] Interestingly, action potential shortening in response to metabolic inhibition is exaggerated in cells from hypertrophied compared to normal ventricles.[47]

Pacemaker Current

The hyperpolarization-activated pacemaker or "funny" current (I_f) is a nonselective cation current that was originally described in automatic tissues such as the sinoatrial node. More recently, I_f has been demonstrated in ventricular cells of several species,[48,49] activating at negative voltages outside the physiological range. The channel genes (HCN family) underlying I_f have recently been cloned,[50] but no studies examining the relative expression of these proteins in normal versus failing human ventricle have been reported to date. Since I_f generates an inward current that drives the membrane voltage toward threshold, it significantly contributes to diastolic depolarization (phase 4) in automatic cells. In rat, I_f density increases with the severity of hypertrophy.[51] In humans, despite a trend toward enhanced I_f in failing myocytes, differences did not reach statistical significance. Furthermore, no differences in the voltage dependence, kinetics, or isoproterenol sensitivity were observed. Nonetheless, the propensity toward an increase in I_f in the setting of reduced I_{K1} may predispose failing ventricular myocytes to enhanced automaticity.

Remodeling of pacemaker currents may contribute to potentially life threatening atrial arrhythmias in HF. In the sinoatrial node (SAN) and atria of the failing dog heart, HCN4 and HCN2 are downregulated and may contribute to SAN dysfunction and atrial arrhythmias in the failing heart.[52]

Sodium Current

Normal impulse formation and conduction in cardiac myocytes depend on I_{Na}. There is compelling evidence that an increase in the late component of this current can also markedly prolong the action potential duration and promote polymorphic ventricular tachycardia (VT), as is the case in the "gain of function" mutations associated with LQT3. Therefore, HF-induced changes in I_{Na} may in fact play an important role in arrhythmias either by disrupting conduction or prolonging repolarization. Studies of I_{Na} in a canine infarct model of HF revealed a significant downregulation of the current, an acceleration of its inactivation properties, and a slowing of its recovery from inactivation in myocytes isolated from the infarct border zone.[53] More recently, in a canine model of repeated microembolization-induced HF, a significant increase in the late component of I_{Na} was demonstrated.[54] Changes in I_{Na} are likely to depend on the etiology of HF (ischemic versus dilated cardiomyopathy) and may have profound implications for arrhythmogenesis given the relative importance of this current to wavefront propagation.

Calcium Homeostasis

L-Type Calcium Current

Heart failure is characterized by depression of developed force, prolongation of relaxation, and blunting of the force–frequency relationship. The fundamental changes in Ca^{2+} handling that develop in ventricular failure are thought to account for abnormalities in excitation–contraction (EC) coupling. However, the cellular and molecular bases of these defects remain controversial. Moreover, intracellular Ca^{2+} and the action potential are intricately linked through Ca^{2+}-mediated cell surface channels and transporters such as the L-type Ca current (I_{Ca-L}), I_K, Ca^{2+}-activated Cl^- current (I_{Ca-Cl}), and the Na^+–Ca^{2+} exchanger (NCX).

The voltage-dependent L-type Ca channel is a multisubunit protein that is ubiquitous in the heart. I_{Ca-L} is the primary source of Ca^{2+} entry, triggering Ca^{2+} release from the sarcoplasmic reticulum (SR), and initiating actin–myosin crossbridge cycling in the heart. The density of I_{Ca-L} has been studied in a number of animal models of ventricular hypertrophy and failure.[55] The severity of ventricular dysfunction appears to influence the density of I_{Ca-L},[9,11] the number of dihydropyridine (DHP) binding sites,[56–59] or both. In general, L-type current is increased in mild-to-moderate hypertrophy and decreased in more severe hypertrophy and failure. Studies of I_{Ca-L} in cells isolated from failing human hearts parallel those in animal models with severe hypertrophy or failure, exhibiting either no change or a decrease in current density[9,11] or DHP binding sites.[59] Moreover, failing myocytes also exhibit attenuated augmentation of I_{Ca-L} by β-adrenergic stimulation[60] and depression of rate-dependent potentiation compared to normal cells.[61]

The basic electrophysiological features of I_{Ca-L} are altered in some studies of HF. The most common change is a significant slowing of the whole-cell current decay rate.[14] This is expected to alter EC coupling and prolong the action potential duration. Such alterations may reflect deficiencies in Ca^{2+} handling as exemplified by a reduction in the peak of the Ca^{2+} transient, causing less Ca^{2+}-induced inactivation of I_{Ca-L}. The mechanism underlying prolonged whole-cell current decay is unknown, but a recent single-channel comparison of I_{Ca-L} in human ventricular myocytes advocates an increase in open channel probability hypothesized to be due to a dephosphorylation defect.[62]

The molecular basis underlying changes in the density of I_{Ca-L} is unknown. In failing human hearts the steady-state level of the α_{1C} mRNA is decreased by Northern blot,[62] but is unchanged by ribonuclease protection assay.[41] It is not known whether there is a change in the level of immunoreactive protein, although a reduction in the number of DHP binding sites has been reported in some studies. Hypertrophy after myocardial infarction in the rat is associated with a reemergence of the α_{1C} fetal gene isoform.[63] Two reports of changes in human Ca channel subunit mRNA exhibit disparate findings. Northern blots of terminally failing left ventricular samples revealed no change in subunit α_{1C} mRNA.[62] In contrast, samples from right ventricular endomyocardial biopsies revealed an inverse relationship between subunit mRNA levels [measured by competitive polymerase chain reaction (PCR)] and LV end diastolic pressure in transplanted hearts.[64]

T-Type Calcium Current

Upregulation or reexpression of the T-type Ca current (I_{Ca-T}) is a prominent feature of several animal models of HF.[65] I_{Ca-T}, which activates at hyperpolarized voltages and may contribute to enhanced automaticity in the heart, is much less prevalent in the adult ventricle than $I_{Ca\text{-}L}$. Normal maturation of cardiomyocytes is associated with loss of $I_{Ca\text{-}T}$, but myocytes grown in primary culture, exposed to insulin-like growth factor (IGF-1) in short-term culture, or isolated from the atria of rats with growth hormone-secreting tumors reexpress this current. Since T-type current has not been detected in cells isolated from either normal or failing human ventricles, it is unlikely to play a major role in progression of human HF and associated arrhythmogenesis.

Calcium Transient

The amplitude of the intracellular Ca^{2+} transient and its rate of decay are reduced in intact preparations[66] and cells[17,31] isolated from failing ventricles (Figure 18–3). These changes result from defective function of the SR, but the precise molecular mechanisms remain controversial. The SR Ca^{2+}-ATPase (SERCA2a) and the Na^+–Ca^{2+} exchanger (NCX) are primary mediators of Ca^{2+} removal from the cytoplasm. SERCA2a is inhibited by dephosphorylated phospholamban (PLB) by direct protein–protein interactions. Ca^{2+} entry into the cell through $I_{Ca\text{-}L}$ stimulates release of Ca^{2+} from the SR through the ryanodine receptor (RyR) in a process known as Ca^{2+}-induced Ca^{2+} release. The level of ventricular RyR mRNA[67] and protein[68] decreases in some studies of terminal human HF.

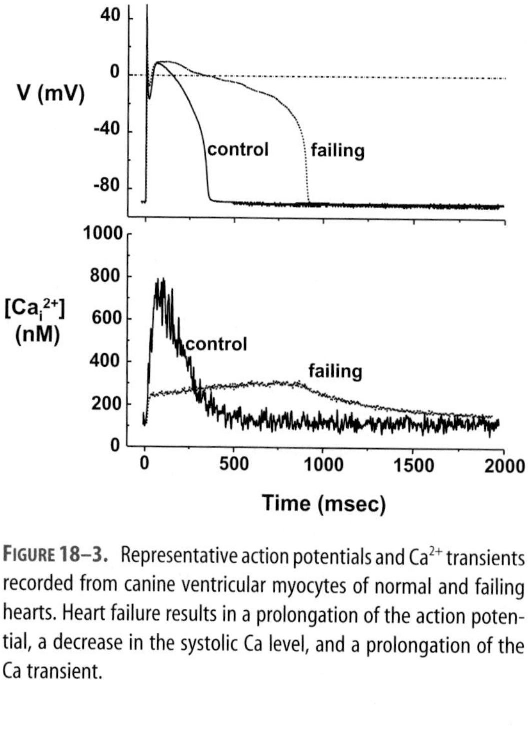

FIGURE 18–3. Representative action potentials and Ca^{2+} transients recorded from canine ventricular myocytes of normal and failing hearts. Heart failure results in a prolongation of the action potential, a decrease in the systolic Ca level, and a prolongation of the Ca transient.

Several studies have demonstrated a reduction in SERCA2a mRNA,[69–72], but fewer have shown a reduction in immunoreactive protein.[17] Despite overwhelming evidence regarding defective Ca^{2+} sequestration by the SR in the failing heart, it remains controversial whether there is a direct change in SERCA pump function.[73] Indeed, SERCA function may in fact be indirectly modulated by changes in the relative expression or function of PLB, which is consistently reduced (at the mRNA level) in failing human hearts.[69,71]

Alterations in the function of the ryanodine receptor (RyR2) in the failing heart have been associated with progression of HF and the generation of ventricular arrhythmias. The Marks laboratory has demonstrated protein kinase A (PKA) hyperphosphorylation of RyR2 with destabilization of the binding of the regulatory protein FKBP12.6, resulting in uncoupled gating and Ca^{2+} leak from the SR.[74] The findings are reminiscent of the changes observed in the inherited arrhythmia syndrome, catecholaminergic polymorphic ventricular tachycardia, associated with mutations in RyR2.[75]

Intracellular Ca^{2+} concentration, $[Ca^{2+}]_i$, is an important modulator of cardiac cellular electrophysiology, affecting the function of a number of ion channels and transporters and increasing the resistance between cells by reducing gap junctional conductance.[76] NCX current importantly contributes to $[Ca^{2+}]_i$ regulation by extruding cytoplasmic Ca^{2+} via an electrogenic exchange for extracellular Na^+. Most studies from hypertrophied and failing hearts have demonstrated an increase in both NCX mRNA and protein,[17,70] suggesting that enhanced NCX function compensates for defective SR removal of Ca^{2+} from the cytoplasm. However, direct studies of NCX function in failing hearts are limited. Na^+-dependent Ca^{2+} flux into sarcolemmal vesicles is enhanced in a human sarcolemmal preparation.[77] In contrast, the Ni^{2+}-sensitive exchanger current is unchanged in the rabbit pacing tachycardia model. In the context of a prolonged Ca^{2+} transient, NCX is likely to play a significant role in reshaping the action potential profile and may do so in a spatially heterogeneous manner.[78] Forward-mode exchanger function (Na^+ in and Ca^{2+} out) compensates for defective SR Ca^{2+} removal at the expense of depleting the releasable pool of Ca^{2+} with repetitive stimulation (flat or negative force–frequency relation). In contrast, reverse mode exchange (Na^+ out and Ca^{2+} in) may provide inotropic support to the failing myocardium. Computer simulations based on the canine pacing tachycardia model suggest that augmentation of reverse mode exchanger function during the early plateau shortens the action potential duration,[79] whereas an overall increase in forward mode function and changes in the decay rate of the L-type Ca current prolong the action potential in HF.

Sodium–Potassium Pump

The Na^+–K^+-ATPase (Na/K pump) transports K^+ into the cell and Na^+ out with a stoichiometry of 2:3, thereby, generating an outward repolarizing current. The Na^+–K^+-ATPase is a heterodimer consisting of α and β subunits, each having three isoforms. The α subunit determines the pump's glycoside sensitivity. Both expression and function of the Na^+–K^+-ATPase are reduced in HF.[80] Such downregulation may have several arrhythmic consequences: (1) reduction in the outward repolarizing current prolongs action potential duration and refractoriness; (2) reduced pump function leads to a rise in intracellular [Na^+], an enhancement of reverse mode NCX, an increase in inward current, and a prolongation of the action potential; and (3) cells with less Na^+–K^+-ATPase activity have greater difficulty handling changes in extracellular [K^+], which may "destabilize" the membrane potential making it more susceptible to spontaneous depolarizations and delayed afterdepolarizations (DADs).[81]

Gap Junctions and Connexins

Gap junction channels are specialized transmembrane proteins that permit electrical and chemical communication between cells.[82] Mammalian gap junction channels, or connexons, are built by the oligomerization of a family of closely related genes encoding connexins (Cx). These are transmembrane proteins consisting of four highly conserved membrane-spanning α-helices, two extracellular loops, and one intracellular loop. Three different connexins have thus far been identified in the mammalian heart: Cx40, Cx43, and Cx45, named for their respective molecular masses. Most cardiovascular disorders are associated with changes in the density and distribution of gap junction proteins, which may translate into functional changes in cell-to-cell coupling.[83] A significant reduction in density and an altered distribution of the major cardiac gap junction protein (Cx43) have been demonstrated in ischemic, hypertrophic, and dilated cardiomyopathies. In fact, not only is Cx43 downregulated, it is redistributed from the intercalated disk to along the entire cell border (lateralization),[84] a pattern observed in early cardiac development. In an experimental model of myocardial infarction, the border zone exhibits lateralization of Cx43 without a change in intercalated disk size. In the pressure overload guinea pig model,[14] a 37% reduction in overall Cx43 protein is observed following the onset of HF, but no change occurs during compensated hypertrophy. The Cx43 content is also significantly lower in adult cardiomyopathic hamster hearts. Furthermore, these proteins are highly regulated and as such are subject to modification by several external factors present in complex cardiovascular diseases, such as failure. For example, de Mello and colleagues suggested that RAAS, through continuous production of angiotensin II, depresses junctional conductance, an effect that is diminished by angiotensin-converting enzyme (ACE) inhibition.[85] The functional consequences of gap junctional downregulation and redistribution on cell-to-cell coupling, conduction, recovery, and arrhythmogenesis are only beginning to be unveiled. Recently, we investigated mechanisms underlying conduction slowing and arrhythmogenesis in the canine tachypacing model of HF.[86] We found that despite a significant reduction of conduction velocity in both ventricles, Cx43 downregulation was limited to the left ventricle, suggesting involvement of additional factors in the mechanism of conduction slowing in this model. We further demonstrated that a

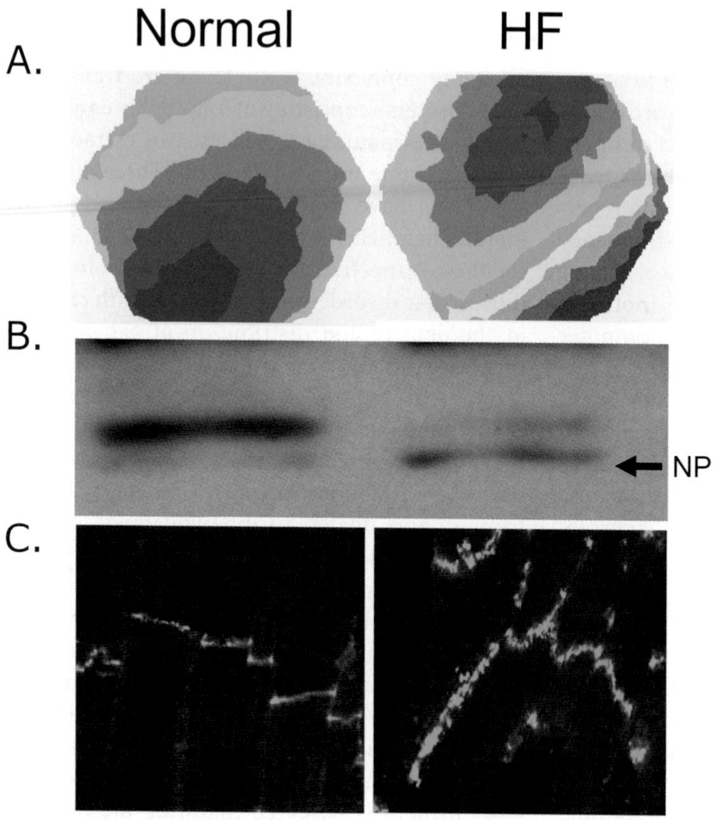

FIGURE 18–4. (A) Depolarization contour maps measured in canine wedge preparations from control and failing hearts that demonstrate conduction slowing in heart failure. (B) Representative western blots of Cx43 in tissue samples from control and failing hearts that indicate an increase in a dephosphorylated isoform of Cx43 (NP, arrow) despite overall reduction of total Cx43 expression in heart failure. (C) Confocal optical sections of tissue isolated from control and failing canine ventricles stained for Cx43, indicating an abundance of Cx43 on lateral cell borders in heart failure.

change in the phosphorylation status of Cx43 and alterations in subcellular localization (lateralization) significantly contribute to conduction slowing in the failing heart (Figure 18–4).

Neurohumoral Modulation of Channel/Transporter Function in Heart Failure

In the face of impaired LV function, the body attempts to maintain circulatory homeostasis through a complex series of neurohumoral changes. Prominently, the SNS and RAAS systems are activated. Activation of the SNS increases both heart rate and contractility and redistributes blood flow centrally by peripheral vasoconstriction. Similarly, the RAAS causes vasoconstriction and increases circulatory volume. These neurohumoral changes are initially adaptive, maintaining systolic function and vital tissue perfusion, but are ultimately deleterious, leading to progression of the HF phenotype. For example, chronic release of catecholamines can be cardiotoxic, resulting in maladaptive changes in adrenergic receptor densities. Volume overload and vasoconstriction produced by chronic activation of both the SNS and RAAS increase myocardial wall stress, which, coupled with increased oxygen demand, raises the potential for progressive myocyte damage and dropout. In addition, the combination of neurohumoral activation and mechanical wall stress activates signal transduction cascades that produce myocyte hypertrophy and lead to an increase in interstitial collagen content. Both consequences are deleterious for systolic and diastolic function of the heart.

Adrenergic signaling in human HF is the subject of extensive study.[87] β_1-, β_2-, and α_1-Adrenergic receptors mediate the effects of increased catecholamines in the heart. β_1 and β_2 receptors are coupled to adenylyl cyclase, which, upon activation, raises cellular cAMP levels.[88] α_1, on the other hand, is coupled by a G protein to phospholipase C (PLC), which hydrolyzes inositol phospholipids increasing cellular inositol 1,4,5-trisphosphate

(IP_3) and diacylglycerol (DAG). Angiotensin II (AT1) receptors are similarly coupled to PLC. Activation of the AT1 or β-adrenergic receptors initiates signal transduction cascades triggering cell growth and altering the level of intracellular Ca^{2+}. Indeed, a byproduct of local catecholamine excess in the heart is an increase in cellular Ca^{2+} load, which may activate phospholipases, proteases, and endonucleases, culminating in cell necrosis or apoptosis and leading to progression of the failing phenotype.

These signaling pathways significantly modulate the function of a number of ion channels and transporters. For example, the net effect of β-adrenergic stimulation is to shorten the ventricular action potential despite an increase in inward current by $I_{Ca\text{-}L}$. This shortening is mediated by a concomitant increase in I_K density and a leftward shift in its activation to more hyperpolarized potentials.[89] α_1-Adrenergic receptor stimulation, on the other hand, inhibits several K currents in the mammalian heart, including I_{to}, I_{K1}, and I_K, thereby prolonging the action potential duration.[23]

Dyssynchronous Mechanical Activation

Mechanical load is another important modulator of myocardial excitability. The effects of altered hemodynamic load may be exaggerated in the failing ventricle. In a rabbit model of doxorubicin-induced HF, increased load produced marked shortening of the action potential duration and enhanced susceptibility to arrhythmia in failing compared to control hearts.[21] The effect of load is likely to be distributed heterogeneously across the ventricular wall or throughout the myocardium, and thus has the potential to increase dispersion of repolarization and vulnerability to arrhythmia. In fact, we recently found that dyssynchronous mechanical activation of the ventricle, even in the absence of overt myocardial failure, resulted in a heterogeneous remodeling of electrical activity between the early activated, low stress anterior wall and the late activated, high stress lateral wall. In short, the lateral wall was associated with a shorter action potential and a slower endocardial conduction velocity compared to the low stress anterior wall.

Ventricular Electrical Remodeling and Arrhythmogenesis in Heart Failure

Sudden death due to ventricular arrhythmias in HF is likely to involve multiple mechanisms. The variability in the reported electrophysiological changes is in part methodological, but also reflects a high degree of heterogeneity in the pathophysiology of the disease. The stage of HF is a crucial determinant of the degree and character of electrical remodeling and arrhythmic risk. Data from clinical trials support this concept. For example, the risk of sudden (presumed arrhythmic) death was proportionately greater in patients with moderate HF (VheFT-I trial). Changes in risk of sudden death with progression of heart disease are likely to be a reflection of dynamic changes in the electrophysiological substrate. We are currently in the process of defining the sequence of events that lead to changes in elecrophysiological properties as HF develops at the multicellular network tissue level, and their underlying molecular mechanisms and changes in gene expression profile at different stages of HF.

Triggered automaticity arising from afterdepolarizations could be enhanced by several electrophysiological changes present in HF. For example, the plateau phase of the action potential is quite labile, a time of high membrane resistance, during which small changes in current can easily tip the balance between abrupt repolarization and maintained depolarization. Therefore, prolongation of action potential duration in HF translates into enhanced repolarization lability and susceptibility to EAD-triggered ventricular arrhythmias. Indeed, ventricular myocytes isolated from failing canine hearts exhibit more spontaneous EADs than those of normal hearts. For example, complex afterdepolarizations and triggered arrhythmias are common in hypertrophied rat ventricular myocardium exposed to K channel blockers and dogs exposed to Ca channel agonists. Moreover, alterations in $I_{Ca\text{-}L}$ density and kinetics predispose to EAD- or DAD-mediated arrhythmias. Finally, changes in the cellular environment such as hypokalemia, hypomagnesemia, and elevated levels of catecholamines may further increase the susceptibility to EAD-mediated arrhythmias.

Altered Ca^{2+} handling in hypertrophy and failure may also contribute to electrical instability. The characteristic slow decay of the Ca^{2+} transient and increased diastolic levels of $[Ca^{2+}]_i$ can predispose to oscillatory release of Ca^{2+} from the SR and DAD-mediated triggered arrhythmias. The slow decay of the Ca^{2+} transient enhances ion flux through the NCX, predisposing patients to late phase 3 EAD-mediated triggered arrhythmias.

Reentrant excitation underlies the vast majority of arrhythmias. In HF, several changes in both myocyte and interstitial compartments, in both the atria and ventricles, create substrates for reentry. In the setting of healed myocardial infarction, macroreentrant circuits arise at the border zone of the infarcted region where ultraslow conduction occurs at least in part as a result of gap junctional remodeling. In the absence of prior infarction, macroreentry is less likely to be involved. Hence patients with nonischemic cardiomyopathy are less likely to be inducible at electrophysiological study. Finally, there are emerging data regarding enhanced spatial and temporal dispersion of repolarization in the failing heart, which predispose patients to nonexcitable gap reentry underlying polymorphic ventricular tachycardia and ventricular fibrillation.

Atrial Electrical Remodeling in Heart Failure

Congestive HF is a major risk factor for the development of atrial fibrillation (AF). Although atrial action potentials are not significantly altered with atrial enlargement due to tricuspid or mitral valve abnormalities, they are remodeled in the setting of LV failure. In the canine tachycardia pacing HF model, several atrial ionic currents are downregulated, including I_{Ks} (by 30%), $I_{Ca,L}$ (by 30%), and I_{to} (by 50%).[90] In contrast, the density of NCX current is substantially increased, as is the expression of NCX protein. A variety of other currents, including I_{K1}, I_{Kr}, and $I_{Ca,T}$, are unchanged. The net effect of this remodeling is to prolong atrial action potentials and increase interatrial and intraatrial dispersion of refractoriness.

Atrial and ventricular ion channels might be expected to respond similarly to comparable stimuli. This, however, is not always the case. For example, chronic rapid pacing of the atrium results in a persistent shortening of the atrial effective refractory period and action potential duration.[91] This then results in shortening of the atrial cardiac wavelength, which acts to maintain the ongoing AF; hence, the paradigm AF begets AF.[92] Finally, despite major differences in atrial remodeling of active membrane properties in the settings of rapid atrial pacing and ventricular pacing-induced HF, both paradigms form clear electrophysiological substrates for a common disease, AF.

Conclusions

The increased risk of arrhythmias and sudden cardiac death in patients with myocardial hypertrophy and HF is secondary to complex remodeling that occurs in both the myocyte and interstitial compartments of the heart. The key components of ventricular myocyte remodeling are the functional expression of a number of ion channels, transporters and receptors that result in action potential prolongation, abnormal Ca^{2+} cycling, and aberrant adrenergic signaling. Remodeling of the extracellular matrix and/or gap junction channels cause abnormalities in impulse conduction as well as an exaggeration in the heterogeneity between cellular electrical properties. The remodeling process creates an electrophysiological substrate that is highly sensitive to triggers for malignant arrhythmias.

References

1. Schocken DD, Arrieta MI, Leaverton PE, Ross EA. Prevalence and mortality rate of congestive heart failure in the United States. *J Am Coll Cardiol* 1992;20:301–306.
2. Ho KK, Anderson KM, Kannel WB, Grossman W, Levy D. Survival after the onset of congestive heart failure in Framingham Heart Study subjects. *Circulation* 1993;88:107–115.
3. Tomaselli GF, Beuckelmann DJ, Calkins HG, Berger RD, Kessler PD, Lawrence JH, Kass D, Feldman AM, Marban E. Sudden cardiac death in heart failure. The role of abnormal repolarization. *Circulation* 1994;90:2534–2539.
4. Chakko CS, Gheorghiade M. Ventricular arrhythmias in severe heart failure: Incidence, significance, and effectiveness of antiarrhythmic therapy. *Am Heart J* 1985;109:497–504.
5. Hallstrom A, Pratt CM, Greene HL, Huther M, Gottlieb S, DeMaria A, Young JB. Relations between

heart failure, ejection fraction, arrhythmia suppression and mortality: Analysis of the Cardiac Arrhythmia Suppression Trial. *J Am Coll Cardiol* 1995;25:1250–1257.

6. Cohn JN, Archibald DG, Ziesche S, Franciosa JA, Harston WE, Tristani FE, Dunkman WB, Jacobs W, Francis GS, Flohr KH, *et al.* Effect of vasodilator therapy on mortality in chronic congestive heart failure. Results of a Veterans Administration Cooperative Study. *N Engl J Med* 1986;314:1547–1552.
7. Myerburg RJ, Gelband H, Nilsson K, Sung RJ, Thurer RJ, Morales AR, Bassett AL. Long-term electrophysiological abnormalities resulting from experimental myocardial infarction in cats. *Circ Res* 1977;41:73–84.
8. Benitah JP, Gomez AM, Bailly P, Da Ponte JP, Berson G, Delgado C, Lorente P. Heterogeneity of the early outward current in ventricular cells isolated from normal and hypertrophied rat hearts. *J Physiol* 1993;469:111–138.
9. Brooksby P, Levi AJ, Jones JV. The electrophysiological characteristics of hypertrophied ventricular myocytes from the spontaneously hypertensive rat. *J Hypertens* 1993;11:611–622.
10. Bryant SM, Shipsey SJ, Hart G. Regional differences in electrical and mechanical properties of myocytes from guinea-pig hearts with mild left ventricular hypertrophy. *Cardiovasc Res* 1997;35:315–323.
11. Cerbai E, Barbieri M, Li Q, Mugelli A. Ionic basis of action potential prolongation of hypertrophied cardiac myocytes isolated from hypertensive rats of different ages. *Cardiovasc Res* 1994;28:1180–1187.
12. Momtaz A, Coulombe A, Richer P, Mercadier JJ, Coraboeuf E. Action potential and plateau ionic currents in moderately and severely DOCA-salt hypertrophied rat hearts. *J Mol Cell Cardiol* 1996;28:2511–2522.
13. Keung EC, Aronson RS. Non-uniform electrophysiological properties and electrotonic interaction in hypertrophied rat myocardium. *Circ Res* 1981;49:150–158.
14. Ryder KO, Bryant SM, Hart G. Membrane current changes in left ventricular myocytes isolated from guinea pigs after abdominal aortic coarctation. *Cardiovasc Res* 1993;27:1278–1287.
15. Hanna N, Cardin S, Leung TK, Nattel S. Differences in atrial versus ventricular remodeling in dogs with ventricular tachypacing-induced congestive heart failure. *Cardiovasc Res* 2004;63:236–244.
16. Qin D, Zhang ZH, Caref EB, Boutjdir M, Jain P, el-Sherif N. Cellular and ionic basis of arrhythmias in postinfarction remodeled ventricular myocardium. *Circ Res* 1996;79:461–473.
17. O'Rourke B, Kass DA, Tomaselli GF, Kaab S, Tunin R, Marban E. Mechanisms of altered excitation-contraction coupling in canine tachycardia-induced heart failure, I: Experimental studies. *Circ Res* 1999;84:562–570.
18. Rozanski GJ, Xu Z, Whitney RT, Murakami H, Zucker IH. Electrophysiology of rabbit ventricular myocytes following sustained rapid ventricular pacing. *J Mol Cell Cardiol* 1997;29:721–732.
19. Kaab S, Nuss HB, Chiamvimonvat N, O'Rourke B, Pak PH, Kass DA, Marban E, Tomaselli GF. Ionic mechanism of action potential prolongation in ventricular myocytes from dogs with pacing-induced heart failure. *Circ Res* 1996;78:262–273.
20. Akar FG, Rosenbaum DS. Transmural electrophysiological heterogeneities underlying arrhythmogenesis in heart failure. *Circ Res* 2003;93:638–645.
21. Pye MP, Cobbe SM. Arrhythmogenesis in experimental models of heart failure: The role of increased load. *Cardiovasc Res* 1996;32:248–257.
22. Litovsky SH, Antzelevitch C. Rate dependence of action potential duration and refractoriness in canine ventricular endocardium differs from that of epicardium: Role of the transient outward current. *J Am Coll Cardiol* 1989;14:1053–1066.
23. Fedida D, Giles WR. Regional variations in action potentials and transient outward current in myocytes isolated from rabbit left ventricle. *J Physiol* 1991;442:191–209.
24. Lukas A, Antzelevitch C. Differences in the electrophysiological response of canine ventricular epicardium and endocardium to ischemia. Role of the transient outward current. *Circulation* 1993;88:2903–2915.
25. Drouin E, Charpentier F, Gauthier C, Laurent K, Le Marec H. Electrophysiologic characteristics of cells spanning the left ventricular wall of human heart: Evidence for presence of M cells. *J Am Coll Cardiol* 1995;26:185–192.
26. Yan GX, Rials SJ, Wu Y, Liu T, Xu X, Marinchak RA, Kowey PR. Ventricular hypertrophy amplifies transmural repolarization dispersion and induces early afterdepolarization. *Am J Physiol Heart Circ Physiol* 2001;281:H1968–1975.
27. Antzelevitch C. The Brugada syndrome: Ionic basis and arrhythmia mechanisms. *J Cardiovasc Electrophysiol* 2001;12:268–272.
28. Furukawa T, Kimura S, Furukawa N, Bassett AL, Myerburg RJ. Potassium rectifier currents differ in myocytes of endocardial and epicardial origin. *Circ Res* 1992;70:91–103.
29. Liu DW, Antzelevitch C. Characteristics of the delayed rectifier current (IKr and IKs) in canine ventricular epicardial, midmyocardial, and

endocardial myocytes. A weaker IKs contributes to the longer action potential of the M cell. *Circ Res* 1995;76:351–365.
30. Ten Eick RE, Zhang K, Harvey RD, Bassett AL. Enhanced functional expression of transient outward current in hypertrophied feline myocytes. *Cardiovasc Drugs Ther* 1993;7(Suppl. 3):611–619.
31. Beuckelmann DJ, Nabauer M, Erdmann E. Alterations of K^+ currents in isolated human ventricular myocytes from patients with terminal heart failure. *Circ Res* 1993;73:379–385.
32. Wettwer E, Amos GJ, Posival H, Ravens U. Transient outward current in human ventricular myocytes of subepicardial and subendocardial origin. *Circ Res* 1994;75:473–482.
33. Nabauer M, Beuckelmann DJ, Uberfuhr P, Steinbeck G. Regional differences in current density and rate-dependent properties of the transient outward current in subepicardial and subendocardial myocytes of human left ventricle. *Circulation* 1996;93:168–177.
34. Xu H, Dixon JE, Barry DM, Trimmer JS, Merlie JP, McKinnon D, Nerbonne JM. Developmental analysis reveals mismatches in the expression of K^+ channel alpha subunits and voltage-gated K^+ channel currents in rat ventricular myocytes. *J Gen Physiol* 1996;108:405–419.
35. Wickenden AD, Kaprielian R, Parker TG, Jones OT, Backx PH. Effects of development and thyroid hormone on K^+ currents and K^+ channel gene expression in rat ventricle. *J Physiol* 1997;504(Pt. 2):271–286.
36. Po S, Snyders DJ, Baker R, Tamkun MM, Bennett PB. Functional expression of an inactivating potassium channel cloned from human heart. *Circ Res* 1992;71:732–736.
37. Dixon JE, Shi W, Wang HS, McDonald C, Yu H, Wymore RS, Cohen IS, McKinnon D. Role of the Kv4.3 K+ channel in ventricular muscle. A molecular correlate for the transient outward current. *Circ Res* 1996;79:659–668.
38. Akar FG, Wu RC, Deschenes I, Armoundas AA, Piacentino V, 3rd, Houser SR, Tomaselli GF. Phenotypic differences in transient outward K^+ current of human and canine ventricular myocytes: Insights into molecular composition of ventricular Ito. *Am J Physiol Heart Circ Physiol* 2004;286:H602–609.
39. Han W, Wang Z, Nattel S. Slow delayed rectifier current and repolarization in canine cardiac Purkinje cells. *Am J Physiol Heart Circ Physiol* 2001;280:H1075–1080.
40. Gidh-Jain M, Huang B, Jain P, el-Sherif N. Differential expression of voltage-gated K+ channel genes in left ventricular remodeled myocardium after experimental myocardial infarction. *Circ Res* 1996; 79:669–675.
41. Kaab S, Dixon J, Duc J, Ashen D, Nabauer M, Beuckelmann DJ, Steinbeck G, McKinnon D, Tomaselli GF. Molecular basis of transient outward potassium current downregulation in human heart failure: A decrease in Kv4.3 mRNA correlates with a reduction in current density. *Circulation* 1998;98: 1383–1393.
42. Koumi S, Backer CL, Arentzen CE. Characterization of inwardly rectifying K+ channel in human cardiac myocytes. Alterations in channel behavior in myocytes isolated from patients with idiopathic dilated cardiomyopathy. *Circulation* 1995;92:164–174.
43. Furukawa T, Bassett AL, Furukawa N, Kimura S, Myerburg RJ. The ionic mechanism of reperfusion-induced early afterdepolarizations in feline left ventricular hypertrophy. *J Clin Invest* 1993;91:1521–1531.
44. Tsuji Y, Opthof T, Kamiya K, Yasui K, Liu W, Lu Z, Kodama I. Pacing-induced heart failure causes a reduction of delayed rectifier potassium currents along with decreases in calcium and transient outward currents in rabbit ventricle. *Cardiovasc Res* 2000;48:300–309.
45. Li GR, Lau CP, Leung TK, Nattel S. Ionic current abnormalities associated with prolonged action potentials in cardiomyocytes from diseased human right ventricles. *Heart Rhythm.* 2004;1:460–468.
46. Martin RL, Koumi S, Ten Eick RE. Comparison of the effects of internal $[Mg^{2+}]$ on IK1 in cat and guinea-pig cardiac ventricular myocytes. *J Mol Cell Cardiol* 1995;27:673–691.
47. Kimura S, Bassett AL, Furukawa T, Furukawa N, Myerburg RJ. Differences in the effect of metabolic inhibition on action potentials and calcium currents in endocardial and epicardial cells. *Circulation* 1991;84:768–777.
48. Cerbai E, Pino R, Porciatti F, Sani G, Toscano M, Maccherini M, Giunti G, Mugelli A. Characterization of the hyperpolarization-activated current, I(f), in ventricular myocytes from human failing heart. *Circulation* 1997;95:568–571.
49. Hoppe UC, Jansen E, Sudkamp M, Beuckelmann DJ. Hyperpolarization-activated inward current in ventricular myocytes from normal and failing human hearts. *Circulation* 1998;97:55–65.
50. Ludwig A, Zong X, Hofmann F, Biel M. Structure and function of cardiac pacemaker channels. *Cell Physiol Biochem* 1999;9:179–186.
51. Cerbai E, Barbieri M, Mugelli A. Occurrence and properties of the hyperpolarization-activated current If in ventricular myocytes from normoten-

sive and hypertensive rats during aging. *Circulation* 1996;94:1674–1681.
52. Zicha S, Fernandez-Velasco M, Lonardo G, L'Heureux N, Nattel S. Sinus node dysfunction and hyperpolarization-activated (HCN) channel subunit remodeling in a canine heart failure model. *Cardiovasc Res* 2005;66:472–481.
53. Pu J, Boyden PA. Alterations of Na^+ currents in myocytes from epicardial border zone of the infarcted heart. A possible ionic mechanism for reduced excitability and postrepolarization refractoriness. *Circ Res* 1997;81:110–119.
54. Undrovinas AI, Maltsev VA, Sabbah HN. Repolarization abnormalities in cardiomyocytes of dogs with chronic heart failure: Role of sustained inward current. *Cell Mol Life Sci* 1999;55:494–505.
55. Hall DG, Morley GE, Vaidya D, Ard M, Kimball TR, Witt SA, Colbert MC. Early onset heart failure in transgenic mice with dilated cardiomyopathy. *Pediatr Res* 2000;48:36–42.
56. Mascelli MA, Lance ET, Damaraju L, Wagner CL, Weisman HF, Jordan RE. Pharmacodynamic profile of short-term abciximab treatment demonstrates prolonged platelet inhibition with gradual recovery from GP IIb/IIIa receptor blockade. *Circulation* 1998;97:1680–1688.
57. Morgan K, Stevens EB, Shah B, Cox PJ, Dixon AK, Lee K, Pinnock RD, Hughes J, Richardson PJ, Mizuguchi K, Jackson AP. Beta 3: An additional auxiliary subunit of the voltage-sensitive sodium channel that modulates channel gating with distinct kinetics. *Proc Natl Acad Sci USA* 2000;97:2308–2313.
58. Vatner DE, Sato N, Kiuchi K, Shannon RP, Vatner SF. Decrease in myocardial ryanodine receptors and altered excitation-contraction coupling early in the development of heart failure. *Circulation* 1994;90:1423–1430.
59. Gengo PJ, Sabbah HN, Steffen RP, Sharpe JK, Kono T, Stein PD, Goldstein S. Myocardial beta adrenoceptor and voltage sensitive calcium channel changes in a canine model of chronic heart failure. *J Mol Cell Cardiol* 1992;24:1361–1369.
60. Ouadid H, Albat B, Nargeot J. Calcium currents in diseased human cardiac cells. *J Cardiovasc Pharmacol* 1995;25:282–291.
61. Piot C, Lemaire S, Albat B, Seguin J, Nargeot J, Richard S. High frequency-induced upregulation of human cardiac calcium currents. *Circulation* 1996;93:120–128.
62. Schroder F, Handrock R, Beuckelmann DJ, Hirt S, Hullin R, Priebe L, Schwinger RH, Weil J, Herzig S. Increased availability and open probability of single L-type calcium channels from failing compared with nonfailing human ventricle. *Circulation* 1998;98:969–976.
63. Gidh-Jain M, Huang B, Jain P, Battula V, el-Sherif N. Reemergence of the fetal pattern of L-type calcium channel gene expression in non infarcted myocardium during left ventricular remodeling. *Biochem Biophys Res Commun* 1995;216:892–897.
64. Hullin R, Asmus F, Ludwig A, Hersel J, Boekstegers P. Subunit expression of the cardiac L-type calcium channel is differentially regulated in diastolic heart failure of the cardiac allograft. *Circulation* 1999;100:155–163.
65. Nuss HB, Houser SR. T-type Ca^{2+} current is expressed in hypertrophied adult feline left ventricular myocytes. *Circ Res* 1993;73:777–782.
66. Gwathmey JK, Copelas L, MacKinnon R, Schoen FJ, Feldman MD, Grossman W, Morgan JP. Abnormal intracellular calcium handling in myocardium from patients with end-stage heart failure. *Circ Res* 1987;61:70–76.
67. Meyer M, Schillinger W, Pieske B, Holubarsch C, Heilmann C, Posival H, Kuwajima G, Mikoshiba K, Just H, Hasenfuss G, *et al.* Alterations of sarcoplasmic reticulum proteins in failing human dilated cardiomyopathy. *Circulation* 1995;92:778–784.
68. Heerdt PM, Holmes JW, Cai B, Barbone A, Madigan JD, Reiken S, Lee DL, Oz MC, Marks AR, Burkhoff D. Chronic unloading by left ventricular assist device reverses contractile dysfunction and alters gene expression in end-stage heart failure. *Circulation* 2000;102:2713–2719.
69. Arai M, Alpert NR, MacLennan DH, Barton P, Periasamy M. Alterations in sarcoplasmic reticulum gene expression in human heart failure. A possible mechanism for alterations in systolic and diastolic properties of the failing myocardium. *Circ Res* 1993;72:463–469.
70. Studer R, Reinecke H, Bilger J, Eschenhagen T, Bohm M, Hasenfuss G, Just H, Holtz J, Drexler H. Gene expression of the cardiac Na(+)-Ca^{2+} exchanger in end-stage human heart failure. *Circ Res* 1994;75:443–453.
71. Schwinger RH, Bohm M, Schmidt U, Karczewski P, Bavendiek U, Flesch M, Krause EG, Erdmann E. Unchanged protein levels of SERCA II and phospholamban but reduced Ca^{2+} uptake and Ca(2+)-ATPase activity of cardiac sarcoplasmic reticulum from dilated cardiomyopathy patients compared with patients with nonfailing hearts. *Circulation* 1995;92:3220–3228.
72. Feldman AM, Weinberg EO, Ray PE, Lorell BH. Selective changes in cardiac gene expression during compensated hypertrophy and the transition to

cardiac decompensation in rats with chronic aortic banding. *Circ Res* 1993;73:184–192.
73. Hasenfuss G. Alterations of calcium-regulatory proteins in heart failure. *Cardiovasc Res* 1998;37: 279–289.
74. Marx SO, Reiken S, Hisamatsu Y, Jayaraman T, Burkhoff D, Rosemblit N, Marks AR. PKA phosphorylation dissociates FKBP12.6 from the calcium release channel (ryanodine receptor): Defective regulation in failing hearts. *Cell* 2000;101:365–376.
75. Wehrens XH, Lehnart SE, Huang F, Vest JA, Reiken SR, Mohler PJ, Sun J, Guatimosim S, Song LS, Rosemblit N, D'Armiento JM, Napolitano C, Memmi M, Priori SG, Lederer WJ, Marks AR. FKBP12.6 deficiency and defective calcium release channel (ryanodine receptor) function linked to exercise-induced sudden cardiac death. *Cell* 2003; 113:829–840.
76. Noma A, Tsuboi N. Dependence of junctional conductance on proton, calcium and magnesium ions in cardiac paired cells of guinea-pig. *J Physiol* 1987;382:193–211.
77. Studer R, Reinecke H, Vetter R, Holtz J, Drexler H. Expression and function of the cardiac Na^+/Ca^{2+} exchanger in postnatal development of the rat, in experimental-induced cardiac hypertrophy and in the failing human heart. *Basic Res Cardiol* 1997; 92(Suppl. 1):53–58.
78. Xiong W, Tian Y, DiSilvestre D, Tomaselli GF. Transmural heterogeneity of Na^+-Ca^{2+} exchange: Evidence for differential expression in normal and failing hearts. *Circ Res* 2005;97:207–209.
79. Winslow RL, Rice J, Jafri S, Marban E, O'Rourke B. Mechanisms of altered excitation-contraction coupling in canine tachycardia-induced heart failure, II: Model studies. *Circ Res* 1999;84:571–586.
80. Seppet EK, Kolar F, Dixon IM, Hata T, Dhalla NS. Regulation of cardiac sarcolemmal Ca^{2+} channels and Ca^{2+} transporters by thyroid hormone. *Mol Cell Biochem* 1993;129:145–159.
81. Nuss HB, Kaab S, Kass DA, Tomaselli GF, Marban E. Cellular basis of ventricular arrhythmias and abnormal automaticity in heart failure. *Am J Physiol* 1999;277:H80–91.
82. Brink PR, Cronin K, Ramanan SV. Gap junctions in excitable cells. *J Bioenerg Biomembr* 1996;28:351–358.
83. Guerrero PA, Schuessler RB, Davis LM, Beyer EC, Johnson CM, Yamada KA, Saffitz JE. Slow ventricular conduction in mice heterozygous for a connexin43 null mutation. *J Clin Invest* 1997;99:1991–1998.
84. Peters NS, Coromilas J, Severs NJ, Wit AL. Disturbed connexin43 gap junction distribution correlates with the location of reentrant circuits in the epicardial border zone of healing canine infarcts that cause ventricular tachycardia. *Circulation* 1997;95:988–996.
85. De Mello W, Altieri P. The role of the renin-angiotensin system in the control of cell communication in the heart: Effects of enalapril and angiotensin II. *J Cardiovasc Pharmacol* 1992;20:643–651.
86. Akar FG, Spragg DD, Tunin RS, Kass DA, Tomaselli GF. Mechanisms underlying conduction slowing and arrhythmogenesis in nonischemic dilated cardiomyopathy. *Circ Res* 2004;95:717–725.
87. Bristow MR. Beta-adrenergic receptor blockade in chronic heart failure. *Circulation* 2000;101:558–569.
88. Vinogradova TM, Zhou YY, Bogdanov KY, Yang D, Kuschel M, Cheng H, Xiao RP. Sinoatrial node pacemaker activity requires Ca(2+)/calmodulin-dependent protein kinase II activation. *Circ Res* 2000;87:760–767.
89. Hartzell HC, Duchatelle-Gourdon I. Regulation of the cardiac delayed rectifier K current by neurotransmitters and magnesium. *Cardiovasc Drugs Ther* 1993;7(Suppl. 3):547–554.
90. Nattel S, Li D. Ionic remodeling in the heart: Pathophysiological significance and new therapeutic opportunities for atrial fibrillation. *Circ Res* 2000;87: 440–447.
91. Allessie MA. Atrial electrophysiologic remodeling: Another vicious circle? *J Cardiovasc Electrophysiol* 1998;9:1378–1393.
92. Wijffels MC, Kirchhof CJ, Dorland R, Allessie MA. Atrial fibrillation begets atrial fibrillation. A study in awake chronically instrumented goats. *Circulation* 1995;92:1954–1968.

19
Ventricular Electrical Remodeling in Compensated Cardiac Hypertrophy

Stephan K.G. Winckels and Marc A. Vos

Introduction

Ventricular hypertrophy (VH) is a structural adaptation of the heart that develops in response to either congenital or acquired pathologies to reduce wall stress.[1] Dominant etiologies are genetic mutations (e.g., in sarcomeric proteins),[2] ischemic disease (less myocardium available to pump blood with a resulting reaction of surviving muscle), valvular disease (increase in volume and/or pressure), and hypertensive heart disease (increase in pressure).[3] Initially, the term remodeling was reserved for structural changes (hypertrophy, dilatation). More recently, it has been recognized that adaptive mechanisms are present on different levels (structural, contractile, and electrical), which collectively ensure that the heart can maintain normal peripheral perfusion (compensated state). In time these so-called ventricular remodeling processes may become maladaptive, progressing into a decompensated state of congestive heart failure (CHF), which has a poor prognosis with high mortality.[4] The position of VH in the course of CHF (Figure 19–1) is still a matter of debate: it may be present as a separate entity or as an intermediate stage of compensation preceding decompensation and heart failure. By itself, left ventricular hypertrophy (LVH) is also a risk factor for mortality.[5,6]

Ventricular electrical remodeling (ER) has been shown to be present in humans, both in compensated LVH and in CHF.[7] The most important and consistently found electrical change is an increase in action potential duration (APD; Figure 19–2 and Tables 19–1 and 19–2), but other changes such as conduction disturbances[8] and altered Ca^{2+} homeostasis[9] have been reported. Ventricular ER in general can lead to a proarrhythmic state with a high risk of sudden cardiac death (SCD), presumably from ventricular tachyarrhythmias (VT).[10]

The aim of the present chapter is, first, to provide a general overview of the current understanding of different repolarization-related electrophysiological changes that occur in compensated LVH and in CHF. For in-depth reviews concerning ER in atria, conduction-related ER, we refer to other publications.[7,11–14] Our second aim is to present the current understanding of the time course of evolution and reversibility of ER in LVH. The clinical observation that ER always coincides with either compensated VH or CHF gave rise to the view that ER is a consequence of either disorder. We will dispute this reasoning as our third aim and refer to ER as a cause of VH.

Defining Electrical Remodeling in Animal Models of Left Ventricular Hypertrophy and Congestive Heart Failure

In this chapter, descriptions concerning electrical remodeling will be restricted to adaptations in ventricular repolarization. Nonuniform lengthening of the APD may increase dispersion of repolarization, either defined as spatial or temporal. These parameters will not be addressed, although

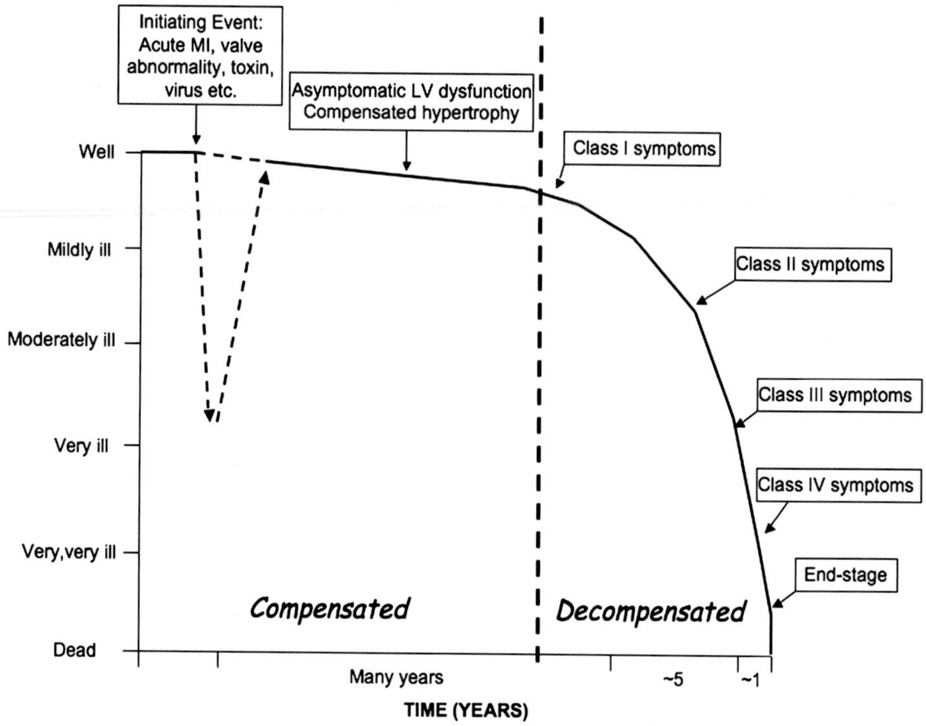

FIGURE 19–1. Graphic representation of the course of heart failure (black line). Health status is depicted (*y*-axis) and followed in time. After an initiating event, well-being drops and may return to a near-normal level as compensatory remodeling mechanisms develop. A period of compensated hypertrophy or asymptomatic left ventricular (LV) dysfunction may follow befor progressive symptoms of decompensation, i.e., CHF, occur. Thi chapter concentrates on the compensated situation, left of th dashed lined. (Adapted with permission from Katz.[69])

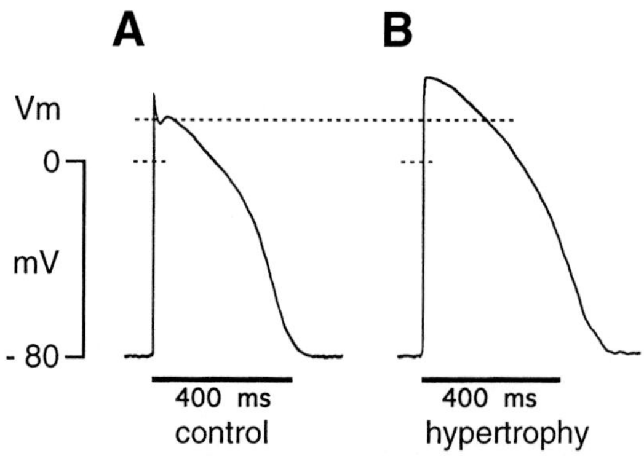

FIGURE 19–2. Action potentials recorded in preparations isolated from superficial (<3 mm deep) subendocardial left ventricular (LV) septum from an undiseased heart (A) and from a patient with aortic stenosis and compensated LV hypertrophy (B). Basic cycle length, 2500 msec; temperature, 35°C. A small notch at phase 1 of the action potential suggested the presence of an I_{to} in undiseased preparations. In diseased preparations, notch was absent, the early plateau phase was higher, and there was a clear action potential prolongation. APD90 repolarization was as follows: undiseased, 384 ± 23 msec ($n = 4$ from two hearts); diseased, 449 ± 11 msec ($n = 59$ from 59 hearts). (Reprinted with permission from Bailly *et al.*[65])

TABLE 19–1. Electrocardiographic and regional parameters.[a]

Reference	Species	Etiology	QT	MAPD
Davey *et al.*[31]	Human	LVH, mixed	N.C.	
Tsuji *et al.*[27]	Rabbit	CAVB + pacing	↑	
Tsuji *et al.*[28]	Rabbit	CAVB + pacing	↑	
Schoenmakers *et al.*[32]	Dog	CAVB	↑	↑
Vos *et al.*[34]	Dog	CAVB	↑	↑
Tsuji *et al.*[28]	Rabbit	Pacing CHF	↓	
Chugh *et al.*[29]	Dog	Pacing CHF		↑
Hsieh *et al.*[63]	Dog	Pacing CHF	↑	↑
Pye and Cobbe[64]	Rabbit	Doxorubicin		N.C./↑
Davey *et al.*[31]	Human	CHF mixed	↑	

[a]Changes in QT (from ECG) and monophasic action potential duration (MAPD) in humans and animal models with either documented compensated ventricular hypertrophy (upper part) or with congestive heart failure (CHF) (lower part). LVH, left ventricular hypertrophy; CAVB, chronic AV block. ↑, ↓, and N.C. indicate upregulation, downregulation, and no change, respectively.

TABLE 19–2. Ventricular cellular action potentials and currents.[a]

Reference	Species	Etiology	Pheno	APD	I_{Na}	I_{CaL}	I_{to}	I_K	I_{K1}
Bailly *et al.*[65]	Human	Mixed	No	↑			N.C.		
Kleiman and Houser[16]	Cat	RVH	Yes					↓	↑
Ten Eick *et al.*[43]	Cat	RVH	No				↑		
Furukawa *et al.*[24]	Cat	Ao banding	No	↑				↓	
Rials *et al.*[17]	Cat	Ao banding	No	↑					
Rials *et al.*[22]	Rabbit	R/N	Yes	↑					
Rials *et al.*[42]	Rabbit	R/N, 3 months	Yes			N.C.	↑		↓
Rials *et al.*[42]	Rabbit	R/N, 6 months	Yes			↓	↑		N.C.
McIntosh *et al.*[41]	Rabbit	Perinephritis	Yes	↑			↓		
Gillis *et al.*[40]	Rabbit	Ao banding	No	↑			↓	N.C.r	↓
Naqvi *et al*[23]	Rabbit	Ao banding	Yes	↑		N.C.			
Tsuji *et al.*[27]	Rabbit	CAVB + pacing	Yes	↑			N.C.	↓r + s	↑
Sipido *et al.*[9]	Dog	CAVB	No			N.C.			
Volders *et al.*[66]	Dog	CAVB	No	↑					
Volders *et al.*[35]	Dog	CAVB	No				N.C.	N.C.r ↓s	N.C.
Antoons *et al.*[46]	Dog	CAVB	No		↓ peak				
Song *et al.*[44]	Dog	Ao banding	Yes			N.C.			
Charpentier *et al.*[21]	Ferret	RVH	No	↑					
Tsuji *et al.*[33]	Rabbit	Pacing CHF	Yes	↑		↓	↓	↓r + s	N.C.
Tsuji *et al.*[28]	Rabbit	Pacing CHF	Yes					N.C.r ↓s	
Kääb *et al.*[37]	Dog	Pacing CHF	Yes			N.C.	↓		↓
O'Rourke *et al.*[45]	Dog	Pacing CHF	Yes	↑		N.C.			
Valdivia *et al.*[47]	Dog	Pacing CHF	No		↓ peak ↑ late				
Zicha *et al.*[30]	Dog	Embolization	Yes		↓ peak				
Rozanski *et al.*[39]	Rabbit	Pacing CHF	Yes	↑		N.C.		↓	N.C.
Valdivia *et al.*[47]	Human	CHF	No		↓ peak ↑ late				
Beuckelmann *et al.*[36]	Human	Mixed CHF	No	↑				↓	↓
Kääb *et al.*[38]	Human	Mixed CHF	Yes				↓		

[a]Changes measured on a cellular level in action potential duration (APD) and ionic currents in humans and animal models with either ventricular hypertrophy (upper part) or with congestive heart failure (CHF) (lower part). A "Yes" in the column "Pheno" indicates that the cited paper includes information on whether hypertrophy or heart failure was present. RVH, right ventricular hypertrophy; Ao banding, aortic banding; R/N, renal artery banding plus contralateral nephrectomy; CAVB, chronic AV block; I_{Na}, Na^+ current, with peak and late indicating peak and late I_{Na}, respectively; I_{CaL}, L-type Ca^{2+} current; I_{to}, transient outward K^+ current; I_K, delayed rectifier K^+ current, with r and s indicating rapid and slow components, respectively; I_{K1}, inward rectifier K^+ current. ↑, ↓, and N.C. indicate upregulation, downregulation, and no change, respectively.

we are aware that they are critically important for arrhythmogenesis.

As electrophysiological data in human hypertrophic cardiac tissue are limited, several animal models of VH have been developed to study the nature of electrical remodeling,[15–18] each with its specific set of advantages and drawbacks. The choice of the animal is very important with respect to extrapolation to the human state. Rats and mice have short action potentials (AP), which lack a plateau and are therefore not useful for studying adaptations in cardiac repolarization.[19] Because the most important change in hypertrophic ER, a prolonged APD, can be mainly attributed to changes in repolarization, models using small rodents are excluded from this overview.

Most animal models of VH are based on mechanical overload, either induced by pressure or by volume. Right VH can be induced in cats[20] and ferrets[21] by pulmonary artery banding. A combination of unilateral nephrectomy and contralateral renal artery banding in rabbits leads to renovascular hypertension with compensated LVH.[22] Aortic banding has been performed in rabbits[23] and cats.[17,24] The canine model of chronic complete atrioventricular block (CAVB) is characterized by ventricular electrical, structural, and contractile remodeling through volume overload.[25] This model is very suitable for studying the development of ventricular ER in a heart with compensated, biventricular hypertrophy and a high incidence of drug-induced torsade de pointes arrhythmias.[26] In rabbits, this bradycardia causes hemodynamic difficulties with a high mortality when no backup pacing is performed.[27] When adequately paced, biventricular hypertrophy without signs of heart failure develops.[28]

Heart failure has been created using rapid (ventricular) pacing in dogs and rabbits[27,29] or with the use of repeated embolizations to create regional ischemia in canines.[30]

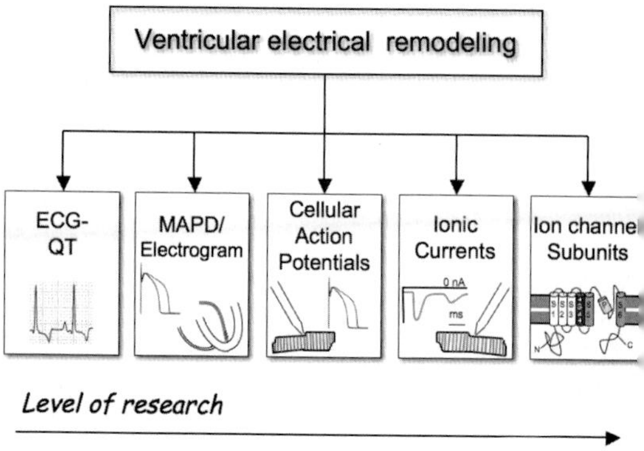

Figure 19–3. Schematic overview of the levels of research o which ventricular electrical remodeling can be described. From le to right, increasingly narrower levels are depicted. ECG, electrc cardiogram; MAPD, monophasic action potential duration.

Aim 1. Electrical Adaptations in Hypertrophied Myocardium

Ventricular electrical remodeling can be described on several levels (Figure 19–3), from electrocardiographic abnormalities to changes in individual ion channel subunits. In between those extremes, changes can also be described by regional measurements involving multiple cardiac myocytes [monophasic action potential duration (MAPD) or electrograms] and individual cellular measurements (APs and ionic currents). In Tables 19–1, 19–2, and 19–3 the electrophysiological changes are summarized at these levels. In each of these tables, adaptations in both compensated LVH an CHF are separately depicted to illustrate similari ties and differences between these two pathologi cal states.

Electrocardiographic and Regional Measurements (Table 19–1)

In clinical practice, surface electrocardiogram (ECGs) are a readily available and easy tool to assess electrical activity and provide informatio concerning ER in the whole heart. As prolongatior of cellular repolarization is reported in many

Table 19–3. Molecular characterization of ion channel subunits.[a]

Reference	Species	Etiology	Pheno	SCN5A	KCNH2	KCNQ1	KCNE1	KV4.3	Kir2.1	Kchip2
Tsuji *et al.*[28]	Rabbit	CAVB + pacing	Yes		↓	↓	↓	N.C.		N.C.
Ramakers *et al.*[48]	Dog	CAVB	No			↓	↓			
Stengl *et al.*[49]	Dog	CAVB	No			↓	N.C.			
Antoons *et al.*[46]	Dog	CAVB	No	↓						
Rose *et al.*[52]	Rabbit	Pacing CHF	No					↓		↓
Tsuji *et al.*[28]	Rabbit	Pacing CHF	Yes		N.C.	↓	↓	↓		
Akar *et al.*[51]	Dog	Pacing CHF	Yes		↑	N.C.	N.C.	↓	N.C.	N.C.
Zicha *et al.*[53]	Dog	Pacing CHF	No					↓		
Zicha *et al.*[30]	Dog	Embolization	Yes	N.C./↓						
Zicha *et al.*[53]	Human	Mixed CHF	No					↓		
Borlak and Thum[50]	Human	Mixed CHF	No	↓	N.C.	↑		↓	↓	

[a]Changes measured on a molecular expression level of ion channel subunits in humans and animal models with either ventricular hypertrophy (uppe part) or with congestive heart failure (CHF) (lower part). A "Yes" in the column "Pheno" indicates that this specific paper includes information on whethe hypertrophy or heart failure was present. CAVB, chronic AV block. ↑, ↓, and N.C. indicate upregulation, downregulation, and no change, respectively.

tudies of VH, QT prolongation would theoretially be the logical ECG representative. Surprisngly little has been reported on QT(c) or MAPD hanges in patients with LVH. One study describng QT in both patients with LVH and patients vith CHF showed no QT(c) increase in LVH atients when compared to controls.[31] In CAVB abbits and dogs an increase in QTc together with n increase in MAP duration (MAPD) has been locumented.[28,32–34] This combined increase in vhole heart and regional repolarization duration s also observed in (models of) CHF (Table 19–1).

Changes in Cellular Action Potentials and onic Currents (Table 19–2)

The ventricular AP is generated by the collaboraion of several ion channels, pumps, and exchangrs, which are selective for an ion and have specific properties (Figure 19–4). The AP produces the lectromechanical coupling that is necessary for ardiac pump function. AP duration depends on he balance of inward, depolarizing, and outward, epolarizing, currents during the plateau phase. A decrease in outward current or an increase in nward current can lead to a prolonged APD.

Based on Table 19–2, it can be concluded that prolongation of APD is consistently seen in a multitude of animal models and patients, independent of proper heart function or heart failure. Despite this similar phenotype of APD prolongation, very diverse and sometimes contradictory changes of ion currents are reported.

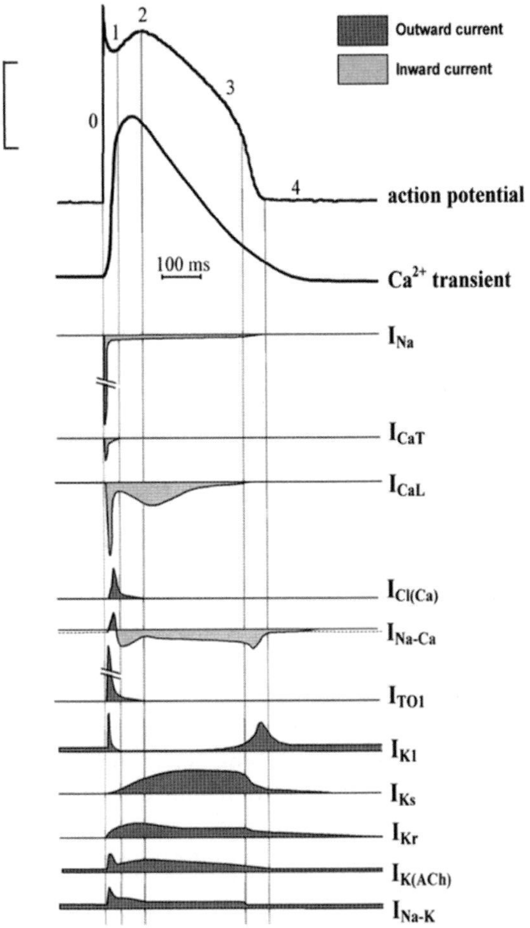

Figure 19–4. Schematic overview of the depolarizing and repolarizing currents that shape the action potential in the normal mammalian ventricle. A schematic of the time course of each of the currents is shown together with the course of the Ca^{2+} transient. (Reprinted from the thesis of Volders.[70])

Repolarizing K^+ Currents

When attempting to explain a prolonged APD, analysis of the repolarizing potassium currents is an obvious starting point. The function of several K^+ currents is altered in LVH/CHF. The most consistent finding in larger mammals with a plateau in the ventricular AP is a downregulation in the density of the delayed rectifier current I_K,[16,24,27,28,35] which is the dominant current to repolarize the cell. Similar observations have been documented in CHF.[28,33,36–39] This current can be divided into a slow (I_{Ks}) and a rapid component (I_{Kr}). In the left ventricle of both rabbits and dogs, I_{Ks} is downregulated,[27,28,35] whereas I_{Kr} is sometimes downregulated[27,28] and sometimes unchanged.[35,40]

Remodeling of other K^+ currents has also been demonstrated, though not with the same consistency (no change or decrease) as changes in I_K. The transient outward K^+ current, I_{to}, responsible for early repolarization and the spike-and-dome morphology (Figure 19–2A), has been found to be both upregulated and downregulated in different reports. In two studies using rabbits with LV pressure overload, a downregulation of I_{to} was found,[40,41] whereas in rabbits with nephrectomy and renal artery banding, an upregulation of the current was described.[42] An upregulation was also observed in the right ventricle of cats with pulmonary banding.[43] In the CAVB models, no change in this current was detected.[27,35]

Similar inconsistencies can be found for the inward rectifier current I_{K1}, which contributes to the terminal phase of repolarization and maintains the resting membrane potential. The important component of I_{K1} for APD prolongation is the outward current at voltages more positive than the equilibrium potential for K^+. The current is upregulated,[16] downregulated,[40] and unchanged.[35] In a study by Rials *et al.*,[42] I_{K1} current density showed a biphasic course: after 3 months of VH, the current was downregulated, but after 6 months no change versus control rabbits was found. The timing of the measurements seems therefore important and needs to be considered when evaluating the results.

Depolarizing Ca^{2+} Currents

During the plateau phase of the AP, the L-type Ca^{2+} current, I_{CaL}, is the most important inward current. During VH, no change in I_{CaL} can be observed in both rabbit and dog models of VH.[9,23,42,44] But again, in long-standing VH, I_{CaL} might be decreased.[42] Also in animal models and patients with CHF, either no change in I_{CaL} is found,[37,39,45] or a downregulation is noticed.[33]

Depolarizing Na^+ Currents

Due to the initial interest in K^+ currents, few reports on I_{Na} in electrical remodeling are present. In one report on CAVB dogs, (peak) I_{Na} is downregulated.[46] This downregulation is also observed in several animal models of CHF[30,47] and in one human study.[47] In addition to this downregulation of peak I_{Na}, the late component of I_{Na} is upregulated in CHF.[47] The latter alteration could contribute to the prolongation of APD and therefore this current is under intense investigation.

Changes in Expression of Ion Channel Subunits (Table 19–3)

Alterations in ion channel subunit expression constitute the feature by which electrical remodeling is present on a molecular level. Downregulation of I_{Ks} on a cellular level is supported by observations of downregulation of the α subunit of that channel, KCNQ1,[28,48,49] and of the β subunit, KCNE1.[28,48] In one report, KCNE1 was unaltered.[4] In CHF this downregulation is not consistently seen, as one report shows a downregulation,[2] another shows an upregulation,[50] and a third shows no change.[51] The α subunit of the ion channel carrying the I_{Kr} current is KCNH2 (hERG). In rabbits with CAVB, molecular expression is down, despite the fact that this current is unchanged (Table 19–2).[28] Also in CHF models, the response of KCNH2 expression is not clear as both an upregulation[51] and no change[28] were found, whereas I_{Kr} was either downregulated[33] or unchanged.[28]

One of the α subunits of the I_{to} channel, Kv4.3 is unchanged in CAVB rabbits,[28] which is in line with the unchanged expression seen in the β subunit KChip2. In CHF, however, this subunit is consistently downregulated, both in animal models[28,51–53] and in humans,[50,53] whereas KChip2 is downregulated or unchanged.

Other channel subunits are less well studied. The α subunit of the cardiac sodium channel SCN5A is downregulated on an mRNA level in one report of VH in dogs due to CAVB, concurring with the finding that this current has a lower amplitude.[46] In CHF this subunit is either downregulated on an mRNA level[50] or unchanged,[3] whereas on a protein level this subunit is downregulated.[30]

Aim 2A. Time Course of Electrical Remodeling and Arrhythmogenesis

Ventricular hypertrophy can be viewed in two ways: as an intermediate step in the progression from asymptomatic LV dysfunction toward overt heart failure (Figure 19–1) or as a separate entity of compensation. In the first view, similar stimuli remain present for a long period (chronic), whereas different signaling pathways are required for the second view. From data presented in this chapter, it becomes apparent that electrical remodeling develops independently of the mechanical endpoint: it is present both in compensated LVH and CHF. This indicates that repolarization-dependent ER is an early adaptation process, which precedes the structural changes. Confirmatory data for this sequence of events came from a rat model of myocardial infarction[54] and from a ransgenic mouse model.[55] Three days after inf-rction, pacing could induce ventricular tachycar-lias in the absence of hypertrophy in the infarcted ats. Also in the CAVB dog, this distinct temporal ehavior between electrical and structural remod-ling can be seen (Figure 19–5). Immediately after AVB, AV dyssynchrony occurs and the ventricles re activated from a new focus with profound radycardia (≤50% of original sinus rate) and an ltered ventricular activation pattern. This reduces ardiac output markedly.[25] At this time point (0 veeks), no ER is present and no arrhythmias can e induced with a drug challenge.[26] In 2 weeks at dioventricular rhythm, several remodeling proc-esses can be seen: the cardiac output is returning o subnormal values[25] probably due to an increase n contractility, +LV dP/dt_{max},[25,56] and an increase n repolarization times (QTc time). Now, 66% of he dogs respond with arrhythmias after adminis-ration of an APD-prolonging drug. At 6 weeks, ardiac output is restored, electrical remodeling is maintained, the contractile parameter (+LV dP/dt_{max}) is decreasing, whereas structural remode-ling, indicated by heart-to-body-weight ratio, is reaching its maximal value. Induction of arrhyth-mia remains high. At 12 weeks of AVB, electrical and structural remodeling are still at their respec-tive maximum levels, while contractile remode-ling is decreasing further, back to control values. Again, the proarrhythmic outcome has not changed, indicating that ER is the dominant factor for the development of drug-induced torsade de pointes.

Whether ER remains stable in time is not completely clear yet. As mentioned in the studies of Rials,[42] time-dependent changes did occur in ion currents, suggesting that some dynamic feature may be active. The discrepancies in (1) changes in ion currents with respect to molecular expression and (2) specific ion currents described within the same model[42] may also be related to the moment of measurement.

Aim 2B. Reversal of Electrical Remodeling

The different remodeling processes do not only have distinct time courses, but also different reversal reactions to interventions (Table 19–4). When sinus rate is restored by biventricular pacing after 8 weeks in electrically remodeled CAVB dogs, LV mass and volume decrease, but QT and LV MAPD remain unaltered.[56] The same reaction was also observed in AVB dogs in which cyclosporin was used to reverse remodeling: VH decreased, but QT did not.[57]

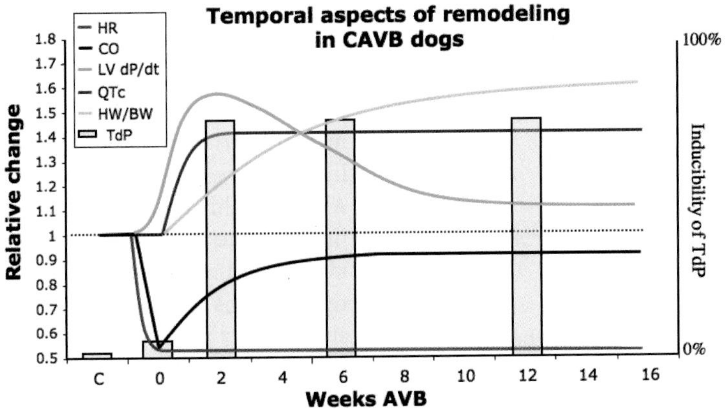

FIGURE 19–5. Time course of the ventricular remodeling in the chronic AV block (CAVB) dog. Relative changes in several parameters are plotted: at control (C) and at 0–16 weeks after induction of AV block (AVB). Bar graphs depict relative inducibility (in percentage) of torsade de pointes arrhythmias (TdP) after an arrhythmogenic challenge. HR, heart rate; CO, cardiac output; LV *dP/dt*, maximum positive slope of the left ventricular systolic pressure; QTc, heart rate corrected QT interval; HW/BW, heart-weight-to-body-weight ratio. Contains data from numerous references.[26,32,34,56,71]

TABLE 19–4. Regression of electrical remodeling.[a]

Reference	Species	Etiology	Intervention	Observed change
Peschar *et al.*[56]	Dog	CAVB	Pacing	LV mass/volume ↓, QT N.C., LV MAPD N.C.
Rials *et al.*[42]	Rabbits	R/N	Captopril	Myocyte size ↓, HW/BW ↓, APD ↓, ion current normalization
Schreiner *et al.*[57]	Dog	CAVB	Cyclosporin	Hypertrophy ↓, QT N.C., arrhythmias ↓
Kurita *et al.*[67]	Human	CAVB	Pacing	QT ↓ at high heart rate in TdP patients, QT N.C. at low rate
Harding *et al.*[68]	Human	Mixed CHF	LVAD	APD ↓, QTc ↓
Xydas *et al.*[58]	Human	Mixed CHF	LVAD	QTc ↓, QRS ↓, LVEDD ↓, myocyte size ↓
Terracciano *et al.*[59]	Human	Mixed CHF	LVAD	APD ↓, myocyte size ↓

[a]Changes measured in remodeling processes after different interventions in humans and animal models with either ventricular hypertrophy (upper part) or with congestive heart failure (CHF) (lower part). CAVB, chronic AV block; R/N, renal artery banding plus contralateral nephrectomy; (M)APD, (monophasic) action potential duration; HW/BW, heart-to-body-weight ratio; TdP, torsade de pointes arrhythmias; LVEDD, left ventricular end diastolic dimension. ↑, ↓, and N.C. indicate upregulation, downregulation, and no change, respectively.

A different observation was made in rabbits with renovascular pressure overload treated with an angiotensin-converting enzyme (ACE) inhibitor: both VH and APD decreased.[42] The regression of ER was also documented by a normalization of ionic currents. In humans with CHF in whom a left ventricular assist device (LVAD) was implanted, reversal of ER and a decrease in myocyte size were seen.[58,59]

A confounding variable in these studies was the time of follow-up to document reversibility. In general, when no regression of ER was seen, follow-up was restricted to shorter periods (6–8 weeks) as compared to the studies in which ER decreased (several months). The time course of reversibility of ER may be longer than that of VH. On the other hand, it is also clear that changes in structure are by no means indications that ER is also adapting. This suggests that ER and VH may be two separate processes that can be modulated (treated) independently.

Aim 3. Electrical Remodeling: Cause or Consequence?

From the distinct time courses of the remodeling processes (Figure 19–5) and the different regression reactions (Table 19–4), the question of whether ER is the cause or the consequence of VH becomes actual again. Unfortunately, there are no studies in large mammals to address this question. Using rodents, the relevance of I_{to} for hypertrophy or contractile adaptations has been investigated. It was shown that I_{to} as the dominant repolarization current plays an important role: (1) Pharmacological or adenovirus-mediated blockade of I_{to} leads to ventricular hypertrophy in neonatal myocytes.[60] (2) Maintaining high expression levels of I_{to} by gene therapy prevented the development of ventricular hypertrophy through the calcineurin pathway[61] in the aortic constriction mice and in neonatal rat cells.[62]

Thus, the proposed sequence could be as follows: reducing I_{to} leads to (1) prolongation of the APD, (2) increased $[Ca^{2+}]_i$, (3) activation of the calcineurin pathway, and (4) ventricular hypertrophy.

Conclusions

Repolarization-dependent electrical remodeling is an early response that is associated with an enhanced susceptibility to ventricular arrhythmias. Electrical remodeling is characterized by an increased ventricular action potential duration. Although this lengthening is a consistent cellular finding, the responsible modifications in both inward and outward currents and in their respective proteins are quite diverse and require further study. Electrical remodeling is not reflected in structural adaptations and occurs independently of whether the mechanical cardiac endpoint is normal, seminormal, or severely depressed.

Acknowledgment. This research was sponsored in part by Netherlands Heart Foundation Grant 1996T103.

References

1. Grossman W, Jones D, McLaurin LP. Wall stress and patterns of hypertrophy in the human left ventricle. *J Clin Invest* 1975;56(1):56–64.
2. Ahmad F, Siedman J, Seidman C. The genetic base for cardiac remodeling. *Annu Rev Genomics Hum Genet* 2005;6:185–216.
3. Stevenson WG, Stevenson LW. Prevention of sudden death in heart failure. *J Cardiovasc Electrophysiol* 2001;12(1):112–114.
4. Levy D, Kenchaiah S, Larson MG, *et al.* Long-term trends in the incidence of and survival with heart failure. *N Engl J Med* 2002;347(18):1397–1402.
5. Brown DW, Giles WH, Croft JB. Left ventricular hypertrophy as a predictor of coronary heart disease mortality and the effect of hypertension. *Am Heart J* 2000;140(6):848–856.
6. Levy D, Garrison RJ, Savage DD, Kannel WB, Castelli WP. Prognostic implications of echocardiographically determined left ventricular mass in the Framingham Heart Study. *N Engl J Med* 1990; 322(22):1561–1566.
7. Tomaselli GF, Marban E. Electrophysiological remodeling in hypertrophy and heart failure. *Cardiovasc Res* 1999;42(2):270–283.
8. Kostin S, Dammer S, Hein S, Klovekorn WP, Bauer EP, Schaper J. Connexin 43 expression and distribution in compensated and decompensated cardiac hypertrophy in patients with aortic stenosis. *Cardiovasc Res* 2004;62(2):426–436.
9. Sipido K, Volders P, De Groot S, *et al.* Enhanced Ca(2+) release and Na/Ca exchange activity in hypertrophied canine ventricular myocytes: Potential link between contractile adaptation and arrhythmogenesis. *Circulation* 2000;102(17):2137–2144.
10. Zipes DP, Wellens HJ. Sudden cardiac death. *Circulation* 1998;98(21):2334–2351.
11. Hill JA. Electrical remodeling in cardiac hypertrophy. *Trends Cardiovasc Med* 2003;13(8):316–322.
12. Richard S, Leclercq F, Lemaire S, Piot C, Nargeot J. Ca2+ currents in compensated hypertrophy and heart failure. *Cardiovasc Res* 1998;37(2):300–311.
13. Dobrev D. Electrical remodeling in atrial fibrillation. *Herz* 2006;31(2):108–112.
14. Severs NJ, Coppen SR, Dupont E, Yeh HI, Ko YS, Matsushita T. Gap junction alterations in human cardiac disease. *Cardiovasc Res* 2004;62(2):368–377.
15. Hasenfuss G. Animal models of human cardiovascular disease, heart failure and hypertrophy. *Cardiovasc Res* 1998;39(1):60–76.
16. Kleiman RB, Houser SR. Outward currents in normal and hypertrophied feline ventricular myocytes. *Am J Physiol* 1989;256(5Pt. 2):H1450–H1461.
17. Rials SJ, Wu Y, Ford N, *et al.* Effect of left ventricular hypertrophy and its regression on ventricular electrophysiology and vulnerability to inducible arrhythmia in the feline heart. *Circulation* 1995; 91(2):426–430.
18. Verduyn S, Vos M, Van der Zande J, Van der Hulst F, Wellens H. Role of interventricular dispersion of repolarization in acquired torsade-de-pointes arrhythmias: Reversal by magnesium. *Cardiovasc Res* 1997;34(3):453–463.
19. Gussak I, Chaitman BR, Kopecky SL, Nerbonne JM. Rapid ventricular repolarization in rodents: Electrocardiographic manifestations, molecular mechanisms, and clinical insights. *J Electrocardiol* 2000; 33(2):159–170.
20. Kleiman RB, Houser SR. Calcium currents in normal and hypertrophied isolated feline ventricular myocytes. *Am J Physiol* 1988;255(6Pt. 2):H1434–H1442.
21. Charpentier F, Baudet S, Le Marec H. Triggered activity as a possible mechanism for arrhythmias in ventricular hypertrophy. *Pacing Clin Electrophysiol* 1991;14(11Pt. 2):1735–1741.
22. Rials SJ, Wu Y, Xu X, Filart RA, Marinchak RA, Kowey PR. Regression of left ventricular hypertrophy with captopril restores normal ventricular action potential duration, dispersion of refractoriness, and vulnerability to inducible ventricular fibrillation. *Circulation* 1997;96(4):1330–1336.
23. Naqvi RU, Tweedie D, MacLeod KT. Evidence for the action potential mediating the changes to contraction observed in cardiac hypertrophy in the rabbit. *Int J Cardiol* 2001;77(2–3):189–206.
24. Furukawa T, Myerburg RJ, Furukawa N, Kimura S, Bassett AL. Metabolic inhibition of ICa, L and IK differs in feline left ventricular hypertrophy. *Am J Physiol* 1994;266(3Pt. 2):H1121–H1131.
25. De Groot S, Schoenmakers M, Molenschot M, Leunissen J, Wellens H, Vos M. Contractile adaptations preserving cardiac output predispose the hypertrophied canine heart to delayed afterdepolarization-dependent ventricular arrhythmias. *Circulation* 2000;102(17):2145–2151.
26. Thomsen MB, Volders PG, Beekman JD, Matz J, Vos MA. Beat-to-beat variability of repolarization determines proarrhythmic outcome in dogs susceptible to drug-induced torsades de pointes. *J Am Coll Cardiol* 2006;48(6):1268–1276.
27. Tsuji Y, Opthof T, Yasui K, *et al.* Ionic mechanisms of acquired QT prolongation and torsades de pointes in rabbits with chronic complete atrioventricular block. *Circulation* 2002;106(15):2012–2018.

28. Tsuji Y, Zicha S, Qi X, Kodama I, Nattel S. Potassium channel subunit remodeling in rabbits exposed to long-term bradycardia or tachycardia: Discrete arrhythmogenic consequences related to differential delayed-rectifier changes. *Circulation* 2006;113(3):345–355.
29. Chugh SS, Johnson SB, Packer DL. Altered response to ibutilide in a heart failure model. *Cardiovasc Res* 2001;49(1):94–102.
30. Zicha S, Maltsev VA, Nattel S, Sabbah HN, Undrovinas AI. Post-transcriptional alterations in the expression of cardiac Na+ channel subunits in chronic heart failure. *J Mol Cell Cardiol* 2004;37(1):91–100.
31. Davey PP, Barlow C, Hart G. Prolongation of the QT interval in heart failure occurs at low but not at high heart rates. *Clin Sci (Lond)* 2000;98(5):603–610.
32. Schoenmakers M, Ramakers C, Van Opstal J, Leunissen J, Londono C, Vos M. Asynchronous development of electrical remodeling and cardiac hypertrophy in the complete AV block dog. *Cardiovasc Res* 2003;59(2):351–359.
33. Tsuji Y, Opthof T, Kamiya K, *et al.* Pacing-induced heart failure causes a reduction of delayed rectifier potassium currents along with decreases in calcium and transient outward currents in rabbit ventricle. *Cardiovasc Res* 2000;48(2):300–309.
34. Vos M, De Groot S, Verduyn S, *et al.* Enhanced susceptibility for acquired torsade de pointes arrhythmias in the dog with chronic, complete AV block is related to cardiac hypertrophy and electrical remodeling. *Circulation* 1998;98(11):1125–1135.
35. Volders P, Sipido K, Vos M, *et al.* Downregulation of delayed rectifier K(+) currents in dogs with chronic complete atrioventricular block and acquired torsades de pointes. *Circulation* 1999;100(24):2455–2461.
36. Beuckelmann DJ, Nabauer M, Erdmann E. Alterations of K+ currents in isolated human ventricular myocytes from patients with terminal heart failure. *Circ Res* 1993;73(2):379–385.
37. Kääb S, Nuss HB, Chiamvimonvat N, *et al.* Ionic mechanism of action potential prolongation in ventricular myocytes from dogs with pacing-induced heart failure. *Circ Res* 1996;78(2):262–273.
38. Kaab S, Dixon J, Duc J, *et al.* Molecular basis of transient outward potassium current downregulation in human heart failure: A decrease in Kv4.3 mRNA correlates with a reduction in current density. *Circulation* 1998;98(14):1383–1393.
39. Rozanski GJ, Xu Z, Whitney RT, Murakami H, Zucker IH. Electrophysiology of rabbit ventricular myocytes following sustained rapid ventricula pacing. *J Mol Cell Cardiol* 1997;29(2):721–732.
40. Gillis AM, Geonzon RA, Mathison HJ, Kulisz E Lester WM, Duff HJ. The effects of barium, dofetilide and 4-aminopyridine (4-AP) on ventricula repolarization in normal and hypertrophied rabbit heart. *J Pharmacol Exp Ther* 1998;285(1):262-270.
41. McIntosh MA, Cobbe SM, Kane KA, Rankin AC Action potential prolongation and potassium currents in left-ventricular myocytes isolated from hypertrophied rabbit hearts. *J Mol Cell Cardio* 1998;30(1):43–53.
42. Rials SJ, Xu X, Wu Y, Marinchak RA, Kowey PR Regression of LV hypertrophy with captopril normalizes membrane currents in rabbits. *Am J Physio* 1998;275(4Pt. 2):H1216–H1224.
43. Ten Eick RE, Zhang K, Harvey RD, Bassett AL Enhanced functional expression of transient outward current in hypertrophied feline myocytes *Cardiovasc Drugs Ther* 1993;7(Suppl. 3):611–619.
44. Song LS, Pi Y, Kim SJ, *et al.* Paradoxical cellular Ca2+ signaling in severe but compensated canine left ventricular hypertrophy. *Circ Res* 2005;97(5) 457–464.
45. O'Rourke B, Kass DA, Tomaselli GF, Kaab S, Tunin R, Marban E. Mechanisms of altered excitation contraction coupling in canine tachycardia-induced heart failure, I: Experimental studies. *Circ Re* 1999;84(5):562–570.
46. Antoons G, Stengl M, Ramakers C, Sipido K, Vos M. Properties of sodium currents in the dog with chronic atrioventricular block (abstract). *J Mol Cel Cardiol* 2005;39(1):195.
47. Valdivia CR, Chu WW, Pu J, *et al.* Increased late sodium current in myocytes from a canine heart failure model and from failing human heart. *J Mo Cell Cardiol* 2005;38(3):475–483.
48. Ramakers C, Vos M, Doevendans P, *et al.* Coordinated down-regulation of KCNQ1 and KCNE1 expression contributes to reduction of I(Ks) in canine hypertrophied hearts. *Cardiovasc Res* 2003 57(2):486–496.
49. Stengl M, Ramakers C, Donker D, *et al.* Temporal patterns of electrical remodeling in canine ventricular hypertrophy: Focus on I(Ks) downregulation and blunted beta-adrenergic activation *Cardiovasc Res* 2006;72(1):90–100.
50. Borlak J, Thum T. Hallmarks of ion channel gene expression in end-stage heart failure. *FASEB J* 2003;17(12):1592–1608.
51. Akar FG, Wu RC, Juang GJ, *et al.* Molecular mechanisms underlying K+ current downregulation in canine tachycardia-induced heart failure.

Am J Physiol Heart Circ Physiol 2005;288(6):H2887–H2896.

2. Rose J, Armoundas AA, Tian Y, *et al.* Molecular correlates of altered expression of potassium currents in failing rabbit myocardium. *Am J Physiol Heart Circ Physiol* 2005;288(5):H2077–H2087.
3. Zicha S, Xiao L, Stafford S, *et al.* Transmural expression of transient outward potassium current subunits in normal and failing canine and human hearts. *J Physiol* 2004;561(Pt. 3):735–748.
4. Huang B, Qin D, El-Sherif N. Early down-regulation of K+ channel genes and currents in the postinfarction heart. *J Cardiovasc Electrophysiol* 2000; 11(11):1252–1261.
5. Hill JA, Karimi M, Kutschke W, *et al.* Cardiac hypertrophy is not a required compensatory response to short-term pressure overload. *Circulation* 2000;101(24):2863–2869.
6. Peschar M, Vernooy K, Vanagt W, Reneman R, Vos M, Prinzen F. Absence of reverse electrical remodeling during regression of volume overload hypertrophy in canine ventricles. *Cardiovasc Res* 2003; 58(3):510–517.
7. Schreiner K, Kelemen K, Zehelein J, *et al.* Biventricular hypertrophy in dogs with chronic AV block: Effects of cyclosporin A on morphology and electrophysiology. *Am J Physiol Heart Circ Physiol* 2004;287(6):H2891–H2898.
8. Xydas S, Rosen RS, Ng C, *et al.* Mechanical unloading leads to echocardiographic, electrocardiographic, neurohormonal, and histologic recovery. *J Heart Lung Transplant* 2006;25(1):7–15.
9. Terracciano CM, Hardy J, Birks EJ, Khaghani A, Banner NR, Yacoub MH. Clinical recovery from end-stage heart failure using left-ventricular assist device and pharmacological therapy correlates with increased sarcoplasmic reticulum calcium content but not with regression of cellular hypertrophy. *Circulation* 2004;109(19):2263–2265.
0. Kassiri Z, Zobel C, Nguyen TT, Molkentin JD, Backx PH. Reduction of I(to) causes hypertrophy in neonatal rat ventricular myocytes. *Circ Res* 2002; 90(5):578–585.
1. Lebeche D, Kaprielian R, del Monte F, *et al.* In vivo cardiac gene transfer of Kv4.3 abrogates the hypertrophic response in rats after aortic stenosis. *Circulation* 2004;110(22):3435–3443.
62. Zobel C, Kassiri Z, Nguyen TT, Meng Y, Backx PH. Prevention of hypertrophy by overexpression of Kv4.2 in cultured neonatal cardiomyocytes. *Circulation* 2002;106(18):2385–2391.
63. Hsieh MH, Chen YJ, Lee SH, Ding YA, Chang MS, Chen SA. Proarrhythmic effects of ibutilide in a canine model of pacing induced cardiomyopathy. *Pacing Clin Electrophysiol* 2000;23(2):149–156.
64. Pye MP, Cobbe SM. Arrhythmogenesis in experimental models of heart failure: The role of increased load. *Cardiovasc Res* 1996;32(2):248–257.
65. Bailly P, Benitah JP, Mouchoniere M, Vassort G, Lorente P. Regional alteration of the transient outward current in human left ventricular septum during compensated hypertrophy. *Circulation* 1997;96(4):1266–1274.
66. Volders P, Sipido K, Vos M, Kulcsar A, Verduyn S, Wellens H. Cellular basis of biventricular hypertrophy and arrhythmogenesis in dogs with chronic complete atrioventricular block and acquired torsade de pointes. *Circulation* 1998;98(11):1136–1147.
67. Kurita T, Ohe T, Marui N, *et al.* Bradycardia-induced abnormal QT prolongation in patients with complete atrioventricular block with torsades de pointes. *Am J Cardiol* 1992;69(6):628–633.
68. Harding JD, Piacentino V 3rd, Gaughan JP, Houser SR, Margulies KB. Electrophysiological alterations after mechanical circulatory support in patients with advanced cardiac failure. *Circulation* 2001; 104(11):1241–1247.
69. Katz AM. *Heart Failure: Pathophysiology, Molecular Biology, and Clinical Management.* Philadelphia: Lippincott Williams & Wilkins, 2000.
70. Volders P. Cellular mechanisms of acquired torsades de pointes in the hypertrophied canine heart; the substrate and the trigger. Thesis. Maastricht, the Netherlands, 1999.
71. Donker D, Volders P, Arts T, *et al.* End-diastolic myofiber stress and ejection strain increase with ventricular volume overload—-Serial in-vivo analyses in dogs with complete atrioventricular block. *Basic Res Cardiol* 2005;100(4):372–382.

20
Physiological and Other Biological Pacemakers

Michael R. Rosen, Peter R. Brink, Ira S. Cohen, and Richard B. Robinson

Introduction

Physiological pacemaking in the heart is the province of the sinus node, in which a family of ionic currents contributes to the pacemaker potential. Of paramount importance in initiating pacemaker function is I_f, an inward current carried by sodium through a family of channels that is hyperpolarization activated and cyclic nucleotide gated (HCN channels). In many settings where physiological pacemaking fails, therapy involves electronic pacing. Because of shortcomings in this otherwise excellent technology, there has been a search for biological alternatives in which either gene or cell therapy is used to decrease outward current or increase inward current to provide pacemaker function. The various technologies used will be summarized as well as directions for optimizing biological pacemaker function and for using them in tandem with electronic units.

Pacemaker Therapy

Pacemaker therapy is an established part of medical practice, such that few of us remember what the world was like before the electronic pacemaker era. As recently as the early 1960s many patients experiencing Adams–Stokes seizures resulting from high degree heart block were given sublingual isoproterenol as therapy. The diagnosis was effectively a death sentence and the therapy was both inconvenient and not very efficacious: every 2h the patient had to take isoproterenol; although it maintained a faster heart rate than that of the baseline idioventricular rhythm it was often arrhythmogenic.[1]

During their infancy implantable electronic pacemakers were clumsy, hockey-puck-sized devices delivering impulses at a fixed rate. While certainly better than preexisting therapy, there were problems: limited battery life, infection and lead dislodgement, and parasystolic competition from the patient's own idioventricular rhythm. In the past 50 years there have been dramatic advances, through demand pacing, atrioventricular (AV) sequential pacing, and through the application of pacing for treating a variety of arrhythmias as well as heart failure. All these advances have been made while modifying the power packs such that their mass is a fraction of that of the original implantable devices.[2]

Why attempt to improve upon this situation? Because as good as they are, electronic pacemakers have limitations. These include poor responsiveness to the demands of exercise and emotion, the requirements of monitoring and maintenance (including at times battery and/or electrode replacement), suboptimal flexibility for pediatric treatment, limited flexibility with regard to electrode placement site, infection, and occasional interference from other devices.[2–4] For these reasons biological pacemakers have become the subject of a concerted research effort. In this chapter we will first consider the physiological pacemaker of the heart, and then will review the field of biological pacemaking.

Physiological Pacemakers

The physiological cardiac pacemaker is the sinus node, which generates a rate and rhythm having great stability under normal circumstances. In addition, the heart makes use of biological redundancy such that a complex backup system is in place. Hence, in addition to the sinus node, there are pacemaker cells in the atrium, AV junction, and Purkinje system, each of which is capable of driving the heart (at progressively lower rates as one proceeds distally from the sinus node through the Purkinje system) in the event that higher pacemaker centers fail.[5]

The key aspects of physiological pacemaker function are summarized in Figure 20–1. The property central to sinoatrial impulse initiation is automaticity, the gradual depolarization of cells during phase 4 of the transmembrane potential until a threshold potential is reached and an action potential is initiated.[6] Phase 4 depolarization begins as the result of an inward current carried by sodium and potassium, and is referred to as I_f (the f stands for "funny," given the observation that this inward current depends on hyperpolarization for its initiation and increases in magnitude with increasingly hyperpolarizing voltage steps).[7] Also contributing inward current during phase 4 are the Na–Ca exchanger and the inward Ca currents, $I_{Ca,L}$ and $I_{Ca,T}$.[6] The sinus node action potential itself is largely Ca dependent (in contrast to the faster-rising Na-dependent action

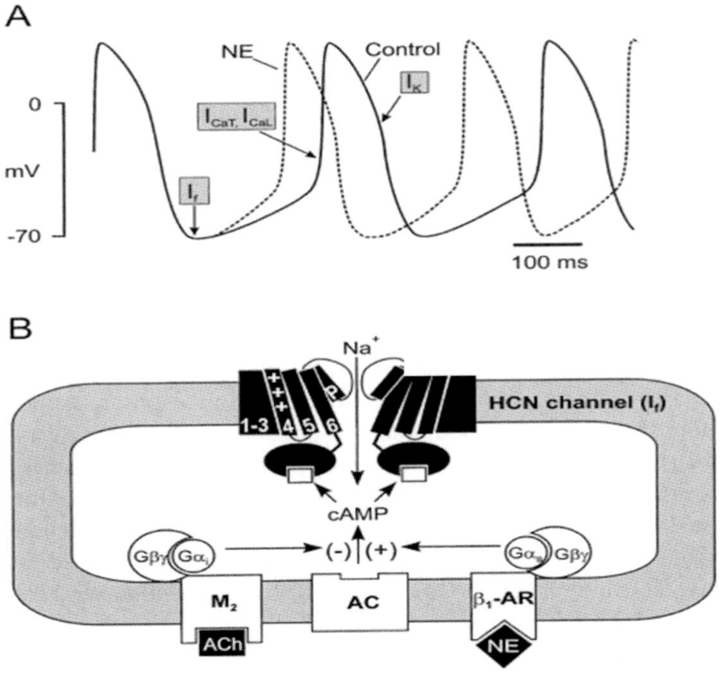

FIGURE 20–1. (A) Representation of sinoatrial node action potential (control: solid lines) and some of the ion channels that contribute to it. I_f is activated on hyperpolarization and provides inward current during phase 4. T- and L-type Ca currents are initiated toward the end of phase 4: the latter also contributes the major current to the upstroke of the action potential. Delayed rectifier current (I_K) is responsible for repolarization. The acceleratory effects of norepinephrine (NE) are shown as broken lines. Note the prominent increase in phase 4, reflecting the actions of NE on I_f. (B) Illustration of the pacemaker channel. There are six transmembrane-spanning domains: when the channel is in the open position, Na is the major carrier of inward ion current. Cyclic AMP binding sites are present near the amino terminus. Also depicted are β_1-adrenergic (B_1-AR) and M2-muscarinic receptors, providing, respectively, norepinephrine and acetylcholine binding sites. Via G protein coupling these regulate adenylyl cyclase (AC) activity, which, in turn, regulates intracellular cAMP levels, determining availability of the second messenger for binding and for channel modulation. (Reprinted from Biel *et al.*,[6] with permission.)

potentials of working myocardium). Repolarizing current is provided via potassium channels, generating an outward current.[6] Hence, a balance between inward and outward currents determines the sinus rate, and any intervention that increases inward or decreases outward current will increase the pacemaker rate.

Just as there is redundancy in pacemaker automaticity at various sites in the heart from sinus node through Purkinje system, there is also redundancy within the node itself. Use of highly selective I_f -blocking drugs such as ivabradine has resulted in about a 30% decrease in heart rate[8]; but the sinus node continues to fire, as the other inward and outward current components are still intact. Hence it is possible to manipulate the ionic determinants of pacemaker current to alter the heart rate without fear that altering a single component will turn off pacemaker function completely.

A key attribute of the sinus node is its autonomic responsiveness. Sympathetic stimulation and/or catecholamine increase phase 4 depolarization and sinus rate; parasympathetic stimulation and/or acetylcholine decrease rate. These properties are attributable to the family of ion channels that underlies the I_f pacemaker current (Figure 20–1). Note that the channel, which has six transmembrane spanning domains, incorporates a cyclic AMP (cAMP) binding site near its carboxy-terminus. The channel, then, is hyperpolarization activated and cyclic nucleotide gated, hence the designation HCN.[6] There are four isoforms of the HCN channel, designated HCN1–4; isoforms 1, 2, and 4 reside in the heart, 4 and 1 are preponderant in the sinus node, and 2 in the myocardium and Purkinje system.

β-Adrenergic catecholamine binds to a β_1-adrenergic receptor and via a G-protein-transduced pathway operates through adenylyl cyclase to break down ATP to cAMP , which then can interact with its HCN channel site to increase pacemaker rate (Figure 20–1). The increase in rate results from an increase in activation kinetics and positive shift along the voltage axis of the current. In contrast, acetylcholine, binding to an M2 muscarinic receptor, utilizes its G-protein-transduced pathway to brake the increase in rate by decreasing cAMP levels. At high concentrations, acetylcholine also increases the potassium current $I_{K,Ach}$ to accelerate repolarization, hyperpolarize the membrane, and suppress phase 4. This further slows the rate of impulse initiation.

Biological Pacemakers

Three situations in which biological materials may be used as opposed to an electronic pacemaker are (1) repair or creation of a sinoatrial node in sick sinus syndrome with intact AV nodal function, (2) creation of a demand ventricular pacemaker in individuals with high degree or complete heart block and atrial fibrillation, and (3) creation of an AV bridge in individuals with normal sinus node function and AV nodal disease (note, this is not a biological pacemaker, but a biological alternative to electronic AV sequential pacing). This presentation will focus on biological pacemakers rather than on AV bridges.

In creating a biological pacemaker we recognize that any intervention that increases inward current or decreases outward current during diastole in an excitable cell might induce pacemaker function. We have characterized what we believe to be the optimal characteristics of a biological pacemaker as follows:[3] It should create a stable physiological rhythm for the life of the patient, require no battery or electrode and no replacement, compete effectively in direct comparison with electronic pacemakers, confer no risk of inflammation/infection or neoplasia, adapt to changes in physical activity and/or emotion with appropriate and rapid changes in heart rate, propagate through an optimal pathway of activation to maximize the efficiency of contraction and cardiac output, and have limited and preferably no arrhythmic potential. We have deliberately set a high bar here because electronic pacemakers provide a standard for excellence as palliative therapy. Indeed, to exceed the success of electronic pacemakers, the biological pacemaker must represent cure, not palliation.

Biological pacemaking has incorporated two general approaches, that of gene therapy and that of cell therapy. Initial studies focused on gene therapy and generated transient successes, in keeping with the episomal delivery of the gene. While gene therapy remains an important field for investigation, cell therapies have also been explored. We will discuss gene and cell therapies sequentially.

Gene Therapy

Initial Attempts at Biological Pacemaking

Initial attempts at biological pacemaking focused on sympathomimetic modulation of existing pacemaker current. Edelberg *et al.*[9] reasoned that since β-adrenergic catecholamines can increase the sinus rate, overexpressing β-adrenergic receptors should enhance the heart rate. Hence, they incorporated the gene encoding the β_2-adrenergic receptor into a plasmid and injected this into porcine atrium *in situ*. Although the transfection was transient, they demonstrated both a faster atrial rate and an enhanced atrial rate response to catecholamine infusion in the injected animals. Concerns about this approach were (1) that therapy would rely on the ability of the existing sinoatrial node (or other endogenous pacemaker) to respond to catecholamine: if the node were in any way damaged or diseased the response might be unpredictable; and (2) catecholamines can be arrhythmogenic.

Miake *et al.* provided the first proof of concept experiments that alteration of ion channel function could create a biological pacemaker.[10] They reasoned that if repolarizing current were reduced, this would permit inward currents to depolarize the membrane during electrical diastole, resulting in a functioning biological pacemaker. To this end, they replaced three amino acid residues in the pore of the Kir2.1 gene that regulates the ion current, I_{K1}, and created a dominant negative construct. This was presumed to form multimeric, nonfunctional channels with endogenously expressed wild-type Kir2.1 and/or 2.2. The construct and green fluorescent protein (GFP) were packaged in a replication-deficient adenoviral vector that was injected into the left ventricular cavity of guinea pigs. After 3–4 days I_{K1} was about 80% reduced in isolated ventricular myocytes, and ventricular ectopic rhythms were seen on ECG.

The major concern about this approach was that diminishing a repolarizing current might excessively prolong repolarization. This concern was borne out in later experiments.[11] An additional problem was that the identity of the inward pacemaker current in the setting of reduced I_{k1} was not known. Preliminary data favored the occurrence of several inward currents and, in addition, it was hypothesized that the likely carrier is the Na–Ca exchanger.[12,13]

Using HCN to Create Biological Pacemakers

Proof of concept that increasing I_f in myocytes would lead to increases in pacemaker rate was provided by our group.[14–16] We elected to overexpress the HCN channel as the biological pacemaker because it not only carries the primary pacemaker current but because I_f activates on hyperpolarization and turns off at depolarized potentials. Therefore it has no effect to prolong action potential duration. After showing in rat ventricular myocytes in culture that I_f could be overexpressed by administering the HCN2 gene using a plasmid as the vector,[14] we questioned whether the channel expressed was autonomically regulated. Here, we infected ventricular myocytes with an adenoviral construct incorporating HCN2 and found cAMP regulation of the current was preserved, similar to that for wild-type I_f.[15] We also found that a β subunit, MiRP1, administered via a plasmid, increased pacemaker current density and the kinetics of exogenously expressed HCN2 in *Xenopus* oocytes.[16] The final *in vitro* experiment involved HCN2 overexpression in neonatal myocytes in culture using an adenoviral vector. The spontaneous rate increased, suggesting a similar approach might result in biological pacemaking *in situ*.[14,15] These results are demonstrated in Figure 20–2.

Our initial attempt at proof of concept *in vivo* involved injecting HCN2 into left atrial myocardium.[17] We used an adenoviral vector incorporating HCN2, with a second adenovirus expressing green fluorescent protein (to facilitate visualization of transfected cells). In terminal experiments we used vagal stimulation to induce sinoatrial slowing and/or AV nodal block, and studied the subsequent escape rhythms. The approach was successful and we pace-mapped the ectopic rhythms to the site of injection of the construct. We then isolated and studied cells from that region, which showed I_f at least 100-fold greater than native current.[17]

Although this approach successfully demonstrated functional escape rhythms, we believed it

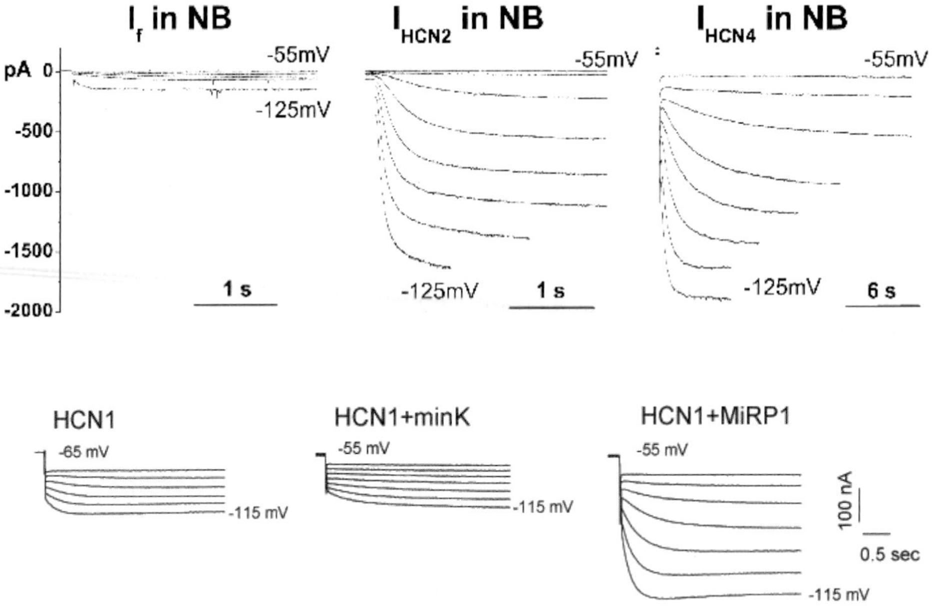

FIGURE 20–2. Top: Representative tracings from newborn (NB) rat ventricular myocytes transfected with HCN genes. Left, native I_f in newborn myocyte; center, transfection with the HCN2 gene; right, transfection with the HCN4 gene. Note the markedly larger currents in the center and right panels as compared to the left panel. Bottom: MiRP1 transfection increases the current in *Xenopus* oocytes transfected with HCN2. Left represents HCN2 alone; center HCN2 plus the β subunit minK; right HCN2 plus the β subunit MiRP1. Note the markedly larger current in the right panel. (Modified from Qu *et al.*[14] and Yu *et al.*,[16] with permission.)

important to test the concept in the ventricle. Hence, under fluoroscopic control, we injected the same construct into the left bundle branch system of intact dogs.[18] We again used vagal stimulation to slow the sinus rate or induce atrioventricular block and found that HCN2-injected dogs developed escape rhythms whose rates were about 25% faster than the idioventricular rates of control or sham-injected (GFP without HCN2) animals (Figure 20–3).[18] We then isolated left bundle branch fibers from the injection site and studied them with microelectrode techniques. They showed an automatic rate significantly faster from those generated at the same sites by tissues from control or sham-injected animals.[18] Current recordings from cells disaggregated from the same sites showed approximately 100-fold overexpression of I_f in HCN2-injected animals. Finally, immunohistochemistry demonstrated increased fluorescence to an anti-HCN2 antibody.

More recent experiments have focused on fine-tuning pacemaker properties using mutant or chimeric constructs. For example, we have used the E324A mutant channel, incorporating a single point mutation at position 324 of the parent mHCN2, and found that this elicits a sequence of complex changes: first, there is less channel and current expression with the mutant than the parent HCN2; however, there is a positive shift of both activation and cAMP responsiveness: the result is expressed as a baseline rate not very different from that with HCN2 alone, but there is a greater rate response to catecholamine.[19] Interventions such as this provide the means to optimize pacemaker constructs, which is a current goal.

Why Seek Alternatives to Gene Therapy?

An obvious advantage of the HCN-based approach to gene therapy is that it not only overexpresses members of the primary pacemaker gene family, but it does not induce excess prolongation of repolarization and it retains the function of autonomic responsiveness. However, there are problems with the viral vector approach: replication-deficient adenoviruses or naked plasmids represent episomal strategies and the construct administered is not incorporated into the cell's genome. Such expression of biological pacemaking is transitory. Moreover, the viral vector induces inflammation and there is also the risk of infection. Finally, some viruses that might be expected to result in genomic incorporation of a pacemaker construct carry an already-demonstrated risk of neoplasia.[3,4] Concerns such as these have led us and others to examine cell therapy approaches to biological pacemaking. These approaches have largely (albeit not exclusively) depended on xenografting human stem cells into animal hearts.

Cell Therapy

Human Embryonic Stem Cells

Research on embryonic stem cells has been proceeding for over 25 years, having been initiated by biologists interested in maturation during early stages of development.[20,21] Research on human embryonic stem cells is far more recent and has not only provided some of the most exciting prospects in science in recent decades,[22] but has unleashed a firestorm of criticism, primarily from religious and social conservatives.[23,24] The result has severely hampered human stem cell research

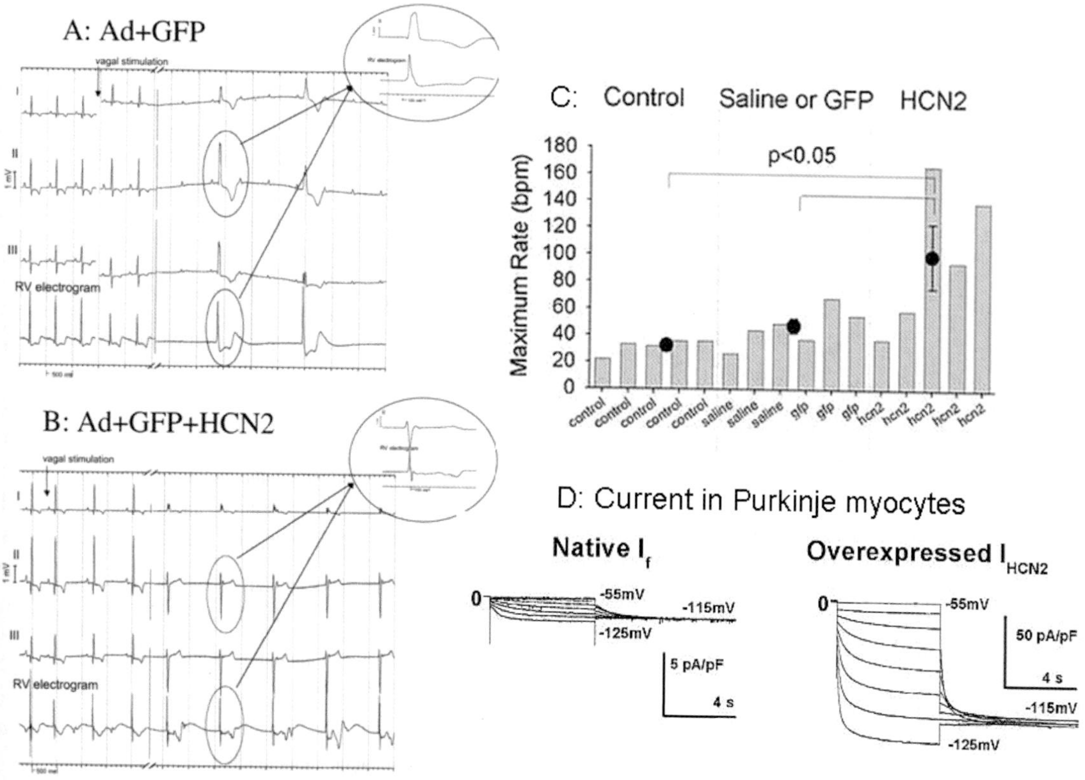

FIGURE 20–3. (A and B) Leads I, II, and III and a right ventricular electrogram (top to bottom) of the ECGs of two different dogs. (A) It was injected with an adenoviral vector carrying green fluorescent protein (GFP) alone. (B) It received the same vector incorporating GFP plus the HCN2 gene. Animals were anesthetized 6 days after injection and the vagi were isolated and stimulated (stimulation is marked by the arrows). The interval between traces is 22 sec in (A) and 5 sec in (B). The animal that received GFP developed an idioventricular rhythm having a slower rate than the animal receiving GFP + HCN2. Insets show the temporal relationship between the lead II QRS complex and the electrogram. (C) Posterior divisions of left bundle branch (construct injection site) were isolated from five control animals that had not been injected, six animals that received GFP, and five animals that received GFP plus HCN2 (each bar represents one animal). Note the rate generated by the bundle branches from the animals receiving HCN2 were significantly greater than those of the other two groups. (D) I_f in a Purkinje myocyte isolated from the left bundle branch of a control animal (left) and one receiving HCN2 (right). The current is markedly greater in the latter (note the vertical gains of 5 pA/pF on the left and 50 pA/pF on the right). (Modified from Plotnikov *et al.*,[18] with permission.)

in the United States and a number of other countries. The major contribution to date in human embryonic stem cell research on biological pacemaking has been provided by the Gepstein group.[25–27] They have used embryonic stem cells to create a cardiogenic line that has been implanted into the hearts of immunosuppressed pigs in complete heart block. Their implantation has resulted in stable idioventricular rhythms that have persisted for months, and whose initiating current appears consistent with I_f.

Yet, questions remain regarding the long-term consistency of function as well as whether the current providing pacemaker function is I_f or a family of currents. A major concern is the need for immunosuppression: most physicians and patients faced with a decision to pace biologically and immunosuppress, versus to pace electronically and not immunosuppress, would elect the latter approach.

Adult Human Mesenchymal Stem Cells

Because of the limitations of gene therapy and concerns about embryonic stem cells we turned to adult mesenchymal stem cells (hMSCs) to provide pacemaker function in the intact heart. hMSCs are multipotent stem cells that are expected to differentiate along mesenchymally derived lineages. Our strategy was to use them as platforms to carry HCN or other genes of interest to regions of the heart. We realized the key property needed for them to be effective platforms for gene delivery would be gap junctional coupling with adjacent myocytes. Without such coupling, the pacemaker signal could not be transmitted. Another complexity of cell implantation is the possibility of rejection by the host animal. We were encouraged here by reports suggesting hMSCs might be immunoprivileged.[28] For this reason, we studied them without the use of immunosuppression.

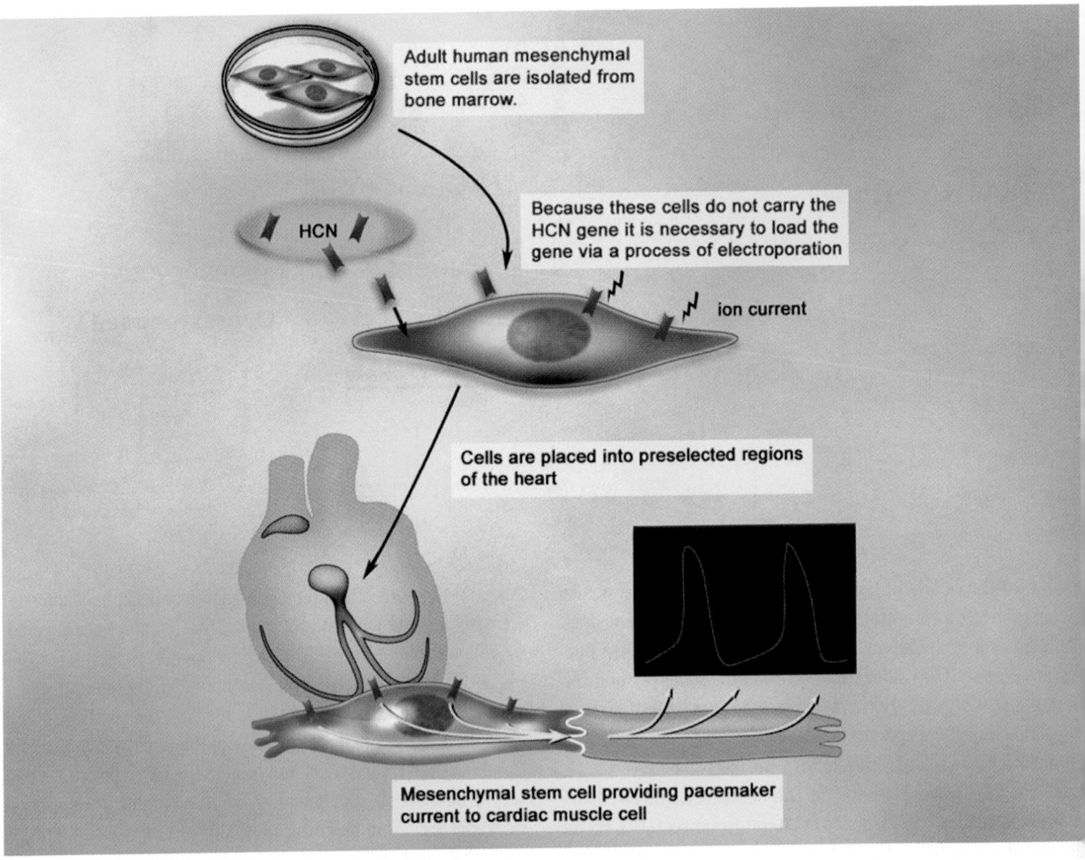

FIGURE 20–4. Experimental plan for hMSC-based pacemaker. See the text for discussion. [Modified from Dougherty M. CUMC Collaborates to Develop Biological Pacemaker. *In Vivo*. Columbia University Medical Center 2004;3(11):6, with permission.]

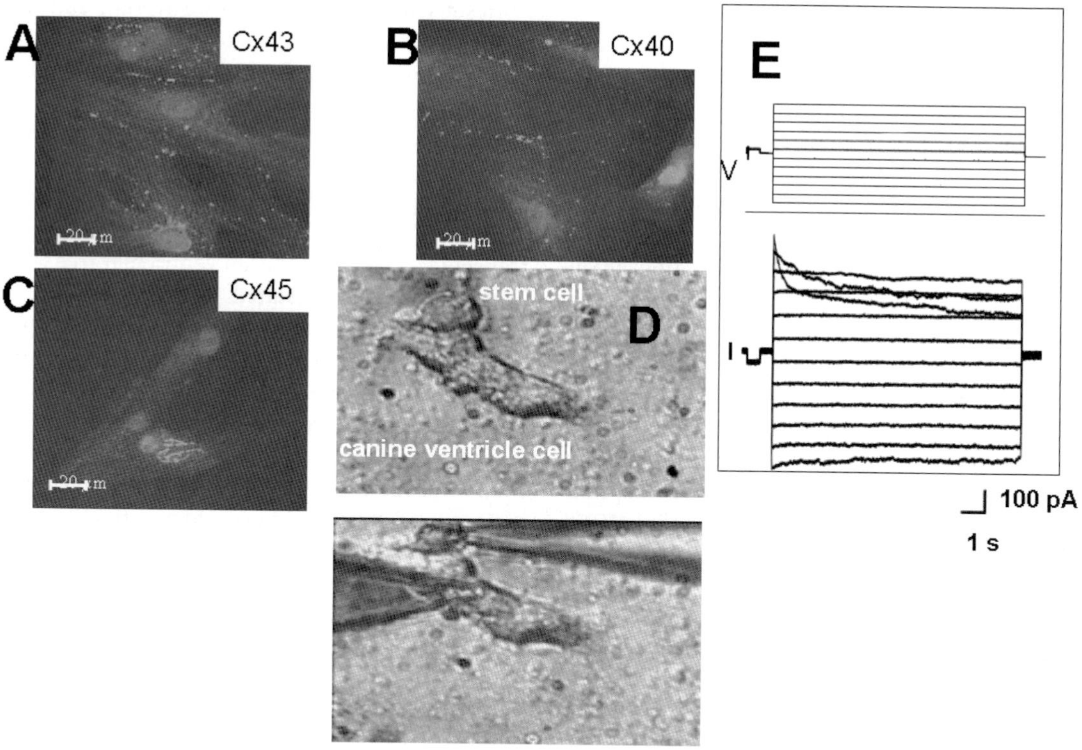

FIGURE 20–5. Immunohistochemical stains for connexin 43 (A), connexin 40 (B), and connexin 45 (C) in hMSCs. Note the punctate staining that is positive for Cx43 and Cx40. There is no staining for Cx45. (D) An hMSC and a canine ventricular myocyte in culture before (above) and after (below) impalement with electrodes. (E) The voltage protocol (V) and the current traces (I) are recorded. Note the asymmetric nature of the currents. (Modified from Valiunas *et al.*,[30] with permission.)

Figure 20–4 summarizes the strategy for working with hMSCs to create biological pacemakers.[3,4] Preliminary gene chip analysis showed no message for HCN2 or HCN4, some message for KCNQ1 (the gene encoding the α subunit for I_{Ks}), and abundant message for the gap junctional protein, connexin43 (Cx43). Heubach *et al.* reported a similar result[29] and performed biophysical studies indicating that hMSCs express a Ca-activated K current, a clofilium-sensitive outward current, and, occasionally, an L-type Ca current.

Our initial experiments *in vitro* tested the coupling of hMSCs to one another, to other cell lines, and to cardiac myocytes.[30] Effective gap junctional coupling was demonstrated physiologically via intercellular dye transfer and by passage of current between cells in a pair. The current traces were asymmetrical, reflecting the presence of Cx43 in myocytes and Cx43 and Cx40 in hMSCs and the formation of heterotypic channels (Figure 20–5).

The critical importance of having functional gap junctions in the cell pairs can be appreciated from the following. In the normal sinus node, cells incorporate a family of ion channel genes that includes the pacemaker gene HCN4.[6] I_f activates on hyperpolarization and initiates diastolic depolarization and action potentials that propagate to the rest of the atrium via low resistance gap junctions. While hMSCs can serve as a platform for HCN genes if appropriately loaded with them, they do not have the complement of channels required for initiating action potentials. Nor do they have the means to hyperpolarize such that overexpressed HCN channels will open. We hypothesized that if the hMSCs coupled to ventricular myocytes, then hyperpolarization of the latter would open the HCN channels in the hMSCs, and the HCN current generated by the stem cells would initiate an action potential in the myocyte.[3] The action potential can then propagate to other cells in the myocardium. Hence, we proposed using two independent cell types, each generating an essential component (the hMSC providing pacemaker current and the myocyte providing the ion channels needed to initiate an action potential). We hypothesized the two cell types might then operate as a single functional unit as suggested in Figure 20–4.

The other advantage of the hMSC was that it allowed us to build a pacemaker without using viral vectors. Rather, we used electroporation, which provides a transfection efficacy approximating 50%.[31] Having loaded hMSCs with HCN2, we demonstrated that the hMSC now generated I_f-like current (Figure 20–6) that responded to cesium and to autonomic modulation in a manner similar to native I_f.

In subsequent experiments we overlaid cultures of rat ventricular myocytes on an island of HCN2 and GFP-loaded hMSCs. These manifested a significantly faster beating rate than control cultures. These tissue culture experiments were predictive of subsequent intact animal studies.[31] Here, we loaded approximately one million hMSCs with HCN2 + GFP or GFP alone and injected them transepicardially into the left ventricular free wall. Vagal stimulation resulted in expression of an idioventricular rhythm at approximately 60 bpm that was pace-mapped to the injection site (Figure 20–7). The rate generated was significantly faster than the rates of hearts that received hMSCs with GFP.[31] We then excised the injected sites and found basophilic cells that stained positively for vimentin (a stain for mesenchymal tissues) and for the human antigen CD44 (Figure 20–7).[31] Abundant gap junctions were also demonstrated immunohistochemically among hMSCs and between hMSCs and muscle cells.[31]

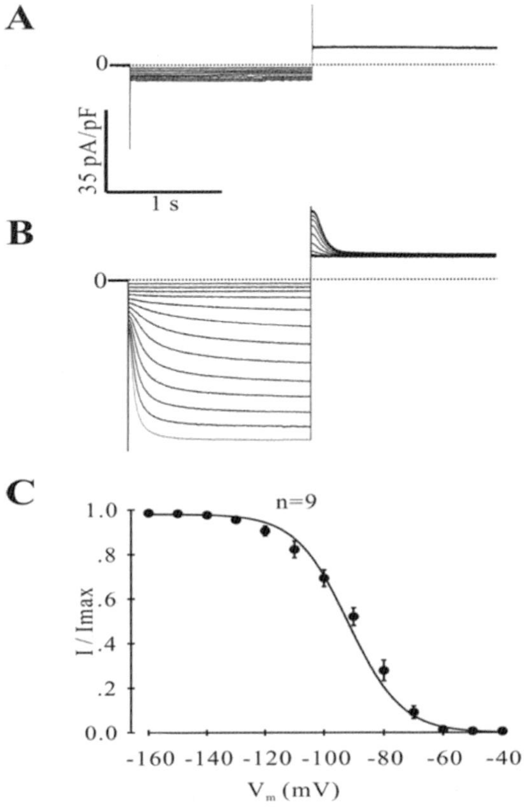

FIGURE 20–6. I_f recorded from a native hMSC (A) and I_{HCN2} from an hMSC in which HCN2 has been overexpressed via electroporation (B). Note the essential absence of I_f in the former. (C) The current–voltage relationship for I_{HCN2} (note the tail currents in the inset), which is seen to activate in a physiologically relevant voltage range. (Reprinted from Potapova *et al.*,[31] with permission.)

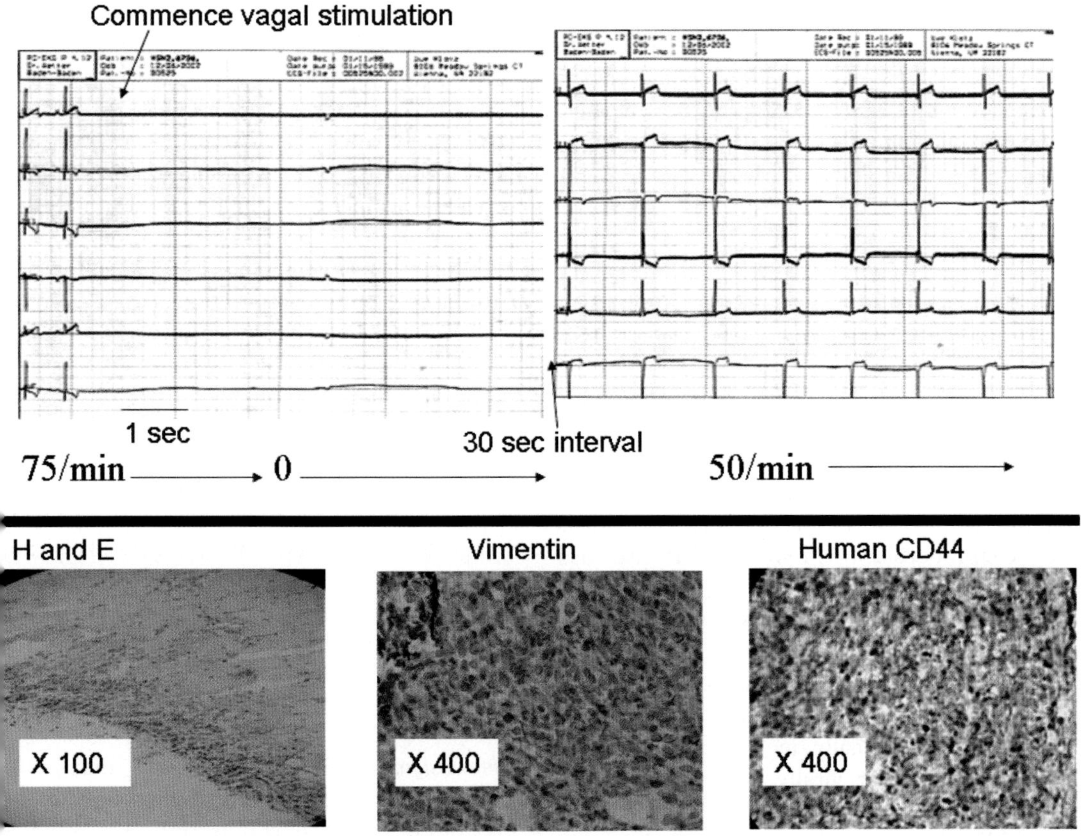

FIGURE 20–7. Expression of hMSC-based biological pacemaker function in canine heart. Upper panels: An experiment in a dog that received hMSCs containing GFP + HCN2 as a left ventricular transepicardial injection 3 days prior to this experiment. On this day, the animal was anesthetized and the vagi were isolated. Vagal stimulation led to a 20-sec period of cardiac arrest after which the escape pacemaker function demonstrated in the center panel was seen. This persisted for 3 min, at which time vagal stimulation was discontinued and a postvagal sinus tachycardia occurred. Subsequently, the origin of pacemaker activity was pace-mapped to the site of injection (data not shown). Lower panels: Histological sections of tissue removed from the injection site. Left: Hematoxylin and eosin stain showing basophilic cells abutting on normal myocardium. Center: Higher magnification of vimentin staining of the interface between the two cell types stained. Note the brown-staining mesenchymal cells overlying the myocytes. Right: The cells were also positive for the CD44 antigen, consistent with their human origin. (Modified from Potapova *et al.*,[31] with permission.)

New Approaches to Biological Pacemaking

This is a fast-developing field and new approaches are rapidly appearing. Among these are the expression of pacemaker genes in fibroblasts and their fusion with myocytes using polyethylene glycol, and the expression of the ion channels needed to generate a complete and automatic action potential in a cell line.[32,33] These and other approaches must be brought along much like the earlier ones to ultimately optimize biological pacemaking.

Another approach is that of tandem pacemaking, which incorporates the paired function of a biological and an electronic pacemaker.[19] Not only will such an approach be essential in any phase 1/phase 2 clinical trial but will probably be used for the first generation of biological pacemakers. Assuming these perform optimally, then the biological component to the pacemaker will provide the dominant and autonomically responsive rhythm to the heart, while conserving the battery life of the electronic component. The electronic component in turn will provide a backup for the biological system should it fail, as well as a means to monitor the function of the biological and electronic components.

What Remains to Be Learned?

There is much that remains in the learning curve regarding biological pacemaking. First, we need to decide on the optimal gene construct to be used for biological pacemaking: will it be one of the wild-type genes, HCN1–4, or a combination? Or will it be some other gene altogether? For example, in recent studies the engineering of a K channel to mimic some of the properties of HCN channels has been reported.[34] We and others are also working with mutant and chimeric genes that may manifest properties of activation, inactivation and autonomic response that are better adapted to biological pacemaking than the wild-type genes.[19,35] It is possible and even likely that those genes that are optimal functionally in hMSCs may differ from those best for virally administered gene therapy.

In addition, although experiments to date have been promising, there is much to learn about viral approaches and about stem cells. For the viruses, inflammation, infection, and the potential for neoplasia remain concerns. Also essential is to understand whether genomic incorporation of the gene construct will be possible, thereby conferring life-long function.

There is a different range of concerns for stem cells. First, will they evolve into other cell lineages? While we would not want to see cartilage or hematopoietic cells in the heart, their evolution into other cell types might not be problematic as long as gap junctional continuity and HCN function persisted. Will they migrate elsewhere in the body? This might create problems regardless of site and may necessitate the incorporation of a "death gene" within the construct.

Although there are concerns relating to inflammation, infection, graft rejection, and neoplasia, preliminary data for hMSCs are encouraging in that they indicate little to no inflammation and no rejection over a 6-week period postimplantation.[36] But long-term studies relating to both the effectiveness of the pacemaker and its potential toxicity are still needed, as is a direct comparison with electronic pacemakers.

Finally, delivery systems for biological pacemakers are a challenge currently being addressed via needle/electrode combinations operating through a catheter or hollow-lumen steerable catheters or combinations of both. The goal here is to tailor placement to the optimal site in any patient while minimizing trauma.

Conclusion

In closing, there are many approaches in what is an active and competitive field. Will we have biological pacemakers? This is highly likely. But which one will be the ultimate construct and how it will be administered and with what success are all matters still to be sorted out.

Acknowledgments. We express our thanks to Laureen Pagan for her careful attention to the preparation of this manuscript. The studies referred to were supported by USPHS-NHLBI Grants HL-28958, HL-67101, GM-55263, DK-60037, and HL-20558, and by Boston Scientific.

References

1. Scherf D, Schott A. *Extrasystoles and Allied Arrhythmias*. Chicago: Year Book Medical Publishers, 1973.
2. Zivin A, Bardy G, Mehra R. Cardiac pacemakers. In: Spooner PM, Rosen MR, Eds. *Foundations of Cardiac Arrhythmias*. New York: Marcel Dekker Inc., 2001:571–598.
3. Rosen MR, Brink, PR, Cohen IS, *et al.* Genes, stem cells and biological pacemakers. *Cardiovasc Res* 2004;64:12–23.
4. Rosen, M. Biological pacemaking: In our lifetime? *Heart Rhythm* 2005;2:418–428.
5. Hope RR, Scherlag BJ, El-Sherif N, *et al.* Hierarchy of ventricular pacemakers. *Circ Res* 1976;39:883–888.
6. Biel M, Schneider A, Wahl C. Cardiac HCN channels: Structure, function, and modulation. *Trends Cardiovasc Med* 2002;12:202–216.

7. Di Francesco D. A study of the ionic nature if the pacemaker current in calf Purkinje fibres. *J Physiol* 1981;314:377–393.
8. Borer JS. Drug Insight: I_f inhibitors as specific heart-rate-reducing agents. *Nat Clin Pract Cardiovasc Med* 2004;1:103–109.
9. Edelberg JM, Huang DT, Josephson ME, *et al.* Molecular enhancement of porcine cardiac chronotropy. *Heart* 2001;86:559–562.
10. Miake J, Marban E, Nuss HB. Gene therapy: Biological pacemaker created by gene transfer. *Nature* 2002;419:132–133.
11. Miake J, Marban E, Nuss HB. Functional role of inward rectifier current in heart probed by Kir2.1 overexpression and dominant-negative-suppression. *J Clin Invest* 2003;111:1529–1536.
12. Silva J, Rudy Y. Mechanism of pacemaking in I(K1)-downregulated myocyte. *Circ Res* 2003;92: 261–263.
13. Miake J, Nuss B. Multiple ionic conductance sustain Ik1-suppressed biopacemaking. *Circulation* 2003; 92:261–263.
14. Qu J, Altomare C, Bucchi A. *et al.* Functional comparison of HCN isoforms expressed in ventricular and HEK293 cells. *Pflugers Arch Eur J Physiol* 2002; 444:597–601.
15. Qu J, Barbuti A, Protas L, *et al.* HNC2 overexpression in newborn and adult ventricular myocytes: Distinct effects on gating and excitability. *Circ Res* 2001;89:E8–14.
16. Yu H, Wu J, Potapova I, *et al.* MinK-related peptide 1: A β subunit for the HCN ion channel subunit family enhances expression and speeds activation. *Circ Res* 2001;88:E84–87.
17. Qu J, Plotnikov AN, Danilo P Jr, *et al.* Expression and function of a biological pacemaker in canine heart. *Circulation* 2003;107:1106–1109.
18. Plotnikov AN, Sosunov EA, Qu J, *et al.* A biological pacemaker implanted in the canine left bundle branch provides ventricular escape rhythms having physiologically acceptable rates. *Circulation* 2004; 109:506–512.
19. Bucchi A, Plotnikov A, Shlapakova I, *et al.* Wild-type and mutant HCN channels in a tandem biological-electronic cardiac pacemaker. *Circulation* 2006;114(10):992–999.
20. vans MJ, Kaufman MH. Establishment in culture of pluripotential cells from mouse embryos. *Nature* 1981;292:154–156.
21. Martin GR. Isolation of pluripotent cell line from early mouse embryos cultured in medium conditioned by teratocarcinoma stem cells. *Proc Natl Acad Sci USA* 1981;78:7634–7638.
22. Gepstein L. Derivation and potential application of human embryonic stem cells. *Circ Res* 2002;91: 866–876.
23. Mooney C. *The Republican War on Science.* New York: Basic Books, 2005.
24. Scott CT. *Stem Cell Now.* New York: Pi Press, 2006: 96.
25. Kehat I, Kenyagin- Karsenti D, Snir M, *et al.* Human embryonic stem cells can differentiate into myocytes with structural and functional properties of cardiomyocytes. *J Clin Invest* 2001;108:407–414.
26. Kehat I, Gepstein A, Spira A, *et al.* High resolution electrophysiological assessment of human embryonic stem cells-derived cardiomyocytes: A novel in vitro model for the study of conduction. *Circ Res* 2002;91:659–661.
27. Kehat, I, Khimovich L, Caspi O, *et al.* Electromechanical integration of cardiomyocytes derived from human embryonic stem cells. *Nat Biotechnol* 2004;22:1282–1289.
28. Liechty KW, MacKenzie TC, Shaaban AF, *et al.* Human mesenchymal stem cells engraft and demonstrate site specific differentiation after in utero implantation in sheep. *Nat Med* 2002;6:1282–1286.
29. Heubach JF, Graf EM, Leutheuser J, *et al.* Electrophysiological properties of the human mesenchymal stem cells. *J Physiol* 2003;554(3):659–672.
30. Valiunas V, Doronin S, Valiuniene L, *et al.* Human mesenchymal stem cells make cardiac connexins and form functional gap junctions. *J Physiol* 2004; 555(3):617–626.
31. Potapova I, Plotnikov A, Lu Z, *et al.* Human mesenchymal stem cell as a gene delivery system to create cardiac pacemakers. *Circ Res* 2004;94:841–859.
32. Cho HC, Kashiwakura Y, Marban E. Creation of biological pacemaking by cell fusion. *Circulation* 2005;112:II-307 (abstract).
33. Cho HC, Kashiwakura Y, Azene E, *et al.* Conversion of non-excitable cells to self contained biological pacemakers. Circulation 2005;112:II-307 (abstract).
34. Kashiwakura Y,Cho HC, Azene E, *et al.* Creation of a synthetic pacemaker channel. *Circulation* 2005; 112:II-93 (abstract).
35. Bucchi A, Plotnikov AN, Shlapakova IN, Danilo P, Brink PR, Cohen IS, Rosen MR, Robinson RB. In vitro evaluation of a chimeric HCN based biological pacemaker predicts in vivo function. *Circulation* 2006;114:11-50.
36. Plotnikov AN, Shlapakova IN, Szabolcs MJ, *et al.* Adult human mesenchymal stem cells carrying HCN2 gene perform biological pacemaker function with no overt rejection for 6 weeks in canine heart. *Circulation* 2005;112:II-221.

Part II
Clinical Rhythmology: Diagnostic Methods and Tools

21
Diagnostic Electrocardiography

Preben Bjerregaard

Introduction

Almost any arrhythmia or conduction disturbance can occur as the sole manifestation of cardiac disease and the diagnosis, therefore, dependst upon a correct interpretation of the electrocardiogram (ECG). As recently pointed out by Shlomo Stern from Tel Aviv, Israel: "The electrocardiogram is still the cardiologist's best friend."[1]

Since Augustus Desire Waller recorded the first human ECG in 1887,[2] and its clinical usefulness was demonstrated by among others Sir Thomas Lewis and Sir James Mackenzie almost 100 years ago, the ECG has remained one of the most important diagnostic tools in medicine in a format that has remained unchanged since Goldberger in 1942[3] added the unipolar amplified extremity leads.

One of the fascinating aspects of the ECG is its diagnostic content, which may be unnoticed for a very long time and then suddenly, when pointed out, become obvious to everyone. Even today new features of ECGs are being discovered that are of prognostic importance or indicate new diseases. Most of them are related to cardiac repolarization.

In the following, a few clinical examples will be given of more recently discovered ECG abnormalities, which have turned out to be hallmarks of new diseases. The cases presented are real life stories from the author's archives. At a time when new diagnostic tests are developed almost on a daily basis, it is becoming more and more difficult to know when to use them and how to interpret the test results. It is then reassuring to know that the ECG is still one of the most valuable diagnostic tools in daily clinical practice, and knowing how to interpret it can be very rewarding.

The following chapters will deal with tools that have been developed to examine various electrocardiographic information in more detail and have therefore become the important next step in the workup of patients at risk. In some cases genetic screening is the only way to establish a diagnosis.

Case 1

Patient #8 (Table 21–1) was sitting in a restaurant when she suddenly collapsed with cardiac arrest. She was resuscitated, but with severe anoxic encephalopathy, and she died 2 weeks later. She had no history of cardiac disease or syncope prior to the event. She had a daughter (patient #16, Table 21–1) who had died suddenly at the age of 8 years while sitting at her desk in a classroom at school. The autopsy of our patient showed no organic cardiac disease or other explanation for her death. The first ECG shortly after admission to the hospital (Figure 21–1A) was interpreted as sinus tachycardia with right bundle branch block (RBBB) and right axis deviation. Even though the QT interval appeared prolonged, it was difficult to assess because of the wide QRS complex and tachycardia. The next day the heart rate was slightly slower and the QRS had normalized (Figure 21–1B). Repolarization changes in V1–V3 suggesting Brugada syndrome were now present, and a

Table 21–1. Family with Brugada syndrome, prolonged QT, and RBBB caused by mutation in the sodium channel gene SCN5A.[a]

		1 Greatgrandfather Seizure episodes for several years SCD while driving at age 51 ECG not available		
Siblings/grandparents				
	2 70-year-old female (wife) Asymptomatic ECG: normal	**3[X]** 72-year-old male, grandfather SCD, myocardial infarction (2006) QTc: 573 msec, RBBB Giant negative T waves V2–V6	**4[X]** 70-year-old male (brother) Asymptomatic QTc: 450 msec ICD	
5[X] 45-year-old male Collapse in college QTc: 466 msec Procainamide positive ICD	**6[X]** 44-year-old female Asymptomatic QTc: 483 msec ICD	**7[X]** 41-year-old male Asymptomatic QTc: 447 msec Brugada type 3 ICD	**8** 40-year-old female SCD (2003) QTc: 480 msec Brugada type 1	**9** 31-year-old male Asymptomatic QTc: 383 msec Brugada type 2 ICD
10 10-year-old female Asymptomatic QTc: 422 msec	**11** 22-year-old female Asymptomatic QTc: 404 msec		**12** 13-year-old male Asymptomatic QTc: 406 msec	**13** 8-month-old male QTc: 402 msec
14 7-year-old female Asymptomatic QTc: 420 msec	**15** 14-year-old female Williams syndrome QTc: 407 msec		**16** 8-year-old female SCD (1993) Ostial ridge left coronary artery	**17** 8-month-old male QTc: 403 msec
18[X] 4-year-old male Asymptomatic QTc: 429 msec ICD	**19** 10-year-old male Asymptomatic QTc: 398 msec			

[a]SCD, sudden cardiac death; ECG, electrocardiogram; ICD, implantable cardioverter defibrillator; RBBB, right bundle branch block; X, mutation carrier (patients #2, 12, 13, and 17 were not screened).

diagnosis of prolongation of the QT interval was made as well. The family was very interested in being ECG tested, and later all had genetic screening as well. Because of a delay in getting the results from genetic screening and the great anxiety in the family, the decision to insert an implantable cardioverter defibrillator (ICD) was made prior to getting the result from the genetic screening. Only patient #5 (Table 21–1) had additional testing done, which included the usual next steps in a patient suspected of having Brugada syndrome, namely, a procainamide challenge test and an electrophysiological (EP) study. They were both positive and in some ways supported the diagnosis of Brugada syndrome in other family members with the Brugada sign in the ECG. Lack of funding (health insurance or private money) prohibited further studies in other family members, and the implanted ICDs were graciously donated by a U.S. ICD manufacturer.

This family illustrates many of the problems we face on a daily basis dealing with primary electrical diseases of the heart, which are inheritable and have a high risk of sudden cardiac death (SCD). Problems exist when the genetic mutation is unknown, and the decision about who should have an ICD is based purely on clinical presentation and electrocardiographic phenomena; other

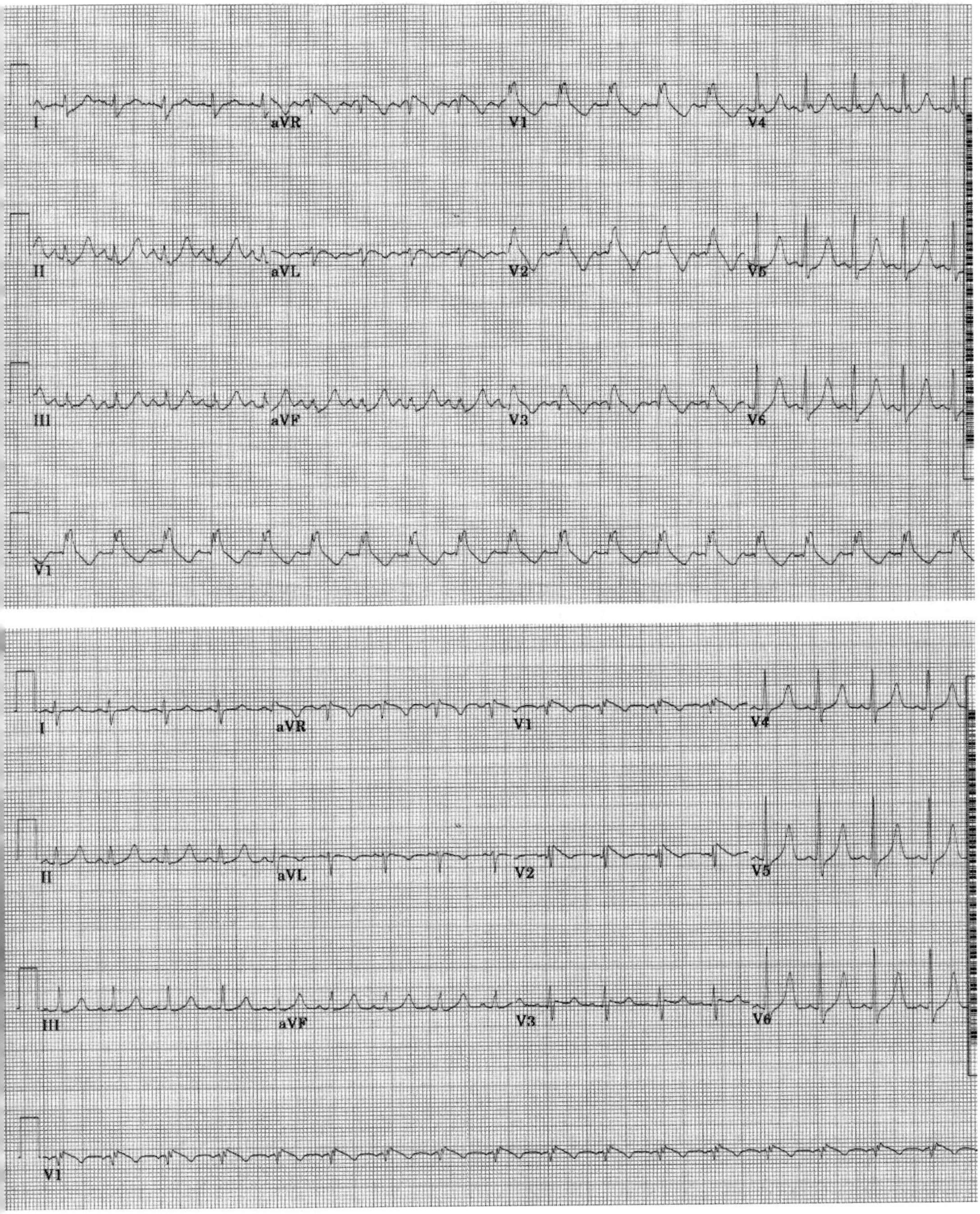

FIGURE 21–1. (A) A 12-lead ECG from patient #8 (Table 21–1) showing sinus tachycardia at a heart rate of 115 beats/min, RBBB, and right axis deviation. (B) A 12-lead ECG from patient #8 (Table 21–1) showing sinus tachycardia at a heart rate of 103 beats/min, right axis deviation, a QT-interval of 388 msec with QTc = 508 msec, and Brugada type 1 changes in V1–V3.

problems may arise when it becomes clear who the carriers of a deadly mutation are.

Patients #3 and #16 (Table 21–1) both illustrate how mistakes can be made in assuming that all patients who die suddenly in a family with an inheritable disease with a high risk of SCD also have the disease or die from it. Patient #3 (Table 21–1) had a very prolonged QT interval and the genetic mutation, but died from an acute myocardial infarction with cardiac arrest. He was resuscitated at home with severe anoxic encephalopathy as a consequence, but underwent cardiac catheterization prior to his death. He had earlier turned down the offer of an ICD. When the death certificate from patient #16 (Table 21–1) was found, it showed a congenital ostial fibrous ridge in the left coronary artery as the possible cause of death. Genetic testing on tissue available from the autopsy 13 years earlier showed no evidence of an SCN5A mutation.

Patient #9 (Table 21–1) illustrates how inconclusive or borderline ECG findings may be overinterpreted when they occur in a patient from a family with a high risk of SCD. This patient received an ICD based upon an ECG with Brugada type 2 changes (Figure 21–2) at the same time as his siblings received one. He was asymptomatic. When the result of the genetic screening became available, it became clear, however, that he was not a carrier. Since the type 2 Brugada sign can be a normal variant and a negative genetic screening for a known mutation can be considered very reliable, it is quite likely that this patient received an ICD he did not need. The patient has decided to keep the device until it needs replacement, at which time the genetic screening will be repeated.

Patient #18 (Table 21–1) is a healthy 4-year-old child with a normal ECG on the day of screening (Figure 21–3). He received an ICD because he was a carrier of the SCN5A mutation. His father (patient #5, Table 21–1) had received an ICD, and because the family was still unsure about the circumstances around the SCD of an 8-year-old girl in the family (patient #16, Table 21–1), they wanted the boy protected against SCD. He was, therefore, provided with an external defibrillator that he carried in a backpack for 2 years without any complications; he now has an implantable defibrillator.

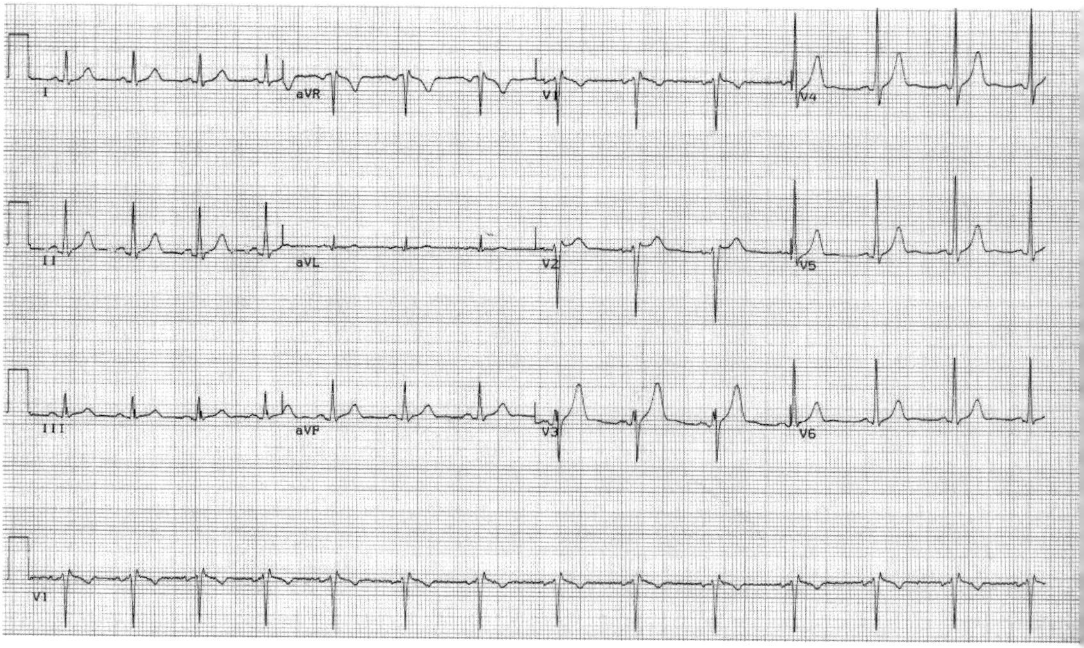

FIGURE 21–2. A 12-lead ECG from patient #9 (Table 21–1) showing sinus rhythm with a normal QT interval, but Brugada type 2 changes in lead V2.

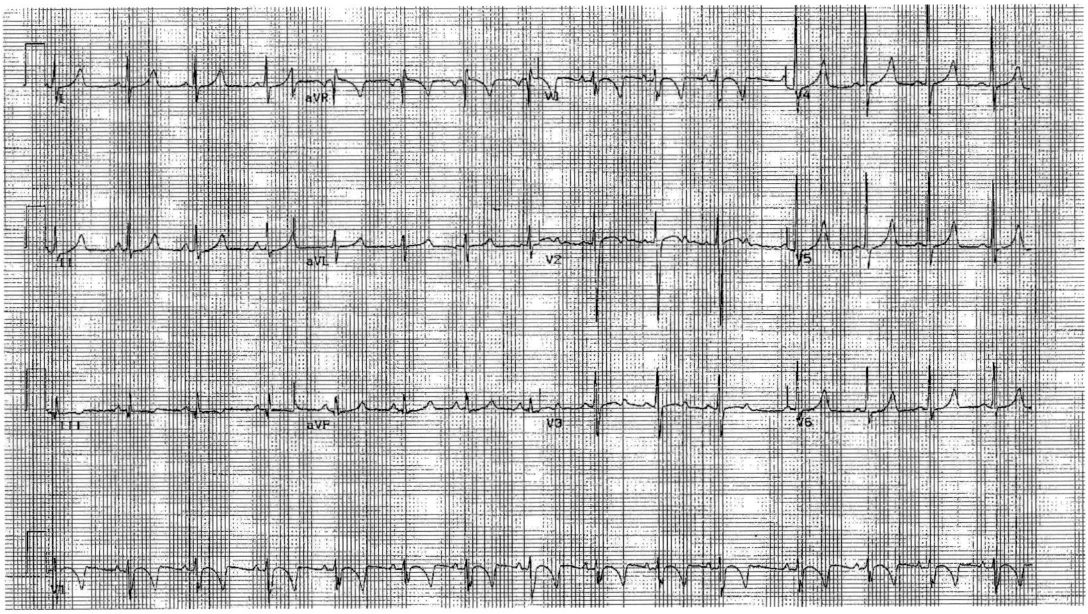

FIGURE 21–3. A 12-lead ECG from patient #18 (Table 21–1) showing normal sinus rhythm at a rate of 88 beats/min, a QT-interval of 360 msec with QTc = 432 msec, and nonspecific T wave abnormalities in V1–V3.

Mutations in the SCN5A gene encoding for the voltage-gated cardiac Na^+ channel have been linked to a variety of clinical entities causing sudden cardiac death, including Brugada sydrome, long QT syndrome, and progressive conduction system disease. While the diseases are distinct, the overall spectrum of related phenotypes is becoming very complex, and phenotype overlapping between these three diseases, as seen in our family, has also been described by others.[4–6]

Case 2

The supervisor in my laboratory with more than 20 years of experience in scanning of Holter recordings hardly believed her eyes when she was watched the nighttime continuous ECG recording of a 16-year-old girl. After a daytime recording with normal sinus rhythm at a maximum heart rate of 110 beats/min and only a few premature ventricular contractions (PVCs) (a few couplets and triplets) the heart rate at 2 AM started to gradually accelerate to rates as high as 180 beats/min, and remained above 100 beats/min for the rest of the night (Figure 21–4). The diary, which was later confirmed by both the patient and her mother, indicated that the patient had been sleeping all night. The next morning the patient had several similar episodes while she was physically active at home. All episodes followed the same pattern. A sudden acceleration in heart rate either as sinus, junctional, or atrial tachycardia was accompanied by ST depression and PVCs, initially isolated and uniform, but later, as the heart rate got faster, becoming multiform with couplets, triplets, and salvos. Occasionally atrial flutter or fibrillation would occur leading to a complex mixture of atrial and ventricular tachyarrhythmias (Figure 21–5). A special feature was bidirectional PVC as couplets (Figure 21–6). The 12-lead ECG, echocardiography, and an EP study in the patient were normal. When a low dose of isoproterenol (0.02 μg/kg/min) was administered, however, the arrhythmias were reproduced.

This clinical picture is very characteristic of catecholaminergic polymorphic ventricular tachycardia (CPVT). The mystery regarding the nightly episodes was solved when the patient informed us about taking 0.125 mg of hyoscyamine sulfate (an

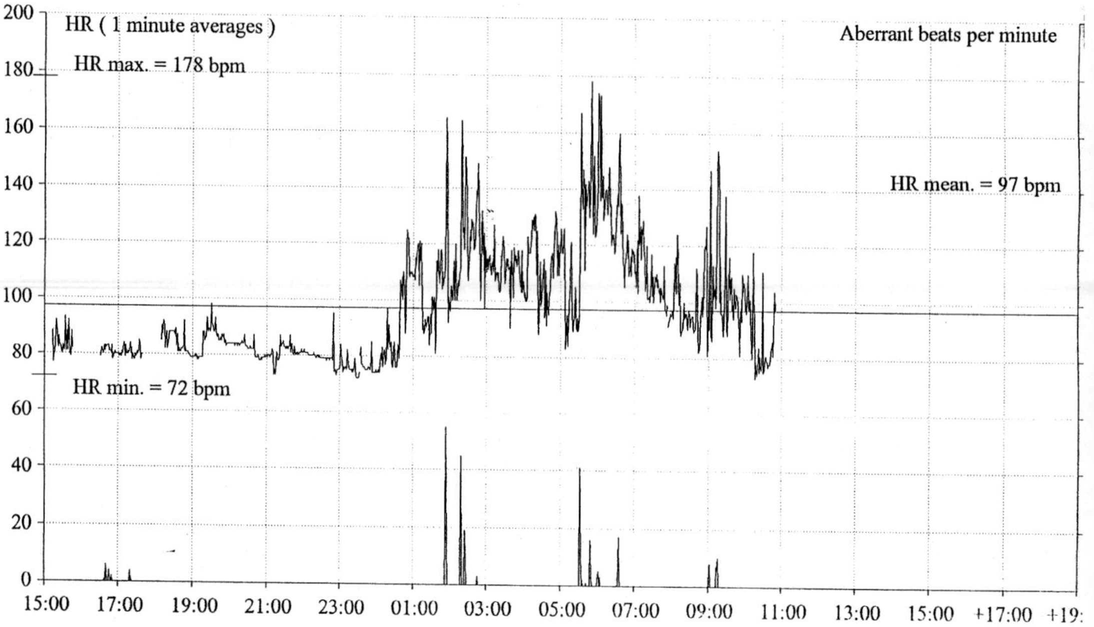

FIGURE 21–4. A 24-h trend of heart rate and number of aberrant beats in patient #7 (Table 21–2).

anticholinergic drug) at bedtime for an abdominal disorder. A Holter recording off the drug showed no arrhythmias during sleep.

The patient (#7, Table 21–2), who is now 25 years of age, presented with a 2-year history of approximately 10 episodes of syncope. They always happened during physical activity or emotional distress, and she would usually lose consciousness completely. She was treated with an ICD and β blocker, and has so far received only one shock by the ICD. She has had two additional syncopal episodes due to her usual tachyarrhythmia, but at a heart rate below the detection rate for ventricular fibrillation (VF) programmed at 220 beats/min. It is usually not feasible to program the detection rate lower, since it will lead to a higher increase in number of shocks, which are unnecessary, since most of the episodes terminate spontaneously. Due to the autosomal dominant inheritance of the disease she was strongly

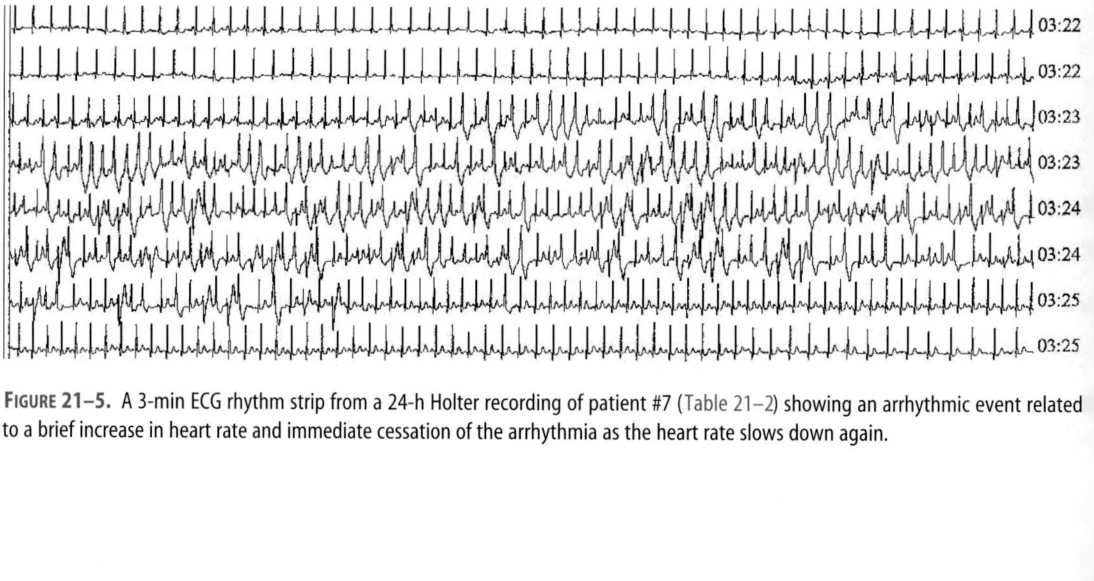

FIGURE 21–5. A 3-min ECG rhythm strip from a 24-h Holter recording of patient #7 (Table 21–2) showing an arrhythmic event related to a brief increase in heart rate and immediate cessation of the arrhythmia as the heart rate slows down again.

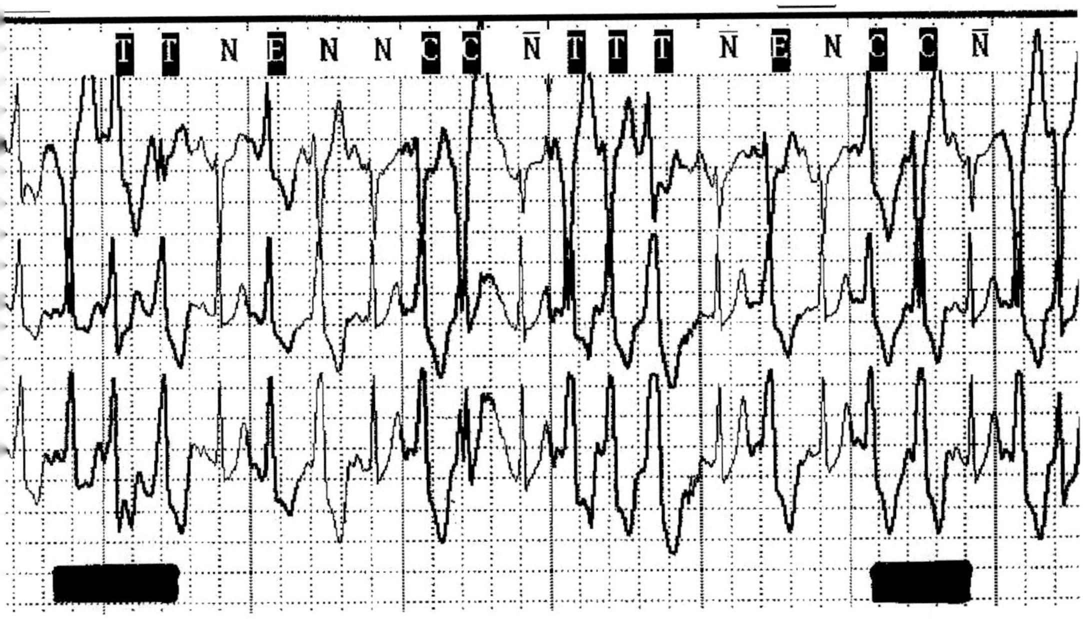

Figure 21–6. A brief ECG rhythm strip from patient #8 (Table 21–2) showing bidirectional PVCs in lead 1, while all the PVCs in leads 2 and 3 are uniform.

Table 21–2. Family with a clinical picture of catecholaminergic polymorphic ventricular tachycardia.[a]

	1 52-year-old greatgrandmother SCD while dancing		
Siblings/grandparent			
	2 62-year-old grandmother Recurrent syncope Normal ECG Positive Holter		3 19-year-old male Recurrent syncope SCD
Siblings/parents			
4 Newborn Congenital heart disease	5 24-year-old mother Recurrent syncope SCD	6 19-year-old female SCD (drowning?)	7 25-year-old mother Recurrent syncope Holter positive
Children			
	8 17-year-old male Recurrent syncope Holter positive ICD	9 17-year-old female Asymptomatic Holter negative	10 3-year-old male Asymptomatic
	11 16-year-old male Recurrent syncope Polydactyly Holter positive ICD		12 2-year-old male Asymptomatic

[a]SCD, sudden cardiac death; ECG, electrocardiogram; ICD, implantable cardioverter defibrillator.

encouraged not to become pregnant. As seen from Table 21–2, patients #10 and #12 are both her children. It is still not known whether they have the disease. They have been asymptomatic and have not yet been investigated further.

Table 21–2 clearly shows the tragic story that unfolded when the patient's family history was revealed. Our patient's mother (patient #2, Table 21–2) had lived with syncopal episodes since she was a teenager, and Holter monitoring clearly showed that she had the same diagnosis as her daughter, She felt some improvement during treatment with a β blocker and opted not to get an ICD. Her brother (patient #3, Table 21–2) started to have syncope at the age of 9 years and had to be taken out of school because some of the other children took advantage of the fact that he would pass out every time they scared him. It could happen several times a day and was considered a benign event, because he always woke up soon after. One time he did not wake up after passing out, and he died at the age of 19 years. The patient's oldest daughter (patient #5, Table 21–2) had collapsed in a skating ring and had serious brain damage after being resuscitated. She was pregnant at the time and gave birth to patient #11 (Table 21–2) while on life support, only to die 2 years later. She had a history of recurrent syncope, but no ECG documentation of arrhythmias prior to her death. Her diagnosis of CPVT was, however, established when both her children were diagnosed with the disease.

Patients #8 and #11 (Table 21–2) were 8 and 9 years old, respectively, when they were first evaluated by ECG and Holter monitoring. They had no history of syncope and been rather healthy. Patient #11 (Table 21–2), who was born while his mother was on life support, was born with syndactyly. A 12-lead ECG was normal in both children. During Holter monitoring patient # 8 (Table 21–2) had only 122 PVCs in a 24-h period, but a diagnosis of CPVT was highly likely due to their relationship to tachycardia and the presence of ventricular bigeminy and eight bidirectional PVCs as couplets in one of the recorded leads (V1-like). In the two other recorded leads all PVCs had the same morphology (Figure 21–6). Patient #11 (Table 21–2) had a total of 208 uniform PVCs during tachycardia with one episode of ventricular trigeminy and quadrigeminy. Despite the lack of symptoms and more complex tachyarrhythmias both were treated with a β blocker and an ICD. Despite high doses of β blocker they have both had arrhythmic events with ICD shocks that in both of them were possibly life-saving. Figure 21–7 shows a VF episode from the ICD of patient #11 (Table 21–2). It shows how ventricular tachycardia degenerates into ventricular flutter, and ventricular fibrillation prior to a 29.8-J shock is delivered and restores a narrow QRS complex rhythm.

The storage of arrhythmic events in implantable pacemakers and defibrillators offers new opportunities for documentation of the sequence of events behind cardiac arrest. Such events were recorded in both patients #8 and #11 (Table 21–2).

The clinical presentation of our patients is very similar to that reported as CPVT by others.[7–11] It is not known at which point in life the disease becomes clinically manifest, but syncope and SCD are rarely seen before the age of 4 years.[9] As a result, ECG recording during tachycardia may have to be repeated several times in a child before the diagnosis can be excluded. The strong relationship between symptoms and physical or emotional stress was very evident in our family as well as in the family presented by Fisher *et al.*[11] where "at times of general excitement (e.g., watching soccer), several members of the family often fainted at the same time."

Nam *et al.*[12] have examined the cellular mechanisms underlying the development of catecholaminergic ventricular tacycardia and have shown that under conditions of defective calcium handling, delayed afterdepolarization-induced extrasystolic activity can serve as a trigger for ventricular tachycardia and VF.

Genetic screening is pending in our family. If it turns out positive, it will be very helpful in making a correct diagnosis, especially in young children who are still asymptomatic. In 2000 Priori *et al.*[13] demonstrated that the cardiac ryanodine receptor gene (*RyR2*) is responsible for CPVT. A recent article by Testes *et al.*[14] accompanied by an editorial by Gussak[15] cautioned against using the clinical picture alone for the diagnosis of CPVT. Out of 11 patients diagnosed clinically with CPVT and referred for genetic screening, only 4 hosted novel CPVT1-associated *RyR2* mutations. Three patients

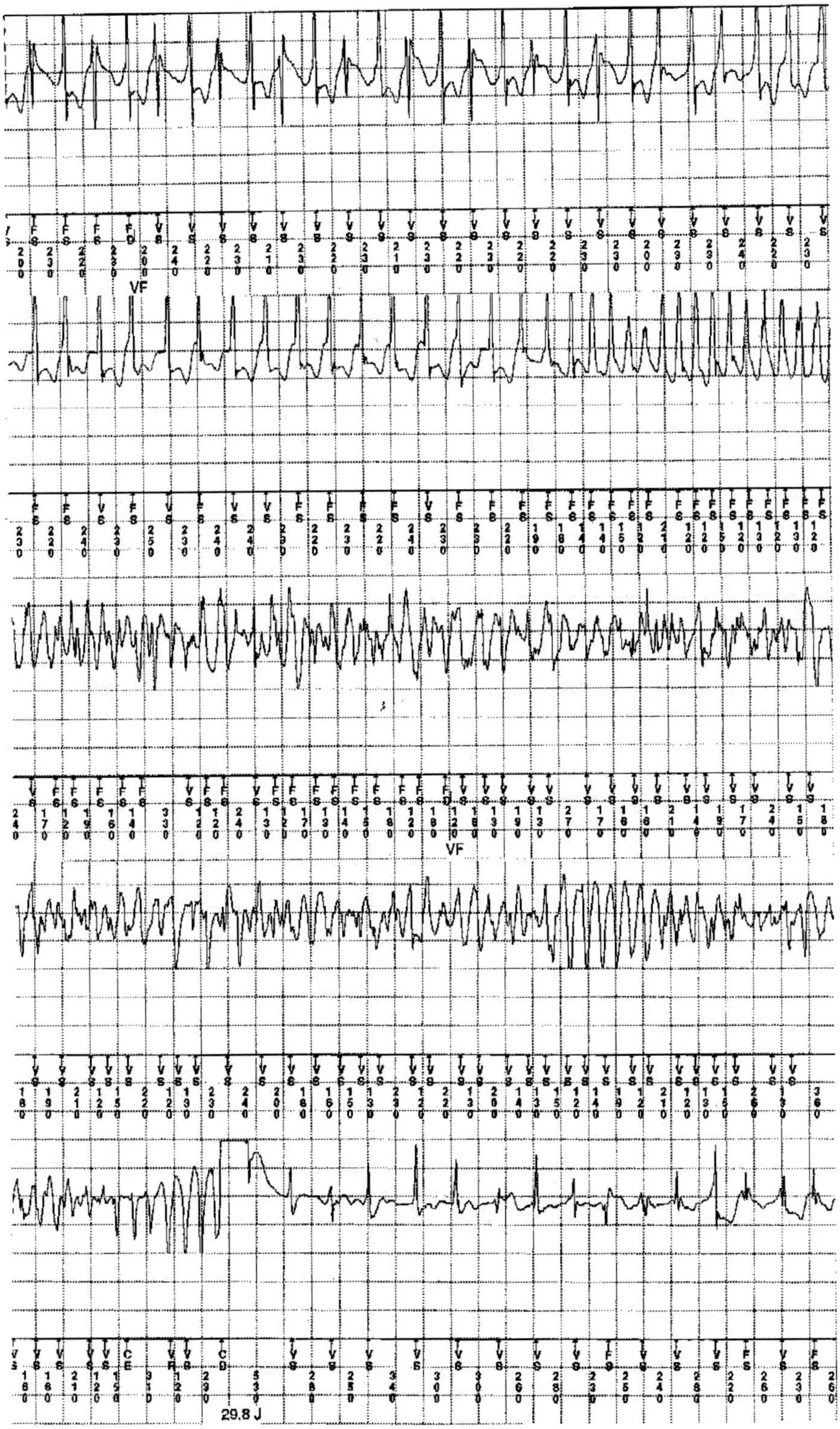

FIGURE 21–7. An arrhythmic episode with loss of consciousness in patient #11 (Table 21–2) retrieved from the memory of his ICD. It shows a gradual increase in heart rate with a bidirectional ventricular tachycardia leading to ventricular flutter and ventricular fibrillation terminated by a 29.8-J shock, which restores a narrow complex rhythm.

had Andersen–Tawil (AT)-associated mutations and one long QT5 (LQT5). Three were genotype negative. None of our patients had prolonged QT interval or abnormal U waves as described in AT syndrome, and none of them had periodic paralysis as also seen in this syndrome. It is of some interest, however, that patient #11 (Table 21–2) had syndactyly, which has been described as a feature of AT syndrome.

This case shows the benefit of obtaining an ECG recording in situations in which patients normally have symptoms, especially when the ECG at baseline is normal. If tachycardia is not present at any point during a 24-h recording, an exercise stress test is helpful. It also shows the importance of meticulously scrutinizing even a few innocent looking PVCs among more than 100,000 beats in a 24-h recording and considering their significance in the context of the clinical picture (patients #8 and #11, Table 21–2). If CPVT is suspected, bidirectional PVCs are a strong clue to the diagnosis. It is important, however, to examine consecutive PVCs in several leads, since bidirectional PVCs in some leads may appear uniform in other leads (Figure 21–6). As also pointed out by Gussak,[15] bidirectional PVCs or ventricular tachycardia characterized by a 180° alternating QRS axis on a beat-to-beat basis are not pathognomonic for CPVT, but are seen in patients with AT syndrome and ARVD2 as well.

Case 3

A 62-year-old African-American female with cor onary artery disease S/P percutaneous trans luminal coronary angioplasty (PTCA) and sten placement in the first obtuse marginal branch o the circumflex coronary artery 3 years earlier pre sented with intermittent chest pain radiating t her left arm, nausea, and dizziness over a 24-h period. Following nitroglycerine and β blocke therapy the patient became pain free. Cardia enzymes were normal. The ECG on admissio showed sinus rhythm with minimal T wave inver sion in leads II, aVF and V3–V4 (Figure 21–8). P waves were missing in V1 and V2 in only som ECG recordings, making it unlikely that this wa a significant finding. During the following 48h while the patient remained asymptomatic an hemodynamically stable, there were dramati changes in the ECG with marked prolongation o the QT interval and major global T wave inversio (Figure 21–9). The patient underwent cardia catheterization showing no coronary artery steno sis greater than 30%, but unexpectedly severe lef ventricular (LV) dysfunction with anterolatera and diaphragmatic hypokinesis and an LV ejec tion fraction of 30%. A remarkable finding was a very slow flow in the left anterior descending cor onary artery. During the catheterization, when an intracoronary injection of adenosine was given in

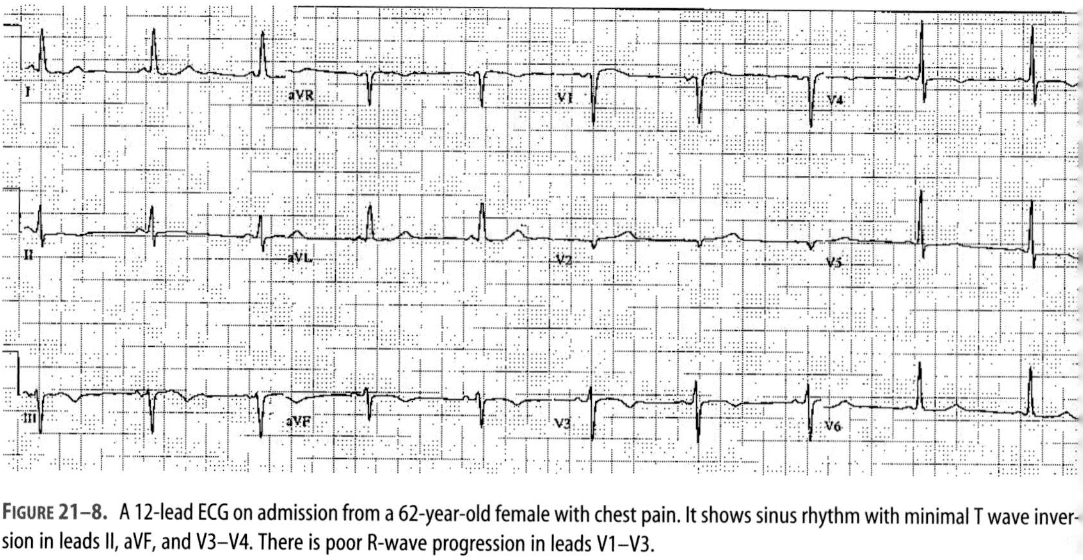

FIGURE 21–8. A 12-lead ECG on admission from a 62-year-old female with chest pain. It shows sinus rhythm with minimal T wave inversion in leads II, aVF, and V3–V4. There is poor R-wave progression in leads V1–V3.

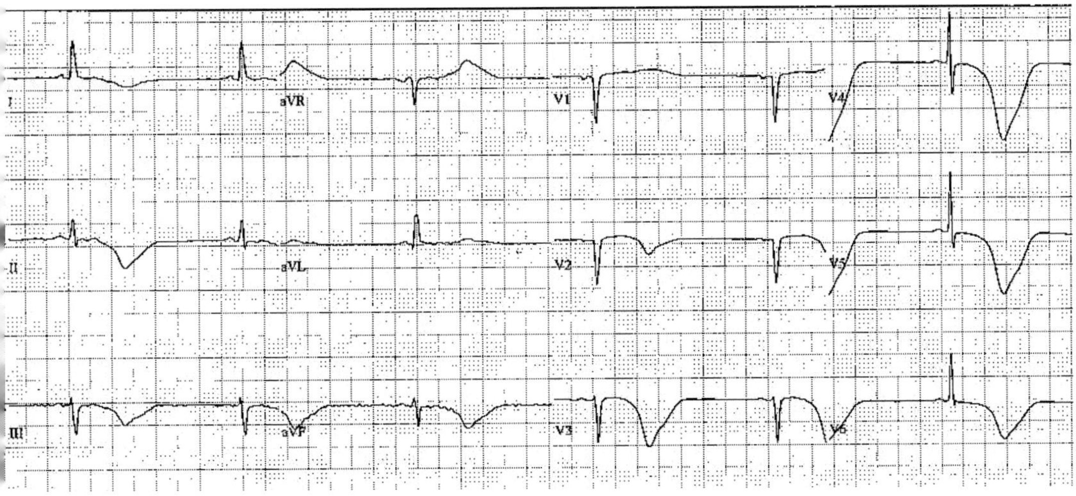

GURE 21–9. A 12-lead ECG 2 days following admission for chest ain in a 62-year-old female. It shows sinus bradycardia at 37 eats/min with a QT interval of 728 msec with QTc = 571 msec and major global T wave inversion. The patient was asymptomatic at the time of the ECG recording.

rder to assess the significance of a stenosis of the ight coronary artery, the patient had a 5-sec pisode of nonsustained VF.

This case represents an electrocardiographic henomenon that lacks an understanding of both he etiology and the cellular electrophysiological nechanism. Major T wave inversions with signifi-ant QT prolongation have been observed in atients following intense emotional distress,[16] erebrovascular accidents,[17,18] severe electrolyte listurbances, and myocardial ischemia,[19] some-imes accompanied by stunning of the myocar-lium. In the latter setting is has been part of a new yndrome called Tako-Tsubo syndrome. It was irst described in Japan in 1991[20] and received its ame from a round-bottomed narrow-necked apanese fishing pot used for trapping octopus. 'he left ventricle in cases of unexplained stunning f the myocardium, which is being reported at an ncreased frequency, often takes the shape of such pot. The syndrome is characterized by transient eft apical and mid-ventricular wall motion abnor-nalities in the absence of acute occlusive coro-ary artery disease.[21,22] The disorder occurs most ommonly in postmenopausal women, and the pisodes are often preceded by an acute increase n psychological or emotional stress. The electro-ardiographic changes have varied, but major lobal T wave changes are often seen. The severe LV dysfunction is usually reversible. We have had such patients referred to us for ICD implantation with the indication based upon a low ejection fraction during the acute phase of the disease, and found LV function to be normal when the patients were examined later. It is, therefore, strongly recommended that no decision about ICD implantation be made before the ECG has normalized and the patient's LV function is reevaluated.

Even though vasospasm and catecholamine cardiotoxicity have both been proposed as possible etiologies of the T wave changes and stunning of the myocardium described above, none of them has been proven. Ibanez and Benezet-Mazuecos in a recent editorial in the *Mayo Clinic Proceedings*[23] have provided strong arguments for the theory that Tako-Tsubo syndrome is an "aborted myocardial infarction" resulting from an acute atherothrombotic event with rapid and complete lysis of the thrombus. Much more work is needed, however, before these interesting cases can be fully explained.

Concluding Remarks

Brugada syndrome, long QT syndrome, catecholaminergic polymorphic ventricular tachycardia, and Tako-Tsubo syndrome are all examples of diseases in which electrocardiographic findings are crucial for a correct diagnosis, and the diagnosis is mainly based upon the ECG. Several other diseases could have been included, and there are many more cases in which a correct diagnosis of arrhythmia in the setting of a known disease can be crucial for the outcome of a patient.

In a recent editorial in the *Journal of Electrocardiology*, J. Willis Hurst[24] raised serious concerns about our current level of teaching electrocardiography in medical schools and to our residents. Long gone are the days when a stethoscope, a chest X-ray, and an ECG were the only tools available for the diagnosis of heart diseases. Due to the excitement over important newer tools such as echocardiography, nuclear cardiology, and cardiac catheterization, electrocardiography has been left out.

I hope that the cases I have presented have shown how fascinating electrocardiography can be, and how an unusual finding may lead to the discovery of a new disease or turn out to be the key to solve the mystery of syncope or SCD in a family over several generations.

As stated by J. Willis Hurst: "Excellent knowledge of electrocardiography is needed now by internists and cardiologists more than any previous time in medical history."

References

1. Stern S. Electrocardiogram. Still the cardiologist's best friend. *Circulation* 2006;113:e753;e756.
2. Waller AG. A demonstration on man of electromotive changes accompanying the heart's beat. *J Physiol* 1887;8:229–234.
3. Goldberger E. A simple indifferent, electrocardiographic electrode of zero potential and a technique of obtaining augmented unipolar, extremity leads. *Am Heart J* 1942;23:483–492.
4. Bezzina C, Veldkamp MW, Van den Berg MP, Postma AV, Rook MB, Viersma J-W, Van Langen IM, Tan-Sindhunata G, Bink-Boelkens TE, Van der Hout AM, Mannens MM, Wilde AA. A Single Na^+ channel mutation causing both long-QT and Brugada syndromes. *Circ Res* 1999;85:1206–1213.
5. Priori SG, Napolitano C, Schwartz PJ, Bloise R, Crotti L, Ronchetti E. The elusive link between LQT3 and Brugada syndrome. The role of flecainide challenge. *Circulation* 2000;102:945–947.
6. Van Den Berg MP, Wilde AAM, Viersma JW, Brouwer J, Haaksma J, Van Der Hout AH, Stolte-Dijkstra I, Bezzina CR, Van Langen IM, Beaufor Krol GCM, Cornel JH, Crijns HJGM. Possibl bradycardic mode of death and successful pac maker treatment in a large family with features c long QT syndrome type 3 and Brugada syndrom *J Cardiovasc Electrophysiol* 2001;12:630–636.
7. Benson DW, Gallagher JJ, Sterba R, Klein G Armstrong BE. Catecholamine induced doub tachycardia: Case report in a child. *Pacing Cli Electrophysiol* 1980;3:96–103.
8. Eldar M, Belhassen B, Hod H, Schuger C Scheinman MM. Exercise-induced double (atria and ventricular) tachycardia: A report of thre cases. *J Am Coll Cardiol* 1989;14:1376–1381.
9. Leenhardt A, Lucet V, Denjoy I, Gray F, Ngo DD, Coumel P. Catecholaminergic polymorphi ventricular tachycardia in children. A 7-yea follow-up of 21 patients. *Circulation* 1995;91 1512–1519.
10. Myrianthefs M, Cariolou M, Eldar M, Minas M Zambartas C. Exercise-induced ventricular arrhyth mias and sudden cardiac death in a family. *Ches* 1997;111:1130–1133.
11. Fisher JD, Krikler D, Hallidie-Smith KA. Familia polymorphic ventricular arrhythmias. A quarte century of successful medical treatment based o serial exercise-pharmacologic testing. *J Am Co Cardiol* 1999;34(7):2015–2022.
12. Nam G-B, Burashnikov A, Antzelevitch C. Cellula mechanisms underlying the development of cate cholaminergic ventricular tachycardia. *Circulatio* 2005;111:2727–2733.
13. Priori SG, Napolitano C, Memmi M, Colombi B Drago F, Gasparini M, DeSimone L, Coltorti F Bloise R, Keegn R, Filho FESC, Vignati G, Benata A, DeLogu A. Clinical and molecular characteriza tion of patients with catecholaminergic polymor phic ventricular tachycardia. *Circulation* 2002;106 69–74.
14. Tester DJ, Arya P, Will M, Haglund CM, Farley AL Makielski JC, Ackerman MJ. Genotypic heteroge neity and phenotypic mimicry among patient referred for catecholaminergic polymorphic ven tricular tachycardia genetic testing. *Heart Rhythm* 2006;3:800–805.
15. Gussak I. Molecular pathogenesis of catecholamin ergic polymorphic ventricular tachycardia: Se matters! *Heart Rhythm* 2006;3:806–807.
16. Ro AS, Gellman J. A case of global T-wave inver sions and impaired left ventricular functioning following intense emotional distress. *Clin Cardio* 2003;26:397.
17. Kacharava AG, Ahmed A, Ware DL. QT changes associated with intracranial hemorrhage. *J Cardiovasc Electrophysiol* 2000;11:1181.

18. Inoko M, Nakashima J, Haruna T, Nakano K, Yanazume T, Nakane E, Kinugawa T, Ohwaki H, Ishikawa M, Nohara R. Serial changes of the electrocardiogram during the progression of subarachnoidal hemorrhage. *Circulation* 2005;112:e331–e332.
19. Rebeiz AG, Al-Khatib SM. A case of severe ischemia-induced QT prolongation. *Clin Cardiol* 2001;24: 750.
20. Dote K, Sato H, Tateishi H, Uchida T, Ishihara M. Myocardial stunning due to simultaneous multivessel coronary spasms: A review of 5 cases. *J Cardiol* 1991;21:203–214.
21. Rosenmann D, Balkin J, Butnaru A, Wanderman K, Klutstein M, Tzivoni D. Transient left ventricular apical ballooning. *Cardiology* 2006;105:124–127.
22. Abi-Saleh B, Iskandar SB, Schoondyke JW, Fahrig S. Tako-Tsubo syndrome as a consequence of transient ischemic attack. *Rev Cardiovasc Med* 2006;7: 37–41.
23. Ibanez B, Benezet-Mazuecos J. Takotsubo syndrome: A Bayesian approach to interpreting its pathogenesis. *Mayo Clin Proc* 2006;81(6):732–735.
24. Hurst JW. Where have all the teachers of electrocardiography gone? *J Electrocardiol* 2006;39:112.

22
Ambulatory Monitoring (Holter, Event Recorders, External, and Implantable Loop Recorders and Wireless Technology)

Rajesh N. Subbiah, Lorne J. Gula, George J. Klein, Allan C. Skanes, Raymond Yee, and Andrew D. Krahn

Introduction

Elucidating the underlying cause of unexplained syncope, palpitations, or other possible arrhythmia-related symptoms is a formidable clinical challenge. Cardiac monitoring supplements the most important "test" in patients with syncope or palpitations, that of a thoughtful history and physical examination.[1,2] Ideally, comprehensive physiological monitoring during spontaneous symptoms would constitute what, at present, is an unattainable gold standard test for establishing a cause. Short of that goal, establishing an accurate symptom–rhythm correlation can often provide a diagnosis.

Ambulatory outpatient monitoring is a powerful diagnostic tool for the evaluation of cardiac arrhythmias. Evolving technologies have provided a wide array of monitoring options for patients suspected of having cardiac arrhythmias, with each modality differing in duration of monitoring, quality of recording, convenience, and invasiveness.

Holter Monitoring

Short-term electrocardiographic monitoring via 3 or, in some cases, 12 surface electrodes is the most common initial investigation in patients who present with syncope or palpitations. Typically this occurs in the emergency room or primary care setting with telemetry and continuous monitoring. The diagnostic yield, however, is generally low. In a pooled analysis by Linzer *et al.*, among patients with symptoms of syncope or presyn cope, there was a 4% correlation between symp toms and arrhythmias with Holter monitoring fo more than 12 h.[3]

The observations on electrocardiographi monitoring must be correlated with the clinica presentation, as findings may be unrelated i observed in the absence of symptoms. The likeli hood of another syncopal episode occurrin during the monitoring period is the major limit ing factor. Presyncope is a more common even during ambulatory monitoring, but is less likel to be associated with an arrhythmia.[4,5] Addition ally, the ubiquity of presyncope as a symptom i the community makes its utility as a surrogate fo syncope relatively uncertain.

Holter monitoring is useful where an arrhyth mic etiology is suggested historically or in unex plained syncope in a patient at relatively high ris for arrhythmia (i.e., underlying structural hear disease or abnormal baseline electrocardiogram) The Holter monitor is a portable battery-operate device that connects to the patient using bipola electrodes and provides recordings from up to 1 electrocardiographic leads. Data are stored in th device using analog or digital storage media. Th data are transformed into a digital format an analyzed using interpretive software. Additiona markers for patient-activated events and tim correlates are included to allow greater diagnosti accuracy. Continuous electrocardiographic moni toring is possible for 24 h to a maximum o 48 h (see Figure 22–1). This may allow the docu mentation of symptomatic and/or asymptomati events.

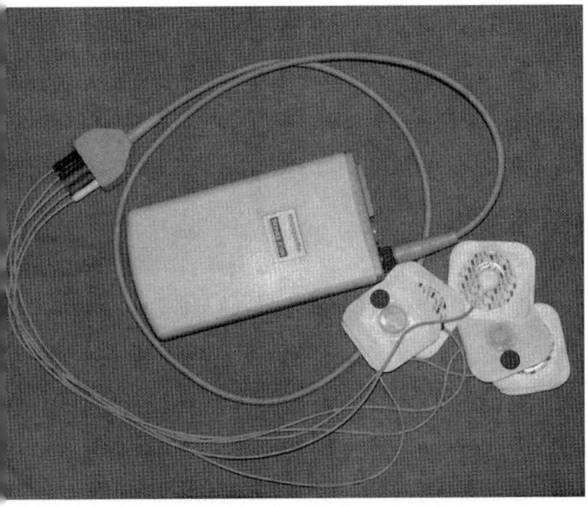

GURE 22–1. Holter monitor. The recording device (center) is orn by the patient using a shoulder strap or belt loop, attaching three to five skin electrodes for continuous monitoring. An event utton (not shown) at the top of the housing of the device is essed in the event of symptoms to mark the recording. See text r discussion.

There are, however, a number of limitations. atients may not experience symptoms or cardiac rrhythmias during the Holter recording. The hysical size of the device may hinder the ability f patients to sleep comfortably or engage in ctivities that precipitate symptoms. Patients are urther inconvenienced because the devices have o be removed while showering or bathing. There s also significant variability in patient documenation of activated events, such that accurate ymptom–rhythm correlation is undermined. It is herefore not surprising that Holter monitoring as a low diagnostic yield. In several large series f patients utilizing 12 h or more of ambulatory nonitoring for investigation of syncope only 4% ad recurrence of symptoms during monitorng.[3,6,7] The overall diagnostic yield of ambulatory r Holter monitoring was 19%. These studies eported symptoms that were not associated with rrhythmias in 15% of cases. The causal relationhip between the arrhythmia and syncope was ncertain. Uncommon asymptomatic arrhythnias such as prolonged sinus pauses, atrioventricular block (such as Mobitz type II block), and onsustained ventricular tachycardia can provide mportant contributions to the diagnosis, often nstigating further investigations to rule out strucural heart disease and other precipitating factors. While these observations necessitate prompt attention, it is important to interpret the results in the clinical context of the syncopal presentation so common causes of syncope such as neurocardiogenic syncope are not unduly excluded.

It is also important to understand that normal ambulatory electrocardiographic monitoring does not exclude an arrhythmic cause for syncope. If the pretest probably is high for an arrhythmic cause, then further investigations such as prolonged monitoring or electrophysiological studies are required. One study has investigated extending the duration of ambulatory Holter monitoring to 72 h.[6] In this study an increase in the number of asymptomatic arrhythmias detected was observed, but not the overall diagnostic yield. In our institution we typically use Holter monitoring for 48 h. It is a noninvasive test that provides information to establish a rhythm profile in patients and the diagnosis in those patients with frequent symptoms. The more frequent the symptoms, the higher the diagnostic yield of Holter monitoring. The apparent modest yield of Holter monitoring presumably reflects the primary care use of the device in patients with frequent symptoms facilitating a symptom–rhythm correlation. This leads to selection bias in the referral population, leading to an apparent nearly futile yield in referred patients who, by definition, have failed short-term monitoring.

Transtelephonic Monitors and External Loop Recorders

Transtelephonic electrocardiographic monitors are recording devices that transmit data via an analog phone line to a base station (Figure 22–2). The received signal is then converted to an interpretable recording that is displayed or printed as a single lead rhythm strip. There are two specific types of devices. The first does not save a recording of the rhythm for later playback and requires the patient to transmit the data "live" to the base station where it can be analyzed. The second type of device, with solid-state memory capacity allowing recording and storage of electrocardiographic signals during symptoms, has replaced the nonrecording units. The electrocardiographic signals are collected prospectively for 1–2 min. The major

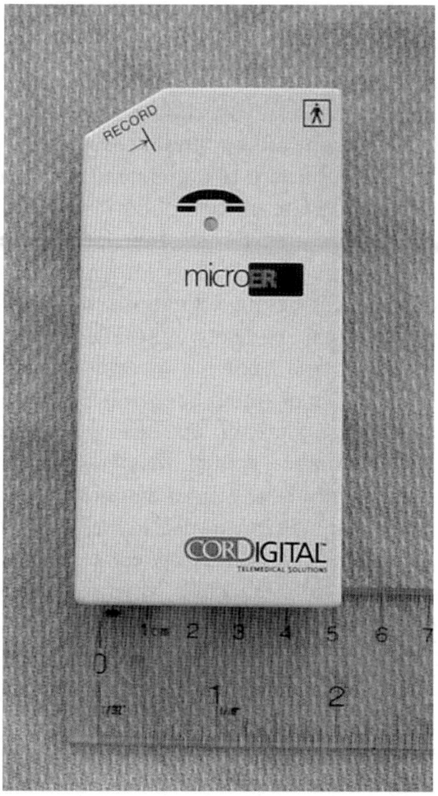

FIGURE 22–2. Transtelephonic monitors. The device is lightweight and portable and is easily placed in a handbag or pocket. Four recording electrodes are present on the back of the device to permit single lead rhythm strip capture. A record button (top left) is pressed in the event of symptoms, and the recorded event is transmitted to a base station over an analog phone line.

limitation with this device is the requirement that symptoms persist long enough for the device to record the event, and the inability to record the events that surround the onset of symptoms.

An external cardiac loop recorder continuously records and stores an external single modified limb lead electrogram with a 4- to 18-min memory buffer (Figure 22–3, left). After the onset of spontaneous symptoms the patient activates the device, which stores the previous 3–6 min of recorded information as well as the following 1–2 min. The device memory is then "frozen." In lay terms, it answers the question: "What just happened?" The captured rhythm strip can subsequently be uploaded and analyzed (Figure 22–4). This system can be used for weeks to months provided weekly

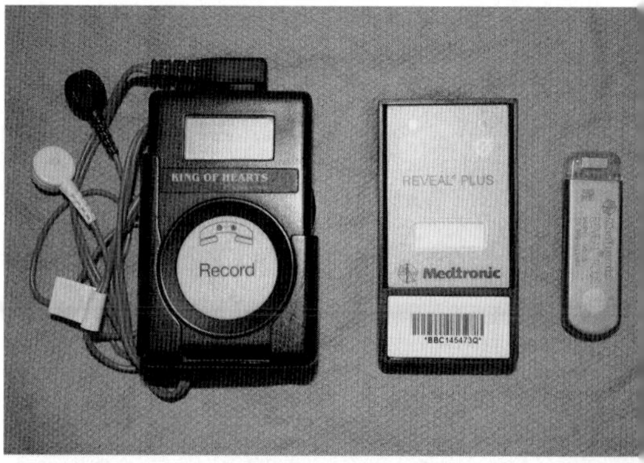

FIGURE 22–3. Loop recorders. An external loop recorder (left) wi cables that attach to the patient. The record button is pressed the event of symptoms to store the previous 9 min and the ensuir 1 min. The phone receiver is also placed over this button to tran mit data over an analog phone line. An implantable loop record (right) and patient activator (center). The patient activator is use to "freeze" symptomatic events that are retrieved with a pac maker programmer. Automatic events can also be captured (s text for discussion).

battery changes are performed. The recordin device is attached with two leads to the chest wa of the patient and needs to be removed for bathin or showering.

Long-term compliance with this device can b challenging because of electrode and skin-relate

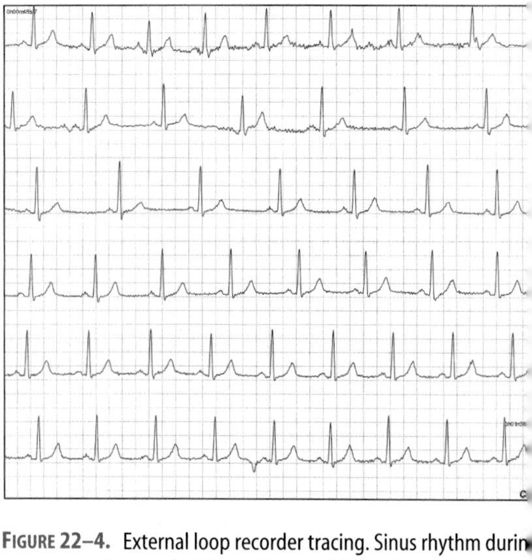

FIGURE 22–4. External loop recorder tracing. Sinus rhythm durin presyncope is recorded in a 43-year-old female with recurrer unexplained syncope and presyncope. The fluctuation in heart rat is suggestive of neurocardiogenic syncope.

roblems and waning of patient motivation in the bsence of symptom recurrence. Linzer *et al.* eported the use of patient-activated loop recorders in 57 patients with syncope and nondiagnostic ndings on history, physical examination, and 2- Holter monitoring.[8,9] A diagnosis was obtained 1 14 of 32 patients who had recurrence of symptoms. Device malfunction, patient noncompliance, or inability to activate the recorder was esponsible for the lack of diagnosis in the remaining 18 patients. Other studies have also reported imilar findings[9,10] and demonstrated that loop ecorders are complementary to 24-h ambulatory lectrocardiographic monitoring. The diagnostic ield for external loop recorders in these three tudies[3,9,10] ranged from 24% to 47%, with the ighest yield in patients with palpitations.

A prospective randomized clinical trial compared the utility of external loop recorders to conentional Holter monitoring in a community-based eferral population with syncope and presynope.[11] Not surprisingly, the ability to obtain a ymptom–rhythm correlation increased from 2% for Holter monitoring to 56% for the external oop recorder ($p < 0.001$), which allowed an ncreased duration of monitoring from 48 h to 4 veeks. A higher diagnostic yield was also obtained mong patients randomized to Holter monitoring vho remained undiagnosed and crossed over to se of a loop recorder. This trial suggests that oop recorders should be considered as first ine technology when attempting to establish a ymptom–rhythm correlation in the initial workup f patients with syncope. Unfortunately, patient r device-related failed activation occurred in 4% of loop recorder patients, limiting their useulness in some patients.[11] Analysis of factors peraining to use of external loop recorders has evealed a particularly low diagnostic yield among atients who are unfamiliar with technology, live lone, or have low motivation for achieving a iagnosis (Gula *et al.*, 2004).[12] More recently, eiffel *et al.* retrospectively compared the results btained by Holter monitoring, loop recording, nd autotriggered loop recording in 600 patients rom a database of approximately 100,000 patients. he autotriggered loop recording approach proided a higher yield of diagnostic events (36%) ompared to loop recording (17%) and Holter nonitoring (6.2%).[13]

The external loop recorder appears to have its greatest role in motivated patients with frequent symptoms in whom spontaneous symptoms are likely to recur within 4–6 weeks. Given that it is noninvasive and cost effective, it should be considered in all patients in whom an arrhythmic cause for syncope is suspected, keeping in mind that the major limitation of this device is the need to continuously wear external electrodes.

Implantable Loop Recorders

The implantable loop recorder (ILR) is a relatively recent investigational tool in undiagnosed syncope that permits prolonged monitoring without external electrodes. It is ideally suited to patients with infrequent recurrent syncope thought to be secondary to an arrhythmic cause. Similar to the external loop recorder, it is designed to correlate physiology with recorded cardiac rhythms, but unlike the external loop recorder, it is implanted and therefore devoid of surface electrodes and accompanying compliance issues. The ILR also monitors much longer time periods than an external loop recorder. Currently the ILR (Medtronic Reveal Plus Model 9526) has a pair of sensing electrodes with 3.7-cm spacing on a small elongated recording device 6 cm long, 2 cm wide, and 0.8 cm thick, weighing 17 g (Figure 22–3 right). The battery life is 18–24 months. The device can be implanted subcutaneously in the chest wall with local anesthetic and antibiotic prophylaxis.

Prior to implantation, cutaneous mapping should be performed to optimize the sensed signal to avoid T wave oversensing, which can falsely be interpreted as a high rate episode. An adequate signal can usually be obtained anywhere in the left hemithorax.[14] The recorded bipolar signal is stored in the device as 21 min of uncompressed or 42 min of compressed signal. A compressed signal is generally used due to marginally better quality than the uncompressed signal, which maximizes memory capability. The patient, along with a spouse, family member, or friend, is instructed in the use of the activator at the time of implant. Once an episode is recorded (i.e., a presyncopal or syncopal event occurs) the memory is "frozen" by the patient or a relative by applying a nonmagnetic hand-held activator (Figure 22–3 center).

The episode is then uploaded for interrogation to a pacemaker programmer (Medtronic 9790). Though heart rate is usually easily discerned, p waves can occasionally be difficult to interpret. The most recent version of the ILR has programmable automatic detection of high and low heart rate episodes, as well as pauses.

A classification system for recorded events has been proposed by Brignole *et al.*[15] (Table 22–1) that assigned the mechanism of syncope according to the pattern of bradycardia recorded during spontaneous syncope. An example of the cardioinhibitory component of neurocardiogenic or vasovagal syncope is illustrated in Figure 22–5. This would be considered a 1A response. Figure 22–6 illustrates a primary bradycardia (1C response), highly suggestive of intrinsic AV node disease. This classification is useful for researc purposes for event classification, and is likely t prove useful in directing therapy once validated

Currently there are several studies establishin the efficacy of ILR in the diagnosis of syncope.[16–] The largest of these studies is a multicenter stud of 206 patients.[19] The majority of patients ha undergone noninvasive and invasive testin including head-up tilt testing and electrophysio logical studies. The etiology of syncope wa arrhythmic in 22% of patients, sinus rhythm wit exclusion of arrhythmia in 42% of patients, an no further episodes occurred in 22% of patients. Bradycardia was the most commonly detecte arrhythmia (17% vs. 6% tachycardia), usuall leading to pacemaker implantation.[19] From thi study, 4% of patients failed to properly activat

Table 22–1. ISSUE classification of detected rhythm from the ILR.[a]

Classification	Sinus rate	AV node	Comment
Asystole (RR > 3 sec)			
1A	Arrest	Normal	Progressive sinus bradycardia until sinus arrest probably vasovagal
1B	Bradycardia	AV block	AV block with associated sinus bradycardia probably vasovagal
1C	Normal or tachycardia	AV block	Abrupt AV block without sinus slowing suggests intrinsic AV node disease
Bradycardia			
2A	Decrease >30%	Normal	Probably vasovagal
2B	HR < 40 for >10 sec	Normal	Probably vasovagal
Minimal HR change			
3A	<10% variation	Normal	Suggests noncardiac cause: unlikely vasovagal
3B	HR increase or decrease10–30%, not <40 or >120 bpm	Normal	Suggests vasovagal
Tachycardia			
4A	Progressive tachycardia	Normal	Sinus acceleration suggests orthostatic intolerance or noncardiac cause
4B	N/A	Normal	Atrial fibrillation
4C	N/A	Normal	Supraventricular tachycardia
4D	N/A	Normal	Ventricular tachycardia

Source: Adapted from Brignole *et al.*[15] with permission.

[a]ILR, implantable loop recorder; AV, atrioventricular; HR, heart rate; bpm, beats per minute; N/A, not applicable.

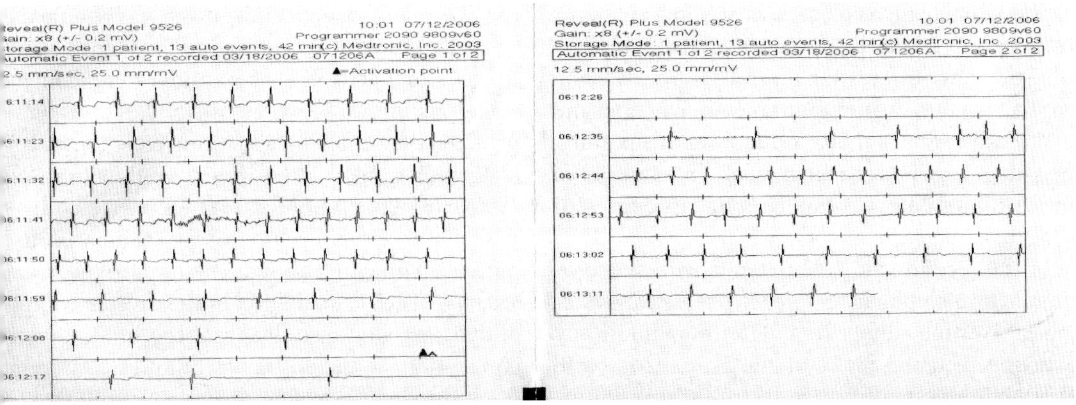

FIGURE 22–5. Automatic event detection from an implantable loop recorder (ILR). This is a typical tracing of an event captured by an ILR during syncope in a patient. The arrow and letter A denote automatic activation when the device detects a 3-sec pause. Each line constitutes 10 sec of a single lead rhythm strip. Note the slowing of the sinus rate prior to onset of a prolonged pause, which resulted in syncope. This is consistent with the diagnosis of neurocardiogenic syncope (ISSUE classification 1A).

the device and thus did not establish a symptom–rhythm correlation. Multivariate modeling did not identify any significant preimplant predictors of subsequent arrhythmia detection other than a weak association with advancing age and bradycardia. No age group had an incidence of bradycardia greater than 30%, suggesting a limited role for empiric pacing in the unexplained syncope population.[19]

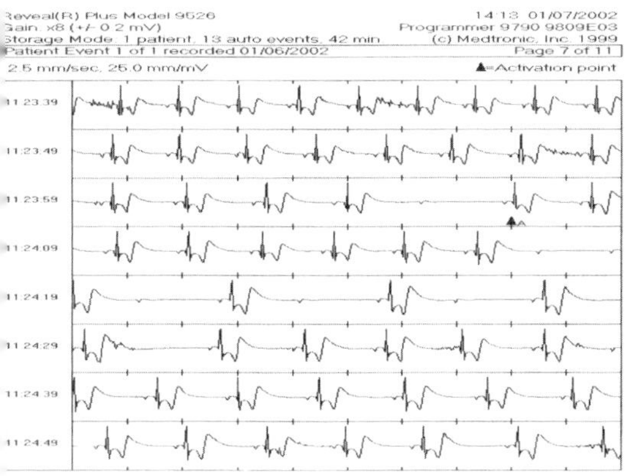

FIGURE 22–6. Manual event detection from an implantable loop recorder (ILR). Manual activation during presyncope in a 73-year-old male with two previous episodes of unexplained syncope. Note that the sinus rate and pr interval are unchanged surrounding the period of 2:1 atrioventricular (AV) conduction. This is classified as a 1C response by the proposed ISSUE classification, suggesting intrinsic AV node disease.

Further studies have highlighted the potential utility of ILR in the diagnosis of syncope. In a group of patients with ongoing seizures despite anticonvulsant therapy, Zaidi *et al.* performed cardiac assessment including head-up tilt testing and carotid sinus massage in all patients, and implantation of an ILR in 10 patients.[20,21] Two of the 10 patients with an ILR had marked bradycardia preceding a seizure: one was due to sinus pauses and the other was due to heart block. Importantly, this study suggested seizures that are atypical in presentation may have a cardiovascular cause in as many as 42% of cases, and cardiovascular assessment including long-term cardiac monitoring with an ILR may play a role in select patients with atypical seizures.

In recent studies[22,23] from the International Study on Syncope of Uncertain Etiology (ISSUE) investigators, ILRs were implanted in three different groups of syncopal patients to assess cardiac rhythm during syncope after conventional testing. The first study involved tilt tests in 111 patients with unexplained syncope, and loop recorders implanted after the tilt test, regardless of result.[23] Syncope recurred in 34% of patients in both the tilt-positive and tilt-negative group, with marked bradycardia or asystole the most common recorded arrhythmia during follow-up (46% and 62%, respectively). The heart rate response during tilt testing did not predict spontaneous heart rate response, with a much higher incidence of asystole than expected based on demographics or tilt response. This study suggests that observations during tilt testing correlate poorly with cardiac rhythm during spontaneous syncope, and that bradycardia is more common in this population than previously recognized. An example of the cardioinhibitory component of vasodepressor syncope is illustrated in Figure 22–5.

In the second study, 52 patients with syncope, bundle branch block, and negative electrophysiological testing underwent ILR implantation.[22] Syncope recurred in 22 of the 52 patients with conduction system disease. Long-term monitoring demonstrated marked bradycardia mainly attributed to complete AV block in 17 patients, while it excluded AV block in 2 patients. Three patients did not properly activate the device after symptoms. This study confirmed that negative electrophysiological testing does not exclude intermittent complete AV block, and that prolonged monitoring or consideration of permanent pacing is reasonable in this population.

The third study examined the spontaneous rhythm in 35 patients with syncope, overt heart disease, and negative electrophysiological testing.[24] The underlying heart disease was predominantly ischemic or hypertrophic cardiomyopathy with moderate left ventricular dysfunction. Although previous studies have suggested that patients with negative electrophysiological testing have a better prognosis, there remains concern regarding risk of ventricular tachycardia in this group. Symptoms recurred in 19 of the 35 patients (54%), with bradycardia in 4, supraventricular tachyarrhythmias in 5, and ventricular tachycardia in only 1 patient. There were no sudden deaths during 16 ± 11 months of follow-up.

A prospective randomized trial compared early use of the ILR for prolonged monitoring to conventional testing in patients undergoing a cardiac workup for unexplained syncope.[18,25] Sixty patients (age 66 ± 14 years) with unexplained syncope were randomized to "conventional" testing with an external loop recorder, tilt test, and electrophysiological study versus prolonged monitoring with an implantable loop recorder with 1 year of monitoring. Patients were excluded if they had a left ventricular ejection fraction less than 35%. If patients remained undiagnosed after their assigned strategy, they were offered crossover to the alternate strategy. A diagnosis was obtained in 14 of 27 patients randomized to prolonged monitoring, compared to 6 of 30 undergoing conventional testing (52% vs. 20%, $p = 0.012$). Overall, prolonged monitoring was more likely to result in a diagnosis than conventional testing (55% vs. 19%, $p = 0.0014$). Bradycardia was detected in 14 patients undergoing monitoring, compared to 3 patients with conventional testing (40% vs. 8%, $p = 0.005$). These data highlight the diverse etiology of syncope, and also illustrate the limitations of conventional diagnostic techniques. Although there is clear selection bias in enrollment of patients referred to an electrophysiologist for workup, this study suggests that tilt testing has a modest yield at best when applied to all patients undergoing investigation for unexplained syncope, and that electrophysiological testing is of very limited utility in patients with preserved left ventricular function.

A recent prospective, multicenter observational study (ISSUE 2) investigated the efficacy of therapies based on ILR diagnosis of recurrent suspected neurocardiogenic syncope.[26] Patients were included in the study if they experienced three or more clinically severe syncopal episodes over 2 years without significant electrocardiographic or cardiac abnormalities. Patients with postural hypotension and carotid sinus syncope were excluded. After the first documented episode of syncope after ILR implantation, the device was interrogated and therapy was prescribed accordingly. The 1-year recurrence rate of syncope in 392 patients was 33%. Among 103 patients with a documented episode, 53 patients were randomized to specific therapy; 47 received a pacemaker due to asystole and 6 received antitachyarrhythmia therapy (catheter ablation, four; implantable defibrillator, one; and antiarrhythmic drug, one) and the remaining 50 patients did not receive specific therapy. The 1-year recurrence rate among the 53 patients assigned to a specific therapy was 10% compared with 41% in the patients without specific therapy. The 1-year recurrence rate in patients with pacemakers was 5%. It was concluded that a strategy based on diagnostic information from early ILR implant, with therapy delayed until documentation of syncope, allows safe, specific, and effective therapy in patients with neurocardiogenic syncope.

When to Choose Prolonged Monitoring

The literature clearly supports the use of the implantable loop recorder in patients with recurrent unexplained syncope who have failed a noninvasive workup and continue to have episodes. This represents a select group that has been referred for further testing, where ongoing symptoms are likely and a symptom–rhythm correlation is a feasible goal. Widespread early use of the ILR is likely to reduce the diagnostic yield as the prevalence of arrhythmias falls, supported by data from the RAST trial.[18,25] The optimal patient for prolonged monitoring with an external or implantable loop recorder has symptoms suspicious for arrhythmia, namely abrupt onset with minimal prodrome, typically brief loss of consciousness, and complete resolution of symptoms within seconds to minutes. Episodes are not necessarily posture related, and may be associated with palpitations. After clinical assessment, including determination of left ventricular function, a decision must be made as to whether the underlying condition is potentially life threatening. We have historically used a left ventricular ejection fraction of 35% as a cutoff for performing electrophysiological testing prior to employing a prolonged monitoring strategy. Primary and secondary prevention trials using implantable defibrillators support this practice. All reports using the ILR have suggested a low incidence of life-threatening arrhythmia or significant morbidity with a prolonged monitoring strategy. This suggests a good prognosis for patients with recurrent unexplained syncope in the absence of left ventricular dysfunction or with negative electrophysiological testing, and attests to the safety of a monitoring strategy. This finding was particularly striking in the negative electrophysiological testing arm of the ISSUE study (see discussion above).

Lastly, syncope resolves during long-term monitoring in almost one-third of patients even in the presence of frequent episodes prior to loop recorder implantation. This suggests that the cause of syncope in some instances is self-limited, or reflects a transient physiologial abnormality. Long-term monitoring strategies may also have a role in the assessment of patients who have infrequent palpitations but are at risk of arrhythmias.

Conclusion

The identification of a cause for presyncope, syncope, or palpitations remains a significant challenge for clinicians despite advances in knowledge pertaining to mechanisms. A careful history and examination are mandatory in the assessment of these patients. However, the accurate correlation of symptoms to rhythm requires the judicious use of these monitoring tools. Ambulatory cardiac monitoring applied as either an external or implantable modality has provided a powerful means to elucidate the etiology of symptoms such as presyncope, syncope, or palpitations. The choice of ambulatory monitoring strategies is determined by the index of suspicion of cardiac arrhythmias, the frequency and nature of symptoms, and, ultimately, by the diagnostic yield of the particular monitoring strategy. For instance, implantable loop recorders have significantly improved the success of obtaining electrocardiographic rhythm data during spontaneous symptoms in patients with recurrent unexplained syncope. The clinician should consider early use of external and implantable loop recorders when an arrhythmia is suspected based on clinical presentation and initial noninvasive testing.

References

1. Sheldon R, Rose S, Ritchie D, Connolly SJ, Koshman ML, Lee MA, Frenneaux M, Fisher M, Murphy W. Historical criteria that distinguish syncope from seizures. *J Am Coll Cardiol* 2002;40:142–148.
2. Alboni P, Brignole M, Menozzi C, Raviele A, Del Rosso A, Dinelli M, Solano A, Bottoni N. Diagnostic value of history in patients with syncope with or without heart disease. *J Am Coll Cardiol* 2001;37:1921–1928.
3. Linzer M, Yang EH, Estes NA, Wang P, Vorperian VR, Kapoor WN. Diagnosing syncope: Unexplained syncope. Clinical Efficacy Assessment Project of the American College of Physicians. *Ann Intern Med* 1997;127:76–86.
4. Kapoor WN. Evaluation and management of the patient with syncope. *JAMA* 1992;268:2553–2560.

5. Krahn AD, Klein GJ, Yee R, Skanes AC. Predictive value of presyncope in patients monitored for assessment of syncope. *Am Heart J* 2001;141:817–821.
6. Bass EB, Curtiss EI, Arena VC, Hanusa BH, Cecchetti A, Karpf M, Kapoor WN. The duration of Holter monitoring in patients with syncope. Is 24 hours enough? *Arch Intern Med* 1990;150:1073–1078.
7. Waktare JE, Malik M. Holter, loop recorder, and event counter capabilities of implanted devices. *Pacing Clin Electrophysiol* 1997;20:2658–2669.
8. Linzer M, Pritchett EL, Pontinen M, McCarthy E, Divine GW. Incremental diagnostic yield of loop electrocardiographic recorders in unexplained syncope. *Am J Cardiol* 1990;66:214–219.
9. Cumbee SR, Pryor RE, Linzer M. Cardiac loop ECG recording: A new noninvasive diagnostic test in recurrent syncope. *South Med J* 1990;83:39–43.
10. Brown AP, Dawkins KD, Davies JG. Detection of arrhythmias: Use of a patient-activated ambulatory electrocardiogram device with a solid-state memory loop. *Br Heart J* 1987;58:251–253.
11. Sivakumaran S, Krahn AD, Klein GJ, Finan J, Yee R, Renner S, Skanes AC. A prospective randomized comparison of loop recorders versus Holter monitors in patients with syncope or presyncope. *Am J Med* 2003;115:1–5.
12. Gula LJ, Krahn AD, Massel D, Skanes A, Yee R, Klein, GJ. External loop recorders: Determinants of diagnostic yield in patients with syncope. *Am Heart J* 2004;147:644–648.
13. Reiffel JA, Schwarzberg R, *et al.* Comparison of autotriggered memory loop recorders versus standard loop recorders versus 24-hour Holter monitors for arrhythmia detection. *Am J Cardiol* 2005;95:1055–1059.
14. Krahn AD, Klein GJ, Yee R, Norris C. Maturation of the sensed electrogram amplitude over time in a new subcutaneous implantable loop recorder. *Pacing Clin Electrophysiol* 1997;20:1686–1690.
15. Brignole M, Moya A, Menozzi C, Garcia-Civera R, Sutton R. Proposed electrocardiographic classification of spontaneous syncope documented by an implantable loop recorder. *Europace* 2005;7(1):14–18.
16. Krahn AD, Klein GJ, Yee R, Norris C. Final results from a pilot study with an implantable loop recorder to determine the etiology of syncope in patients with negative noninvasive and invasive testing. *Am J Cardiol* 1998;82:117–119.
17. Krahn AD, Klein GJ, Yee R, Takle-Newhouse T, Norris C. Use of an extended monitoring strategy in patients with problematic syncope. Reveal Investigators. *Circulation* 1999;99:406–410.
18. Krahn AD, Klein GJ, Yee R, Skanes AC. Randomized assessment of syncope trial: Conventional diagnostic testing versus a prolonged monitoring strategy. *Circulation* 2001;104:46–51.
19. Krahn AD, Klein GJ, Fitzpatrick A, Seidl K, Zaidi A, Skanes A, Yee R. Predicting the outcome of patients with unexplained syncope undergoing prolonged monitoring. *Pacing Clin Electrophysiol* 2002;25:37–41.
20. Zaidi A, Clough P, Mawer G, Fitzpatrick A. Accurate diagnosis of convulsive syncope: Role of an implantable subcutaneous ECG monitor. *Seizure* 1999;8:184–186.
21. Zaidi A, Clough P, Cooper P, Scheepers B, Fitzpatrick AP. Misdiagnosis of epilepsy: Many seizure-like attacks have a cardiovascular cause. *J Am Coll Cardiol* 2000;36:181–184.
22. Brignole M, Menozzi C, Moya A, Garcia-Civera R, Mont L, Alvarez M, Errazquin F, Beiras J, Bottoni N, Donateo P. Mechanism of syncope in patients with bundle branch block and negative electrophysiological test. *Circulation* 2001;104:2045–2050.
23. Moya A, Brignole M, Menozzi C, Garcia-Civera R, Tognarini S, Mont L, Botto G, Giada F, Cornacchia D. Mechanism of syncope in patients with isolated syncope and in patients with tilt-positive syncope. *Circulation* 2001;104:1261–1267.
24. Menozzi C, Brignole M, Garcia-Civera R, Moya A, Botto G, Tercedor L, Migliorini R, Navarro X. Mechanism of syncope in patients with heart disease and negative electrophysiologic test. *Circulation* 2002;105:2741–2745.
25. Krahn AD, Klein GJ, Yee R, Hoch JS, Skanes AC. Cost implications of testing strategy in patients with syncope: Randomized assessment of syncope trial. *J Am Coll Cardiol* 2003;42:495–501.
26. Brignole M, Sutton R, *et al.* Early application of an implantable loop recorder allows effective specific therapy in patients with recurrent suspected neurally mediated syncope. *Eur Heart J* 2006;27:1085–1092.

23 Signal Averaged Electrocardiogram

Gioia Turitto, Raushan Abdula, David Benson, and Nabil El-Sherif

Introduction

The term "signal averaged electrocardiogram" (SAECG) encompasses any technique that results in an improvement of the signal-to-noise ratio, thus allowing analysis of signals that are too small to be detected by routine measurement. Among such signals are those arising from areas of slow and inhomogeneous conduction in diseased ventricular myocardium [usually referred to as late potentials (LPs)]. These potentials are small because the activation front is slow and fractionated, or the mass of tissue undergoing depolarization is small, or both. Late potentials are of clinical relevance because they may identify a substrate for reentrant ventricular excitation.[1]

Important technical advances in the field of SAECG were made in the early 1980s and included the introduction and refinement of filtering techniques, the selection of bipolar orthogonal leads and their combination into a vector magnitude for maximal sensitivity, as well as the use of computer algorithms to identify QRS offset and provide numerical values for signals in the terminal part of the QRS.[2,3] In 1991, a Task Force of the American College of Cardiology, the American Heart Association, and the European Society of Cardiology published standards for acquisition and analysis of LPs and attempted to define clinical indications for the SAECG.[4] The recommended applications consisted of risk stratification for future arrhythmic events and sudden cardiac death (SCD) in survivors of myocardial infarction (MI), and prediction of malignant ventricular tachyarrhythmias in patients with coronary artery disease and syncope, or asymptomatic nonsustained ventricular tachycardia (VT). Other groups of patients with organic heart disease in whom the SAECG has been utilized for risk stratification for SCD include patients with idiopathic dilated cardiomyopathy, hypertrophic cardiomyopathy, right ventricular cardiomyopathy, etc. The original recommendations of the Task Force were updated by an American College of Cardiology Expert Consensus Document.[5]

This chapter will review the technical aspects as well as the clinical relevance of the SAECG for risk stratification of SCD.

Technical Aspects of the Signal Averaged Electrocardiogram

Time-Domain Analysis

Electrocardiogram (ECG) data acquisition consists of several steps: proper recording, amplification, digitization, identification and alignment of the signal of interest, time-ensemble averaging, and filtering.[6,7] Typically, 200–600 cardiac cycles are acquired. The QRS selection process uses a cross-correlation algorithm, where each detected QRS is compared to a preselected template. A correlation coefficient of >0.98 is typically required for a good match; this allows rejection of abnormal QRS such as ventricular premature complexes or noisy beats. Time-ensemble averaging is used because the signal of interest, i.e., the QRS, is repetitive, while much of the interfering noise (environmental noise, electromyographic noise, etc.) is random. Thus, time-ensemble averaging results in an improved signal-to-noise ratio. Filtering is also applied to reduce the residual noise and improve identification of LPs. A bidirectional

Butterworth filter has been recommended for analysis of LPs.[2] By using this filter, the first part of the QRS is bandpass filtered, and then the second part of the QRS as well as the ST segment are filtered in reverse time, starting from the end of the data and moving toward the middle of the QRS. A bipolar orthogonal lead system is used to optimize the recording of LPs because of their unknown distribution on the body surface. The three leads are processed separately, and then combined into a vector magnitude of the form $\sqrt{X^2 + Y^2 + Z^2}$ and used for subsequent analysis. Bandpass filtering of the SA vector magnitude may further discriminate LPs from noise. Early studies of the frequency signature of LPs showed that they contained predominantly high frequencies, and filters that eliminate low frequencies may expose LPs more clearly. Commercial SAECG systems apply bandpass filtering with a low-pass setting of 250 Hz and a high-pass setting of 25–40 Hz. Computer algorithms are utilized to identify QRS onset and offset. These algorithms depend on the signal-to-noise ratio.[2] Once the QRS offset is defined, time-domain analysis of the SAECG mainly consists of the determination of three parameters: the duration of the filtered QRS complex (QRSD), the duration of low-amplitude signals of <40 μV, i.e., the time that the filtered QRS voltage remains below 40 μV (LAS40), and the root mean square voltage of the terminal 40 msec of the QRS (RMS40). The ad hoc Task Force recommended that for adequate LP analysis, a low noise level of <1 μV with a 25-Hz high-pass cutoff or <0.7 μV with a 40-Hz high-pass cutoff be obtained.[4] The Task Force also recognized that the definition of an LP and the scoring of an SAECG as normal or abnormal have not been standardized. Representative criteria indicate that an LP exists (using a 40-Hz high-pass filter) when (1) QRSD is >114 msec, (2) LAS40 is >38 msec, and (3) RMS40 is <20 μV[4] (Figure 23–1). Time-domain

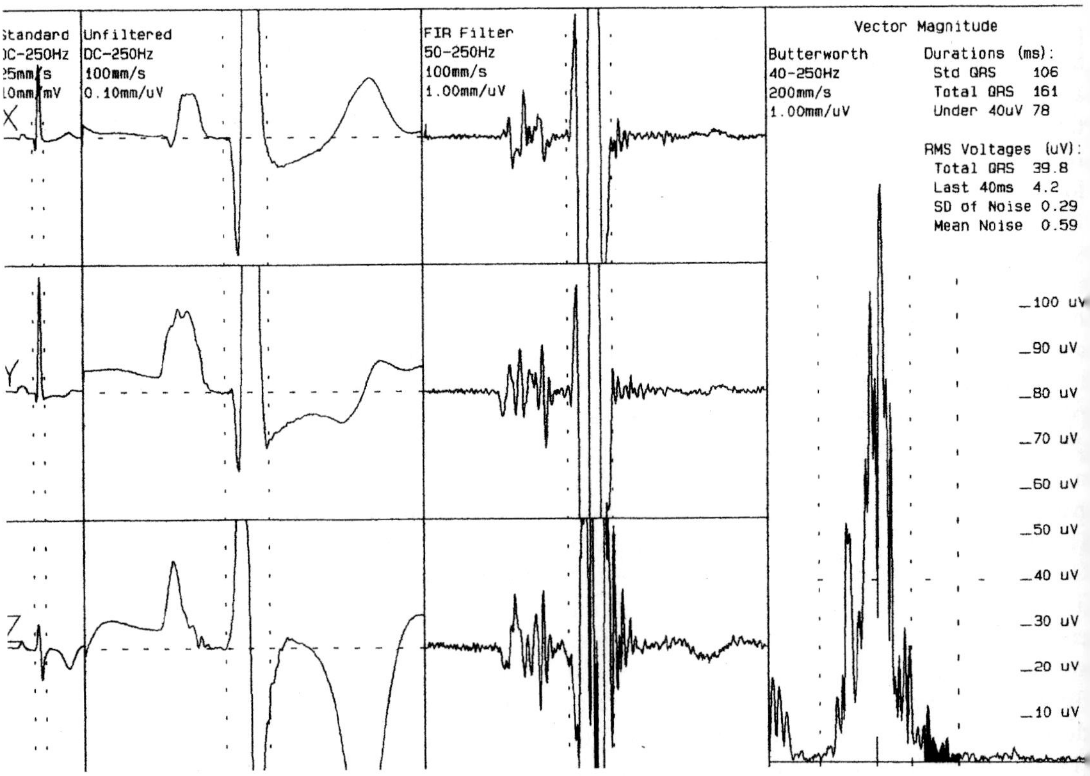

FIGURE 23–1. Example of abnormal time-domain analysis of the SAECG. Filtered QRS duration and duration of low-amplitude signals are prolonged, while voltage of the terminal QRS is decreased, at a filter setting of 40–250 Hz. Total QRS, high-frequency QRS duration; under 40 μV, duration of low-amplitude signals <40 μV; RMS, root mean square; last 40 ms, RMS voltage of the terminal 40 msec of the QRS.

analysis remains the mainstay for SAECG analysis, due to its proven diagnostic accuracy and high reproducibility.[7]

More recently, the ambulatory ECG has been proposed to record and examine the SAECG for risk stratification of post-MI patients.[8,9] The prognostic value of SAECGs obtained from ambulatory (Holter) ECG recordings was found to compare favorably to that of conventional SAECGs.

Frequency-Domain Analysis

Techniques for frequency-domain analysis were devised to overcome some of the limitations of time-domain analysis, namely the inability to detect abnormal and delayed conduction within the QRS complex, or in the presence of intraventricular conduction defects. The rationale for frequency-domain analysis is the observation that the QRS, LPs, and ST segment waveforms in the SAECG have different spectral characteristics. Various techniques have been described under different names, including spectrotemporal mapping, spectral turbulence analysis, wavelet decomposition analysis, and acceleration spectrum analysis.[10–15] At the present time, none of these techniques has gained widespread acceptance, due to their lack of standardization, suboptimal reproducibility, and the lack of convincing evidence that frequency-domain analysis results in a greater diagnostic and prognostic accuracy than conventional time-domain analysis.

Table 23–1. Prevalence of an abnormal SAECG in normal subjects and in postinfarction patients with or without malignant ventricular tachyarrhythmias.[a]

	Prevalence (%)	
Study groups	Time domain	Frequency domain
Normal subjects	0–10	4
Recent MI (<2 weeks), no VTA	14–29	26
Remote MI (≥1 month), no VTA	18–33	23
Remote MI (≥1 month), VTA	52–90	73–92

Source: Reproduced from Cain,[5] with permission from the American College of Cardiology Foundation.

[a]SAECG, signal averaged electrocardiogram; MI, myocardial infarction; VTA, ventricular tachyarrhythmias.

Clinical Applications of the Signal Averaged Electrocardiogram

Risk Stratification in the Postinfarction Period

The prevalence of an abnormal SAECG in normal subjects, and in patients with prior MI with or without ventricular tachyarrhythmias, is shown in Table 23–1.[5] The reported wide range in the prevalence of LPs following MI may be related to differences in the diagnostic criteria for LPs, as well as in the time of recording of the SAECG,[16–18] and the site of MI.[19] El-Sherif *et al.* showed that the prevalence of an abnormal SAECG recording varied widely in the first 60 days after MI.[17,18] An abnormal recording 6–30 days after MI had the most significant relation to arrhythmic events occurring in the first year post-MI.[18] Late potentials became progressively less frequent following hospital discharge.[16,17] In a study by Gomes *et al.*, LPs were more common in patients with inferior MI compared to patients with anterior MI.[19] This could be related to the fact that the inferoposterior segments of the left ventricle depolarize later than the anteroseptal and anterior segments. Thus, in patients with inferior MI, delayed regional activation is likely to outlast normal ventricular depolarization and appear as LPs after the QRS offset. On the other hand, in patients with anterior MI, the abnormal myocardial region is activated early during the QRS complex, resulting in partial obscuring of LPs.

Risk stratification of survivors of MI has been successfully performed with time-domain analysis of the SAECG. Several prospective studies have confirmed the increased likelihood of malignant ventricular tachyarrhythmias and SCD in post-MI patients with an abnormal SAECG.[18–29] A previous review analyzed studies in which the SAECG was performed in approximately 5000 patients within 1 month of MI (usually at the time of hospital discharge), with an average follow-up of 13 months.[30] The SAECG was abnormal in 29% of patients, while arrhythmic events occurred in 7% of patients. The positive predictive accuracy of the SAECG was low (mean: 17%, range: 8–29), while its negative predictive accuracy was high (mean: 96%, range: 81–99). Because of the low predictive accuracy of the test, no intervention is justified in post-MI patients based solely on the presence of

Table 23–2. Prognostic value of the SAECG for serious arrhythmic events after myocardial infarction.[a]

Studies (*n*)	22
Patients (*n*)	9883
Follow-up (months)	22
Arrhythmic events (%)	7.2
Sensitivity (%)	62
Specificity (%)	77
Positive predictive accuracy (%)	19
Relative risk	4.8
Odds ratio	5.7

Source: Reproduced from Bailey *et al.*,[29] with permission from the American College of Cardiology Foundation.
[a]SAECG, signal averaged electrocardiogram.

an abnormal SAECG.[5] The prognostic value of the SAECG in post-MI patients was also reviewed by Bailey *et al.* in a meta-analysis of almost 10,000 patients.[29] This showed the high sensitivity and specificity of the test, as well as its low positive predictive accuracy (Table 23–2).[29]

A multicenter NIH-sponsored substudy of the Cardiac Arrhythmia Suppression Trial (CAST) was conducted to define the best predictive criteria of time-domain SAECG in the post-MI period.[26] A total of 1158 patients were recruited and followed for an average of 10 ± 3 months. Forty-five patients (4%) suffered serious arrhythmic events (nonfatal VT or SCD). A Cox regression analysis with six SAECG variables indicated that a filtered QRS duration at 40 Hz ≥ 120 msec was the most predictive criterion of arrhythmic events (Table 23–3). An abnormal SAECG, defined as a QRS duration at 40 Hz ≥120 msec, was present in 12% of the study population. The positive, negative, and total predictive accuracy of an abnormal SAECG were 17%, 98%, and 88%, respectively.[26]

Table 23–3. Prognostic value of the SAECG after myocardial infarction in the CAST Substudy.[a]

Variable	χ^2	Probability
QRSD/25 Hz	32.4	0.0000
RMS40/25 Hz	4.1	0.0433
LAS/25 Hz	23.8	0.0000
QRSD/40 Hz	37.1	0.0000
RMS40/40 Hz	4.5	0.0344
LAS/40 Hz	10.3	0.0001

Source: Reproduced from El-Sherif *et al.*,[26] with permission from the American College of Cardiology Foundation.
[a]SAECG, signal averaged electrocardiogram; CAST, Cardiac Arrhythmia Suppression Trial; LAS, duration of low-amplitude signals of <40 μV; QRSD, high-frequency filtered QRS duration; RMS40, root mean square voltage of the terminal 40 msec of the QRS. All parameters were measured at high-pass filter settings of 25 Hz and 40 Hz.

Several studies have shown that the predictive value of the SAECG could be increased by combining its results with other clinical data, such as left ventricular ejection fraction (LVEF), degree of ventricular ectopy, and heart rate variability.[18–22,25,27,29] More recently, the prognostic value of T wave alternans, LPs on the SAECG, and LVEF was prospectively studied in 102 patients with acute MI.[31] T wave alternans was present in 50 patients (49%), LPs in 21 patients (21%), and LVEF <40% in 28 patients (27%). During a follow-up period of 13 ± 6 months, symptomatic arrhythmic events occurred in 15 patients (15%). The event rate was significantly higher in patients with one or more abnormal tests. When the sensitivity, specificity, and predictive accuracy of the three risk stratifiers, alone or in combination, were tested, the highest positive predictive value (50%) was obtained with the combined assessment of LPs and T wave alternans (Table 23–4).[31]

Bailey *et al.* surveyed the literature to estimate prediction values for five common tests for major arrhythmic events (MAE) after MI.[29] They identified 44 studies on SAECG, heart rate variability, ventricular arrhythmias on ambulatory ECG, LVEF, and electrophysiology study. Their meta-analysis used receiver-operating characteristic curves to estimate mean values for sensitivity and specificity for each test and 95% confidence limits (Figure 23–2). Therefore, it may be feasible to stratify as many as 90% of post-MI patients into "high risk" (>30%) and "low risk" (<3%) categories using combinations of four noninvasive tests (Table 23–5).[29] With this approach, the first step would be performance of both SAECG and LVEF. If the two tests were both negative or both positive (as would be true for 64.2% of the patients), further testing would not be done, as the 2-year probability of V-MAE would be very low in the former situation (2.2%), and high enough in the latter situation (38.7%) to warrant consideration of implantable cardioverter defibrillator (ICD) implantation. The second step would be performance of a 24-h ambulatory ECG in the 35.8% of patients who had only a positive SAECG or only a low LVEF, resulting in an intermediate risk for

TABLE 23–4. Predictive value and univariate Cox analysis of different noninvasive risk stratifiers for arrhythmic events following myocardial infarction.[a]

	Sensitivity (%)	Specificity (%)	PPV (%)	NPV (%)	Total PV (%)	RH (95% CI)	*p* value
TWA	93	59	28	98	64	16.8 (2.2–127.8)	0.0006
LPs	53	85	38	91	80	5.7 (2.1–15.7)	0.0008
EF	60	78	32	92	75	4.7 (1.7–13.2)	0.004
TWA + LPs	53	91	50	92	85	8.6 (3.1–23.9)	0.0001
TWA + EF	60	84	39	92	80	6.3 (2.3–17.8)	0.0005
LPs + EF	40	86	33	89	79	3.8 (1.4–10.8)	0.001
TWA + LPs + EF	40	91	43	90	83	5.5 (2.0–15.5)	0.001

Source: Reproduced from Ikeda *et al.*,[31] with permission from the American College of Cardiology Foundation.

[a]CI, confidence interval; EF, left ventricular ejection fraction; LPs, late potentials on the SAECG; NPV, negative predictive value; PPV, positive predictive value; PV, predictive value; RH, relative hazard; TWA, T wave alternans.

V-MAE (10.6% over 2 years). If the ambulatory ECG and heart rate variability were both normal or both abnormal (25%), no further testing would be needed, because in the former situation, the posterior probability would still be below the original prior probability, despite having either an abnormal SAECG or a low LVEF, and in the latter case, the posterior probability would again be

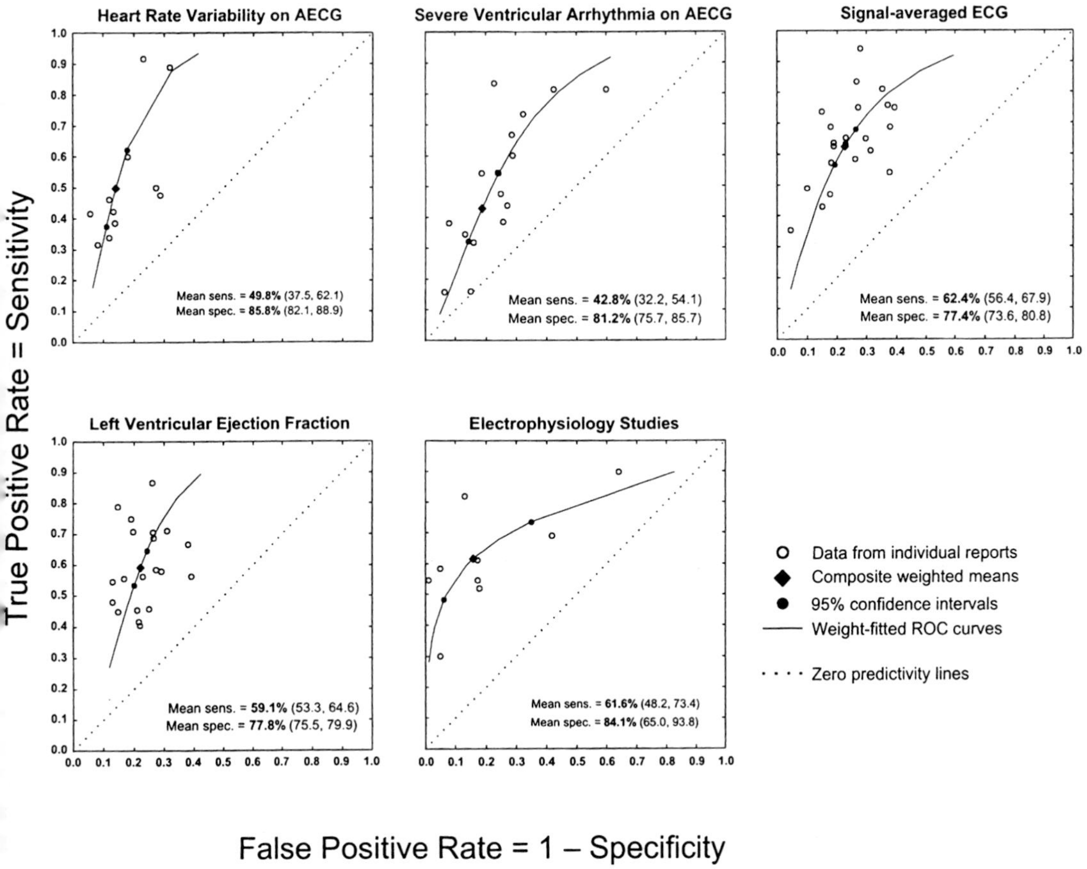

FIGURE 23–2. Receiver operator curves (ROC) for five risk stratifiers for major arrhythmic events after myocardial infarction. Mean values for sensitivity and specificity and 95% confidence intervals for each test are shown. AECG, ambulatory electrocardiogram. (Reproduced from Bailey *et al.*,[29] with permission from the American College of Cardiology Foundation.)

TABLE 23–5. Staged application of tests for prediction of major arrhythmic events following myocardial infarction.[a,b]

Test combination	Results of tests	Proportion of population (%)	Probability of MAE over 2 years (%)
Stage 1 = SAECG and LVEF	Both negative	56.6	2.2
	Only one positive	35.8	10.6
	Both positive	7.6	38.7
Stage 2 = AECG (SVA and HRV) performed on "only one positive" patient of stage 1	Both negative	23.3	4.7
	Only one positive	10.8	17.5
	Both positive	2.6	48.2

Source: Reproduced from Bailey *et al.*,[29] with permission from the American College of Cardiology Foundation.

[a]Based on a 2-year prior probability of 7.9%.

[b]MAE, major arrhythmic events; SAECG, signal averaged electrocardiogram; AECG, ambulatory (Holter) ECG; HRV, heart rate variability; LVEF, left ventricular ejection fraction; SVA, serious ventricular arrhythmias on ambulatory (Holter) ECG.

high enough to warrant consideration of ICD implantation. As a result of this noninvasive approach, approximately 90% of patients would be accurately risk stratified into low-risk (80%) and high-risk (10%) groups for MAE, while the unstratified group would include only 10% of post-MI patients.

A recently noted limitation of risk stratification studies in post-MI patients may be the reduced ability to predict arrhythmic events in patients who underwent revascularization procedures, such as thrombolysis or primary coronary angioplasty or stenting, at the onset of MI. This may be related to the lower incidence of arrhythmic events with the contemporary, aggressive treatment of MI, including reperfusion strategies and pharmacotherapy (i.e., β blockers).[32–34] In this setting, the prognostic value of LPs may be diminished.[32–34]

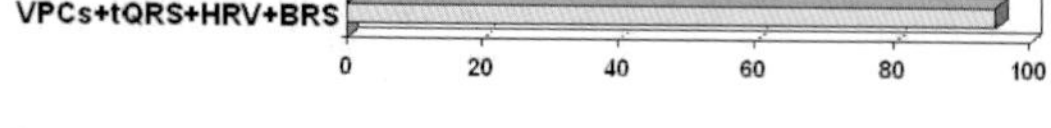

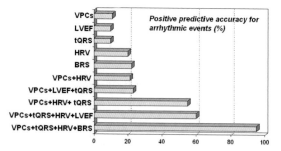

FIGURE 23–3. Positive predictive accuracy of a battery of noninvasive risk stratifiers, alone or in combination, in the postinfarction period. BRS, baroreflex sensitivity; HRV, heart rate variability; LVEF, left ventricular ejection fraction; tQRS, high-frequency QRS duration on the SAECG; VPCs, ventricular premature complexes during ambulatory (Holter) ECG. (Modified from Camm and Fei,[25] with permission.)

This review of the literature suggests that sensitivities and specificities for the most commonly used noninvasive tests for risk stratification of SCD in post-MI patients, including the SAECG, are relatively low. No one test is satisfactory alone for accurately predicting risk. Combinations of tests in stages may result in an improvement of the positive predictive accuracy of noninvasive risk stratifiers, as shown in Figure 23–3. Large prospective studies to develop a robust prediction model are still warranted.

Risk Stratification in Patients with Ischemic Cardiomyopathy

The SAECG was initially utilized to predict the outcome of programmed ventricular stimulation in patients with coronary artery disease and asymptomatic nonsustained VT.[30] In a study from Turitto *et al.*, LPs proved to be the single most accurate predictor for the induction of sustained monomorphic VT in 105 patients with nonsustained VT.[35] In this study, concordance between the results of programmed stimulation and those f the SAECG was observed in 84% of cases. The argest subgroup consisted of patients who had a ormal SAECG and no induced sustained monomorphic VT (70%). In these patients, the spontaeous arrhythmia may be due to mechanisms ther than reentry. The group with both abnormal AECG and induced sustained VT accounted for 4% of cases. The results of the two tests were iscordant in the remaining 16% of cases. This nay be explained by electrophysiological limitaions of both programmed stimulation and SAECG echniques.[35] Subsequent studies have shown that he SAECG may also predict the results of programmed stimulation in patients with nonischemic ilated cardiomyopathy.[36,37]

The prognostic significance of the SAECG was tudied in patients with ischemic or nonischemic ardiomyopathy.[38–43] The most recent and compelling data on the predictive accuracy of the AECG in patients with coronary artery disease, rior MI, left ventricular dysfunction, and asymptomatic nonsustained VT originated from the AECG substudy of the Multicenter UnSustained 'achycardia Trial (MUSTT).[40] In this large, prospective, multicenter study, SAECG data from 268 patients were entered in a Cox proportional azards modeling to examine individual and joint elations between SAECG parameters and arrhythnic death or cardiac arrest (primary end point), ardiac death, and total mortality. In all patients, SAECG quantitative variables were processed at 40 to 250 Hz and included filtered QRSD, RMS40, and LAS40. First, to assess the prognostic content of a "normal" versus "abnormal" SAECG, the SAECG parameters were analyzed as continuous variable and as dichotomized at standard cut points. A QRSD >114 msec was the single most powerful independent predictor of the primary end point and cardiac death, and was, thus, defined as an abnormal SAECG (Table 23–6).[40] The SAECG variables remained significant predictors after adjustment for prognostic clinical and treatment factors. Second, to illustrate the ability of the SAECG to stratify risk, patients were divided by QRSD [>114 msec (abnormal SAECG) versus ≤114 msec (normal SAECG)] and Kaplan–Meier survival curves were generated for each outcome (Figure 23–4).[40] With an abnormal SAECG, the 5-year rates of the primary end point (28% versus 17%, $p = 0.0001$), cardiac death (37% versus 25%, $p = 0.0001$), and total mortality (43% versus 35%, $p = 0.0001$) were significantly higher. The combination of LVEF <30% and abnormal SAECG identified a particularly high-risk subset that constituted 21% of the total population. Thirty-six percent and 44% of patients with this combination experienced arrhythmic events or cardiac death, respectively, during a 5-year follow-up. On the other hand, 13% and 20% of patients without this combination experienced arrhythmic events or

Table 23–6. Multivariate analysis of SAECG quantitative values as predictors of outcome in the MUSTT SAECG Substudy.[a]

	Arrhythmic death/ cardiac arrest		Cardiac death	
Predictor	χ^2	p	χ^2	p
Continuous variables				
Filtered QRS duration	29.2	<0.001	34.0	<0.001
RMS voltage	14.3	0.004	17.0	<0.001
Duration of LAS	14.3	0.59	0.2	0.62
Dichotomous variables				
Filtered QRS duration(>114 vs. ≤114 msec)	23.1	<0.001	20.8	<0.001
RMS voltage (<20 vs. ≥20 μV)	0.3	0.59	0.1	0.73
Duration of LAS (<38 vs ≥38 msec)	1.6	0.21	0.3	

Source: Reproduced from Gomes *et al.*,[40] with permission from the American Heart Association.
[a]SAECG, signal averaged electrocardiogram; MUSTT, Multicenter UnSustained Tachycardia Trial; LAS, low-amplitude signals of <40 μV; RMS, root mean square voltage of the terminal 40 msec of filtered QRS. SAECG parameters were analyzed at 40–250 Hz filter setting.

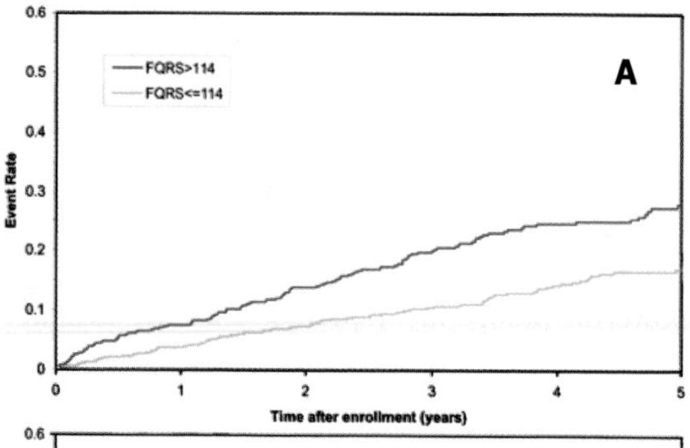

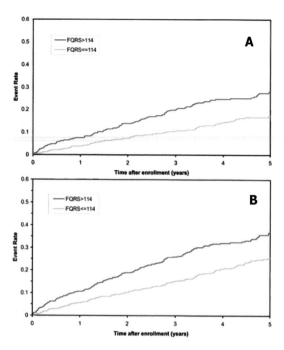

FIGURE 23–4. Kaplan–Meier estimates of arrhythmic death or cardiac arrest (A) and cardiac death (B) by SAECG result in the MUSTT substudy. $p < 0.001$ between groups; fQRS, high-frequency QRS duration. (Reproduced from Gomes *et al.*,[40] with permission from the American Heart Association.)

cardiac death, respectively, during a 5-year follow-up. It was concluded that an abnormal SAECG (defined as a filtered QRS duration >114 msec) is a strong predictor for both arrhythmic events and cardiac mortality in patients with ischemic cardiomyopathy. The noninvasive combination of an abnormal SAECG and reduced LVEF may have utility in selecting high-risk patients for intervention, such as ICD implantation.[40]

Risk Stratification in Patients with Nonischemic Dilated Cardiomyopathy

Studies investigating the prognostic value of the SAECG in nonischemic dilated cardiomyopathy are relatively scarce.[39,41–43] In an early study by Mancini *et al.*, the SAECG was found to be a predictor of survival in 114 patients with dilated cardiomyopathy.[41] Freedom from adverse events (VT, death) was significantly higher in patients with normal SAECG than in those with abnormal recording or with bundle branch block. Fauchier *et al.* reached similar conclusions in a more recen report, which identified the SAECG as a powerf predictor of all-cause cardiac death in 131 patient with idiopathic dilated cardiomyopathy, inde pendent of the presence of sustained ventricula tachyarrhythmia or bundle branch block.[42] Th heterogeneity of the study population with respec to the presence of spontaneous ventricular tach yarrhythmias and bundle branch block, as well a the empirical use of antiarrhythmic drugs, whic could have influenced both the results of th SAECG and clinical outcome, may explain the dis crepancies between these reports and other serie which did not find any correlation between a abnormal SAECG and prognosis in patients wit dilated cardiomyopathy.[39,43]

Turitto *et al.* performed SAECG and pro grammed ventricular stimulation in a group of 8 subjects with nonischemic dilated cardiomyopa thy and spontaneous nonsustained VT, who ha a mean follow-up of 22 months.[39] Survival analysi with a Cox proportional hazards model demon strated that no test result was significantly asso ciated with arrhythmic events or total cardia mortality.[39] When 2-year survival analysis wa based on the results of the SAECG, there were n significant differences in arrhythmia-free surviva or cumulative survival between patients with o without abnormal SAECG (Figure 23–5). A

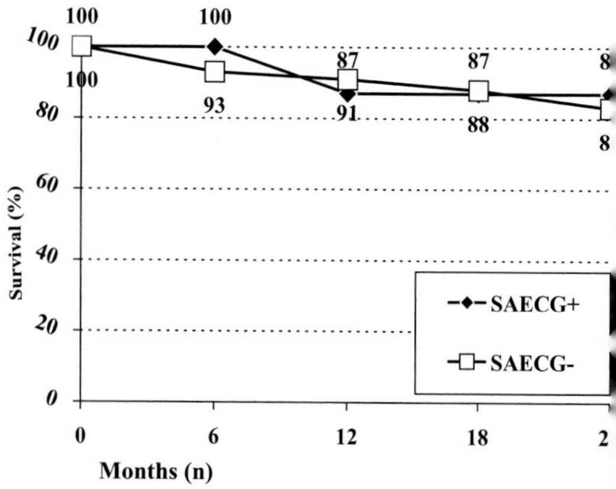

FIGURE 23–5. Two-year actuarial survival curves for arrhythmi events in 80 patients with nonischemic dilated cardiomyopath classified by SAECG results. SAECG+, abnormal recording; SAECG– normal recording. Data are expressed as mean value standar error. (Reproduced from Turitto *et al.*,[39] with permission from th American College of Cardiology Foundation.)

important finding in this study was that the presence of a normal SAECG and lack of inducibility of sustained monomorphic VT did not portend a favorable prognosis in patients with nonischemic dilated cardiomyopathy and spontaneous nonsustained VT.[39]

In the Marburg Cardiomyopathy Study, arrhythmia risk stratification was performed prospectively in 343 patients with idiopathic dilated cardiomyopathy.[43] This included analysis of LVEF by echocardiography, SAECG, arrhythmias on ambulatory ECG, QTc dispersion, heart rate variability, baroreflex sensitivity, and T wave alternans. During 52 ± 21 months of follow-up, major arrhythmic events, defined as sustained VT, ventricular fibrillation, or SCD, occurred in 46 patients (13%). On multivariate analysis, LVEF was the only significant arrhythmia risk predictor in patients with sinus rhythm, with a relative risk of 2.3 per 10% decrease of ejection fraction (95% CI, 1.5–3.3; $p = 0.0001$). In patients with atrial fibrillation, multivariate Cox analysis identified LVEF and absence of β blocker therapy as the only significant arrhythmia risk predictors. In addition, SAECG, baroreflex sensitivity, heart rate variability, and T wave alternans did not appear to be helpful for arrhythmia risk stratification in this population.[43] These results strongly support the recommendation that novel risk stratification strategies be sought in patients with nonischemic dilated cardiomyopathy.

Miscellaneous Applications

Hypertrophic Cardiomyopathy

There are limited data on the prevalence and prognostic value of the SAECG in patients with hypertrophic cardiomyopathy. In two studies from the group of McKenna, there was low prevalence of abnormal SAECG and lack of correlation with SCD.[44,45]

Arrhythmogenic Right Ventricular Cardiomyopathy

An abnormal SAECG is frequently seen in patients with right ventricular cardiomyopathy, and LPs have been listed as a minor diagnostic criterion for this disease.[46] The prevalence of LPs varies from 14% to 83% (mean: 62%) in patients with right ventricular cardiomyopathy.[30,47–51] This wide range is probably related to the variable anatomic extent of the disease, with a lower proportion of abnormal recordings in localized forms and a higher proportion in more advanced stages and in patients with documented VT.[51] Abnormal SAECG results may also be obtained in 4–16% of family members of patients with right ventricular cardiomyopathy.[48,49,51]

"Primary Electrical Disease"

This term refers to ventricular tachyarrhythmias occurring in the absence of documented structural heart disease. The exclusion of unrecognized right ventricular cardiomyopathy is important, especially in patients with right-sided VT (left bundle branch block configuration). It is possible that the SAECG may have a role in identifying patients with concealed focal structural abnormalities of the right ventricle.[50] The value of the SAECG in patients with "idiopathic" VT was investigated by Mehta *et al.*[52] They performed right and left ventricular endomyocardial biopsies, SAECG, and programmed ventricular stimulation in 38 patients with VT and no evidence of structural heart disease. Late potentials had a moderate sensitivity for abnormal biopsy findings and inducible VT (63% and 37%, respectively), but a high specificity for these variables (84% and 100%, respectively). In another study, Leclercq and Coumel enrolled 132 patients with "idiopathic" VT.[47] Further testing revealed underlying heart disease in 26 of the patients, including 13 with right ventricular cardiomyopathy. LPs were present in 81% of the patients with heart disease and only in 4% of those with normal hearts, yielding a sensitivity of 86% and a specificity of 96% for detecting clinically silent arrhythmogenic cardiomyopathies. Recent studies suggested that LPs may be of value for risk stratification of patients with the Brugada syndrome.[53–55]

Conclusions

The SAECG is an established noninvasive test for risk stratification for SCD, especially in survivors of MI. It has a very high negative predictive accuracy but a relatively low positive predictive accuracy. Improved risk stratification may be accomplished if this test is utilized as part of an algorithm in conjunction with other risk stratifiers. For this purpose, new ambulatory monitoring devices utilizing digital recordings with a high sampling rate may permit the simultaneous analysis of several noninvasive parameters (e.g., LPs, heart rate variability, T wave alternans) from the same recording.

At the present time, the major limitation of the SAECG, as well as other noninvasive risk markers, is that their low positive predictive value seems to preclude their wide application for selection of patients at risk for SCD, who may be candidates for ICD implantation.

References

1. El-Sherif N, Gough WB, Restivo M. Electrophysiologic correlates of ventricular late potentials. In: El-Sherif N, Turitto G, Eds. *High-Resolution Electrocardiography*. Mount Kisco, NY: Futura Publishing Co., Inc., 1992:279–298.
2. Simson MB. Use of signals in the terminal QRS complex to identify patients with ventricular tachycardia after myocardial infarction. *Circulation* 1981;64:235–241.
3. Scherlag BJ, Lazzara R. High-resolution electrocardiography: Historical perspectives. In: El-Sherif N, Turitto G, Eds. *High-Resolution Electrocardiography*. Mount Kisco, NY: Futura Publishing Co., Inc., 1992:3–20.
4. Breithardt G, Cain ME, El-Sherif N, Flowers NC, *et al.* Standards for analysis of ventricular late potentials using high-resolution or signal-averaged electrocardiography: A statement by a Task Force Committee of the European Society of Cardiology, the American Heart Association, and the American College of Cardiology. *J Am Coll Cardiol* 1991;17: 999–1006.
5. Cain ME. Signal-averaged electrocardiography. ACC Expert Consensus Document. *J Am Coll Cardiol* 1996;27:238–249.
6. Caref EB, Turitto G, Ibrahim BB, *et al.* Role of bandpass filters in optimizing the value of signal-averaged electrocardiogram as a predictor of the results of programmed stimulation. *Am J Cardiol* 1989;64:16–26.
7. Vazquez R, Caref EB, Torres F, Reina M, Ortega F, El-Sherif N. Short-term reproducibility of time domain, spectral temporal mapping, and spectral turbulence analysis of the signal-averaged electrocardiogram in normal subjects and patients wit acute myocardial infarction. *Am Heart J* 1995;130 1011–1019.
8. Steinbigler P, Haberl R, Bruggeman T, *et al.* Postinfarction risk assessment for sudden cardiac deat using late potential analysis of the digital Holte electrocardiogram. *J Cardiovasc Electrophysio* 2002;13:1227–1232.
9. Roche F, DaCosta A, Karnib I, *et al.* Arrhythmi risk stratification after myocardial infarction usin ambulatory electrocardiography signal averaging *Pacing Clin Electophysiol* 2002;25:791–798.
10. Cain ME, Ambos HD, Markham J, Lindsay BD Arthur RM. Diagnostic implications of spectral an temporal analysis of the entire cardiac cycle i patients with ventricular tachycardia. *Circulatio* 1991;83:1637–1648.
11. Haberl R, Jilge G, Putler R, Steinbeck G. Spectra mapping of the electrocardiogram with Fourie transform for identification of patients with sustained ventricular tachycardia and coronary arter disease. *Eur Heart J* 1989;10:316–322.
12. Kelen GJ, Henkin R, Starr A-M, Caref EB Bloomfield D, El-Sherif N. Spectral turbulenc analysis of the signal-averaged electrocardiogran and its predictive accuracy for inducible sustaine monomorphic ventricular tachycardia. *Am Cardiol* 1991;67:965–975.
13. Hnatkova K, Kulakowski P, Staunton A, Camm AJ Malik M. Wavelet decomposition of the signal averaged electrocardiogram used for the risk stratification after acute myocardial infarction. In *Computers in Cardiology*. Los Alamitos, CA: IEEE Computer Society Press, 1994:673–676.
14. Chan EKY. Acceleration spectrum analysis: A nove quantitative method for frequency domain analysi of the signal-averaged electrocardiogram. *An Noninvasive Electrocardiol* 1996;1:306–315.
15. Vazquez R, Caref EB, Torres F, Reina M Guerrero JA, El-Sherif N. Reproducibility o time-domain and three different frequency-domain techniques for the analysis of the signal-averaged electrocardiogram. *J Electrocardiol* 2000 33:99–105.
16. Kuchar L, Thorburn CW, Sammel NL. Late potentials detected after myocardial infarction: Natura history and prognostic significance. *Circulatio* 1986;74:1280–1289.
17. Turitto G, Caref EB, Macina G, Fontaine JM, Ursel SN, El-Sherif N. Time course of ventricular arrhythmias and the signal-averaged electrocardiogram i the post-infarction period: A prospective study o correlation. *Br Heart J* 1988;60:17–21.
18. El-Sherif N, Ursell SN, Bekheit S, *et al.* Prognosti significance of the signal-averaged ECG depends o

the time of recording in the postinfarction period. *Am Heart J* 1989;118:256–264.
9. Gomes AJ, Winters SL, Martinson M, *et al.* The prognostic significance of quantitative signal-averaged variables relative to clinical variables, site of myocardial infarction, ejection fraction and ventricular premature beats: A prospective study. *J Am Coll Cardiol* 1989;13:377–384.
0. Kuchar DL, Thorburn CW, Sammel NL. Prediction of serious arrhythmic events after myocardial infarction: Signal-averaged electrocardiogram, Holter monitoring, radionuclide ventriculography. *J Am Coll Cardiol* 1987;9:531–538.
1. Gomes JA, Winters SL, Stewart D, *et al.* A new noninvasive index to predict sustained ventricular tachycardia and sudden death in the first year after myocardial infarction based on signal-averaged electrocardiogram, radionuclide ejection fraction and Holter monitoring. *J Am Coll Cardiol* 1987;10: 349–357.
2. Cripps T, Bennett D, Camm J, *et al.* Prospective evaluation of clinical assessment, exercise testing and signal-averaged electrocardiogram in predicting outcome after acute myocardial infarction. *Am J Cardiol* 1988;62:995–999.
3. Ahuja RK, Turitto G, Ibrahim BB, Caref EB, El-Sherif N. Combined time-domain and spectral turbulence analysis of the signal-averaged ECG improves its predictive accuracy in postinfarction patients. *J Electrocardiol* 1994;27(Suppl.):202–206.
4. Denes P, El-Sherif N, Katz R, *et al.* Prognostic significance of signal-averaged electrocardiogram after thrombolytic therapy and/or angioplasty during acute myocardial infarction (CAST Substudy). *Am J Cardiol* 1994;74:216–220.
5. Camm AJ, Fei L. Risk stratification after myocardial infarction. *Pacing Clin Electophysiol* 1994;17(Pt. 2):401–416.
6. El-Sherif N, Denes P, Katz R, *et al.* Definition of the best prediction criteria of the time domain signal-averaged electrocardiogram for serious arrhythmic events in the postinfarction period. *J Am Coll Cardiol* 1995;25:908–914.
7. Reinhardt L, Makijarvi M Fetsch T, *et al.* Noninvasive risk modeling after myocardial infarction. *Am J Cardiol* 1996;78:627–632.
8. De Chillou C, Sadoul N, Bizeau O, *et al.* Prognostic value of thrombolysis, coronary artery patency, signal-averaged electrocardiography, left ventricular ejection fraction, and Holter electrocardiographic monitoring for life-threatening ventricular arrhythmias after a first acute myocardial infarction. *Am J Cardiol* 1997;80:852–858.
9. Bailey JJ, Berson AS, Handelsman H, Hodges M. Utility of current risk stratification tests for predicting major arrhythmic events after myocardial infarction. *J Am Coll Cardiol* 2001;38:1902–1911.
30. Turitto G, Sorgato A, Alakhras M., El-Sherif N. QRS Averaging. In: Zareba W, Maison-Blanche P, Locati EH, Eds. *Noninvasive Electrocardiology in Clinical Practice*. Armonk, NY: Futura Publishing Co., Inc., 2001:49–69.
31. Ikeda T, Sakata T, Takami M, *et al.* Combined assessment of T-wave alternans and late potentials used to predict arrhythmic events after myocardial infarction. A prospective study. *J Am Coll Cardiol* 2000;35:722–730.
32. Hohnloser SH, Franck P, Klingenheben T, Zabel M, Just H. Open infarct artery, late potentials, and other prognostic factors after acute myocardial infarction in the thrombolytic era. A prospective trial. *Circulation* 1994;90:1747–1756.
33. Huikuri HV, Tapanainen JM, Lindgren K, *et al.* Prediction of sudden cardiac death after myocardial infarction in the beta-blocking era. *J Am Coll Cardiol* 2003;42:652–658.
34. Bauer A, Guzik P, Barthel P, *et al.* Reduced prognostic power of ventricular late potentials in post-infarction patients of the reperfusion era. *Eur Heart J* 2005;26:755–761.
35. Turitto G, Fontaine JM, Ursell SN, Caref EB, Henkin R, El-Sherif N. Value of the signal-averaged electrocardiogram as a predictor of the results of programmed stimulation in nonsustained ventricular tachycardia. *Am J Cardiol* 1988;61:1272–1278.
36. Turitto G, Ahuja R, Bekheit S, Caref EB, Ibrahim B, El-Sherif N. Incidence and prediction of induced ventricular tachyarrhythmias in idiopathic dilated cardiomyopathy. *Am J Cardiol* 1994;73:770–773.
37. Turitto G, Rao S, Caref EB, El-Sherif N. Time- and frequency-domain analysis of the signal averaged electrocardiogram in patients with ventricular tachycardia and ischemic versus non-ischemic dilated cardiomyopathy. *J Electrocardiol* 1994; 27(Suppl.):213–218.
38. Turitto G, Fontaine JM, Ursell S, Caref EB, Bekheit S, El-Sherif N. Risk stratification and management of patients with organic heart disease and nonsustained ventricular tachycardia: Role of programmed stimulation, left ventricular ejection fraction and the signal averaged electrocardiogram. *Am J Med* 1990;88:1–35N–41N.
39. Turitto G, Ahuja RK, Caref EB, *et al.* Risk stratification for arrhythmic events in patients with nonischemic dilated cardiomyopathy and nonsustained ventricular tachycardia: Role of programmed ventricular stimulation and the signal-averaged electrocardiogram. *J Am Coll Cardiol* 1994;24: 1523–1528.

40. Gomes JA, Cain ME, Buxton AE, Josephson ME, Lee KL, Hafley GE. Prediction of long-term outcomes by signal-averaged electrocardiography in patients with unsustained ventricular tachycardia, coronary artery disease, and left ventricular dysfunction. *Circulation* 2001;104:436–441.
41. Mancini DM, Wong KL, Simson MB. Prognostic value of an abnormal signal-averaged electrocardiogram in patients with nonischemic congestive cardiomyopathy. *Circulation* 1993;87:1083–1092.
42. Fauchier L, Babuty D, Cosnay P, Poret P, Rouesnel P, Fauchier JP. Long-term prognostic value of time domain analysis of signal-averaged electrocardiography in idiopathic dilated cardiomyopathy. *Am J Cardiol* 2000;85:618–623.
43. Grimm W, Christ M, Bach J, Muller HH, Maisch B. Noninvasive arrhythmia risk stratification in idiopathic dilated cardiomyopathy: Results of the Marburg Cardiomyopathy Study. *Circulation* 2003; 108:2883–2891.
44. Cripps TR, Counihan PJ, Frenneaux MP, Ward DE, Camm AJ, McKenna WJ. Signal-averaged electrocardiography in hypertrophic cardiomyopathy. *J Am Coll Cardiol* 1990;15:956–961.
45. Kulakowski P, Counihan PJ, Camm AJ, McKenna WJ. The value of time and frequency domain, and spectral temporal mapping analysis of the signal-averaged electrocardiogram in identification of patients with hypertrophic cardiomyopathy at increased risk of sudden death. *Eur Heart J* 1993; 14:941–950.
46. McKenna WJ, Thiene G, Nava A, *et al.*, on behalf of the Task Force of the Working Group Myocardial and Pericardial Disease of the European Society of Cardiology and of the Scientific Council on Cardiomyopathies of the International Society and Federation of Cardiology, supported by the Schoepfer Association. Diagnosis of arrhythmogenic right ventricular dysplasia/cardiomyopathy. *Br Heart J* 1994;71:215–218.
47. Leclercq JF, Coumel P. Late potentials in arrhyt mogenic right ventricular dysplasia. Prevalenc diagnostic and prognostic values. *Eur Heart J* 199 14(Suppl. E):80–83.
48. Oselladore L, Nava A, Buja F, *et al.* Signal-average electrocardiography in familial form of arrhyt mogenic right ventricular cardiomyopathy. *Am Cardiol* 1995;75:1038–1041.
49. Hermida J-S, Minassian A, Jarry G, *et al.* Famili incidence of late ventricular potentials and electr cardiographic abnormalities in arrhythmogen right ventricular dysplasia. *Am J Cardiol* 199 79:1375–1380.
50. Corrado D, Nava A, Buja G, *et al.* Familial cardi myopathy underlies syndrome of right bund branch block, ST segment elevation and sudde death. *J Am Coll Cardiol* 1996;27:443–448.
51. Nasir K, Rutberg J, Tandri H, Berger R, Tomase G, Calkins H. Utility of SAECG in arrhythmogen right ventricle dysplasia. *Ann Noninvasive Electr cardiol* 2003;8:112–120.
52. Mehta D, McKenna WJ, Ward DE, Davies M Camm AJ. Significance of signal-averaged electr cardiography in relation to endomyocardial biops and ventricular stimulation studies in patients wit ventricular tachycardia without clinically appare heart disease. *J Am Coll Cardiol* 1989;14:372–379.
53. Ikeda T, Sakurada H, Sakabe K, *et al.* Assessme of noninvasive markers in identifying patients risk in the Brugada syndrome: Insight into risk str tification. *J Am Coll Cardiol* 2001;37:1628–1634.
54. Ajiro Y, Hagiwara H, Kasanuki H. Assessment markers for identifying patients at risk for lif threatening arrhythmic events in Brugada syr drome. *J Cardiovasc Electrophysiol* 2005;16:52–53
55. Ikeda T, Takami M, Sugi K, Mizusawa Y, Sakura H, Yoshino H. Noninvasive risk stratification subjects with a Brugada-type electrocardiogra and no history of cardiac arrest. *Ann Noninvasi Electrocardiol* 2005;10:396–403.

24

leart Rate Variability: Measurements and Risk Stratification

i Gang and Marek Malik

ntroduction

eart rate variability (HRV) describes the tempo-l variation in the intervals between consecutive eart beats in sinus rhythm. It is the intervals etween consecutive beats that are being analyzd ather than the heart rate per se (Figure 24–1). RV assesses cardiac autonomic tone at the level f the sinus node and has been used as a measure f cardiac autonomic modulation. The compo-ents of HRV provide measurement of the degree f autonomic modulations rather than of the level f autonomic tone.[1] A very early investigation of RV was performed in 1965 by Hon and Lee who valuated fetal heart rate pattern preceding fetal eath.[2] Later in the 1970s Ewing *et al.* developed set of bedside tests to assess autonomic neu-opathy in diabetic patients including evaluation f RR interval variation.[3] Wolf's report in 1977 is e first clinical observational study of the associ-tion between HRV and hospital mortality in atients after acute myocardial infarction (MI).[4] 1 1981 Akselrod *et al.* assessed HRV using power pectrum analysis and demonstrated that sympa-etic and parasympathetic nervous activities ade a frequency-specific contribution to the eart rate power spectrum.[5] In the late 1980s leiger *et al.* reported that reduced HRV pre-icted increased mortality after acute MI.[6] The ndings are well supported by numerous late tudies.[7,8] Since then HRV has been used in wide reas for the purpose of risk stratification and iagnosis while this chapter will focus on the pplication of HRV to risk stratification in adult atients with cardiac disorders, in particular, on the relation of HRV to sudden cardiac death (SCD).

Methodology and Indices of Heart Rate Variability Measurement

Despite the efforts of the Task Force of the North American Society of Pacing and Electrophysiol-ogy and the European Society of Cardiology to unify and standardize the methodology for HRV measurements, there has been no consensus so far on the best method and/or index of HRV for clini-cal use in different settings. Methods for quantify-ing HRV have generally been categorized as time domain, frequency (spectral) domain, geometric, and nonlinear analysis. Heart rate turbulence (HRT) can also be considered a measure of the variability in heart rate.

Traditionally, HRV analysis has been per-formed on the 24-h Holter monitoring electrocar-diograms (ECGs) or short-term (usually 5–20 min) ECG recordings at rest or during maneuver. Taking advantage of the storage function of an implantable cardioverter defibrillator (ICD), it has recently become possible to evaluate HRV on heart rate recordings retrieved from ICD memory; in particular, HRV patterns can be evaluated on specific time windows before the onset of ven-tricular tachyarrhythmias and under control conditions.[9] Furthermore, long-term continuous HRV can be analyzed from an implanted cardiac resynchronization device.[10,11] Recommended by the Committee[12] in 1996, two types of recordings should be used whenever possible: (1) short-term

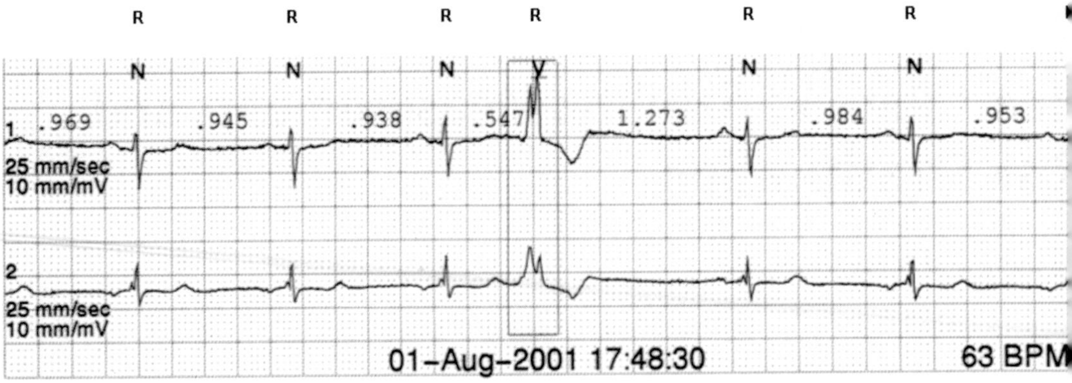

Figure 24–1. A strip of a 24-h Holter ECG recording obtained from a patient with a history of myocardial infarction, showing the N–N/R–R intervals. The individual N–N intervals were automatically measured (in seconds) and labeled, which are the basis for the analysis of heart rate variability (HRV). The ECG strip al shows a single ventricular ectopic beat, which should not included in the HRV calculation.

recordings of 5 min made under physiologically stable conditions processed by frequency-domain methods and/or (2) nominal 24-h recordings processed by time-domain methods. To obtain reliable results, the long-term recording analyzed by the time-domain methods should contain at least 18 h of analyzable ECG data that include the whole night. It is essential to perform visual check and manual corrections of individual RR intervals and QRS complex classifications for statistical time- domain or frequency-domain methods.[12]

Time-Domain Analysis

In time-domain analysis, the intervals between consecutive normal-to-normal beats are measured over a purposely predefined time period of ECG recordings. A set of statistical indices can be calculated from the intervals directly or indirectly:

Statistical Methods[12]

1. *SDNN* is the standard deviation of all normal-to-normal (NN) intervals. It is the simplest variable to calculate and the most commonly used HRV index. Though it can be obtained from 5-min to 24-h recordings, its measurement depends on the length of the recording period. Thus, it is inappropriate to compare SDNN measures derived from recordings of different length.[12] SDNN reflects all the cyclic components responsible fo variability in the period of recording and est mates overall HRV.

2. *SDANN* is the standard deviation of th 5-min average NN intervals. It is affected b editing error or arrhythmias less than SDNN, thu providing a "smoothed out" version of SDNN an an estimate of long-term fluctuation of hea rate.

3. *SDNN index* is the mean of the 5-min stan dard deviation of NN intervals calculated ove 24 h. The SDNN index reflects the average of var ability in NN intervals that occurs within a 5-mi period.

4. *NN50* and *pNN50*. NN50 is the absolu count of differences between successive NN inte vals > 50 msec, while pNN50 is the proportion o differences > 50 msec in the total number of N intervals. Both NN50 and pNN50 are measures o short-term variation, estimating high-frequenc variation in heart rate.

5. *RMSSD* is the root mean square of successiv differences between adjacent NN intervals. It is measure of short-term variation and estimate high-frequency variation in heart rate. It has bee demonstrated to have better statistical properti compared to *pNN50*.

6. *SDAAM* is the standard deviation of the 5 min median atrial-to-atrial depolarization inte vals derived from implanted cardiac electroni devices.[10,11]

eometric Methods

his method calculates the sample density distri-ution of NN interval durations or sample density istribution of differences between adjacent NN tervals, such as HRV triangular index (HRVi),[7] iangular index NN (TINN), and Lorenz plot of N intervals. The HRVi is the integral of the ensity distribution (the number of all NN inter-al) divided by the maximum of the density dis-ibution. It has been well accepted as a powerful sk stratifier in post MI. HRVi is dependent on e length of the bin, more influenced by the lower an the higher frequencies. Its major advantage es in their relative insensitivity to the analytical uality of the series of NN intervals;[12–14] while ajor disadvantage is the need for a reasonable umber of NN intervals to construct the geomet-c pattern, at least 20-min recording is required, referable 24 h. The HRVi expresses overall HRV easured over 24 h and strongly correlated with DNN, if they are derived from long-term record-ngs of adequate quality.

Of various time-domain HRV variables, SDNN, DANN, RMSSD, and HRVi were recommended y the Task Force Committee in 1996.[12]

requency-Domain Analysis

)f various spectral methods, most commonly sed methods to transform signals into the fre-uency domain are based on fast Fourier trans-orm (FFT) and autoregressive analysis to calculate ower spectral density (PSD; msec^2/Hz), which rovides basic information on how power (vari-nce) distributes as a function of frequency. Sim-licity of algorithm and high processing speed are he main advantages of FFT, while autoregressive nalysis is superior for its smoother spectral com-onents, easy postprocessing of the spectrum, nd accurate estimation of PSD. Its disadvantage s the need for verification of the suitability of the hosen model and its complexity. Both of these nathematical methods yield similar results.[12]

pectral Components

rom short-term recordings, three spectral com-onents can be distinguished in the calculated pectrum, which included high-frequency (HF), ow-frequency (LF), and very-low-frequency (VLF) components. From spectral analysis performed on long-term recordings, an additional spectral component, ultralow frequency (ULF), may be distinguished. In addition, total power and LF/HF ratio are commonly calculated from the spectral results of both short-term and long-term recordings. The spectrum can be divided into three or four bands, usually in the following frequency ranges: ULF ≤ 0.003 Hz, VLF 0.003–0.04 Hz (≤0.04 Hz if calculated from short-term recording), LF 0.04–0.15 Hz, and HF 0.15–0.4 Hz.

For an accurate spectral analysis of HRV, mechanisms modulating the heart rate should not change during the ECG recording time; however, it cannot be considered stationary during the 24-h period for the physiological mechanism of heart rate modulations responsible for LF and HF power components.[15] Thus, it is recommended that short-term recordings free of ectopy, missing data, and noise for frequency-domain analysis should be used. It should always be strictly determined whether the spectral analysis is performed on short-term or long-term ECGs, and normalized units should always be quoted with absolute values of the LF and HF power in order to describe completely the distribution of power in spectral components.[12]

Heart rate variability represents the most promising quantitative markers of autonomic activity. Although the physiological basis of HRV components cannot be simplified as has frequently been described, it is commonly accepted that the HF component reflects the efferent vagal activity, the LF component is affected by both sympathetic and parasympathetic activities,[5] while the LF/HF ratio is often used as a proxy for the sympathovagal balance. The physiological basis for ULF and VLF is rather less clear than the HF and LF components. Analysis of transient physiological phenomena by specific methods remains a challenging research topic.

Reference Values

There have been so far no well-accepted "normal values" of HRV measures available for use in various clinical settings. As no recent report is found concerning the reference values of all HRV indices in large normal populations, Table 24–1

Table 24–1. Reference values of traditional measures of heart rate variability in healthy subjects aged 40–69 years.[16]

Variable	Unit	Normal value (mean ± SD)	Variable	Unit	Normal value (mean ± SD)
Time domain analysis of nominal 24 h			Spectral analysis of stationary supine 5-min recording		
SDNN	msec	141 ± 39	Total power	$msec^2$	3466 ± 1018
SDANN	msec	127 ± 35	LF	$msec^2$	1170 ± 416
RMSSD	msec	27 ± 12	HF	$msec^2$	975 ± 203
HRV triangular index		37 ± 15	LF	nu	54 ± 4
			HF	nu	29 ± 3
			LF/HF ratio		1.5–2.0

HF, high-frequency power; HRV, heart rate variability; LF, low-frequency power; nu, normalized unit; RMSSD, the root mean square of successive differences between adjacent normal-to-normal intervals; SD, standard deviation; SDANN, the standard deviation of the 5-min average normal-to-normal intervals; SDNN, the standard deviation of all normal-to-normal intervals.

lists the reference values of standard time-domain and frequency-domain measures of HRV reported in 1995 by Bigger *et al.*[16]

Nonlinear Methods

The nonlinear methods differ from traditional HRV analysis because they are not designed to assess the magnitude of variability, but rather the quality, scaling, complexity, and correlation properties of the signal. Several algorithms have been developed to describe nonlinear characteristics of HRV signals.[17–22] Commonly processed indices of nonlinear methods include the exponent β of the 1/f slope for long-term analysis and the scaling exponent α for short-term recordings, which provide measures of the presence or absence of fractal correlation properties of RR intervals at different time scales and reflect the complexity of heart rate behavior. Power-law slope,[23,24] approximate entropy (ApEn)[20] and detrended fluctuation analysis,[18] and Poincaré plots[20,25] are other nonlinear measures of HRV often used in clinical studies. There has been great progress in the nonlinear method over the past decade and a variety of nonlinear variables reflecting different aspects of HRV have been investigated in patient populations.[18,20,22,24,26,27] More recently, an increasing number of studies have been reported regarding its value in risk stratification,[24,28] particularly i[n] identifying patients at risk for SCD.[22,29] Howeve[r] the computing programs for nonlinear analysi[s] are currently not available on commercial system[s] Indices of exponent α or β do not correspond wit[h] conventional time or frequency domain parame[-] ters from ambulatory Holter recordings. Th[e] optimum nonlinear measures remain to be deter[-] mined. The standard measures and consente[d] reference values are also lacking.

Other Techniques for Analyzing Behavior of Heart Rate

A variety of analytical techniques used for evalu[-] ating heart rate behavior have been reported i[n] recent years including wavelet transform-base[d] approaches,[30–32] prevalent low-frequency oscilla[-] tion,[33] and other more complicated models.[3] Further technical and clinical studies in larg[e] populations of both healthy subjects and patient[s] are required before their research or clinica[l] value can be established for these techniques Very recently, a novel technique evaluating hear[t] rate deceleration capacity has been developed The heart rate deceleration capacity quantifie[s] the characterizations of deceleration-relate[d] modulation, and has been tested in post-M[I] populations.[35]

ability and Reproducibility of Heart ate Variability Measurements

rly studies suggested great stability of HRV easures derived from 24-h ambulatory monitor-g in normal subjects,[36,37] in patients after MI,[38] d in patients with ventricular arrhythmia.[39] In rmal older subjects, repeated HRV analysis owed that HRV measures remained stable over months if their activity level was not changed.[40] tak *et al.* prospectively evaluated HRV and RT at about 10 days and 12 months after MI in 0 consecutive patients; they found that HRV creased significantly over the observation period hile there were no significant changes in HRT.[41] milarly, Jokinen *et al.* reported traditional meas-ements of HRV improved significantly between 7 days and 12 months after MI, whereas the ope of HRT remained stable.[42] Jokinen *et al.* also und a significant change in HRT onset.[42] In the me group of patients, the fractal HR dynamics mained unchanged.[42] Data regarding the stabil-y and reproducibility of nonlinear methods are nited.

tervention and Factors of Heart ate Variability Modifications

n early experiment in post-MI dogs showed that blockers did not modify HRV,[43] while later clin-al studies demonstrated the beneficial effect of blockers on HRV.[44–51] The Beta-blocker Heart ttack Trial (BHAT), an HRV study, revealed at 6-week propranolol therapy improved HF ower and blunted the morning increase in the F/HF ratio in 88 patients with acute MI, but ere was no change in the placebo groups (n = 6).[44] Airaksinen *et al.* reported that β blockers ttenuated the initial vagal activation associated ith acute coronary occlusion in 116 patients ndergoing elective one-vessel coronary angi-plasty.[45] Most studies found that β blocker erapy induced a significant increase in HRV easures related to parasympathetic activity in atients with chronic heart failure (CHF),[46–49] ven in advanced heart failure.[50,51] Some ntiarrhythmic drugs associated with increased ortality can reduce HRV.[52–54] In the substudy of the European Myocardial Infarct Amiodarone Trial (EMIAT), depressed HRV identified post-MI patients who might benefit from prophylactic treatment with amiodarone.[55] The effects of hormone replacement therapy on cardiac autonomic modulation in postmenopausal women have been inconsistent.[56,57] Depression was associated with lower HRV.[58] Sertraline (an antidepressant) may facilitate the rate of recovery of SDNN in depressed acute MI survivors.[59] Spironolactone was found to improve HRV in CHF patients (n = 28), with particular effects during the morning hours.[60] Scopolamine increased HRV but low-dose scopolamine did not prevent ventricular fibrillation (VF) caused by acute myocardial ischemia in post-MI dogs.[61]

Post-MI patients who had received thrombolytic treatment showed early and better improvement of HRV than those who did not.[62,63] Patients with acute MI who had a successful thrombolysis had higher HRV measures compared to those who had failed therapy, and this finding was independent of infarction site.[64] Heart rate variability measurements were significantly depressed and were associated with myocardial ischemic episodes in patients after coronary artery bypass grafting (CABG) surgery.[65,66] More recently it has been reported that cardiac resynchronization therapy (CRT) significantly modified HRV (SDANN, SDAAM) and lack of HRV improvement after CRT identified patients at higher risk for major cardiovascular events.[10,11,67] In long-term heavy smokers, HRV values were significantly lower and the LF/HF ratio was higher compared to nonsmokers.[68] Smoking cessation significantly decreased heart rate, and increased all 24-h time- and frequency-domain indexes of HRV.[69] In normal older adults exercise training increased total HRV.[40] Aerobic training in sedentary subjects modified HRV toward vagal dominance.[70] In addition, SDANN and HF values may increase after weight loss.[71] Stress management significantly increased HRV in patients with stable coronary artery disease (CAD) compared with patients under usual care.[72]

Many but not all interventions associated with increased HRV are also associated with better survival rates.[61,73] Data on modification of HRV are limited because the effects of most factors on HRV modification are not established.

Heart Rate Variability in Risk Stratification of Cardiac Patients

Heart Rate Variability in Patients after Myocardial Infarction

Despite incomplete understanding of the physiological significance of HRV parameters, this methodology is of substantial utility in identifying patients with increased cardiac mortality, particularly in the survivors of an acute MI. The association between reduced HRV and increased mortality in post-MI has been intensively investigated in the past 2 decades.[6,7,74,75] Its value for risk stratification in post-MI populations has been established,[12] and further confirmed by many later studies. Copie *et al.* reported that HRV < 17 U had a 40% sensitivity, 86% specificity, and 20% positive predictive accuracy for predicting cardiac death in 579 survivors of acute MI followed up for ≥2 years.[76] Power law regression parameters were demonstrated as powerful predictors of death of any cause or arrhythmic death in 715 patients with recent MI.[23] Both traditional and nonlinear HRV were independently associated with mortality after MI[77] even in the fibrinolytic era.[78] A multiparametric HRV analysis better predicted increased risk of arrhythmia than the standard measurement of global HRV in acute MI survivors.[28] In 1998[79] and 2001[80] La Rovere *et al.* demonstrated more conclusively that both HRV and baroreflex sensitivity predicted cardiac and arrhythmic death among 1284 post-MI patients in the Autonomic Tone and Reflexes After Myocardial Infarction (ATRAMI) study. Recent studies using other HRV techniques also confirmed the value of HRV assessment in risk stratification of post-MI patients.[22,33,35,81] Very recently, impaired heart rate deceleration capacity has been shown to be a powerful predictor of mortality after MI and was more accurate than the conventional measures of HRV. Stratification by dichotomized deceleration capacity was especially powerful in patients with left ventricular ejection fraction (LVEF) > 30%.[35]

Heart Rate Variability in Relation to Coronary Artery Disease

In 1995, Huang *et al.* investigated HRV in 52 patients with unstable angina, 52 patients with acute MI, and 41 normal subjects. They found that all time-domain and frequency-domain measures of HRV were reduced in patients with acute coronary syndromes compared to normal controls ($p < 0.001$). There was no significant difference in HRV measures between patients with unstable angina and acute MI. In patients with unstable angina who stabilized after admission, HRV increased over the second 24 h of monitoring. In contrast, HRV was further depressed in patients who had episodes of chest pain or transient ST-segment depression during the second 24 h.[82] The association of HRV with angina or MI was confirmed by late reports.[21,83] Tsuji *et al.* investigated the association of reduced HRV with risk for new cardiac events (angina, MI, CAD death, or CHF) in a community-based population ($n = 2501$ eligible) from the Framingham Heart Study with follow-up of a mean of 3.5 years. After adjustment for other relevant risk factors, all time- and frequency-domain measures except the LF/HF ratio were significantly associated with risk for a cardiac event ($p = 0.0016$–0.0496). One standard deviation decrement in SDNN was associated with a hazard ratio of 1.47 for new cardiac events.[83] Reduced HRV predicted CAD events and CAD mortality in patients with angina[82,84] and in postmenopausal women.[85] Depressed HRV before and after CABG was associated with worse postoperative outcome. The data remain limited concerning the association of HRV measurements with severity of disease and the evolution of HRV with development of a coronary event. More evidence from large prospective studies is required to ascertain the predictive value of HRV measurements for new coronary events in CAD and its clinical implications.

Heart Rate Variability in Patients with Chronic Heart Failure

Over the past decade, numerous studies have showed that CHF is associated with autonomic dysfunction, which can be quantified by measuring HRV. UK-HEART prospectively examined the value of HRV as an independent predictor of death in 433 outpatients with CHF (age 62 ± 9. years old; NYHA functional class I to III; mean LVEF, 0.41 ± 0.17) over a mean follow-up of 48 ± 161 days. The annual mortality rate for the study opulation in the SDNN subgroups was 5.5% for 100 msec, 12.7% for 50–100 msec, and 51.4% for 50 msec of SDNN. Reduced SDNN values identi-ied patients at increased risk of death and pre-licted death from progressive CHF better than ther conventional clinical measurements.[86] Late tudies confirmed that patients with reduced DNN were at significantly increased risk of SCD r all-cause mortality.[87,88] The HRT slope was also ound to have independent prognostic value for leath from decompensated HF.[89] However, in CHF patients with the most severe functional mpairment, HRV indexes may not provide inde-endent prognostic information.[90] More recently, a Rovere *et al.* convincingly demonstrated that educed short-term LF power during controlled reathing predicted SCD in patients with CHF ndependent of many other clinical variables.[91] Their finding was supported by a later report of Guzzetti *et al.*[92]

Adamson *et al.* demonstrated the prognostic value of long-term continuous HRV measure-ments from an implantable device in 288 patients with CHF. Continuous HRV was measured as SDAAM sensed by the device. An SDAAM < 50 msec averaged over 4 weeks was associated with increased mortality risk (hazard ratio 3.20, $p = 0.02$). The SDAAM was persistently lower over the entire follow-up period in patients who required hospitalization or died. This study shows the potential value of evaluating continuous long-term SDAAM for clinical management in patients with CHF.[11]

Heart Rate Variability, Ventricular Tachyarrhythmias, and Sudden Cardiac Death

There is experimental[93] and epidemiological evidence of an association between depressed HRV and SCD,[22,29,91,92,94–96] even though the pathophysiological link of this association is still not completely understood. Table 24–2 presents a summary of selected studies assessing the predictive value of HRV for SCD. An early observation showed that survivors of sudden cardiac arrest ($n = 16$) had reduced LF and HF spectral power, whereas nonsurvivors ($n = 5$) had a loss of both LF and HF power.[94] A later investigation in 575 survivors of acute MI demonstrated that depressed HRV ($p < 0.001$) and ventricular tachycardia runs ($p < 0.05$) at the time of hospital discharge predicted arrhythmic death over a 2-year follow-up.[96] Huikuri *et al.* found that only reduced α_1 (<0.75) was identified as an independent predictor of arrhythmic death ($n = 75$) with an adjusted relative risk of 1.4 (95% CI 1.1–1.7, $p < 0.05$) in a substudy of the DIAMOND trial consisting of 446 survivors of acute MI with an LVEF ≤35%.[22] The prognostic power of altered HRV as a predictor of SCD in the general population was reported later by the same primary investigators.[29] Reduced α_1 (<1.0) predicted SCD ($n = 29$) with an adjusted relative risk of 4.3 (95% CI 2.0–9.2, $p < 0.001$) independent of other predictors in 325 subjects aged ≥65 years.[29] In CHF, depressed HRV was demonstrated to predict the risk of SCD.[91,92] However, HRV (SDNN) failed to predict sustained ventricular tachycardia (VT), VF, or SCD ($n = 38$) during a follow-up of 52 ± 21 months in a prospective observational study including 263 patients with idiopathic cardiomyopathy.[97]

Early studies observed a temporal relation between reduction or alteration of HRV and the onset of ventricular tachyarrhythmias based on data from 24-h Holter recordings.[26,98–100] All frequency-domain measures of HRV were significantly reduced before onset of spontaneous episodes of VT, and the ratio between LF and HF increased substantially before the episodes ($p = 0.05$).[98] Nonlinear methods revealed alterations in RR-interval dynamics before spontaneous onset of ventricular tachyarrhythmias.[26] A case–control study showed that reduced HRV (SDNN and nonlinear method) was associated with susceptibility to VF but not with stable monomorphic VT in post-MI patients.[25] Based on HRV analysis from 10-min high-resolution ECG, Perkiomaki *et al.* showed that only α_1 was an independent predictor of ICD shock or death with a hazard ratio 1.20 (95% CI 1.03–1.39) for every 0.10 decrease in α_1 ($p = 0.020$) in 55 patients with impaired left ventricular function and an ICD of various indications.[101] Bikkina *et al.* reported that short-term HRV from an 11-beat strip of ECG recorded before electrophysiological study was significantly lower in subjects with inducible VT ($n = 12$) compared to those without clinical or electrocardiographic evidence of VT ($n = 20$).[102]

TABLE 24–2. Heart rate variability and sudden cardiac death: summary of selected studies.

Study	Study population (*N*)	Study design	HRV method	Main parameter investigated	Main findings of the study
Bigger *et al.*[8]	Recent MI (*N* = 715)	Observational; 4-year follow-up	Holter recording; FD analysis	ULF, VLF, LF, HF	VLF strongly associated with SCD
Algra *et al.*[95]	Subjects who had Holter ECG (*N* = 245 SCD, 467 control)	Observational; 2-year follow-up	24-h Holter recording; TD analysis	Short-term RR variation <25 msec	Relative risk for SCD 3.0 (95% confidence interval 2.1–5.0)
Hartikainen *et al.*[96]	Recent MI (*N* = 575)	Observational; 2-year follow-up	24-h Holter recording; geometric method	HRV triangular index	Depressed HRV independently predicted arrhythmic death
Perkiomaki *et al.*[25]	PMI, CA (*N* = 30) PMI, VT (*N* = 30)	Case control	Holter recording; TD analysis, Poincaré plot analysis	SDNN and Poincaré plot	Low HRV is related to susceptibility to VF not to stable monomorphic VT
Shusterman *et al.*[99]	CA, VF, VT (*N* = 53)	Observational	Holter recording; TD and FD analysis	HF, LF, LF/HF, SDNN, RMSSD	LF, LF/HF ratio decreased significantly before the onset of VT
Huikuri *et al.*[22]	Recent MI and impaired LVF (*N* = 446)	Observational; follow-up of 685 ± 386 days	Holter recording; TD and FD analysis, fractal analysis	Exponents α_1 and α_2 and exponent β	Reduced α_1 predicted arrhythmic death better than others
Pruvot *et al.*[9]	PMI with ICD (*N* = 58)	Observational	ICD recording; FD analysis	TF, VLF, HF, LF	Reduction in HRV before VTA onset
Markikallio *et al.*[29]	Age ≥ 65 years (*N* = 325)	Observational; 10-year follow-up	24-h Holter; conventional and fractal scaling measures	Short-term fractal scaling exponent	Reduced α_1 as independent predictor of SCD
La Rovere *et al.*[91]	CHF (*N* = 444)	Observational; 3-year follow-up	8-min ECG recording; TD and FD analysis	LF	Reduced LF as independent predictor of SCD
Guzzetti *et al.*[92]	CHF (*N* = 330)	Observational; 3-year follow-up	24-h Holter; TD and FD analysis	VLF, LF	Reduced nighttime LF linked to SCD independently
Grimm *et al.*[97]	Idiopathic DCM (*N* = 263)	Observational; follow-up of 52 ± 21 months	24-h Holter recording; TD analysis	SDNN	HRV was not predictive of major arrhythmic events

CA, cardiac arrest; CHF, chronic heart failure; DCM, dilated cardiomyopathy; FD, frequency domain; HF, high-frequency power; HRV, heart rate variability; ICD, implantable cardioverter defibrillator; LF, low-frequency power; LVF, left ventricular function; MI, myocardial infarction; nu, normalized unit; PMI, post-myocardial infarction; RMSSD, the root mean square of successive differences between adjacent normal-to-normal intervals; SCD, sudden cardiac death; SD, standard deviation; SDANN, the standard deviation of the 5-min average normal-to-normal intervals; SDNN, the standard deviation of all normal-to-normal intervals; TD, time domain; TF, total power; ULF, ultralow-frequency power; VLF, very low-frequency power; VF, ventricular fibrillation; VT, ventricular tachycardia; VTA, ventricular tachyarrhythmias.

The recent availability of ICDs that can record and retrieve R–R intervals preceding an arrhythmic event provides a unique opportunity to accurately analyze the behavior of heart rate before onset of ventricular tachyarrhythmias.[9,103,104] A significant reduction in HRV was found before onset of ventricular arrhythmias compared with control conditions suggesting a state of sympathetic excitation preceding ventricular arrhythmic events.[9] Although others failed to detect significant differences in short-term HRV (time- and frequency-domain analysis and nonlinear methods) immediately before the arrhythmic events using the ECG data stored in ICD, they observed that the heart rate and frequency of ectopic beats were significantly increased before onset of VT or VF.[104] These findings suggest a shift of autonomic balance toward sympathetic predominance and reduced vagal tone before onset of ventricular arrhythmic events that may reflect a transient electrical instability favoring the onset of ventricular tachyarrhythmias in patients with cardiac disorders.

Heart Rate Variability in Patients with Other Cardiac Disorders

In patients with cardiac hypertrophy of various etiology, reduced HRV was found to be independently associated with the extent of cardiac hypertrophy.[105] Preserved HRV identified patients with nonischemic dilated cardiomyopathy at lower risk of mortality as suggested by the results from the trial of Defibrillators in Non-Ischemic Cardiomyopathy Treatment Evaluation (DEFINITE), which included 274 participants.[106] In patients who had undergone total correction of tetralogy of Fallot, HRV assessment was applied to stratify patients at risk of life-threatening arrhythmias by analyzing the status of the adrenergic nervous system and HRV differentiated patients with and without severe postoperative ventricular arrhythmias.[107] The role of HRV in the diagnosis and therapeutic decision making in AF has not yet been established, while it has been shown that HRV analysis is a promising technique for assessing the interplay of sympathetic and parasympathetic activity before the onset of AF. Hogue *et al.* demonstrated using logistic regression analysis that increased heart rate and decreased ApEn were independently associated with AF in post- CABG patients based on the averaged values for the three 20-min intervals preceding the onset of AF, suggesting such HRV assessment may provide useful information for risk stratification or investigation of mechanisms in postoperative AF.[20] Diminished circadian variation in HRV before CABG may indicate a propensity for AF.[108] More studies are needed to confirm these findings. In elderly people, Huikuri *et al.* found that 24-h HRV (power-law relationship) independently predicted cardiac death in a random sample of 347 subjects aged ≥65 years who were followed up for 10 years.[24] A recent ECG study in postmenopausal women from the Women's Health Initiative confirmed that reduced HRV remained one of the dominant risk predictors for coronary heart disease (CHD) mortality.[85]

Summary and Further Work in Heart Rate Variability Research

Heart rate variability has considerable potential in assessing the role of autonomic nervous system fluctuations in normal healthy individuals and in patients with various cardiovascular and noncardiovascular disorders.[12] Over the past decade HRV studies have enhanced our understanding of physiological phenomena, the actions of medications, and disease mechanisms.

Heart rate variability has become an established risk stratifier for arrhythmic events and mortality in post-MI populations,[12] but reduced HRV alone has only moderate sensitivity and specificity. In combination with other major risk factors, e.g., LVEF, HRV can identify cardiac patients at particularly high risk of mortality, and the positive predictive accuracy of HRV can be improved up to 33–58%.[8,109] Compared to assessment of left ventricular function, HRV as a risk stratifier is superior with respect to predicting arrhythmic events and sudden death. A multiparametric approach combining HRV parameters from all domains may provide better prediction of arrhythmic risk compared with the standard measures of global HRV in post-MI patients.[28] The association of reduced HRV with susceptibility to life-threatening tachyarrhythmias has been confirmed by most published studies. Increasing evidence suggests that nonlinear heart rate dynamics may have significant prognostic power for stratifying patients at high risk of SCD. A majority of clinical studies indicate that HRV is of important prognostic value in patients with CHF[86,91,92] and that depressed HRV identifies patients at significantly increased risk of cardiac mortality.

The area of HRV behavior before the onset of life-threatening ventricular tachyarrhythmias offers exciting possibilities for further research to explore the predictive power for the timing of the onset of fatal ventricular tachyarrhythmia and the mechanism to initiate the events. Rapid developments in technology have made it possible to capture electrocardiographic data from implantable cardiac devices in or out of the hospital, which will facilitate HRV research and the further development of computing algorithms. The specificity and predictive accuracy of altered HRV in predicting imminent or future fatal arrhythmic events are still low for clinical risk assessment in cardiac patients. More evidence for the predictive value of HRV measurements in ventricular tachyarrhythmias and SCD is required by carefully designed clinical studies/trials to evaluate its clinical applicability. It is also important to conduct well-designed intervention trials in patients with abnormal autonomic function to reveal the potential clinical role of HRV using either conventional or novel methods. Although there is growing awareness that nonlinear analysis of HRV may improve the predictive accuracy of Holter monitoring ECG in post-MI patients, more clinical studies in a large population are needed to confirm the findings. It is promising to explore other novel techniques characterizing the behavior of heart rate from long-term ECG recordings[33,35] and applications in other cardiac populations. It is clear that HRV assessment by conventional and nonlinear methods is a useful research tool for documenting alterations in autonomic modulation in relation to arrhythmic events and providing prognostic information in patients with cardiac disorders. However, the clinical application of HRV assessment using any technique has not been established for monitoring the behavior of HRV in individual patients. More research is needed to identify the optimal approach and algorithm of HRV assessment for future application of HRV in clinical practice.

References

1. Malik M, Camm AJ. Components of heart rate variability—what they really mean and what we really measure. *Am J Cardiol* 1993;72:821–822.
2. Hon EH, Lee ST. Electronic evaluations of the fetal heart rate patterns preceding fetal death: Further observations. *Am J Obstet Gynecol* 1965;87:814–826.
3. Ewing DJ, Martyn CN, Young RJ, *et al.* The value of cardiovascular autonomic function tests: 10 years experience in diabetes. *Diabetes Care* 1985;8:491–498.
4. Wolf MM, Varigos GA, Hunt D, *et al.* Sinus arrhythmia in acute myocardial infarction. *Med J Aust* 1978;2:52–53.
5. Akselrod S, Gordon D, Ubel FA, *et al.* Power spectrum analysis of heart rate fluctuation: A quantitative probe of beat-to-beat cardiovascular control. *Science* 1981;213:220–222.
6. Kleiger RE, Miller JP, Bigger JT Jr, *et al.* Decreased heart rate variability and its association with increased mortality after acute myocardial infarction. *Am J Cardiol* 1987;59:256–262.
7. Malik M, Farrell T, Cripps T, *et al.* Heart rate variability in relation to prognosis after myocardial infarction: Selection of optimal processing techniques. *Eur Heart J* 1989;10:1060–1074.
8. Bigger JT Jr, Fleiss JL, Steinman RC, *et al.* Frequency domain measures of heart period variability and mortality after myocardial infarction. *Circulation* 1992;85:164–171.
9. Pruvot E, Thonet G, Vesin JM, *et al.* Heart rate dynamics at the onset of ventricular tachyarrhythmias as retrieved from implantable cardioverter-defibrillators in patients with coronary artery disease. *Circulation* 2000;101:2398–2404.
10. Adamson PB, Kleckner KJ, VanHout WL, *et al.* Cardiac resynchronization therapy improves heart rate variability in patients with symptomatic heart failure. *Circulation* 2003;108:266–269.
11. Adamson PB, Smith AL, Abraham WT, *et al.* Continuous autonomic assessment in patients with symptomatic heart failure: Prognostic value of heart rate variability measured by an implanted cardiac resynchronization device. *Circulation* 2004;110:2389–2394.
12. Task Force of the European Society of Cardiology and the North American Society of Pacing and Electrophysiology. Heart rate variability: Standards of measurement, physiological interpretation and clinical use. *Circulation* 1996;93:1043–1065.
13. Malik M, Cripps T, Farrell T, *et al.* Prognostic value of heart rate variability after myocardial infarction: A comparision of different data processing methods. *Med Biol Eng Comput* 1989;27:603–611.
14. Malik M, Xia R, Odemuyiwa O, *et al.* Influence of the recognition artefact in automatic analysis of long-term electrocardiograms on time-domain measurement of heart rate variability. *Med Biol Eng Comput* 1993;31:539–544.
15. Furlan R, Guzzetti S, Crivellaro W, *et al.* Continuous 24-hour assessment of the neural regulation of systemic arterial pressure and RR variabilities in ambulant subjects. *Circulation* 1990;81:537–547.
16. Bigger JT Jr, Fleiss JL, Steinman RC, *et al.* RR variability in healthy, middle-aged persons compared with patients with chronic coronary heart disease or recent acute myocardial infarction. *Circulation* 1995;91:1936–1943.

17. Lombardi F, Sandrone G, Mortara A, *et al.* Linear and nonlinear dynamics of heart rate variability after acute myocardial infarction with normal and reduced left ventricular ejection fraction. *Am J Cardiol* 1996;77:1283–1288.
18. Ho KK, Moody GB, Peng CK, *et al.* Predicting survival in heart failure case and control subjects by use of fully automated methods for deriving nonlinear and conventional indices of heart rate dynamics. *Circulation* 1997;96:842–848.
19. Makikallio TH, Seppanen T, Airaksinen KE, *et al.* Dynamic analysis of heart rate may predict subsequent ventricular tachycardia after myocardial infarction. *Am J Cardiol* 1997;80:779–783.
20. Hogue CW Jr, Domitrovich PP, Stein PK, *et al.* RR interval dynamics before atrial fibrillation in patients after coronary artery bypass graft surgery. *Circulation* 1998;98:429–434.
21. Makikallio TH, Ristimae T, Airaksinen KE, *et al.* Heart rate dynamics in patients with stable angina pectoris and utility of fractal and complexity measures. *Am J Cardiol* 1998;81:27–31.
22. Huikuri HV, Makikallio TH, Peng CK, *et al.* Fractal correlation properties of R-R interval dynamics and mortality in patients with depressed left ventricular function after an acute myocardial infarction. *Circulation* 2000;101:47–53.
23. Bigger JT Jr, Steinman RC, Rolnitzky LM, *et al.* Power law behavior of RR-interval variability in healthy middle-aged persons, patients with recent acute myocardial infarction, and patients with heart transplants. *Circulation* 1996;93:2142–2151.
24. Huikuri HV, Makikallio TH, Airaksinen KE, *et al.* Power-law relationship of heart rate variability as a predictor of mortality in the elderly. *Circulation* 1998;97:2031–2036.
25. Perkiomaki JS, Huikuri HV, Koistinen JM, *et al.* Heart rate variability and dispersion of QT interval in patients with vulnerability to ventricular tachycardia and ventricular fibrillation after previous myocardial infarction. *J Am Coll Cardiol* 1997;30:1331–1338.
26. Huikuri HV, Seppanen T, Koistinen MJ, *et al.* Abnormalities in beat-to-beat dynamics of heart rate before the spontaneous onset of life-threatening ventricular tachyarrhythmias in patients with prior myocardial infarction. *Circulation* 1996;93:1836–1844.
27. Pikkujamsa SM, Makikallio TH, Sourander LB, *et al.* Cardiac interbeat interval dynamics from childhood to senescence: Comparison of conventional and new measures based on fractals and chaos theory. *Circulation* 1999;100:393–399.
28. Voss A, Hnatkova K, Wessel N, *et al.* Multiparametric analysis of heart rate variability used for risk stratification among survivors of acute myocardial infarction. *Pacing Clin Electrophysiol* 1998;21:186–192.
29. Makikallio TH, Huikuri HV, Makikallio A, *et al.* Prediction of sudden cardiac death by fractal analysis of heart rate variability in elderly subjects. *J Am Coll Cardiol* 2001;37:1395–1402.
30. Chen SW. A wavelet-based heart rate variability analysis for the study of nonsustained ventricular tachycardia. *IEEE Trans Biomed Eng* 2002;49:736–742.
31. Tan BH, Shimizu H, Hiromoto K, *et al.* Wavelet transform analysis of heart rate variability to assess the autonomic changes associated with spontaneous coronary spasm of variant angina. *J Electrocardiol* 2003;36:117–124.
32. Toledo E, Gurevitz O, Hod H, *et al.* Wavelet analysis of instantaneous heart rate: A study of autonomic control during thrombolysis. *Am J Physiol Regul Integr Comp Physiol* 2003;284:R1079–R1091.
33. Wichterle D, Simek J, La Rovere MT, *et al.* Prevalent low-frequency oscillation of heart rate: Novel predictor of mortality after myocardial infarction. *Circulation* 2004;110:1183–1190.
34. Barbieri R, Matten EC, Alabi AA, *et al.* A point-process model of human heartbeat intervals: New definitions of heart rate and heart rate variability. *Am J Physiol Heart Circ Physiol* 2005;288:H424–H435.
35. Bauer A, Kantelhardt JW, Barthel P, *et al.* Deceleration capacity of heart rate as a predictor of mortality after myocardial infarction: Cohort study. *Lancet* 2006;367:1674–1681.
36. Kleiger RE, Bigger JT, Bosner MS, *et al.* Stability over time of variables measuring heart rate variability in normal subjects. *Am J Cardiol* 1991;68:626–630.
37. Van Hoogenhuyze D, Weinstein N, Martin GJ, *et al.* Reproducibility and relation to mean heart rate of heart rate variability in normal subjects and in patients with congestive heart failure secondary to coronary artery disease. *Am J Cardiol* 1991;68:1668–1676.
38. Kautzner J. Reproducibility of heart rate variability measurement. In: Malik M, Camm AJ, Eds. *Heart Rate Variability.* Armonk, NY: Futura; 1995:165–171.
39. Bigger JT Jr, Fleiss JL, Rolnitzky LM, *et al.* Stability over time of heart period variability in patients with previous myocardial infarction and ventricular arrhythmias. The CAPS and ESVEM investigators. *Am J Cardiol* 1992;69:718–723.

40. Stein PK, Ehsani AA, Domitrovich PP, *et al.* Effect of exercise training on heart rate variability in healthy older adults. *Am Heart J* 1999;138:567–576.
41. Ortak J, Weitz G, Wiegand UK, *et al.* Changes in heart rate, heart rate variability, and heart rate turbulence during evolving reperfused myocardial infarction. *Pacing Clin Electrophysiol* 2005; 28(Suppl. 1):S227–S232.
42. Jokinen V, Tapanainen JM, Seppanen T, *et al.* Temporal changes and prognostic significance of measures of heart rate dynamics after acute myocardial infarction in the beta-blocking era. *Am J Cardiol* 2003;92:907–912.
43. Adamson PB, Huang MH, Vanoli E, *et al.* Unexpected interaction between beta-adrenergic blockade and heart rate variability before and after myocardial infarction. A longitudinal study in dogs at high and low risk for sudden death. *Circulation* 1994;90:976–982.
44. Lampert R, Ickovics JR, Viscoli CJ, *et al.* Effects of propranolol on recovery of heart rate variability following acute myocardial infarction and relation to outcome in the Beta-Blocker Heart Attack Trial. *Am J Cardiol* 2003;91:137–142.
45. Airaksinen KE, Ikaheimo MJ, Niemela MJ, *et al.* Effect of beta blockade on heart rate variability during vessel occlusion at the time of coronary angioplasty. *Am J Cardiol* 1996;77:20–24.
46. Pousset F, Copie X, Lechat P, *et al.* Effects of bisoprolol on heart rate variability in heart failure. *Am J Cardiol* 1996;77:612–617.
47. Goldsmith RL, Bigger JT, Bloomfield DM, *et al.* Long-term carvedilol therapy increases parasympathetic nervous system activity in chronic congestive heart failure. *Am J Cardiol* 1997;80: 1101–1104.
48. Lin JL, Chan HL, Du CC, *et al.* Long-term beta-blocker therapy improves autonomic nervous regulation in advanced congestive heart failure: A longitudinal heart rate variability study. *Am Heart J* 1999;137:658–665.
49. Mortara A, La Rovere MT, Pinna GD, *et al.* Nonselective beta-adrenergic blocking agent, carvedilol, improves arterial baroflex gain and heart rate variability in patients with stable chronic heart failure. *J Am Coll Cardiol* 2000;36:1612–1618.
50. Aronson D, Burger AJ. Effect of beta-blockade on heart rate variability in decompensated heart failure. *Int J Cardiol* 2001;79:31–39.
51. Lin LY, Lin JL, Du CC, *et al.* Reversal of deteriorated fractal behavior of heart rate variability by beta-blocker therapy in patients with advanced congestive heart failure. *J Cardiovasc Electrophysiol* 2001;12:26–32.
52. Zuanetti G, Latini R, Neilson JM, Schwartz P Ewing DJ. Heart rate variability in patien with ventricular arrhythmias: Effect of antiarrhyth mic drugs. Antiarrhythmic Drug Evaluatio Group (ADEG). *J Am Coll Cardiol* 1991;17:604 612.
53. Lombardi F, Torzillo D, Sandrone G, *et al.* Beta blocking effect of propafenone based on spectra analysis of heart rate variability. *Am J Cardi* 1992;70:1028–1034.
54. Bigger JT Jr, Rolnitzky LM, Steinman RC, *et a* Predicting mortality after myocardial infarctio from the response of RR variability to antiarrhyth mic drug therapy. *J Am Coll Cardiol* 1994;2 733–740.
55. Malik M, Camm AJ, Janse MJ, *et al.* Depresse heart rate variability identifies postinfarctio patients who might benefit from prophylacti treatment with amiodarone: A substudy of EMIA (The European Myocardial Infarct Amiodaron Trial). *J Am Coll Cardiol* 2000;35:1263–1275.
56. Rosano GM, Patrizi R, Leonardo F, *et al.* Effect c estrogen replacement therapy on heart rate varia bility and heart rate in healthy postmenopaus women. *Am J Cardiol* 1997;80:815–817.
57. Fernandes EO, Moraes RS, Ferlin EL, *et a* Hormone replacement therapy does not affect th 24-hour heart rate variability in postmenopausa women: Results of a randomized, placebo controlled trial with two regimens. *Pacing Cli Electrophysiol* 2005;28(Suppl. 1):S172–S177.
58. Carney RM, Blumenthal JA, Stein PK, *et al.* Depres sion, heart rate variability, and acute myocardia infarction. *Circulation* 2001;104:2024–2028.
59. McFarlane A, Kamath MV, Fallen EL, *et al.* Effec of sertraline on the recovery rate of cardiac auto nomic function in depressed patients after acut myocardial infarction. *Am Heart J* 2001;142:617 623.
60. Yee KM, Pringle SD, Struthers AD. Circadian vari ation in the effects of aldosterone blockade o heart rate variability and QT dispersion in conges tive heart failure. *J Am Coll Cardiol* 2001;37:1800 1807.
61. Hull SS Jr, Vanoli E, Adamson PB, *et al.* D increases in markers of vagal activity imply pro tection from sudden death? The case of scopo lamine. *Circulation* 1995;91:2516–2519.
62. Lind P, Hintze U, Moller M, *et al.* Thrombolyti therapy preserves vagal activity early after acut myocardial infarction. *Scand Cardiovasc J* 200 35:92–95.
63. Kelly PA, Nolan J, Wilson JI, *et al.* Preservation o autonomic function following successful reper fusion with streptokinase within 12 hours of th

onset of acute myocardial infarction. *Am J Cardiol* 1997;79:203–205.

64. Zabel M, Klingenheben T, Hohnloser SH. Changes in autonomic tone following thrombolytic therapy for acute myocardial infarction: Assessment by analysis of heart rate variability. *J Cardiovasc Electrophysiol* 1994;5:211–218.
65. Wu ZK, Vikman S, Laurikka J, *et al.* Nonlinear heart rate variability in CABG patients and the preconditioning effect. *Eur J Cardiothorac Surg* 2005;28:109–113.
66. Laitio TT, Makikallio TH, Huikuri HV, *et al.* Relation of heart rate dynamics to the occurrence of myocardial ischemia after coronary artery bypass grafting. *Am J Cardiol* 2002;89:1176–1181.
67. Fantoni C, Raffa S, Regoli F, *et al.* Cardiac resynchronization therapy improves heart rate profile and heart rate variability of patients with moderate to severe heart failure. *J Am Coll Cardiol* 2005;46:1875–1882.
68. Barutcu I, Esen AM, Kaya D, *et al.* Cigarette smoking and heart rate variability: Dynamic influence of parasympathetic and sympathetic maneuvers. *Ann Noninvasive Electrocardiol* 2005;10: 324–329.
69. Stein PK, Rottman JN, Kleiger RE. Effect of 21 mg transdermal nicotine patches and smoking cessation on heart rate variability. *Am J Cardiol* 1996;77: 701–705.
70. Tulppo MP, Hautala AJ, Makikallio TH, *et al.* Effects of aerobic training on heart rate dynamics in sedentary subjects. *J Appl Physiol* 2003;95:364–372.
71. Karason K, Molgaard H, Wikstrand J, *et al.* Heart rate variability in obesity and the effect of weight loss. *Am J Cardiol* 1999;83:1242–1247.
72. Blumenthal JA, Sherwood A, Babyak MA, *et al.* Effects of exercise and stress management training on markers of cardiovascular risk in patients with ischemic heart disease: A randomized controlled trial. *JAMA* 2005;293:1626–1634.
73. Vanoli E, Cerati D, Pedretti RF. Autonomic control of heart rate: Pharmacological and nonpharmacological modulation. *Basic Res Cardiol* 1998; 93(Suppl. 1):133–142.
74. Casolo GC, Stroder P, Signorini C, *et al.* Heart rate variability during the acute phase of myocardial infarction. *Circulation* 1992;85:2073–2079.
75. Bigger JT Jr, Fleiss JL, Rolnitzky LM, *et al.* The ability of several short-term measures of RR variability to predict mortality after myocardial infarction. *Circulation* 1993;88:927–934.
76. Copie X, Hnatkova K, Staunton A, *et al.* Predictive power of increased heart rate versus depressed left ventricular ejection fraction and heart rate variability for risk stratification after myocardial infarction. Results of a two-year follow-up study. *J Am Coll Cardiol* 1996;27:270–276.
77. Stein PK, Domitrovich PP, Huikuri HV, *et al.* Traditional and nonlinear heart rate variability are each independently associated with mortality after myocardial infarction. *J Cardiovasc Electrophysiol* 2005;16:13–20.
78. Zuanetti G, Neilson JM, Latini R, *et al.* Prognostic significance of heart rate variability in post-myocardial infarction patients in the fibrinolytic era. The GISSI-2 results. Gruppo Italiano per lo Studio della Sopravvivenza nell' Infarto Miocardico. *Circulation* 1996;94:432–436.
79. La Rovere MT, Bigger JT Jr, Marcus FI, *et al.* Baroreflex sensitivity and heart-rate variability in prediction of total cardiac mortality after myocardial infarction. ATRAMI (Autonomic Tone and Reflexes After Myocardial Infarction) Investigators. *Lancet* 1998;351:478–484.
80. La Rovere MT, Pinna GD, Hohnloser SH, *et al.* Baroreflex sensitivity and heart rate variability in the identification of patients at risk for life-threatening arrhythmias: Implications for clinical trials. *Circulation* 2001;103:2072–2077.
81. Tapanainen J, Thomsen P, Kober L, *et al.* Fractal analysis of heart rate variability and mortality after an acute myocardial infarction. *Am J Cardiol* 2002;90:347–352.
82. Huang J, Sopher SM, Leatham E, *et al.* Heart rate variability depression in patients with unstable angina. *Am Heart J* 1995;130:772–779.
83. Tsuji H, Larson MG, Venditti FJ, *et al.* Impact of reduced heart rate variability on risk for cardiac events. The Framingham Heart Study. *Circulation* 1996;94:2850–2855.
84. Forslund L, Bjorkander I, Ericson M, *et al.* Prognostic implications of autonomic function assessed by analyses of catecholamines and heart rate variability in stable angina pectoris. *Heart* 2002;87: 415–422.
85. Rautaharju PM, Kooperberg C, Larson JC, *et al.* Electrocardiographic abnormalities that predict coronary heart disease events and mortality in postmenopausal women: The Women's Health Initiative. *Circulation* 2006;113:473–480.
86. Nolan J, Batin PD, Andrews R, *et al.* Prospective study of heart rate variability and mortality in chronic heart failure: Results of the United Kingdom heart failure evaluation and assessment of risk trial (UK-heart). *Circulation* 1998;98: 1510–1516.
87. Bilchick KC, Fetics B, Djoukeng R, *et al.* Prognostic value of heart rate variability in chronic congestive heart failure (Veterans Affairs' Survival

Trial of Antiarrhythmic Therapy in Congestive Heart Failure). *Am J Cardiol* 2002;90:24–28.
88. Boveda S, Galinier M, Pathak A, *et al.* Prognostic value of heart rate variability in time domain analysis in congestive heart failure. *J Interv Card Electrophysiol* 2001;5:181–187.
89. Moore RK, Groves DG, Barlow PE, *et al.* Heart rate turbulence and death due to cardiac decompensation in patients with chronic heart failure. *Eur J Heart Fail* 2006;8(6):585–590.
90. Makikallio TH, Huikuri HV, Hintze U, *et al.* Fractal analysis and time- and frequency-domain measures of heart rate variability as predictors of mortality in patients with heart failure. *Am J Cardiol* 2001;87:178–182.
91. La Rovere MT, Pinna GD, Maestri R, *et al.* Short-term heart rate variability strongly predicts sudden cardiac death in chronic heart failure patients. *Circulation* 2003;107:565–570.
92. Guzzetti S, La Rovere MT, Pinna GD, *et al.* Different spectral components of 24 h heart rate variability are related to different modes of death in chronic heart failure. *Eur Heart J* 2005;26:357–362.
93. Hull SS Jr, Evans AR, Vanoli E, *et al.* Heart rate variability before and after myocardial infarction in conscious dogs at high and low risk of sudden death. *J Am Coll Cardiol* 1990;16:978–985.
94. Dougherty CM, Burr RL. Comparison of heart rate variability in survivors and nonsurvivors of sudden cardiac arrest. *Am J Cardiol* 1992;70:441–448.
95. Algra A, Tijssen JG, Roelandt JR, *et al.* Contribution of the 24 hour electrocardiogram to the prediction of sudden coronary death. *Br Heart J* 1993;70:421–427.
96. Hartikainen JE, Malik M, Staunton A, *et al.* Distinction between arrhythmic and nonarrhythmic death after acute myocardial infarction based on heart rate variability, signal-averaged electrocardiogram, ventricular arrhythmias and left ventricular ejection fraction. *J Am Coll Cardiol* 1996; 28:296–304.
97. Grimm W, Christ M, Sharkova J, *et al.* Arrhythmia risk prediction in idiopathic dilated cardiomyopathy based on heart rate variability and baroreflex sensitivity. *Pacing Clin Electrophysiol* 2005; 28(Suppl. 1):S202–S206.
98. Huikuri HV, Valkama JO, Airaksinen KE, *et al.* Frequency domain measures of heart rate variability before the onset of nonsustained and sustained ventricular tachycardia in patients with coronary artery disease. *Circulation* 1993;87:1220–1228.
99. Shusterman V, Aysin B, Gottipaty V, *et al.* Autonomic nervous system activity and the spontaneous initiation of ventricular tachycardia. ESVEM Investigators. Electrophysiologic stud versus electrocardiographic monitoring trial. *Am Coll Cardiol* 1998;32:1891–1899.
100. Makikallio TH, Koistinen J, Jordaens L, *et a* Heart rate dynamics before spontaneous onset o ventricular fibrillation in patients with heale myocardial infarcts. *Am J Cardiol* 1999;83:880 884.
101. Perkiomaki JS, Zareba W, Daubert JP, *et al.* Fracta correlation properties of heart rate dynamics an adverse events in patients with implantable cardi overter-defibrillators. *Am J Cardiol* 2001;88:17–22
102. Bikkina M, Alpert MA, Mukerji R, *et al.* Dimin ished short-term heart rate variability predict inducible ventricular tachycardia. *Chest* 1998;11 312–316.
103. Lombardi F, Porta A, Marzegalli M, *et al.* Hear rate variability patterns before ventricular tachy cardia onset in patients with an implantable car dioverter defibrillator. Participating Investigator of ICD-HRV Italian Study Group. *Am J Cardic* 2000;86:959–963.
104. Nemec J, Hammill SC, Shen WK. Increase in hear rate precedes episodes of ventricular tachycardi and ventricular fibrillation in patients wit implantable cardioverter defibrillators: Analysi of spontaneous ventricular tachycardia databas *Pacing Clin Electrophysiol* 1999;22:1729–1738.
105. Alter P, Grimm W, Vollrath A, *et al.* Heart rat variability in patients with cardiac hypertrophy– relation to left ventricular mass and etiology. *A Heart J* 2006;151:829–836.
106. Rashba EJ, Estes NA, Wang P, *et al.* Preserve heart rate variability identifies low-risk patient with nonischemic dilated cardiomyopathy: Result from the DEFINITE trial. *Heart Rhythm* 2006; 281–286.
107. Daliento L, Folino AF, Menti L, *et al.* Adrenergi nervous activity in patients after surgical correc tion of te tralogy of Fallot. *J Am Coll Cardic* 2001;38:2043–2047.
108. Jideus L, Ericson M, Stridsberg M, *et al.* Dimin ished circadian variation in heart rate variabilit before surgery in patients developing postopera tive atrial fibrillation. *Scand Cardiovasc J* 2001;3 238–244.
109. Farrell TG, Bashir Y, Cripps T, *et al.* Risk stratifica tion for arrhythmic events in postinfarctio patients based on heart rate variability, ambula tory electrocardiographic variables and the signal averaged electrocardiogram. *J Am Coll Cardi* 1991;18:687–697.

25
Surface Mapping and Magnetoelectrocardiography

Satsuki Yamada

Introduction

The most reliable predictor for sudden cardiac death is reduced systolic function of the left ventricle. There is no established single noninvasive electrophysiological parameter for detecting high risk patients for sudden cardiac death, although a combination of several parameters might be useful. The electrocardiogram (ECG) is widely used as a standard diagnostic tool, but there are certain limitations, as some ECGs may not provide sufficient information required for clinical decision as in patients with baseline ECG abnormalities, e.g., with ventricular hypertrophy, ischemic heart disease, or use of certain medications. Patients with a normal or nonspecific ECG, in spite of latent cardiac disease, are less likely to be hospitalized and consequently suffer adverse events, including increased mortality.[1] Therefore, it is essential to have additional diagnostic tools to increase the probability of detecting individuals who are likely to suffer from adverse cardiac events.

A magnetocardiogram (MCG) is a body surface mapping technique that detects cardiac magnetic fields and especially weak electrophysiological phenomena that could be missed by an ECG. The advantages of MCGs over traditional ECGs are increased sensitivity to small signals, lack of distortion from conductivity in body tissues, and presentation of direct current (DC) component signals and primary currents. This review will highlight the basic principles and recent advantages of magnetocardiography, and clinical application of an MCG for detecting arrhythmic substrates related to sudden cardiac death. Areas of future basic and clinical research are also discussed.

Basic Principles of Magnetocardiograms

Biomagnetic Fields

A changing electric field produces a magnetic field, as Hans C. Ørsted found that a compass needle placed by chance near a wire carrying electrical current swings (electromagnetism) (Table 25–1). This principle also applies to the currents associated with the electrophysiological phenomena in the human body. Action potentials originating in myocardial cells create electrical currents and thus both electric and magnetic fields occur. At the body surface, the cardiac electric fields are measured by ECGs and by body surface potential mappings, while the cardiac magnetic fields are measured by MCGs.

Although the cardiac magnetic field is the strongest of all biomagnetic fields, the cardiac magnetic field (adult heart 10^{-10} T, fetal heart 10^{-12} T) is a million times weaker than the earth's magnetic field (10^{-5} T) and a thousand times weaker than the magnetic fields associated with urban noise (approximately 10^{-7} T) (Figure 25–1).[2,3] Therefore, picking up these weak physiological signals in a noisy environment is one of the primary issues in MCG studies. To improve the signal-to-noise ratio, current MCG systems use superconducting quantum interference devices

TABLE 25–1. History of magnetocardiogram.[a]

Year	MCG	ECG and others
Eleventh century	Compasses in China (detection of the earth's magnetic field)	
1820	Discovery of electromagnetism (Ørsted)	
		ECG in humans (Waller, 1887) ECG system by Einthoven (1903) Fetal ECG (Cremer, 1906) ECG in sinus rhythm, AF, and VF (Lewis 1901–11) Percutaneous transfemoral catheterization (Seldinger, 1953) Echocardiogram (Edler and Hertz, 1953)
1963	Detection of the cardiac magnetic fields (Baule)	
1970	Single-channel MCG system using SQUID (Cohen)	EP study (Wellens, 1971) MR (Lauterbur, 1974)
1980s	Multichannel MCG system using DC SQUID	
1990s	High-temperature SQUID MCG system without a magnetically shielded room	Catheter ablation in WPW syndrome by radiofrequency current (Jackman, 1991)

[a]AF, atrial fibrillation; DC, direct current; ECG, electrocardiogram; EP, electrophysiological; MCG, magnetocardiogram; MR, magnetic resonance; SQUID, superconducting quantam interference device; WPW syndrome, Wolff–Parkinson–White syndrome; VF, ventricular fibrillation.

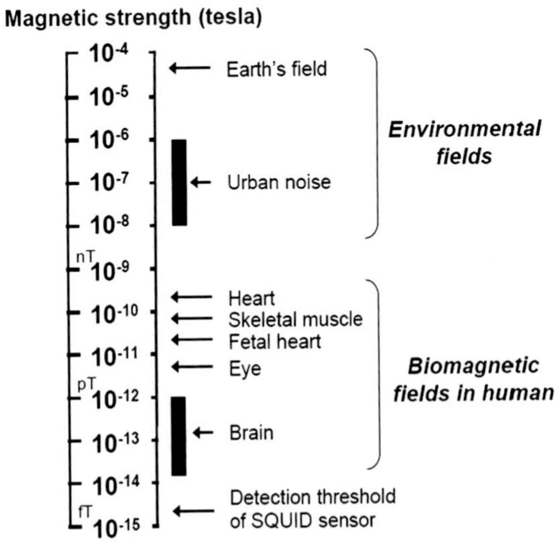

FIGURE 25–1. Biomagnetic fields. fT, femtotesla; nT, nanotesla; pT, picotesla; SQUID, superconducting quantum interference device.

(SQUIDs, minimal detection threshold of 10^{-15} T), a gradiometer, a magnetically shielded room, filtering, and signal averaging.

Advantages of Magnetocardiograms over Electrocardiograms

Both ECGs and MCGs provide information originating from the same phenomena (cardiac electrophysiological activity) by using different methods, i.e., ECGs detect the electrical fields using electrodes, while MCGs measure the magnetic fields using SQUID sensors. Therefore, signals show similar patterns in the two kinds of mappings (Figure 25–2). Waveforms of atrial activation, ventricular depolarization, and ventricular repolarization are called P, QRS, and T waves, respectively, in both mappings. The conduction time also shows significant linear correlation between ECGs and MCGs.

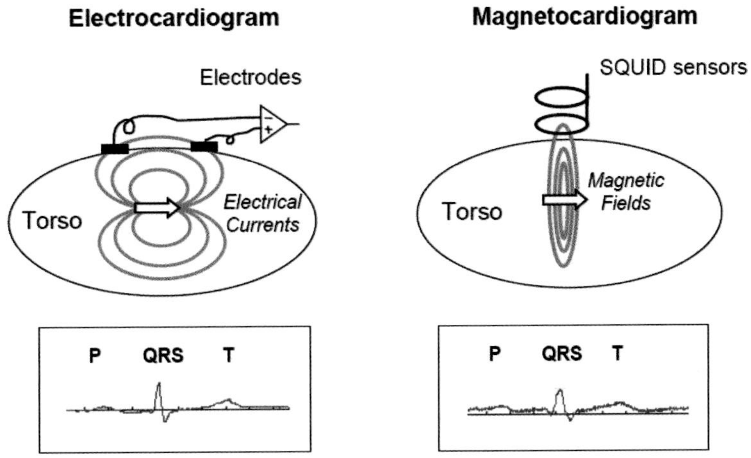

FIGURE 25–2. Relationship between signals and sensors in electrocadiography and that in magnetocardiography. One heart beat was simultaneously recorded by electrocardiography (lead II, left bottom) and magnetocardiography (approximately V1 position, right bottom) in the same subject, a 60-year-old healthy male. SQUID, superconducting quantum interference device.

Both MCGs and ECGs are body surface mappings and not direct-contact mappings of the heart and share many similarities. However, MCGs have some advantages over ECGs (Table 25–2), related to several signal-modifying variables between the heart and sensors at the body surface.[4] First, MCGs constitute a completely noninvasive system measuring the spontaneous magnetic fields that accompany the heartbeat. There is no need for electrodes, radiation, or stimulation procedures in MCGs, whereas ECGs need patch or needle electrodes. Not needing direct contact to the body confers the second advantage; skin electrode interference does not exist in MCGs. A third advantage is that MCGs are less affected by conductivities of body tissues than are ECGs. Fluids and fat surrounding the heart reduce signal strength in ECGs but not in MCGs. These three advantages make MCGs uniquely valuable in fetal diagnosis. Moreover, DC components are not filtered in MCGs and this advantage makes them valuable for analyzing baseline shifts in cardiac ischemia. With respect to spatial components, the cardiac magnetic fields are measured as vectors in MCGs, while cardiac electrical fields are scalar values in ECGs. The DC components plus vector

TABLE 25–2. Advantages of magnetocardiogram.[a]

	12-lead ECG	BSPM	MCG	EPS
Advantage				
1. Effects of body tissues on conductivities	High	High	Low	Low
2. Contact to skin or heart required	Yes, noninvasive	Yes, noninvasive	No	Yes, invasive
3. Skin-electrode or tissue-electrode interference	Yes	Yes	No	Yes
4. Components of volume currents	High	High	Low	Low
5. Direct current filtering required	Yes	Yes	No	Yes
6. Use for fetal study	Yes, low	Yes, low	Yes, high	No
7. Spatial resolution	Low	Intermediate	Intermediate	High
8. Imaging technology	Low	High	High	High
9. Diagnosis/treatment	Diagnosis	Diagnosis	Diagnosis	Diagnosis/treatment
Disadvantage				
1. Environmental noise	Low	Low	High	Low
2. Portability	Yes, high	Yes, intermediate	No	No
3. Costs	Low	Intermediate	High	High
4. Clinical evidence	High	Intermediate	Low	High

[a]BSMP, body surface potential mapping; ECG, electrocardiogram; EPS, electrophysiological study; MCG, magnetocardiogram.

analysis make the baseline value of zero closer to "absolute zero" in MCGs compared to the baseline in ECGs. Because of these advantages, MCGs can provide unique and additional information when ECGs are not practical or not sensitive enough. Examples of phenomena successfully examined using MCGs are fetal arrhythmias (see the section on Fetal Magnetocardiograms), differentiation between primary and secondary ST-T changes, at-rest abnormalities in stable angina pectoris (see the section on Ischemic Heart Disease), and His potentials recording (see the section on Arrhythmias). In addition to the advantages of MCGs over ECGs (at the same recording position), current MCG systems have multiple channels (up to 64) and a variety of computer-based analyzing methods.[4,5]

Measurements of Cardiac Magnetic Fields

Magnetocardiogram System

The MCG system is composed of sensors, computers for data processing, and a magnetically shielded system. Sensors are placed in a cooling system called a "Dewar" (or "cryostat"; arrow in Figure 25–3A) to maintain superconductance. Because MCG systems have not been internationally standardized, their gradiometers (a first order or up to a third order), sensors, number of measuring points (1 to up to 64), measuring areas, and shielding systems (with or without a shielding room, passive or active shield) differ between laboratories. In Japan, a 64-channel MCG system (Hitachi MC-6400 model, Fukuda Denshi, Japan; Figure 25–3A and B) was officially approved by the Japanese Ministry of Health, Labor, and Welfare in 2002, and was commercialized in 2003 as the first system in Japan. In the United States, Model CMI-2409 (nine-channel system, Cardiomag Imaging, USA) was approved by the Food and Drug Administration as the first system in the United States. Biomagnetic Technologies Inc. (USA), CTF Systems Inc. (Canada), Neuromag Ltd. (Finland), Advanced Technologies Biomagnetics (Italy), Donier GmbH (Germany), Siemens AG (Germany), and Philips GmbH (Germany) also do or did offer commercially available MCG or magnetoencephalography systems.

Measurements

Spatial Components of the Cardiac Magnetic Fields

The cardiac magnetic fields are measured as vector markers consisting of three spatial components,

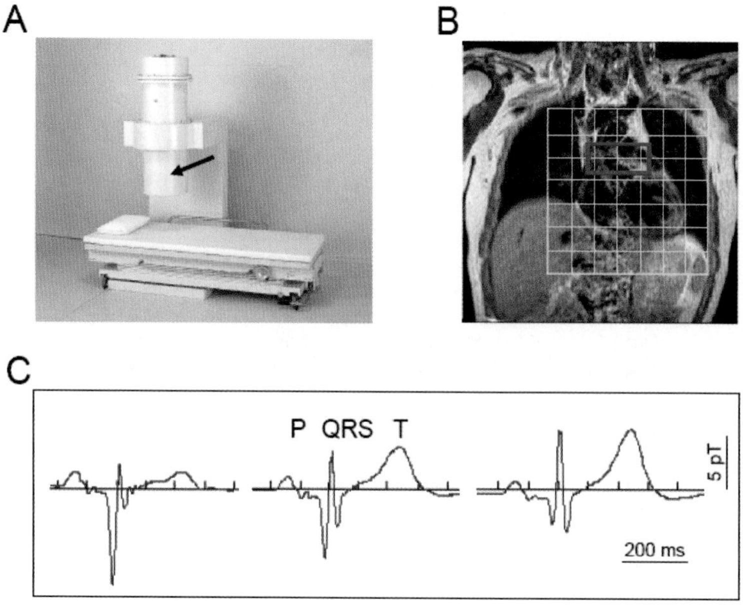

FIGURE 25–3. A 64-channel magnetocardiographic system. (A) Overview of the system (arrow indicates a Dewar). (B) A measuring area of 8 by 8 matrix (sensor interval, 2.5 cm; a measuring area, 17.5 by 17.5 cm) superimposed on a magnetic resonance image. (C) Signals (normal-component cardiac magnetic fields) at 3 (red area in B) out of 64 channels. pt, picotesla.

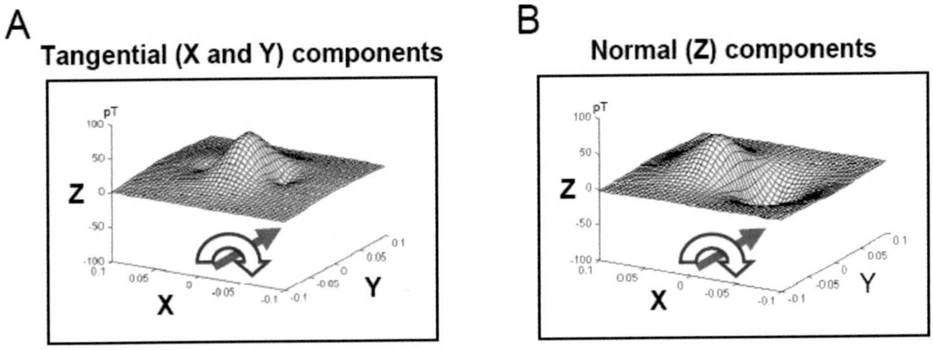

FIGURE 25–4. Spatial components of cardiac magnetic fields. Magnetic fields (curved arrow) show clockwise rotation along the electrical currents (straight arrow). The magnetic strength just above the magnetic source is the maximum in the tangential (or X and Y) components (A), while it is "zero" in the normal (or Z) components (B). pT, picotesla.[44]

called the X, Y, and Z components, corresponding to the horizontal, longitudinal, and vertical components, respectively, in the anterior–posterior view (Figure 25–4). As magnetic fields show clockwise rotation along the electrical currents, the magnetic strength just above the magnetic source is the maximum in the tangential (or X and Y) components (Figure 25–4A), while it is "zero" transitioning from positive to negative in the normal (or Z) components, as the electrical voltage above the electrical source is zero in ECGs or in body surface potential mappings (Figure 25–4B). The normal-component MCG was developed first, but now both normal- and tangential-component MCGs are commercially available. The advantages of the normal-component MCG are (1) less disturbance by volume (or secondary) currents, (2) it is a compact system because sensor numbers can be halved, compared with the tangential system, and (3) it is easy to compare with ECG or body surface potential mapping. The main advantage of the tangential-component MCG is that foci and mechanisms of electrophysiological phenomena can be directly analyzed without mathematical models (see the section on Arryhthmias).

Measurements of the Cardiac Magnetic Fields Using Magnetocardiograms

Special attention must be paid to reduce environmental noise when measuring biomagnetic fields. Ideally, MCG systems should be set up in a room that is magnetically shielded and isolated from major sources of environmental noise, such as electronic devices with motors and the transportation systems, e.g., the detection limit was less than a few femto (10^{-15}) tesla/$\sqrt{Hz}$ when the cardiac magnetic fields are measured in a magnetically shielded room at subway level.[6] Accessories producing magnetic noise, such as watches, cellular phones, and coins, must be kept away from the sensors. And patients with an implanted pacemaker are excluded because pacemakers produce a large amount of magnetic noise. Patients with a prior history of cardiac surgery or stenting for coronary revascularization, who thus have magnetic noise originating from wires, clips, prosthetic valves, or stents, may have a large amount of noise, but most of them are still good candidates for MCGs. Applicants need not remove their clothes for MCG measurement because clothes do not affect magnetic fields and because SQUID sensors placed in a Dewar do not have to be in direct contact with the skin.

The 64-channel MCG system reduces examination time because the 17.5-cm^2 measuring area is large enough to cover the four chambers of the heart (Figure 25–3B) and because this system can simultaneously record the signals in all 64 channels plus the ECG signals from limb leads. One examination including two measurements (anterior–posterior and posterior–anterior projections) is usually completed within 15 min. A system with a smaller measuring area would require multiple measurements to cover the four chambers.

Analysis

Measured data are sent to network computers and are analyzed by several methods: grid maps investigating the spatial distribution of the cardiac magnetic fields (Figure 25–3C), overlapped waveforms, isomagnetic field maps (see the section on Arrhythmias, Figures 25–5A and B), and integral values (see the section on Ischemic Heart Disease). Filtering (standard filter: 0.1–100 Hz), baseline correction, signal averaging (see the section on Arrhythmias, Figure 25–5B), and time frequency analysis (see the section on Arrhythmias, Figure 25–8) are used according to the noise level.

Spatial and Temporal Accuracy of Magnetocardiograms

The accuracy of MCG is affected by many factors: the signal-to-noise ratio, the numbers and intervals of sensors,[7] the distance from the magnetic source to the sensor, the clinical or simulated study, models, and the comparison tools. In general, the spatial error of MCGs is one-third to one-half that of ECGs.[4] The spatial accuracy of the 64-channel system (sensor arrangement: an 8-by-8 matrix in a 2.5-cm interval, with a total measuring area of 17.5 by 17.5 cm; minimum sampling interval: 0.5 msec, 2 kHz) is 1.4 ± 0.7 mm in simulation, whereas it is approximately 1 cm in clinical cases.[7] Conduction times on MCGs have a linear correlation with those on intracardiac electrode recordings.[6]

Clinical Utility for Detecting High-Risk Patients for Sudden Cardiac Death

Fetal Magnetocardiograms

Fetal death (≥20 weeks gestation) annually affects 27,000 cases in the United States, at approximately 7.0 per 1000 live births.[8] Fetal arrhythmias, such as atrioventricular conduction block, supraventricular tachycardia, and long QT syndrome, especially complicated with hydrops fetalis, are a significant risk for fetal death.[9] Indeed, atrioventricular nodal reentry or atrioventricular reciprocating tachycardia in individuals without structural heart disease, which is not life-threatening in adults, can be fatal in a fetus or neonate, because fetuses and neonates are more vulnerable to tachycardia-induced heart failure. However, the natural course of fetal arrhythmias is still not completely understood. There has been no reliable tool for detecting fetal arrhythmias and no placebo-controlled study for the treatment of fetal arrhythmias.

One of the promising areas for MCGs is prenatal diagnosis of electrophysiological abnormalities in congenital cardiac diseases, because the advantages of MCGs, such as no need for electrodes and less interference by tissue conductivities, become more valuable (Table 25–2). Fetal MCGs are unaffected by vernix caseosa and by amniotic fluid and are reliable throughout the second and third trimesters of pregnancy, whereas fetal ECGs measured on the maternal abdomen

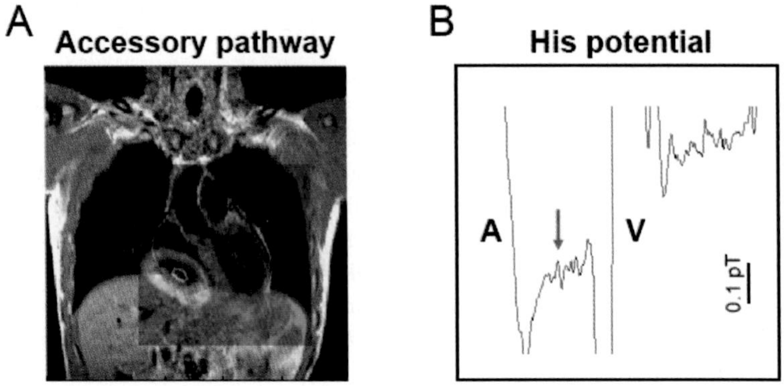

FIGURE 25–5. Clinical application of magnetocardiograms: arrhythmias. (A) A location of an accessory pathway diagnosed by magnetocardiography was superimposed on magnetic resonance imaging. (B) His potential (arrow) was recorded between atrial (A) and ventricular (V) potentials. pT, picotesla.[6,7]

are reliable only before week 27 of gestation.[10] M-mode, pulse Doppler, and tissue velocity imaging of echocardiography are well recognized methods for detecting fetal arrhythmias.[11] Fetal MCGs can also be applied to cases with poor echocardiographic imaging.[12] Moreover, fetal MCGs can provide (1) direct information on ventricular repolarization abnormalities[13] and (2) clear differentiation between atrial and ventricular components, thus (3) enabling diagnosis of arrhythmic mechanisms with an accuracy similar to postnatal ECGs,[14] while a fetal ECG or echocardiogram focuses mainly on the diagnosis of heart rhythm.

Fetal MCGs have three main goals: (1) observation of fetal well-being, normal development, or growth restriction, (2) detection and diagnosis of arrhythmias, and (3) evaluation of the efficacies of therapies, if needed.

Normal Cardiac Development Evaluated by Fetal Magnetocardiograms

In fetal MCGs, electrical activity of the fetus can be measured at the maternal abdominal wall from week 15 of gestation in some cases to week 20 with approximately 100% reliability.[15] Echocardiographic screening before MCG measurement helps to understand the position of the fetus and to identify the best recording point.

Normal values of fetal MCGs change according to gestational age. A multicenter study with a registration of 582 healthy fetuses reported that the durations of the P wave and QRS complex increase linearly with gestational age, suggesting concomitant increases in cardiac mass and cardiac dimension.[15] The PQ interval and T wave are independent of fetal age.

Fetal Arrhythmias

Prenatal diagnosis is not only of academic interest, but is also useful for the management of high-risk pregnancies. Clinical cases of long QT syndrome,[16–18] supraventricular tachycardia,[14] atrial flutter, atrioventricular conduction block,[19] and cardiac hypertrophy[20] have all been prenatally diagnosed using MCGs.

Supraventricular Tachycardia in the Fetus

The etiology of supraventricular tachycardia is different between newborns and adults. In neonates, atrioventricular reciprocating tachycardia in Wolff–Parkinson–White syndrome is more common, and atrioventricular nodal reentry is less common, compared to adults. Although the etiology of supraventricular tachycardia in the fetus is considered to be similar to neonates, the differential diagnosis between the two tachycardias is difficult in neonates through conventional tools.

Wakai *et al.* analyzed 96 episodes of supraventricular tachycardias in eight fetuses (17–31 weeks of gestation, two with and six without delta waves) using MCG.[14] Their study showed that MCG could differentiate P, QRS, and T waves during both sinus rhythm (100–155 bpm) and tachycardia (185–305 bpm), and thus could diagnose their mechanisms with the same accuracy as postnatal ECGs. They also reported unique properties of fetal arrhythmias suggesting autonomic influences: (1) a variety of initiation and termination patterns, (2) reentrant premature atrial complexes as the most common pattern of initiation, compared with a spontaneous atrial premature complex in adults, (3) transient bradycardia as the most common pattern of the termination, spontaneous block in adults, and (4) a strong association between episodes of supraventricular tachycardia and fetal trunk movement.

Long QT Syndrome in the Fetus

Although QT prolongation and certain T wave abnormalities are well recognized risk factors for ventricular tachyarrhythmia and sudden cardiac death at all ages after birth,[21] their incidence and association with fetal death have not been established.

Wakai *et al.* assessed the QT interval and T wave alternans in 120 fetuses (78 normal pregnancies, 43 fetal arrhythmias, 14–39 weeks gestation) using fetal MCG.[13] Their study showed that rate-corrected QT intervals (= $QT/\sqrt{RR}$ interval) in normal sinus rhythm match Bazzet's formula for adults, independent of gestational age. However, QT prolongation was prominent in fetuses with poor outcomes and often accompanied by T wave alternans. They reported a case of *in utero* pharmacological treatment for a hydropic fetus with torsade de pointes and atrioventricular conduction block associated with long QT syndrome, suggesting that MCG-guided pharmacological treatment might be a therapeutic option for fetal arrhythmias.[17]

Ischemic Heart Disease

Ischemic heart disease is the major cause of sudden cardiac death. In this section, we will focus on MCG challenges to develop highly sensitive detection of cardiac injury or arrhythmic substrates in ischemic heart disease.

Detection of Baseline Shift in Cardiac Ischemia

Both MCGs and ECGs differ in the concept of the baseline or zero level. One of the reasons is that direct currents are filtered in ECGs but not in MCGs. The ECG baseline is determined as the PR segment[22] or the TP segment,[23] while the MCG baseline is determined on an absolute scale measured by the SQUID sensors. In other words, amplitudes in ECGs are based on an external voltage standard rather than an absolute scale.[23] Proposing that MCG would be better than ECG for determining the baseline value, Cohen and colleagues investigated the mechanism of ST changes during cardiac ischemia.[24–26] Subendocardial ischemia causes depression of the ST segment in ECGs, while transmural ischemia causes ST elevation. But it is not clear when ST elevation occurs or whether an injury current flows only during the ST segment or during both baseline and ST segments. Cohen *et al.* first investigated ST elevation after coronary occlusion in dog models in 1975[24] and then investigated ST depression during exercise in patients with stable angina pectoris in 1983.[26] They found that cardiac ischemia changed both the baseline and ST segments, shifting them in opposite directions. During acute coronary occlusion, the size of the baseline shift was approximately equal to that of the ST segment change, but in angina pectoris it was about 70% the size of the ST segment shift. An MCG baseline shift was not observed in left bundle branch block or early depolarization, a normal variant of ST change.[25] It was concluded from these results that ST elevation during acute coronary occlusion is a secondary result of a primary injury current that is interrupted during the ST interval.[24]

Measuring DC components to directly identify injury currents is challenging. It would enable us to detect cardiac damage in individuals with baseline cardiac disease (i.e., new myocardial infarction in cardiac hypertrophy, in bundle branch block, or in manifest Wolff–Parkinson–White syndrome). As Cohen *et al.* reported,[24–26] MCG has the potential to measure them, but has not succeeded in clinical situations mainly because of the difficulty in separating DC components of cardiac magnetic fields from low-frequency noises near DC.

Currently, other MCG parameters, such as current density vector, signal morphology, conduction time, amplitude ratio, and dipole analysis, have been proposed to detect cardiac ischemia, mainly under stress tests. The sensitivity and specificity of QT prolongation or QT dispersion on MCG are 85% and 68%, respectively,[27] and that of vector analysis in acute coronary syndrome are 93% and 95%.[28] A combination of several MCG parameters might improve the accuracy of diagnosis.

At-Rest Phase Abnormalities in Angina Pectoris

The first indications of ischemic heart disease are subjective symptoms and ST changes on ECGs. Both of these parameters, however, differ between individuals. About half of the patients with new onset myocardial infarction have no symptoms before the onset. Abnormalities in the ECG are observed in 70–90% of angina pectoris patients during exercise tests, but in only about 50% of angina pectoris patients at rest.[29] Clinical tools to identify ischemic heart disease in at-rest individuals and in the asymptomatic phases are thus limited.

We calculated the MCG integral value[30–32] with ischemic heart disease (myocardial infarction without myocardial viability, angina pectoris with myocardial variability, and controls) at rest hypothesizing that a combination of two parameters, ST changes (voltage) and QT intervals (conduction time), would be more sensitive in detecting ventricular repolarization abnormalities, compared with a single parameter. Indeed, the sensitivity of MCG integral values for detecting ischemic heart disease under exercise test is superior to that of ECG (MCG 82% versus ECG 47%).[33]

Comparing the infarction and the control groups, we found that both their ECG and MCG showed differences: the infarction patients had longer QT intervals on their ECG and had smaller integral values on their MCG. Comparing angina pectoris patients with controls, a new finding is that the integral values on MCG of the angina pectoris patients were smaller than those on the MCG of the controls, while ECG parameters (QT interval, QT dispersion, and ST changes) did not differ.[4,30,32] This study revealed that the MCG of unstressed and asymptomatic individuals with angina pectoris have potential abnormalities. Moreover, the MCG integral values decreased more in the myocardial infarction group than in the angina pectoris group, and they increased after coronary intervention, thus indicating that integral values in MCG can reflect myocardial viability and treatment effects.

A Future Risk of Arrhythmic Events in Myocardial Infarction

An implantable cardioverter defibrillator (ICD) is the first line therapy for preventing sudden cardiac death among patients with left ventricular dysfunction. However, a low rate of appropriate ICD therapy (<40% in MADIT-II or in SCD-HeFT) suggests an urgent need for more accurate predictors. T wave alternans, late potential in signal-averaged ECG, and MCG are the candidates. In MCG, after several retrospective studies,[34] a prospective study was reported by Korhonen *et al.*[35] They first showed that intra-QRS fragmentation in MCG, which correlates with slow conduction in intraoperative cardiac mapping,[36] increased in patients with an old myocardial infarction with a prior history of ventricular tachycardia. Then, they utilized intra-QRS fragmentation in MCG as a predictor of future cardiac events. Intra-QRS fragmentation has some advantages over T wave alternans or signal-averaged ECG. First, intra-QRS fragmentation has broader applications as populations with atrial fibrillation, bundle branch block, or β blocker therapy are good candidates, while they are not for signal-averaged ECG or T wave alternans. Second, intra-QRS fragmentation examines abnormalities within the QRS complex, not only in late potentials.

Among 158 patients with acute myocardial infarction and left ventricular dysfunction (mean follow-up of 50 months), increased intra-QRS fragmentation in MCG predicted both arrhythmic events and all-cause mortality, whereas QRS duration in ECG predicted only all-cause mortality. In multivariate analysis, intra-QRS fragmentation in MCG was the strongest predictor of arrhythmic events with a hazard ratio of 5.1 (95% confidence interval 1.7–15.9) (left ventricular ejection fraction less than 30%: hazard ratio 3.1, 95% confidence interval 1.1–8.8). The combined criteria of intra-QRS fragmentation and low ejection fraction had 50% positive and 91% negative predictive values for arrhythmic events, suggesting that MCG analysis could provide prognostic information in addition to ventricular dysfunction.[35]

Ventricular Abnormalities in Nonischemic Heart Disease

Case studies in individuals with cardiac hypertrophy due to pressure overload[37] or due to congenital heart disease,[38] cardiomyopathy,[39] Kawasaki disease,[40] diabetes mellitus,[41] or heart transplantation[34] have been reported using MCGs.

As a trial for noninvasive detection of graft rejection after heart transplantation, high sensitivity and specificity were reported in MCGs (an increase in current dipole strength attributed to changes in intramyocardial impedance: sensitivity 91% and specificity 93% for acute rejections; an increase in an approximately 90-Hz component during QRS complex: sensitivity 83% and specificity 84% for chronic rejections).[34]

Arrhythmias

To detect arrhythmic substrates that cause sudden cardiac death, MCGs and electrophysiological (EP) studies are compared in this section, which first discusses detection of arrhythmic foci. As previously described (see the section on Analysis), the spatial accuracy of the multichannel MCG system is 0.5–2.0 cm in the analysis of the location of accessory pathways in Wolff–Parkinson–White syndrome (Figure 25–5A). This result is applied to an electrophysiological phenomena that can be approximated by a single-dipole model, such as a premature complex,[7] an accessory pathway,[7,42,43] and a His potential (Figure 25–5B). The MCGs are more sensitive in detecting His potentials than other body surface mappings of cardiac activities.

To reduce noise, signal averaging was done in these analyses, but signal averaging can obscure physiological signals. The topic in the latter part of this section is beat-to-beat analysis using tangential components in MCGs.[44,45] This analytical method covers the whole sequence of a heart beat and all mechanisms of arrhythmias, from automaticity to reentry.

His Potential Recording in Magnetocardiograms

The origin of atrioventricular conduction block cannot be determined without an invasive electrophysiological study because the amplitude of a His potential is too small to record on standard ECGs. We investigated the feasibility of measuring His potentials on MCG by using 2-min signal averaging (101 ± 36 beats).[6] In 14 out of 22 patients (64%), a spike potential was recorded between the atrial and the ventricular components (Figure 25–5B). His ventricular intervals in the MCG were significantly correlated with those in the EP studies ($R = 0.81$, $p < 0.01$). A statistically significant relation between His ventricular intervals measured on the body surface and those determined in an EP study has not been demonstrated in previous reports.

Conduction Delay

A conduction delay predisposes the heart to cardiac arrhythmias, but ECGs show less information about the atria compared with the ventricles (Figure 25–6). We previously reported that MCGs are superior in detecting local conduction delays in the early stage of paroxysmal atrial fibrillation, while ECGs detect conduction delays originating from broader areas in advanced stages of paroxysmal atrial fibrillation.[46] Based on these preliminary data, we prospectively followed patients with ischemic heart disease and no prior history of atrial fibrillation.[47] They were divided into two groups according to P wave duration on MCG (patients with P wave < 115 msec and those with ≥115 msec). There was no significant difference in ECG parameters between the two groups. Prolonged P wave duration on MCG identified those with a low ejection fraction and ventricular dilatation. During a mean follow-up of 2.1 years, prolonged P wave patients on MCG had a higher incidence of atrial fibrillation (18% versus 0%) and heart failure hospitalization (45% versus 9%), compared with the control group.

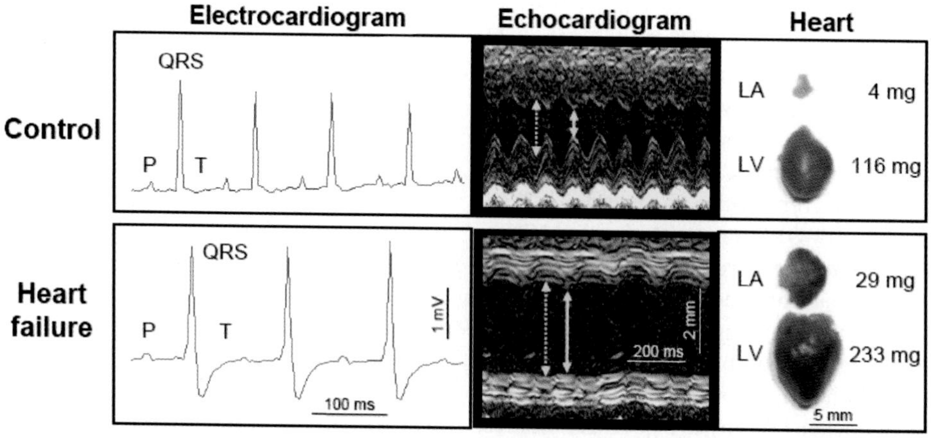

FIGURE 25–6. Arial remodeling in pressure overload-induced heart failure. The heart failure mouse induced by transverse aortic constriction (bottom) had a 2-fold increase in left ventricular (LV) weight and a 7-fold increase in left atrial (LA) weight (right), compared with a control mouse (top). Electrocardiogram (left) in the heart failure mouse showed an increase of QRS amplitude, prolongation of PQ, QRS, and QT intervals, and ST-T changes, which were compatible with ventricular remodeling confirmed by echocardiography (middle) and autopsy (right). In spite of a clear difference in QRS-T components between the two mice, the P wave in ECG was not representative of atrial enlargement and hypertrophy. Therefore, more sensitive tools for detecting atrial remodeling are required. Dot arrow, left ventricular diastolic dimension; solid arrow, left ventricular systolic dimension.

Atrial Fibrillation

Atrial tachyarrhythmias are divided into three clinical diagnoses (atrial tachycardia, atrial flutter, and atrial fibrillation) and have three mechanisms (reentry, automaticity, and triggered activity). The clinical diagnosis of arrhythmic mechanisms is currently based on EP studies because ECG-based diagnosis does not show a 1:1 correspondence with the mechanisms. To identify mechanisms noninvasively, we made a two-step algorithm using MCG. The first step is to visualize electrical currents through an MCG animation. Reentrant circuit numbers (single or multiple) and size (macro- or microreentry) are screened through the animation. The second step is a time frequency analysis that can reveal regular activity under a random pattern.

Mechanisms of Tachyarrhythmias: Automaticity, Macroreentry, or Microreentry

We animated MCG by editing isomagnetic field maps (the tangential components of the cardiac magnetic fields) with a minimal interval of 1 msec.[45] The cardiac magnetic fields (red areas in Figure 25–7) showed a single peak during sinus rhythm or atrial premature complex, a large circuit during atrial flutter due to macroreentry along the tricuspid annulus, and a disorganized pattern during atrial fibrillation. When atrial fibrillation shifted to atrial flutter, the disorganized pattern fused to a single pattern, and then evolved into a circle. During common atrial flutter, atrial activation showed counterclockwise rotation in the animation. This study showed how the pattern of the cardiac magnetic fields reflects the kind of atrial activation in the right atrium: a circular pattern for atrial flutter and a disorganized pattern for atrial fibrillation. Notably, unique information through MCG is that the magnetic fields show three patterns (disorganized multiple peaks, a single peak, and a weak circular pattern) when atrial fibrillation shifts to common atrial flutter. Further studies are required to use MCG to differentiate atrial activation in the right atrium from that in the left atrium and to classify additional patterns of atrial flutter.

The MCG animation can also be applied to analyze reentrant circuits during ventricular tachycardia. The magnetic sources show a circular pattern during atrial flutter because its macroreentrant circuit is almost round and parallel to the SQUID sensors, while those during ventricular tachycardia in ischemic heart disease may show a more complicated pattern because of its smaller and three-dimensionally complex reentrant circuit.

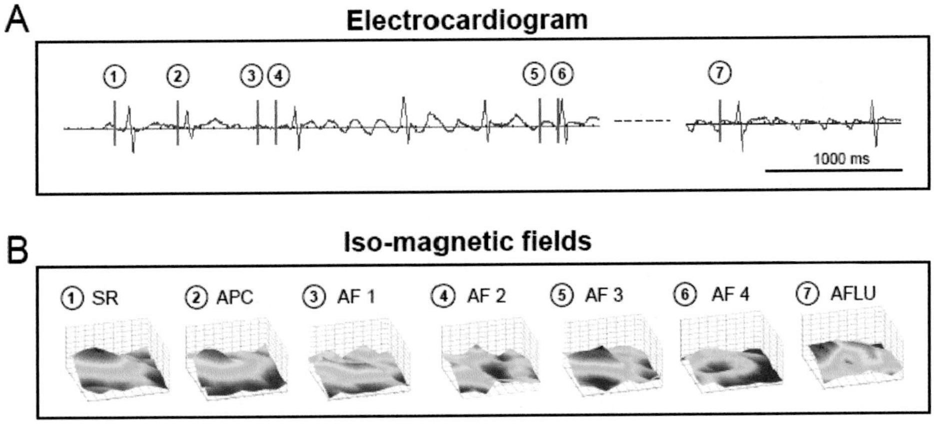

FIGURE 25–7. Paroxysmal atrial flutter. Initiation of paroxysmal atrial flutter was simultaneously recorded by electrocardiography (A) and magnetocardiography (B). The cardiac magnetic fields (red or yellow areas in B) showed a single peak during sinus rhythm (SR, 1 in B) or atrial premature complex (APC, 2 in B), a large circuit during atrial flutter (AFLU) due to macroreentry along the tricuspid annulus (7 in B), and a disorganized pattern during atrial fibrillation (AF, 3 and 4 in B). When AF shifted to AFLU, the disorganized pattern fused to a single pattern (5 in B), and then evolved into a circle (6 in B).[45]

Mechanisms of Tachyarrhythmias: Reentry with or Without Focal Automaticity

As the next step, we classified disorganized patterns hypothesizing that regular signals are amplified through time frequency, while irregular signals are reduced. Time-frequency analysis showed multiple peaks at a high field strength ($0.2–0.6 \times 10^{-12}$ pT), which were clearly isolated from the other peak in the MCG of a patient with focal automatic atrial tachycardia (Figure 25–8A left), and showed a broad distribution at a range of 6–10 Hz at a low field strength (0.1–0.15 pT) in the MCG of a patient with multiple reentrant wavelets (arrow in Figure 25–8A right). These two patterns could not be differentiated as a quantitative parameter by ECG or MCG animation. Time-frequency analysis also shows patterns that differ between partial atrial standstill[48] and total atrial standstill (Figure 25–8B). The studies reviewed in this section suggest that MCGs could be used to detect local atrial conduction delay, risk for new onset atrial fibrillation with subsequent heart failure hospitalization, mechanisms of atrial arrhythmias, and degree of atrial electrical remodeling. Thus MCGs may provide key information for determining which strategies to use in the treatment of atrial fibrillation (e.g., pharmacological or nonpharmacological therapy, rhythm control or rate control).

Future Direction of Magnetocardiograms

Understanding and measurement of magnetic fields have existed for centuries as early navigators used the earth's magnetic fields to guide them in the navigation of the earth and sea (Table 25–1).

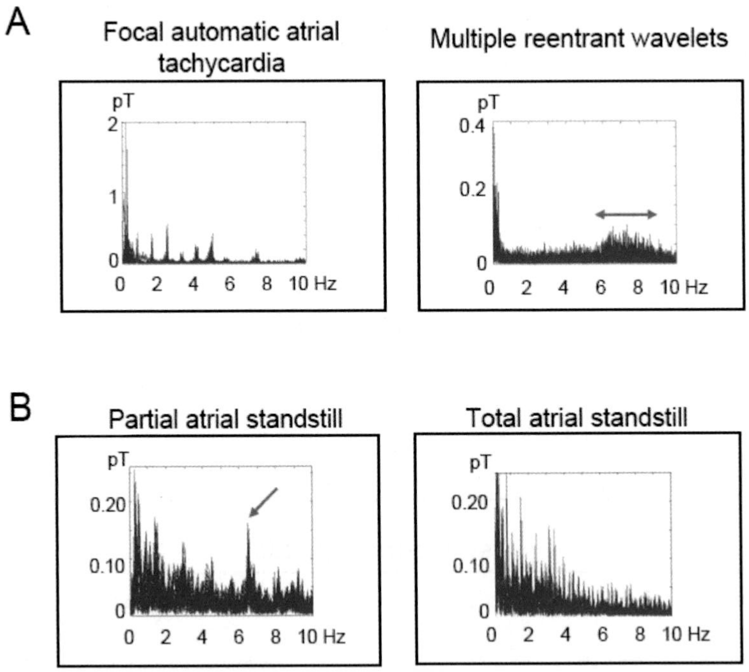

FIGURE 25–8. Magnetocardiographic time-frequency components. A disorganized pattern in isomagnetic field maps during atrial tachyarrhythmias was classified by time-frequency components as regular signals are amplified through time-frequency analysis, while irregular signals are reduced. Time-frequency analysis showed multiple peaks, which were clearly isolated from other peaks in a patient with focal automatic atrial tachycardia (A left), and showed a broad distribution at a range of 6–10 Hz at a low field strength (arrow in A right) in a patient with multiple reentrant wavelets. Among chronic atrial fibrillation with no f wave on the electrocardiogram, the magnetocardiogram detected a high-frequency component (6 Hz, arrow in B left) in a patient with partial atrial standstill, but did not in a patient with total atrial standstill (B right). pT, picotesla.[4,48]

The cardiac magnetic field was detected much later and was first described by Baule and McFee in 1963.[49] Over the years, advances have been made in the field of magnetocardiography[50–53] and it has been developed as a potentially useful diagnostic tool with multichannel recordings. Recent reports provide further evidence confirming MCG as a practical and useful tool for providing supplemental information to other diagnostic modalities including ECG for optimal patient care.

The most important advantage of MCGs over ECGs is that they are more sensitive to small signals. The studies reviewed here suggest that MCGs could be used to detect ischemic heart disease in people who have no symptoms and show no ECG abnormalities and to noninvasively obtain information useful for determining treatment strategies (existence of cardiac ischemia or viability in ischemic heart disease, risk for future cardiac events, mechanisms of tachyarrhythmias, degree of electrical remodeling, etc.). If this is the case, MCGs can be a powerful tool in preventing sudden cardiac death.

One factor limiting the clinical use of MCGs is that their utility has not yet been established. There are very few animal studies[54] and few clinical studies in a large population or from the prospective approach. Other than ECGs, there are few clinical data with which MCGs can be compared, especially data in basic medicine. The potential benefits of MCGs and the most effective way to use them in clinical medicine have therefore not been understood. A second limiting factor is that MCG systems and parameters have not been standardized.[55] The cost effectiveness of MCG must also be improved.

The search for future uses of MCGs is ongoing. One is in three-dimensional diagnosis combined with electrophysiological, anatomical,[4] and metabolic information.[56] These kinds of information are currently obtained in different images, but a combined image helps provide a comprehensive understanding of a given pathophysiology. Another approach is a therapeutic one. EP studies using nonmagnetic catheters under MCG monitoring[57,58] might reduce radiation time allowing for less invasive ablation procedures to treat arrhythmias.

In conclusion, MCGs, body surface mapping of the cardiac magnetic fields measured using SQUID sensors, can be used in clinical diagnosis when ECGs are not practical or noninformative, such as in fetal cardiac assessment, ischemic heart disease, and arrhythmias. Establishing their utility will require further studies in both basic and clinical approaches.

Body Surface Potential Mappings

Body surface potential mappings have been proposed to diagnose arrhythmic foci and dispersion of ventricular repolarization.[59,60] However, data on body surface potential mapping is mainly based on small, nonrandomized clinical studies or on simulation models, therefore its utility for detecting a risk for sudden cardiac death has not been established.

References

1. Pope JH, Aufderheide TP, Ruthazer R, *et al.* Missed diagnosis of acute cardiac ischemia in the emergency department. *N Engl J Med* 2000;342:1163–1170.
2. Williamson SJ, Kaufmann L. Biomagnetism. Sources and their detection. *J Magnetism Magn Mater* 1981;22:147–160.
3. Nowak H. Biomagnetic instrumentation. In: Andrä A, Nowak H, Eds. *Magnetism in Medicine. A Handbook.* Berlin: Wiley-VCH, 1998:88–135.
4. Yamada S, Yamaguchi I. Magnetocardiograms in clinical medicine: Unique information on cardiac ischemia, arrhythmias, and fetal diagnosis. *Intern Med* 2005;44:1–19.
5. Yamaguchi I, Tsukada K, Eds. *Magnetocardiogram Interpretation: A Basic Manual.* Tokyo: Corona, 2006:125–147.
6. Yamada S, Kuga K, On K, Yamaguchi I. Noninvasive recording of His potential using magnetocardiograms. *Circ J* 2003;67:622–624.
7. Yamada S, Tsukada K, Miyashita T, *et al.* Noninvasive diagnosis of arrhythmic foci by using magnetocardiograms: Method and accuracy of magneto-anatomical mapping system. *J Arrhythmia* 2000;16:580–586.
8. Barfield WD. Racial/ethical trends fetal mortality–United States, 1990–2000. *MMWR Morb Mortal Wkly* 2004;53:529–532.
9. Wren C. Cardiac arrhythmias in the fetus and newborn. *Semin Fetal Neonatal Med* 2006;11:182–190.

10. Lewis MJ. Review of electromagnetic source investigations of the fetal heart. *Med Eng Phys* 2003; 25:801–810.
11. Rein AJJT, O'Donnell C, Geva T, *et al.* Use of tissue velocity imaging in the diagnosis of fetal cardiac arrhythmias. *Circulation* 2002;106:1827–1833.
12. Comani S, Liberati M, Mantini D, *et al.* Characterization of fetal arrhythmias by means of fetal magnetocardiography in three cases of difficult ultrasonographic imaging. *Pacing Clin Electrophysiol* 2004;27:1647–1655.
13. Zhao H, Strasburger JF, Cuneo BF, *et al.* Fetal cardiac repolarization abnormalities. *Am J Cardiol* 2006;98:491–496.
14. Wakai RT, Strasburger JF, Li Z, Deal BJ, Gotteiner NL. Magnetocardiographic rhythm patterns at initiation and termination of fetal supraventricular tachycardia. *Circulation* 2003;107:307–312.
15. Stinstra J, Golbach E, van Leeuwen P, *et al.* Multicentre study of fetal cardiac time intervals using magnetocardiography. *Br J Obstet Gynaecol* 2002;109:1235–1243.
16. Hamada H, Horigome H, Asaka M, *et al.* Prenatal diagnosis of long QT syndrome using fetal magnetocardiography. *Prenat Diagn* 1999;19:677–680.
17. Cuneo BF, Ovadia M, Strasburger JF, *et al.* Prenatal diagnosis and in utero treatment of torsades de pointes associated with congenital long QT syndrome. *Am J Cardiol* 2003;91:1395–1398.
18. Ménendez T, Achenbach S, Beinder E, *et al.* Prenatal diagnosis of QT prolongation by magnetocardiography. *Pacing Clin Electrophysiol* 2000;23: 1305–1307.
19. Li Z, Strasburger JF, Cuneo BF, *et al.* Giant fetal magnetocardiogram P waves in congenital atrioventricular block. A marker of cardiovascular compensation? *Circulation* 2004;110:2097–2102.
20. Horigome H, Shiono J, Shigemitsu S, *et al.* Detection of cardiac hypertrophy in the fetus by approximation of the current dipole using magnetocardiography. *Pediatr Res* 2001;50:242–245.
21. Schwartz PJ, Stramba-Badiale M, Segantini A, *et al.* Prolongation of the QT interval and the sudden infant death syndrome. *N Engl J Med* 1998;338: 1709–1714.
22. Wang K, Asinger RW, Marriott HJ. ST-segment elevation in conditions other than acute myocardial infarction. *N Engl J Med* 2003;349:2128–2135.
23. Mirvis DM. The normal electrocardiogram. In: Mirvis DM, Ed. *Electrocardiography. A Physiologic Approach.* St. Louis, MO: C.V. Mosby, 1993: 102–112.
24. Cohen D, Kaufman LA. Magnetic determination of the relationship between the S-T segment shift and the injury current produced by coronary artery occlusion. *Circ Res* 1975;36:414–424.
25. Savard P, Cohen D, Lepeschkin E, Cuffin BN Madias JE. Magnetic measurement of S-T and T-Q segment shifts in humans. Part I: Early repolarization and left bundle branch block. *Circ Res* 1983; 53:264–273.
26. Cohen D, Savard P, Rifkin RD, Lepeschkin E Strauss WE. Magnetic measurement of S-T and T-Q segment shifts in humans. Part II: Exercise-induced ST segment depression. *Circ Res* 1983;53:274–279.
27. Van Leeuwen P, Hailer B, Lange S, Donker D Grönemeyer D. Spatial and temporal changes during QT interval in the magnetic field of patients with coronary artery disease. *Biomed Tech* 1999; 44:139–142.
28. Park JW, Hill PM, Chung N, Hugenholtz PG, Jung F. Magnetocardiography predicts coronary artery disease in patients with acute chest pain. *Ann Noninvasive Electrocardiol* 2005;10:312–323.
29. Gersh BJ, Braunwald E, Bonow RO. Chronic coronary artery disease. In: Braunwald E, Zipes DP, Libby P, Eds. *Heart Disease. A Textbook of Cardiovascular Medicine*, 6th ed. Philadelphia, PA: WB Saunders, 2001:1272–1352.
30. Tsukada K, Miyashita T, Kandori A, *et al.* An isointegral mapping technique using magnetocardiogram, and its possible use for diagnosis of ischemic heart disease. *Int J Card Imaging* 2000;16:55–66.
31. Yamada S, Tsukada K, Miyashita T, Yamaguchi I. Calculating integral values of the cardiac magnetic field is more sensitive to repolarization abnormalities than conducting electrocardiograms. *Comput Cardiol* 2000;27:371–373.
32. Yamada S, Tsukada K, Miyashita T, Watanabe S, Yamaguchi I. Evaluating ventricular repolarization abnormalities in the at-rest phase in ischemic heart disease by using magnetocardiograms. *Biomed Tech* 2001;46:47–49.
33. Kanzaki H, Nakatani S, Kandori A, Tsukada K, Miyatake K. A new screening method to diagnose coronary artery disease using multichannel magnetocardiogram and simple exercise. *Basic Res Cardiol* 2003;98:124–132.
34. Stroink G, Moshage W, Achenbach S. Cardiomagnetism. In: Andrä A, Nowak H, Eds. *Magnetism in Medicine. A Handbook.* Berlin: Wiley-VCH, 1998: 136–189.
35. Korhonen P, Husa T, Tietrala I, *et al.* Increased intra-QRS fragmentation in magnetocardiography as a predictor of arrhythmic events and mortality in patients with cardiac dysfunction after myocardial infarction. *J Cardiovasc Electrophysiol* 2006;17: 396–401.

36. Korhonen P, Pesola K, Jarvinen A, *et al.* Relation of magnetocardiographic arrhythmia risk parameters to delayed ventricular conduction in postinfarction ventricular tachycardia. *Pacing Clin Electrophysiol* 2002;25:1339–1345.
37. Nomura M, Fujino K, Katayama M, *et al.* Analysis of the T wave of the magnetocardiogram in patients with essential hypertension by means of isomagnetic and vector arrow maps. *J Electrocardiol* 1988; 21:174–182.
38. Terada Y, Mitsui T, Sato M, Horigome H, Tsukada K. Right ventricular volume unloading evaluated by tangential magnetocardiography *Jpn J Thorac Cardiovasc Surg* 2000;48:16–23.
39. Shiono J, Horigome H, Matsui A, *et al.* Detection of repolarization abnormalities in patients with cardiomyopathy using current vector mapping technique on magnetocardiogram. *Int J Cardiovasc Imaging* 2003;19:163–170.
40. Shiono J, Horigome H, Matsui A, *et al.* Evaluation of myocardial ischemia in Kawasaki disease using an integral map on magnetocardiogram. *Pacing Clin Electrophysiol* 2002;25:915–921.
41. Brockmeier K, Schmitz L, Wiegand S, *et al.* High-pass-filtered magnetocardiogram and cardiomyopathy in patients with type 1 diabetes mellitus. *J Electrocardiol* 1997;30:293–300.
42. Weismuller P, Abraham-Fuchs K, Schneider S, *et al.* Biomagnetic noninvasive localization of accessory pathways in Wolff-Parkinson-White syndrome. *Pacing Clin Electrophysiol* 1991;14:1961–1965.
43. Weismuller P, Abraham-Fuchs K, Schneider S, *et al.* Magnetocardiopgraphic noninvasive localization of accessory pathways in the Wolff-Parkinson-White syndrome by a multichannel system. *Eur Heart* 1992;13:616–622.
44. Tsukada K, Haruta Y, Adachi A, *et al.* Multichannel SQUID system detecting tangential components of the cardiac magnetic field. *Rev Sci Instrum* 1995; 66:5085–5091.
45. Yamada S, Tsukada K, Miyashita T, Kuga K, Yamaguchi I. Noninvasive, direct visualization of macro-reentrant circuits by using magnetocardiograms: Initiation and persistence of atrial flutter. *Europace* 2003;5:343–350.
46. Yamada S, Tsukada K, Miyashita T, *et al.* The superiority of magnetocardiograms over electrocardiograms for detecting conduction delay in the right atrium. *Pacing Clin Electrophysiol* 2003;26(Pt. II): 1048.
47. Yamada S, Tsukada K, Miyashita T, *et al.* Magnetocardiogram is a useful noninvasive tool to identify patients at high risk of atrial fibrillation and heart failure hospitalization. In: Halgren E, Ahlfors S, Hämäläinen M, Cohen D, Eds. *Biomag 2004 Proceedings of the 14th International Conference on Biomagnetism.* Boston, August 8–12, 2004:422.
48. Yamada S, Tsukada K, Miyashita T, Oyake Y, Kuga K, Yamaguchi I. Noninvasive diagnosis of partial atrial standstill using magnetocardiograms. *Circ J* 2002;66:1178–1180.
49. Baule G, McFee R. Detection of the magnetic field of the heart. *Am Heart J* 1963;66:95–96.
50. Baule GM, McFee R. The magnetic heart vector. *Am Heart J* 1970;79:223–236.
51. Cohen D, Norman JC, Molokhia F, Hood W Jr. Magnetocardiography of direct currents: S-T segment and baseline shifts during experimental myocardial infarction. *Science* 1971;172:1329–1333.
52. Barry WH, Fairbank WM, Harrison DC, *et al.* Measurement of the human magnetic heart vector. *Science* 1977;198:1159–1162.
53. Karp PJ, Katila TE, Saarinen M, Siltanen P, Varpula TT. The normal human magnetocardiogram. II. A multipole analysis. *Circ Res* 1980;47:117–130.
54. Brisinda D, Caristo ME, Fenici R. Contactless magnetocardiographic mapping in anesthetized Wistar rats: Evidence of age-related changes of cardiac electrical activity. *Am J Physiol Heart Circ Physiol* 2006;291:H368–H378.
55. Franz MR. Magnetism: The last resort? *J Cardiovasc Electrophysiol* 2001;12:778–779.
56. Mäkelä T, Pham QC, Clarysse P, *et al.* A 3-D model-based registration approach for the PET, MR and MCG cardiac data fusion. *Med Image Anal* 2003;7:377–389.
57. Feniti, R, Pesola K, Mäkijärvi M, *et al.* Nonfluoroscopic localization of an amagnetic catheter in a realistic torso phantom by magnetocardiographic and body surface potential mapping. *Pacing Clin Electrophysiol* 1998;21(Pt. II):2485–2491.
58. Feniti, R, Pesola K, Korhonen P, *et al.* Magnetocardiographic pacemapping for nonfluoroscopic localization of intracardiac electrophysiology catheters. *Pacing Clin Electrophysiol* 1998;21(Pt. II):2492–2499.
59. De Ambroggi L, Negroni MS, Monza E, Bertoni T, Schwartz PJ. Dispersion of ventricular repolarization in the long QT syndrome. *Am J Cardiol* 1991; 68:614–620.
60. Freedman RA, Fuller MS, Greenberg GM, *et al.* Detection and localization of prolonged epicardial electrograms with 64-lead body surface signal-averaged electrocardiography. *Circulation* 1991;84: 871–883.

26
Microvolt T Wave Alternans: Mechanisms and Implications for Prediction of Sudden Cardiac Death

Ganiyu O. Oshodi, Lance D. Wilson, Ottorino Costantini, and David S. Rosenbaum

Introduction

Sudden cardiac death (SCD) accounts for greater than 50% of all cardiac deaths every year in the United States alone.[1] While therapy with an implantable cardioverter defibrillator (ICD) is effective in treating the ventricular tachyarrhythmias most often responsible for SCD, it remains difficult to identify the population that derives the most benefit from this therapy. Recent studies have focused solely on a reduced left ventricular ejection fraction (LVEF) as a criteria for selecting patients who benefit from implantation of an ICD.[2,3] However, LVEF, as a measure of contractility, is a dynamic measurement that changes over time and poorly defines the electrical substrate that leads to SCD.[4] Moreover, the absolute risk reduction derived from ICD therapy in the primary prevention studies based on a low LVEF alone is small (~2.5%/year), and the rate of appropriate device therapy is ~5–7% per year. Based on the current paradigm for risk stratification for SCD, it would be necessary to implant approximately 15–20 ICDs to save one life. With these considerations in mind, it is highly desirable to have accurate and reliable tests that improve risk stratification for SCD.

Among other risk stratification tests, microvolt T wave alternans (TWA) has emerged as a simple and cost-effective[5] tool to better define the electrical substrate of patients with a known cardiomyopathy, and to identify patients at the highest and lowest risk of ventricular tachyarrhythmias. In this chapter, we will review the mechanisms underlying its development, its measurement, and its potential use as a clinical tool for screening and identifying patients at risk for SCD.

Definition and History of T Wave Alternans

Cardiac alternans was first recognized as pulsus alternans by Traube in 1872, and was associated with poor outcomes.[6] More recently, TWA, defined as beat-to-beat oscillations in the amplitude of the T wave that occur on an every-other-beat basis, has been recognized as a marker of increased risk for ventricular tachyarrhythmias.

Visible TWA occurs when oscillations in T wave amplitude are large enough to be discerned on the surface electrocardiogram (ECG); it was first reported in dogs by Hering.[7] Lewis then reported the same phenomenon in humans, concluding that it increased the risk of adverse events.[8] T wave alternans was subsequently reported in a range of clinical conditions, including HIV cardiomyopathy,[9] long QT syndrome,[10] coronary vasospasm,[11] acute myocardial infarction,[12] Prinzmetal's angina,[13] antiarrhythmic drug therapy,[14] alcoholism,[15] and electrolyte imbalance.[16] Even though visible TWA is associated with ventricular arrhythmias, it is quite rare (0.1% incidence).[17]

In the 1980s the spectral analysis method was developed for the detection and quantification of TWA, which is not visible on the surface ECG (i.e., "microvolt-level" alternans). This work confirmed a close relationship between TWA and cardiac electrical instability.[18,19] In 1994, Rosenbaum *et al.*[20] reported, for the first time in humans, a relationship between TWA and susceptibility to ventricular arrhythmias by demonstrating a strong correlation between a positive TWA test and inducible ventricular tachycardia by electrophysiological studies (EPS). In addition, TWA was equivalent to EPS in predicting arrhythmia-free survival, and the risk of developing life-threatening ventricular arrhythmias was increased 13-fold in patients with positive TWA tests.

Initially, atrial pacing was used to achieve the elevation in heart rate necessary to elicit TWA, but exercise soon became the preferred method for eliciting TWA.[21,22] This led to the ability to use TWA as a simple, inexpensive, and noninvasive test to risk stratify patients at risk for SCD.

Basic Cellular Mechanisms of Repolarization Alternans

Cellular Basis for Electrocardiographic T Wave Alternans

There is compelling evidence that TWA results from beat-to-beat alternations in the time course of membrane repolarization at the cellular level (Vm-ALT).[23–26] Alternations in cellular action potential shape and duration were initially observed from single ventricular sites using microelectrodes[27–29] and contact electrodes.[30–33] However, the mechanisms linking cellular alternans to electrocardiographic TWA were definitively established through detailed measurements of the time course of membrane voltage (Vm) throughout the ventricle at a time when TWA was elicited on the surface ECG. These studies were performed using high-resolution optical mapping techniques in a guinea pig model of pacing-induced TWA.[23–25] Importantly, TWA in this model exhibits characteristics of TWA in humans[20]: (1) TWA was induced reproducibly above a critical heart rate threshold, (2) the magnitude of alternans was titratable and persists at a steady state (i.e., does not require abrupt rate change), (3) TWA affected primarily the peak of the T wave rather than the ST segment or QRS complex, (4) TWA was a consistent (actually requisite) precursor to ventricular fibrillation (VF), and (5) the guinea pig possesses action potential and calcium handling properties that are comparable to humans.[34] These finding suggested that disorders that produce TWA in heart disease arise from abnormalities of intracellular processes. These studies also demonstrated that TWA on the ECG actually corresponds to substantially greater alternans of repolarization at the myocyte level.[23] This may explain why the detection of very subtle ("microvolt-level") TWA has physiological and prognostic significance in patients.

Cellular, Subcellular, and Molecular Basis for Repolarization Alternans

The Restitution Hypothesis

It was originally hypothesized that Vm-ALT at the cellular level may be caused by incomplete recovery (from deactivation or inactivation) on alternating beats of one or more ionic currents that govern repolarization.[27,28,35–37] This may explain why T wave alternans in patients[20,38] and experimental animals[19,23] occurs above a heart rate threshold that is significantly lower in subjects that are vulnerable to ventricular arrhythmias. It is well recognized from studies in single cells that cellular repolarization and action potential duration (APD) are highly sensitive to the timing of a premature stimulus[39] because the major voltage-gated ion channels that govern repolarization such as I_{kr}, I_{ks}, I_{to}, and I_{Ca} all exhibit time-dependent activation.[40] Hence, APD shortens in an exponential fashion as the premature coupling interval is progressively shortened. The membrane ionic and intracellular processes that control the extent of APD shortening following a premature stimulus are collectively referred to as APD restitution.[30,39,41] The "restitution hypothesis" states that Vm-ALT occurs when the slope of the APD restitution curve is >1, which has been taken as evidence that sarcolemmal mechanisms, rather than calcium cycling or other cellular mechanisms, determine Vm-ALT.[42–46] Restitution is presumed to cause cellular alternans since, at a constant cycle length, APD prolongation during one beat is necessarily followed by a short diastolic interval, which, according to restitution, will shorten APD on the following beat, which will then lengthen the diastolic interval causing repeated long–short–long APD cycles.

The role of restitution in the mechanism of cellular alternans was suggested in numerous studies.[41,47] However, although a variety of sarcolemmal currents can exhibit alternating-type activity including I_{to},[48] I_{Ca},[49] and I_{kr},[50] few have been definitively shown to be mechanistically responsible for producing Vm-ALT.[51] Moreover, although the "restitution hypothesis" for cellular alternans has been primarily demonstrated in modeling studies, it has not been well supported experimentally.[26,52]

The Calcium Cycling Hypothesis

There are convincing data for a primary role of sarcoplasmic reticulum (SR) calcium (Ca) cycling in the mechanism of Vm-ALT.[26,31,53–60] Inhibiting calcium cycling by blocking the ryanodine receptor (RyR), I_{Ca}, or by depleting SR calcium stores with caffeine, eradicates Vm-ALT.[54,56,57,61,62] However, because of the interdependence of membrane voltage (Vm) and intracellular Ca, which are under tight regulatory control, sorting out the mechanistic relationship between beat-to-beat alternations in calcium cycling and cellular ionic currents in the development of cellular Vm-ALT presents a difficult "chicken and egg" problem. Vm-ALT can cause alternans of the Ca transient (Ca-ALT) by several mechanisms,[63,64] and conversely, Ca-ALT can cause Vm-ALT.[65,66] However, the seminal observations of Chudin *et al.*[67] that beat-to-beat alternation of calcium transient amplitude is similarly induced under current-clamp (where Vm-ALT occurs) and voltage-clamp (i.e., where Vm-ALT is prevented) conditions proved that Ca-ALT is not dependent on Vm-ALT, and strongly supported the notion that cellular alternans arises from SR calcium cycling.

Dual voltage-calcium imaging was recently used to generate an independent line of evidence supporting a primary role of calcium cycling rather than APD restitution in the mechanism of Vm-ALT.[26] The guinea pig model of TWA includes an epicardial gradient of APD restitution, thus providing an opportunity to determine if myocytes with steepest restitution slopes are most susceptible to Vm-ALT. However, when compared to Vm-ALT resistant myocytes, Vm-ALT-susceptible myocytes failed to exhibit steep restitution or prolonged APD.[26] Instead, Vm-ALT-susceptible myocytes had the slowest time constant for diastolic calcium reuptake and greatest propensity for rate-dependent cytosolic calcium accumulation, strongly suggesting that calcium cycling, rather than restitution properties, dictates Vm-ALT.[26] Similar finding were observed in isolated ventricular myocytes.[52]

The subcellular mechanisms of Ca-ALT have been experimentally explored in intact heart preparations, where it has been demonstrated that Vm-ALT-susceptible myocytes express significantly less SERCA2a (a protein responsible for SR Ca reuptake)[23,68,69] and RyR (the protein largely responsible for SR calcium release)[68] compared to Vm-ALT-resistant myocytes, suggesting a molecular basis for cellular alternans.[68] Experiments performed in normal myocytes subjected to pharmacological inhibition of either RyR or SERCA2a have also demonstrated, at least conceptually, that dysfunction of either of these key calcium cycling proteins can cause Ca-ALT.[68,70,71] These findings support the contention that calcium cycling proteins in general, and two general properties of SR calcium handling, calcium release and reuptake, are directly implicated in the mechanism of alternans of calcium handling.

According to the aforementioned discussion, it is generally believed that cellular alternans occurs when the heart rate exceeds the ability of the Ca cycling machinery to maintain Ca homeostasis on a beat-by-beat basis. So what are the mechanisms for generating beat-to-beat alternans of membrane repolarization in response to alternans of Ca transients? This is a critical question because Vm-ALT produces T wave alternans and cardiac arrhythmogenesis. Two likely electrogenic sarcolemmal currents that are sensitive to cytosolic Ca, and therefore can alternate Vm during Ca-ALT, are I_{Ca} and the N^+/Ca^{2+} exchanger (NCX). During alternans, alternating large and small Ca releases will prolong or shorten APD, respectively, when forward mode NCX is the predominant electrogenic mechanism. This is sometimes referred to as "electromechanically concordant" or "positive Ca-Vm coupling" alternans.[65,66] Conversely, when I_{Ca} is the predominant electrogenic current, large or small Ca releases will shorten or lengthen APD, respectively, by Ca-dependent inactivation of I_{Ca}. This will produce "electromechanically discordant" or "negative coupling" alternans.[65,66]

Mechanism Linking Repolarization Alternans to the Genesis of Arrhythmias

Mechanism of Discordant Alternans Between Cells

The development of spatially discordant alternans (i.e., Vm-ALT occurring with opposite phase between neighboring cells) is the key to the link between cellular alternans and cardiac arrhythmogenesis. When Vm-ALT is initiated, it occurs with identical phase (APD either prolongs or shortens simultaneously in all cells) in all cells of a particular region of the ventricular myocardium (i.e., concordant alternans, Figure 26–1B, left). However, as illustrated in Figure 26–1B (right), after a premature impulse (*) or change in pacing rate above a critical heart rate threshold, Vm-ALT switches phase in some cells (site B) but not others (site A), such that some cells undergo a prolongation of APD while other populations of cells undergo APD shortening on the same beat (i.e., Dis-ALT).[23,24] Although it is unclear why neighboring cells under apparently identical conditions would respond differently with respect to their alternans phase, two fundamental mechanisms for Dis-ALT have been proposed. (1) Discordance arises based on intrinsic differences in calcium handling and/or repolarization properties between cells.[23] However, experimental evidence for this is limited.[72] (2) Computer simulations of homogeneous tissue predict that conduction velocity restitution alone, or interacting with spatial heterogeneities of repolarization, can potentially explain Dis-ALT.[38,42,73,74]

The fact that a properly timed premature stimulus applied during cellular alternans changes the magnitude or phase of APD alternans implicates restitution as a possible mechanism in Dis-ALT. In addition, as the kinetics of APD restitution are heterogeneous between myocytes located in different regions of the ventricle, it could be postulated that a properly timed premature stimulus

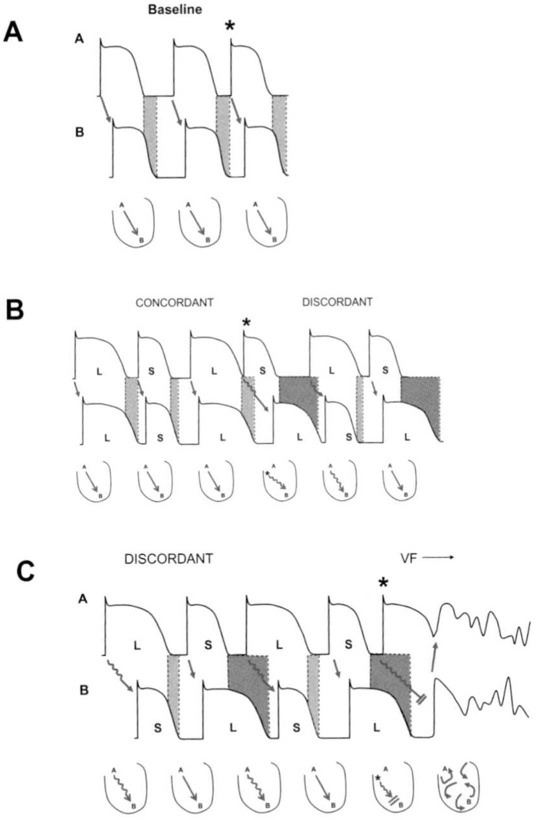

FIGURE 26–1. Mechanisms of discordant alternans and ventricular fibrillation (VF) induced by discordant alternans. L indicates a long APD, while S indicates a short APD. Action potential propagation between two ventricular sites, A and B, is shown. A premature beat is represented by the asterisk (*). A detailed explanation of these mechanisms is presented in the text.

may change the phase of APD alternans in some regions but not others; this is, by definition, a requirement for Dis-ALT.[28,35] Recently, a mechanism of Dis-ALT based on conduction/repolarization dynamics was proposed.[65] As demonstrated in Figure 26–1A, at slower heart rates where no alternans is present, a premature beat (*) will propagate between ventricular sites (site A to site B) with normal conduction velocity; when dispersion of repolarization (grey bar) is normal the premature beat propagates into fully repolarized myocardium. However, as shown in Figure 26–1B, during concordant alternans, a properly timed premature beat (or abrupt increase in heart rate) will propagate slowly into partially repolarized myocardium (i.e., in the wake of enhanced dispersion of repolarization, red bar). The slowing in the conduction prolongs the diastolic interval between the next beats in the downstream myocardium (at site B). Due to APD restitution, downstream action potentials will be prolonged, causing a switch in phase of APD relative to the upstream (site A) action potentials. This produces Dis-ALT.

Recent computer modeling studies have suggested an alternative mechanism for Dis-ALT.[45] According to these simulations, although Dis-ALT can arise, as suggested above, if sufficient heterogeneities of APD restitution are present in myocardium, Dis-ALT is also produced even in the absence of spatial heterogeneity of APD restitution, provided that significant restitution of conduction velocity was present.[45] Restitution of conduction velocity arises because conduction slows progressively as the coupling interval of a premature stimulus is progressively shortened. In computer simulations, if a tightly coupled premature stimulus causes marked conduction slowing [for example, Figure 26–1B, premature beat (*)], a spatial heterogeneity of diastolic intervals is introduced such that each cell is operating on a different point of its APD restitution curve. Under these circumstances, Dis-ALT can arise because the premature stimulus changes the phase of some cells but not others, depending on where on the APD restitution curve the premature impulse arrives. However, it remains unclear how to extrapolate modeling findings to the intact heart, which, unlike computer models, is not homogeneous and is composed of considerable electrophysiological and structural complexities. Moreover, in contrast to these simulations, experimental studies suggest that in normal myocardium, restitution of conduction velocity is minimal relative to APD restitution, because premature stimulus-induced conduction slowing leads to block or fails to capture myocardium before substantial slowing of conduction velocity occurs.[23,75] In experimental studies, the pattern of Dis-ALT is also independent of the pacing site, further supporting the role of APD gradients rather than conduction restitution in the mechanism of Dis-ALT. Clearly, as illustrated in Figure 26–1, mechanisms of Dis-ALT involving restitution of conduction velocity and APD heterogeneities are not mutually exclusive. It is possible that heterogeneity of APD restitution between myocytes plays a critical role in Dis-ALT, but under circumstances where conduction velocity is slowed (e.g., by myocardial disease or drugs), restitution of conduction velocity may play an additive role. For example, flecainide can evoke local activation sequence alternans[76] or ST segment alternans[77] that precedes VF. In addition, as heterogeneities of cellular calcium cycling in myocytes can explain spatial differences in susceptibility to Vm-ALT, these same heterogeneities could also explain the development of Dis-ALT. Moreover, it is quite likely that spatial heterogeneities of repolarization and calcium cycling are interrelated.[57]

An additional mechanism contributing to susceptibility to Dis-ALT has been proposed related to intracellular uncoupling.[24] Cardiac myocytes are connected via gap junctions that allow the flow of ionic current between cells. In general, electrotonic coupling between cells acts to homogenize repolarization. In contrast, cell-to-cell uncoupling tends to unmask intrinsic differences in cellular electrophysiological properties.[78] Cell-to-cell uncoupling will have an important effect on spatial heterogeneity of repolarization [79,80] and any tendency for neighboring myocytes to alternate with opposite phase because of differences in APD restitution will be opposed by electrotonic coupling between these regions. In a guinea pig model of alternans, introduction of a structural barrier to electrotonically uncouple neighboring cells greatly facilitated the development of Dis-ALT.[24] Conversely, disease or drug-induced uncoupling between cells may promote Dis-ALT.

Discordant Alternans Is a Mechanism of Arrhythmogenesis

A novel mechanism linking cellular alternans to reentrant arrhythmogenesis was recently described.[23] The transformation from concordant alternans to Dis-ALT (Figure 26–1B) has significant consequences for the spatial organization of repolarization across the ventricle. As shown in Figure 26–1B (right), during discordant alternans marked spatial dispersion of repolarization emerges (red bars). Discordant alternans also produces a substrate by which conduction block and reentrant excitation can be easily initiated by a premature stimulus (Figure 26–1C). When an impulse (*) propagates (from site A) into still depolarized myocardium (i.e., in the wake of enhanced dispersion of repolarization after the long beat, red bar in site B), conduction block, initiating reentrant excitation can occur (Figure 26–1C, VF). Consequently, Dis-ALT is the key to the mechanism linking TWA to cardiac arrhythmogenesis, and in fact in an experimental model of alternans, VF never occurred without Dis-ALT. The same paradigm was used to explain the initiation of a variety of arrhythmias including polymorphic and monomorphic ventricular tachycardia (VT), as the resultant arrhythmias were determined by structural discontinuities in the tissue, but in each case discordant alternans was required to initiate reentry.[24] Therefore, discordant alternans amplifies physiological heterogeneities of repolarization present at baseline into pathophysiological heterogeneities of sufficient magnitude to produce conduction block and reentrant excitation.[23–25]

Measurement of T Wave Alterans in Patients

The measurement of TWA is based on the principle that the magnitude of TWA increases with increasing heart rate. In a given subject, TWA develops at a specific heart rate and is usually reproducible and sustained above that heart rate threshold.[21] In patients with cardiac electrical instability, TWA develops at slower heart rates than in normal subjects. Thus, the heart rate at which TWA appears is an important determinant of whether a test is positive or negative.[81,82]

The test involves an ECG recording made during rest, exercise, and recovery. T wave alternans is a low-frequency, low-amplitude signal; therefore, noise reduction is paramount. Multi-contact, noise-reducing electrodes attenuate myopotentials, and mild skin abrasion ensures reduced impedance at the skin–electrode interface. The exercise portion of the test should produce a gradual and controlled elevation in heart rate, particularly in the range of 100–110 bpm.[82] This is important because TWA that develops above 110 bpm is not considered clinically significant. Since the TWA test is heart rate dependent rather than workload dependent, it can be a submaximal stress test, and manual control of the treadmill to achieve the required heart rate may be the best "exercise protocol." The modified Bruce or Naughton exercise protocols may also be used depending on the subject's functional capacity, and a bicycle exercise protocol has been described.[21] In general, a subject should exercise with a goal of achieving a heart rate of at least 120 bpm. Detailed descriptions of TWA measurement and the techniques used for noise reduction have been published.[83,84]

Interpretation of T Wave Alternans Tests

Sustained alternans is defined as TWA that is >1.9 μV in amplitude, lasts longer than a minute, and persists above a patient-specific heart rate threshold. Comprehensive rules and criteria for interpretation have been published.[85] Figure 26–2 describes an algorithm for interpretation based on three simple concepts. If sustained TWA is present and the onset heart rate (OHR) is ≤110 bpm, the test is positive. If sustained alternans is absent, or if it develops above the 110 bpm threshold, *and* the test is clearly absent at a heart rate ≥105 bpm, the test is negative. Finally, if the patient cannot reach a heart rate of 105 bpm, or if there is a "gap" in the ability to interpret the test during the critical heart rate period (100–110 bpm), the test is considered indeterminate. An example of the latter scenario would be a test in which TWA develops at a heart rate >110 bpm, but frequent premature ventricular contractions (PVCs) or noise obscure the test such that it is possible to be sure the test is negative only up to a heart rate of 90 bpm.

We recently enhanced these criteria to improve reproducible interpretation of the TWA test for use in the Alternans Before Cardioverter Defibrillator (ABCD) Trial.[86] These enhancements include interpreting a test as; 1. Positive if TWA is present during a predominant (not necessarily the entire test) portion of the test while heart rate remains above the patient-specific threshold for TWA. 2. Negative no matter how dense the ventricular ectopy if there is no TWA for more than 1 min of artifact-free time while heart rates >105 bpm, and 3. Indeterminate if there is no TWA at heart rates

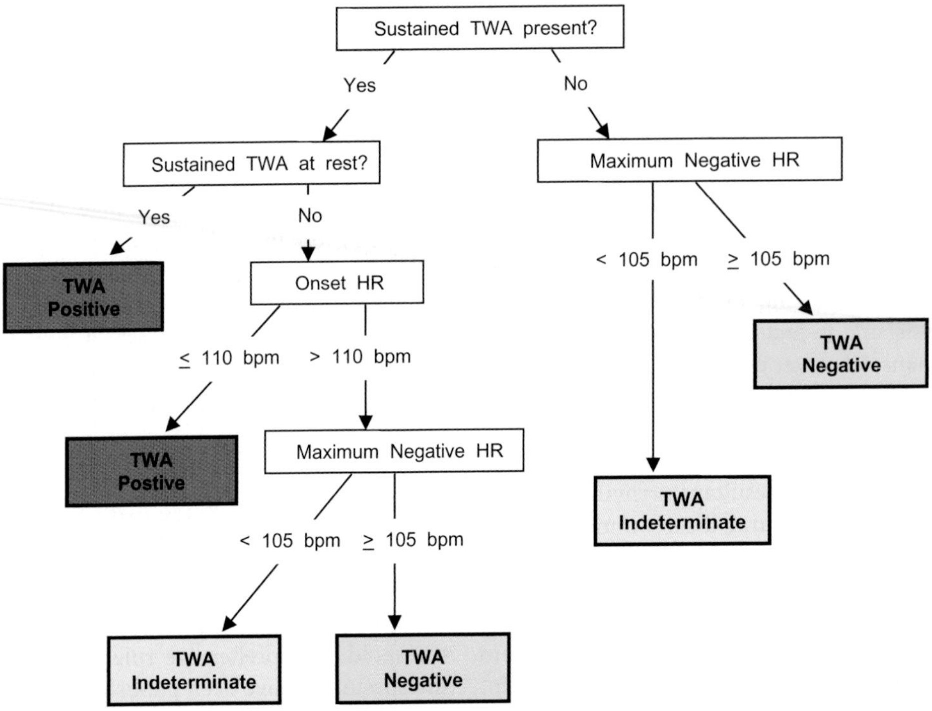

FIGURE 26–2. Flow chart used to classify TWA tests. See the text for discussion. HR, heart rate; TWA, microvolt T wave alternans; HRT, positive HR threshold; Neg HRT, negative HR threshold.

>105 bpm (i.e. ruling out a positive test), and when noise or PVCs obscure interpretation in the critical heart rate range of 100–110 bpm (i.e. can not rule out a negative test).

The role of indeterminate tests, which occur in 20–30% of cases,[85] in risk stratification is controversial. Recent data[87–89] have grouped positive and indeterminate tests into an "abnormal" group, as indeterminate tests are at least as predictive of poor cardiovascular outcomes as positive ones (Figure 26–3).[90] This approach is intuitive as the majority of tests are "indeterminate" from excessive ectopic ventricular beats or the inability to achieve a heart rate of at least 105 bpm. If the test is "indeterminate" because of excessive noise, it should be immediately repeated as approximately 50% of such tests will become either positive or negative. In a meta-analysis on the utility of TWA,[91] 8 of 19 studies included indeterminate results in the outcome analysis. Sensitivity testing did not reveal any difference in the overall utility of TWA whether the indeterminate tests were included as abnormal or were excluded from the analysis. Finally, TWA is currently a qualitative

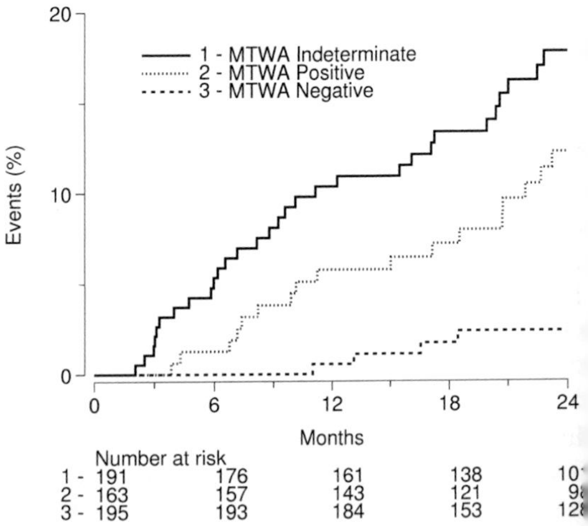

FIGURE 26–3. Kaplan–Meier event-free survival of patients with an indeterminate, a positive, and a normal TWA. The "indeterminate" tests had at least as high an event rate as the positive tests. This was substantiated in patients with frequent ventricular ectopy and an inability to reach a target heart rate, but not in patients who had a high noise level as a reason for indeterminacy. (Reproduced from Hohnloser *et al.*,[89] with permission.)

test. However, there are some data suggesting that the magnitude of the alternans voltage[92] and the onset heart rate[93] of TWA may have additive value in predicting adverse cardiovascular events.

Signal Processing for Detection of T Wave Alternans

The spectral analysis or frequency domain method[19] for measuring TWA is based on the concept that TWA occurs at a specific frequency of 0.5 cycles/beat (every other beat). Using spectral analysis, changes in the T wave that occur at the alternans frequency can be easily detected and separated from changes that occur at other frequencies that are regarded as noise.

The algorithm for the spectral analysis method of measuring TWA has been described in detail[83] and is illustrated in Figure 26–4. First, a 128-beat sequence of QRS complexes is selected for analysis and the QRS complexes are aligned such that each point on the T wave corresponds to the same point on all the subsequent T waves (Figure 26–4A). A point is then selected on the T wave (t), and the voltage is measured for that point on each T wave. The voltage for that selected point in each beat forms a beat series (Figure 26–4B). A power spectrum for all the frequencies of alteration for that point is then created using the fast Fourier transform. The same process is repeated for all the points on the T wave and the spectra are averaged.

T wave alternans, which is usually not evident on examination of the beat series, becomes evident on spectral analysis as a peak in voltage fluctuation occurring at the 0.5 cycles/beat frequency (Figure 26–4C). Voltage fluctuations at other frequencies are due to other sources such as respiration, movement, myopotentials, or baseline drift of the ECG signal. The noise level is measured from frequencies adjacent to the TWA frequency (0.45–0.49 cycles/beat), the designated noise band. The alternans power (measured in μV^2) is the difference between the power at the alternans frequency (0.5 cycles/beat) and the power at the noise frequency band. The alternans voltage or V_{alt} (measured in μV) is the square root of the alternans power. An alternans voltage of >1.9 μV is considered abnormal.

An important feature of the spectral analysis method is that an estimate of the statistical significance of the TWA measurement can be obtained (the K score), and is defined as the ratio of the alternans power to the standard deviation of the noise level in the noise band. A K score of >3 is considered significant.

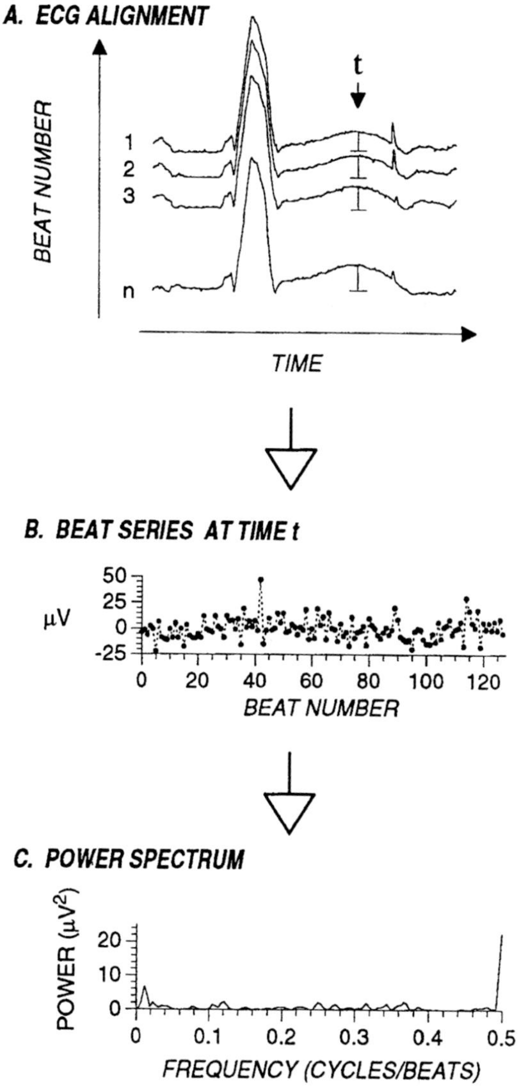

FIGURE 26–4. Algorithm used to measure microvolt-level electrical alternans from the surface ECG. (A) Sequentially recorded ECG complexes are aligned about their QRS complexes using cross-correlation. Beat-to-beat fluctuations of ECG amplitude are measured separately for each point of the ECG. In this example, a point of the ECG located at a time, *t*, is evaluated for electrical alternans. (B) Beat-to-beat fluctuations in the amplitude of point *t* are represented as a beat series. (C) The power spectrum is calculated from the fast Fourier transform of the beat series shown in (B). (Reproduced from Rosenbaum *et al.*,[83] with permission.)

Alternative Methods for Measuring T Wave Alternans

Alternative methods of measuring TWA have been suggested, such as the modified moving average (MMA) method.[94,95] This method uses a Holter-based system to acquire the ECG data and an averaging technique to compare odd and even T wave voltages for signal processing. Another method that has been described is the complex demodulation method.[96] These methods do not fully account for fluctuations outside of the alternans frequency (especially non-random noise) and require further validation.

Clinical Utility of T Wave Alternans

The utility of TWA testing in predicting the risk of SCD was established in several observational studies and in different populations. Although case studies and small series describe its use in patients with long QT syndrome, arrhythmogenic right ventricular dysplasia,[97] hypertrophic cardiomyopathy,[98] and Brugada syndrome, these do not constitute, for now, an established area of clinical utility.

The majority of the data have been collected in patients with reduced LVEF, either due to coronary disease or to a nonischemic dilated cardiomyopathy. An abnormal TWA test has been shown to be predictive of an increased risk of ventricular arrhythmias or total mortality in both patient groups.[87–89,99–101] However, the positive predictive value (PPV) of the test is 15–25% at 1–2 years of follow-up. This is similar to other risk stratifiers including LVEF alone and EPS. However, the greatest strength of TWA testing lies in its high negative predictive value (NPV), which is above 95% in almost all studies.[89,91,99,102] This is true for patients with coronary disease, but also for those with nonischemic cardiomyopathy, a group for whom other risk stratifiers, including EPS, performed poorly. Bloomfield *et al.*[99] followed 549 patients with LVEF ≤40% with both ischemic or nonischemic cardiomyopathy for an average of 20 months, and reported that patients with an abnormal TWA test were more than five times more likely to die or have a sustained ventricular arrhythmia than patients with a negative test. A normal TWA test had an NPV of 97.5% for the primary endpoint of total mortality or sustained ventricular tachyarrhythmia (Figure 26–5). Confirming these data, a recent meta-analysis by Gehi *et al.*[91] involving 19 studies and 2608 subjects showed NPV and PPV of 97.2% and 19.3%, respectively. The average follow-up was 21 months and indeterminate results were excluded from the analysis. Subgroup analysis from this meta-analysis showed that there was no significant difference in the NPV of different clinical subgroups. However, the PPV varied significantly depending on the patient's clinical situation. For instance, the PPV was lowest in the primary prevention of SCD for postmyocardial infarction (MI) patients regardless of LVEF (6%) and highest in patients with a history of a prior ventricular tachyarrhythmic event (51%). This is not surprising, as it would be expected that patients who have already experienced a tachyarrhythmic event would have the arrhythmogenic substrate that causes an abnormal TWA. Interestingly, the PPV of patients with depressed LVEF [i.e., the congestive heart failure (CHF) population that clinicians are most interested in risk stratifying for SCD] was fairly high (25.5%), with no significant difference between ischemic and nonischemic cardiomyopathy.

The Bloomfield study, the Gehi meta-analysis, and all prior studies suggest that patients who

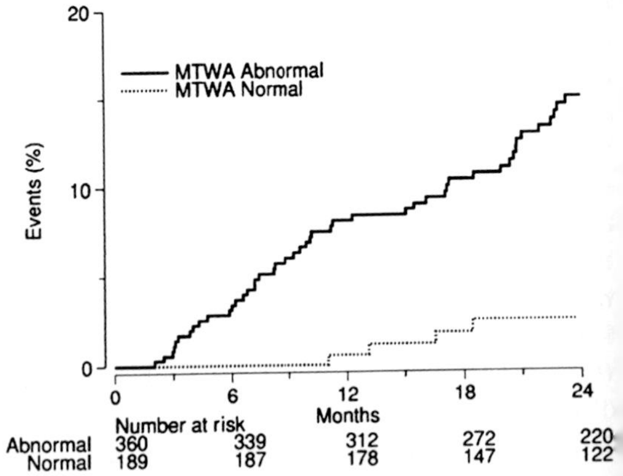

FIGURE 26–5. Kaplan–Meier mortality curves for patients with normal versus abnormal microvolt T wave alternans (TWA) test results. In 2 years of follow-up, only four events occurred in the 189 patients with a normal TWA test; 47 events occurred in the group with an abnormal TWA test. Abnormal TWA tests comprise positive tests ($n = 162$, 2-year event rate 12.3%) and indeterminate tests ($n = 198$, 2-year event rate 17.5%). (Reproduced from Momiyama *et al.*,[98] with permission.)

have a normal TWA test have a very low risk of SCD or significant ventricular tachyarrhythmias. In today's climate of implanting ICDs in all patients at risk, i.e., those with an LVEF of ≤0.35, such a high NPV may allow clinicians to identify patients at lowest risk of SCD who may safely forego ICD therapy. In addition, some clinicians are currently reluctant to refer patients for ICD therapy based on a low LVEF alone because of device complications and recalls, inappropriate shocks, patient comorbidities, and concerns regarding health care economics. Since TWA testing is simple and noninvasive it would allow clinicians a simple means to risk stratify patients with a low LVEF further. This may be repeated either at regular intervals, or with changes in clinical status,[103,104] to assess for dynamic changes in arrhythmogenic substrate over time.

The cost effectiveness of such a strategy was recently investigated by Chan *et al.*[5] who studied MADIT II like patients with ischemic cardiomyopathy and LVEF ≤0.30. In addition to finding that TWA is a significant independent predictor for all-cause (HR of 2.24, $p < 0.002$) mortality, it was concluded that risk stratification with TWA testing, in addition to a low LVEF, significantly improved the cost effectiveness of ICD implantation.

T wave alternans testing should be performed when the arrhythmogenic substrate is stable. In patients with recent myocardial infarction, studies suggest that the test should be done at least 2 weeks after the MI. Ikeda *et al.* showed that in 850 patients undergoing TWA testing at least 2 weeks after their infarct, TWA independently predicted SCD or ventricular fibrillation with a hazard ratio of 5.9 and an NPV of 99%.[105] In contrast, in a study by Tapanainen *et al.* when TWA testing was performed within 2 weeks after an infarct, many tests were incomplete due to the inability of the patients to exercise.[106] Even though the NPV of the test was preserved (99%), there was no increased risk of adverse cardiovascular events with a positive TWA, as there were a large number of indeterminate tests.

When compared to other noninvasive risk stratification tests used to predict SCD, TWA has been shown to be superior,[88,107,108] including signal averaged electrocardiogram (SAECG),[108,109] baroreflex sensitivity (BRS), QT dispersion, QRS duration,[110] nonsustained ventricular tachycardia on a 24-h Holter monitor, and heart rate variability. In fact, Hohnloser *et al.* found TWA to be the only independent predictor of ventricular tachycardia or ventricular fibrillation in 95 patients undergoing ICD implantation for secondary prophylaxis of SCD.[107] This held true for established risk stratifiers such as LVEF and EPS. We recently completed the ABCD trial,[86] a multicenter prospective trial that has enrolled 566 patients with ischemic cardiomyopathy and nonsustained ventricular tachycardia. The overall objective of the study is to determine if strategies incorporating noninvasive TWA to guide ICD therapy could improve the therapeutic efficacy of SCD prevention. All patients systematically underwent EPS and TWA testing, and were followed longitudinally for the primary endpoint of ICD therapy or SCD. This trial will allow the clinician to compare strategies to guide ICD therapy for primary prevention of SCD including comparing EPS alone versus TWA alone as risk stratifiers. In fact, using TWA as an initial screening tool and combining it in some patients with other noninvasive tests, or with EPS may improve the predictive value of TWA alone.[105,108] Recently, Rashba *et al.* demonstrated, in 144 patients with ischemic cardiomyopathy referred for EPS, that TWA was the only noninvasive independent predictor of death, ventricular tachyarrhythmic event, or appropriate ICD shocks. Interestingly, a negative EPS increased the already high NPV of TWA further.[111]

Limitations of the T Wave Alternans Test

Because TWA testing requires elevating heart rate ≥105 bpm, the test is "indeterminate" in patients who cannot achieve this target heart rate, whether due to intrinsic heart disease, medication, or decreased functional capacity from any cause. Interestingly, it has been suggested that heart rate elevation for TWA testing may be accomplished using pharmacotherapy, such as dobutamine.[112] In addition, the TWA test is also "indeterminate" when frequent ectopy obscures the beat-to-beat variations in the T wave. As discussed above, patients with decreased functional capacity and frequent ventricular ectopy have inherently a higher mortality, and it therefore makes sense for these TWA tests to be considered abnormal.

Similarly, in patients with permanent atrial fibrillation, because of the heart rate irregularity, and in patients dependent on ventricular pacing, because of the profound changes in repolarization, the TWA test cannot be performed.

Effect of Medications on T Wave Alternans Testing

Despite varying effects of medications on TWA, the test retains a significant predictive value for ventricular tachyarrhythmias.[113–115] In a study of patients with dilated cardiomyopathy given class I, III, and IV antiarrhythmic medications, TWA was shown to have a better predictive value than LVEF for the occurrence of ventricular tachyarrhythmias.[116]

Whether to do a TWA test on or off β blockers has been a matter of controversy. Since these agents have been shown to reduce the magnitude of TWA,[103,104,113,117] patients on β blockers may be less likely to have a positive test. Some investigators have suggested that this correlates with the ability of β blockers to reduce cardiovascular mortality.[104,113,117] Other experts feel that to assess risk more accurately, and to decrease the heart rate indeterminate tests, the β blocker should be withheld prior to the test. However, TWA has successfully predicted cardiovascular events in patients taking β blockers,[101,107] and our current thinking is that patients should be tested on the medical therapy that they are chronically taking to assess their risk of SCD accurately. The effects of class I antiarrhythmic drugs such as procainamide[118] and class III drugs such as sotalol and amiodarone[104,119,120] have been studied in small numbers of patients. All drugs seem to reduce the magnitude of TWA, but the significance of this is unclear.

References

1. Zheng ZJ, Croft JB, Giles WH, *et al.* Sudden cardiac death in the United States, 1989 to 1998. *Circulation* 2001;104:2158–2163.
2. Bardy GH, Lee KL, Mark DB, *et al.* Amiodarone or an implantable cardioverter-defibrillator for congestive heart failure. *N Engl J Med* 2005;352: 225–237.
3. Moss AJ, Zareba W, Hall WJ, *et al.* Prophylactic implantation of a defibrillator in patients with myocardial infarction and reduced ejection fraction. *N Engl J Med* 2002;346:877–883.
4. Myerburg RJ, Kessler KM, Castellanos A. Sudden cardiac death: Epidemiology, transient risk, and intervention assessment. *Ann Intern Med* 1993; 119:1187–1197.
5. Chan PS, Stein K, Chow T, *et al.* Cost-effectiveness of a microvolt T-wave alternans screening strategy for implantable cardioverter-defibrillator placement in the MADIT-II-eligible population. *J Am Coll Cardiol* 2006;48:112–121.
6. Traube L. Ein Fall von Pulsus Bigeminus nebst Bemerkungen uber die Leberschwellungen bei Klappenfehlern und uber acute Leberatrophie. *Berlin Klin Wochenschr* 1872;9:185–188.
7. Hering HE. Experimentelle studien an Saugerthierien uber das elektrocardiogramm. II. Mittheilung. *Z Exp Pathol Ther* 1910;7:363–378.
8. Lewis T. Notes upon alternation of the heart. *Q J Med* 1910;4:141–144.
9. Kent S, Ferguson M, Trotta R, *et al.* T wave alternans associated with HIV cardiomyopathy, erythromycin therapy, and electrolyte disturbances. *South Med J* 1998;91:755–758.
10. Schwartz PJ, Malliani A. Electrical alternation of the T-wave: Clinical and experimental evidence of its relationship with the sympathetic nervous system and with the long Q-T syndrome. *Am Heart J* 1975;89:45–50.
11. Cheng TC. Electrical alternans: An association with coronary artery spasm. *Arch Intern Med* 1983;143:1052–1053.
12. Puletti M, Curione M, Righetti G, *et al.* Alternans of the ST-segment and T-wave in acute myocardial infarction. *J Electrocardiol* 1980;13:297–300.
13. Kleinfeld MJ, Rozanski JJ. Alternans of the ST-segment in Prenzmetal's angina. *Circulation* 1977;55:574–577.
14. Bardaji A, Vidal F, Richart C. T wave alternans associated with amiodarone. *J Electrocardiol* 1993; 26:155–157.
15. Reddy CVR, Kiok JP, Khan RG, *et al.* Repolarization alternans associated with alcoholism and hypomagnesemia. *Am J Cardiol* 1984;53:390–391.
16. Shimoni Z, Flateau E, Schiller D, *et al.* Electrical alternans of giant U waves with multiple electrolyte abnormalities. *Am J Cardiol* 1984;54:920–921.
17. Kalter HH, Schwartz ML. Electrical alternans. *NY State J Med* 1948;98:1164–1166.
18. Adam D, Smith J, Akselrod S, *et al.* Fluctuations in T-wave morphology and susceptibility to ventricular fibrillation. *J Electrocardiol* 1984;17:209–218.

19. Smith JM, Clancy EA, Valeri R, *et al.* Electrical alternans and cardiac electrical instability. *Circulation* 1988;77:110–121.
20. Rosenbaum DS, Jackson LE, Smith JM, *et al.* Electrical alternans and vulnerability to ventricular arrhythmias. *N Engl J Med* 1994;330:235–241.
21. Hohnloser SH, Klingenheben T, Zabel M, *et al.* T wave alternans during exercise and atrial pacing in humans. *J Cardiovasc Electrophysiol* 1997;8:987–993.
22. Estes NAMI, Michaud G, Zipes DP, *et al.* Electrical alternans during rest and exercise as predictors of vulnerability to ventricular arrhythmias. *Am J Cardiol* 1997;80:1314–1318.
23. Pastore JM, Girouard SD, Laurita KR, *et al.* Mechanism linking T-wave alternans to the genesis of cardiac fibrillation. *Circulation* 1999;99:1385–1394.
24. Pastore JM, Rosenbaum DS. Role of structural barriers in the mechanism of alternans-induced reentry. *Circ Res* 2000;87:1157–1163.
25. Walker ML, Rosenbaum DS. Repolarization alternans: Implications for the mechanism and prevention of sudden cardiac death. *Cardiovasc Res* 2003;57:599–614.
26. Pruvot EJ, Katra RP, Rosenbaum DS, *et al.* Role of calcium cycling versus restitution in the mechanism of repolarization alternans. *Circ Res* 2004;94:1083–1090.
27. Kleinfeld M, Stein E. Electrical alternans of components of the action potential. *Am Heart J* 1968;75:528–530.
28. Rubenstein DS, Lipsius SL. Premature beats elicit a phase reversal of mechanoelectrical alternans in cat ventricular myocytes: A possible mechanism for reentrant arrhythmias. *Circulation* 1995;91:201–214.
29. Karagueuzian HS, Khan SS, Hong K, *et al.* Action potential alternans and irregular dynamics in quinidine-intoxicated ventricular muscle cells: Implications for ventricular proarrhythmia. *Circulation* 1993;87:1661–1672.
30. Franz MR, Swerdlow CD, Liem LB, *et al.* Cycle length dependence of human action potential duration in vivo. *J Clin Invest* 1988;82:972–979.
31. Hirayama Y, Saitoh H, Atarashi H, *et al.* Electrical and mechanical alternans in canine myocardium in vivo: Dependence on intracellular calcium cycling. *Circulation* 1993;88:2894–2902.
32. Kurz RW, Mohabir R, Ren X-L, *et al.* Ischaemia induced alternans of action potential duration in the intact heart: Dependence on coronary flow, preload, and cycle length. *Eur Heart J* 1993;14:1410–1420.
33. Sutton PMI, Taggart P, Lab M, *et al.* Alternans of epicardial repolarization as a localized phenomenon in man. *Eur Heart J* 1991;12:70–78.
34. Bers DM. Excitation-contraction coupling and cardiac contractile force. In: Bers DM, Ed. *Cardiac Inotrophy and Ca Mismanagement,* 2nd ed. Dordrecht, The Netherlands: Kluwer Academic Publishers, 2001:273–331.
35. Dilly SG, Lab MJ. Electrophysiological alternans and restitution during acute regional ischemia in myocardium of anesthetized pig. *J Physiol (Lond)* 1988;402:315–333.
36. Murphy CF, Lab MJ, Horner SM, *et al.* Regional electromechanical alternans in anesthetized pig hearts: Modulation by mechanoelectric feedback. *Am J Physiol Heart Circ Physiol* 1994;267:H1726–H1735.
37. Kurz RW, Ren XL, Franz MR. Dispersion and delay of electrical restitution in the globally ischaemic heart. *Eur Heart J* 1994;15:547–554.
38. Bellavere F, Ferri M, Guarini L, *et al.* Prolonged QT period in diabetic autonomic neuropathy: A possible role in sudden cardiac death? *Br Heart J* 1988;59:379–383.
39. Boyett MR, Jewell BR. A study of the factors responsible for rate-dependent shortening of the action potential in mammalian ventricular muscle. *J Physiol (Lond)* 1978;285:359–380.
40. Carmeliet E. Repolarization and frequency in cardiac cells. *J Physiol (Paris)* 1977;73:903–923.
41. Elharrar V, Surawicz B. Cycle length effect on restitution of action potential duration in dog cardiac fibers. *Am J Physiol Heart Circ Physiol* 1983;244:H782–H792.
42. Watanabe MA, Fenton FH, Evans SJ, *et al.* Mechanisms for discordant alternans. *J Cardiovasc Electrophysiol* 2001;12:196–206.
43. Rashba EJ, Osman AF, MacMurdy K, *et al.* Influence of QRS duration on the prognostic value of T wave alternans. *J Cardiovasc Electrophysiol* 2002;13:770–775.
44. Garfinkel A, Kim YH, Voroshilovsky O, *et al.* Preventing ventricular fibrillation by flattening cardiac restitution. *Proc Natl Acad Sci USA* 2000;97:6061–6066.
45. Qu Z, Garfinkel A, Chen P, *et al.* Mechanisms of discordant alternans and induction of reentry in simulated cardiac tissue. *Circulation* 2000;102:1664–1670.
46. Riccio ML, Koller ML, Gilmour RF Jr. Electrical restitution and spatiotemporal organization during ventricular fibrillation. *Circ Res* 1999;84:955–963.

47. Watanabe M, Otani NF, Gilmour RF Jr. Biphasic restitution of action potential duration and complex dynamics in ventricular myocardium. *Circ Res* 1995;76:915–921.
48. Lukas A, Antzelevitch C. Differences in the electrophysiological response of canine ventricular epicardium and endocardium to ischemia: Role of the transient outward current. *Circulation* 1993; 88:2903–2915.
49. Konta T, Ikeda K, Yamaki M, *et al.* Significance of discordant ST alternans in ventricular fibrillation. *Circulation* 1990;82:2185–2189.
50. Luo C, Rudy Y. A model of the ventricular cardiac action potential: Depolarization, repolarization, and their interaction. *Circ Res* 1991;68:1501–1526.
51. Hua F, Gilmour RF Jr. Contribution of IKr to rate-dependent action potential dynamics in canine endocardium. *Circ Res* 2004;94:810–819.
52. Goldhaber JI , Xie LH, Duong T, *et al.* Action potential duration restitution and alternans in rabbit ventricular myocytes: The key role of intracellular calcium cycling. *Circ Res* 2005;96:459–466.
53. Davey P, Bryant S, Hart G. Rate-dependent electrical, contractile and restitution properties of isolated left ventricular myocytes in guinea-pig hypertrophy. *Acta Physiol Scand* 2001;171:17–28.
54. Lab MJ, Lee JA. Changes in intracellular calcium during mechanical alternans in isolated ferret ventricular muscle. *Circ Res* 1990;66:585–595.
55. Lee HC, Mohabir R, Smith N, *et al.* Effect of ischemia on calcium-dependent fluorescence transients in rabbit hearts containing Indo-1: Correlation with monophasic action potentials and contraction. *Circulation* 1988;78:1047–1059.
56. Saitoh H, Bailey J, Surawicz B. Alternans of action potential duration after abrupt shortening of cycle length: Differences between dog Purkinje and ventricular muscle fibers. *Circ Res* 1988;62: 1027–1040.
57. Saitoh H, Bailey J, Surawicz B. Action potential duration alternans in dog Purkinje and ventricular muscle fibers. *Circulation* 1989;80:1421–1431.
58. Spencer CI, Mörner SEJN, Noble MIM, *et al.* Effects of nifedipine and low [Ca^{2+}] on mechanical restitution during hypothermia in guinea pig papillary muscles. *Basic Res Cardiol* 1993;88:111–119.
59. Miller WL, Sgura FA, Kopecky SL, *et al.* Characteristics of presenting electrocardiograms of acute myocardial infarction from a community-based population predict short- and long-term mortality. *Am J Cardiol* 2001;87:1045–1050.
60. Laurita KR, Singal A, Pastore JM, Rosenbaum DS. Spatial heterogeneity of calcium transients may explain action potential dispersion during T-wav alternans. *Circulation* 1998;98(Suppl. I):I-18 (abstract).
61. Hirata Y, Kodama I, Iwamura N, *et al.* Effects c verapamil on canine Purkinje fibers and ventricu lar muscle fibers with particular reference to th alternation of action potential duration after sudden increase in driving rate. *Cardiovasc Re* 1979;13:1–8.
62. Narayan P, McCune SA, Robitaille P-ML, *et a* Mechanical alternans and the force-frequenc relationship in failing rat hearts. *J Mol Cell Cardio* 1995;27:523–530.
63. Bouchard RA, Clark RB, Giles WR. Effect of action potential duration on excitation contraction coupling in rat ventricular myocytes Action potential voltage-clamp measurements *Circ Res* 1995;76:790–801.
64. Stern MD. Theory of excitation-contractio coupling in cardiac muscle. *Biophys J* 1992;63 497–517.
65. Weiss JN, Karma A, Shiferaw Y, *et al.* From pulsu to pulseless: The saga of cardiac alternans. *Cir Res* 2006;98:1244–1253.
66. Sato D, Shiferaw Y, Garfinkel A, *et al.* Spatiall discordant alternans in cardiac tissue: Role o calcium cycling. *Circ Res* 2006;99:520–527.
67. Chudin E, Goldhaber JI, Weiss J, *et al.* Intracellu lar Ca2 dynamics and the stability of ventricula tachycardia. *Biophys J* 1999;77:2930–2941.
68. Wan X, Laurita KR, Pruvot E, *et al.* Molecular cor relates of repolarization alternans in cardiac myo cytes. *J Mol Cell Cardiol* 2005;39:419–428.
69. Laurita KR, Katra R, Wible B, *et al.* Transmura heterogeneity of calcium handling in canine. *Cir Res* 2003;92:668–675.
70. Diaz ME, O'Neill SC, Eisner DA. Sarcoplasmi reticulum calcium content fluctuation is the ke to cardiac alternans. *Circ Res* 2004;94:650–656.
71. Hüser J, Wang YG, Sheehan KA, *et al.* Functiona coupling between glycolysis and excitation contraction coupling underlies alternans in ca heart cells. *J Physiol (Lond)* 2000;524:795–806.
72. Chinushi M, Kozhevnikov D, Caref EB, *et al* Mechanism of discordant T wave alternans i the in vivo heart. *J Cardiovasc Electrophysiol* 2003 14:632–638.
73. Podrid PJ, Fuchs T, Candinas R. Role of the sym pathetic nervous system in the genesis of ventricu lar arrhythmia. *Circulation* 1990;82:I-103–I-113.
74. Cao JM, Qu ZL, Kim YH, *et al.* Spatiotempora heterogeneity in the induction of ventricula fibrillation by rapid pacing: Importance of car diac restitution properties. *Circ Res* 1999;84:1318-1331.

75. Laurita KR, Girouard SD, Rudy Y, *et al.* Role of passive electrical properties during action potential restitution in the intact heart. *Am J Physiol Heart Circ Physiol* 1997;273:H1205–H1214.
76. Watanabe T, Yamaki M, Kubota I, *et al.* Relation between activation sequence fluctuation and arrhythmogenicity in sodium-channel blockade. *Am J Physiol Heart Circ Physiol* 1999;277:H971–H977.
77. Tachibana H, Yamaki M, Kubota I, *et al.* Intracoronary flecainide induces ST alternans and reentrant arrhythmia on intact canine heart–A role of 4-aminopyridine-sensitive current. *Circulation* 1999;99:1637–1643.
78. Suzuki K, Murtuza B, Smolenski RT, *et al.* Cell transplantation for the treatment of acute myocardial infarction using vascular endothelial growth factor-expressing skeletal myoblasts. *Circulation* 2001;104:I207–1212.
79. Poelzing S, Akar FG, Baron E, *et al.* Heterogeneous connexin43 expression produces electrophysiological heterogeneities across ventricular wall. *Am J Physiol Heart Circ Physiol* 2004;286:H2001–H2009.
80. Poelzing S, Rosenbaum DS. Altered connexin43 expression produces arrhythmia substrate in heart failure. *Am J Physiol Heart Circ Physiol* 2004;287: H1762–H1770.
81. Turitto G, Caref EB, El-Attar G, *et al.* Optimal target heart rate for exercise-induced T-wave alternans. *Ann Noninvasive Electrocardiol* 2001;6: 123–128.
82. Kavesh NG, Shorofsky SR, Sarang SE, *et al.* Effect of heart rate on T wave alternans. *J Cardiovasc Electrophysiol* 1998;9:703–708.
83. Rosenbaum DS, Albrecht P, Cohen RJ. Predicting sudden cardiac death from T wave alternans of the surface electrocardiogram: Promise and pitfalls. *J Cardiovasc Electrophysiol* 1996;7:1095–1111.
84. Magnano AR, Holleran S, Ramakrishnan R, *et al.* Autonomic nervous system influences on QT interval in normal subjects. *J Am Coll Cardiol* 2002;39:1820–1826.
85. Bloomfield DM, Hohnloser SH, Cohen RJ. Interpretation and classification of microvolt T wave alternans tests. *J Cardiovasc Electrophysiol* 2002;13:502–512.
86. Costantini O, Hohnloser SH, Kirk MM, Lerman BB, Baker JH II, Barathi S, Dettmer MM, Rosenbaum DS, for the ABCD Investigators. The Alternans Before Cardioverter Defibrillator (ABCD) Trial. Late Breaking Clinical Trials Session, American Heart Association, November 2006.
87. Chow T, Keriakes D, Bartone C, *et al.* Prognostic utility of microvolt T-wave alternans in risk stratification of patients with ischemic cardiomyopathy. *J Am Coll Cardiol* 2006;47:1820–1827.
88. Hohnloser SH, Klingenheben T, Bloomfield D, *et al.* Usefulness of microvolt T-wave alternans for prediction of ventricular tachyarrhythmic events in patients with dilated cardiomyopathy: Results from a prospective observational study. *J Am Coll Cardiol* 2003;41:2220–2224.
89. Hohnloser SH, Ikeda T, Bloomfield DM, *et al.* T-wave alternans negative coronary patients with low ejection and benefit from defibrillator implantation. *Lancet* 2003;362:125–126.
90. Kaufman ES, Bloomfield DM, Steinman RC, *et al.* "Indeterminate" microvolt T-wave alternans tests predict high risk of death or sustained ventricular arrhythmias in patients with left ventricular dysfunction. *J Am Coll Cardiol* 2006;48:1399–1404.
91. Gehi AK, Stein RH, Metz LD, *et al.* Microvolt T-wave alternans for the risk stratification of ventricular tachyarrhythmic events: A meta-analysis. *J Am Coll Cardiol* 2005;46:75–82.
92. Klingenheben T, Ptaszynski P, Hohnloser SH. Quantitative assessment of microvolt T-wave alternans in patients with congestive heart failure. *J Cardiovasc Electrophysiol* 2005;16:620–624.
93. Kitamura H, Ohnishi Y, Okajima K, *et al.* Onset heart rate of microvolt-level T-wave alternans provides clinical and prognostic value in nonischemic dilated cardiomyopathy. *J Am Coll Cardiol* 2002;39:295–300.
94. Nearing BD, Verrier RL. Modified moving average analysis of T-wave alternans to predict ventricular fibrillation with high accuracy. *J Appl Physiol* 2002;92:541–549.
95. Verrier RL, Nearing BD, La Rovere MT, *et al.* Ambulatory electrocardiogram-based tracking of T wave alternans in postmyocardial infarction patients to assess risk of cardiac arrest or arrhythmic death. *J Cardiovasc Electrophysiol* 2003;14:705–711.
96. Nearing B, Huang AH, Verrier RL. Dynamic tracking of cardiac vulnerability by complex demodulation of the T-wave. *Science* 1991;252:437–440.
97. Kinoshita O, Tomita T, Hanaoka T, *et al.* T-wave alternans in patients with right ventricular tachycardia. *Cardiology* 2003;100:86–92.
98. Momiyama Y, Hartikainen J, Nagayoshi H, *et al.* Exercise-induced T-wave alternans as a marker of high risk in patients with hypertrophic cardiomyopathy. *Jpn Circ J* 1997;61:650–656.
99. Bloomfield DM, Bigger JT, Steinman RC, *et al.* Microvolt T-wave alternans and the risk of death or sustained ventricular arrhythmias in patients with left ventricular dysfunction. *J Am Coll Cardiol* 2006;47:456–463.

100. Sarzi Braga S, Vaninetti R, Laporta A, *et al.* T wave alternans is a predictor of death in patients with congestive heart failure. *Int J Cardiol* 2004;93:31–38.
101. Klingenheben T, Zabel M, D'Agostino RB, *et al.* Predictive value of T-wave alternans for arrhythmic events in patients with congestive heart failure. *Lancet* 2000;356:651–652.
102. Baravelli M , Salerno-Uriarte D, Guzzetti D, *et al.* Predictive significance for sudden death of microvolt-level T wave alternans in New York Heart Association class II congestive heart failure patients: A prospective study. *Int J Cardiol* 2005;105:53–57.
103. Murata M, Harada M, Shimizu A, *et al.* Effect of long-term beta-blocker therapy on microvolt-level T-wave alternans in association with the improvement of the cardiac sympathetic nervous system and systolic function in patients with non-ischemic heart disease. *Circ J* 2003;67:821–825.
104. Klingenheben T, Grönefeld G, Li YG, *et al.* Effect of metoprolol and *d,l*-sotalol on microvolt-level T-wave alternans–Results of a prospective, double-blind, randomized study. *J Am Coll Cardiol* 2001;38:2013–2019.
105. Ikeda T, Saito H, Tanno K, *et al.* T-wave alternans as a predictor for sudden cardiac death after myocardial infarction. *Am J Cardiol* 2002;89:79–82.
106. Tapanainen JM, Still AM, Airaksinen KEJ, *et al.* Prognostic significance of risk stratifiers of mortality, including T wave alternans, after acute myocardial infarction: Results of a prospective follow-up study. *J Cardiovasc Electrophysiol* 2001;12:645–652.
107. Hohnloser SH, Klingenheben T, Li YG, *et al.* T wave alternans as a predictor of recurrent ventricular tachyarrhythmias in ICD recipients: Prospective comparison with conventional risk markers. *J Cardiovasc Electrophysiol* 1998;9:1258–1268.
108. Gold MR, Bloomfield DM, Anderson KP, *et al.* A comparison of T-wave alternans, signal averaged electrocardiography and programmed ventricular stimulation for arrhythmia risk stratification. *J Am Coll Cardiol* 2000;36:2247–2253.
109. Armoundas AA, Rosenbaum DS, Ruskin JN, *et al.* Prognostic significance of electrical alternans versus signal averaged electrocardiography in predicting the outcome of electrophysiological testing and arrhythmia-free survival. *Heart* 1998;80:251–256.
110. Bloomfield DM, Steinman RC, Namerow PB, *et a* Microvolt T-wave alternans distinguishes betwee patients likely and patients not likely to bene from implanted cardiac defibrillator therapy: solution to the Multicenter Automatic Defibrill tor Implantation Trial (MADIT) II conundru *Circulation* 2004;110:1885–1889.
111. Rashba EJ, Osman AF, Macmurdy K, *et a* Enhanced detection of arrhythmia vulnerabili using T wave alternans, left ventricular ejectio fraction, and programmed ventricular stimul tion: A prospective study in subjects with chron ischemic heart disease. *J Cardiovasc Electrophysi* 2004;15:170–176.
112. Caffarone A, Martinelli A, Valentini P, *et a* T wave alternans detection during exercise stres test and during dobutamine stress. A comparati study in patients with a recent myocardial infar tion. *Ital Heart J* 2001;2:265–270.
113. Komiya N, Seto S, Nakao K, *et al.* The influenc of beta-adrenergic agonists and antagonists o T-wave alternans in patients with and witho ventricular tachyarrhythmia. *Pacing Clin Electr physiol* 2005;28:680–684.
114. Kaufman ES, Mackall JA, Julka B, *et al.* Influenc of heart rate and sympathetic stimulation o arrhythmogenic T wave alternans. *Am J Physi Heart Circ Physiol* 2000;279:H1248–H1255.
115. Ohkubo K, Watanabe I, Okumura Y, *et al.* Intra venous administration of class I antiarrhythmi drug induced T wave alternans in an asympto matic Brugada syndrome patient. *Pacing Cli Electrophysiol* 2003;26:1900–1903.
116. Sakabe K, Ikeda T, Sakata T, *et al.* Predicting th recurrence of ventricular tachyarrhythmias fro T-wave alternans assessed on antiarrhythmi pharmacotherapy: A prospective study in patient with dilated cardiomyopathy. *Ann Noninvasiv Electrocardiol* 2001;6:203–208.
117. Rashba EJ, Cooklin M, MacMurdy K, *et a* Effects of selective autonomic blockade on T-wav alternans in humans. *Circulation* 2002;105:837 842.
118. Kavesh NG, Shorofsky SR, Sarang SE, *et a* The effect of procainamide on T wave alternans *J Cardiovasc Electrophysiol* 1999;10:649–654.
119. Tan HL, Wilde AAM. T wave alternans afte sotalol: Evidence for increased sensitivity t sotalol after conversion from atrial fibrillation t sinus rhythm. *Heart* 1998;80:303–306.
120. Kaszala K, Kenigsberg DN, Krishnan SC Drug-induced T wave alternans. *J Cardiovas Electrophysiol* 2006;17:332.

27 Invasive Electrophysiologic Testing: Role in Sudden Death Prediction

Jan Nemec and Win-Kuang Shen

Introduction

The placement of intracardiac catheters to assess the risk of arrhythmia dates back nearly 40 years. The discovery by Wellens *et al.*[1] in 1972 that clinical ventricular tachycardia (VT) in patients with prior myocardial infarction (MI) could be initiated by programmed ventricular stimulation (PVS) generated real enthusiasm about the technique. In the 1980s, many cardiologists would have labeled PVS the most precise and perhaps the most important tool for risk stratification of patients at risk for sudden cardiac death (SCD). Selection of antiarrhythmic treatment on the basis of suppression of VT inducibility was reasonably believed to represent a scientific approach to management of life-threatening arrhythmias.

Although we learned from subsequent studies that reality is more complicated, which led to a more circumscribed role for invasive electrophysiologic testing, it is still a useful and widely used tool for risk stratification in many situations. The role of programmed ventricular stimulation in risk stratification is best defined in patients with prior MI. This topic is the focus of this chapter. The available information on the use of PVS in other conditions is also reviewed, as are two invasive electrophysiological techniques unrelated to PVS: (1) HV interval measurement and (2) induction of atrial fibrillation in Wolff–Parkinson–White (WPW) patients, because they are occasionally being used to predict potentially life-threatening arrhythmias.

Programmed Ventricular Stimulation

Coronary Artery Disease

Most VTs in patients with prior MI are due to reentry, as evidenced by the ability to induce clinical sustained monomorphic VT (SMVT) by PVS. The inducibility of life-threatening clinical arrhythmia in a controlled laboratory setting has enhanced the understanding of the mechanisms leading to SCD in these patients. A hypothesis formulated in the 1970s was that two factors must be present for ventricular tachyarrhythmia to occur: a substrate and a trigger. The substrate was believed to be a fixed anatomical obstacle (e.g., a scar after prior MI) that created conditions for reentry. The clinical trigger initiating reentry was believed to be a ventricular extrasystole. In the catheterization laboratory, the role of the clinical trigger is played by a premature stimulus delivered by a catheter. In this paradigm, the substrate is relatively fixed, whereas the clinical trigger is stochastic if not random.

The implications of this paradigm resulted in widespread use of PVS based on the following assumptions:

1. Most instances of SCD after MI are related to ventricular tachyarrhythmia, either VT or ventricular fibrillation (VF), and many instances of VF result from degeneration of organized VT.
2. Patients with an anatomical substrate that allows sustained reentry VT can be identified by PVS, even if they have never had clinical

arrhythmia; these patients are at higher risk of SCD than are other post-MI patients.

3. After these patients are identified, effective pharmacological treatment can be determined by testing VT inducibility after administration of antiarrhythmic medications.

By and large, the first and second assumptions withstood the test of time with important amendments, whereas the last one was found to be incorrect. Nevertheless, these assumptions did provide a believable mechanistic framework for SCD risk stratification and for management of high-risk patients.

Reproducibility of Clinical Sustained Monomorphic Ventricular Tachycardia by Programmed Ventricular Stimulation

Multiple protocols can be used to induce VT by PVS. In the first PVS report, Wellens *et al.*[1] used a single extrastimulus from a single right ventricular (RV) site. It soon became apparent that the sensitivity of the method is increased with additional extrastimuli and another RV sit Josephson[2] reported that PVS can elicit VT in 95 of patients with coronary artery disease (CAD who present with SMVT. About 10% of VTs ca be induced only by stimulation from the left ven tricle (LV).[3,4]

At present, the details of PVS continue to diffe among different institutions, but a protocol simila to the one used in the Multicenter Unsustaine Tachycardia Trial (MUSTT)[5] is used most fre quently (Figure 27–1), because outcome data ar available from this large study. Stimulation fron both the RV apex and the RV outflow tract, but no from the LV, would usually be performed. Thi stimulation protocol would typically involve stim ulation with an eight-beat drive train (cycle length 600 and 400 msec), followed by one extrastimulus then two, and finally three extrastimuli. The cou pling interval of the last extrastimulus is graduall shortened until an effective refractory period i reached. Subsequently, the coupling interval of th preceding extrastimuli is shortened until an effec tive refractory period is reached for the first extras

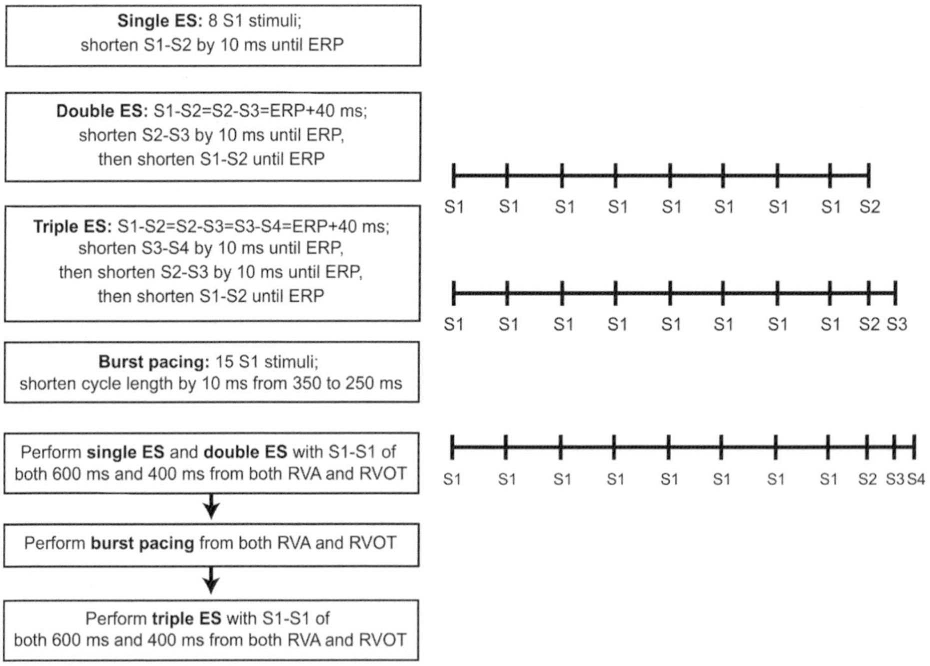

FIGURE 27–1. Simplified protocol of programmed ventricular stimulation used in the Multicenter Unsustained Tachycardia Trial. Variants of this protocol are common in clinical practice. ERP, effective refractory period; ES, extrastimulus or extrastimuli; RVA, righ ventricular apex; RVOT, right ventricular outflow tract. (Modifie from Buxton *et al.*,[5] with permission.)

mulus. A simplified protocol, starting with three xtrastimuli and simultaneously shortening all oupling intervals, has been proposed but has not een widely adopted.[6] Other stimulation protocols clude delivery of extrastimuli during sinus hythm and use of short–long–short sequences.[7] rotocols including PVS during categolamine dministration have been described, but isoroterenol infusion does not appear to facilitate nduction of reentry VT in CAD.[8]

In about one-third of patients, a nonclinical entricular arrhythmia is induced during PVS. his may be either an SMVT of a different (usually horter) cycle length than the VT observed clinially or a polymorphic VT or VF. The likelihood f induction of nonclinical SMVT and appears to e similar to induction of polymorphic VT or VF or that with a PVS protocol using three extrasmuli, but the latter is more likely to require the hird extrastimulus (S4)[9] and short coupling interals.[10] Since induction of polymorphic ventricular rrhythmia may be a nonspecific outcome (see elow) and often requires direct current cardioersion, many operators do not test coupling ntervals shorter than 180 or 200 msec to minimize induction of nonclinical arrhythmias. In a tudy of 52 patients with 57 documented clinical 'Ts, all clinical VTs were induced with coupling ntervals of 180 msec or longer.[10]

Although it is customary to stimulate ventricuar myocardium at twice the diastolic threshold rectangular pulses of 1 or 2 msec), the increase in he stimulation current does not appear to subtantially increase the sensitivity of the study.[11–13] n most studies, the immediate and short-term eproducibility of PVS results appears to be exellent with respect to SMVT induction.[14–17] For xample, Rosenbaum *et al.*[17] reported 98% reproducibility of SMVT induction during the same tudy.

ncreased Risk of Sudden Cardiac Death in 'atients with Inducible Ventricular Tachycardia

The reproducible induction of clinically documented VT led to a question about the risk of rrhythmia in patients with inducible SMVT vithout prior clinical VT. These patients harbor he substrate for ventricular arrhythmia with espect to the substrate and trigger concept. It was natural to investigate the use of VT inducibility as a marker of cardiac arrest risk and effectiveness of treatment with antiarrhythmic drugs (AADs). Several well-designed studies demonstrated that in patients with prior MI and decreased LV function, induction of SMVT during PVS is indeed associated with increased risk of future arrhythmic events and overall mortality. Moreover, this risk was found to be even higher in patients whose VT inducibility could not be abolished by AADs.

Wilber *et al.*[18] studied 166 patients with prior resuscitated cardiac arrest, mostly in the setting of CAD, with PVS. Ventricular arrhythmia (sustained or nonsustained monomorphic VT, polymorphic VT, or VF) was induced in 79%. In 72% of these patients, the arrhythmia was no longer induced with AAD treatment. The prognosis for these patients was significantly better with respect to both arrhythmic and total mortality than for those in whom suppression of VT or VF induction was not accomplished (Figure 27–2). This difference was especially marked in patients with poor systolic LV function. Similar results have been reported by Steinbeck *et al.*,[19] who performed PVS in 170 patients (mostly with CAD) who had preexisting ventricular arrhythmia or high-risk syncope. Ventricular arrhythmia was induced in 115 patients who were randomized to treatment with metoprolol or serial AAD testing; metoprolol

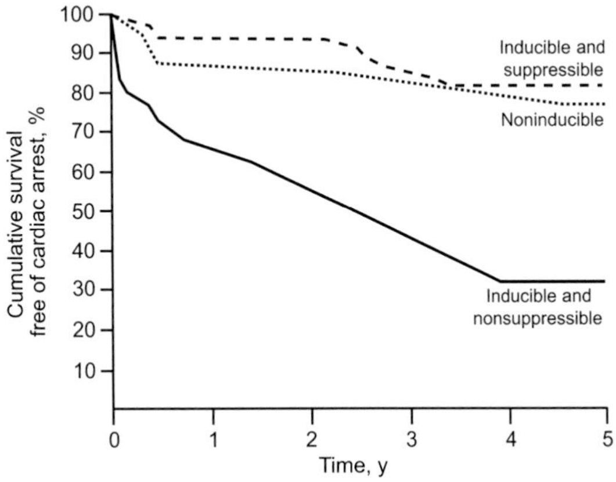

FIGURE 27–2. Proportion of patients free of death and cardiac arrest. The event rate was significantly ($p < 0.001$) higher in patients with inducible ventricular tachycardia that could not be suppressed with antiarrhythmic drug (AAD) treatment than in noninducible and suppressible patients. (Modified from Wilber *et al.*,[18] with permission.)

was used in noninducible patients. The recurrence rate of arrhythmia was again significantly lower in noninducible patients than in inducible patients treated with metoprolol ($p < 0.01$). Among the patients randomized to AAD, the rates of arrhythmia recurrence and overall mortality were higher for those whose arrhythmia could not be suppressed.

The results of the large MUSTT[20] study fully confirmed the role of PVS in risk stratification. This trial enrolled 2202 patients with clinically significant CAD (mostly prior MI), an LV ejection fraction (LVEF) of less than 40%, and nonsustained VT. These patients underwent PVS and, if VT was induced (as was the case in 34.8%), they were randomized either to AAD treatment guided by repeated PVS or to no AAD treatment. An implantable cardioverter defibrillator (ICD) could be used if VT remained inducible despite AAD treatment. The patients with no VT inducible at baseline were not randomized, but were instead followed in a registry. This design allowed comparisons of the rate of overall mortality as well as of the rate of cardiac arrest off treatment between patients with and without inducible VT. The results demonstrated that the patients with inducible VT had a higher risk of arrhythmic events (36% vs. 24% over 5 years; $p = 0.005$).[21] This difference could not be explained by baseline characteristics of the two populations.

An unresolved issue in PVS is the prognostic importance of VF or polymorphic VT. In the MUSTT study, induction of SMVT with three extrastimuli was considered a positive result, whereas VF, VT with a cycle length of less than 220 msec, or polymorphic VT was considered relevant only if induced with one or two extrastimuli.[5] However, the prognostic importance of polymorphic VT induction has not been analyzed separately. Some light has been shed on this question by the retrospective analysis of results from the Multicenter Automatic Defibrillator Implantation Trial II (MADIT-II).[22] This trial randomized 1232 patients with prior MI and LVEF of less than 30% to ICD implantation or standard medical treatment. Most of the 742 patients randomized to ICD implantation underwent PVS by a protocol similar to that of MUSTT.[18] Interestingly, the increased rate of arrhythmic events (as determined by appropriate ICD treatment) in inducible patients did not reach statistical significance, b this difference became significant (odds rati 1.56; $p < 0.02$) when only the patients with SMV during the PVS were classified as "positive." Th finding suggests that VF induction in this patie group has limited prognostic value, in accordan with older data.[19,23–25] However, dissenting opi ions[26] have been expressed, and current guid lines support ICD implantation in patients wi inducible VF.[27]

Another area of controversy concerns t optimal timing of PVS with respect to acute M Although PVS performed before hospital di charge does appear to carry prognostic sign ficance,[23,28] the inducibility rate decreas significantly between 2 and 20 weeks after an MI, and the predictive value of VT induction regar ing future arrhythmic events is better for the la study.[30]

Results of Treatment with Antiarrhythmic Drugs

The data summarized above confirmed that V induction in patients with an MI scar is indee associated with increased arrhythmic and tot mortality. They also showed that suppression VT inducibility with an AAD is associated wit better prognosis. However, the natural conclusio that these findings justify AAD selection based o suppression of VT induction during PVS turne out to be incorrect. The first serious doubts abo AAD effectiveness after an MI were raised by th unexpected results of the Cardiac Arrhythmi Suppression Trial (CAST)[31] and the Cardia Arrhythmia Suppression Trial II (CAST-II) studies. Although administration of the class antiarrhythmics in these trials was not based o the results of PVS, it was nevertheless of concer that these agents, which often effectively sup pressed VT inducibility, turned out to marked increase mortality in patients with a prior MI.

Two studies published in the early 1990s weak ened the case for AAD selection on the basis c PVS results. The Electrophysiologic Study Versu Electrocardiographic Monitoring (ESVEM) trial was designed to compare serial PVS and seri Holter monitoring for selection of AAD therap This trial enrolled patients with prior documente or probable ventricular arrhythmia. Of 242 pati ents randomized for a PVS-based approach, a effective" treatment (with respect to suppression f VT inducibility) was found in 108 (45%). Neverıeless, the rate of death due to arrhythmia in this roup was 10% in 1 year, hardly an acceptable uccess rate. The issue was examined more directly ı the Cardiac Arrest in Seattle: Conventional 'ersus Amiodarone Drug Evaluation (CASCADE) rial,[34] which randomized 228 patients with prior ardiac arrest to treatment based on a combiation of PVS-guided AAD testing and Holter ıonitoring versus empirical treatment with amidarone. The patients treated with amiodarone ad significantly higher arrhythmia-free survival han patients treated with PVS-based therapy 78% vs. 52% at 2 years; $p < 0.001$).

The question of whether antiarrhythmic treatent on the basis of PVS results is efficacious was nally settled by the MUSTT study.[20,21] The atients assigned to PVS-guided treatment indeed ad a slightly lower incidence of arrhythmic and verall mortality than patients who were randmized to no antiarrhythmic treatment. However, his difference was solely due to dramatically ower mortality (both arrhythmic and total) in atients who were treated with ICD implantation; he mortality in patients assigned to "effective" AADs was actually somewhat higher than that in atients receiving no antiarrhythmic treatment Figure 27–3).

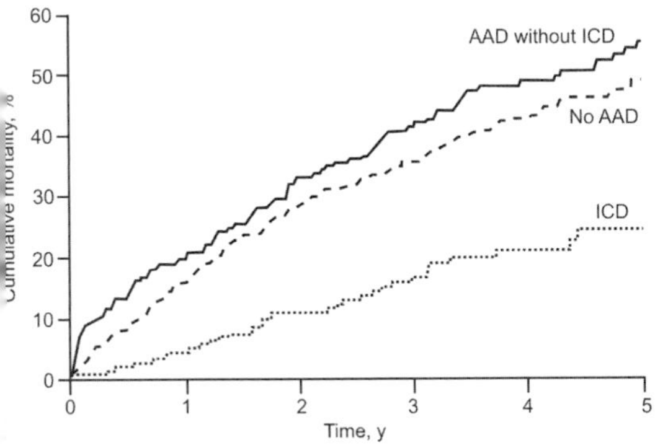

FIGURE 27–3. Mortality rates in the Multicenter Unsustained Tachycardia Trial were significantly lower ($p < 0.001$) in patients who received implantable cardioverter defibrillator (ICD) treatment, whereas patients treated with antiarrhythmic drug (AADs) selected on the basis of programmed ventricular stimulation results did not have decreased mortality compared with patients who received no treatment with antiarrhythmic medication. (Modified from Buxton *et al.*,[20] with permission.)

Thus, it is well established, although somewhat paradoxical, that patients for whom an AAD suppresses VT induction do have a better prognosis, although treatment with the same drug in these patients does not decrease mortality and is probably harmful. The mechanistic explanation for this finding is uncertain, but it is possible that any protective effect of AADs in the MUSTT, CASCADE, and ESVEM studies on the ventricular arrhythmia induced during PVS may be outweighed by the proarrhythmic effects of these AADs. Many of these patients were treated with class I agents, which may be particularly harmful in patients with myocardial ischemia, because they can facilitate phase-2 reentry.[35] One way or the other, the implications for management of high-risk patients are straightforward in the current era of wide availability of ICDs.

Current Role of Programmed Ventricular Stimulation in Risk Stratification after Myocardial Infarction

Although PVS is not useful in the selection of AADs, inducible VT is a well-validated prognostic factor in CAD patients. Along with LVEF and ventricular ectopy, it remains a widely used clinical tool. Specifically, it is used to guide the decision about ICD implantation in the following patients:

1. Patients who have remote MI, an LVEF of 30–35%, and nonsustained VT. If SMVT is induced, then ICD implantation is recommended on the basis of the results of the Multicenter Automatic Defibrillator Implantation Trial (MADIT).[36] For similar patients with an LVEF of less than 30%, ICD implantation would be recommended without the need for PVS, on the basis of the MADIT-II study.[37] Similarly, PVS would often not be considered necessary for patients with stable congestive heart failure despite adequate treatment, based on the results of the Sudden Cardiac Death in Heart Failure Trial (SCD-HeFT).[38] Nevertheless, the absolute survival benefit associated with ICD implantation is substantially higher in the MADIT patients (about 12% per year) than in the MADIT-II or SCD-HeFT populations (about 3% and 1.5% per year, respectively).
2. Patients with clinically significant CAD, an LVEF of 30–40%, and nonsustained VT. On the

basis of the MUSTT data, ICD implantation would usually be indicated in patients with inducible SMVT. As described above, positive PVS increases mortality by about 50% in untreated patients. Again, ICD implantation in the MUSTT study was associated with substantial survival benefit, similar to that of MADIT patients.

3. Patients with prior MI and unexplained syncope. Regardless of LVEF, most physicians would advise ICD placement in patients with SMVT induced by PVS, although this practice is not based on the results of a randomized trial.[27] For patients with LVEF of less than 40% or bundle branch block, the usefulness of PVS is supported by published data.[39,40]

Valvular and Congenital Heart Disease

Little systematic information has been published on the role of PVS in patients who have valvular heart disease. Because of the relatively low risk of SCD after successful valve replacement,[41] these patients rarely undergo PVS unless they present with ventricular arrhythmia. Martinez-Rubio *et al.*[42] retrospectively reported PVS results for 97 patients with valvular disease who presented with VT, VF, or syncope. Although the reproducibility of clinical arrhythmia during PVS was relatively poor (32 of 58 patients presenting with VT), SMVT inducibility was associated with a significantly increased risk of future SCD, VT, or VF ($p < 0.002$). As with CAD, the risk of recurrence of arrhythmia remained high, although use of some AADs suppressed VT inducibility on serial testing.

Ventricular arrhythmias and SCD are important problems in patients who have undergone otherwise successful surgical correction of congenital heart disease. The role of PVS in this population is best characterized in patients after correction of tetralogy of Fallot; SMVT frequently develops in these patients, who are also prone to SCD, because of reentry around the right ventriculotomy scar. The degree of risk correlates with certain clinical parameters, including QRS duration, pulmonary regurgitation, and age.[43] A retrospective multicenter study examined the predictive value of PVS in patients several years after repair of tetralogy of Fallot.[44] Sustained VT (monomorphic or polymorphic) was induced in 87 of 252 (34.5%) patients, and its presence was a major predictor of future ventricular arrhythmia or SCD (relative risk, 5.8; $p < 0.001$); this relationship was strong even after correcting for QRS duration and other established clinical risk factors. However, the question of which patients need PVS after repair of tetralogy of Fallot has yet to be settled. In a retrospective study of a mixed population with congenital heart disease (130 patients; 33% with tetralogy of Fallot), VT induction during PVS also carried a significant risk of clinical VT or SCD; however, the sensitivity was less than perfect.[45]

Idiopathic Dilated Cardiomyopathy

Patients with idiopathic dilated cardiomyopathy (DCM) are at risk for SCD,[38] and SMVT may develop because of reentry. In some patients, SMVT can be reproduced during PVS, and it can sometimes be successfully treated with radiofrequency ablation (RFA)[46–48] (with very high success in the specific case of bundle-branch reentry VT).[49] Despite this fact, results of several smaller studies suggest that the role of PVS in DCM is limited. The rate of SMVT inducibility in patients without clinically documented sustained VT seems quite low (10–15%).[50–52] More importantly, negative results of PVS do not necessarily imply a benign prognosis with respect to SCD.[53,54] Treatment of patients who have DCM with AAD suppressing VT inducibility does not guarantee a low risk of future arrhythmia.[55,56] Whether inducible VT is even associated with a worse prognosis in DCM patients has been contested.[57] Most instances of SCD in patients with DCM may not involve stable reentry around an anatomical obstacle; limited clinical and experimental evidence supports this possibility.[58,59]

Hypertrophic Cardiomyopathy

Sudden death in hypertrophic cardiomyopathy (HCM) is often related to ventricular arrhythmia, and several clinical and noninvasive risk factors have been identified in this population.[60,61] Programmed ventricular stimulation (PVS) can induce VT in about one-third of HCM patients with high-risk clinical characteristics;[62] most VTs are polymorphic, whereas SMVT can be elicited by PVS in less than 10% of patients with inducible VT.[62–64] In one study, VT inducibility orrelated with high-risk clinical characteristics, nd in a kindred with mutation in the gene for α-opomyosin, it was associated with a high degree f LV hypertrophy.[65] Fananapazir *et al.*[66] reported strong association between VT induction (their rotocol included LV stimulation in addition to vo RV sites) and future cardiac arrest or clinical 'T (14 of 82 vs. 3 of 148; $p < 0.002$); prior cardiac rrest was the only other independent predictor f arrhythmic events in their population of 230 ICM patients. Nevertheless, PVS is rarely per-ormed today for risk stratification of HCM atients; instead, LV thickness, nonsustained VT uring Holter monitoring, and historical infor-nation are used widely.[67]

ther Conditions Associated with Ventricular achycardia due to Reentry

eplacement of large areas of myocardium with a car or another nonexcitable tissue can occasion-lly form a substrate for VT reentry in several ncommon cardiac conditions, including arrhyth-nogenic RV dysplasia, idiopathic LV aneurysms,[68] hagasic cardiomyopathy, and cardiac sarcoido-is. These conditions may resemble scarring after rior MI rather than the interstitial fibrosis or nyocardial disarray often associated with DCM or ICM, and PVS can be useful in the identification f patients at risk for VT.

In arrhythmogenic RV dysplasia, replacement f RV (and, less commonly, LV) myocardium ith fatty or fibrous tissue can give rise to SMVT r, occasionally, to primary VF. Although the eproduction of VT (usually due to reentry in the V) and its treatment with RFA[69–71] have been eported, the actual value of PVS for risk stratifi-ation continues to be disputed. Corrado *et al.*[72] eported 132 high-risk patients with arrhyth-nogenic RV dysplasia (10% had prior cardiac rrest and 62% had sustained VT) who underwent VS and ICD implantation. No significant differ-nce was found in the rate of appropriate ICD herapy in patients with inducible versus non-nducible VT, although multiple clinical factors nd LVEF were associated with appropriate treat-nent for rapid VT or VF. At this moment, use of VS as a risk-stratification method in asympto-natic patients with arrhythmogenic RV dysplasia s not supported by clinical data.

Chronic Chagas disease frequently produces myocardial scarring and reentry VT, which can occasionally be targeted with RFA. Induction of VT by PVS in these patients correlates with the presence of sustained VT.[73] In most patients, the VT circuit is located in the inferolateral LV. In a prospective study of 78 patients with cardiac Chagas disease, SMVT was present in 32%; its presence predicted subsequent arrhythmias as well as cardiac death.[74]

Cardiac involvement in sarcoidosis may result in atrioventricular (AV) conduction disturbance or VT. The latter most commonly arises from the LV and may be occasionally associated with an LV aneurysm.[75–77] In the absence of large studies, the relevant medical literature consists of case reports or small series.[78,79] The reentry mechanism of VT related to sarcoidosis has been demonstrated in many cases,[79,80,81] but its induction during PVS may not be a reliable indicator of arrhythmic risk, since the substrate can change depending on disease activity.[79,82]

Primary Electrical Disease

Although ventricular tachyarrhythmias in primary electrical disease (congenital long QT syndrome, Brugada syndrome, catecholaminergic polymorphic VT, short QT syndrome, and idiopathic VF) do not seem to involve reentry around an anatomical obstacle, attempts have been made to use PVS for risk stratification. Bhandari *et al.*[83] performed PVS in 15 high-risk patients with long QT syndrome, including LV stimulation in nine subjects. No sustained VT or VF was induced in any of these patients, although nonsustained VT of six or more beats was observed in 40%. The induction of nonsustained VT had no influence on prognosis.

Sustained polymorphic VT or VF can be induced with three extrastimuli in many patients with Brugada syndrome; the rate of VF induction is significantly higher than in healthy control subjects (14 of 21 vs. 0 of 25), and the RV effective refractory period is shorter.[84] Induction of VF is relatively reproducible in a given patient,[84] but the prognostic value of this phenomenon remains hotly debated. Brugada *et al.*[85] reported a large, prospective, multicenter study of 408 patients with asymptomatic Brugada syndrome who underwent

PVS. Ventricular fibrillation was induced in about 40%, and its inducibility was the strongest predictor of future SCD or resuscitated VF (relative risk, 8.33; $p < 0.001$). It was also reported that inducible VF in a population consisting of both symptomatic and asymptomatic patients predicted future arrhythmic events and was more common in the symptomatic patients.[86,87]

However, this conclusion has been hotly disputed by other groups: Priori *et al.*[88] studied 200 patients with Brugada syndrome, of whom 86 underwent PVS; VF or polymorphic VT was induced in 66%. Although both prior syncope and spontaneous Brugada pattern on a surface electrocardiogram predicted future cardiac arrest, the rate of cardiac arrest did not differ among inducible and noninducible patients. Similar findings were reported by Eckardt *et al.*,[89] who studied 212 symptomatic and asymptomatic patients with Brugada syndrome, of whom 186 underwent PVS; VF was induced in 50%. Although PVS was more often positive in symptomatic patients (63% vs. 39%; $p < 0.001$), the rate of future arrhythmias was extremely low in asymptomatic patients (1 of 123, with mean follow-up of 34 months), and the PVS results were not helpful in risk stratification. In a smaller study, Kanda *et al.*[90] performed PVS in 34 patients with Brugada syndrome, inducing VF in 22. The inducible patients had more pronounced intraventricular conduction disturbance and a higher incidence of late potentials on a signal-averaged electrocardiogram, but had a cardiac event rate similar to that of noninducible patients.

The reason for the difference between the results reported by Brugada *et al.*[85–87] and the other groups is uncertain. The prognostic value of PVS results may have been missed in the negative studies because of their smaller size. However, the rate of arrhythmic events in initially asymptomatic patients reported by Brugada *et al.*[85] is an order of magnitude higher than that reported for one of the negative studies,[89] which may indicate a real difference between patients in different registries.

Limitations and Complications of Programmed Ventricular Stimulation

The current role of PVS in the management of arrhythmic risk in CAD patients is more circumscribed than envisaged in the 1980s, partly becaus[e] of the recognition of the limitations of the substrate and trigger concept. The abnormalities predisposing CAD patients to SCD may be mor[e] dynamic than implied by the concept of a stabl[e] scar allowing reentry. The risk of arrhythmia i[s] modified by ischemia, medications, and autonomic and hemodynamic factors. For example hospitalization for heart failure or for coronar[y] events was a strong risk factor for appropriat[e] ICD discharge in the MADIT-II population.[9] These "nonanatomical" variables probably pla[y] an even more dominant role in cardiac disease[s] characterized by the absence of large scars an[d] functional reentry.

Despite more than 30 years of research, questions remain about certain aspects of PVS technique and interpretation, such as the implication[s] of induced VF, ventricular flutter, or polymorphic VT. Even in a population with mostly stabl[e] CAD, the power of PVS to risk stratify patient[s] is modest (50% relative increase of arrhythmi[c] risk in MUSTT). Programmed ventricular stimulation should be indicated and interprete[d] according to the Bayesian principle. The absolut[e] level of risk associated with inducible VT i[s] highest in patients who have elevated pretest risk as determined by decreased LVEF, ventricula[r] ectopy, nonsustained VT, or congestive hear[t] failure. However, ICD implantation without PV[S] is preferable for patients at highest risk, whos[e] probability of arrhythmic events remains high even after negative PVS.[92] With the increase[d] availability and implantation safety of ICDs, thi[s] population has expanded considerably durin[g] the past decade.

The diagnostic information obtainable by PV[S] should be weighed against the risks of the procedure. Potential complications include bleeding vascular injury, venous thrombosis, and cardia[c] perforation. The limited data in the medical literature suggest that PVS is quite safe. For example in a large series from a single institution, the complication rate was 1.1% in 2524 electrophysiological studies without RFA.[93] The risk was somewha[t] higher in elderly (≥65 years) compared with youn[g] (<65 years) patients (2.2% vs. 0.5%), and systemi[c] disease was identified as another predictor [of] complications. A higher diagnostic yield has bee[n] reported in the elderly population.[94,95] In genera[l] ıost of the reported complications have been ıinor.

‌isk Stratification in Patients with Volff–Parkinson–White Syndrome

'atients with antegrade conduction through an ccessory pathway have a finite but low risk of CD due to VF induced by preexcited AF. In about alf of patients with aborted SCD, VF is the first ıanifestation of WPW syndrome.[96] Although the ossibility of SCD preventable by RFA in a typially young and otherwise healthy patient with VPW is disturbing, available data suggest that ıis is a rare event; in two population-based tudies of WPW patients, none[97] and two[98] cases f SCD were reported during 740 and 1338 years f follow-up, respectively, which suggests an nnual mortality of about 0.1%. No deaths ccurred in patients asymptomatic at diagnosis, ho accounted for about half of both populations. lthough RFA would typically be performed in ıe majority of symptomatic patients, the approriate management of truly asymptomatic patients still being debated. Several attempts have been ıade to risk stratify WPW patients using an invaive electrophysiological study (as well as nonıvasive markers).

Three retrospective reports compared properes of the accessory pathway in patients with rior VF and other WPW patients.[99–101] The shortst RR interval during induced AF appeared to be ıe best discriminator in both studies [180 vs. 40 msec ($p < 0.001$) in the paper by Klein *et al.*[100]]. 'atients with the shortest RR interval of more ıan 260 msec are at low risk,[101] but this cutoff oint has poor positive predictive value. Supression of accessory pathway conduction by ıtravenous procainamide can be assessed noninasively.[99,101–104] However, in at least one report, 0 mg/kg of intravenous procainamide suppressed ntegrade pathway conduction in some patients ith a history of VF, which falsely indicated a low isk.[101] Similar considerations apply to the loss of reexcitation during sinus tachycardia induced y exercise.[103,105]

In summary, the use of invasive electrophysioogical study for assessment of SCD risk in WPW atients is limited, mainly because of the current high success rate of RFA, which also has a low rate of complications. Nearly all adult symptomatic patients are offered RFA regardless of SCD risk. For the truly asymptomatic patient, the risk–benefit ratio of RFA is uncertain, but both the risks and the benefits are likely to be of small magnitude.

HV Interval and Infrahisian Block as Risk Factors for Complete Heart Block and Sudden Death

Prolongation of the HV interval is an indicator of disease of the His–Purkinje system. Scheinman *et al.*[106] reported that among patients with bundle branch block and symptoms of possible arrhythmias, the HV interval was significantly longer in patients with documented heart block as the cause of their symptoms. In a subsequent prospective study of 121 patients with conduction disturbance on a surface electrocardiogram and a fairly frequent history of syncope (36%), an HV interval of more than 70 msec was associated with a higher rate of progression to second- or third-degree heart block (21% over 18 months) compared with patients with an HV interval of less than 70 msec (1.3%; $p < 0.001$). Rates of sudden death, total mortality, and heart failure were also higher in the former group.[107] However, McAnulty *et al.*[108] reported a low incidence of new complete heart block (about 1% per year) in a large prospective study of 554 patients who had bifascicular block. There was no significant difference between the patients with or without prolongation of the HV interval. In this study, syncope was a better predictor than HV interval of the development of complete heart block. Age and heart failure, but not HV interval, were associated with total mortality. In another large prospective study of patients with bifascicular block (517 patients; mean follow-up, 3.4 years), 39% of patients had an HV interval of more than 55 msec. These patients had a significantly higher incidence of AV block during follow-up than patients with a normal HV interval (28% vs. 12% over 7 years; $p < 0.001$).[109] Again, total mortality and the sudden death rate were both higher in patients with prolongation of the HV interval. However, these findings may not be related to the increased rate of bradycardic arrest due to AV block, because these patients also had a higher rate of heart failure, angina, and structural heart disease. It is likely that the HV interval is to some degree a marker of the severity of heart disease.

Nonfunctional infrahisian block during atrial pacing occurs less frequently than prolongation of the HV interval (about 3% of patients with bifascicular block), although some patients with this phenomenon have a normal HV interval.[108,110] It appears to be associated with a high risk of future AV block, especially in symptomatic patients (about 50% in a 5-year period).[110,111]

Some patients with a normal HV interval may, in fact, have conduction system disease, which is manifested by a subsequently documented high-grade infrahisian AV block. In some of these patients, abnormal HV conduction may be elicited by administration of a sodium channel blocker (typically procainamide at an intravenous dose of 10 mg/kg). Infrahisian AV block or marked HV interval prolongation may develop, and is considered an abnormal response.[112,113] However, little prognostic information is available for these patients. This phenomenon occurs rarely (about 3%) in patients with a normal HV interval.[114]

Currently, an electrophysiological study would rarely be indicated for the sole reason of measuring the HV interval, given the relatively low positive predictive value of prolongation of the HV interval for high-grade AV block. The negative predictive value is also less than ideal in patients with bundle branch block and syncope.[115] However, marked HV interval prolongation or infrahisian block during atrial pacing may justify pacemaker placement in a patient with syncope but no other abnormality.[27] Also, measurement of the HV interval may be of value in some patients who have hereditary neuromuscular diseases and a high pretest probability of conduction system disease.[116]

References

1. Wellens HJ, Schuilenburg RM, Durrer D. Electrical stimulation of the heart in patients with ventricular tachycardia. *Circulation* 1972;46:216–226.
2. Josephson, ME. *Clinical Cardiac Electrophysiology: Techniques and Interpretations*, 2nd ed. Philadelphia: Lea & Febiger, 1993.
3. Lin HT, Mann DE, Luck JC, *et al.* Prospective comparison of right and left ventricular stimulatio for induction of sustained ventricular tachycardi *Am J Cardiol* 1987;59:559–563.
4. Michelson EL, Spielman SR, Greenspan AM, *et a* Electrophysiologic study of the left ventricle: Indications and safety. *Chest* 1979;75:592–596.
5. Buxton AE, Fisher JD, Josephson ME, *et al.* Prevention of sudden death in patients with coronar artery disease: The Multicenter Unsustaine Tachycardia Trial (MUSTT). *Prog Cardiovasc D* 1993;36:215–226.
6. Hummel JD, Strickberger SA, Daoud E, *et a* Results and efficiency of programmed ventricula stimulation with four extrastimuli compared wit one, two, and three extrastimuli. *Circulation* 199 90:2827–2832.
7. Denker S, Lehmann MH, Mahmud R, *et al.* Facilitation of macroreentry within the His-Purkinj system with abrupt changes in cycle length. *Circulation* 1984;69:26–32.
8. Niebauer M, Daoud E, Goyal R, *et al.* Use of isoproterenol during programmed ventricular stimulation in patients with coronary artery diseas and nonsustained ventricular tachycardia. *Am Heart J* 1996;131:516–518.
9. Morady F, DiCarlo L, xWinston S, *et al.* A prospective comparison of triple extrastimuli an left ventricular stimulation in studies of ventricular tachycardia induction. *Circulation* 1984;7 52–57.
10. Morady F, DiCarlo LA Jr, Baerman JM, *et al.* Comparison of coupling intervals that induce clinica and nonclinical forms of ventricular tachycardi during programmed stimulation. *Am J Cardi* 1986;57:1269–1273.
11. Brugada P, Wellens HJ. Comparison in the sam patient of two programmed ventricular stimulation protocols to induce ventricular tachycardi *Am J Cardiol* 1985;55:380–383.
12. Kennedy EE, Rosenfeld LE, McPherson CA, *et a* Mechanisms and relevance of arrhythmias induce by high-current programmed ventricular stimulation. *Am J Cardiol* 1986;57:598–603.
13. Weissberg PL, Broughton A, Harper RW, *et a* Induction of ventricular arrhythmias by programmed ventricular stimulation: A prospectiv study on the effects of stimulation current o arrhythmia induction. *Br Heart J* 1987;58:489 494.
14. de Buitleir M, Morady F, DiCarlo LA Jr, *et a* Immediate reproducibility of clinical and nonclinical forms of induced ventricular tachycardi *Am J Cardiol* 1986;58:279–282.

15. Lombardi F, Stein J, Podrid PJ, *et al.* Daily reproducibility of electrophysiologic test results in malignant ventricular arrhythmia. *Am J Cardiol* 1986;57:96–101.
16. McPherson CA, Rosenfeld LE, Batsford WP. Day-to-day reproducibility of responses to right ventricular programmed electrical stimulation: Implications for serial drug testing. *Am J Cardiol* 1985;55:689–695.
17. Rosenbaum MS, Wilber DJ, Finkelstein D, *et al.* Immediate reproducibility of electrically induced sustained monomorphic ventricular tachycardia before and during antiarrhythmic therapy. *J Am Coll Cardiol* 1991;17:133–138.
18. Wilber DJ, Garan H, Finkelstein D, *et al.* Out-of-hospital cardiac arrest: Use of electrophysiologic testing in the prediction of long-term outcome. *N Engl J Med* 1988;318:19–24.
19. Steinbeck G, Andresen D, Bach P, *et al.* A comparison of electrophysiologically guided antiarrhythmic drug therapy with beta-blocker therapy in patients with symptomatic, sustained ventricular tachyarrhythmias. *N Engl J Med* 1992; 327:987–992.
20. Buxton AE, Lee KL, Fisher JD, *et al.*, Multicenter Unsustained Tachycardia Trial Investigators. A randomized study of the prevention of sudden death in patients with coronary artery disease. *N Engl J Med* 1999;341:1882–1890.
21. Buxton AE, Lee KL, DiCarlo L, *et al.* Multicenter Unsustained Tachycardia Trial Investigators. Electrophysiologic testing to identify patients with coronary artery disease who are at risk for sudden death. *N Engl J Med* 2000;342:1937–1945.
22. Daubert JP, Zareba W, Hall WJ, *et al.* Predictive value of ventricular arrhythmia inducibility for subsequent ventricular tachycardia or ventricular fibrillation in Multicenter Automatic Defibrillator Implantation Trial (MADIT) II patients. *J Am Coll Cardiol* 2006;47:98–107.
23. Bhandari AK, Widerhorn J, Sager PT, *et al.* Prognostic significance of programmed ventricular stimulation in patients surviving complicated acute myocardial infarction: A prospective study. *Am Heart J* 1992;124:87–96.
24. Mittal S, Hao SC, Iwai S, *et al.* Significance of inducible ventricular fibrillation in patients with coronary artery disease and unexplained syncope. *J Am Coll Cardiol* 2001;38:371–376.
25. Bourke JP, Young AA, Richards DA, *et al.* Reduction in incidence of inducible ventricular tachycardia after myocardial infarction by treatment with streptokinase during infarct evolution. *J Am Coll Cardiol* 1990;16:1703–1710.
26. Link MS, Saeed M, Gupta N, *et al.* Inducible ventricular flutter and fibrillation predict for arrhythmia occurrence in coronary artery disease patients presenting with syncope of unknown origin. *J Cardiovasc Electrophysiol* 2002;13:1103–1108.
27. Gregoratos G, Abrams J, Epstein AE, *et al.* ACC/AHA/NASPE 2002 Guideline Update for Implantation of Cardiac Pacemakers and Antiarrhythmia Devices: Summary article. A report of the American College of Cardiology/American Heart Association Task Force on Practice Guidelines (ACC/AHA/NASPE Committee to Update the 1998 Pacemaker Guidelines). *J Am Coll Cardiol* 2002;40:1703–1719.
28. Richards DA, Cody DV, Denniss AR, *et al.* Ventricular electrical instability: A predictor of death after myocardial infarction. *Am J Cardiol* 1983;51:75–80.
29. Bhandari AK, Au PK, Rose JS, *et al.* Decline in inducibility of sustained ventricular tachycardia from two to twenty weeks after acute myocardial infarction. *Am J Cardiol* 1987;59:284–290.
30. Nogami A, Aonuma K, Takahashi A, *et al.* Usefulness of early versus late programmed ventricular stimulation in acute myocardial infarction. *Am J Cardiol* 1991;68:13–20.
31. Echt DS, Liebson PR, Mitchell LB, *et al.* Mortality and morbidity in patients receiving encainide, flecainide, or placebo: The Cardiac Arrhythmia Suppression Trial. *N Engl J Med* 1991;324:781–788.
32. The Cardiac Arrhythmia Suppression Trial II Investigators. Effect of the antiarrhythmic agent moricizine on survival after myocardial infarction. *N Engl J Med* 1992;327:227–233.
33. Mason JW, Electrophysiologic Study Versus Electrocardiographic Monitoring Investigators. A comparison of electrophysiologic testing with Holter monitoring to predict antiarrhythmic-drug efficacy for ventricular tachyarrhythmias. *N Engl J Med* 1993;329:445–451.
34. The CASCADE Investigators. Randomized antiarrhythmic drug therapy in survivors of cardiac arrest (the CASCADE Study). *Am J Cardiol* 1993; 72:280–287.
35. Krishnan SC, Antzelevitch C. Flecainide-induced arrhythmia in canine ventricular epicardium: Phase 2 reentry? *Circulation* 1993;87:562–572.
36. Moss AJ, Hall WJ, Cannom DS, *et al.*, Multicenter Automatic Defibrillator Implantation Trial Investigators. Improved survival with an implanted defibrillator in patients with coronary disease at high risk for ventricular arrhythmia. *N Engl J Med* 1996;335:1933–1940.

37. Moss AJ, Zareba W, Hall WJ, *et al.* Prophylactic implantation of a defibrillator in patients with myocardial infarction and reduced ejection fraction. *N Engl J Med* 2002;346:877–883.
38. Bardy GH, Lee KL, Mark DB, *et al.* Amiodarone or an implantable cardioverter-defibrillator for congestive heart failure. *N Engl J Med* 2005;352:225–237.
39. Brembilla-Perrot B, Suty-Selton C, Houriez P, *et al.* Value of non-invasive and invasive studies in patients with bundle branch block, syncope and history of myocardial infarction. *Europace* 2001; 3:187–194.
40. Brembilla-Perrot B, Suty-Selton C, Alla F, *et al.* Risk factors for cardiac mortality in cases of syncope with previous history of myocardial infarction [French]. *Arch Mal Coeur Vaiss* 2003; 96:1181–1186.
41. Gohlke-Barwolf C, Peters K, Petersen J, *et al.* Influence of aortic valve replacement on sudden death in patients with pure aortic stenosis. *Eur Heart J* 1988;9(Suppl. E):139–141.
42. Martinez-Rubio A, Schwammenthal Y, Schwammenthal E, *et al.* Patients with valvular heart disease presenting with sustained ventricular tachyarrhythmias or syncope: Results of programmed ventricular stimulation and long-term follow-up. *Circulation* 1997;96:500–508.
43. Gatzoulis MA, Balaji S, Webber SA, *et al.* Risk factors for arrhythmia and sudden cardiac death late after repair of tetralogy of Fallot: A multicentre study. *Lancet* 2000;356:975–981.
44. Khairy P, Landzberg MJ, Gatzoulis MA, *et al.* Value of programmed ventricular stimulation after tetralogy of Fallot repair: A multicenter study. *Circulation* 2004;109:1994–2000.
45. Alexander ME, Walsh EP, Saul JP, *et al.* Value of programmed ventricular stimulation in patients with congenital heart disease. *J Cardiovasc Electrophysiol* 1999;10:1033–1044.
46. Soejima K, Stevenson WG, Sapp JL, *et al.* Endocardial and epicardial radiofrequency ablation of ventricular tachycardia associated with dilated cardiomyopathy: The importance of low-voltage scars. *J Am Coll Cardiol* 2004;43:1834–1842.
47. Hsia HH, Callans DJ, Marchlinski FE. Characterization of endocardial electrophysiological substrate in patients with nonischemic cardiomyopathy and monomorphic ventricular tachycardia. *Circulation* 2003;108:704–710.
48. Hsia HH, Marchlinski FE. Characterization of the electroanatomic substrate for monomorphic ventricular tachycardia in patients with nonischemic cardiomyopathy. *Pacing Clin Electrophysiol* 2002; 25:1114–1127.
49. Caceres J, Jazayeri M, McKinnie J, *et al.* Sustained bundle branch reentry as a mechanism of clinical tachycardia. *Circulation* 1989;79:256–270.
50. Gonska BD, Bethge KP, Kreuzer H. Programmed ventricular stimulation in coronary artery disease and dilated cardiomyopathy: Influence of the underlying heart disease on the results of electrophysiologic testing. *Clin Cardiol* 1987;10:294–304.
51. Turitto G, Ahuja RK, Caref EB, *et al.* Risk stratification for arrhythmic events in patients with nonischemic dilated cardiomyopathy and nonsustained ventricular tachycardia: Role of programmed ventricular stimulation and the signal-averaged electrocardiogram. *J Am Coll Cardiol* 1994;24:1523–1528.
52. Becker R, Haass M, Ick D, *et al.* Role of nonsustained ventricular tachycardia and programmed ventricular stimulation for risk stratification in patients with idiopathic dilated cardiomyopathy. *Basic Res Cardiol* 2003;98:259–266.
53. Grimm W, Hoffmann J, Menz V, *et al.* Programmed ventricular stimulation for arrhythmia risk prediction in patients with idiopathic dilated cardiomyopathy and nonsustained ventricular tachycardia. *J Am Coll Cardiol* 1998;32:739–745.
54. Brilakis ES, Shen WK, Hammill SC, *et al.* Role of programmed ventricular stimulation and implantable cardioverter defibrillators in patients with idiopathic dilated cardiomyopathy and syncope. *Pacing Clin Electrophysiol* 2001;24:1623–1630.
55. Milner PG, Dimarco JP, Lerman BB. Electrophysiological evaluation of sustained ventricular tachyarrhythmias in idiopathic dilated cardiomyopathy. *Pacing Clin Electrophysiol* 1988;11:562–568.
56. Poll DS, Marchlinski FE, Buxton AE, *et al.* Sustained ventricular tachycardia in patients with idiopathic dilated cardiomyopathy: Electrophysiologic testing and lack of response to antiarrhythmic drug therapy. *Circulation* 1984;70:451–456.
57. Turitto G, Ahuja RK, Bekheit S, *et al.* Incidence and prediction of induced ventricular tachyarrhythmias in idiopathic dilated cardiomyopathy. *Am J Cardiol* 1994;73:770–773.
58. Pogwizd SM, McKenzie JP, Cain ME. Mechanisms underlying spontaneous and induced ventricular arrhythmias in patients with idiopathic dilated cardiomyopathy. *Circulation* 1998;98:2404–2414.
59. Pogwizd SM. Nonreentrant mechanisms underlying spontaneous ventricular arrhythmias in a model of nonischemic heart failure in rabbits. *Circulation* 1995;92:1034–1048.
60. Elliott PM, Poloniecki J, Dickie S, *et al.* Sudden death in hypertrophic cardiomyopathy: Identifi

cation of high risk patients. *J Am Coll Cardiol* 2000;36:2212–2218.
61. Maron BJ, Shen WK, Link MS, *et al.* Efficacy of implantable cardioverter-defibrillators for the prevention of sudden death in patients with hypertrophic cardiomyopathy. *N Engl J Med* 2000; 342:365–373.
62. Fananapazir L, Tracy CM, Leon MB, *et al.* Electrophysiologic abnormalities in patients with hypertrophic cardiomyopathy: A consecutive analysis in 155 patients. *Circulation* 1989;80:1259–1268.
63. Watson RM, Schwartz JL, Maron BJ, *et al.* Inducible polymorphic ventricular tachycardia and ventricular fibrillation in a subgroup of patients with hypertrophic cardiomyopathy at high risk for sudden death. *J Am Coll Cardiol* 1987;10:761–774.
64. Zhu DW, Sun H, Hill R, *et al.* The value of electrophysiology study and prophylactic implantation of cardioverter defibrillator in patients with hypertrophic cardiomyopathy. *Pacing Clin Electrophysiol* 1998;21:299–302.
65. Hedman A, Hartikainen J, Vanninen E, *et al.* Inducibility of life-threatening ventricular arrhythmias is related to maximum left ventricular thickness and clinical markers of sudden cardiac death in patients with hypertrophic cardiomyopathy attributable to the Asp175Asn mutation in the alpha-tropomyosin gene. *J Mol Cell Cardiol* 2004; 36:91–99.
66. Fananapazir L, Chang AC, Epstein SE, *et al.* Prognostic determinants in hypertrophic cardiomyopathy: Prospective evaluation of a therapeutic strategy based on clinical, Holter, hemodynamic, and electrophysiological findings. *Circulation* 1992;86:730–740.
67. Behr ER, Elliott P, McKenna WJ. Role of invasive EP testing in the evaluation and management of hypertrophic cardiomyopathy. *Card Electrophysiol Rev* 2002;6:482–486.
68. Yamashiro S, Kuniyoshi Y, Miyagi K, *et al.* Two cases of ventricular tachycardia with congenital left ventricular malformation in an adult. *Ann Thorac Cardiovasc Surg* 2004;10:42–46.
69. Marchlinski FE, Zado E, Dixit S, *et al.* Electroanatomic substrate and outcome of catheter ablative therapy for ventricular tachycardia in setting of right ventricular cardiomyopathy. *Circulation* 2004;110:2293–2298.
70. Pezawas T, Stix G, Kastner J, *et al.* Ventricular tachycardia in arrhythmogenic right ventricular dysplasia/cardiomyopathy: Clinical presentation, risk stratification and results of long-term follow-up. *Int J Cardiol* 2006;107:360–368.
71. Ellison KE, Friedman PL, Ganz LI, *et al.* Entrainment mapping and radiofrequency catheter ablation of ventricular tachycardia in right ventricular dysplasia. *J Am Coll Cardiol* 1998;32:724–728.
72. Corrado D, Leoni L, Link MS, *et al.* Implantable cardioverter-defibrillator therapy for prevention of sudden death in patients with arrhythmogenic right ventricular cardiomyopathy/dysplasia. *Circulation* 2003;108:3084–3091.
73. Sarabanda AV, Sosa E, Simoes MV, *et al.* Ventricular tachycardia in Chagas' disease: A comparison of clinical, angiographic, electrophysiologic and myocardial perfusion disturbances between patients presenting with either sustained or nonsustained forms. *Int J Cardiol* 2005;102: 9–19.
74. Silva RM, Tavora MZ, Gondim FA, *et al.* Predictive value of clinical and electrophysiological variables in patients with chronic chagasic cardiomyopathy and nonsustained ventricular tachycardia. *Arq Bras Cardiol* 2000;75:33–47.
75. Toda G, Iliev, II, Kawahara F, *et al.* Left ventricular aneurysm without coronary artery disease, incidence and clinical features: Clinical analysis of 11 cases. *Intern Med* 2000;39:531–536.
76. Jain A, Starek PJ, Delany DL. Ventricular tachycardia and ventricular aneurysm due to unrecognized sarcoidosis. *Clin Cardiol* 1990;13:738–740.
77. Grollier G, Galateau F, Scanu P, *et al.* Cardiac sarcoidosis responsible for localized left ventricular ectasia and refractory ventricular tachycardia: Anatomoclinical study [French]. *Arch Mal Coeur Vaiss* 1990;83:561–564.
78. Furushima H, Chinushi M, Sugiura H, *et al.* Ventricular tachyarrhythmia associated with cardiac sarcoidosis: Its mechanisms and outcome. *Clin Cardiol* 2004;27:217–222.
79. Aizer A, Stern EH, Gomes JA, *et al.* Usefulness of programmed ventricular stimulation in predicting future arrhythmic events in patients with cardiac sarcoidosis. *Am J Cardiol* 2005;96:276–282.
80. Noda T, Suyama K, Shimizu W, *et al.* Ventricular tachycardia with figure eight pattern originating from the right ventricle in a patient with cardiac sarcoidosis. *Pacing Clin Electrophysiol* 2004;27: 561–562.
81. Chinushi M, Mezaki T, Aoki Y, *et al.* Demonstration of transient entrainment in monomorphic sustained ventricular tachycardia associated with cardiac sarcoidosis. *Jpn Circ J* 2000;64:635–637.
82. Mezaki T, Chinushi M, Washizuka T, *et al.* Discrepancy between inducibility of ventricular tachycardia and activity of cardiac sarcoidosis: Requirement of defibrillator implantation for the

inactive stage of cardiac sarcoidosis. *Intern Med* 2001;40:731–735.
83. Bhandari AK, Shapiro WA, Morady F, *et al.* Electrophysiologic testing in patients with the long QT syndrome. *Circulation* 1985;71:63–71.
84. Gasparini M, Priori SG, Mantica M, *et al.* Programmed electrical stimulation in Brugada syndrome: How reproducible are the results? *J Cardiovasc Electrophysiol* 2002;13:880–887.
85. Brugada J, Brugada R, Brugada P. Determinants of sudden cardiac death in individuals with the electrocardiographic pattern of Brugada syndrome and no previous cardiac arrest. *Circulation* 2003; 108:3092–3096.
86. Brugada P, Geelen P, Brugada R, *et al.* Prognostic value of electrophysiologic investigations in Brugada syndrome. *J Cardiovasc Electrophysiol* 2001;12:1004–1007.
87. Brugada P, Brugada R, Mont L, *et al.* Natural history of Brugada syndrome: The prognostic value of programmed electrical stimulation of the heart. *J Cardiovasc Electrophysiol* 2003;14:455–457.
88. Priori SG, Napolitano C, Gasparini M, *et al.* Natural history of Brugada syndrome: Insights for risk stratification and management. *Circulation* 2002;105:1342–1347.
89. Eckardt L, Probst V, Smits JP, *et al.* Long-term prognosis of individuals with right precordial ST-segment-elevation Brugada syndrome. *Circulation* 2005;111:257–263.
90. Kanda M, Shimizu W, Matsuo K, *et al.* Electrophysiologic characteristics and implications of induced ventricular fibrillation in symptomatic patients with Brugada syndrome. *J Am Coll Cardiol* 2002;39:1799–1805.
91. Singh JP, Hall WJ, McNitt S, *et al.* Factors influencing appropriate firing of the implanted defibrillator for ventricular tachycardia/fibrillation: Findings from the Multicenter Automatic Defibrillator Implantation Trial II (MADIT-II). *J Am Coll Cardiol* 2005;46:1712–1720.
92. Buxton AE, Lee KL, Hafley GE, *et al.* Relation of ejection fraction and inducible ventricular tachycardia to mode of death in patients with coronary artery disease: An analysis of patients enrolled in the multicenter unsustained tachycardia trial. *Circulation* 2002;106:2466–2472.
93. Chen SA, Chiang CE, Tai CT, *et al.* Complications of diagnostic electrophysiologic studies and radiofrequency catheter ablation in patients with tachyarrhythmias: An eight-year survey of 3,966 consecutive procedures in a tertiary referral center. *Am J Cardiol* 1996;77:41–46.
94. Wagshal AB, Schuger CD, Habbal B, *et al.* Invasiv electrophysiologic evaluation in octogenarians: I age a limiting factor? *Am Heart J* 1993;126:1142 1146.
95. Voss F, Lu J, Schreiner KD, *et al.* Evaluation c syncope in geriatric patients: Normal values complications and outcome of invasive electro physiological study [German]. *Z Kardiol* 2000;89 1026–1031.
96. Timmermans C, Smeets JL, Rodriguez LM, *et a.* Aborted sudden death in the Wolff-Parkinson White syndrome. *Am J Cardiol* 1995;76:492 494.
97. Goudevenos JA, Katsouras CS, Graekas G, *et a.* Ventricular pre-excitation in the general population: A study on the mode of presentation an clinical course. *Heart* 2000;83:29–34.
98. Munger TM, Packer DL, Hammill SC, *et a.* A population study of the natural history o Wolff-Parkinson-White syndrome in Olmste County, Minnesota, 1953–1989. *Circulation* 1993 87:866–873.
99. Attoyan C, Haissaguerre M, Dartigues JF, *et a.* Ventricular fibrillation in Wolff-Parkinson-Whit syndrome: Predictive factors [French]. *Arch Ma Coeur Vaiss* 1994;87:889–897.
100. Klein GJ, Bashore TM, Sellers TD, *et al.* Ventricular fibrillation in the Wolff-Parkinson-White syndrome. *N Engl J Med* 1979;301:1080–1085.
101. Fananapazir L, Packer DL, German LD, *et al.* Procainamide infusion test: Inability to identif patients with Wolff-Parkinson-White syndrom who are potentially at risk of sudden death. *Circulation* 1988;77:1291–1296.
102. Boahene KA, Klein GJ, Sharma AD, *et al.* Valu of a revised procainamide test in the Wolff Parkinson-White syndrome. *Am J Cardiol* 1990 65:195–200.
103. Gaita F, Giustetto C, Riccardi R, *et al.* Stress an pharmacologic tests as methods to identif patients with Wolff-Parkinson-White syndrom at risk of sudden death. *Am J Cardiol* 1989;64 487–490.
104. Wellens HJ, Braat S, Brugada P, *et al.* Use of procainamide in patients with the Wolff-Parkinson White syndrome to disclose a short refractor period of the accessory pathway. *Am J Cardio* 1982;50:1087–1089.
105. Medeiros A, Iturralde P, Guevara M, *et al.* Sudde death in intermittent Wolff Parkinson White syndrome [Spanish]. *Arch Cardiol Mex* 2001;71 59–65.
106. Scheinman M, Weiss A, Kunkel F. His bundl recordings in patients with bundle branch bloc

and transient neurologic symptoms. *Circulation* 1973;48:322–330.

07. Scheinman MM, Peters RW, Modin G, *et al.* Prognostic value of infranodal conduction time in patients with chronic bundle branch block. *Circulation* 1977;56:240–244.

08. McAnulty JH, Rahimtoola SH, Murphy E, *et al.* Natural history of "high-risk" bundle-branch block: Final report of a prospective study. *N Engl J Med* 1982;307:137–143.

09. Dhingra RC, Palileo E, Strasberg B, *et al.* Significance of the HV interval in 517 patients with chronic bifascicular block. *Circulation* 1981;64:1265–1271.

10. Dhingra RC, Wyndham C, Bauernfeind R, *et al.* Significance of block distal to the His bundle induced by atrial pacing in patients with chronic bifascicular block. *Circulation* 1979;60:1455–1464.

11. Petrac D, Radic B, Birtic K, *et al.* Prospective evaluation of infrahisal second-degree AV block induced by atrial pacing in the presence of chronic bundle branch block and syncope. *Pacing Clin Electrophysiol* 1996;19:784–792.

112. Twidale N, Heddle WF, Ayres BF, *et al.* Clinical implications of electrophysiology study findings in patients with chronic bifascicular block and syncope. *Aust N Z J Med* 1988;18:841–847.

113. Twidale N, Heddle WF, Tonkin AM. Procainamide administration during electrophysiology study: Utility as a provocative test for intermittent atrioventricular block. *Pacing Clin Electrophysiol* 1988;11:1388–1397.

114. Girard SE, Munger TM, Hammill SC, *et al.* The effect of intravenous procainamide on the HV interval at electrophysiologic study. *J Interv Card Electrophysiol* 1999;3:129–137.

115. Brignole M, Menozzi C, Moya A, *et al.* Mechanism of syncope in patients with bundle branch block and negative electrophysiological test. *Circulation* 2001;104:2045–2050.

116. Lazarus A, Varin J, Babuty D, *et al.* Long-term follow-up of arrhythmias in patients with myotonic dystrophy treated by pacing: A multicenter diagnostic pacemaker study. *J Am Coll Cardiol* 2002;40:1645–1652.

28
Provocative Testing in Inherited Arrhythmias

Wataru Shimizu and Michael J. Ackerman

Introduction

Heritable channelopathies that include congenital long QT syndrome (LQTS), Brugada syndrome (BrS), and catecholaminergic polymorphic ventricular tachycardia (CPVT) affect an estimated 1 in 2000 persons, may present with syncope or sudden cardiac death, and often elude detection by standard 12-lead electrocardiography (ECG). In LQTS, an estimated 40% of genetically affected subjects have "concealed" LQTS with a normal or borderline heart rate corrected QT interval (QTc) at rest. A significant proportion of patients with BrS has concealed BrS with no evidence of a type 1 Brugada electrocardiographic pattern at rest. Every patient with CPVT has a normal resting ECG. Provocative testing with catecholamines and pharmacological testing with sodium channel blockers are critical diagnostic tests in the evaluation of these channelopathies and can help unmask LQTS, BrS, and CPVT in their concealed state. The role of these provocative tests in the evaluation of inherited arrhythmia syndromes will be reviewed in this chapter.

Congenital Long QT Syndrome

Congenital LQTS is characterized by QT prolongation in the electrocardiogram (ECG) and its trademark dysrhythmia of polymorphic ventricular tachycardia known as torsade de pointes (TdP).[1] The clinical diagnosis of LQTS is mainly based on the resting QTc, cardiac events such as syncope, aborted cardiac arrest, and sudden cardiac death, and a family history of apparent LQTS.[2] However, the electrocardiographic diagnosis at baseline has long been expected to miss some patients affected by congenital LQTS (so called concealed LQTS) as evidenced by syncopal events occurring among family members with a "normal" QT interval.[3] Since 1995, when the first two genes responsible for LQTS were identified, molecular genetic studies have revealed a total of 10 forms of congenital LQTS caused predominantly by cardiac channel mutations or mutations involving key β or auxiliary subunits.[4] Among the 10 genetic subtypes, LQT1, LQT2, and LQT3 constitute the majority of genotyped LQTS and approximately 75% of all LQTS.[5] With these molecular illuminations, this entity of concealed or low pentrant LQTS has been proved genetically. Vincent *et al.* reported that 5 (6%) of 82 mutation carriers from three LQT1 families had a normal QT interval.[6] Priori *et al.* conducted molecular screening in nine families with apparently sporadic cases of LQTS, demonstrating a very low penetrance (38%, 9/24 patients).[7] Swan and co-workers reported that the sensitivity and specificity for identifying genotype-positive patients were 53 and 100%, respectively, in an LQT1 family with a specific *KCNQ1* mutation (D188N).[8] More recently, a large study of genotyped LQTS by Priori *et al.* showed that the percentage of genetically affected patients with a normal QTc was significantly higher in the LQT1 (36%) than in the LQT2 (19%) or the LQT3 (10%) syndromes.[9] Overall, these findings strongly suggest the need for novel tools to unveil concealed mutation carriers of LQTS, especially those with type 1 LQTS (LQT1). The identification of patients with concealed LQTS affords the opportunity to initiate potentially life-saving pharmacotherapies and healthstyle modifications.

Many but not all patients with congenital LQTS suffer from cardiac events such as syncope and/or sudden cardiac death during physical exercise or mental stress. Therefore, provocative testing using catecholamine infusion or exercise has long been used to unmask concealed forms of congenital LQTS, before genetic screening became available.[10]

The Epinephrine QT Stress Test in Long QT Syndrome

Infusion of isoproterenol, a β-adrenergic agonist, or epinephrine, an α + β-adrenergic agonist, has been reported to be useful as a provocative test in LQTS more than two decades ago.[10] The heart rate is usually increased to more than 100 beats/min by isoproterenol, especially by the use of a bolus injection, which often makes it difficult to measure the QT interval precisely due to an overlap of the next P wave on the terminal portion of the T wave. Prior to the discovery of the distinct genetic subtypes of LQTS, the responses to either epinephrine or isoproterenol were extremely heterogeneous and were deemed impossible to interpret; as a result, epinephrine QT stress testing disappeared from the diagnostic work-up of LQTS. Now, however, the heterogeneous response is understood to stem from the underlying genetic heterogeneity and the gene-specific responses to epinephrine can be exploited to expose different types of LQTS in its otherwise concealed state, particularly type 1 LQTS (LQT1). Although isoproterenol is still used occasionally, recent major insights have been gleaned from using epinephrine and are reviewed in more detail below. In contrast to provocation studies using catecholamines, Viskin and colleagues have shown that sudden heart rate oscillations precipitated by intravenous administration of adenosine may expose some patients with concealed LQTS, although genotype-specific responses have not been demonstrated.[11] Compared to controls, patients with LQTS exhibited an exaggerated increase in the QT interval during adenosine-induced bradycardia.

The two major protocols developed for epinephrine QT stress testing include the escalating-dose protocol by Ackerman's group (the Mayo protocol)[12] and the bolus injection followed by brief continuous infusion by Shimizu's group (Shimizu protocol).[13] Both protocols are extremely useful and safe, and overall are well tolerated. Each protocol has some advantages and disadvantages with respect to the other.

Incremental, Escalating Epinephrine Infusion (Mayo Protocol)

Ackerman and co-workers have used a 25-min incremental, escalating infusion protocol (0.025–0.3 μg/kg/min) in the LQT1, LQT2, and LQT3 patients and in the genotyped-negative patients (Figure 28–1A).[12,14,15] With epinephrine infusion at a low dose of ≤0.1 μg/kg/min, the median change of the QT interval was 78 msec in LQT1, −4 msec in LQT2, −58 msec in LQT3, and −23 msec in the genotype-negative patients (Figure 28–1B). They found a paradoxic QT prolongation, defined as a 30-msec increase in the QT (not QTc) interval during low-dose epinephrine infusion, specific in the LQT1 patients (92%), but not in the LQT2 (13%), the LQT3 (0%), and the genotype-negative patients (18%). The paradoxic QT prolongation had a sensitivity of 92.5%, specificity of 86%, positive predictive value of 76%, and negative predictive value of 96% for LQT1 vs. non-LQT1 status (Table 28–1), and provides a presumptive, pregenetic clinical diagnosis of type 1 LQTS (LQT1).

The major advantages of this escalating infusion protocol are better patient tolerance and a lower incidence of false-positive responses. On the other hand, this protocol seems less effective in exposing patients with LQT2 compared to the bolus protocol by Shimizu *et al.* described below. However, this disadvantage is reported to be partially overcome by focusing on the change of T wave morphology during low-dose epinephrine infusion. Khositseth *et al.* reported that the epinephrine-induced notched T wave was more indicative of LQT2 status.[15]

Bolus Injection followed by Brief Continuous Infusion (Shimizu Protocol)

The bolus protocol by Shimizu and co-workers was developed on the basis of a differential

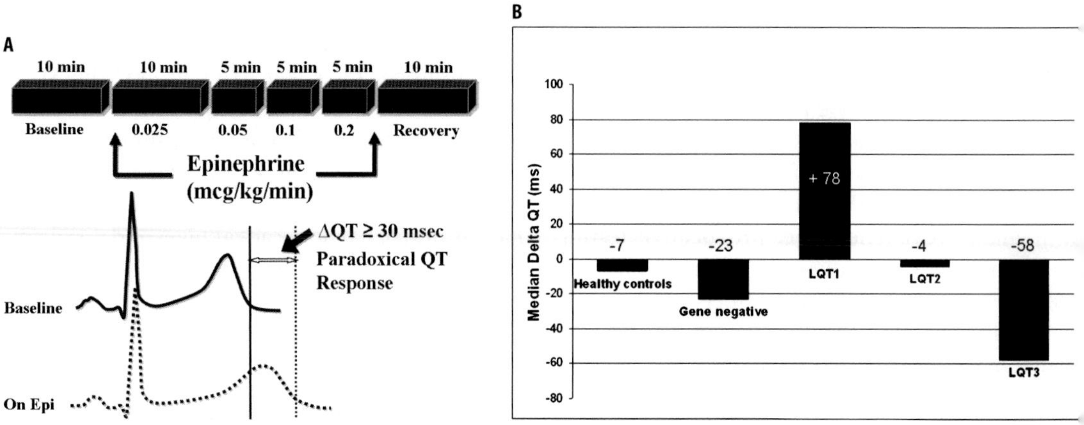

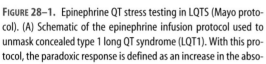

FIGURE 28–1. Epinephrine QT stress testing in LQTS (Mayo protocol). (A) Schematic of the epinephrine infusion protocol used to unmask concealed type 1 long QT syndrome (LQT1). With this protocol, the paradoxic response is defined as an increase in the absolute QT interval by ≥30 msec during infusion of low-dose epinephrine (≤0.1 μg/kg/min). (B) Summary of the low-dose epinephrine-absolute QT response performed in over 200 subjects at the Mayo Clinic.

response of action potential duration (APD) and QT interval to sympathetic stimulation with isoproterenol between the experimental LQT1, LQT2, and LQT3 models employing arterially perfused canine left ventricular wedge preparations.[16] Persistent prolongation of the APD and QT interval at steady-state conditions of isoproterenol infusion was reported in the LQT1 model. Under normal conditions, β-adrenergic stimulation is expected to increase the net outward repolarizing current due to a larger increase of outward currents, including the Ca^{2+}-activated slow component of the delayed rectifier potassium current (I_{Ks}) and the Ca^{2+}-activated chloride current ($I_{Cl(Ca)}$), than that of an inward current, the Na^+/Ca^{2+} exchange current ($I_{Na\text{-}Ca}$), resulting in an abbreviation of APD and the QT interval. A defect in I_{Ks} as seen in LQT1 could account for failure of β-adrenergic stimulation to abbreviate APD and the QT interval, resulting in a persistent and paradoxic QT prolongation under sympathetic stimulation. In the LQT2 model, isoproterenol infusion was reported to initially prolong but then abbreviate APD and the QT interval probably due to an initial augmentation of $I_{Na\text{-}Ca}$ and a subsequent stimulation of I_{Ks}. In contrast to the LQT1 and LQT2 models, isoproterenol infusion constantly abbreviated APD and the QT interval as a result of a stimulation of I_{Ks} in the LQT3 model, because an inward late I_{Na} was augmented in this genotype. Therefore, the bolus protocol of epinephrine testing was expected not only to unmask concealed patients with LQTS but also to presumptively diagnose the three most common subtypes, LQT1, LQT2, and LQT3, by monitoring the temporal course of the QTc to epinephrine at peak effect following bolus injection and at steady-state effect during continuous infusion.

TABLE 28–1. Validity of the epinephrine QT stress test (Mayo protocol) at a QT ≥ 30 msec.

ΔQT[a]	LQT1	Non-LQT1	Predictive value
ΔQT ≥ 30 msec	37	12	Positive predictive value = 76%
ΔQT < 30 msec	3	73	Negative predictive value = 96%
	Sensitivity = 92.5%	Specificity = 86%	

[a]Δ, the change (delta) in the QT interval (epinephrine minus baseline).

Clinical data using the bolus protocol suggested that sympathetic stimulation produces genotype-specific responses of the QTc interval in patients with LQT1, LQT2, and LQT3 (Figure 28–2).[17,18] Epinephrine remarkably prolonged the QTc interval at peak effect when the heart rate is maximally increased (1–2 min after the bolus injection), and the QTc remained prolonged during steady-state epinephrine effect (3–5 min) in patients with LQT1.[17,18] As an aside, this steady-state effect likely correlates with the paradoxic QT response seen with the Mayo protocol. The QTc was also prolonged at peak epinephrine effect (during bolus)

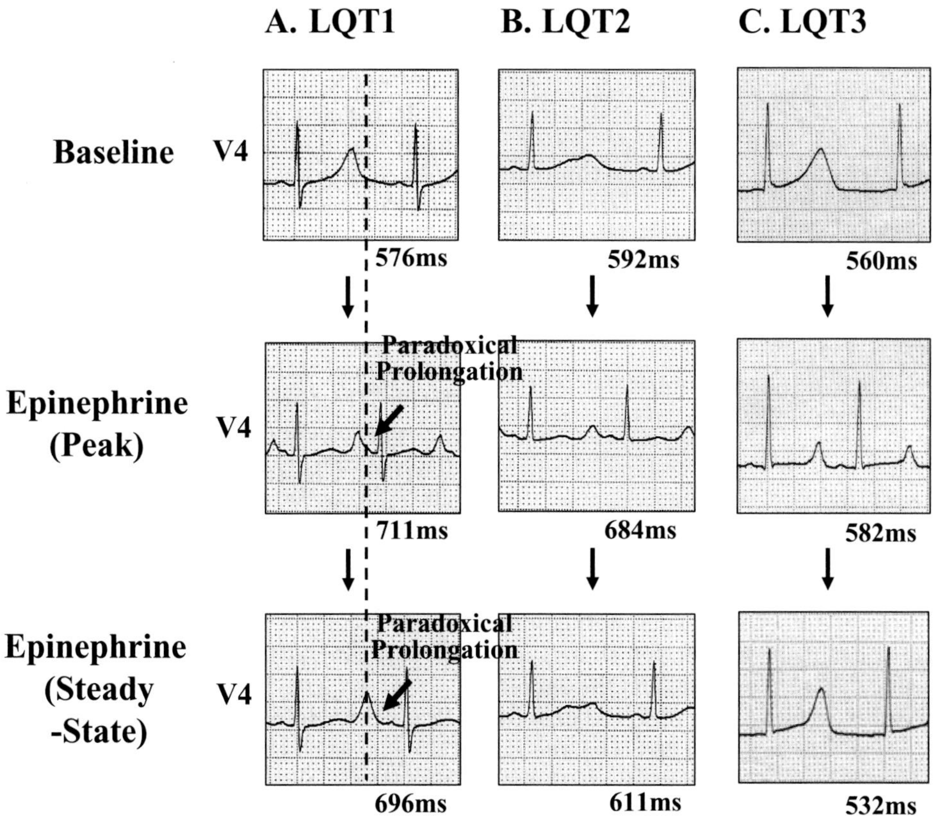

FIGURE 28–2. Differential temporal course of the heart rate corrected QT interval (QTc) to epinephrine QT stress testing in LQT1, 2, and 3 (Shimizu protocol). The V4 lead ECGs under baseline conditions and at peak and steady-state epinephrine effects in LQT1 (A), LQT2 (B), and LQT3 (C) patients using the Shimizu bolus and infusion protocol are shown. The corrected QT interval (QTc) was prominently prolonged from 576 to 711 msec at peak epinephrine effect, and remained prolonged at steady state (696 msec) in the patient with LQT1. It is noteworthy that paradoxic QT prolongation was seen both at peak and steady-state epinephrine effects (arrows). In the patient with LQT2, the QTc was also dramatically prolonged from 592 to 684 msec at peak, but returned to the baseline level at steady state (611 msec). It was much less prolonged (560 to 582 msec) at peak in the LQT3 patient than in either the LQT1 or LQT2 patient, and returned below the baseline level at steady state (532 msec).

in patients with LQT2, but returned to close to baseline levels at the steady-state epinephrine effect.[18] In contrast, the QTc was less prolonged at the peak epinephrine effect in the LQT3 patients than in the LQT1 or LQT2 patients, and was abbreviated below baseline levels at the steady-state epinephrine effect.[18] The responses of the corrected T_{peak}–T_{end} interval reflecting transmural dispersion of repolarization (TDR) approximately paralleled those of the QT interval,[19] supporting the cellular basis for genotype-specific triggers for cardiac events.

By using the steady-state epinephrine effect, Shimizu *et al.* reported an improvement in clinical electrocardiographic diagnosis (sensitivity) from 68% to 87% in the 31 patients with LQT1 and from 83% to 91% in the 23 patients with LQT2, but not in the 6 patients with LQT3 (from 83% to 83%).[18] The bolus protocol of epinephrine effectively predicts the underlying genotype of the LQT1, LQT2, and LQT3 (Figure 28–3).[18] The prolongation of QTc ≥35 msec at steady-state epinephrine effect could differentiate LQT1 from LQT2, LQT3, or control patients with a predictive accuracy ≥90 %. The prolongation of QTc ≥80 msec at peak epinephrine effect could differentiate LQT2 from LQT3 or control patients with a predictive accuracy of 100%.

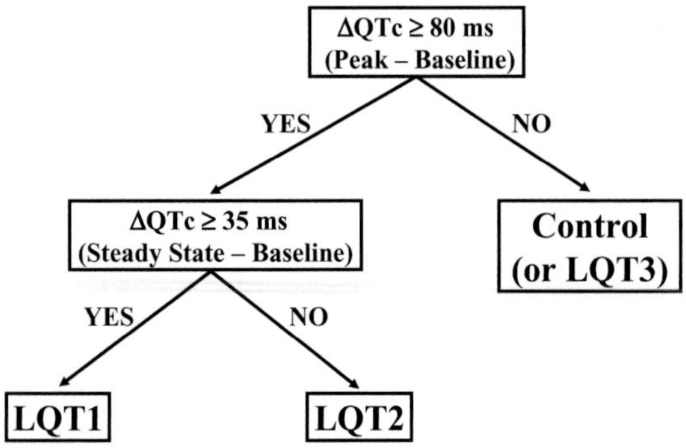

FIGURE 28–3. A flow chart to predict genotype with epinephrine QT stress testing (Shimizu Protocol).

Whether utilizing the Mayo protocol or the Shimizu protocol, the responses to epinephrine should be viewed as diagnostic only, not prognostic. Induction of TdP or ventricular fibrillation is extremely uncommon. In over 400 studies conducted using the Mayo protocol and the Shimizu protocol respectively, we have observed only two episodes of TdP (10 beats and 20 beats) and one episode of macroscopic T wave alternans. In addition, these gene-specific responses are attenuated by β blockers. If a patient displays, epinephrine-induced bradycardia rather than the expected increase in heart rate, then the study should be terminated, a diagnostic interpretation should not be rendered, and a period of monitored beta blocker washout should be considered.

Importantly, the diagnostic profiles gleaned from one protocol should *not* be applied to the other protocol. For example, using the Mayo protocol, we have observed healthy volunteers display a QTc of 600 msec ($\Delta QTc = 140$ msec) during epinephrine infusion due to a negligible change in the absolute QT interval but a brisk chronotropic response. This response could be viewed as either an LQT1 (steady-state) or LQT2 (peak) response if the Shimizu algorithm was erroneously applied (Figure 28–3) in the setting of the Mayo protocol (Figure 28–1A). Here, it is critical to remember that the key determinant is epinephrine-mediated changes in the QT interval for the Mayo protocol and epinephrine-mediated changes in the QTc for the Shimizu protocol. Finally, a caveat regarding epinephrine-accentuated U waves is in order as erroneous inclusion of such U waves during epinephrine infusion underlies some of the false positives.

Since molecular diagnosis is still unavailable to many institutes and requires high costs and is time consuming, a clinical diagnosis of concealed LQTS by the epinephrine QT stress test can direct proper counseling and facilitate the initiation of preventive measures such as QT drug avoidance. Furthermore, a presumptive, pregenetic diagnosis of either LQT1, LQT2, or LQT3 based upon the response to epinephrine can guide gene-specific treatment strategies. Finally, since 25% of LQTS remains genetically elusive, the identification of patients with LQTS and an LQT1-like response to epinephrine, for example, may lead to the identification of novel LQTS-causing susceptibility genes.

Brugada Syndrome

Brugada syndrome is characterized by coved-type ST-segment elevation in the right precordial electrocardiographic leads (V1–V3) and an episode of ventricular fibrillation (VF) in the absence of structural heart disease.[20] However, the ST segment elevation is dynamic and is often concealed, and is reported to be accentuated just before and after episodes of ventricular fibrillation (VF).[21] A variety of antiarrhythmic drugs and autonomic agents have been reported to provoke typical ST-segment elevation.[22] Experimental studies have suggested that an intrinsically prominent transient outward current (I_{to})-mediated action potential (AP) notch and a subsequent loss of AP dome in the epicardium, but not in the endocardium, of the right ventricular outflow tract give rise to a transmural voltage gradient, resulting in a typical ST-segment elevation in leads V1–V3.[23] Because the maintenance of the AP dome is determined by the balance of currents active at the end of phase 1 of the AP (principally I_{to} and the L-type calcium current [$I_{Ca\text{-}L}$]), any interventions that increase outward currents (e.g., I_{to}, I_{Ks}, I_{Kr}) or decrease inward currents (e.g., $I_{Ca\text{-}L}$, fast I_{Na}) at the end of phase 1 of the AP can accentuate ST-segment elevation, thus producing the Brugada phenotype.

Provocative Testing with Sodium Channel Blockers

Among the interventions above, sodium channel blockers effectively amplify or unmask ST-segment elevation, and are used as a provocative test in patients with concealed BrS showing transient or no spontaneous ST-segment elevation.[24,25] Among the sodium channel blockers, the class IC drugs (flecainide, 2 mg/kg in 10 min, iv; pilsicainide 1 mg/kg in 10 min, iv) produce the most pronounced ST-segment elevation due to strong use-dependent blocking of fast I_{Na} secondary to their slow dissociation from the sodium channels.[24] Pilsicainide, a pure class IC drug developed in Japan, seems to induce ST-segment elevation more than flecainide, which is widely used throughout the world. (Figure 28–4). Induction of ventricular arrhythmias by pilsicainide was reported to be less rare than anticipated.[26] In other words, caution should be exercised when using pilsicainide in BrS drug challenge testing because of the increased potential for false-positive responses. Further studies with genetic data as the golden standard will be required to evaluate the true sensitivity and specificity of the provocative testing with each sodium channel blocker. Class IA antiarrhythmic drugs (ajmaline, procainamide, disopyramide, cibenzoline, etc.), which exhibit less use-dependent block of fast I_{Na} due to faster

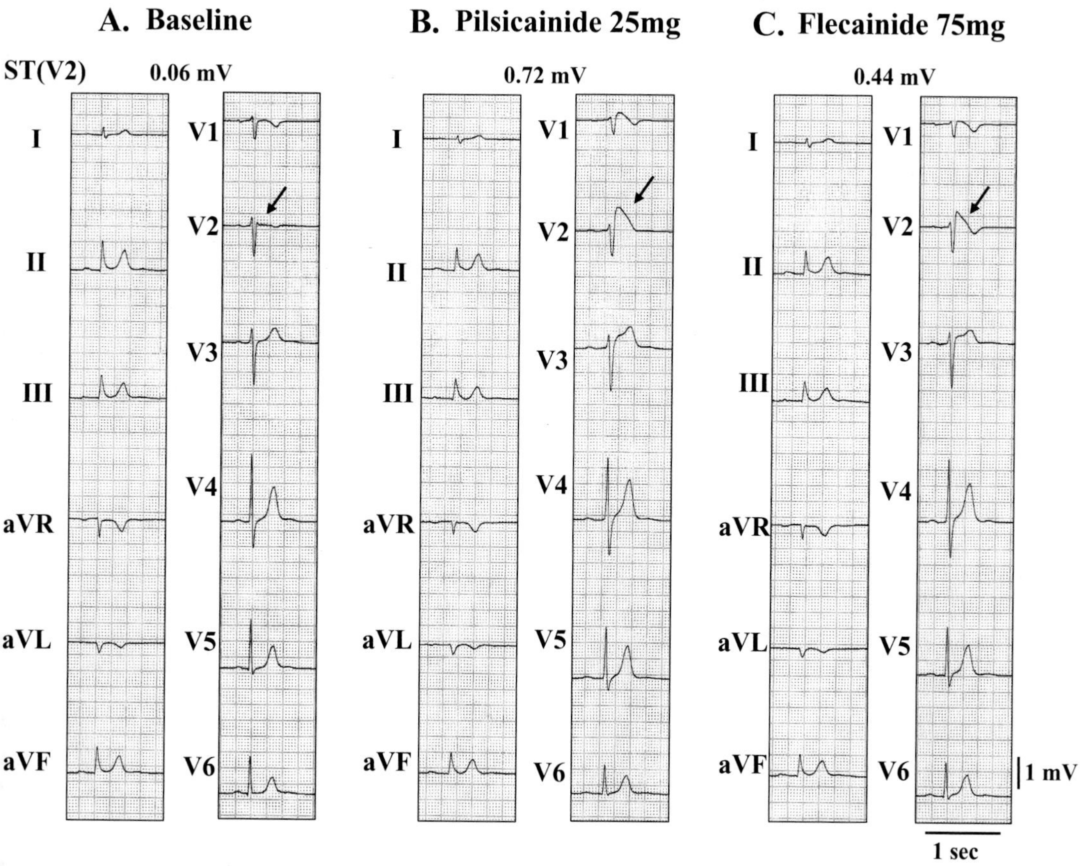

FIGURE 28–4. Effects of class IC sodium channel blockers on the ST segment in a patient with concealed Brugada syndrome. At baseline condition (A, arrow), no significant ST-segment elevation in leads V1–V3 was observed. Both pilsicainide (B, arrow) and flecainide (C, arrow) induced Type 1 coved ST-segment elevation; however, a smaller dose of pilsicainide injection (25 mg) produced more prominent ST-segment elevation than that by flecainide injection (75 mg) in lead V2 (0.72 vs. 0.44 mV).

dissociation of the drug, show a weaker ST-segment elevation than class IC drugs[22,24,25] (Figure 28–5B and C). Ajmaline (1 mg/kg, in 5 min, iv) has been frequently used and is reported to be safer with malignant ventricular arrhythmias in only 1.3% of the patients tested.[27] Wolpert *et al.* reported that ajmaline induced or enhanced Type 1 ST-segment elevation more frequently than flecainide, and that this was due to greater inhibition of I_{to} by flecainide.[28] Disopyramide (2 mg/kg in 10 min, iv) and procainamide (10 mg/kg, in 10 min iv) show weaker accentuation of the ST-segment elevation due to their smaller effect on fast I_{Na} and mild to moderate action to block I_{to} (Figure 28–5C).[22,24,25] Class IB drugs (mexiletine, lidocaine etc.) dissociate from the sodium channel rapidly and therefore have little or no effect on fast I_{Na} at moderate and slow heart rates, and thus are unable

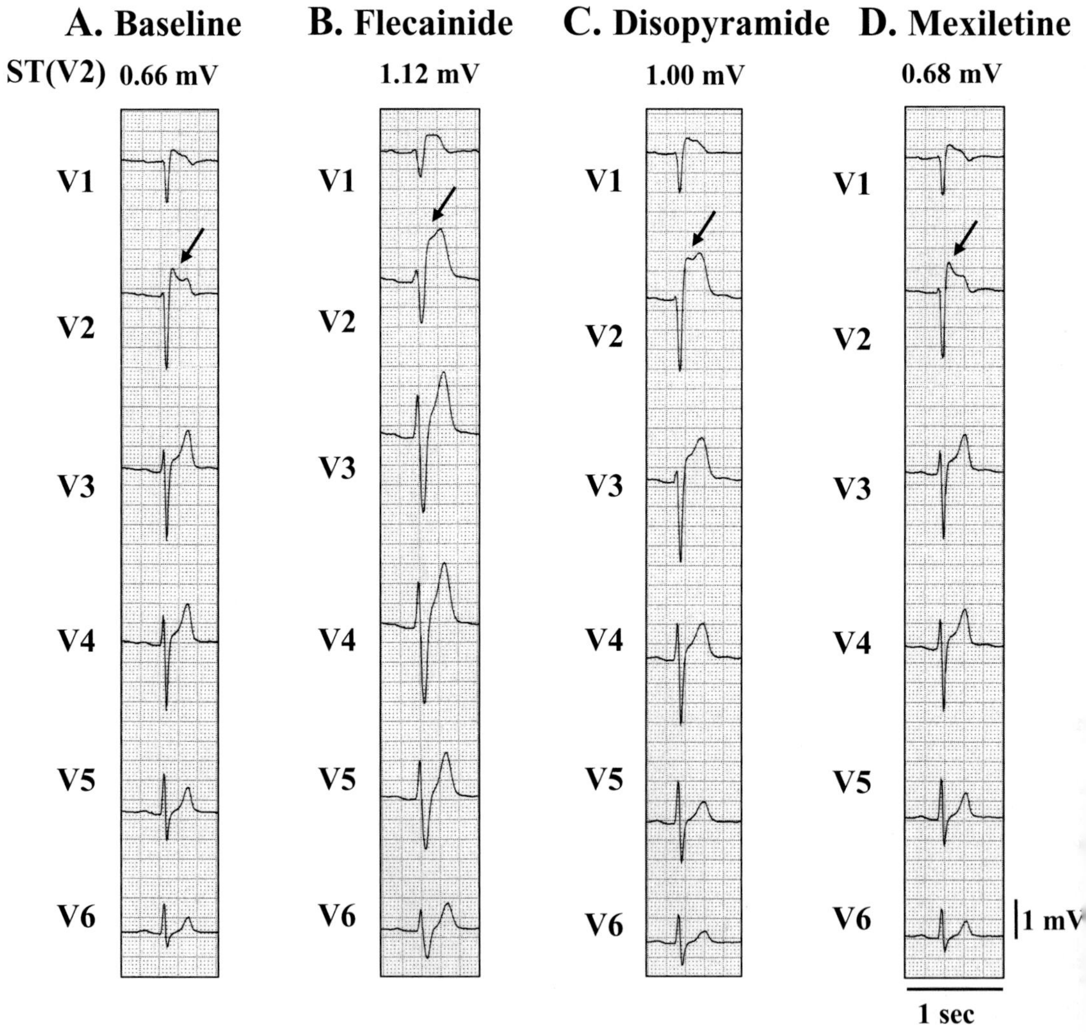

FIGURE 28–5. Effects of different sodium channel blockers on ST-segment elevation in a patient with Brugada syndrome. Six precordial lead electrocardiograms at baseline condition (A), after 100 mg flecainide injection (class IC drug) (B), after 100 mg disopyramide injection (class IA drug) (C), and after 125 mg mexiletine injection (class IB drug) are shown. At baseline conditions (A, arrow), Type 2 saddleback ST-segment elevation was seen in lead V2 (0.66 mV). Flecainide more remarkablly accentuated the ST-segment elevation (1.12 mV) than disopyramide (1.00 mV) (B and C, arrows), while mexiletine had no effect on the ST-segment elevation (0.68 mV) (D, arrow).

TABLE 28–2. Drugs used to unmask the Brugada syndrome.

Flecainide	2 mg/kg/10 min, iv (400 mg, po)
Pilsicainide	1 mg/kg/10 min, iv
Ajmaline	1 mg/kg/5 min, iv
Disopyramide	2mg/kg in 10 min, iv
Procainamide	10 mg/kg/10 min, iv

to cause ST-segment elevation[24] (Figure 28–5D). The recommended dosage of each sodium channel blocker is listed in Table 28–2.[29]

Practice of Testing with Sodium Channel Blockers

The definition of a positive provocative test is a development of the diagnostic Type 1 Brugada ECG (an increase in the absolute J wave amplitude of >0.2 mV with or without right bundle branch block in at least one of the V1–V3 leads) in the case of a Type 2, Type 3, or negative ECG at baseline. The test is considered positive upon an increase in the ST-segment elevation by >0.2 mV. The test does *not* add to the diagnostic value in patients with spontaneous and constant Type 1 Brugada ECG. The test should be monitored with a continuous 12-lead electrocardiographic recording (a speed of 10 mm/sec can be used to monitor throughout the test period, interposed with recordings at 25 or 50 mm/sec), and cardiopulmonary resuscitation facilities and isoproterenol infusion should be at hand. The endpoint of the test is when (1) the diagnostic Type 1 Brugada ECG develops, (2) the ST segment in Type 2 ECG increases by ≥0.2 mV, (3) ventricular or other arrhythmias develop, or (4) the QRS widens to ≥130% of baseline. Particular caution should be exercised in patients with a preexisting atrial and/or ventricular conduction disturbance (e.g., suspected cases of progressive cardiac conduction defect) or in the presence of wide QRS, wide P waves, or prolonged PR intervals (infranodal conduction disease) so as to avoid the risk of precipitating complete AV block.

Catecholaminergic Polymorphic Ventricular Tachycardia

Unlike LQTS and BrS in which the cardinal feature is often evident on the resting 12-lead ECG, this diagnostic test is *always* normal in CPVT. Phenotypically, CPVT mimics LQTS, particularly LQT1, with exercise-induced syncope, seizures, or sudden death, but in the setting of a structurally normal heart *and* a normal 12-lead ECG.[30,31] Approximately two-thirds of CPVT stems from mutations in the *RyR2*-encoded ryanodine receptor/calcium release channel (CPVT1). One possible clue for CPVT1 may be the presence of marked bradycardia.[32] However, the hallmark signature of CPVT is exercise-induced or catecholamine-induced bidirectional ventricular tachycardia.[33] Presently, it is not clear whether catecholamine provocation testing is additive to standard exercise stress testing or whether isoproterenol (more commonly used for CPVT) is superior to epinephrine.

Practically speaking, when faced with a patient presenting with exercise-induced syncope or exercise-induced aborted cardiac arrest and a normal ECG (QTc = 430 msec), the differential diagnosis includes both concealed LQT1 and CPVT. As such, we advocate using the epinephrine QT stress test (either the previously discussed Mayo or Shimizu protocols). Remember that significant epinephrine-induced ventricular ectopy is extremely uncommon in LQTS and occasional premature ventricular contractions (PVCs) and even couplets are not informative. If there is paradoxic QT lengthening, then concealed LQT1 is the presumptive clinical diagnosis. On the other hand, if there is epinephrine-induced bidirectional ventricular tachycardia, then CPVT is likely. Suspicion for CPVT should be raised and CPVT-directed genetic testing initiated for lesser degrees of epinephrine-induced ventricular ectopy such as epinephrine-induced nonsustained ventricular tachycardia, TdP in the absence of paradoxic QT lengthening, and possibly even PVCs in bigeminy during epinephrine infusion. One caveat to remember is that bidirectional ventricular tachycardia can also be seen in *KCNJ2*-mediated Andersen–Tawil syndrome.[34]

Acknowledgments. Dr. W. Shimizu was supported by the Uehara Memorial Foundation, Japan Research Foundation for Clinical Pharmacology, Ministry of Education, Culture, Sports, Science and Technology Leading Project for Biosimulation, and health sciences research grants (H18-Research on Human Genome- 002) from the Ministry of Health, Labour and Welfare, Japan. Dr. Ackerman's research program was supported by the National Institutes of Health (HD42569), the American Heart Association (Established Investigator Award), the Doris Duke Charitable Foundation (Clinical Scientist Development Award), the CJ Foundation for SIDS, and the Dr. Scholl Foundation.

References

1. Schwartz PJ, Periti M, Malliani A. The long QT syndrome. *Am Heart J* 1975;89:378–390.
2. Schwartz PJ, Moss AJ, Vincent GM, Crampton RS. Diagnostic criteria for the long QT syndrome: An update. *Circulation* 1993;88:782–784.
3. Moss AJ, Schwartz PJ, Crampton RS, Locati E, Carleen E. The long QT syndrome: A prospective international study. *Circulation* 1985;71:17–21.
4. Shimizu W. The long QT syndrome: Therapeutic implications of a genetic diagnosis. *Cardiovasc Res* 2005;67:347–356.
5. Priori SG, Napolitano C, Schwartz PJ, Grillo M, Bloise R, Ronchetti E, Moncalvo C, Tulipani C, Veia A, Bottelli G, Nastoli J. Association of long QT syndrome loci and cardiac events among patients treated with beta-blockers. *JAMA* 2004;292:1341–1344.
6. Vincent GM, Timothy KW, Leppert M, Keating M. The spectrum of symptoms and QT intervals in carriers of the gene for the long-QT syndrome. *N Engl J Med* 1992;327:846–852.
7. Priori SG, Napolitano C, Schwartz PJ. Low penetrance in the long-QT syndrome. Clinical impact. *Circulation* 1999;99:529–533.
8. Swan H, Saarinen K, Kontula K, Toivonen L, Viitasalo M. Evaluation of QT interval duration and dispersion and proposed clinical criteria in diagnosis of long QT syndrome in patients with a genetically uniform type of LQT1. *J Am Coll Cardiol* 1998;32:486–491.
9. Priori SG, Schwartz PJ, Napolitano C, Bloise R, Ronchetti E, Grillo M, Vicentini A, Spazzolini C, Nastoli J, Bottelli G, Folli R, Cappelletti D. Risk stratification in the long-QT syndrome. *N Engl J Med* 2003;348:1866–1874.
10. Schechter E, Freeman CC, Lazzara R. Afterdepolarizations as a mechanism for the long QT syndrome: Electrophysiologic studies of a case. *J Am Coll Cardiol* 1984;3:1556–1561.
11. Viskin S, Rosso R, Rogowski O, Belhassen B, Levitas A, Wagshal A, Katz A, Fourey D, Zeltser D, Oliva A, Pollevick GD, Antzelevitch C, Rozovski U. Provocation of sudden heart rate oscillation with adenosine exposes abnormal QT responses in patients with long QT syndrome: A bedside test for diagnosing long QT syndrome. *Eur Heart J* 2006;27:469–475.
12. Ackerman MJ, Khositseth A, Tester DJ, Hejlik JB, Shen WK, Porter CB. Epinephrine-induced QT interval prolongation: A gene-specific paradoxical response in congenital long QT syndrome. *Mayo Clin Proc* 2002;77:413–421.
13. Noda T, Takaki H, Kurita T, Suyama K, Nagaya N, Taguchi A, Aihara N, Kamakura S, Sunagawa K, Nakamura K, Ohe T, Horie M, Napolitano C, Towbin JA, Priori SG, Shimizu W. Gene-specific response of dynamic ventricular repolarization to sympathetic stimulation in LQT1, LQT2 and LQT3 forms of congenital long QT syndrome. *Eur Heart J* 2002;23:975–983.
14. Vyas H, Hejlik J, Ackerman MJ. Epinephrine QT stress testing in the evaluation of congenital long-QT syndrome: Diagnostic accuracy of the paradoxical QT response. *Circulation* 2006;113:1385–1392.
15. Khositseth A, Hejlik J, Shen WK, Ackerman MJ. Epinephrine-induced T-wave notching in congenital long QT syndrome. *Heart Rhythm* 2005;2:141–146.
16. Shimizu W, Antzelevitch C. Differential response to beta-adrenergic agonists and antagonists in LQT1, LQT2 and LQT3 models of the long QT syndrome. *J Am Coll Cardiol* 2000;35:778–786.
17. Shimizu W, Noda T, Takaki H, Kurita T, Nagaya N, Satomi K, Suyama K, Aihara N, Kamakura S, Echigo S, Nakamura K, Sunagawa K, Ohe T, Towbin JA, Napolitano C, Priori SG. Epinephrine unmasks latent mutation carriers with LQT1 form of congenital long QT syndrome. *J Am Coll Cardiol* 2003;41:633–642.
18. Shimizu W, Noda T, Takaki H, Nagaya N, Satomi K, Kurita T, Suyama K, Aihara N, Sunagawa K, Echigo S, Miyamoto Y, Yoshimasa Y, Nakamura K, Ohe T, Towbin JA, Priori SG, Kamakura S. Diagnostic value of epinephrine test for genotyping LQT1, LQT2 and LQT3 forms of congenital long QT syndrome. *Heart Rhythm* 2004;1:276–283.
19. Shimizu W, Tanabe Y, Aiba T, Inagaki M, Kurita T, Suyama K, Nagaya N, Taguchi A, Aihara N, Sunagawa K, Nakamura K, Ohe T, Towbin JA, Priori SG, Kamakura S. Differential effects of β-blockade on dispersion of repolarization in absence and presence of sympathetic stimulation between

LQT1 and LQT2 forms of congenital long QT syndrome. *J Am Coll Cardiol* 2002;39:1984–1991.

20. Brugada P, Brugada J. Right bundle branch block, persistent ST segment elevation and sudden cardiac death: A distinct clinical and electrocardiographic syndrome: A multicenter report. *J Am Coll Cardiol* 1992;20:1391–1396.
21. Matsuo K, Shimizu W, Kurita T, Inagaki M, Aihara N, Kamakura S. Dynamic changes of 12-lead electrocardiograms in a patient with Brugada syndrome. *J Cardiovasc Electrophysiol* 1998;9:508–512.
22. Miyazaki T, Mitamura H, Miyoshi S, Soejima K, Aizawa Y, Ogawa S. Autonomic and antiarrhythmic drug modulation of ST segment elevation in patients with Brugada syndrome. *J Am Coll Cardiol* 1996;27:1061–1070.
23. Yan GX, Antzelevitch C. Cellular basis for the Brugada syndrome and other mechanisms of arrhythmogenesis associated with ST segment elevation. *Circulation* 1999;100:1660–1666.
24. Shimizu W, Antzelevitch C, Suyama K, Kurita T, Taguchi A, Aihara N, Takaki H, Sunagawa K, Kamakura S. Effect of sodium channel blockers on ST segment, QRS duration, and corrected QT interval in patients with Brugada syndrome. *J Cardiovasc Electrophysiol* 2000;11:1320–1329.
25. Brugada R, Brugada J, Antzelevitch C, Kirsch GE, Potenza D, Towbin JA, Brugada P. Sodium channel blockers identify risk for sudden death in patients with ST-segment elevation and right bundle branch block but structurally normal hearts. *Circulation* 2000;101:510–515.
26. Morita H, Morita ST, Nagase S, Banba K, Nishii N, Tani Y, Watanabe A, Nakamura K, Kusano KF, Emori T, Matsubara H, Hina K, Kita T, Ohe T. Ventricular arrhythmia induced by sodium channel blocker in patients with Brugada syndrome. *J Am Coll Cardiol* 2003;42:1624–1631.
27. Rolf S, Bruns HJ, Wichter T, Kirchhof P, Ribbing M, Wasmer K, Paul M, Breithardt G, Haverkamp W, Eckardt L. The ajmaline challenge in Brugada syndrome: Diagnostic impact, safety, and recommended protocol. *Eur Heart J* 2003;24:1104–1112.
28. Wolpert C, Echternach C, Veltmann C, Antzelevitch C, Thomas GP, Spehl S, Streitner F, Kuschyk J, Schimpf R, Haase KK, Borggrefe M. Intravenous drug challenge using flecainide and ajmaline in patients with Brugada syndrome. *Heart Rhythm* 2005;2:254–260.
29. Antzelevitch C, Brugada P, Borggrefe M, Brugada J, Brugada R, Corrado D, Gussak I, Lemarec H, Nademanee K, Perez Riera AR, Shimizu W, Schulze-Bahr E, Tan H, Wilde A. Brugada syndrome. Report of the Second Consensus Conference. Endorsed by the Heart Rhythm Society and the European Heart Rhythm Association. *Circulation* 2005;111:659–670.
30. Leenhardt A, Lucet V, Denjoy I, Grau F, Ngoc DD, Coumel P. Catecholaminergic polymorphic ventricular tachycardia in children. A 7-year follow-up of 21 patients. *Circulation* 1995;91:1512–1519.
31. Priori SG, Napolitano C, Memmi M, Colombi B, Drago F, Gasparini M, DeSimone L, Coltorti F, Bloise R, Keegan R, Cruz Filho FE, Vignati G, Benatar A, DeLogu A. Clinical and molecular characterization of patients with catecholaminergic polymorphic ventricular tachycardia. *Circulation* 2002;106:69–74.
32. Postma AV, Denjoy I, Kamblock J, Alders M, Lupoglazoff JM, Vaksmann G, Dubosq-Bidot L, Sebillon P, Mannens MM, Guicheney P, Wilde AA. Catecholaminergic polymorphic ventricular tachycardia: RYR2 mutations, bradycardia, and follow up of the patients. *J Med Genet* 2005;42:863–870.
33. Cerrone M, Colombi B, Santoro M, di Barletta MR, Scelsi M, Villani L, Napolitano C, Priori SG. Bidirectional ventricular tachycardia and fibrillation elicited in a knock-in mouse model carrier of a mutation in the cardiac ryanodine receptor. *Circ Res* 2005;96:1031–1032.
34. Tester DJ, Arya P, Will M, Haglund CM, Farley AL, Makielski JC, Ackerman MJ. Genotypic heterogeneity and phenotypic mimicry among unrelated patients referred for catecholaminergic polymorphic ventricular tachycardia genetic testing. *Heart Rhythm* 2006;3:800–805.

29
Novel Predictors of Sudden Cardiac Death

Sumeet S. Chugh

Introduction

Despite recent advances in resuscitation science, survival from sudden cardiac arrest (SCA) remains low, and sudden cardiac death (SCD) remains a public health problem of significant proportions. Estimates of the annual incidence of SCD in the United States range from 200,000 to 400,000.[1–4] Currently, severe left ventricular (LV) dysfunction is the best available predictor of SCD risk and is the major indication for primary prevention with the implantable cardioverter defibrillator (ICD).[5–8] Based on this indication, it is estimated that there will be at least 50,000 potential ICD recipients per year among the U.S. Medicare population alone, which is likely to translate into $3–5 billion per year for implantation and follow-up of ICDs.[9] However, using severe LV dysfunction as the criterion for a prophylactic ICD, it takes approximately 10 ICD recipients to save one life during an intermediate follow-up period, indicating that there is significant scope for enhancement of risk stratification.[5,8] Therefore, there is a need to extend beyond the LV ejection fraction, and to identify novel predictors of SCD. This chapter will discuss the utility and limitations of severe LV systolic dysfunction as a risk predictor of SCD, other predictors in the process of being evaluated, and finally, the promise that new genomic predictors may also contribute to the process of SCD risk stratification. Wherever possible, predictors of SCD will be discussed in the context of the overall population, as opposed to population subgroups that can have variable risk.

Left Ventricular Dysfunction and Sudden Cardiac Death in the General Population

Severe LV dysfunction was identified as an important prognosticating factor for SCD over two decades ago,[10] leading to its use as the major criterion for the design and conduct of the prospective randomized ICD trials.[5–8,11] Severe LV dysfunction clearly predicts risk of SCD, but its effectiveness as a determinant of risk, particularly in the context of primary prevention, has recently been debated because of two kinds of observations. First, among recipients of primary prevention ICDs, appropriate ICD therapies may be delivered in less than 30% of ICD recipients over an intermediate (4–5 years) follow-up. This has led to an active discussion regarding the cost-effectiveness of the ICD when the LV ejection fraction is employed for risk stratification.[12] Second, it had been hypothesized that patients with severely decreased LV dysfunction who present to health care providers as a high-risk group (as a result of symptoms or following survival from cardiac arrest) may comprise a small proportion of overall SCD cases.[13] We and others have observed this hypothesis to indeed be true in the general population.[14–16] In a recently published population-based analysis from the Oregon Sudden Unexpected Death Study (Ore-SUDS), severe LV dysfunction was a significant predictor, but was found to affect only a third of all SCD cases in the community. In fact, we observed that at least 65% of overall SCD cases would have not

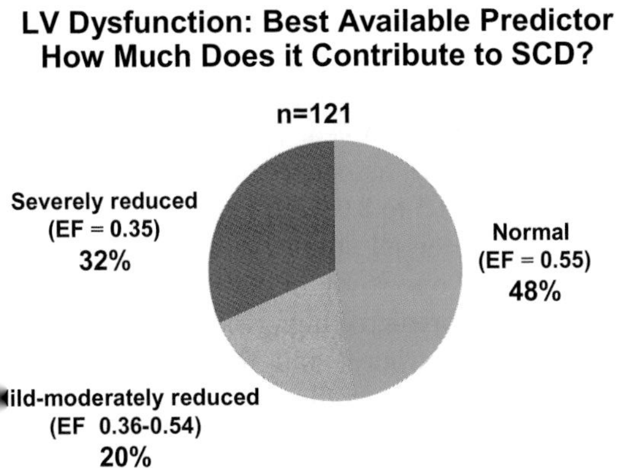

GURE 29–1. In a community-based study, only 30% of sudden ardiac death cases evaluated prior to death had severe LV ysfunction. At least 65% of overall sudden cardiac death cases ould not have met the current criteria for ICD implantation.

net the criteria for prophylactic ICDs by the urrent guidelines (Figure 29–1).[16] Almost half of ll SCD cases had normal LV function and the emaining 20% had either mildly or moderately lecreased [LV ejection fraction (LVEF) >0.35 and <0.50] LV systolic function. Similar observations ave been made in a community-based study in Maastricht, the Netherlands.[14,15] Among 200 cases of SCD with an assessment of LV function availa-ble, 101 (51%) had normal LVEF, defined as >0.50, and 38 (19%) had severely reduced LVEF, defined as ≤ 0.30. Despite the fact that the Netherlands tudy was limited to patients 20–75 years old while Ore-SUDS included all ages, the findings are very similar on either continent. While severe LV lysfunction remains a valuable contributor to isk stratification, the above findings emphasize he significant need to extend beyond the EF and identify novel predictors that could be used ndependently or in combination with the LVEF.

Other Known Predictors of Sudden Cardiac Death

In addition to severe LV dysfunction, current predictors of increased SCD risk that are incorpo-rated in stratification of risk for SCD are limited to a small subset of relatively rare conditions such as hypertrophic obstructive cardiomyopathy and the long QT and Brugada syndromes.[13,17] There-fore, in the general population, determinants of SCD risk may presently be undefined for the majority of cases. This lack of information regard-ing SCD risk markers in the general population is a significant and critical gap in our knowledge of SCD.[3] However, there are potential predictors that have been discussed in the literature and are currently either areas of active investigation or definitely warrant being investigated.

Prolonged Ventricular Repolarization

The link between the prolonged corrected QT interval (QTc) and increased risk of fatal arrhyth-mogenesis is well established by the detailed investigation of the rare monogenic, long QT syn-dromes that constitute a human model for this causative association.[18–21] Howeve, the Rotterdam study reported that QTc was independently asso-ciated with SCD even in a cohort of unrelated individuals.[22] In a cohort of 6693 patients followed for 2 years, patients without evidence of cardiac dysfunction and QTc >440 msec had a 2.3-fold higher risk of SCD compared to those with QTc <440 msec. This association was independent of age, gender, history of myocardial infarction (MI), heart rate, and drug use. A more recent analysis from the same cohort reports that prolonged QTc was an independent risk factor for SCD in older adults followed for 6.7 years.[23,24] QTc was also found to be a predictor of increased overall cardiovascular morbidity and mortality in several cohort studies.[25–29] The potential of prolonged cardiac repolarization as a stratifier of risk among unrelated individuals in the general population clearly merits further evaluation.

Diabetes Mellitus

There are a relatively small number of studies in which the independent role of diabetes mellitus (DM) in enhancing risk of SCD has been investi-gated. However, the results are intriguing as well as consistent. The "Paris Prospective Study I" conducted a longitudinal follow-up of >6000 middle-aged, healthy male Parisian civil servants, over 23 years. A distinction was made between the 120 SCDs and 192 deaths from acute myocardial infarction (MI) that occurred over this time period. In a multivariate analysis, DM independently conferred the highest risk for SCD [relative risk (RR) 2.2] compared to all other variables (age, body mass index, tobacco use, history, heart rate, systolic pressure, and cholesterol and triglyceride levels).[30,31] Similar findings were reported from the U.S. Nurses Study and the Physicians Health Study populations[32,33] as well as a retrospective clinical database analysis from a health cooperative in Seattle.[34] While these findings clearly implicate DM as an important factor in the pathogenesis of SCD, the relationship has not been evaluated in prospective, community-wide studies of SCD. In addition, little is known about the specific ways in which DM-related mechanisms contribute to the pathogenesis of SCD. However, several mechanisms have been postulated. DM increases risk of coronary artery disease (CAD), a condition that is commonly found in association with SCD. In addition, there may be DM-specific accelerated forms of atherosclerosis with enhanced thrombogenicity.[35] Evidence is accumulating for the existence of a distinct form of cardiac dysfunction that has been termed "diabetic cardiomyopathy".[36,37] An intriguing and universal finding among diabetics is their propensity to have a greater prevalence of abnormal prolongation of the QT interval from the electrocardiogram (ECG).[38] Earlier clinical studies have also reported a good correlation between prolonged QTc and overall cardiac mortality in diabetics.[39,40] Several studies have found a significant association between diabetic autonomic dysfunction and prolongation of the QTc.[41–44] Given the recently confirmed status of prolonged QTc as a marker of SCD risk in a large, community-based cohort, this parameter has potential for increased significance among diabetics.

Left Ventricular Hypertrophy

The presence of left ventricular hypertrophy (LVH) is a strong independent risk factor for future cardiac events and all-cause mortality. A recent meta-analysis of 20 studies (48,545 participants) highlighted the strong relationship between LVH and overall adverse outcome, emphasizing the clinical importance of detecting this entity.[45] The adjusted risk of future cardiovascular morbidity associated with baseline LVH ranged from 1.5 to 3.5, with a weighted mean risk ratio of 2. for all studies combined. The adjusted risk of all cause mortality associated with baseline LVH ranged from 1.5 to 8.0, with a weighted mean risk ratio of 2.5 for all studies combined. With the exception of one study in dialysis patients, LVH consistently predicted high risk, independently of examined covariates, and irrespective of race, presence or absence of hypertension or coronary disease, or between clinical and epidemiological samples.[45] Studies at the bench would also suggest that LVH constitutes a significant substrate for genesis of ventricular arrhythmias. Prolonged action potential duration is a salient feature of LVH, independent of cause.[46–49] This may lead to the phenomena of early afterdepolarizations and triggered activity as well as increased dispersion of repolarization that can sustain torsades de pointes ventricular arrhythmia.[50–53] In addition the myocardial fibrosis and myofibrillar disarray observed in LVH predispose to discontinuities in conduction by disrupting intercellular coupling.[54–56] This remodeling of the interstitium in LVH also affects distribution of gap junctions and properties of ion channel excitation and recovery also leading to inhomogeneities of sympathetic nervous system innervation and altered mechanical and electrical loading properties.[55,57–59] It has been postulated that subjects with LVH are in a prothrombotic state and therefore at increased risk for acute coronary thrombosis and SCD.[60,61] Finally, there is evidence to suggest that a subgroup of patients with LVH will eventually develop severe LVD. There is a lack of clinical investigations that have examined the possibility of an independent association between LVH and SCD. The overall risk of SCD appears to be increased in subjects with LVH, independent of the etiology of LVH. An analysis from the Framingham Heart Study observed an independent association between LVH and SCD among patients who had risk factors for CAD.[62]

This study examined 60 SCDs that occurred among 3661 subjects after up to 14 years of follow-up. It was found that LVH (determined by echocardiography) increased the risk of SCA independent of coronary artery disease risk factors with an HR of 2.16. In this study, there was limited informaon regarding the mode of death and whether atients had actually developed significant CAD. lowever, with a minimum estimated prevalence f LVH ranging between 20 and 50% among atients with CAD,[63–65] patients with LVH may epresent a large subgroup of the population at sk for SCA. Recent postmortem evaluations of atients with SCD and CAD have revealed stable laque morphology without evidence of acute oronary syndromes, suggesting that a primary lectrical event and not coronary ischemia may ave been the terminal event leading to SCD.[66,67] iven that the majority of fatal arrhythmias re ventricular tachyarrhythmias,[68] a causal link ith LVH can be readily postulated. Therefore, VH may have significant potential to extend isk stratification for SCD beyond the LV ejection raction.

)besity

wo recent cohort studies have suggested that besity confers increased risk for SCD, independ-nt of other comorbidities such as DM and CAD. n an initial analysis from the Paris Prospective I ohort study restricted to middle-aged males, ody mass index (BMI) was an independent risk actor for SCD.[31] In the Nurses Health Study, cohort of 121,701 U.S. women followed for over 0 years, obese women (BMI $\geq 30\,kg/m^2$) had a .6-fold increased risk of SCD, compared to vomen with a BMI $<25\,kg/m^2$.[32] When DM and ypertension were excluded as terms in the mul-ivariate model, this risk was 2.5-fold (95% CI, .7–3.7). However, the relationship between obe-ity and SCD has been evaluated only in restricted ge/gender/occupation cohorts. The role of besity as a determinant of SCD among the general opulation needs to be further investigated. First bserved in the United States, the epidemic of besity has now become pandemic, spreading to ther industrialized nations as well as the devel-ping world.[69–71] In the United States, approxi-nately 70% of adults are presently classified as verweight or obese compared with less than 25%, 0 years ago.[72,73] A significant rise in the percent-ge of men and women in the severely obese and norbidly obese group is particularly disturbing.[74] A recent analysis from the U.S. Centers for Disease Control (CDC) indicated that obesity currently accounts for over 300,000 deaths annually in the United States and in the near future will overtake tobacco abuse as the leading preventable cause of death.[75,76]

Socioeconomic Status and Sudden Cardiac Death

While socioeconomic factors are likely to have significant effects on incidence of SCA,[2,77,78] until recently this association had not been evaluated in a prospective, population-based manner. In addition, most studies of primary cardiac arrest limit evaluation to those subjects who undergo resuscitation. As a result, the 40–50% of overall SCA cases that are unwitnessed or do not undergo attempted resuscitation may not be included in most existing analyses. In the ongoing Ore-SUDS,[79] we performed a 2-year prospective evaluation of the potential relationship between socioeconomic status and occurrence of SCA evaluating both address of residence as well as specific geographic location of cardiac arrest.[80] Analysis was conducted for both witnessed and unwitnessed SCA cases. In this investigation of all cases of SCA in a large urban and suburban U.S. county (population 670,000), the incidence of SCA based on address of residence was 30–80% higher among residents of neighborhoods in the lowest socioeconomic status quartile compared to neighborhoods in the highest socioeconomic status quartile. The gradient of socioeconomic status was significantly steeper for patients under age 65 years vs. over 65 years. Identical as well as significant effects were observed based on geographic location of SCA. Given that automated external defibrillators (AEDs) are likely to have a significant beneficial impact on survival from out-of-hospital SCA,[81,82] these findings would suggest that for the placement of AEDs in the community, neighborhood SES should be taken into consideration. In the long term, there are likely to be multiple factors that result in the observed association between socioeconomic status and SCA, and these merit further evaluation. Risk factors for CAD such as lack of physical activity, smoking, hyperlipidemia, hypertension, obesity, and DM are more common among individuals with lower socioeconomic status.[78,83,84] A study conducted in the UK found that the incidence of out-of-hospital SCA was significantly higher in areas of socioeconomic deprivation, but the same was not true for overall CAD.[85] A contributory role of psychosocial factors as direct triggers of ventricular arrhythmias and consequent SCA has also been postulated.[77]

Genetic Contributions to Sudden Cardiac Death

Two large retrospective cohort studies have provided evidence that genetic factors influence susceptibility to SCD. Friedlander *et al.*[86] analyzed the potential association with SCA in a cohort of men and women attended by first responders in King County, Washington (235 cases and 374 controls). The second study, conducted in Paris,[31] analyzed deaths in a cohort of 7746 asymptomatic middle aged males followed for a mean of 23 years, using retrospective autopsy and clinical data analyses to classify cardiac deaths as either SCD or MI. Multivariate analyses indicated that the occurrence of SCD in a parent results in a 1.6- to1.8-fold increase in SCD susceptibility despite controlling for conventional risk factors for CAD (e.g., cholesterol subfractions, blood pressure, obesity, and smoking). In a very limited number of cases in the Paris study, where there was a history of both maternal and paternal SCD events ($n = 19$), the relative risk in offspring was ~9 ($p = 0.01$), indicating an additive genetic model. The familial incidence of SCD in the Paris study segregated independently of familial incidence of death due to acute MI. Given this evidence of significant genetic contribution to SCD, the next logical step is to identify culprit gene defects that could be used for screening and identification of the high-risk patient. The difficulty in accomplishing this goal is that of the approximately 30,000 genes that may exist in humans, less than 10% have been identified and assigned one or more functions.[87] As a result, the number of genes that we can currently implicate in fatal arrhythmogenesis is very small, with most of the genome being unexplored in this regard. We therefore need to identify candidate genes using approaches that will incorporate scanning of the whole genome.

There are two other significant issues that nee to be resolved before we can perform a search fo candidate genes.[87] Both deal with the comple nature of the SCD phenotype. First, most patient with SCD have multiple associated disease condi tions such as CAD, DM, obesity, and heart failure Each one of such conditions may also involv genes that are specific for that condition but ma not be involved in SCD. Therefore genes that con tribute to the occurrence of SCD have to be sepa rated from genes that lead to associated conditions Second, even for the so-called "monogenic syn dromes" such as the long QT syndrome, there may be additional modifier genes that are in volved.[88,89] For the complex phenotype of overal SCD, it is quite likely that for an individual patient screening may have to be conducted for a pane of genes instead of a single gene. With new tool for analyzing the genome being developed at a rapid pace, methodologies for identification o new SCD genetic targets are also a moving target For this purpose, traditional candidate gene approaches have a limited possibility of success especially for non-Mendelian diseases and com plex traits such as SCD[87] In theory, it is possible that candidates that are linked to monogenic con ditions such as the long QT syndrome could also have some role in fatal arrhythmogenesis among unrelated individuals in the general population However, initial attempts to test this hypothesi have not had a significant yield. In the ongoing Oregon Sudden Unexpected Death Study[79], the potential role of SCN5A allelic variants (also implicated in long QT syndrome 3) in determin ing risk of SCD was evaluated among patients with CAD using a case–control design. Nonsyn onymous as well as synonymous single nucleotide polymorphisms in the coding regions were evenly distributed between cases and controls and there fore did not confer increased risk of SCD in thi population of primarily white subjects with CAD and SCA[16] Recently an interesting association has been reported between familial short QT interva and increased risk of fatal arrhythmia,[90–92] but this has not been evaluated among unrelated individ uals in the general population. Furthermore, reg ulatory mutations at sites distant from a known and identified gene can have a significant effect[93] on development of a disease phenotype. Conse quently, alternative approaches that use a very igh-resolution map of single nucleotide polymorphisms (SNPs)[94] to search for associations, inkage disequilibrium, or a small shared genomic egment among affected individuals are likely to e necessary.

Proof of concept has recently been published or a cardiac phenotype and a novel gene using he technique of whole genome association.[95] A ommon gene variant in NOS1AP1 (regulator of euronal nitric oxide synthase) that modulates ardiac repolarization (i.e., the QT interval) was dentified from a large sample population of unreated individuals by comparing the genomes of atients with relatively long QT intervals to those vith shorter QT intervals.[95] While genes for SCD using population-based approaches have not yet een identified, this is likely to be investigated in he very near future.[87]

Summary and Conclusions

Predictors of SCD are likely to be diverse and mulifactorial. While the LVEF is a valuable predictor of SCD, the majority of individuals in the general opulation who suffer from SCD do not appear to ave severe LV systolic dysfunction. As a consequence, there is a significant need to extend eyond the LVEF and identify novel predictors of SCD. This review has discussed several clinical redictors that appear to have promise, but a nore detailed evaluation will be required, particularly in large population-based investigations. The availability of potential genetic predictors is mminent, but these will also require validation in nultiple populations before they can find utility n day-to-day clinical risk stratification. For risk tratification of SCD to be comprehensive, factors as diverse as genomics and socioeconomic status nay have to be taken into consideration.

References

1. Cobb LA, Fahrenbruch CE, Olsufka M, Copass MK. Changing incidence of out-of-hospital ventricular fibrillation, 1980–2000. *JAMA* 2002;288(23):3008–3013.
2. Escobedo LG, Zack MM. Comparison of sudden and nonsudden coronary deaths in the United States. *Circulation* 1996;93(11):2033–2036.
3. Myerburg RJ. Scientific gaps in the prediction and prevention of sudden cardiac death. *J Cardiovasc Electrophysiol* 2002;13(7):709–723.
4. Zheng ZJ, Croft JB, Giles WH, Mensah GA. Sudden cardiac death in the United States, 1989 to 1998. *Circulation* 2001;104(18):2158–2163.
5. Bardy GH, Lee KL, Mark DB, Poole JE, Packer DL, Boineau R, *et al.* Amiodarone or an implantable cardioverter-defibrillator for congestive heart failure. *N Engl J Med* 2005;352(3):225–237.
6. Buxton AE, Lee KL, Fisher JD, Josephson ME, Prystowsky EN, Hafley G. A randomized study of the prevention of sudden death in patients with coronary artery disease. Multicenter Unsustained Tachycardia Trial Investigators. *N Engl J Med* 1999;341(25):1882–1890.
7. Moss AJ, Hall WJ, Cannom DS, Daubert JP, Higgins SL, Klein H, *et al.* Improved survival with an implanted defibrillator in patients with coronary disease at high risk for ventricular arrhythmia. Multicenter Automatic Defibrillator Implantation Trial Investigators. *N Engl J Med* 1996;335(26):1933–1940.
8. Moss AJ, Zareba W, Jackson Hall W, Klein H, Wilber DJ, Cannom DS, *et al.* Prophylactic implantation of a defibrillator in patients with myocardial infarction and reduced ejection fraction. *N Engl J Med* 2002;346(12):877–883.
9. Jauhar S, Slotwiner DJ. The economics of ICDs. *N Engl J Med* 2004;351(24):2542–2544.
10. Moss AJ. Prognosis after myocardial infarction. *Am J Cardiol* 1983;52(7):667–669.
11. The Antiarrhythmics versus Implantable Defibrillators (AVID) Investigators. A comparison of antiarrhythmic-drug therapy with implantable defibrillators in patients resuscitated from near-fatal ventricular arrhythmias. *N Engl J Med* 1997; 337(22):1576–1583.
12. Stevenson LW. Implantable cardioverter-defibrillators for primary prevention of sudden death in heart failure: Are there enough bangs for the bucks? *Circulation* 2006;114(2):101–103.
13. Myerburg RJ, Mitrani R, Interian A Jr, Castellanos A. Interpretation of outcomes of antiarrhythmic clinical trials: Design features and population impact. *Circulation* 1998;97(15):1514–1521.
14. de Vreede-Swagemakers JJ, Gorgels AP, Dubois-Arbouw WI, van Ree JW, Daemen MJ, Houben LG, *et al.* Out-of-hospital cardiac arrest in the 1990's: A population-based study in the Maastricht area on incidence, characteristics and survival. *J Am Coll Cardiol* 1997;30(6):1500–1505.
15. Gorgels AP, Gijsbers C, de Vreede-Swagemakers J, Lousberg A, Wellens HJ. Out-of-hospital cardiac

arrest–the relevance of heart failure. The Maastricht Circulatory Arrest Registry. *Eur Heart J* 2003;24(13):1204–1209.
16. Stecker EC, Vickers C, Waltz J, Socoteanu C, John BT, Mariani R, *et al.* Population-based analysis of sudden cardiac death with and without left ventricular systolic dysfunction: Two-year findings from the Oregon Sudden Unexpected Death Study. *J Am Coll Cardiol* 2006;47(6):1161–1166.
17. DiMarco JP. Implantable cardioverter-defibrillators. *N Engl J Med* 2003;349(19):1836–1847.
18. Curran ME, Splawski I, Timothy KW, Vincent GM, Green ED, Keating MT. A molecular basis for cardiac arrhythmia: HERG mutations cause long QT syndrome. *Cell* 1995;80(5):795–803.
19. Keating MT, Sanguinetti MC. Molecular and cellular mechanisms of cardiac arrhythmias. *Cell* 2001;104(4):569–580.
20. Moss AJ, Schwartz PJ, Crampton RS, Tzivoni D, Locati EH, MacCluer J, *et al.* The long QT syndrome. Prospective longitudinal study of 328 families. *Circulation* 1991;84(3):1136–1144.
21. Splawski I, Tristani-Firouzi M, Lehmann MH, Sanguinetti MC, Keating MT. Mutations in the hminK gene cause long QT syndrome and suppress IKs function. *Nat Genet* 1997;17(3):338–340.
22. Algra A, Tijssen JG, Roelandt JR, Pool J, Lubsen J. QTc prolongation measured by standard 12-lead electrocardiography is an independent risk factor for sudden death due to cardiac arrest. *Circulation* 1991;83(6):1888–1894.
23. Moss AJ. QTc prolongation and sudden cardiac death: The association is in the detail. *J Am Coll Cardiol* 2006;47(2):368–369.
24. Straus SM, Kors JA, De Bruin ML, van der Hooft CS, Hofman A, Heeringa J, *et al.* Prolonged QTc interval and risk of sudden cardiac death in a population of older adults. *J Am Coll Cardiol* 2006; 47(2):362–367.
25. Dekker JM, Schouten EG, Klootwijk P, Pool J, Kromhout D. Association between QT interval and coronary heart disease in middle- aged and elderly men. The Zutphen Study. *Circulation* 1994;90(2): 779–785.
26. Elming H, Holm E, Jun L, Torp-Pedersen C, Kober L, Kircshoff M, *et al.* The prognostic value of the QT interval and QT interval dispersion in all-cause and cardiac mortality and morbidity in a population of Danish citizens. *Eur Heart J* 1998;19(9):1391–1400.
27. Goldberg RJ, Bengtson J, Chen ZY, Anderson KM, Locati E, Levy D. Duration of the QT interval and total and cardiovascular mortality in healthy persons (The Framingham Heart Study exper ence). *Am J Cardiol* 1991;67(1):55–58.
28. Karjalainen J, Reunanen A, Ristola P, Viitasalo M QT interval as a cardiac risk factor in a middle age population. *Heart* 1997;77(6):543–548.
29. Schouten EG, Dekker JM, Meppelink P, Kok F Vandenbroucke JP, Pool J. QT interval prolonga tion predicts cardiovascular mortality in an appa ently healthy population. *Circulation* 1991;84(4 1516–1523.
30. Balkau B, Jouven X, Ducimetiere P, Eschwege E Diabetes as a risk factor for sudden death. *Lanc* 1999;354(9194):1968–1969.
31. Jouven X, Desnos M, Guerot C, Ducimetiere I Predicting sudden death in the population: Th Paris Prospective Study I. *Circulation* 1999;99(15 1978–1983.
32. Albert CM, Chae CU, Grodstein F, Rose LM Rexrode KM, Ruskin JN, *et al.* Prospective study c sudden cardiac death among women in the Unite States. *Circulation* 2003;107(16):2096–2101.
33. Albert CM, Mittleman MA, Chae CU, Lee IM, Hen nekens CH, Manson JE. Triggering of sudden deat from cardiac causes by vigorous exertion. *N Engl Med* 2000;343(19):1355–1361.
34. Jouven X, Lemaitre RN, Rea TD, Sotoodehnia N Empana JP, Siscovick DS. Diabetes, glucose leve and risk of sudden cardiac death. *Eur Heart* 2005;26(20):2142–2147.
35. Beckman JA, Creager MA, Libby P. Diabetes an atherosclerosis: Epidemiology, pathophysiology and management. *JAMA* 2002;287(19):2570–2581.
36. Fang ZY, Prins JB, Marwick TH. Diabetic cardiomy opathy: Evidence, mechanisms, and therapeuti implications. *Endocr Rev* 2004;25(4):543–567.
37. Govind S, Saha S, Brodin LA, Ramesh SS, Arvin SR, Quintana M. Impaired myocardial functiona reserve in hypertension and diabetes mellitu without coronary artery disease: Searching for th possible link with congestive heart failure in th myocardial Doppler in diabetes (MYDID) Study II *Am J Hypertens* 2006;19(8):851–857.
38. Veglio M, Borra M, Stevens LK, Fuller JH, Perin PC The relation between QTc interval prolongatio and diabetic complications. The EURODIAB IDDM Complication Study Group. *Diabetologia* 1999 42(1):68–75.
39. Cardoso CR, Salles GF, Deccache W. QTc interva prolongation is a predictor of future strokes i patients with type 2 diabetes mellitus. *Strok* 2003;34(9):2187–2194.
40. Rana BS, Lim PO, Naas AA, Ogston SA, Newto RW, Jung RT, *et al.* QT interval abnormalities ar

often present at diagnosis in diabetes and are better predictors of cardiac death than ankle brachial pressure index and autonomic function tests. *Heart* 2005;91(1):44–50.

1. Lloyd-Mostyn RH, Watkins PJ. Defective innervation of heart in diabetic autonomic neuropathy. *Br Med J* 1975;3(5974):15–17.

2. Nesto RW. Correlation between cardiovascular disease and diabetes mellitus: Current concepts. *Am J Med* 2004;116(Suppl. 5A):11S–22S.

3. Pourmoghaddas A, Hekmatnia A. The relationship between QTc interval and cardiac autonomic neuropathy in diabetes mellitus. *Mol Cell Biochem* 2003;249(1–2):125–128.

4. Veglio M, Chinaglia A, Borra M, Perin PC. Does abnormal QT interval prolongation reflect autonomic dysfunction in diabetic patients? QTc interval measure versus standardized tests in diabetic autonomic neuropathy. *Diabet Med* 1995;12(4):302–306.

5. Vakili BA, Okin PM, Devereux RB. Prognostic implications of left ventricular hypertrophy. *Am Heart J* 2001;141(3):334–341.

6. Cameron JS, Myerburg RJ, Wong SS, Gaide MS, Epstein K, Alvarez TR, *et al.* Electrophysiologic consequences of chronic experimentally induced left ventricular pressure overload. *J Am Coll Cardiol* 1983;2(3):481–487.

7. Cerbai E, Barbieri M, Li Q, Mugelli A. Ionic basis of action potential prolongation of hypertrophied cardiac myocytes isolated from hypertensive rats of different ages. *Cardiovasc Res* 1994;28(8):1180–1187.

8. Nordin C, Siri F, Aronson RS. Electrophysiologic characteristics of single myocytes isolated from hypertrophied guinea-pig hearts. *J Mol Cell Cardiol* 1989;21(7):729–739.

9. Tomita F, Bassett AL, Myerburg RJ, Kimura S. Diminished transient outward currents in rat hypertrophied ventricular myocytes. *Circ Res* 1994; 75(2):296–303.

0. Ben-David J, Zipes DP, Ayers GM, Pride HP. Canine left ventricular hypertrophy predisposes to ventricular tachycardia induction by phase 2 early afterdepolarizations after administration of BAY K 8644. *J Am Coll Cardiol* 1992;20(7):1576–1584.

1. Furukawa T, Bassett AL, Furukawa N, Kimura S, Myerburg RJ. The ionic mechanism of reperfusion-induced early afterdepolarizations in feline left ventricular hypertrophy. *J Clin Invest* 1993;91(4): 1521–1531.

2. Qin D, Zhang ZH, Caref EB, Boutjdir M, Jain P, el-Sherif N. Cellular and ionic basis of arrhythmias in postinfarction remodeled ventricular myocardium. *Circ Res* 1996;79(3):461–473.

53. Wolk R. Arrhythmogenic mechanisms in left ventricular hypertrophy. *Europace* 2000;2(3):216–223.

54. Severs NJ. Gap junction alterations in the failing heart. *Eur Heart J* 1994;15(Suppl. D):53–57.

55. Spach MS, Boineau JP. Microfibrosis produces electrical load variations due to loss of side-to-side cell connections: A major mechanism of structural heart disease arrhythmias. *Pacing Clin Electrophysiol* 1997;20(2Pt. 2):397–413.

56. Weber KT, Brilla CG, Campbell SE. Regulatory mechanisms of myocardial hypertrophy and fibrosis: Results of in vivo studies. *Cardiology* 1992; 81(4–5):266–273.

57. El-Sherif N, Scherlag BJ, Lazzara R, Hope RR. Re-entrant ventricular arrhythmias in the late myocardial infarction period. 1. Conduction characteristics in the infarction zone. Circulation 1977;55(5): 686–702.

58. El-Sherif N, Turitto G. Risk stratification and management of sudden cardiac death: A new paradigm. *J Cardiovasc Electrophysiol* 2003;14(10): 1113–1119.

59. Luke RA, Saffitz JE. Remodeling of ventricular conduction pathways in healed canine infarct border zones. *J Clin Invest* 1991;87(5):1594–1602.

60. Lip GY, Blann AD, Beevers DG. Prothrombotic factors, endothelial function and left ventricular hypertrophy in isolated systolic hypertension compared with systolic-diastolic hypertension. *J Hypertens* 1999;17(8):1203–1207.

61. Varughese GI, Lip GY. Is hypertension a prothrombotic state? *Curr Hypertens Rep* 2005;7(3): 168–173.

62. Haider AW, Larson MG, Benjamin EJ, Levy D. Increased left ventricular mass and hypertrophy are associated with increased risk for sudden death. *J Am Coll Cardiol* 1998;32(5):1454–1459.

63. East MA, Jollis JG, Nelson CL, Marks D, Peterson ED. The influence of left ventricular hypertrophy on survival in patients with coronary artery disease: Do race and gender matter? *J Am Coll Cardiol* 2003;41(6):949–954.

64. Ghali JK, Liao Y, Simmons B, Castaner A, Cao G, Cooper RS. The prognostic role of left ventricular hypertrophy in patients with or without coronary artery disease. *Ann Intern Med* 1992;117(10): 831–836.

65. Sukhija R, Aronow WS, Kakar P, Levy JA, Lehrman SG, Babu S. Prevalence of echocardiographic left ventricular hypertrophy in persons with systemic hypertension, coronary artery disease, and

peripheral arterial disease and in persons with systemic hypertension, coronary artery disease, and no peripheral arterial disease. *Am J Cardiol* 2005;96(6):825–826.

66. Burke AP, Farb A, Liang YH, Smialek J, Virmani R. Effect of hypertension and cardiac hypertrophy on coronary artery morphology in sudden cardiac death. *Circulation* 1996;94(12):3138–3145.
67. Burke AP, Farb A, Pestaner J, Malcom GT, Zieske A, Kutys R, *et al.* Traditional risk factors and the incidence of sudden coronary death with and without coronary thrombosis in blacks. *Circulation* 2002;105(4):419–424.
68. Bayes de Luna A, Coumel P, Leclercq JF. Ambulatory sudden cardiac death: Mechanisms of production of fatal arrhythmia on the basis of data from 157 cases. *Am Heart J* 1989;117(1):151–159.
69. Mokdad AH, Ford ES, Bowman BA, Dietz WH, Vinicor F, Bales VS, *et al.* Prevalence of obesity, diabetes, and obesity-related health risk factors, 2001. *JAMA* 2003;289(1):76–79.
70. Mokdad AH, Serdula MK, Dietz WH, Bowman BA, Marks JS, Koplan JP. The spread of the obesity epidemic in the United States, 1991–1998. *JAMA* 1999;282(16):1519–1522.
71. Roth J, Qiang X, Marban SL, Redelt H, Lowell BC. The obesity pandemic: Where have we been and where are we going? *Obes Res* 2004;12(Suppl. 2): 88S–101S.
72. Flegal KM, Carroll MD, Ogden CL, Johnson CL. Prevalence and trends in obesity among US adults, 1999–2000. *JAMA* 2002;288(14):1723–1727.
73. Manson JE, Bassuk SS. Obesity in the United States: A fresh look at its high toll. *JAMA* 2003;289(2): 229–230.
74. Flegal KM, Carroll MD, Kuczmarski RJ, Johnson CL. Overweight and obesity in the United States: Prevalence and trends, 1960–1994. *Int J Obes Relat Metab Disord* 1998;22(1):39–47.
75. Mokdad AH, Marks JS, Stroup DF, Gerberding JL. Actual causes of death in the United States, 2000. *JAMA* 2004;291(10):1238–1245.
76. Mokdad AH, Marks JS, Stroup DF, Gerberding JL. Correction: Actual causes of death in the United States, 2000. *JAMA* 2005;293(3):293–294.
77. Hemingway H, Malik M, Marmot M. Social and psychosocial influences on sudden cardiac death, ventricular arrhythmia and cardiac autonomic function. *Eur Heart J* 2001;22(13):1082–1101.
78. Mensah GA, Mokdad AH, Ford ES, Greenlund KJ, Croft JB. State of disparities in cardiovascular health in the United States. *Circulation* 2005; 111(10):1233–1241.
79. Chugh SS, Jui J, Gunson K, Stecker EC, John BT Thompson B, *et al.* Current burden of sudde cardiac death: Multiple source surveillance versu retrospective death certificate-based review in large U.S. community. *J Am Coll Cardiol* 2004 44(6):1268–1275.
80. Reinier K, Stecker EC, Vickers C, Gunson K Jui J, Chugh SS. Incidence of sudden cardia arrest is higher in areas of low socioeconomi status: A prospective two year study in a larg United States community. *Resuscitation* 2006 70(2):186–192.
81. Hallstrom AP, Ornato JP, Weisfeldt M, Travers A Christenson J, McBurnie MA, *et al.* Public-acces defibrillation and survival after out-of-hospita cardiac arrest. *N Engl J Med* 2004;351(7):637–646.
82. Hazinski MF, Idris AH, Kerber RE, Epstein A Atkins D, Tang W, *et al.* Lay rescuer automate external defibrillator ("public access defibrilla tion") programs: Lessons learned from an interna tional multicenter trial: Advisory statement fron the American Heart Association Emergency Cardi ovascular Committee; the Council on Cardiopul monary, Perioperative, and Critical Care; and th Council on Clinical Cardiology. *Circulation* 2005 111(24):3336–3340.
83. Jaglal SB, Goel V. Social inequity in risk of coronar artery disease in Ontario. *Can J Cardiol* 1994;10(4) 439–443.
84. Rozanski A, Blumenthal JA, Davidson KW, Saal PG, Kubzansky L. The epidemiology, pathophysiol ogy, and management of psychosocial risk factor in cardiac practice: The emerging field of behavio ral cardiology. *J Am Coll Cardiol* 2005;45(5):637 651.
85. Soo L, Huff N, Gray D, Hampton JR. Geographica distribution of cardiac arrest in Nottinghamshire *Resuscitation* 2001;48(2):137–147.
86. Friedlander Y, Siscovick DS, Weinmann S, Austi MA, Psaty BM, Lemaitre RN, *et al.* Family histor as a risk factor for primary cardiac arres *Circulation* 1998;97(2):155–160.
87. Arking DE, Chugh SS, Chakravarti A, Spooner PM Genomics in sudden cardiac death. *Circ Res* 2004 94(6):712–723.
88. Benhorin J, Moss AJ, Bak M, Zareba W, Kaufma ES, Kerem B, *et al.* Variable expression of long QT syndrome among gene carriers from families wit five different HERG mutations. *Ann Noninvasiv Electrocardiol* 2002;7(1):40–46.
89. Crotti L, Lundquist AL, Insolia R, Pedrazzini M Ferrandi C, De Ferrari GM, *et al.* KCNH2-K897T is a genetic modifier of latent congenital long-QT syndrome. *Circulation* 2005;112(9):1251–1258.

0. Bellocq C, van Ginneken AC, Bezzina CR, Alders M, Escande D, Mannens MM, *et al.* Mutation in the KCNQ1 gene leading to the short QT-interval syndrome. *Circulation* 2004;109(20):2394–2397.
1. Gaita F, Giustetto C, Bianchi F, Wolpert C, Schimpf R, Riccardi R, *et al.* Short QT syndrome: A familial cause of sudden death. *Circulation* 2003;108(8): 965–970.
2. Gussak I, Brugada P, Brugada J, Wright RS, Kopecky SL, Chaitman BR, *et al.* Idiopathic short QT interval: A new clinical syndrome? *Cardiology* 2000; 94(2):99–102.
93. Lettice LA, Horikoshi T, Heaney SJ, van Baren MJ, van der Linde HC, Breedveld GJ, *et al.* Disruption of a long-range cis-acting regulator for Shh causes preaxial polydactyly. *Proc Natl Acad Sci USA* 2002;99(11):7548–7553.
94. Lander ES. The new genomics: Global views of biology. *Science* 1996;274(5287):536–539.
95. Arking DE, Pfeufer A, Post W, Kao WH, Newton-Cheh C, Ikeda M, *et al.* A common genetic variant in the NOS1 regulator NOS1AP modulates cardiac repolarization. *Nat Genet* 2006;38(6): 644–651.

30
Genetic Testing

David J. Tester and Michael J. Ackerman

Introduction

Through advances in molecular medicine, the previous several decades of research have elucidated the fundamental genetic substrates underlying over 4000 genetic disorders, most of which are rare. Currently nearly 1000 genetic tests (www.genetest.org) are available clinically and are offered by more than 600 diagnostic laboratories worldwide. In addition, numerous genetic tests are available on a research basis.

Genetic disease is more common then once believed. In fact, genetic abnormalities are a major cause of illness and death. It is estimated that by 25 years of age, 80 per 1000 live births (8%) will suffer from a genetically based disorder.[1] This genetic load is accounted for by multifactorial disorders (4.64%), congenital anomalies with a genetic etiology (2.66%), single gene disorders (0.36%), chromosome abnormalities (0.18%), and disorders of unknown genetic etiology (0.12%). However, these values may represent an underestimate of the true prevalence of genetic involvement in disease. Many disorders once thought to be nongenetic are now understood to be multifactorial diseases with contributions from various genetic and environmental factors. Disorders of mild genetic conditions may go unrecognized. Disorders of low penetrance and variable expressivity may go undiagnosed in asymptomatic yet genetically affected individuals.

Within the field of molecular cardiac electrophysiology, the previous decade of research has elucidated the fundamental genetic substrates underlying many arrhythmogenic disorders associated with sudden cardiac death including long QT syndrome (LQTS), Andersen–Tawil syndrome (ATS), Timothy syndrome, short QT syndrome (SQTS), catecholaminergic polymorphic ventricular tachycardia (CPVT), Brugada syndrome (BrS), familial atrioventricular (AV) block, and atrial fibrillation. In addition, the molecular underpinnings for cardiomyopathic processes vulnerable to sudden arrhythmic death, such as dilated cardiomyopathy, hypertrophic cardiomyopathy, left ventricular noncompaction syndrome, and arrhythmogenic right ventricular cardiomyopathy, are now understood in greater detail. Genetic testing for several of these heritable channelopathies and cardiomyopathies are currently available through specialized clinical and/or research-based laboratories.

The purpose of this chapter is to provide the reader with a basic understanding of molecular genetics and genetic testing in the setting of cardiac electrophysiological disorders. First we will present a primer on fundamental molecular genetics including the organization of the human genome, transfer of genetic information, different modes of inheritance, and types of mutations in human genetic disease. Next, we will explore techniques utilized in genetic testing. And finally, we will tackle the important issues of genetic testing including clinical versus research-based testing, benefits of genetic testing, limitations to genetic testing, interpretation of the genetic test, role of genetic counselors, and ethical, legal, and societal implications.

'rimer on Molecular Genetics

ieneral Organization and Structure of the Iuman Genome

'hrough a multinational effort, the Human ienome Project was completed in February 2001 .shering in the molecular millennium providing he architectural blueprints of most genes in the .uman genome. The human genome represents he total genetic information or DNA content in .uman cells and is distributed among 46 chromo- omes: 22 autosomal pairs and two sex (X and Y) hromosomes.[2,3] Each chromosome contains ightly packaged linear double-stranded DNA. 'he 24 unique chromosomes are distinguished by hromosome banding techniques (karyotype nalysis) and are classified largely according o their size. The organization of the genomic)NA is rather complex. Much of the genome is nade up of single-copy DNA with precise DNA equences represented only once per genome. The emaining portion of the genome consists of everal classes of repetitive DNA, including DNA vhose sequences are repeated either perfectly or vith some variation. The human genome contains :.9 billion base pairs of genetic information ontaining the molecular blueprints for some 5,000 genes whose highly coordinated expres- ion renders us human. In contrast, the genome f the *Drosophila melanogaster* fruit fly consists f 120 million base pairs and 13,600 genes. Though he human genome contains less than three times s many genes as the fruit fly, the genes are more omplex and create a larger number of protein roducts through alternate splicing of the coding equences within the genes. Now, let us examine he basic structure of the DNA molecule and the asic hereditary element called the gene.

3asic Structure of DNA and the Basic Iereditary Element, the Gene

n 1953, Drs. Watson and Crick described the asic structure of the molecular essence of life: the leoxyribonucleic acid or DNA molecule. DNA is polymeric nucleic acid macromolecule com- osed of "building blocks" called deoxyribonucle- tides of which there are four types: adenine (A), uanine (G), thymine (T), and cytosine (C).[2,3] The DNA molecule is essentially nucleotides that are polymerized into long polynucleotide chains. DNA is said to be a double-stranded molecule made up of two antiparallel complementary strands that are held together by noncovalent (loosely held) hydrogen bonds between complementary bases where A and T always form complementary base pairs and G and C always pair (Figure 30–1). DNA in its native state forms a double helix that resembles a right-handed spiral staircase. DNA segments that store genetic information in the form of a genetic code are called genes (Figure 30–2).

Approximately 30% of the genome is spanned by genes; however, less than 2% of the genomic DNA is actually made up of protein-encoding segments within genes called exons. In between the exons are intervening DNA sequences called introns, which are not a part of the genetic code.

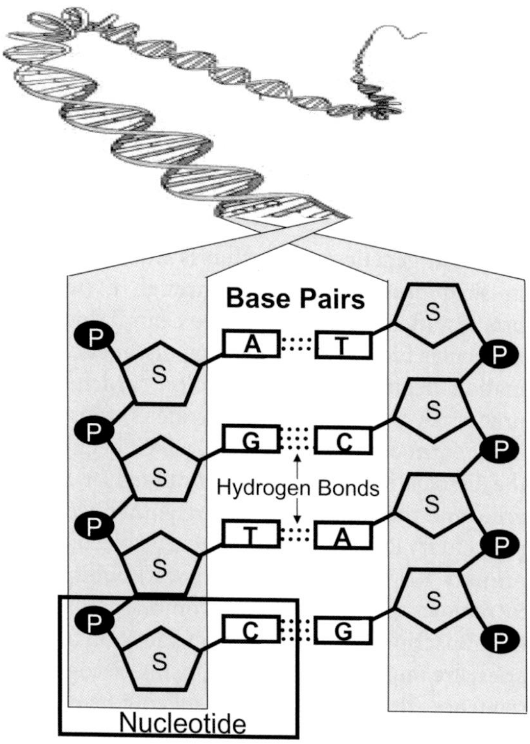

FIGURE 30–1. Depicted is the general organization of DNA, illustrating complementary base pairing via hydrogen bonds between cytosine (C) and guanine (G) and between adenine (A) and thymine (T). As defined by the box, a single nucleotide consist of a phosphate (P) group, deoxyribose sugar (S), and a base (A, C, G, or T).

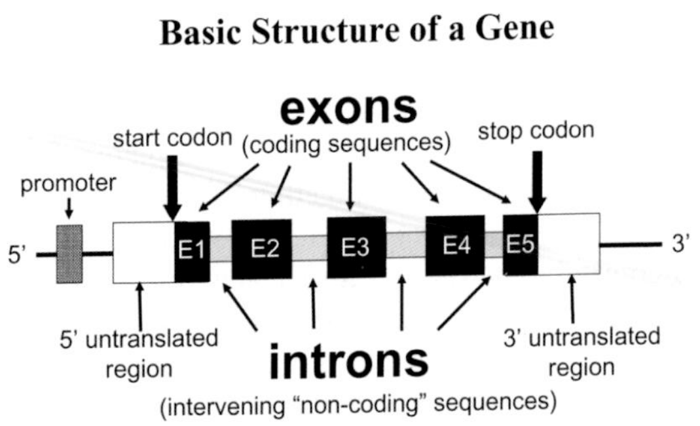

Figure 30–2. The basic structure of a gene consisting of DNA segments (exons) that encode for a protein product is shown. Between the exons are intervening sequences called introns. At the 5′ end of the gene is a regulatory element called the promoter, which initiates transcription. At the 5′ and 3′ ends are "untranslated" regions that are considered a part of the first and last exons, respectively. These sequences are not a part of the genetic code, but may contain additional regulatory elements. To begin translation of the genetic message, as encoded by the gene, is a start codon, and to terminate the message is a stop codon.

Usually upstream (20–100 bp) from the first exon is a regulatory element called the promoter, which controls transcription of the hereditary message as defined by the gene sequence.

Transfer of Genetic Information

Inherited genetic information is transferred to a finished product (protein) through a two-step process often referred to as the central dogma of molecular biology. This passage of genetic information begins with transcription, which is the process by which the genetic code is transcribed in the form of messenger RNA, which begins with the dissociation of the double-stranded DNA molecule and formation of a newly synthesized complementary RNA (ribonucleic acid) molecule. This primary RNA molecule undergoes RNA splicing to remove the noncoding intronic regions from the transcript. Within the intron and exon boundaries are highly conserved splicing recognition sequences that allow the RNA splicing machinery to know precisely were to cleave the sequence in order to remove the noncoding regions (introns) and bring the coding sequences (exons) together. If these sites are disrupted, certain consequences such as splicing errors can occur.

Next, translation involves the decoding of the mRNA-encrypted message and assembly of the intended polypeptide (protein) that will serve a biological function. Polypeptides are polymers of linear repeating units called amino acids. The assembly of a polypeptide or protein is governed by a triplet genetic code, or codon (three consecutive bases), of which there are 64 types that encode for 20 unique amino acids. One codon, ATG, encodes for the amino acid methionine and is always the first codon (start codon) to start the message. Each codon in the linear mRNA is decoded sequentially to give a specific sequence of amino acids that are covalently linked through peptide bonds and ultimately constitute a protein. Three codons, TAA, TAG, and TGA, serve as stop codons that terminate the linearization of the peptide and signal a release of the finish product. The genetic code is redundant in that more than one codon can encode for the same amino acid. For example, often when varying the nucleotide at the third position (wobble position) in a codon, the message does not become altered.

Each of the 20 amino acids has a unique side chain that provides its characteristic properties. Some amino acids are considered nonpolar and hydrophobic (water fearing), while others are polar and hydrophilic (water loving). Some amino acids are negatively charged and have acidic properties, while others are positively charged and have basic properties. It is the unique sequence in which these amino acids occur within a protein that dictates its structural and functional properties. Substituting an amino acid in a protein for an amino acid with different properties could alter the overall function of that protein and provide a pathogenic substrate for disease.

The standard nomenclature for numbering nucleotides and codons within a gene begins with the A of the start codon (ATG) representing nucleotide 1 and ATG as codon 1. Generally, only consecutive nucleotides constituting the coding region of the gene are numbered. Intronic nucleotides are numbered relative to either the first or last nucleotide in the exon preceding or following the intron. For example, the LQT1-associated KCNQ1 splice error mutation M159sp (exon 2, nucleotide substitution: 477 +5 G>A) results from a G-to-A substitution in the intron, five nucleotides following exon 2, where nucleotide 477 is the last nucleotide in the exon. This substitution results in a splicing error following the last codon of the exon [159 encoding for a methionine (M)].[4]

Genetics of Disease: Modes of Inheritance

Inherited variation in the genome is the basis of human and medical genetics. Reciprocal forms of genetic information at a specific locus (location) along the genome are called alleles.[3] An allele can correspond to a segment of DNA or even a single nucleotide. The normal version of genetic information is often considered the "wild-type" or "normal" allele. A large majority of the human genome represents a single version of genetic information. The DNA from one individual is mostly made up of the same exact nucleotide sequence from another individual. However, there are numerous small sections of sequence or even single nucleotides that vary from one individual to another. These normal variations at distinct loci in the DNA sequence are called polymorphisms.

Some polymorphisms are quite common and others represent rare forms of the genetic information. In medical genetics, a disease-causing mutation refers to a variation in DNA sequence that embodies an abnormal allele and is not found in the normal population but subsists only in the disease population. If an individual has a pair of identical alleles, one paternal (from father) and one maternal (from mother), that person is said to be homozygous for that allele. When the alleles are different, that person is said to be heterozygous for that specific allele. The terms genotype and phenotype are used to refer to an individual's genetic or DNA sequence composition at a particular loci or at a combined body of loci (genotype) and to an individual's observed clinical expression of disease (phenotype) in terms of a morphological, biochemical, or molecular trait, respectively.

Genetic disorders are characterized by their patterns of transmission within families (Figure 30–3). There are four basic modes of inheritance: autosomal dominant, autosomal recessive, X-linked dominant, and X-linked recessive.[3] These patterns of inheritance are based largely on two factors: (1) the type of chromosome (autosome or

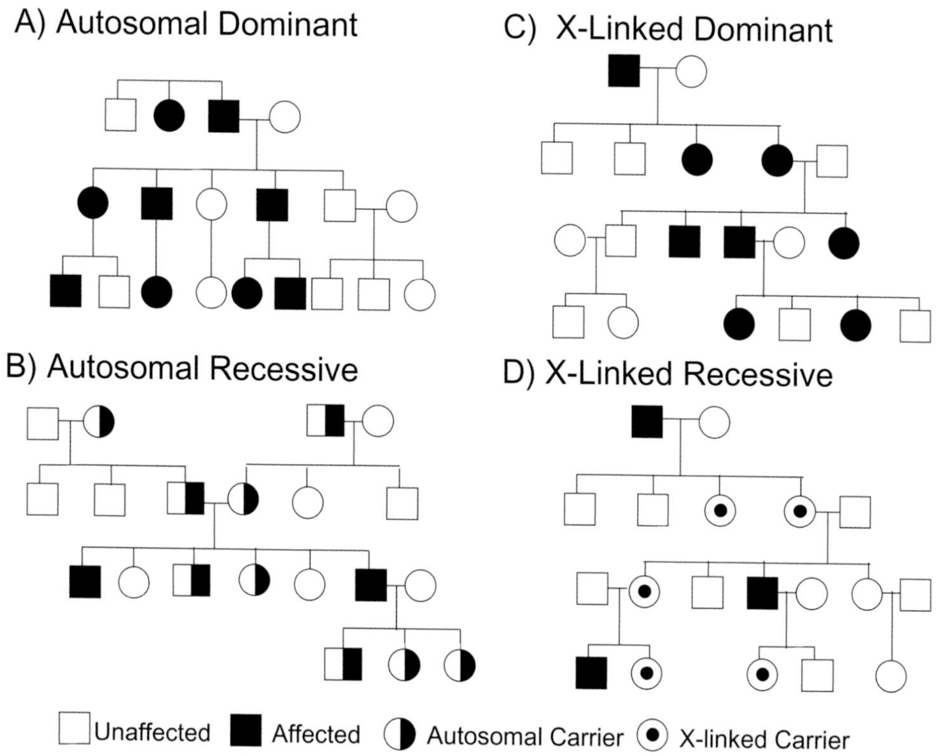

FIGURE 30–3. Pedigrees exemplifying four different modes of inheritance in human genetic disorders are illustrated: (A) autosomal dominant, (B) autosomal recessive, (C) X-linked dominant, and (D) X-linked recessive.

X-chromosome) on which the gene locus is located and (2) whether the phenotype is expressed only when both chromosomes of a pair carry an abnormal allele (recessive) or the phenotype can be expressed when just one chromosome harbors the mutant allele (dominant).

Many genetic disorders appearing monogenic are often found to be genetically heterogeneous once completely analyzed. Genetically heterogeneous disorders have a related clinical phenotype but arise from multiple different genotypes. Genetic heterogeneity may be a consequence of different mutations at the same locus (gene) or a result of mutations at different loci (genes) or both.

In many genetic disorders, the abnormal phenotype can be clearly differentiated form the normal one. However, in some disorders, the abnormal phenotype is completely absent in individuals hosting the disease-causing mutation while other individuals show extremely variable expression of phenotype in terms of clinical severity, age at onset, and response to therapy. Penetrance is the likelihood that a gene will have any expression; when the frequency of phenotypic expression is less than 100%, the gene is said to show reduced or incomplete penetrance (Figure 30–4). Expressivity refers to the level of expression of the phenotype, and when the manifestations of the phenotype in individuals who have the same genotype are diverse, the phenotype is said to exhibit variable expressivity (Figure 30–4). Reduced penetrance and variable expressivity create a significant challenge for the appropriate diagnosis, pedigree interpretation, and risk stratification for the disorder.

Genetic disorders are often subcategorized into three major groups: chromosome disorders, single gene disorders, and multifactorial disorders.

Incomplete Penetrance and Variable Expressivity

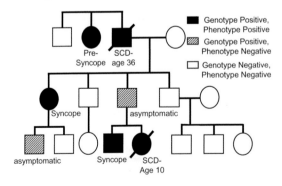

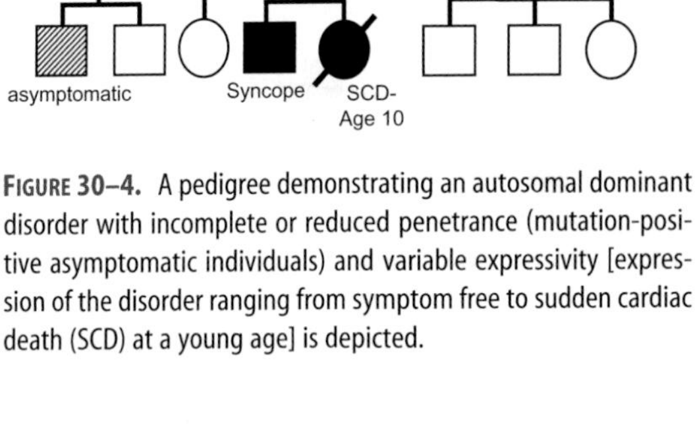

FIGURE 30–4. A pedigree demonstrating an autosomal dominant disorder with incomplete or reduced penetrance (mutation-positive asymptomatic individuals) and variable expressivity [expression of the disorder ranging from symptom free to sudden cardiac death (SCD) at a young age] is depicted.

Types of Mutations in Human Genetic Disease

Like many genomes, the DNA of the human genome is fairly stable but not immutable. Instead, it is susceptible to an assortment of different types of germline (heritable) and somatic anomalies (i.e., mutations). In general, mutations can be classified into three categories: genome mutations, chromosome mutations, and gene mutations (Figure 30–5).[3] Genome mutations entail the abnormal segregation of chromosomes during cell division. Trisomy 21 (Down syndrome) would be an example of this type of mutation where the abnormal cells contain three copies of chromosome 21 instead of two copies found in a normal cell (Figure 30–5A). Using the "encyclopedia" analogy, trisomy 21 would be similar to having an extra volume, whereas Turner's syndrome (XO) with its omitted Y chromosome would be equivalent to a missing volume. Next, chromosome mutations involve the structural breakage and rearrangement of chromosomes during cell division.

In addition, major portions of a particular chromosome may be missing (deleted) or inserted (Figure 30–5B). Patients with chromosome 22 microdeletion syndrome, for example, have variable size deletions involving the long arm of one of the #22 chromosomes (22q11.2). Such a genetic perturbation would be analogous to a specific volume of the encyclopedia having several chapters torn from the book.

Finally, gene mutations involve the alterations at the nucleotide level and disrupt the normal function of a single gene product (Figure 30–5C). Such single gene mutations are classified into three essential categories: nucleotide substitu-

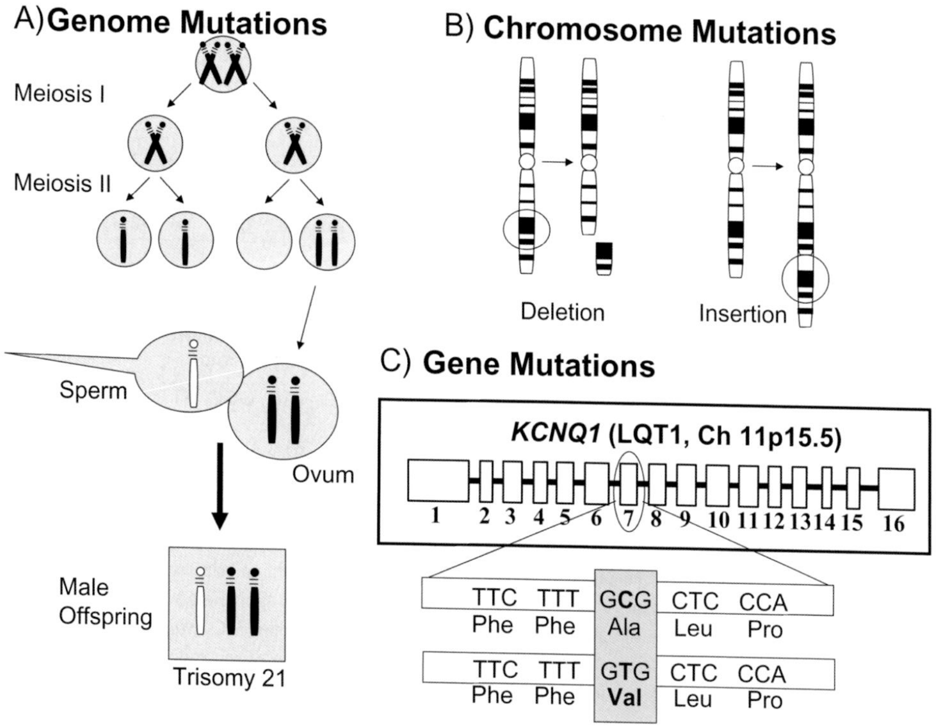

FIGURE 30–5. There are three major categories of mutations in human genetic disease. (A) Genome mutations involve the abnormal segregation of chromosomes during cell division. (B) Chromosome mutations are mutations in which major portions of chromosomes may be deleted or duplicated. (C) Gene mutations involve changes at the nucleotide level and disrupt the normal function of a single gene product.

tions, deletions, and insertions. Single nucleotide substitutions are most common and may represent a transition or a transversion. Transitions are substitutions of a purine (A or G) for a purine or a pyrimidine (C or T) for a pyrimidine. Transversions are substitutions of a purine for a pyrimidine or vice versa.

If a single nucleotide substitution occurs in the coding region (exon), the consequence may be either a synonymous (silent) mutation whereby a different codon still specifies the same amino acid or a nonsynonymous mutation whereby the altered codon dictates a different amino acid or terminates further protein assembly (i.e., introduces a premature stop codon) (Figure 30–6). The term "missense" mutation is also used to indicate a single nucleotide substitution that changes one of the protein's amino acids (Figure 30–6C). Importantly, a missense mutation may or may not result in a functionally perturbed protein. The functional consequence of a missense mutation depends on the differences in biochemical properties between the amino acids that are being exchanged and/or the location in the protein at which the exchange occurs. Again, turning to the "encyclopedia" analogy, the substitution of a single letter (for example "se**t**" and "se**x**") has a potential meaning-altering effect within a sentence. A "nonsense" mutation refers to a nonsynonymous mutation resulting in an exchange of an amino acid for a stop codon (Figure 30–6D). This type of mutation, results in a truncated (shortened) gene product at the location of the new stop codon. Again, depending on where in the protein a nonsense mutation occurs, the functional effects could range from no appreciable difference to functional lethality (a nonfunctioning protein).

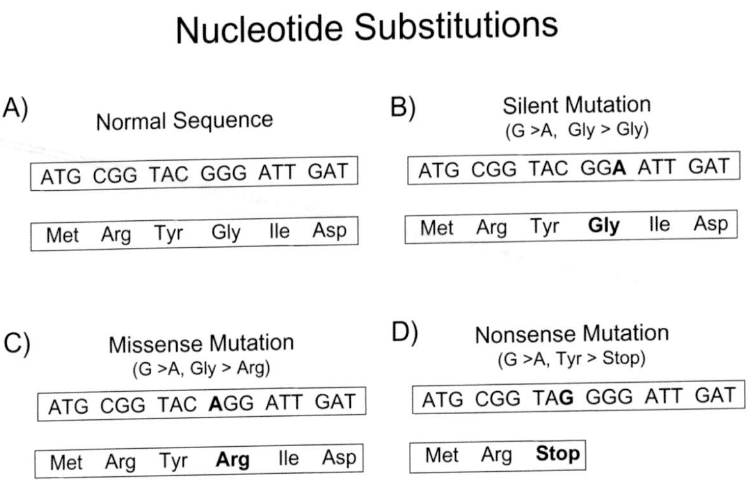

FIGURE 30–6. Examples of nucleotide substitutions. (A) Both the normal DNA and amino acid sequences. (B) A synonymous (silent) mutation. Comparing the sequence to the normal sequence (A) we see that the G>A nucleotide substitution results in a GGA codon that encodes for the same amino acid (glycine, Gly) as the reciprical codon (GGG) in the normal sequence. (C) A nonsynonymous (missense) mutation. Here a G>A nucleotide substitution results in a codon (AGG) that encodes for a different amino acid than the normal codon (GGG). Here the normal amino acid glycine (Gly) is replaced by a new amino acid arginine (Arg). (D) A nonsynonymous (nonsense) mutation. Here a C-to-G nucleotide substitution alters the normal codon (TAC), which encodes for the amino acid tyrosine (Tyr), to give a new codon (TAG), which encodes for a STOP. This mutation leads a truncated protein.

Base substitutions occurring in the intron (noncoding) can result in an altered gene product as well (Figure 30–7). The normal process by which intronic sequences are cleaved from newly transcribed RNA to give a mature messenger RNA product is reliant on specific nucleotide sequences located at the intron/exon (acceptor site) and exon/intron (donor site) boundaries. Base substitutions within these highly conserved regions can result in inappropriate splicing of the immature RNA. In some cases, entire exons can be deleted or entire introns may be included in the mature messenger RNA.

Gene mutations may also involve deletions and insertions. As their names indicate, deletions are subtractions of nucleotides from the normal DNA sequence and insertions are additions of nucleotides to the normal sequence. Both deletions and insertions can be as small as a single nucleotide or as large as several hundreds of nucleotides in length. Most of these exonic insertions and deletions alter the "reading frame" of translation at the point of the deletion/insertion and give rise to a new sequence of amino acids in the finished product, a so-called "frameshift" mutation (Figure 30–8A). Many frameshift mutations result not

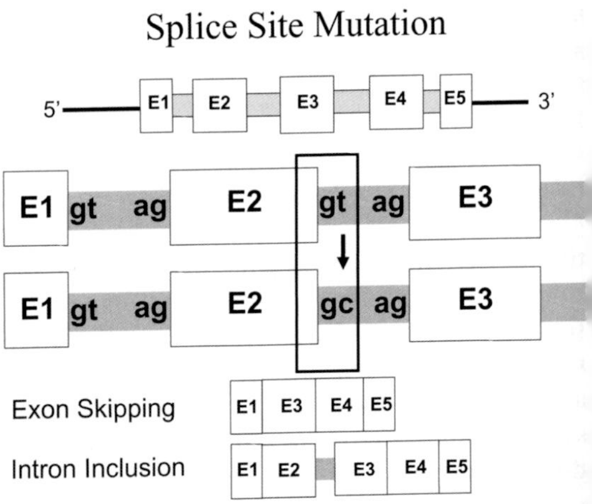

FIGURE 30–7. Splice site mutations. A schematic representation of a five-exon gene (E1–E5) is depicted. Exons are represented by white boxes. Intronic sequences are illustrated in gray. Within the intron and exon boundaries are highly conserved splicing recognition sites as shown in the black box. These particular sequences allow the RNA splicing machinery to know precisely where to cleave the sequence in order to remove the noncoding (introns) regions and bring the coding (exons) sequences together. A DNA alteration (T-to-C) that occurs within the splice recognition sequence as shown here can result in either exon skipping, where in this example exon 2 has been deleted, or intron inclusion, where intron 2 is now included in the transcript.

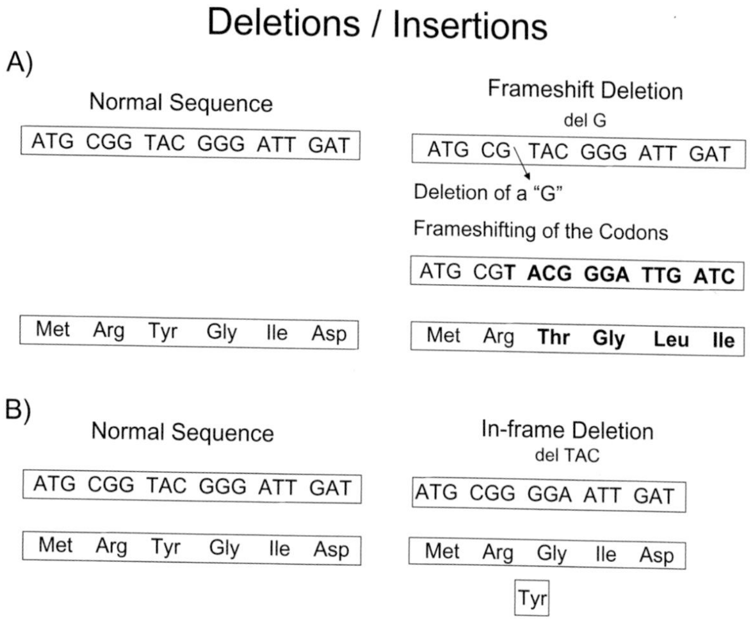

Figure 30–8. Deletion mutation. (A) A frameshift mutation. With the deletion of a single nucleotide, in this case a G in the second codon, a shift of the reading frame occurs. Note how the sequence of amino acids has been altered from this point forward. Although not illustrated here, frameshift mutations resulting from either a deletion or insertion of nucleotides often lead to a premature stop codon and thus a truncated protein. (B) An in-frame deletion mutation. Here we see that the deletion of three nucleotides (TAC) has led to the deletion of a single amino acid (tyrosine, Tyr) in the protein. The remaining amino acid sequence is left unaltered. Three nucleotide insertions (not shown) can have a similar affect, whereby an amino acid is inserted into the protein product.

only in an altered amino acid sequence from the point of the insertion or deletion, but also in a different product length from the normal gene product. Frameshifts often create a new stop codon, which give rise to either a shorter or longer gene product depending on the location of the new stop codon. In-frame deletions and insertions can occur when the number of nucleotides affected is a multiple of three (Figure 30–8B). Perhaps, the most common pathogenic in-frame mutation known occurs in cystic fibrosis. Here, a three-bp deletion in the cystic fibrosis conductance regulator (CFTR) gene that results in an altered gene product missing a single amino acid (phenylalanine at amino acid position 508) accounts for nearly 70% of cystic fibrosis.

Importantly, not all nucleotide alterations (mutations) create a new gene product that causes or modifies a clinical disease state. A DNA sequence variation/change that may (nonsynonymous) or may not (synonymous) alter the encoded protein is called a common polymorphism if present in at least 1% of the normal population. Although not pathogenic or disease causing, nonsynonymous single nucleotide polymorphisms can indeed be *functional* polymorphisms and exert a significant effect on how endogenous and exogenous triggers are handled. Functional polymorphisms are sought to explain the human variation observed with therapeutic and side effect profiles of pharmaceutical agents ("Pharmacogenomics") or to rationalize the heterogeneous expression of disease in families harboring the same, presumptive disease-causing mutation (i.e., "modifier genes").

Techniques Used in Genetic Testing at the Single Gene Level

Biological Material Used for Genetic Testing

In general, for either the research-based or clinical genetic tests, 5–15 ml of blood obtained from venipuncture placed in ethylenediamine tetraacetic acid (EDTA)-containing tubes ("purple top") is requested as the source of genomic DNA for genetic testing. Alternatively, DNA isolated from a buccal (mouth cheek) swab can also be adequate, particularly for confirmatory testing of family relatives. However, such sampling may not yield a sufficient amount of DNA for comprehensive mutational analysis. The clinically available LQTS/BrS genetic test, for example, is currently arranged for analysis from blood-derived genomic DNA rather than buccal swab sampling. Umbilical cord blood may be acquired at the time of birth for newborn screening. In cases of autopsy-negative sudden unexplained death, a cardiac channel molecular autopsy can be completed on EDTA blood if isolated.[5] Alternatively, genomic DNA can be extracted from a piece of frozen tissue. The tissue requested is typically left ventricle myocardium, although any organ (liver, spleen, thymus) with a high nucleus-to-cytoplasm ratio will suffice. Both research-based and clinical genetic testing require a signed and dated informed consent accompanying the samples to be tested.

Polymerase Chain Reaction

The identification of gene mutations typically involves the polymerase chain reaction (PCR) technique used to amplify many copies of a specific region of DNA sequence within the gene of interest. Generally, 20–25 bp forward and reverse oligonucleotide primers are designed to be com plementary to reciprocal intronic DNA sequence flanking the exon (amino acid encoding) of inter est in order to produce PCR products (200–400 bp in length) containing the desired exon to be ana lyzed. When analyzing large exons, overlapping PCR products may need to be designed. It i critical that primers be designed properly in thi mutation detection process as false negative secondary to poor primer design and possibl allelic drop-out can occur (Figure 30–9). For ex ample, in LQTS, the differential amplification o a single allele due to the prevention of prime annealing during PCR (termed allelic dropout was reported recently as a mechanism underlying false-negative genetic test results.[6]

Briefly, a genomic DNA sample isolated fron blood or tissue is pooled with both the forwarc and reverse amplification primer specific for th region of desired amplification (usually an entir

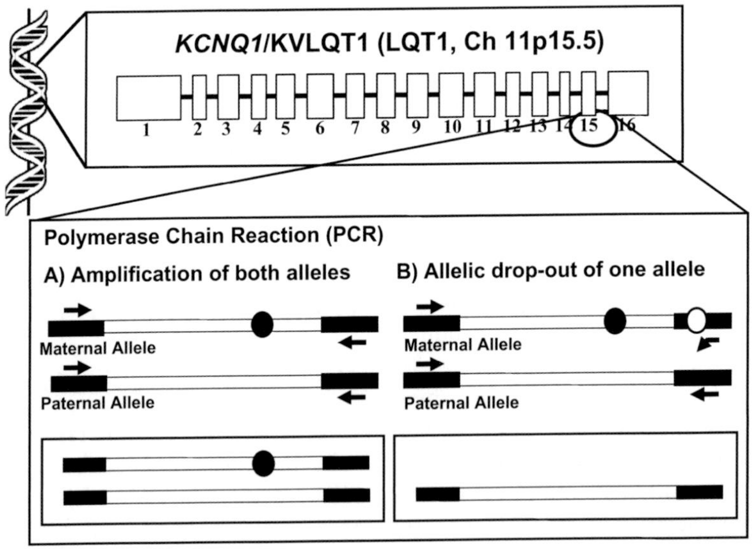

FIGURE 30–9. Allelic drop-out: a possible mechanism explaining false-negative results. To understand how allelic drop-out can cause false negative results, we first need to explore the general design of how PCR is performed for mutation analysis using genomic DNA. By focusing on LQTS-associated exon 15 of *KCNQ1*, we can see how a PCR reaction is first designed to amplify both the maternal and paternal alleles. By designing a forward and reverse primer complementary to flanking intronic DNA sequences, PCR products containing the desired exon can be produced. (A) If a mutation exists on one of the alleles as depicted here with a black circle, then PCR amplification of this sample would generate products containing the mutation tha could be easily detected by most mutation detection platforms such as DHPLC. (B) However, if a single nucleotide polymorphism or SNP (white circle) is localized to the same allele as the muta tion (black circle) and is within the sequence complementary to the 3′ end of the primer such that the primer annealing is dis rupted, then amplification of that allele would not occur and the mutation would be missed. This in essence defines allelic drop-out.

exon) along with a reaction mixture containing dinucleotides (dATP, dCTP, dGTP, and dTTP) or "DNA building blocks" and a DNA polymerase. The reaction mixture is subjected to cycling (typically 30–40 cycles) of specific temperatures designed to denature (95°C) double-stranded DNA, allow for primer annealing (typically at 55–62°C), and extend (72°C) the new synthesized DNA strand. A well-optimized PCR reaction will yield millions of copies of only the specific sequence of interest. These PCR products can be used in numerous downstream molecular techniques.

Intermediate Mutation Detection: Denaturing High-Performance Liquid Chromotagraphy

Polymerase chain reaction amplification is often followed by the use of an intermediate mutation detection platform such as single-stranded conformational polymorphism (SSCP) or denaturing high-performance liquid chromatography (DHPLC). These methods are used to inform the investigator of the presence or absence of a DNA sequence change in the samples examined. Denaturing high-performance liquid chromatography is one of the most sensitive and accurate technologies for the discovery of unknown gene mutations.[7,8] It is based on the creation and separation of double-stranded DNA fragments containing a mismatch in the base pairing between the "wild-type" and "mutant" DNA strands, known as heteroduplex DNA. In general, PCR products are subjected to denaturing (heating) and reannealing (cooling) in order to create heteroduplex (mismatch) and homoduplex (perfect match) molecular species (Figure 30–10A). If a sample harbors a heterozygous mutation, then heteroduplex and homoduplex fragments will be produced following denaturing and reannealing. If a sample is "wild-type" or homozygous, then only homoduplex fragments will be produced. The crude PCR products are injected on a solid phase column that is heated to a specific temperature (individually optimized for each specific PCR product) that allows partial denaturing of the DNA sequence of interest. A linear acetonitrile gradient based on the size of the PCR product is applied to the column to flush the DNA strands and propel the PCR products through a UV detector resulting in a chromatogram showing the sample's elution profile. This elution profile is highly reproducible under optimal conditions. Since heteroduplex species are less thermodynamically stable than homoduplexes, these double-stranded complexes will begin to unravel at the elevated temperature and elute from the column prior to their homoduplex or "wild-type" counterparts, thus producing an elution profile that is unique from the "wild-type" profile, and allowing for detection of mutation hosting samples. Specifically, PCR products containing heterozygote mutations result in the presence of profiles with "shouldering" or additional "peaks" as compared to "wild-type" samples (Figure 30–10B).

Direct DNA Sequencing

While intermediate mutation detection platforms alert the investigator of which samples contain mutations, direct DNA sequencing must be used to decipher the precise underlying DNA change(s). Usually, PCR products to be sequenced are purified from the unincorporated amplification primers and dinucleotides (dNTP) using either an enzymatic or filter column-based method. Pure PCR products are then subjected to sequencing using a single oligonucleotide primer (typically the same forward amplification primer used in the original PCR reaction) and a sequencing reaction mixture containing a sequencing DNA polymerase, dinucleotides (dNTP), and dye-labeled dideoxynucleotides (ddATP–green, ddCTP–blue, ddGTP–black, and ddTTP–red). This composite of sequencing reaction components and PCR product templates is cycled through a series of temperatures similar to that seen in a typical PCR reaction. Resulting sequencing products are then separated according to size by gel-based or capillary-based electrophoresis and a sequencing chromatogram is created (Figure 30–10C).

Review and comparison of the resulting sequence chromatograms and the published "wild-type" DNA and amino acid sequence for the gene/protein of interest will make it possible to determine whether the underlying DNA change is protein altering and potentially pathogenic or a nonpathogenic normal variant. It is imperative that extreme caution be exercised with respect to the assignment of a variant as a pathogenic

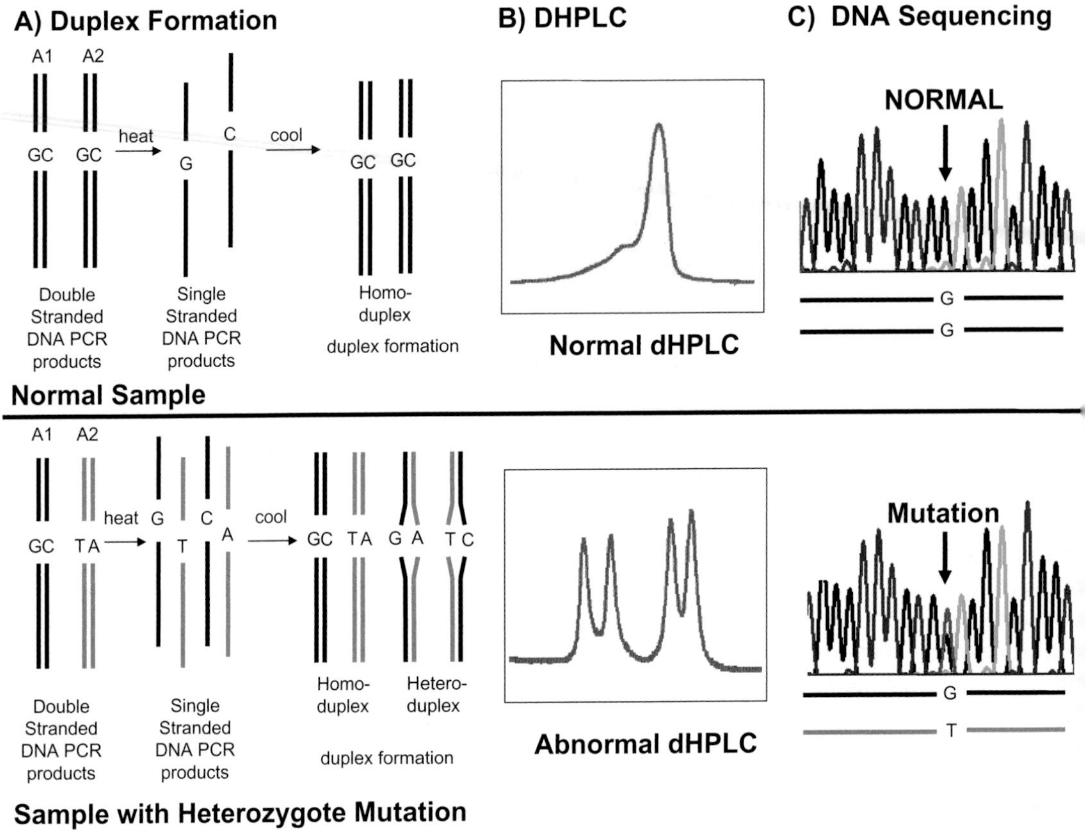

Figure 30–10. Mutation detection process of PCR, DHPLC, and DNA sequencing. Mutation detection by DHPLC relies on heteroduplex (mismatch) and homoduplex (perfect match) formation by heating and cooling both DNA alleles (A1 and A2) and then separating such types by ion-exchange chromatography resulting in (B) DHPLC elution profiles that vary from normal profiles. (C) DNA sequencing is then used to resolve the underlying heterozygote DNA change.

mutation. Ethnic matched controls must be performed. To illustrate this need, recently the first comprehensive determination of the spectrum and prevalence of nonsynonymous single nucleotide polymorphisms (i.e., amino acid substitutions) in the five LQTS-associated cardiac ion channel genes in approximately 800 healthy control subjects from four distinct ethnic groups was performed.[9,10] Approximately 2–5% of healthy individuals were found to host a rare amino acid-altering variant. Some of these variants observed in the normal population may represent subclinical disease modifiers or simply benign background noise.

In this three-step approach, (1) PCR amplification, (2) DHPLC heterozygote analysis, and (3) DNA sequencing, only samples believed to contain a DNA alteration are further analyzed by DNA sequencing. In some cases, the use of an intermediate mutation detection platform such as DHPLC is bypassed for direct DNA sequencing of all samples examined. Though this direct approach to mutational analysis is presently more expensive, it may accelerate mutation detection.

Candidate gene mutational analyses remain labor intensive and expensive. A profound genetic heterogeneity underlies each of the heritable arrhythmia syndromes. Clinical molecular diagnostic testing awaits a next-generation mutation detection platform. Whether “Diagnostic Gene Chips” represent such a platform remains to be seen.

Genetic Testing in Electrical Diseases of the Heart and Sudden Cardiac Death

The study of cardiac channelopathies embodies a relatively new discipline among heart rhythm specialists and allied professionals. In 1995, the discipline of cardiac channelopathies originated with the discovery that defective cardiac channels were at the heart of congenital LQTS.[11,12] Besides LQTS, the channelopathies include SQTS, BrS, ATS, Timothy syndrome, CPVT, progressive cardiac conduction disease, familial atrial fibrillation, idiopathic ventricular fibrillation, and some cases of autopsy-negative sudden unexplained death during infancy, childhood, adolescence, and beyond. Over the past decade, genetic testing for these cardiac channelopathies has been performed in select research laboratories worldwide. Such genetic testing has been conducted principally for the purpose of discovery and genotype–phenotype correlations (to advance the science), and has provided an important tool for improved diagnosis, risk stratification, and management of patients.

The fundamental pathogenic mechanisms responsible for these disorders have been elucidated at least in part and marked genetic and clinical heterogeneity is a common theme with multiple genes and allelic variants responsible for the underlying mechanisms discovered (http://www.fsm.it/cardmoc/). Phenotype–genotype correlations have exposed the distinguishing features of each genetic variant. Consequently, each channelopathy consists of multiple genetic forms that manifest with specific clinical characteristics. For example, LQTS is no longer thought of as a single disorder, but rather a family of multiple related disorders with a common feature of prolonged QT interval on a 12-lead surface electrocardiogram (ECG), yet have distinct characteristics in terms of severity, prognosis, risk stratification, and response to treatment depending on the underlying genetic cause.[13]

Notably, the cardiac channelopathies necessitate a comprehensive approach that is not predicated a priori on a specific set of mutations. This stems from the fact that many families affected by a channelopathy have their own private mutation not to be identified in another unrelated family. Until saturation of all possible disease-causing mutations is accomplished, conversion to diagnostic gene chips annotated with specific mutations will not be possible, and a sequencing-based approach as described above will be required.

Genetic Testing in a Clinical Versus Research Setting

Typically, research laboratories indicate that 6–24 months is the expected time frame within which research subjects learn of a positive result; in some cases research participants have been the direct beneficiary of the testing, with results sometimes provided 1–2 years after submission of a blood sample. However, in some research settings, patients may never be informed of either a positive or negative genetic test result. Genetic testing in the research environment often relies on assays developed in-house rather than on commercially available kits approved by the Food and Drug Administration (FDA).[14] In the research setting, genetic tests are often available before analytical validity and clinical validity are established, and the same level of proper quality control mechanisms found in a clinical laboratory regulated by the Centers for Medicaid and Medicare Services (CMS) through Clinical Laboratory Improvement Amendments (CLIA) requirements may not be in place. Some cardiac channelopathies like LQTS have made the quantum leap from research mode to the highly regulated clinical environment.

In May 2004 the first CLIA-approved, commercial genetic test to detect cardiac channel mutations was released by Genaissance Pharmaceuticals (now Clinical Data). Their diagnostic test, Familion®, provides either comprehensive mutational analysis of five cardiac channel genes implicated in LQTS or an *SCN5A*-targeted test for BrS. The clinically available genetic test to detect cardiac channel abnormalities is a high-throughput, automated, direct DNA sequencing-based assay. In a comprehensive mutational analysis for the five cardiac channel genes implicated in LQTS, the genetic test involves analysis of approximately 75 amplicons and over 12 kb of genetic material. In addition, each amplicon is interrogated with 4-fold redundancy to maximize diagnostic accuracy associated with this comprehensive surveillance.

Rather than reporting results to the research participant after a long period of time as with research testing efforts, results (both positive and negative) from the clinical genetic test are reported to the ordering physician within approximately 4 weeks.

Benefits of Genetic Testing for These Cardiac Conditions

The genetic test can (1) elucidate the exact molecular basis in cases of a strongly suspected channelopathy, (2) establish a definitive molecular diagnosis when the clinical probability is inconclusive such as in "borderline" LQTS, (3) confirm or exclude the presence of a disease-causing mutation in pre-symptomatic family members, and (4) help personalize treatment recommendations and management of a patient's specific channelopathy by characterization of the precise genotype.[15,16]

Current Limitations in Genetic Testing for Arrhythmia Syndromes

Clinical genetic testing is increasingly becoming available for all of the heritable arrhythmia syndromes. In the case of LQTS, approximately 25% of families with a strong clinical probability of LQTS will have a negative genetic test result. Therefore, it is vital to recognize that a negative test result can not fully exclude the diagnosis as a stand alone test. However, in cases where the clinical index of suspicion is intermediate at best, a negative test result may be used as another piece of impartial evidence that has failed to establish the diagnosis. The BrS genetic test is only for the single gene (*SCN5A*) that has been associated with the syndrome. However, *SCN5A* BrS-causing mutations are found in only approximately 20% of families satisfying the clinical diagnosis of BrS. While *KCNJ2* mutations account for over half of ATS and *RyR2* mutations account for over half of CPVT, these genetic tests are still largely conducted in research laboratories, although commercial clinical testing is becoming available.

Who Should Undergo Genetic Testing for Cardiac Channelopathies?

All patients or family members for whom a clinical diagnosis of a channelopathy is suspected should undergo genetic testing from either a commercially available test or via research laboratories depending on the suspected diagnosis. From a clinical test perspective, any patient and his or her first-degree relatives with a suspected clinical diagnosis of LQTS should be offered clinical genetic testing. This testing may also be warranted for patients with unexplained, exertional syncope or drug-induced QT prolongation/torsade de pointes who do not meet full diagnostic criteria for LQTS. Patients suspected of having BrS could undergo clinical genetic testing as long as it is recognized that the yield from the currently available test is approximately 20%. In addition, surviving relatives of an individual suffering a sudden unexplained death even in the setting of a negative family history of cardiac events may benefit from genetic testing. In CPVT and LQTS, for example the sudden death of a relative may be the leading event in these potentially lethal familial disorders.

Interpretation of Genetic Testing Results

The patient and family suspected of having a cardiac channelopathy should be evaluated and managed by a heart rhythm specialist with specific expertise in this discipline. Because of issues associated with incomplete penetrance and variable expressivity, the results of the genetic test must be interpreted cautiously and incorporated into the overall diagnostic evaluation for these disorders. The assignment of a specific variant as a true pathogenic disease-causing mutation will require vigilant scrutiny. If the cardiologist or cardiac channelologist lacks expertise with regard to the pathogenetic basis of these disorders, it may be beneficial to have an appropriately trained genetic counselor as part of the team to be involved in the communication process with the patient concerning the implications of genetic testing and genetic test results. A family history comprising at least three generations should be taken at the onset of the clinical evaluation of the patient and used as an evaluation for referral for further genetic testing and counseling. However, given the multitude of genotype–phenotype considerations specific to these disorders, it seems reasonable to expect that the cardiologist/channelologist should be the primary physician responsible for directing the patient's care.

Family Matters: Ethical, Legal, and Societal Implications

Patients should be well informed of the implications of genetic testing and in no way should be coerced into providing a DNA sample for analysis. Full disclosure should be given as to the intent of either the research or clinical genetic test, the results of the analysis, and who will have access to the results. Genetic information should be considered private and personal information with the potential for mishandling.[17,18] Disclosure of confidential information to third parties, such as insurance companies or employers, can have consequences to the patient in the form of genetic discrimination. Legislation is advancing to protect patients from potential misuse of genetic information.

Genetic testing is becoming increasingly understood as both a family and individual experience.[19] Although genetic testing is performed on genetic material isolated from an individual, the individual's decision to undergo genetic testing and the individual's test results may have profound implications for other family members, especially if disorders associated with sudden cardiac death are involved. Under current guidelines, only the index case or legal guardian, if the index case is a minor, may be informed of the genetic test results, and the decision/responsibility to inform unsuspecting relatives of the potential for genetic predisposition for sudden cardiac death lies solely with the informed patient. To what degree moral or even legal obligations should be placed on the informed family member to be responsible for disclosing potentially life-saving genetic information to uninformed and unaware relatives who may be at risk for a potentially lethal cardiac event is debatable. For example, should an individual with a family history of sudden cardiac death be held accountable if he or she has been informed of the identification of their family's LQTS mutation yet fails to inform a family member who subsequently experiences sudden cardiac death?

With the increase in availability of genetic testing, a wider distribution of the potential benefits, such as certainty of diagnosis, increased psychological well-being, and greater awareness of prophylactic treatment and risk stratification, may be achieved. However, it may also contribute to an increase in risks associated with genetic testing including depression, anxiety, guilt, stigmatization, discrimination, family conflict, and unnecessary or inappropriate use of risk-reducing strategies.[19]

Conclusions

Advances in molecular medicine are rapidly propelling the field of cardiac electrophysiology into the realm of genetic testing. As novel genes are discovered, the compendium of available genetic tests will surely increase. To be sure, it is our hope that through the discovery of new underlying mechanisms of disease and further refinement of our existing knowledge of these genetic disorders, we can in the words of Dr. Charles W. Mayo, "heal the sick and advance the science."

References

1. Baird PA, Anderson TW, Newcombe HB, Lowry RB. Genetic disorders in children and young adults: A population study. *Am J Hum Genet* 1988;42(5): 677–693.
2. Strachan T, Read A. *Human Molecular Genetics*, 2nd ed. New York: Wiley-Liss, 1999.
3. Nussbaum RL, McInnes RR, Willard HF, Eds. *Thompson and Thompson Genetics in Medicine*, 6th ed. Philadelphia, PA: W.B. Saunders Co, 2001: 51–94.
4. Tester DJ, Will ML, Haglund CM, Ackerman MJ. Compendium of cardiac channel mutations in 541 consecutive unrelated patients referred for long QT syndrome genetic testing. *Heart Rhythm* 2005; 2(5):507–517.
5. Tester DJ, Ackerman MJ. The role of molecular autopsy in unexplained sudden cardiac death. *Curr Opin Cardiol* 2006;21(3):166–172.
6. Tester DJ, Cronk LB, Carr JL, *et al.* Allelic dropout in long QT syndrome genetic testing: A possible mechanism underlying false negative results. *Heart Rhythm* 2006;3(7):815–821.
7. Ning L, Moss A, Zareba W, *et al.* Denaturing high-performance liquid chromatography quickly and reliably detects cardiac ion channel mutations in long QT syndrome. *Genet Test* 2003;7(3):249–253.
8. Spiegelman JI, Mindrinos MN, Oefner PJ. High-accuracy DNA sequence variation screening by DHPLC. *BioTechniques* 2000;29(5):1084–1090, 1092.

9. Ackerman MJ, Tester DJ, Jones GS, Will ML, Burrow CR, Curran ME. Ethnic differences in cardiac potassium channel variants: Implications for genetic susceptibility to sudden cardiac death and genetic testing for congenital long QT syndrome. *Mayo Clinic Proc* 2003;78(12):1479–1487.
10. Ackerman MJ, Splawski I, Makielski JC, *et al.* Spectrum and prevalence of cardiac sodium channel variants among black, white, Asian, and Hispanic individuals: Implications for arrhythmogenic susceptibility and Brugada/long QT syndrome genetic testing.[see comment]. *Heart Rhythm* 2004;1(5):600–607.
11. Curran ME, Splawski I, Timothy KW, Vincent GM, Green ED, Keating MT. A molecular basis for cardiac arrhythmia: HERG mutations cause long QT syndrome. *Cell* 1995;80(5):795–803.
12. Wang Q, Shen J, Li Z, *et al.* Cardiac sodium channel mutations in patients with long QT syndrome, an inherited cardiac arrhythmia. *Hum Mol Genet* 1995;4(9):1603–1607.
13. Napolitano C, Bloise R, Priori SG. Gene-specific therapy for inherited arrhythmogenic diseases. *Pharmacol Ther* 2006;110(1):1–13.
14. Constantin CM, Faucett A, Lubin IM. A primer on genetic testing. *J Midwifery Womens Health* 2005; 50(3):197–204.
15. Tester DJ, Ackerman MJ. Genetic testing for cardiac channelopathies: Ten questions regarding clinical considerations for heart rhythm allied professionals. *Heart Rhythm* 2005;2(6):675–677.
16. Priori SG, Napolitano C. Role of genetic analyses in cardiology: Part I: Mendelian diseases: Cardiac channelopathies. *Circulation* 2006;113(8): 1130–1135.
17. Thomas SM. Society and ethics–the genetics of disease. *Curr Opin Genet Dev* 2004;14(3):287–291.
18. Lea DH, Williams J, Donahue MP. Ethical issues in genetic testing. *J Midwifery Womens Health* 2005; 50(3):234–240.
19. Van Riper M. Genetic testing and the family. *J Midwifery Womens Health* 2005;50(3):227–233.

Part III
Heritable Cardiac Channelopathies, Primary Electrical Diseases, and Clinical Syndromes

Celebrating the Challenge of Cardiac Arrhythmias

Jeffrey A. Towbin

The field of cardiac arrhythmias has matured dramatically over the past 15 years, initially spurred on by the studies performed on the genetics of arrhythmia disorders. Once the genetic basis of disorders such as the long QT syndrome (LQTS) and Brugada syndrome (BrS) was discovered to occur due to disruption in ion channel encoding genes, basic electrophysiologists joined the fray, opening up a new area of study with significant clinical relevance. This book is a result of such bedside-to-bench collaboration.

Today, the genetic foundation of arrhythmia disorders is known to be based on disruption of a "final common pathway," now called ion channelopathies. In addition to LQTS and BrS, catecholaminergic polymorphic ventricular tachycardia (CPVT), short QT syndrome (SQTS), atrial fibrillation (AF), and Wolf–Parkinson–White (WPW) syndrome have, at least in part, been defined genetically. Overlap disorders including arrhythmogenic right ventricular dysplasia/cardiomyopathy (ARVD/C), dilated cardiomyopathy (DCM), Andersen–Tawil syndrome, and Timothy syndrome are also defined, with ion channel disruption central to the clinical features or secondarily dysfunctional.

These new genetic and biophysical discoveries have opened up several new sciences as well. Drug discovery now requires analysis of potential effects on channel function. Pharmacogenomics is also the key to new approaches to medical therapy of "old" disorders. The concepts of gene-targeted therapies have grown out of this work. The pioneering work by Arthur Moss, Peter Schwartz, G. Michael Vincent, and others on the use of mexilitine and other similar therapies in LQT3, a gain-of-function persistent sodium channel leak treated with a sodium channel blocking agent, as well as the use of potassium supplementation in other forms of treatments to be devised have caused a reawakening to older therapies during studies of outcomes in patients treated with classic modalities such as β blockers and have resulted in newer approaches such as internal cardioverter defibrillator (ICD) implantation. In addition, fee-for-service genetic testing has finally become available for clinical use.

In the chapters that follow, an excellent group of assembled authors outline the current state of knowledge in the area of arrhythmias, as well as novel new concepts that are likely to define the future of diagnosis and treatment of these high-risk disorders. This has been an exciting field and, as demonstrated in this book by Gussak and Antzelevitch, the best is yet to come.

31 Congenital Long QT Syndrome

Michael J. Ackerman, Anant Khositseth, David J. Tester, and Peter J. Schwartz

Introduction

Once considered an extremely rare yet lethal arrhythmogenic peculiarity, congenital long QT syndrome (LQTS) is understood today as a primary cardiac arrhythmia syndrome ("cardiac channelopathy") that is both far more common and, overall, much less lethal than previously recognized. Clinically, LQTS is often characterized by prolongation of the heart rate corrected QT interval (QTc) on a 12-lead surface electrocardiogram (ECG) and is associated with syncope, seizures, and sudden cardiac death due to ventricular arrhythmias (Torsade des pointes, TdP) usually following a precipitating event such as exertion, extreme emotion, or auditory stimulation. The molecular breakthroughs of the 1990s, led in large measure by the research laboratories of Drs. Mark Keating and Jeffrey Towbin in conjunction with LQTS registries containing meticulously phenotyped patients directed by Drs. Arthur Moss and Peter Schwartz, revealed the fundamental molecular underpinnings of LQTS—namely, defective cardiac channels.[1]

Maturing from the decade of research-based genetic testing, LQTS genetic testing is now a routine, commercially available molecular diagnostic test. Nevertheless, the cornerstone of the clinical evaluation for LQTS remains a time honored careful personal/family history evaluation and meticulous inspection of the electrocardiogram (ECG) to detect either overt prolongation of the QT interval or suspicious T wave abnormalities. Once patients exhibit the clinical and/or genetic substrate for LQTS, it is critical to delineate whether they possess a substrate that resembles a "ticking time bomb" waiting for the necessary trigger to detonate, or perhaps a "dud" destined for asymptomatic longevity.

In this chapter, we will first present some case vignettes followed by a review of the historical background, epidemiology and prevalence, molecular genetics, and clinical presentations of LQTS. Next, we will explore unique genotype—phenotype relationships that help define the various forms of LQTS. We will then offer a detailed outline for the diagnostic evaluation and clinical management of LQTS, including current treatment strategies involving current and potential pharmacotherapies, device therapy with implantable cardioverter defibrillators (ICD), and surgery involving the left cardiac sympathetic denervation (LCSD) procedure. Lifestyle recommendations, prevention, and competitive sport issues will be reviewed. Finally, we will conclude with clinical pearls derived from a dissection of the case vignettes.

Case Vignettes

Case #1: Do I or Do I Not Have Long QT Syndrome, That Is the Question?

JPA is a 15-year-old male referred for a second opinion and possible ICD implantation following the diagnosis of LQT1. At a preparticipation sports physical, an innocent murmur was heard, an ECG was obtained, and a QTc of 440 msec was oted. The patient fainted once in the setting of aving his blood drawn. His family history was ompletely negative. No ECGs were performed n the parents. Holter monitoring revealed a QTc maximum of 501 msec occurring at 2:30 AM. An epinephrine QT stress test using the Mayo ontinuous infusion protocol demonstrated a 00 msec increase in the QTc during low-dose pinephrine. Genetic testing revealed a rare amino cid substitution in the *KCNQ1*-encoded I_{Ks} potasium channel localizing to the C-terminus of the hannel. The patient was diagnosed with LQT1, laced on once-a-day atenolol β blocker therapy, nd restricted from all competitive sports; a recommendation for sudden death primary prevenion with an ICD has been rendered.

Case #2: Oh Great, an Infant with LQT3, Now What Do I Do?

MA is a healthy asymptomatic newborn female born to a mother with genetically proven LQT3. The family history is significant for a nocturnal udden death involving a maternal aunt at age 40. The initial newborn ECG shows a QTc of 420 msec. Would you perform any additional tests or dismiss s normal?

Case #3: Doctor Please Do Something, My Defibrillator Keeps Shocking Me

LA is a 32-year-old female with symptomatic LQT2, a QTc of 550 msec, and a positive family istory of multiple premature sudden deaths. Despite adequate β blocker therapy with nadolol, she continues to receive frequent ventricular ibrillation-terminating ICD therapies. What therapeutic strategy would you consider next?

These three cases highlight several aspects in he clinical evaluation, risk stratification, and management of LQTS. The approach to each case will be summarized at the chapter's conclusion.

Historical Background

Congenital LQTS was first described by Anton Jervell and Fred Lange-Nielsen in 1957 in a Norwegian family in which four of six children had prolonged QT interval, congenital sensorineural hearing loss, and recurrent syncope during exercise or emotion; three of them died suddenly at ages 4, 5, and 9 years.[2] The QT prolongation on the electrocardiogram (ECG) was obvious and the inheritance pattern appeared to be autosomal recessive. A similar clinical syndrome of sudden death during exercise and emotion, but with normal hearing and autosomal dominant inheritance, was first described separately by Romano[3] and Ward[4] in the early 1960s after observing families with similar presentations including prolongation of the QT interval, syncope, and sudden death. These two inherited forms of LQTS with different modes of inheritance have become known, respectively, as the Jervell and Lange-Nielsen syndrome (JLNS) and the Romano–Ward syndrome (RWS).

Epidemiology and Prevalence

The prevalence of congenital LQTS in the United States is speculated to be approximately 1 in 5000 persons,[5] causing hundreds to thousands of sudden deaths in children, adolescents, and young adults each year.[6] However, the latest data from Italy presented in 2005 suggest the incidence may be as high as 1 in 2000–3000 live births.[7] In addition, LQTS is one of the most common causes of autopsy-negative sudden unexplained death.[8]

Romano–Ward syndrome is the most common inherited form of LQTS, accounting for over 99% of cases, and is transmitted as an autosomal dominant trait, whereby each child of an affected parent has a 50% chance of inheriting the abnormal allele and males and females are equally affected. In contrast to RWS, JLNS is associated with congenital deafness and is extremely rare. Males and females are also equally affected. Initially understood exclusively as an autosomal recessive disorder, JLNS is now known to be a syndrome in which the auditory phenotype (deafness) is autosomal recessive, but the cardiac phenotype is autosomal dominant.[9] Thus, technically, both parents of a child with JLNS actually have RWS, albeit curiously with a generally mild/negligible cardiac phenotype.

Molecular Genetics

With respect to its pathogenic mechanisms, hundreds of mutations in 10 distinct LQTS susceptibility genes have been identified so far and principally involve either loss-of-function potassium channel mutations or gain-of-function sodium channel mutations (Figure 31–1). The majority of all genotyped LQTS and 75% of all clinically robust LQTS are a pure "channelopathy" stemming from mutations involving cardiac channel α subunits: *KCNQ1*-encoded I_{Ks} potassium channel (LQT1, 30–35%), the *KCNH2*-encoded I_{Kr} potassium channel (LQT2, 25–30%), or the *SCN5A*-encoded I_{Na} sodium channel (LQT3, 5–10%).

Rare subtypes stem from perturbations in key cardiac channel interacting proteins [I_{Ks}, I_{Kr}, or I_{Na} β subunits (LQT5, LQT6, LQT10)] or structural membrane scaffolding proteins such as ankyrin B (LQT4) or caveolin 3 (LQT9). Complex, multisystem syndromes that include abnormal repolarization have been included as variants of LQTS. These syndromes include Andersen–Tawil syndrome (ATS1, also annotated as LQT7), due in part to mutations in the *KCNJ2*-encoded Kir2.1 potassium channel, and Timothy syndrome (TS1, also annotated as LQT8), due to mutations in the L-type calcium channel α subunit. This chapter will focus mostly on the clinically pure forms of LQTS, particularly the three most common subtypes, LQT1–3.

Clinical Presentations

The clinical manifestations of LQTS range from a lifelong asymptomatic course in some cases to premature sudden cardiac death during infancy in others. As a simple rule of thumb, approximately 50% of patients with genetic evidence of LQTS will never have a symptom attributable to LQTS, and a significant proportion (ranging from 10% to 50% depending on genotype) of those with genetic LQTS do not show overt QT prolongation.[5,10,11] Patients failing to display QT prolongation at rest are said to have *concealed LQTS*. While risk of an LQTS-precipitated event generally increases with increasing QTc, it is nevertheless possible to experience sudden cardiac death as a sentinel event despite having concealed LQTS (i.e., normal resting QTc). This is fortunately quite uncommon. The most common presenting symptoms are recurrent syncope, seizures, and sudden cardiac death (Figure 31–2). These events are due to the hallmark feature of LQTS, namely polymorphic ventricular tachyarrhythmias, called TdP, which are most often self-terminating. Rarely,

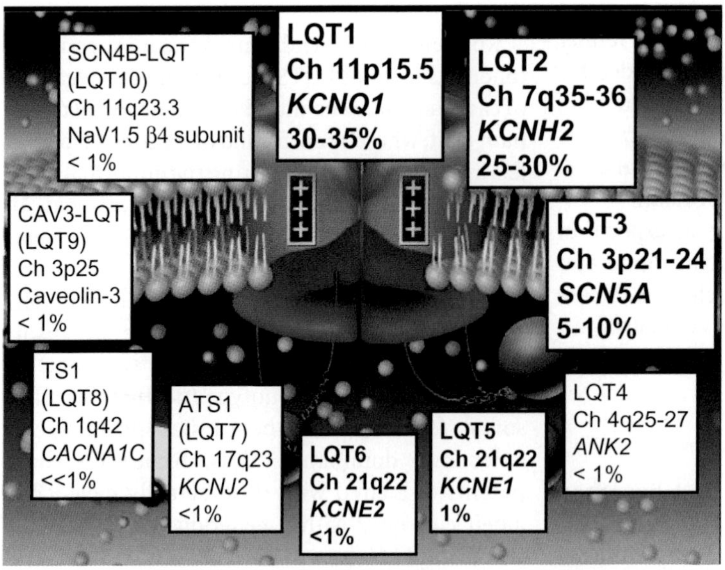

Figure 31–1. Compendium of LQTS-susceptibility genes.

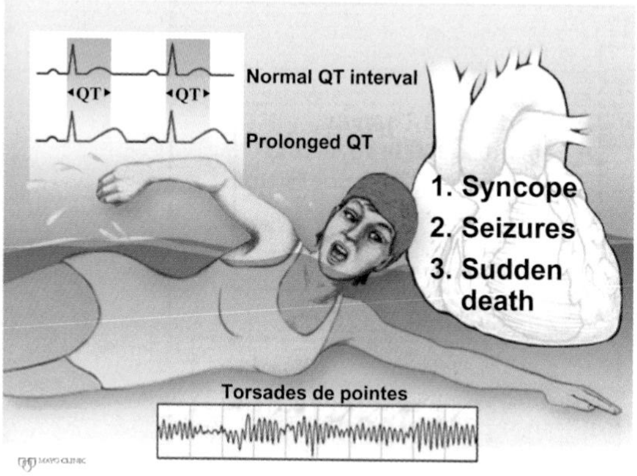

FIGURE 31–2. Summary of the key clinical features of LQTS.

TdP continue to degenerate, yielding ventricular fibrillation and sudden death. Overall, less than 5% of patients with LQTS will present with a sentinel event of sudden death or aborted cardiac arrest. Conversely, less than half of LQTS sudden death victims experienced a prior warning episode of syncope.

Syncope is the most frequent symptom, occurring commonly between age 5 and 15 years. Among symptomatic probands, 50% experience their first cardiac event by 12 years of age, and by 40 years of age the proportion increases to almost 90%.[12] In general, approximately 50% of patients present with activity- or emotion-related symptoms—primarily syncope, seizures, or palpitations. The majority of cardiac events are related to physical activity or emotional stress. To be certain, a "fight-flight-fright"-triggered faint must be considered potentially ominous until proven otherwise, and a meticulous LQTS evaluation must be conducted. In fact, new data from the LQTS Registry indicate that recent syncope is the most significant harbinger of future sudden death, greater than genotype and degree of QT prolongation.[13] Thus, it is critically important to properly distinguish an ordinary vasovagal faint from a possibly torsadogenic one.

In general, and without consideration of the underlying LQTS-causing genotype, the risk of the first cardiac event in males is typically higher in childhood and decreases after puberty, perhaps due in part to regression of QTc duration.[14,15] On the other hand, during adolescence and adulthood, females appear more vulnerable to LQTS-related cardiac events. In addition, females are at significant risk for cardiac events during the postpartum period. In fact, Rashba and colleagues reported nearly 10% of female probands experienced their first cardiac events during the postpartum period.[16]

Genotype–Phenotype-Specific Correlations

Some of the phenotypic heterogeneity in LQTS is now understood because of the underlying genetic heterogeneity, particularly with respect to gene-specific triggers for cardiac events.[17] Figure 31–3 summarizes some of the genotype-specific features observed in LQT1, LQT2, and LQT3.

LQT1 Phenotype

Patients with the most common genetic subtype (LQT1) predominantly have exertional-triggered symptoms. Interestingly, swimming appears to be a gene-specific arrhythmogenic trigger associated almost exclusively with LQT1.[18,19] With few exceptions to date, all LQTS patients, with either a personal history or an extended family history of a near drowning, have a defective *KCNQ1* gene facilitating strategic genotyping.[19] The common triggers other than swimming include running, startle, anger, and fright. LQT1 mutations cause a defective I_{Ks} channel that is responsive to adrenergic stimulation, so the usual shortening of QT in response to increased heart rate is impaired and QTc progressively lengthens during exercise and early recovery. The common ECG finding in LQT1 is prolonged T wave duration or a broad-based T wave pattern.[20,21]

LQT2 Phenotype

Auditory stimuli, such as a telephone ringing or an alarm clock sounding, is a common trigger in LQTS, and often indicates the presence of a *KCNH2* (LQT2) defect.[22] Additionally, there is a relatively gene-specific molecular basis underlying cardiac events during the postpartum period in LQTS.[23] Postpartum cardiac events were found to be more common in LQT2 (16%) than

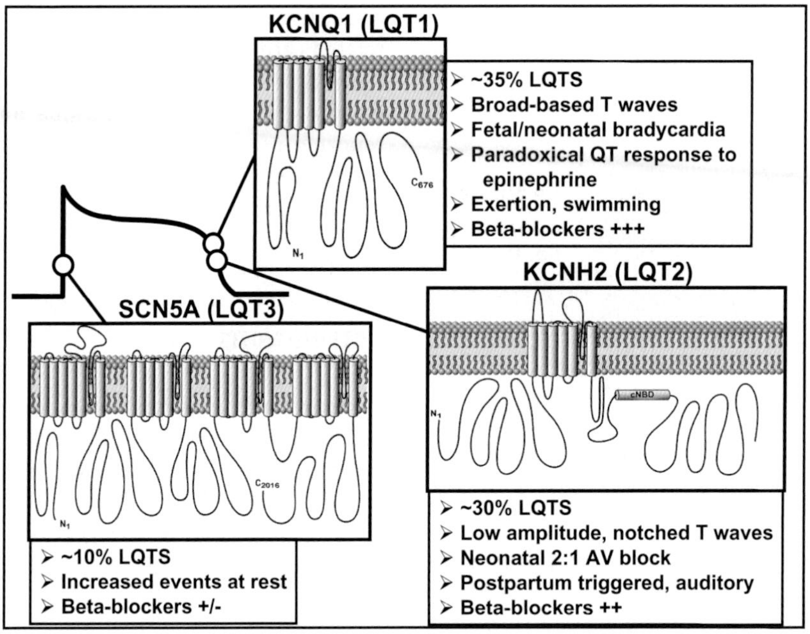

FIGURE 31–3. Summary of the key genotype-phenotype correlations.

in LQT1(<1%).[23,24] Fifteen percent of LQT2-associated cardiac events occur during rest or sleep. The finding of bifid T waves in the inferior and lateral leads is characteristic of LQT2.[25]

LQT3 Phenotype

Sleep/rest-triggered events seem most common in patients harboring the defective sodium channel Nav1.5 encoded by *SCN5A*.[17,26] In LQT3, *SCN5A* mutations impair inactivation of I_{Na}, causing repetitive reopenings throughout the action potential and persistent inward current, resulting in prolongation of the action potential duration and QT interval.[27]

The underlying genotype has a profound influence on the clinical course.[28] Families with LQT1 and LQT2 comprise approximately 60–70% of LQTS and have a much higher risk of cardiac events than patients with LQT3. However, the "lethality" of a given cardiac event appears to be greatest in LQT3. Fortunately, *SCN5A*-based LQTS (LQT3) is approximately 10-fold less common than the potassium channel LQTS subtypes.

Diagnostic Evaluation

Schwartz *et al.* proposed the first diagnosti criteria for LQTS in 1985, which include QTc > 440 msec, stress-induced syncope, an family members with LQTS as major criteria an congenital deafness, episodes of T wave alternans low heart rate (in children), and abnorma ventricular repolarization as minor criteria.[2] However, the more recent understanding of th "overlap zone" between LQTS and health has rendered this cutoff value of 440 msec a major limitation of the original "Schwartz criteria."

A modified "Schwartz score" containing nev criteria and a point system based upon a range o QTc values and the clinical/family history was formulated in 1993 (Table 31–1).[30] The "Schwart score," recently modified for what concerns th points necessary for a "high clinical probability o LQTS," ranges from 0 to 9 and contains thre diagnostic probabilities: ≤1 point, low probabilit of LQTS; 2 or 3 points, intermediate probability o LQTS; and ≥3.5 points, high probability of LQTS.[3] The Schwartz criteria provide a very useful guid

ABLE 31–1. Schwartz/Moss score for long QT syndrome (LQTS) agnostic criteria.

Variable		Points
ECG findings		
QTc msec[a]	≥ 480	3
	460–470	2
	450 (in males)	1
Torsade de pointes		2
T wave alternans (macroscopic)		1
Notched T wave in three leads		1
Low heart rate for age[b]		0.5
Clinical history		
Syncope[c]		
With stress		2
Without stress		1
Congenital deafness		0.5
Family history[d]		
Family members with definite LQTS[e]		1
Unexplained sudden cardiac death < age 30 years among immediate family members		0.5

QTc calculated using Bazett's formula (QTc = QT/square root RR).
Mutually exclusive.
Resting heart rate below the second percentile for age.
The same family member cannot be counted in both.
Definite LQTS is defined by an LQTS score ≥3.5.

or contemplating a clinical diagnosis of LQTS with the positive predictive value of a modified "Schwartz score" ≥3.5 approaching 100%.

Importantly, however, the Schwartz criteria should be used *only* for the diagnosis of clinically evident LQTS. By definition, these criteria *cannot* identify the patients or family members with concealed LQTS. This critical point stems from the observation that a significant proportion of LQTS is concealed and that the penetrance, defined as the ratio between patients with a manifest clinical phenotype (QT prolongation, symptoms, etc.) and the total number of family member carriers of the mutation identified in the LQTS proband, may be as low as 25%. Although the clinical risk of the patient with concealed LQTS is much lower than the patient with manifest LQTS, the risk of an untoward cardiac event is not zero and, hence, it is essential to correctly identify all family members. Thus, in the evaluation of first-degree relatives of a definitely affected LQTS proband, it is no longer acceptable to exclude LQTS among individuals based upon an equivocal QTc or a low Schwartz score. Instead, genotyping, for the estimated 75% of families who possess an LQTS-causing mutation, is the only definitive diagnostic test for the rest of the family.

Symptomatic patients, who have an ECG with a borderline (440–460 msec) or normal QTc, will have a borderline or questionable (score of 2 or 3) LQTS diagnosis based on clinical criteria. In this situation, serial ECGs should be performed since the QTc value in LQTS patients may vary from time to time. Furthermore, a careful inquiry about family history of sudden death as well as screening ECGs from other family members may be informative. In addition, stress testing using exercise protocols or the epinephrine QT stress test may be helpful in exposing LQTS, particularly LQT1.

The 12-Lead Electrocardiogram

The 12-lead ECG remains the cornerstone in the LQTS clinical diagnosis and the principal screening tool. The hallmark ECG feature of LQTS includes prolongation of the QTc as measured by Bazett's formula (QTc = QT interval/square root of RR interval).[32] The QT interval is defined as the time interval between the onset of QRS and the end of the T wave. This value is corrected for the heart rate by dividing it by the square root of the preceding RR interval (Bazett's QTc formula). Note, with a heart rate of 60 beats per minute (RR interval = 1 sec), the QTc equals the QT interval. More rapid heart rates cause the calculated QTc to increase relative to the measured QT interval.

Lead II is generally the accepted lead for QTc calculation because the inscription of the T wave is usually discrete.[33] Alternatively, the lateral precordial leads V5 and V6 are sometimes quite informative.[33,34] When sinus arrhythmia is present, an average QTc from the entire lead II strip (at least three consecutive determinations) must be determined.[26,35] Simply taking the longest observed QTc will result in too many false-positive classifications.

It is vital that the ECG be directly visualized and QTc manually calculated by a physician with expertise in LQTS. The computer-calculated QTc is *not* acceptable in the evaluation of LQTS. Independent manual calculation is mandatory. Unfortunately, Viskin and colleagues have shown that humans are not much better than a computer when it comes to accurately calculating the

QT interval. Compared to "QT aficionados" who made significant QTc miscalculations <5% of the time, heart rhythm specialists and general cardiologists often failed to correctly calculate the QTc (>60% and >75% of the time, respectively).[36]

Even when the QTc has been calculated accurately, the abundance of concealed LQTS and misconceptions about the normal distribution of the QTc have posed a serious diagnostic challenge (Figure 31–4). Before the molecular revelations in LQTS, a QTc of ≥440 msec (males) and ≥460 msec (females) was considered prolonged.[37] Subsequently, Vincent *et al.*[26] examined the QTc distribution in three families with LQT1 and found that no genotype-positive individuals had a QTc ≤410 msec and no unaffected (genotype negative) persons had a QTc ≥470 msec in men or ≥480 msec in women, and that significant numbers of patients were erroneously classified using the 440 msec cutoff. From a screening standpoint, if a QTc of 460 msec is used as a cutoff point, the positive predictive value is 92% and the negative predictive value is 94%.[5] Again for screening purposes, we advocate designating QTc values ≥470 msec as "prolonged" to maximize both the positive and negative predictive values as a screening test. Such a single cutoff value will tend, however, to yield slightly more false positives among females than males after puberty when women tend to have a slightly longer QTc.

Figure 31–4 depicts the distribution of QTc values among healthy postpubertal adult men and women as well as the QTc distribution seen for all

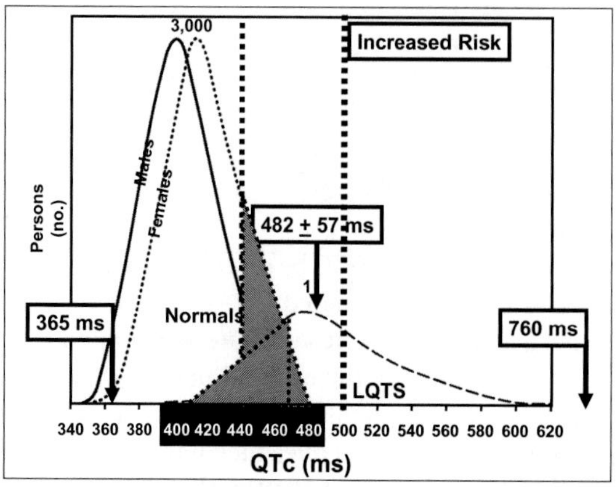

FIGURE 31–4. QTc distribution in health and LQTS.

genotype-positive patients evaluated in Mayo Clinic's LQTS clinic. Despite our "indoor track record" of a genotyped LQT1 family member with a QTc of 365 msec, the interpretation of a QTc < 400 msec is statistically easy—normal, no LQTS—with virtually 100% negative predictive value. On the other end, a QTc ≥ 480 msec almost always indicates repolarization pathology due to either acquired or congenital LQTS. Even beyond this threshold, however, it is important to remember that although rarely, this is an area in which healthy individuals (generally women) without LQTS can still reside. More importantly, the overlap zone (400–480 msec) is where great consternation occurs. Here, the physician must understand the normal QTc distribution in healthy subjects versus the 1 in 3000 LQTS-affected persons. For example, an asymptomatic patient with a negative family history and a screening QTc of 450 msec has >500:1 odds favoring normalcy rather than concealed LQTS.

Complicating matters further is the observation that LQTS individuals with a "normal" ECG (i.e., "low-penetrant" LQTS or "concealed" LQTS) can indeed, albeit uncommonly, have cardiac events, including sudden death. Approximately 10% of genotype-positive index cases presented for LQTS genetic testing with a QTc ≤ 440 msec.[38] These observations have transformed this extensive "overlap zone" into the "nightmare zone." Thus, although the risk for sudden death in a patient with a QTc < 440 msec remains exceedingly rare, the presence of a normal QTc in a genotype-positive LQTS patient must *not* be interpreted as a risk-free marker. As will be discussed later in the treatment section, such genotype-positive, phenotype-negative patients must be advised of simple, potentially life-saving preventive measures including avoidance of medications that prolong the QT interval. Understanding this QTc overlap zone is foundational to the LQTS evaluation and constitutes one of the major misunderstandings in the clinical evaluation of LQTS.

T-U Wave Abnormalities and T Wave Alternans

Besides manually calculating the QTc and understanding the QTc overlap zone, sleuth-like inspection of the morphology of the T waves should also ɜ conducted in an LQTS evaluation (Figure 1–5). Unusual T waves, wide-based slowly generated, notched, bifids, biphasic, low-amplitude umps and bumps on the downslope limb, indisnct termination due to U waves, sinusoidal oscil- tion, or simply a delayed inscription of normally ppearing T waves, may lead to the diagnosis of QTS despite a normal or borderline QTc.[21] These wave abnormalities may be evident particularly the lateral precordial leads. However, caution ust be exercised with concluding LQT-suspi- ous T wave peculiarities based upon changes in e precordial leads of V2 and V3. In addition, the wave morphology may be somewhat gene spe- fic, providing another piece of evidence permit- ng strategic genotyping.[20,39] Patients with LQT3 nd to have a late-appearing T wave clearly dis- nct from the low-amplitude, moderately delayed wave observed in LQT2. Both of these T wave rofiles are different from the broad-based, pro- nged T wave pattern seen in LQT1.[20,21] However, e classic LQT3-like T wave pattern can often be een in patients with LQT1.

Previously, Lupoglazoff and colleagues classi- ed a notched T wave as a grade 1 (G1) notch hen it occurred at or below the apex whatever e amplitude, and as grade 2 (G2) when the pro- uberance occurred above the apex.[40] G2 notches ppear more specific and often indicate LQT2. Iowever, baseline ECG showing G2 notches is not commonly found. Recently, Khositseth *et al.*[41] reported G2 notching elicited during low-dose epinephrine may unmask some patients with concealed LQT2. The mandate for careful inspection of T wave morphology is 2-fold: (1) unmask a patient with concealed LQTS, i.e., a normal resting QTc with a peculiar T wave, and (2) provide a possible starting point for the mutational analysis based upon the suggested ECG pattern.

Besides QTc and T wave morphology, macrovoltage and microvoltage T wave alternans (TWA) and QT dispersion (QTd) may be informative. T wave alternans is characterized by beat-to-beat alternation of the morphology, amplitude, and/or polarity of the T wave and is a marker of major electrical instability and regional heterogeneity of repolarization and is likely to be associated with an increased risk of cardiac events.[42,43] QT dispersion is defined as the difference between the maximal and minimal QT intervals in the 12 standard leads and may reflect spatial repolarization.[44] It has been described as an arrhythmic marker for LQTS. There is evidence that QTd is increased in LQTS patients compared to normal controls.[45,46] Moenning and colleagues have confirmed the finding that a significant and independent difference in QTd between mutation carriers and unaffected family members exists.[47] However, a cutoff value of QTd to distinguish LQTS from health is not available.

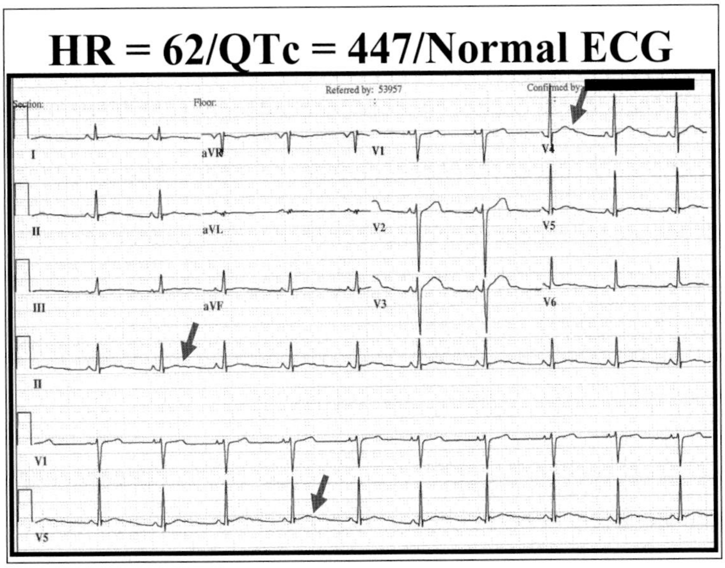

IGURE 31–5. Example of T wave sleuthng: 12-lead ECG in proband with LQT2, orderline QT prolongation, and abnormal wave morphology.

Holter Monitoring

In patients with a nondiagnostic QTc, Holter monitoring may aid in the evaluation of LQTS. Again, caution must be exercised with interpreting Holters in a patient with an equivocal history and a borderline QTc. Presently, the normal distribution of 24-h maximal QTc values is poorly understood, and concerns have been raised regarding the filter settings in Holter recordings and, hence, the precision/accuracy of Holter QT intervals. Critically, a Holter-recorded maximum QTc exceeding 500 msec does not equal LQTS. Instead, the value of repeated Holter recordings lies in capturing the appearance of T wave patterns (such as T wave notching) that might suggest LQTS in patients with borderline QT prolongation and an uncertain clinical diagnosis.[40]

Exercise Testing

Exercise testing may enhance the diagnostic accuracy of the LQTS evaluation, as inadequate shortening of QTc with increasing heart rate has been observed.[48] Swan *et al.*[49] studied 19 LQTS patients and 19 healthy controls undergoing exercise testing. During the recovery phase of exercise, the QT interval lengthened abnormally and the inhomogeneity of repolarization increased in LQTS. LQT2 patients had less QT interval shortening than LQT3 patients in response to increasing heart rate.[50] Moreover, LQT1 patients displayed a diminished chronotropic response and exaggerated prolongation of the QT interval after exercise. In contrast, the QT interval shortens more in LQT2 than in LQT1 patients when the heart rate increases and the sinus nodal rate response is normal.[51] The majority of these studies have been conducted in LQTS patients having a diagnostic QTc at rest. Provocative testing is most needed, however, in exposing the patient with concealed LQTS. Here, exercise testing may help identify such a patient, especially the patient with LQT1, by detecting inadequate QT adaptation during heart rate increase and during the recovery phase.

It is important to note that exercise-induced ventricular ectopy is uncommon in LQTS. In fact, induction of premature ventricular contractions in bigeminy or as couplets and, of course, bidirectional ventricular tachycardia should prompt su picion for a mimicker of LQTS, namely catech laminergic polymorphic ventricular tachycardia

Macrovoltage TWA at rest or during exercis epinephrine QT stress testing is abnormal an prognosticates increased risk. However, exercis induced macrovoltage TWA is extremely rare an we have seen epinephrine-induced macrovoltag TWA in only 1 of the past 300 epinephrine Q stress tests.[52] On the other hand, after conductin nearly 100 microvoltage T wave studies usin either the epinephrine QT stress test or treadmi stress testing, we cannot assign any clinical utilit to this test. In fact, we have discontinued micr voltage T wave testing in both of our Long Q Syndrome clinics.

Epinephrine QT Stress Test

The epinephrine QT stress test has proven to be powerful diagnostic tool to unmask conceale LQTS, particularly LQT1. Whether using th Shimizu protocol or the Ackerman/Mayo proto col, the primary finding that points to LQT involves a paradoxic lengthening of the QT (Shimizu protocol) or the absolute QT interva (Ackerman/Mayo protocol) during infusion o epinephrine.[52,53] When present, a tentative diag nosis of LQT1 is rendered (75% positive predic tive value) and β blocker therapy is initiated whil waiting for confirmation by genetic testing. Given a 96% negative predictive value, this test i also performed in patients hosting a novel LQT1 associated mutation to provide an *in vivo* physi ological challenge of the patient's I_{Ks} pathway Such testing provides independent conformatio for the pathogenicity of the newly discovere mutation. Importantly, β blockers significantl confound the interpretation of the epinephrin QT stress test. The reader is directed to Chapte 28 (this volume) by Shimizu and Ackerman, whic details catecholamine stress testing in the eva luation heritable arrhythmia syndromes wit particular focus on the epinephrine QT stres test.

Molecular Genetic Testing

The discipline of cardiac channelopathies bega on March 10, 1995, with tandem publications b e Keating laboratory in *Cell* that revealed LQTS be a disease of the cardiac channels.[55,56] These undational discoveries permitted research-ased genetic testing for LQTS over the ensuing ecade. In August 2004, akin to the evolution om research testing to clinical testing for its ster channelopathy, cystic fibrosis, LQTS genetic sting completed its maturation as Genaissance harmaceuticals (now Clinical Data, Inc.), based New Haven, CT, introduced the FAMILION™ inical diagnostic genetic test involving a com-rehensive open reading frame analysis of the anslated exons for the genes associated with QT1, LQT2, LQT3, LQT5, and LQT6.

When there is no doubt about the clinical diag-osis, the genetic test will be positive about 75% f the time.[38,57,58] Identification of the specific QTS-associated mutation then assists with geno-ype-guided therapy and provides the gold stand-rd diagnostic marker for the unambiguous enetic classification of all relatives. An estimated -10% of LQTS probands have spontaneous ermline mutations (sporadic) and 5–10% of atients who are genotype positive have more ian one mutation.[57–60] Like patients with JLNS autosomal recessive LQTS plus deafness), this ubset of patients with multiple mutations tends have a more severe phenotype.[60] These obser-ations emphasize the critical importance of omprehensive genetic testing rather than a "find-nd-stop" approach.

To be sure, a negative genetic test *must not* esult in removal of the diagnosis in a patient with high probability/definite "Schwartz score." emember, 20–25% of patients with clinically efinite LQTS will have a negative genetic test. On he other hand, there appears to be an abundance f patients for whom the diagnosis of LQTS may ave been assigned prematurely based upon ather soft criteria. In this setting, a negative enetic test result that objectively and unemotion-lly *rules out* at least 75% of LQTS may be a useful iece of data for a specialist to help the patient/ amily move away from the diagnosis. Among atients referred for LQTS genetic testing despite n intermediate probability "Schwartz score," 4% had a positive genetic test enabling their tatus to be elevated from diagnostic ambiguity borderline LQTS) to diagnostic certainty.[39] inally, the physician must be aware that the LQTS genetic test has an estimated 5% false-positive rate.[61,62] That is, approximately 5% of healthy individuals are positive for a rare genetic variant in these LQTS-susceptibility genes. These rare variants tend to localize to the N- and C-termini of the LQT1- and LQT2-associated potassium channels and to the N-terminus, C-terminus, and cytoplasmic interdomain linkers of the *SCN5A*-encoded sodium channel (LQT3). Thus, it is critical that the physician carefully synthesize all components of the diagnostic evaluation. This meticulous, comprehensive approach is vital to ensure that the wisest recommendations are rendered.

Management

When LQTS was estimated to affect 1:20,000 persons, the disease was viewed as a "death sentence" with an untreated annual mortality of 5–10%. Akin to the "tip of the iceberg" phenomenon, LQTS has become much more common (1 in 3000) and much less severe (overall annual mortality ~1%) over the past half century since its original description in 1957.

Risk Stratification

The issue of risk stratification in LQTS is clinically important. The phenotypic expression of LQTS varies profoundly from asymptomatic longevity to premature sudden cardiac death despite medical therapy. The great challenge is to try to discern which of these divergent outcomes is most likely in each of our patients. Occurrence of an LQTS-related cardiac event like syncope before 5 years of age suggests a serious LQTS phenotype, and syncope occurring in the first year of life is associated with an extremely poor prognosis.[63]

Overall, among LQTS patients, the risk of cardiac events is higher in males until puberty and higher in females during adulthood.[15] Events tend to occur earlier in males than females, and males who are still asymptomatic at age 20 years may be considered at lower risk (lowest in LQT1) for manifesting cardiac events.[15,64] Even if event free for the first 20 years of life, females continue to have a discernible risk for cardiac events in adulthood and may be at increased vulnerability to an arrhythmic event during the postpartum period.[16]

Among the known LQTS genotypes, patients with LQT1 appear to be more "frequent fainters," but patients with LQT3 appear to have the highest lethality rate per cardiac event.[17,28] The frequency of cardiac events including syncope, aborted cardiac arrest, and sudden death was highest in LQT1 (60% of patients), moderate LQT2 (40%), and lowest in LQT3 (18%).[28] Since the rate of death was the same in each of these three genotypes, the percentage of lethal events was highest in LQT3 patients. The JLNS is associated with very early clinical manifestations and a poorer prognosis than autosomal dominant Romano–Ward LQTS.[9,65] Patients with JLNS due to compound homozygous/heterozygous mutations involving *KCNQ1* (JLN1) have a significantly greater risk than patients with JLN2 due to mutations involving *KCNE1*.[65] Patients with the very rare form of LQTS with syndactyly, now known as type 1 Timothy syndrome secondary to mutations in the L-type calcium channel, have a very poor prognosis.[66,67]

A history of recurrent cardiac arrest increases the probability of sudden cardiac death at follow-up.[68] Perhaps more than any other risk factor, syncope should be viewed as a strong sudden death warning sign.[13] This observation now elevates to the level of critical importance the proper distinction between vasovagal syncope and torsadogenic syncope, less the trend toward early ICD therapy be accelerated even further. A negative family history for sudden cardiac death cannot be regarded as a predictor of favorable outcomes. On the other hand, a family history of sudden cardiac arrest may not indicate an increased risk for the affected relatives left behind.

A markedly prolonged QT interval (i.e., QTc > 600 msec) is associated with a greater risk for cardiac events, but only a minority of LQTS patients manifest such a QTc.[12,33] More recently, QTc values > 500 msec[64] or 530 msec[13] have been indicated as proarrhythmic cutoff values. Despite a discernible relationship between clinical risk and degree of QT prolongation, there does not appear to be a *no risk* QTc. Patients with LQTS but a QTc persistently <440 msec comprise the near zero risk category.[33]

T wave notching or humps appear to be more common in symptomatic patients and may be of prognostic significance.[69] QT dispersion >100 mse and a lack of shortening following a β blocke therapy are associated with high risk of recurrer cardiac events.[46] Beat-to-beat repolarization labil ity may identify patients with sudden cardia death and predict arrhythmia-free survival. Various methods quantifying T wave morpholog have been developed based on observations tha T wave morphology is a reflection of repolariza tion wavefront in the myocardium.[71] The T wav spectral variance (TWSV) index, a new metho to assess beat-to-beat variability of the T wav revealed increased heterogeneity of repolariza tion in patients prone to both VT and VF.[72] Macro scopic TWA on the 12-lead ECG is a marker c severe electrical instability in LQTS.[42,43] Howeve quantitation of the actual risk of sudden cardia death associated with TWA is still uncertain, an visible TWA is an infrequent sighting in the LQT evaluation.[63] Nonetheless, it can be used appro priately as a marker of persisting electrical insta bility and risk despite current therapy. Ther appears to be no role or justification, especially i children, for invasive electrophysiology studies i LQTS risk stratification as most LQTS patient are not inducible during programmed electrica stimulation.[73]

Using catecholamine provocation with dob utamine instead of exercise stress testing, Neme *et al.*[74] demonstrated that μV-TWA occurred a lower heart rates in patients with LQTS tha in healthy people. However, catecholamine provoked μV-TWA failed to identify high-ris subjects. In contrast, the investigators describe and quantified macroscopic nonalternating, beat to-beat lability in T wave amplitude and mor phology during catecholamine stress testing wit dobutamine.[75] This lability was quantified using newly derived T wave lability index (TWLI) base on a determination of the root mean square o the differences in T wave amplitude at each iso chronic point. The TWLI was significantly highe in LQTS and marked T wave lability (TWLI ≥ 0.095) was detected in all three LQTS genotype (10/23), but in no control subjects. Importantly all high-risk patients having either a history o out-of-hospital cardiac arrest or syncope plus a least one sudden death in the family had TWLI ≥ 0.095. Future studies are necessary to determin whether such catecholamine-provoked T wav ability identifies patients harboring high-risk genetic substrates.

Treatment Recommendations

Today, there is uniform agreement that all symptomatic patients with LQTS require treatment because the risk of mortality without treatment is unacceptably too high. However, with the growing, but often unjustified attitude to move away from time tested β blocker therapy to more aggressive and more definitive, sudden death preventative, ICD therapy, the treatment plan for the symptomatic patient must be individualized. Here, the perceived risk–benefit ratios should be explained carefully to the patients. Given the potential morbidities associated with lifelong ICD therapy in a young person, the patients should be educated sufficiently to be able to have a say in the final decision. In general, there is probably universal agreement that an episode of aborted cardiac arrest, whether occurring while on medical therapy or not, warrants an ICD.

On the other hand, the need to treat asymptomatic patients is debatable. In 1993, Garson *et al.*[33] reported that cardiac arrest was the sentinel event in 9% of patients with LQTS. Furthermore, 12% of patients who were asymptomatic at the time of diagnosis later developed symptoms, including sudden death in 4%. This provided a cogent argument for the universal treatment of all patients with LQTS, both symptomatic and asymptomatic. More recently, Priori *et al.*[76] suggested that all *young asymptomatic* patients should be treated because sudden death as the sentinel event has been documented too frequently. Ackerman[5] recommended that after a patient with LQTS has been diagnosed, all first-degree relatives must be screened, a cardiologist must be involved in the care of families with LQTS, symptomatic patients must be treated, and treatment options must be considered carefully in asymptomatic patients.

We recommend that pharmacotherapy be strongly considered in *most asymptomatic* patients unless the patient is >30 years old, male, with LQT1 or the QTc is < 440 msec.

To be sure, many patients with LQTS harbor a long QT "dud" rather than a "ticking time bomb" and are destined for asymptomatic longevity. In fact, there are many LQTS patients who require *no* therapy. However, until clinical testing reveals the virtually "no risk" patient, near universal treatment will continue to be the prudent recommendation. Debate will continue over when an asymptomatic patient is no longer young and has "outgrown" his or her LQTS risk such that no medical therapy is necessary. All LQTS investigators have a collection of patients who had their sentinel event occur in their 30s, 40s, 50s, and even 60s such that suggesting any age as a cutoff in the decision for prophylactic therapy in an asymptomatic patient seems arbitrary. Besides, this may be a mute point as the standard therapy for LQTS, i.e., β blocker therapy, has been found to prolong life in older persons independent of its protective effect in LQTS, providing an "excuse"/"rationale" for a universal treatment recommendation.

The ultimate goal for the treatment of LQTS is to prevent sudden cardiac death secondary to a long QT heart that degenerates into polymorphic ventricular tachycardia and fails to spontaneously convert back to normal sinus rhythm. Currently, the treatment options for inherited LQTS include β blocker therapy, ICD, continuous pacing, a surgical procedure involving a left cervical sympathetic denervation surgery (LCSD), and genotype-directed therapy.

Pharmacotherapy

β Blocker therapy remains the front line therapy for most LQTS, particularly type 1 and type 2 LQTS.[29,68] Although not a randomized study, β blockers appear to decrease mortality from 71% in historical controls to 6% in a treated group.[77] A study from the Pediatric Electrophysiology Society demonstrated that β blockers were effective in decreasing symptoms, ventricular arrhythmias, and sudden death.[33] A large retrospective study involving 869 LQTS patients of whom 69% were symptomatic treated with β blocker revealed a marked beneficial effect with a significant reduction in cardiac events including sudden death with mortality below 2%.[68]

It is generally thought that all β blockers are equally protective, with propranolol 2–4 mg/kg/day, nadolol 0.5–2.0 mg/kg/day, metoprolol 0.5–1.0 mg/kg/day, and atenolol 0.5–1.0 mg/kg/day being most commonly used. These are significant doses of β blockers, and a commonly observed mistake is inadequate dosing (homeopathic doses). When prescribing different β blockers, the total dose, dosing schedule, and adverse effects need to be considered. Propranolol and nadolol are nonselective β blockers, whereas atenolol and metoprolol are relatively cardioselective β blockers. Propranolol has a short half-life and requires frequent dosing. Moreover, it causes side effects involving the central nervous system. Atenolol is more popular than propranolol in treatment of LQTS due to fewer side effects, decreased blood–brain barrier penetration, and longer half-life. However, one study suggested atenolol may not be sufficiently protective for the treatment of LQTS, especially a once-a-day dosing, so it recommended twice-a-day dosing of atenolol if chosen.[78] In general, we recommend (1) either nadolol or propranolol in children, adolescents, and adults, (2) liquid propranolol until the patient is able to swallow pills, and (3) nadolol, propranolol, or metoprolol during pregnancy (the preferred β blocker among obstetricians is metoprolol). Although the data are limited, we have concluded that atenolol is not as protective as the other β blockers. At minimum, the practice of once-a-day dosing of atenolol is not pharmacokinetically justified.

Other pharmacotherapeutic strategies including calcium channel blockers and potassium channel openers should be considered unproven in LQTS and should not represent "stand alone" therapies. Patients with severe symptoms including appropriate ICD therapies refractory to both β blocker therapy and surgical denervation are probably the only candidates for calcium channel blockers such as verapamil or potassium channel openers such as nicorandil.

Device Therapy: Pacemakers and Implantable Cardioverter Defibrillators

Pacemaker Therapy

Viskin *et al.*[79] demonstrated that the majority of spontaneous arrhythmias in congenital LQTS are pause dependent (TdP is usually preceded by sudden decrements in cycle length). Overall, LQTS patients have slower resting heart rates than normal subjects, particularly in LQT3 patients. Moreover, β blocker therapy can cause profoun bradycardia and sinus pauses. For these reason cardiac pacing in conjunction with β blocke therapy has been shown to be beneficial i preventing pause-dependent TdP, especially i patients with LQT2.[80–82] However, cardiac pacin should be considered as an adjunct to β blocke therapy, not as a sole therapy, in treatment o LQTS patients who have preexisting atrioven tricular (AV) block or evidence of pause-depend ent arrhythmias. Moreover, concomitant β blocke therapy and continuous pacing have failed to sig nificantly reduce the sudden death risk in high risk patients.[81] In conclusion, cardiac pacing is possible adjuvant therapy to β blocker therapy i patients with bradycardia, AV block, and pause dependent TdP as seen in LQT2, or in LQT patients. In practice, we have seldom implante only a pacemaker. Instead, if the patient is per ceived to be at significant risk and a pacemake appears indicated, an implantable defibrillato pacemaker is the preferred device therapy.

Implantable Cardioverter Defibrillator Therapy

Contrary to the seemingly current and pervasiv trend embracing ICD therapy as frontline therap in LQTS, <10% of the patients seen in our respec tive LQTS clinics have an ICD. The majority ar being managed successfully without an ICD. Th ICD represents one of the twentieth century' greatest medical advances, and when used appro priately, it is both life saving and life changin When used indiscriminantly, it is only life chang ing and in some instances dramatically so. Figur 31–6 summarizes the indications for ICD therap in our LQTS clinics. There is almost universa agreement with the recommendation for ICD therapy as secondary prevention following a aborted cardiac arrest.[83–85]

In terms of the ICD as primary prevention, th various risk–benefit scenarios must be considere carefully. The motivation for primary preventio ICD therapy is the correct recognition that β blockers significantly reduce but do not eliminat the risk for sudden death.[13,68] Although emotion ally compelling and currently cited as a class II indication for ICD therapy, there is no evidenc to indicate that a positive family history of sudde death is an independent risk factor for thos

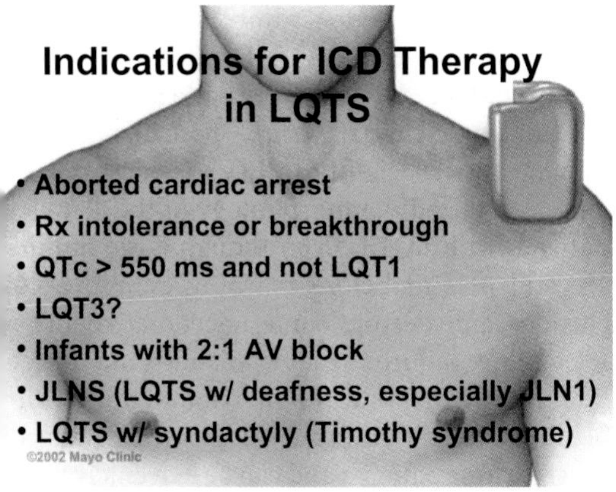

Indications for ICD Therapy in LQTS
• Aborted cardiac arrest
• Rx intolerance or breakthrough
• QTc > 550 ms and not LQT1
• LQT3?
• Infants with 2:1 AV block
• JLNS (LQTS w/ deafness, especially JLN1)
• LQTS w/ syndactyly (Timothy syndrome)
©2002 Mayo Clinic

FIGURE 31–6. Summary of indications for ICD therapy in LQTS.

enetically affected family members and relatives who are still living. Risk factors that warrant consideration of an ICD include (Figure 31–6) (1) yncope despite adequate β blocker therapy,[13] (2) ntolerance of primary pharmacotherapy, (3) evere QT prolongation (QTc > 550 msec) and not QT1 genotype,[85,86] (4) LQT3 genotype,[28,68,87] (5) nfants with 2:1 AV block,[33] (6) JLNS, especially atients with type 1 JLNS,[65] and (7) LQTS with yndactyly (Timothy syndrome).[67] In practice, if n ICD seems indicated, we generally proceed with a single-lead system unless a need for pacing herapy has already been declared (i.e., pause-ependent TdP, severe bradycardia). The majority of our implanted devices are still single-lead CDs. In some cases, surgical denervation might e considered an alternative to primary prevention ICD therapy or the next step in the patient eceiving appropriate ventricular fibrillation-erminating ICD therapies.

eft Cardiac Sympathetic Denervation

he concept of imbalance in cardiac sympathetic nnervation in LQTS[88] (overactivity of the left stellate ganglion and decreased right stellate ganglion ctivity) contributed to left cardiac sympathetic lenervation (LCSD) surgery. Its main rationale was and is the unquestionable evidence that left-ided cardiac sympathetic nerves have a very high rrhythmogenic potential.[88,89] There has not been randomized, controlled clinical trial to systematically evaluate the efficacy of LCSD. However, Moss *et al.*[89] first reported successful LCSD in a single symptomatic LQTS patients refractory to β blockers.

Recently, Schwartz *et al.*[90] reported the results of the LCSD in 147 LQTS patients with an average QTc of 543 ± 65 msec; 99% of them were symptomatic and 48% had experienced cardiac arrest. After LCSD, 46% of these patients became asymptomatic, syncope occurred in 31%, aborted cardiac arrest in 16%, and sudden death in 7%. The 5-year mortality for high-risk patients with syncope only prior to surgery was only 3% and was confined to those continuing to have a QTc > 500 msec 6 months after surgery. It was concluded that the LCSD is associated with a significant, long-term reduction in the frequency of aborted cardiac arrest and syncope and should be considered in all LQTS patients who experience syncope despite β blocker therapy and in those who have arrhythmia storms and shocks with an ICD.[31]

In the absence of a head-to-head trial randomizing high-risk patients to either ICD or LCSD therapy, a decision to proceed initially with LCSD therapy for the perceived high-risk patient (primary prevention) rather than ICD therapy will likely rely on the surgical expertise with respect to this surgical denervation procedure. Among experienced surgeons, mortality associated with LCSD should be near zero, and morbidity (Horner's syndrome with ptosis of the left eyelid) should be <3%. Compared to the complications associated with ICD therapy including inappropriate therapies, lead fractures, and infections, the overall morbidity is much less and the impact on quality of life may be much better with LCSD. Presently, among leading LQTS centers in the United States, LCSD remains reserved for patients having the most malignant expressions of their LQTS, typically patients experiencing multiple ventricular fibrillation-terminating ICD therapies.

Gene-Specific Therapy

Patients with LQT1

Due to the fact that life-threatening cardiac events occur during sympathetic activation in 90% of cases,[17] patients with LQT1 are effectively protected by the use of antiadrenergic interventions. In LQT1, β blocker therapy is the most effective.[86]

If syncope recurs despite β blocker therapy, LCSD is effective.[90] The majority of patients with LQT1 will not require ICD therapy.[31]

Patients with LQT2

In LQT2, β blockers are effective, although more breakthroughs occur among patients with LQT2 compared to LQT1.[13,68] Attempts to augment serum potassium via supplementation and spironolactone therapy have been shown to attenuate the QT interval both acutely and long term.[91,92] However, given the lack of outcome data and the extremely poor patient tolerability due to side effects, this strategy has gained little traction. The corollary is important, however, namely that keen attention should be given during medical illnesses (vomiting and diarrhea) that could decrease serum potassium significantly thereby increasing the potential for an LQT-triggered cardiac event. The recent demonstration of a relatively LQT2-specific, pause-dependent TdP mechanism may prompt consideration for dual chamber ICD/PM therapy in the high-risk patient with LQT2.[82] Presently, we generally advise single-lead ICD therapy for the high-risk patient.

Patients with LQT3

The management of patients with LQT3 is complex and difficult. Fortunately, LQT3 accounts for only 5–10% of the families seen in LQTS clinics. Strong evidence indicates that β blocker therapy is not sufficient in patients with LQT3, because of a 14–17% incidence of cardiac arrest/sudden death.[17,68,93] In fact, β blockers appear to be proarrhythmic in *in vitro* models of LQT3.[87] β Blocker therapy should be viewed as insufficient for patients with LQT3.

Sodium channel blockade represents a rational approach for a gene-specific therapy in LQT3, since most LQT3-causing mutations precipitate an increase in late sodium current via the Nav1.5 sodium channel. In an arterially perfused canine left ventricular wedge preparation pharmacologically mimicking LQT1–3, the sodium channel blocker mexiletine effectively reduced dispersion and prevented TdP in both LQT2 and LQT3 models.[94] Mexiletine also abbreviated the action potential duration of M cells more than that of epicardium and endocardium, thus diminishin transmural dispersion and the effect of isoprote enol to induce TdP in LQT1 models.[95]

Clinically, Schwartz *et al.*[50] first demonstrate that mexiletine significantly shortened the QT and normalized the morphology of the T wave i patients with LQT3. Even though large number are still needed before reaching definitive con clusions and despite some anecdotal reports of mexiletine failures, the available data sugge that mexiletine (always in conjunction with blockers) has a significant QT shortening effect i most of these patients and can be extremely usefu especially in the management of newborns wit life-threatening forms of LQT3. Besides mexilet ine, flecainide has been studied in families wit LQT3 and has been shown to attenuate the QT also.[96,97] However, flecainide also blocks the I_K current and in some patients with LQT3, flecain ide has mimicked some of the Brugada syndrom patterns.[98]

In practice, we assess the degree of QTc short ening produced by oral mexiletine and if signi ficant (≥50 msec), we continue with mexiletine based pharmacotherapy. However, althoug attenuating the QTc seems like an antiarrhythmi intervention, there are no data that currentl exist to demonstrate that mexiletine eithe decreases the number of syncopal events o improves survival. Thus, for now, it is very rea sonable to seriously consider concomitant ICD therapy for most patients with LQT3. For asymp tomatic infants and small children, the risks of a ICD likely outweigh the benefits. Here, a strateg of mexiletine, monitoring, LCSD, and an auto matic external defibrillator (AED) may be mor prudent.

Lifestyle Modification and Sports Participation in LQTS

Besides the aforementioned consideration regarding active therapy, there are several pre ventative health measures for the patient/famil that receives a life changing diagnosis of LQTS First, patients should be reminded of the impor tance of healthy sleep and dietary habits. A die rich in potassium cannot hurt. In contrast hypokalemia can potentially precipitate an LQT elated event. Therefore, careful attention to ydration and electrolyte replenishment during llnesses (vomiting, diarrhea, etc.) that can deplete otassium is prudent. A potassium supplement ould be considered, particularly for patients with QT2, although it is difficult to push potassium evels harder without the concomitant use of nedications that facilitate retention of potassium. Regarding supplements or complimentary alter- ative medicines, caution should be exercised vith products containing amphetamine-like gents or cesium.[99] While a healthy weight should e sought, aggressively fast and excessive weight oss has been associated with QT prolongation nd in theory could precipitate a cardiac event in patient with congenital LQTS. Grapefruit juice, specially purple grapefruit juice, contains a hemical that inhibits the I_{Kr} potassium channel ncoded by *KCNH2*, akin to the mechanism of early all Food and Drug Administration (FDA)- pproved medications associated with drug- nduced QT prolongation.[100]

Second, patients with LQTS in general and QT2 in particular should be advised to remove/ ninimize sources of loud noise in their environ- nent (such as alarm clocks and telephones), espe- ially while sleeping.[17,18,31] Third, for the patient/ amily with LQTS, the AED should be viewed as kin to the epinephrine pen for patients with life- hreatening allergies. Fourth, patients with LQTS hould have a disease identification card/bracelet vith them at all times. It is important that adult amily members are instructed on how to perform hump-version, which in LQTS may terminate TdP, restoring sinus rhythm, prior to initiating CPR.

Perhaps most importantly, patients should onsult their doctor before taking any medica- ions. At a minimum, all patients with LQTS *must* void drugs known to aggravate the QT interval s a drug-mediated side effect (www.qtdrugs.org). Occasionally, the patient will need a medicine that s on the "QT Hit List" and the physician and atient must carefully consider the risks and ben- efits. If there is a reasonable alternative medica- ion with similar efficacy, then the decision is imple.

However, there are several scenarios that are not so straightforward including (1) treatment of asthma with albuterol, (2) treatment of concomitant depression with selective serotonin reuptake inhibitors, and (3) treatment of concomitant attention deficit disorder with ritalin or other attention deficit-hyperactivity disorder therapies. In each case, the physician must weigh carefully the evidence for this potential side effect and determine, in the context of treating the whole person, what constitutes the best risk–benefit decision.

Finally, the single greatest impact on lifestyle pertains to the issue of sports participation. For patients diagnosed during their adolescent years, it is probably an underestimate to call this impact "huge." According to the 2005 Bethesda Guidelines, competitive sports should be prohibited in patients with *symptomatic* LQTS even if treated with either pharmacotherapy or ICD therapy.[101] The guidelines also suggest the possibility of liberalizing the restrictions in patients with genotype-positive but phenotype-negative LQTS. Suffice it to say this is an extraordinarily complex issue. If we took inventory of every activity of daily living associated with a LQT-triggered event seen in our LQTS clinics, we would have to restrict almost every activity: sleeping, waking, eating, brushing teeth, watching TV, etc.

Indeed, it seems prudent to recommend avoiding "competitive" sports as competition brings together the key triggers that threaten the long QT heart, the "fight-flight-fright" response.[102] Furthermore, such recommendations seem particularly appropriate in patients with LQT1 where exercise and activities such as swimming seem to be key arrhythmogenic triggers. However, there are known, predictable health outcomes for the obese, sedentary individual and encouraging an active, normal life for LQTS patients should be the goal. As our patients hear our admonitions to stay fit with "mild to moderate recreational physical activity" they astutely perceive the logical inconsistency behind prohibiting competitive sports while permitting recreational activities and wonder to what extent potential liability considerations are driving this recommendation. Ideally, we would prefer to see the risks and benefits laid out in excruciating detail and to help each patient/ family draw their own conclusions regarding a reasonable risk exposure.

Case Vignettes Revisited

Case #1: Do I or Do I Not Have Long QT Syndrome, That Is the Question?

JPA is a 15-year-old male referred for a second opinion and possible ICD implantation following the diagnosis of LQT1. At a preparticipation sports physical, an innocent murmur was heard, an ECG was obtained, and a QTc of 440 msec was noted. The patient fainted once in the setting of having his blood drawn. His family history was completely negative. No ECGs were performed on the parents. Holter monitoring revealed a QTc maximum of 501 msec occurring at 2:30 AM. An epinephrine QT stress test using the Mayo continuous infusion protocol demonstrated a 100 msec increase in the QTc during low-dose epinephrine. Genetic testing revealed a rare amino acid substitution in the KCNQ1-encoded I_{Ks} potassium channel localizing to the C-terminus of the channel. The patient was diagnosed with LQT1, placed on once-a-day atenolol β blocker therapy, and restricted from all competitive sports; a recommendation for sudden death primary prevention with an ICD has been rendered.

This case reflects the hazards of diagnostic miscues in the evaluation of LQTS. First, just on the clinical presentation, his QTc of 440 msec should represent normalcy with an odds ratio of about 1000:1 rather than the capture of a patient with concealed LQTS. Second, ECGs of the parents of an index case should be viewed as obligatory in the evaluation of LQTS. Third, a Holter QTc > 500 msec is per se of very modest value. Fourth, using the Mayo epinephrine QT stress test, an increase in QTc can be totally normal. Again, the LQT1 profile with this test is a paradoxic increase in the *absolute QT interval*. Fifth, the genetic test must be interpreted carefully and incorporated into the entire diagnostic work-up. In this context, the genetic test was likely a false positive, which can occur in approximately 5% of healthy subjects.

Now, even if the diagnosis of concealed LQT1 were correct, the physician's management plan was equally amiss. First, atenolol may not be sufficiently protective in LQTS and certainly should not be dosed in a once-a-day fashion if the goal is for 24-h coverage. Second, the latest Bethesda Conference guidelines would support lifting of the competitive sports ban in patients with concealed LQTS. Finally, despite being an all too common recommendation, prophylactic ICD therapy should be viewed as excessive for the management of concealed LQT1. Unfortunately, our LQTS clinics are replete with this exact case scenario. In fact, 40% of patients coming to Mayo Clinic's LQTS clinic with a diagnosis of LQTS have left without the diagnosis.[103]

Case #2: Oh Great, an Infant with LQT3, Now What Do I Do?

JMA is a healthy asymptomatic newborn female born to a mother with genetically proven LQT3. The family history is significant for a nocturnal sudden death involving a maternal aunt at age 40. The initial newborn ECG shows a QTc of 420 msec. Would you perform any additional tests or dismiss as normal?

First, a one time ECG is unreliable for a determination of LQTS. Second, once a LQTS genotype has been established in a family, the screening ECG is unacceptable as a test to exclude the diagnosis. Here, the infant should have the family-specific mutation test performed. If negative, then the evaluation is over and the infant can be dismissed as normal. If positive, however, then the approach to an infant with *concealed* LQT3 likely favors monitoring only.

Case #3: Doctor Please Do Something, My Defibrillator Keeps Shocking Me

LLA is a 32-year-old female with symptomatic LQT2, a QTc of 550 msec, and a positive family history of multiple premature sudden deaths. Despite adequate β blocker therapy with nadolol, she continues to receive frequent ventricular fibrillation-terminating ICD therapies. What therapeutic strategy would you consider next?

Possible "out-of-desperation" additional pharmacotherapeutic strategies include calcium channel blockers, mexiletine, ranolazine, nicorandil, and/or spironolactone with potassium supplementation. However, the most definitive therapy would be the left cardiac sympathetic denervation (LCSD) procedure, which can be performed extrapleurally, without opening the chest.

in less than 1 h. Performed correctly, this procedure is not associated with Horner's syndrome and the degree of left ptosis, if present, is minimal (1–2 mm). For this malignant subset of LQTS, the potential benefit of this surgical intervention is extremely high.

References

1. Moss AJ, Schwartz PJ. 25th anniversary of the International Long-QT Syndrome Registry: An ongoing quest to uncover the secrets of long-QT syndrome. *Circulation* 2005;111(9):1199–1201.
2. Jervell A, Lange-Nielsen F. Congenital deaf-mutism, functional heart disease with prolongation of the QT interval, and sudden death. *Am Heart J* 1957;54(1):59–68.
3. Romano C GG, Pongiglione R. Aritmie cardiache rare dell'eta'pediatrica. II. Accessi sincopali per fibrillazione ventricolare parossistica. *Clin Peditr (Bologna)* 1963;45:656–683.
4. Ward OC. A new familial cardiac syndrome in children. *J Irish Med Assoc* 1964;54:103–106.
5. Ackerman MJ. The long QT syndrome: Ion channel diseases of the heart. *Mayo Clin Proc* 1998;73(3): 250–269.
6. Vincent GM. The molecular genetics of the long QT syndrome: Genes causing fainting and sudden death. *Annu Rev Med* 1998;49:263–274.
7. Crotti L S-BM, Pedrazzini M, Ferrandi C, Insolia R, Goulene K, Salice P, Mannarino S, Schwartz PJ. Prevalence of the long QT syndrome. *Circulation* 2005;112(Suppl. II):660.
8. Tester DJ, Ackerman MJ. Postmortem long QT syndrome genetic testing for sudden unexplained death in the young. *J Am Coll Cardiol* 2007;16; 49(2):240–246.
9. Goldenberg I, Moss AJ, Zareba W, *et al.* Clinical course and risk stratification of patients affected with the Jervell and Lange-Nielsen syndrome. *J Cardiovasc Electrophysiol* 2006;17:1161–1168.
10. Moss AJ. Long QT syndromes. *Curr Treat Options Cardiovasc Med* 2000;2(4):317–322.
11. Schwartz PJ. Clinical applicability of molecular biology: The case of the long QT syndrome. *Curr Control Trials Cardiovasc Med* 2000;1(2):88–91.
12. Moss AJ, Schwartz PJ, Crampton RS, *et al.* The long QT syndrome. Prospective longitudinal study of 328 families. *Circulation* 1991;84(3):1136–1144.
13. Hobbs JB, Peterson DR, Moss AJ, *et al.* Risk of aborted cardiac arrest or sudden cardiac death during adolescence in the long-QT syndrome. *JAMA* 2006;296(10):1249–1254.
14. Lehmann MH, Timothy KW, Frankovich D, *et al.* Age-gender influence on the rate-corrected QT interval and the QT-heart rate relation in families with genotypically characterized long QT syndrome. *J Am Coll Cardiol* 1997;29(1):93–99.
15. Locati EH, Zareba W, Moss AJ, *et al.* Age- and sex-related differences in clinical manifestations in patients with congenital long-QT syndrome: Findings from the International LQTS Registry. *Circulation* 1998;97(22):2237–2244.
16. Rashba EJ, Zareba W, Moss AJ, *et al.* Influence of pregnancy on the risk for cardiac events in patients with hereditary long QT syndrome. LQTS Investigators. *Circulation* 1998;97(5):451–456.
17. Schwartz PJ, Priori SG, Spazzolini C, *et al.* Genotype-phenotype correlation in the long-QT syndrome: Gene-specific triggers for life-threatening arrhythmias. *Circulation* 2001;103:89–95.
18. Moss AJ, Robinson JL, Gessman L, *et al.* Comparison of clinical and genetic variables of cardiac events associated with loud noise versus swimming among subjects with the long QT syndrome. *Am J Cardiol* 1999;84(8):876–879.
19. Ackerman MJ, Tester DJ, Porter CJ. Swimming, a gene-specific arrhythmogenic trigger for inherited long QT syndrome. *Mayo Clin Proc* 1999;74(11): 1088–1094.
20. Moss AJ, Zareba W, Benhorin J, *et al.* ECG T-wave patterns in genetically distinct forms of the hereditary long QT syndrome. *Circulation* 1995;92(10): 2929–2934.
21. Zhang L, Timothy KW, Vincent GM, *et al.* Spectrum of ST-T-wave patterns and repolarization parameters in congenital long-QT syndrome: ECG findings identify genotypes. *Circulation* 2000;102 (23):2849–2855.
22. Wilde AA, Jongbloed RJ, Doevendans PA, *et al.* Auditory stimuli as a trigger for arrhythmic events differentiate HERG- related (LQTS2) patients from KVLQT1-related patients (LQTS1). *J Am Coll Cardiol* 1999;33(2):327–332.
23. Khositseth A, Tester DJ, Will ML, Bell CM, Ackerman MJ. Identification of a common genetic substrate underlying postpartum cardiac events in congenital long QT syndrome. *Heart Rhythm* 2004;1:60–64.
24. Heradien MJ, Goosen A, Crotti L, *et al.* Does pregnancy increase cardiac risk for LQT1 patients with the KCNQ1-A341V mutation? *J Am Coll Cardiol* 2006;48:1410–1415.
25. Lehmann MH, Suzuki F, Fromm BS, *et al.* T wave "humps" as a potential electrocardiographic marker of the long QT syndrome. *J Am Coll Cardiol* 1994;24(3):746–754.

26. Vincent GM, Timothy KW, Leppert M, Keating M. The spectrum of symptoms and QT intervals in carriers of the gene for the long-QT syndrome. *N Engl J Med* 1992;327(12):846–852.
27. Dumaine R, Wang Q, Keating MT, *et al.* Multiple mechanisms of Na+ channel-linked long-QT syndrome. *Circ Res* 1996;78(5):916–924.
28. Zareba W, Moss AJ, Schwartz PJ, *et al.* Influence of genotype on the clinical course of the long-QT syndrome. International Long-QT Syndrome Registry Research Group. *N Engl J Med* 1998;339 (14):960–965.
29. Schwartz PJ. Idiopathic long QT syndrome: Progress and questions. *Am Heart J* 1985;109(2): 399–411.
30. Schwartz PJ, Moss AJ, Vincent GM, Crampton RS. Diagnostic criteria for the long QT syndrome. An update. *Circulation* 1993;88(2):782–784.
31. Schwartz PJ. The congenital long QT syndromes from genotype to phenotype: Clinical implications. *J Intern Med* 2006;259(1):39–47.
32. Bazett HC. An analysis of the time-relations of electrocardiograms. *Heart* 1920;7:353–370.
33. Garson A Jr, Dick M 2nd, Fournier A, *et al.* The long QT syndrome in children. An international study of 287 patients. *Circulation* 1993;87(6):1866–1872.
34. Garson A Jr, Kertesz NJ, Towbin JA. Improved electrocardiographic identification of the long QT syndrome. *J Am Coll Cardiol* 2001;37(Suppl. A): 467A.
35. Allan WC, Timothy K, Vincent GM, Palomaki GE, Neveux LM, Haddow JE. Long QT syndrome in children: The value of rate corrected QT interval and DNA analysis as screening tests in the general population. *J Med Screen* 2001;8(4):173–177.
36. Viskin S, Rosovski U, Sands AJ, *et al.* Inaccurate electrocardiographic interpretation of long QT: The majority of physicians cannot recognize a long QT when they see one. [See comment.] *Heart Rhythm* 2005;2(6):569–574.
37. Moss AJ, Schwartz PJ, Crampton RS, Locati E, Carleen E. The long QT syndrome: A prospective international study. *Circulation* 1985;71(1):17–21.
38. Tester DJ, Will ML, Haglund CM, Ackerman MJ. Effect of clinical phenotype on yield of long QT syndrome genetic testing. *J Am Coll Cardiol* 2006;47(4):764–768.
39. Vincent GM, Timothy K, Fox J, Zhang L. The inherited long QT syndrome: From ion channel to bedside. *Cardiol Rev* 1999;7(1):44–55.
40. Lupoglazoff JM, Denjoy I, Berthet M, *et al.* Notched T waves on Holter recordings enhance detection of patients with LQt2 (HERG) mutations. *Circulation* 2001;103(8):1095–1101.
41. Khositseth A, Hejlik J, Shen WK, Ackerman M Epinephrine-induced T-wave notching in cor genital long QT syndrome. *Heart Rhythm* 2005; 141–146.
42. Schwartz PJ, Malliani A. Electrical alternation (the T-wave: Clinical and experimental evidence (its relationship with the sympathetic nervou system and with the long Q-T syndrome. *A Heart J* 1975;89(1):45–50.
43. Zareba W, Moss AJ, le Cessie S, Hall WJ. T wav alternans in idiopathic long QT syndrome. *J A Coll Cardiol* 1994;23(7):1541–1546.
44. Napolitano C, Priori SG, Schwartz PJ. Significanc of QT dispersion in the long QT syndrome. *Pro Cardiovasc Dis* 2000;42(5):345–350.
45. Day CP, McComb JM, Campbell RW. QT disper sion: An indication of arrhythmia risk in patient with long QT intervals. *Br Heart J* 1990;63(6):342 344.
46. Priori SG, Napolitano C, Diehl L, Schwartz PJ. Dis persion of the QT interval. A marker of therapeu tic efficacy in the idiopathic long QT syndrom *Circulation* 1994;89(4):1681–1689.
47. Moennig G, Schulze-Bahr E, Wedekind H, *et a* Clinical value of electrocardiographic parameter in genotyped individuals with familial long Q syndrome. *Pacing Clin Electrophysiol* 2001;24(4P 1):406–415.
48. Vincent GM, Jaiswal D, Timothy KW. Effects c exercise on heart rate, QT, QTc and QT/QS2 in th Romano-Ward inherited long QT syndrome. *Ar J Cardiol* 1991;68(5):498–503.
49. Swan H, Toivonen L, Viitasalo M. Rate adaptatio of QT intervals during and after exercise in chi dren with congenital long QT syndrome. *Eu Heart J* 1998;19(3):508–513.
50. Schwartz PJ, Priori SG, Locati EH, *et al.* Long Q syndrome patients with mutations of the SCN5 and HERG genes have differential responses t Na+ channel blockade and to increases in hear rate. Implications for gene-specific therapy. *Circu lation* 1995;92(12):3381–3386.
51. Swan H, Viitasalo M, Piippo K, Laitinen P, Kontul K, Toivonen L. Sinus node function and ventricu lar repolarization during exercise stress test i long QT syndrome patients with KvLQT1 an HERG potassium channel defects. *J Am Co Cardiol* 1999;34(3):823–829.
52. Ackerman MJ, Khositseth A,Tester, DJ, Hejlik Shen WK, Porter CJ. Epinephrine-induced Q interval prolongation: A gene-specific paradoxica response in congenital long QT syndrome. *May Clin Proc* 2002;77(5):413–421.
53. Shimizu W, Noda T, Takaki H, *et al.* Epinephrin unmasks latent mutation carriers with LQT1 form

of congenital long-QT syndrome. *J Am Coll Cardiol* 2003;41(4):633–642.
54. Vyas H, Hejlik J, Ackerman MJ. Epinephrine QT stress testing in the evaluation of congenital long-QT syndrome: Diagnostic accuracy of the paradoxical QT response. *Circulation* 2006;113(11): 1385–1392.
55. Curran ME, Splawski I, Timothy KW, Vincent GM, Green ED, Keating MT. A molecular basis for cardiac arrhythmia: HERG mutations cause long QT syndrome. *Cell* 1995;80(5):795–803.
56. Wang Q, Shen J, Splawski I, *et al.* SCN5A mutations associated with an inherited cardiac arrhythmia, long QT syndrome. *Cell* 1995;80(5):805–811.
57. Tester DJ, Will ML, Haglund CM, Ackerman MJ. Compendium of cardiac channel mutations in 541 consecutive unrelated patients referred for long QT syndrome genetic testing. *Heart Rhythm* 2005; 2:507–517.
58. Napolitano C, Priori SG, Schwartz PJ, *et al.* Genetic testing in the long QT syndrome: Development and validation of an efficient approach to genotyping in clinical practice. [See comment.] *JAMA* 2005;294(23):2975–2980.
59. Splawski I, Shen J, Timothy KW, *et al.* Spectrum of mutations in long-QT syndrome genes. KVLQT1, HERG, SCN5A, KCNE1, and KCNE2. *Circulation* 2000;102(10):1178–1185.
60. Westenskow P, Splawski I, Timothy KW, Keating MT, Sanguinetti MC. Compound mutations: A common cause of severe long-QT syndrome. *Circulation* 2004;109:1834–1841.
61. Ackerman MJ, Tester DJ, Jones G, Will MK, Burrow CR, Curran M. Ethnic differences in cardiac potassium channel variants: Implications for genetic susceptibility to sudden cardiac death and genetic testing for congenital long QT syndrome. *Mayo Clinic Proc* 2003;78:1479–1487.
62. Ackerman MJ, Splawski I, Makielski JC, *et al.* Spectrum and prevalence of cardiac sodium channel variants among black, white, Asian, and Hispanic individuals: Implications for arrhythmogenic susceptibility and Brugada/long QT syndrome genetic testing. *Heart Rhythm* 2004;1:600–607.
63. Priori SG, Aliot E, Blomstrom-Lundqvist C, *et al.* Task Force on Sudden Cardiac Death of the European Society of Cardiology. *Eur Heart J* 2001;22(16): 1374–1450.
64. Priori SG, Schwartz PJ, Napolitano C, *et al.* Risk stratification in the long-QT syndrome. *N Engl J Med* 2003;348:1866–1874.
65. Schwartz PJ, Spazzolini C, Crotti L, *et al.* The Jervell and Lange-Nielsen syndrome: Natural history, molecular basis, and clinical outcome. *Circulation* 2006;113(6):783–790.
66. Marks ML, Trippel DL, Keating MT. Long QT syndrome associated with syndactyly identified in females. *Am J Cardiol* 1995;76(10):744–745.
67. Splawski I, Timothy KW, Sharpe LM, *et al.* Cav1.2 calcium channel dysfunction causes a multisystem disorder including arrhythmia and autism. *Cell* 2004;119:19–31.
68. Moss AJ, Zareba W, Hall WJ, *et al.* Effectiveness and limitations of beta-blocker therapy in congenital long-QT syndrome. *Circulation* 2000;101 (6):616–623.
69. Malfatto G, Beria G, Sala S, Bonazzi O, Schwartz PJ. Quantitative analysis of T wave abnormalities and their prognostic implications in the idiopathic long QT syndrome. *J Am Coll Cardiol* 1994;23(2): 296–301.
70. Atiga WL, Calkins H, Lawrence JH, Tomaselli GF, Smith JM, Berger RD. Beat-to-beat repolarization lability identifies patients at risk for sudden cardiac death. *J Cardiovasc Electrophysiol* 1998; 9(9):899–908.
71. Zareba W. New electrocardiographic indices of risk stratification. *J Electrocardiol* 2001;34:332.
72. Steinbigler P, Haberl R, Nespithal K, Spiegl A, Schmucking I, Steinbeck G. T wave spectral variance: A new method to determine inhomogeneous repolarization by T wave beat-to-beat variability in patients prone to ventricular arrhythmias. *J Electrocardiol* 1998;30(Suppl.):137–144.
73. Bhandari AK, Shapiro WA, Morady F, Shen EN, Mason J, Scheinman MM. Electrophysiologic testing in patients with the long QT syndrome. *Circulation* 1985;71(1):63–71.
74. Nemec J, Ackerman, MJ, Tester D, Hejlik J, Shen WK. Catecholamine provoked microvoltage T wave alternans in genotyped long QT syndrome. *Pacing Clin Electrophysiol* 2003;26(8):1660–1667.
75. Nemec J, Hejlik JB, Shen WK, Ackerman MJ. Catecholamine-induced T-wave lability in congenital long QT syndrome: a novel phenomenon associated with syncope and cardiac arrest. *Mayo Clin Proc* 2003;78:40–50.
76. Priori SG, Maugeri FS, Schwartz PJ. The risk of sudden death as first cardiac event in asymptomatic patients with the long QT syndrome. *Circulation* 1998;98(Suppl. I):777 (abstract).
77. Schwartz PJ. The long QT syndrome. *Curr Probl Cardiol* 1997;22(6):297–351.
78. Chatrath R, Bell CM, Ackerman MJ. Beta-blocker therapy failures in symptomatic probands with genotyped long-QT syndrome. *Pediatr Cardiol* 2004;25(5):459–465.
79. Viskin S, Fish R, Zeltser D, *et al.* Arrhythmias in the congenital long QT syndrome: How often is

torsade de pointes pause dependent? *Heart* 2000; 83(6):661–666.
80. Eldar M, Griffin JC, Van Hare GF, *et al.* Combined use of beta-adrenergic blocking agents and long-term cardiac pacing for patients with the long QT syndrome. *J Am Coll Cardiol* 1992;20(4):830–837.
81. Dorostkar PC, Eldar M, Belhassen B, Scheinman MM. Long-term follow-up of patients with long-QT syndrome treated with beta- blockers and continuous pacing. *Circulation* 1999;100(24):2431–2436.
82. Tan HL, Bardai A, Shimizu W, *et al.* Genotype-specific onset of arrhythmias in congenital long-QT syndrome: Possible therapy implications. *Circulation* 2006;114:2096–2103.
83. Chatrath R, Porter CJ, Ackerman MJ. Role of transvenous implantable cardioverter-defibrillators in preventing sudden cardiac death in children, adolescents, and young adults. *Mayo Clin Proc* 2002;77:226–231.
84. Zareba W, Moss AJ, Daubert JP, Hall WJ, Robinson JL, Andrews M. Implantable cardioverter defibrillator in high-risk long QT syndrome patients. *J Cardiovasc Electrophysiol* 2003;14:337–341.
85. Monnig G, Kobe J, Loher A, *et al.* Implantable cardioverter-defibrillator therapy in patients with congenital long-QT syndrome: A long-term follow-up. *Heart Rhythm* 2005;2(5):497–504.
86. Villain E, Denjoy I, Lupoglazoff JM, *et al.* Low incidence of cardiac events with B-blocking therapy in children with long QT syndrome. *Eur Heart J* 2004;25:1405–1411.
87. Shimizu W, Antzelevitch C. Differential effects of beta-adrenergic agonists and antagonists in LQT1, LQT2 and LQT3 models of the long QT syndrome. *J Am Coll Cardiol* 2000;35(3):778–786.
88. Schwartz PJ, Locati E. The idiopathic long QT syndrome: Pathogenetic mechanisms and therapy. *Eur Heart J* 1985;6(Suppl. D):103–114.
89. Moss AJ, McDonald J. Unilateral cervicothoracic sympathetic ganglionectomy for the treatment of long QT interval syndrome. *N Engl J Med* 1971; 285(16):903–904.
90. Schwartz PJ, Priori SG, Cerrone M, *et al.* Left cardiac sympathetic denervation in the management of high-risk patients affected by the long-QT syndrome. *Circulation* 2004;109(15):1826–1833.
91. Compton SJ, Lux RL, Ramsey MR, *et al.* Genetically defined therapy of inherited long-QT syndrome. Correction of abnormal repolarization by potassium. *Circulation* 1996;94(5):1018–1022.
92. Etheridge SP, Compton SJ, Tristani-Firouzi M, Mason JW. A new oral therapy for long QT syndrome: Long-term oral potassium improves repolarization in patients with HERG mutations. *J Am Coll Cardiol* 2003;42:1777–1782.
93. Priori SG, Napolitano C, Schwartz PJ, *et al.* Association of long QT syndrome loci and cardiac events among patients treated with B-blockers. *JAMA* 2004;292:1341–1344.
94. Shimizu W, Antzelevitch C. Sodium channel block with mexiletine is effective in reducing dispersion of repolarization and preventing torsade des pointes in LQT2 and LQT3 models of the long-QT syndrome. *Circulation* 1997;96(6):2038–2047.
95. Shimizu W, Antzelevitch C. Cellular basis for the ECG features of the LQT1 form of the long-QT syndrome: Effects of beta-adrenergic agonists and antagonists and sodium channel blockers on transmural dispersion of repolarization and torsade de pointes. *Circulation* 1998;98(21):2314–2322.
96. Moss AJ, Windle JR, Hall WJ, *et al.* Safety and efficacy of flecainide in subjects with long QT-3 syndrome (DeltaKPQ mutation): A randomized, double-blind, placebo-controlled clinical trial. *Ann Noninvasive Electrocardiol* 2005;10(4Suppl.):59–66.
97. Khan IA, Gowda RM. Novel therapeutics for treatment of long-QT syndrome and torsade de pointes. *Int J Cardiol* 2004;95(1):1–6.
98. Priori SG, Napolitano C, Schwartz PJ, Bloise R, Crotti L, Ronchetti E. The elusive link between LQT3 and Brugada syndrome: The role of flecainide challenge. *Circulation* 2000;102:945–947.
99. Vyas H, Johnson J, Houlihan R, Bauer BA, Ackerman MJ. Acquired long QT syndrome secondary to cesium chloride supplement. *J Altern Complement Med* 2006;12(10):1011–1014
100. Fitzgerald PT, Ackerman MJ. Drug-induced torsades de pointes: The evolving role of pharmacogenetics. *Heart Rhythm* 2005;2:S30–S37.
101. Zipes DP, Ackerman MJ, Estes NA 3rd, Grant AO, Myerburg RJ, Van Hare G. Task Force 7: Arrhythmias. *J Am Coll Cardiol* 2005;45:1354–1363.
102. Maron BJ, Isner JM, McKenna WJ. 26th Bethesda conference: Recommendations for determining eligibility for competition in athletes with cardiovascular abnormalities. Task Force 3: Hypertrophic cardiomyopathy, myocarditis and other myopericardial diseases and mitral valve prolapse. *J Am Coll Cardiol* 1994;24(4):880–885.
103. Taggart NW, Haglund CM, Tester DJ, Ackerman MJ. Diagnostic miscues in congenital long QT syndrome. *Circulation* 2007;115:2613–2620.

32 Brugada Syndrome: Clinical and Genetic Aspects

Paola G. Meregalli, Hanno L. Tan, and Arthur A.M. Wilde

Introduction

After its recognition in 1992[1] as a distinct clinical entity, Brugada syndrome has increasingly been recognized worldwide as an important cause of sudden cardiac death (SCD) at a young age, in the absence of structural cardiac abnormalities. Patients affected with Brugada syndrome are at risk for SCD from fast polymorphic ventricular tachycardia (VT)/ventricular fibrillation (VF), especially at rest.[2] Brugada syndrome is characterized by a typical electrocardiographic (ECG) pattern consisting of ST segment elevation in the right precordial leads and in leads positioned in the upper intercostal spaces,[3–5] (Figure 32–1). The large number of case reports and clinical/experimental studies lately published about Brugada syndrome indicate its increasing weight and interest for its still not completely known aspects, such as the underlying pathophysiological mechanism, its genetic background, and its prognosis and treatment.

The pathophysiological mechanism underlying this syndrome remains controversial,[6] with two predominant theories regarding the typical ECG features and the genesis of the arrhythmias: (1) a repolarization disorder, i.e., unequal expression of the transient outward potassium current I_{to} between the epicardium and the other transmural layers,[7–10] or (2) a depolarization disorder,[11–13] i.e., a delay in the onset of the action potential in the region of the right ventricle outflow tract (RVOT).[14–16]

In 2002 a First Consensus Report was published to define the diagnostic criteria for this syndrome.[17] Three repolarization patterns of ST-segment elevation (with two different shapes) were recognized as potential manifestations of Brugada syndrome. The coved-type morphology (type I) is characterized by a coved-shaped J wave elevation ≥2 mm, followed by a negative T wave. A type I ECG is required for the diagnosis, while a saddleback-shaped ST elevation or a coved-type <1 mm (types II–III) are indeterminate forms that necessitate pharmacological challenge[17] (Figure 32–2).

The diagnosis is posed when a type I ECG, spontaneously or after provocation with sodium channel blockers, is present in more than one right precordial lead in the absence of structural abnormalities, and in association with one of the following conditions: (1) documented VF or polymorphic VT, (2) a family history of SCD at a young age or a type I ECG in family members, (3) otherwise unexplained syncope, or (4) inducibility of VT/VF with programmed electrical stimulation (EPS).[17,18] Spontaneous occurrence of a type I ECG has prognostic implications, representing a condition with increased risk for malignant arrhythmias and, if present in conjunction with Brugada syndrome-associated symptoms, conferring an indication for implantation of an implantable cardioverter defibrillator (ICD).[19,20]

Risk stratification and indications for ICD implantation are extensively discussed in the Second Consensus Report paper, published in 2005.[18] This topic and other important aspects to consider in the interpretation of ECG patterns in Brugada syndrome are presented later in this chapter.

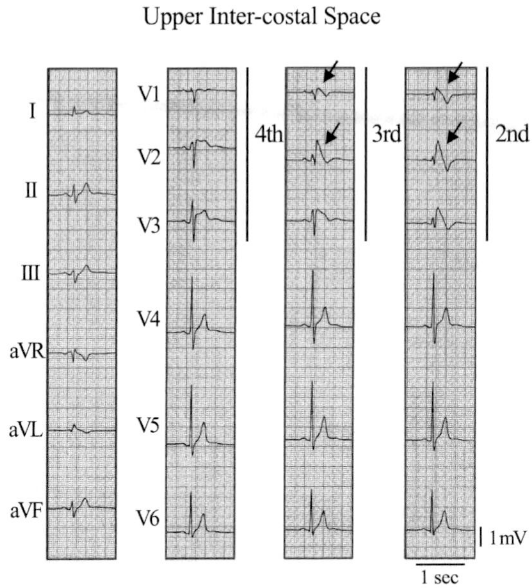

FIGURE 32–1. Four ECG traces of a resuscitated Brugada syndrome patient showing most severe ST-T abnormalities in leads positioned over the second and third intercostal space (right two panels) where a coved-type ECG is present (arrows). Intermediate ST-T abnormalities (saddleback-type) are recorded in the fourth intercostal space (leads V2–V3). Calibrations are given. (Courtesy of Dr. Wataru Shimizu.)

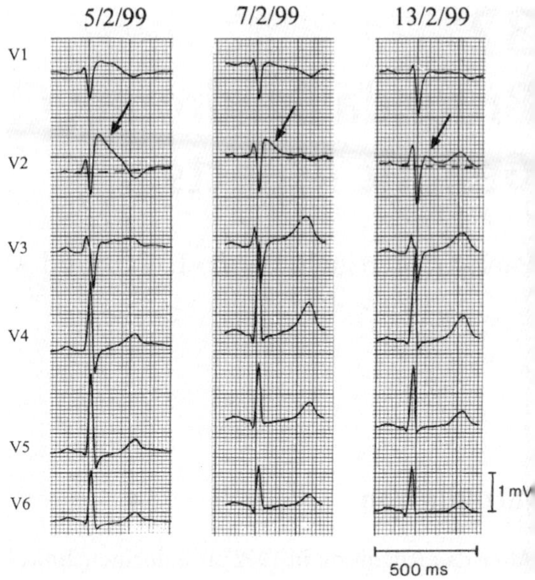

FIGURE 32–2. Precordial leads ECG of a resuscitated patient with three types of ST segment elevation described in Brugada syndrome. Within a few days the ECG changed from type I (left panel) to type II (middle) and type III (right panel). For explanation see text. The arrows indicate the J waves. Calibrations are given. (Modified from Wilde *et al.*[17])

Brugada syndrome is inherited as an autosomal dominant trait. In 1998, it was linked to mutations in the SCN5A gene, encoding the α subunit of the cardiac sodium channel protein.[21] Up to now, more than 80 mutations correlating with the Brugada syndrome phenotype have been found (inherited Arrhythmia Database: http://www.fsm.it/cardmoc/) (Figure 32–3). It is estimated that SCN5A mutations account for 20–30% of all Brugada syndrome cases. Discovery of new genes is still ongoing.

A linkage to a second locus on chromosome 3 was demonstrated in a large Brugada syndrome family and direct sequencing of that region led very recently to the identification of a novel mutation in the glycerol-3-phosphate dehydrogenase 1-like gene (GPD1L).[22,23] The exact function of the product of the GPD1L gene is still unknown, but most likely the mutant protein causes Brugada syndrome through a reduction in Na^+ inward current,[23] as well as the other Brugada-linked SCN5A mutations.[24]

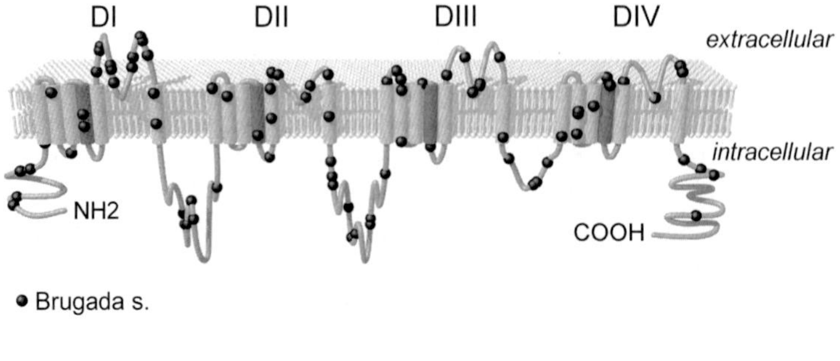

FIGURE 32–3. Representation of the α subunit of the voltage-gated SCN5A sodium channel showing the locations of the mutations associated with Brugada syndrome (circle). (Courtesy of Dr Andre Linnenbank, Department of Experimental Cardiology, AMC, The Netherlands.)

General Clinical Properties

Demography and Clinical Presentation

Since its recognition as a distinct subgroup of idiopathic VF in 1992, Brugada syndrome has been increasingly described worldwide, although its exact prevalence remains unclear and can vary significantly in different regions of the world.[25,26] It is endemic in East and Southeast Asia, where it underlies the sudden unexplained nocturnal death syndrome (SUNDS),[27] and is also particularly prevalent in Japan, the Philippines, and Thailand, being the leading cause of sudden death among young men.[28,29] In China and Korea, the reported incidence is lower.[30–32] In Europe, Brugada syndrome has beenextensively described,[19,33] with the exception of the Scandinavian countries,[34] and its prevalence is estimated at 5–50 cases per 10,000 inhabitants.[35,36] Conversely, the occurrence of Brugada-type ECG in the United States seems to be very uncommon.[37,38]

Arrhythmic events in Brugada syndrome can occur at all ages, from childhood to the elderly (range 2–77 years),[1,31,39,39a,40] with a peak around the fourth decade.[41] It is estimated that Brugada syndrome causes 4–12% of all SCD, and up to 20% among patients without identifiable structural abnormalities.[42]

The clinical presentation is heterogeneous, and may include palpitations, dizziness, syncope, and (aborted) sudden death, but many subjects remain asymptomatic.[43,44]

Sudden death results from fast polymorphic VT originating from the RVOT,[45] degenerating into VF.[1,2,46] Ventricular arrhythmias and (aborted) sudden death in Brugada syndrome—distinct from arrhythmogenic right ventricular cardiomyopathy (ARVC)—typically occur at rest when the vagal tone is augmented,[47] and often at night.[48,49] Self-terminating VT may provoke (recurrent) syncope and may explain why patients experience agonal respiration at night after which they wake up.[50–54] An estimated 80% of patients with documented VT/VF have a history of syncope.[33] The clinical presentation with sustained monomorphic VT, although uncommon, has also been described.[55–57] Data obtained from stored electrograms of ICDs have demonstrated that although premature ventricular complexes (PVCs) in patients affected with Brugada syndrome are rare,[58] their prevalence increases prior to spontaneous VF.[59] These PVCs appear to have the same morphology as the first VT beat, and different VT episodes are initiated by similar PVCs in the same subject.[59,60] They show a left bundle branch block (LBBB) morphology[61] and endocardial mapping localized their origin in the RVOT.[62] Further confirmation of the role of these initiating PVCs and of the RVOT derives from the clinical benefit resulting from their elimination via catheter ablation.[62]

No significant variations in QTc intervals precede spontaneous VF episodes.[1,59]

The occurrence of supraventricular tachycardia is also more prevalent and episodes of atrial flutter/fibrillation are often documented[1,63–68] with an estimated prevalence of 10–30%.[48,69] Given that a history of atrial arrhythmias correlates with VT/VF inducibility during EPS, and that ST segment elevation correlates with the onset of atrial fibrillation episodes,[48] Brugada syndrome patients with paroxysmal atrial arrhythmias may constitute a population at higher risk with a more advanced disease state,[70] but these data are still limited.[71]

A salient property in the clinical manifestation of Brugada syndrome is the higher disease prevalence in males (70–80% of all affected subjects), particularly in regions where this syndrome is endemic, despite equal genetic transmission among both genders.[28,35,41] That a role in gender disparity could be played by sex hormones, in particular by testosterone, was suggested by the demonstration that castration attenuated ST elevations in two asymptomatic male Brugada syndrome patients[72] and by the revelation that men affected with Brugada syndrome have significantly higher levels of testosterone than age-matched control subjects.[73] A possible explanation for this phenomenon, derived from clinical[74] and experimental studies,[75,76] is that sex hormones may modulate potassium currents (e.g., I_{to}) during the early repolarization phase of the cardiac action potential.

Genetic Aspects

In 1998, Brugada syndrome was linked to mutations in the SCN5A gene, encoding the pore-forming α subunit of the human cardiac sodium channel protein.[21] The SCN5A gene is situated on chromosome 3p21 and encodes a large protein of 2016 amino acid residues.[77] Every α subunit contains four homologous domains, each composed of six segments, and is assembled with two ancillary β subunits to form the voltage-dependent cardiac sodium channel. This channel belongs to a family with different isoforms and different biophysical properties according to its tissue distribution.[78] In the heart, it is responsible for the rapid initiating phase of the action potential and thus plays an important role in impulse formation and propagation through the cardiac conduction system and muscle.

In recent years more than 80 SCN5A gene mutations (inherited Arrhythmia Database: http://www.fsm.it/cardmoc/) have been described in patients with the Brugada syndrome phenotype, alone or in combination with long QT syndrome type 3 and/or progressive cardiac conduction defects, diseases in which SCN5A mutations may also be present[20,79–82] (Figure 32–3).

Functional studies have previously been performed with mutant proteins from at least 20 different SCN5A mutations. The common effect of SCN5A mutations associated with Brugada syndrome is reduction in sodium current (I_{Na}) resulting from failure of expression of the mutant sodium channel in the cell membrane (trafficking) or changes in its functional properties (gating), resulting from (1) a shift in the voltage and time dependence of I_{Na} activation and/or inactivation, (2) enhanced entry into an intermediate state of inactivation from which the channel recovers more slowly, and (3) accelerated inactivation.[24,81,83,84]

The reduction in I_{Na} caused by the mutant sodium channels in Brugada syndrome is in agreement with the clinical observation that sodium channel blockers accentuate ST segment abnormalities in affected subjects.[85] Moreover, this finding concurs with the demonstration that Brugada syndrome patients who carry an SCN5A mutation have significantly more conduction disorders than noncarriers.[86,87]

Despite the increasing number of SCN5A mutations recognized in Brugada syndrome, the proportion of clinically diagnosed Brugada syndrome patients who carry an SCN5A mutation is estimated to be around 30%, suggesting that the genetic basis of Brugada syndrome is heterogeneous.[33] Other genes still await identification; possible candidates are genes that modulate currents active during early repolarization phases of the action potential, such as I_{to}, the calcium current $I_{Ca\text{-}L}$ and potassium delayed rectifier currents I_{Ks} and I_{Kr},[88] as well as genes encoding adrenergic receptors, cholinergic receptors, ion-channel interacting proteins, transcriptional factors, and transporters.[89,90]

Recently, a novel mutation in the GPD1L gene on chromosome 3p22–24 has been described, linked to the Brugada syndrome phenotype in a large family.[22,23] This gene encodes a protein whose function in the heart still remains unknown, but the mutant protein, when studied in cell lines, was responsible for a diminished inward sodium current, similar to the other SCN5A mutations in Brugada syndrome studied so far.[23,24]

Of interest, SCN5A mutations are also implicated in LQT3 and Lev-Lenègre disease,[79,81,82] and some SCN5A mutations may cause a combination of Brugada syndrome and LQT3 or Lev-Lenègre disease within the same family or even within the same individual.[91,92] While LQT3-associated SCN5A mutations generally increase I_{Na}, those associated with Lev-Lenègre disease reduce it, similar to those in Brugada syndrome.[81]

Though SCN5A mutations account, so far, for 30% of all affected patients,[33,35] genetic testing is recommended during work-up in Brugada syndrome to support the clinical diagnosis, to identify affected relatives, and to better elucidate the genotype–phenotype relationship in Brugada syndrome.

Electrocardiographic Characteristics

Typical electrocardiographic abnormalities have represented, since its first description, the fundamental aspect in the recognition of subjects affected by Brugada syndrome.[1,2] Particular attention was given to the presence of a (incomplete) right bundle branch block (RBBB), accompanied by ST segment elevation in the right precordial leads, not related to ischemia, electrolyte imbalance, and structural heart disease.[4] At present, diagnosis of Brugada syndrome revolves around characteristic ST segment elevations in leads

V1–V3 and in leads positioned at the superior intercostal spaces, whereas the presence of an RBBB is no longer required.[17]

A total of three ECG repolarization patterns were described as potential manifestations of Brugada syndrome: type I ECG, referred to as coved-type, is the one illustrated in 1992 during the first description of the Brugada syndrome and consists of >2 mm J point elevation, followed by a downsloping ST segment and a negative T wave; type II ECG, called the saddleback type, also shows an elevated J point (>2 mm) with a gradually descending ST segment that does not reach the baseline and gives rise to a positive or biphasic T wave; type III ECG could be any of the previously described morphologies and is characterized by a smaller magnitude of ST segment elevation (≤1 mm) (Figure 32–2). The presence of a type I ECG is required for the diagnosis.[17]

Important considerations and cautions in the interpretation of the ECG in diagnosing Brugada syndrome have to be taken into account. First, the ST segment in Brugada syndrome is typically highly dynamic, exhibiting profound day-to-day variations in amplitude and morphology, even within the same patient.[93,94] This may contribute to possible bias and underestimation of the prevalence of Brugada syndrome. An interindividual variation of the ST segment can also be observed between members of the same family who carry the same SCN5A mutation. The magnitude of the ST segment elevation does not differ between SCN5A mutation carriers and nonmutation carriers in Brugada syndrome.[86]

Second, many agents and conditions are reported to significantly influence ST segment elevation in Brugada syndrome. Sodium channel blockers,[95] α-adrenoreceptor agonists, and cholinergic stimulation (increased vagal tone) provoke an augmentation of ST segment elevation, while α-adrenoreceptor blockade and β-adrenoreceptor stimulation with isoprenaline reduce the amount of ST segment abnormalities.[14,96] Since accentuation of ST elevation immediately preceding episodes of VF has been extensively reported,[14,48,66,97] all these drugs also strongly modulate susceptibility to arrhythmias.

Some clinically relevant aspects derive from these observations. (1) A variety of Na^+ channel blockers are utilized as diagnostic tools for unmasking concealed forms of Brugada syndrome.[85,98] (2) Use of any Na^+ channel blocker and other medications able to provoke ST elevation must be avoided in patients with Brugada syndrome[85,95] (Table 32–1). Particular attention must be also given to clinical management surrounding general anesthesia of patients affected with Brugada syndrome.[30,99–102] (3) Administration of isoprenaline, a β-adrenoreceptor agonist, can be effectively used in case of repetitive VT and arrhythmic storms in Brugada syndrome patients.[103,104]

Another important modulating factor is body temperature. Several case reports revealed that febrile illness[105–107] or prolonged contact with hot water[108] could precipitate arrhythmic events in Brugada syndrome patients. It is also our personal experience that asymptomatic Brugada patients with a normal basal ECG can, during an episode of fever, display typical ECG changes with different amounts of ST segment elevations up to the appearance of a type-I pattern (Figure 32–4). In 1999 Dumaine *et al.* discovered that the changes in Na^+ channel gating properties, induced by the SCN5A mutant T1620, were more prominent at higher temperature (32°C compared to room temperature),[109] which supports the notion that the consequences of possessing a certain SCN5A mutation or a mutation in other genes responsible for Brugada syndrome can be manifested only

Table 32–1. Medications to avoid in patients affected with Brugada syndrome.

Medications to be avoided in Brugada syndrome patients
Sodium channel blockers
Class I antiarrhythmic drugs (flecainide, ajmaline, propafenone, pilsicainide, procainamide, disopyramide, cibenzoline)[85,95]
Local anesthetics (lidocaine, bupivacaine)[178]
Carbamazepine, phenothiazine[167]
Tricyclic and tetracyclic antidepressants[164–168]
α-Adrenergic stimulation (norepinephrine, methoxamine)[100]
Medications to be used with caution in Brugada syndrome patients
β-Adrenergic blockers[96,100]
Calcium antagonists, nondihydropyridines (verapamil, diltiazem)[100,161,162]
Nitrates[66]
General anesthetics/antagonism of anesthesia[30,99–102]
Muscarinic drugs (i.e., neostigmine)[30,96,100]

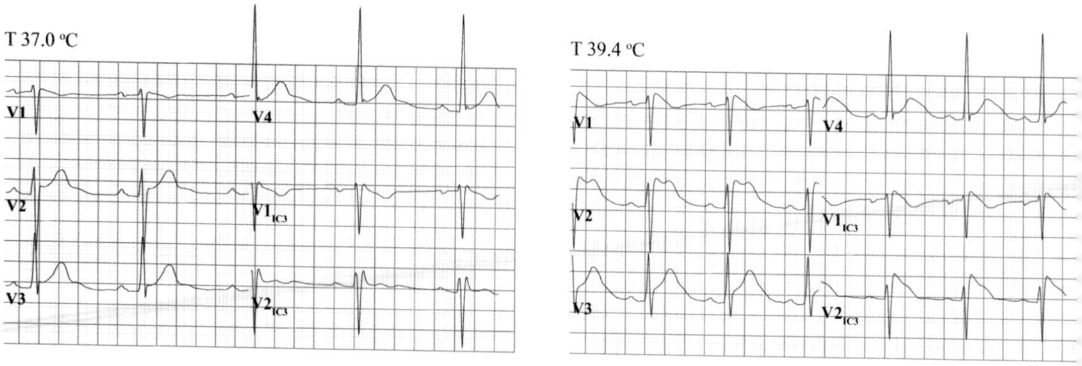

Figure 32–4. An ECG recorded at normal temperature and during fever in a male subject affected with Brugada syndrome. Leads $V1_{IC3}$ and $V2_{IC3}$ are positioned above V1 and V2, respectively, in the third intercostal space. This patient had multiple syncopes during fever with documented VF. Screening of SCN5A was negative. During fever, we recorded ST segment elevation with the appearance of type I in leads V1, $V1_{IC3}$ and $V2_{IC3}$, and type II in lead V2 (right panel), while ECGs of the same patient during normothermia display only minimal ST segment elevation (left panel).

during fever or in a hot climate. For this reason, appropriate treatment of fever illnesses is strongly recommended in all patients with Brugada syndrome.[39a] Also, activities and conditions that may provoke augmentation of body temperature must be discouraged.[90,108]

Importance of Positioning of the Precordial Leads and New Electrocardiographic Parameters

The signature ST elevations in Brugada syndrome are usually observed in leads V1–V3, with rare occurrences in inferior or lateral limb leads.[110–112] More strikingly, leads positioned cranially from V1 and V2 in the third ($V1_{IC3}$ and $V2_{IC3}$) or second ($V1_{IC2}$ and $V2_{IC2}$) intercostal spaces often produce the most severe abnormalities, both in the presence and absence of pharmacological challenge,[5,113,114] as also demonstrated with body surface mapping.[3,115] The use of 87-lead body surface maps permitted us to demonstrate that in 7/28 Brugada patients the typical ECG pattern was located at the level of the RVOT (second and third intercostals space), while conventional leads V1 and V2 registered only minimal ST segment elevation. Conversely, investigation of the more cranial leads in 40 control subjects did not reveal any significant ST elevation either at baseline or after disopyramide.[3] In a recently performed clinical investigation into the diagnostic value of flecainide testing in unmasking SCN5A-related Brugada syndrome, 45% (21/47) of the subjects with a positive response under flecainide were identified after a type I ECG had exclusively occurred in leads positioned over the third intercostal space.[116] Therefore, it is our opinion that ECG investigation in these more cranial leads should be performed whenever a case of Brugada syndrome is suspected.[116,117]

Recently, attention has also been paid to the recognition of other ECG criteria, in addition to the amount of J point elevation that may aid in identifying subjects at risk for sudden death. There are two new ECG parameters. (1) S wave width in leads II and III, to be considered a mirror image of the electrical activity taking place in the RVOT, a core area in the pathophysiology of Brugada syndrome;[6] these S waves were significantly wider in the individuals with a positive response to flecainide than in the negative responders.[116] (2) S wave width in lead V1 ≥ 0.08 sec was shown to be a good predictor of arrhythmic events in Brugada syndrome patients.[118] Spontaneous ECG fluctuations measured on separate days in Brugada syndrome patients are also associated with the highest risk of arrhythmic events and can be used as a noninvasive method for risk stratification, as well as the presence of late potentials on signal-averaged ECGs.[119,120]

Other Electrocardiographic Features in Brugada Syndrome

Brugada syndrome has habitually been accompanied by RBBB, thought atypical because of the absence of a wide S wave in the left lateral leads.[35] The presence of a RBBB is no longer considered necessary for the diagnosis,[17] though a widening of the QRS complex is frequently observed in patients affected by Brugada syndrome.[116,118]

Actually, signs of conduction defects are found at all levels (Figure 32–5), particularly in patients carrying an SCN5A mutation[86,87]: QRS axis deviation,[1,112,121,122] P wave enlargement,[116] and PQ prolongation, presumably reflecting prolonged His-ventricular conduction time.[1,35,86,123] Moreover, sinus node dysfunction[122,124,125] and atrioventricular (AV) node dysfunction[86,95,126] have been extensively reported. In contrast, QTc duration generally is within the normal range,[17,35,70] but it may be occasionally prolonged.[1]

In a recently studied cohort, the presence of an SCN5A mutation greatly influenced the phenotype, with more exhibition of clinically relevant conduction defects (first degree AV block, complete RBBB, LBBB, hemiblocks) in SCN5A carriers than in noncarriers,[87] independent of the amount of ST segment elevation.

Drug Test

Pharmacological challenges utilize intravenous administration of sodium channel blockers, i.e., class IA (except quinidine) and IC, but not class IB[96] antiarrhythmic drugs. They are used to unmask concealed forms of Brugada syndrome because of their capacity to provoke/exaggerate ST segment changes.[85,95,127–129] Provocation tests are required when ST segment elevation is not initially present or when type II or III ECG patterns are seen.[17] However, provocation challenges are not recommended and could even be harmful in the presence of a spontaneous type I ECG.[18,130]

The diagnostic yield and safety of such tests, when performed with ajmaline or flecainide, have been recently reported in genotyped populations. Ajmaline (1 mg/kg body weight; 10 mg/min) was the most powerful drug,[131] with a higher sensitivity (80%) and specificity (94%)[132] than flecainide (2 mg/Kg; max 150 mg) (sensitivity 77%, specificity 80%) (Figure 32–6).[116] They have also proven to be safe in large series of patients[116] when conducted according to the guidelines of the European Society of Cardiology.[17] In particular, drug infusion must be discontinued when a type I ECG is reached or when PVCs/(non)sustained VT occur or when QRS duration increases by more than 30% of the basal value. If not, life-threatening ventricular tachyarrhythmias may develop[45,130] (Figure 32–6).

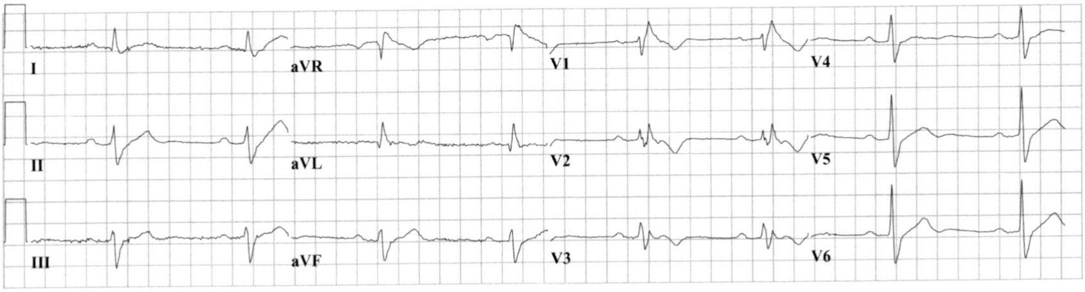

Figure 32–5. Twelve-lead ECG recorded at basal condition in a 49-year-old male subject who suffered from aborted sudden death. In addition to an ST segment elevation in V1, signs of conduction disorders are present, including sinus bradycardia, PQ interval prolongation, left QRS axis deviation, and widening of the QRS complex with an RBBB configuration, suggestive of Brugada syndrome.

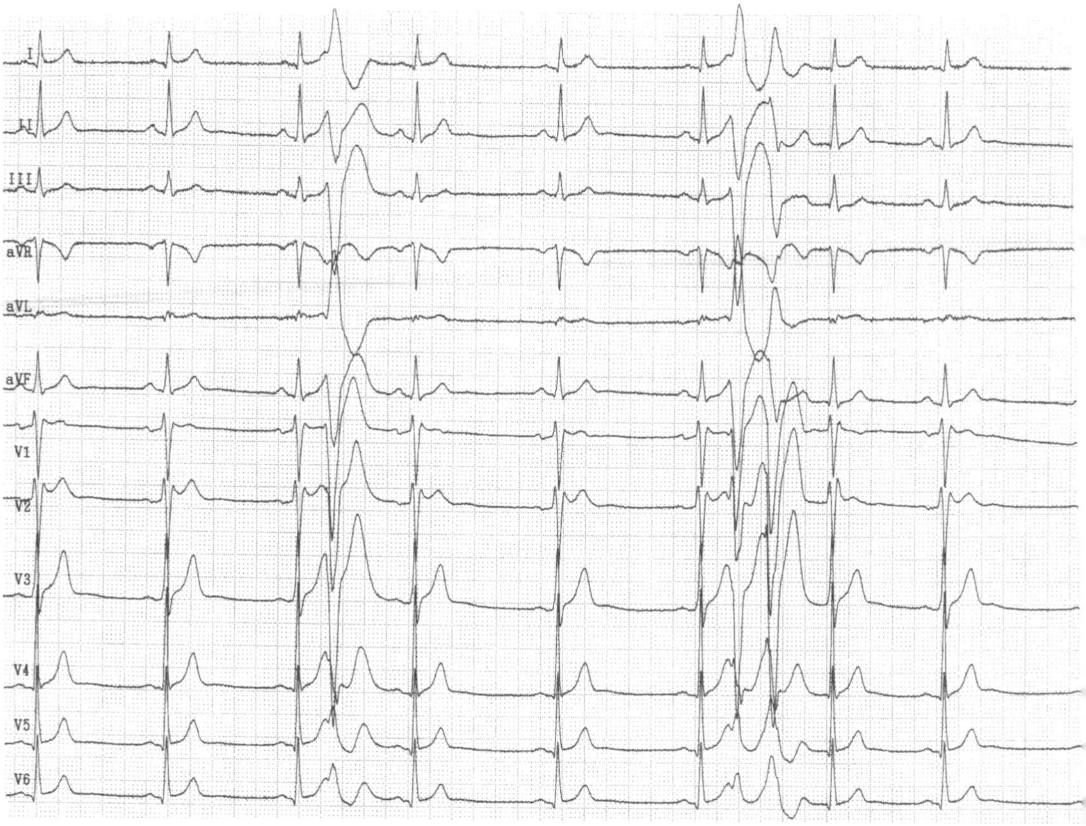

FIGURE 32–6. An ECG recorded after intravenous infusion of 80 mg flecainide in a 45-year-old male subject showing a saddle-back ST segment elevation in leads V1 and V2 (type II) and the appearance of premature ventricular beats, isolated and in couples, from the right ventricular outflow tract. The ectopic beats show a short coupling interval. Flecainide challenge was performed to pose the diagnosis of Brugada syndrome after an aborted sudden death.

Interestingly, the presence of an SCN5A mutation seems to increase the risk of arrhythmias during infusion with sodium channel blockers.[130]

Structural Abnormalities

A central characteristic of Brugada syndrome is the absence of clear structural abnormalities.[1,2]

Nonetheless, there has been evidence that Brugada syndrome may represent a mild form of right ventricle cardiomyophaty, not apparent with routine diagnostic tools.[123,133] Similarities with ARVC were pointed out, especially by Italian researchers,[123,134] and were strengthened by the discovery of an SCN5A mutation in a family with ARVC.[135] The ability to detect slight structural abnormalities has become greater with electron beam computed tomography (CT) scan and cardiac magnetic resonance imaging (MRI). These methods have revealed RV wall motion abnormalities and RVOT enlargement in two series of Brugada syndrome patients (these studies included control subjects).[136–138] More recently, 18 Brugada syndrome patients underwent biventricular endomyocardial biopsies, which revealed changes compatible with myocarditis (n = 14) or with right ventricular cardiomyopathy (n = 4), although the hearts appeared normal at noninvasive evaluation (no control group in this study).[139] Interestingly an SCN5A mutation was found in all the four patients with cardiomyopathic changes.

These findings demonstrate a link between unctional and structural abnormalities and also upport the hypothesis that sodium channel nutations themselves may induce subtle strucural derangements and myocardial cell death. This hypothesis has been tested in transgenic dult mice with SCN5A haploinsufficiency where significant amount of cardiac fibrosis was ound[140] and is supported by the clinical observaion that certain SCN5A defects were associated vith fibrosis in the conduction system and in the entricular myocardium.[141]

Differential Diagnosis in Brugada Syndrome

A number of clinical conditions that are also accompanied by ST segment elevation should be arefully ruled out before the diagnosis of Brugada yndrome is made (Table 32–2).

Relatively common causes of ST segment elevaion include (1) early repolarization syndrome;[8] 2) acute myocardial infarction, isolated right entricular infarction, or left ventricular aneuysm;[142–144] (3) Prinzmetal's angina, which may also coexist with Brugada syndrome;[145,146] (4) elecrolyte disturbances, such as hyperkalemia and hypercalcaemia;[147,148] (5) acute pericarditis/myocarditis;[149] (6) RBBB or LBBB and left ventricular hypertrophy;[150] and (7) ECG recorded after electrical cardioversion.[17]

More rarely, ST segment elevation may occur under the following conditions: (1) acute pulmonary embolism/acute aortic dissection;[151,152] (2) ARVC;[134,153] (3) long QT syndrome type III;[154] (4) hypothermia;[155] (5) Duchenne muscular dystrophy and Friedreich's ataxia;[156,157] (6) central and autonomic nervous system abnormalities;[158,159] and (7) mechanical compression of the RVOT by a mediastinal tumor.[160]

Furthermore, a variety of drugs and intoxications can lead to a Brugada-like ST segment elevation (Table 32–1). This group also includes cardiac antiischemic medication, such as calcium channel blockers or nitrates, and medications used to provoke/antagonize anesthesia.[100,161,162]

Finally, tricyclic or tetracyclic antidepressant medications as well as selective serotonin reuptake inhibitors and cocaine should be mentioned. All these drugs have been reported to cause a Brugada-like ST segment elevation[163–167] and tricyclic antidepressants have been reported to provoke VF, even when used in normal dosages.[168]

TABLE 32–2. Abnormalities associated with Brugada-like ST segment elevation.[a]

Conditions that can lead to ST segment elevation, mimicking Brugada syndrome
Early repolarization syndrome[8]
Cocaine intoxication[163]
Acute myocardial infarction or isolated right ventricular infarction[142,143]
Prinzmetal's angina[145,146]
Hyperkalemia and hypercalcemia[147,148]
Acute pericarditis/myocarditis[149]
RBBB or LBBB and left ventricular hypertrophy[150]
Acute aortic dissection/acute pulmonary embolism[151,152]
Arrhythmogenic right ventricular cardiomyopathy[134,179]
Long QT syndrome type III[154]
Hypothermia[155]
Duchenne muscular dystrophy[156]
Friedreich's ataxia[157]
Various central and autonomic nervous system abnormalities[158,159]
Mechanical compression of the RVOT by a mediastinal tumor[160]

[a]RBBB, LBBB, right and left bundle branch block; RVOT, right ventricle outflow tract.

Therapy

The most effective prevention of sudden death in patients affected by Brugada syndrome who suffered from (aborted) cardiac arrest or syncope or are considered at high risk for ventricular arrhythmias are ICDs.[19,20] Recommendations for ICD implantations are discussed in the Second Consensus Report about Brugada syndrome.[18]

Quinidine is the only oral agent that has been proven to normalize the ST segment[169] and to be effective in suppressing arrhythmic events in patients with Brugada syndrome (both spontaneous events and inducible VT/VF during EPS);[170,171] neither β-blockers nor amiodarone have proven to be effective.[4,172]

Risk Stratification

The prognosis of Brugada syndrome patients is still being debated. While it is accepted that patients with aborted sudden death or those who have had symptoms such as dizziness, syncope, or nocturnal agonal respiration should receive an ICD, conflicting data exist regarding risk stratification and therapeutic options in asymptomatic individuals. Brugada *et al.* reported a high incidence of cardiac death or documented VF (8%) in a large series of asymptomatic patients ($n = 190$) with a Brugada syndrome ECG (mean follow up 2 years).[19,173]

In contrast, a multicenter study in Italy conducted by Priori *et al.* showed that asymptomatic patients have a very good prognosis (no arrhythmic events during a mean follow up of 33 months in 30 asymptomatic patients)[33] and similar results were found by Eckardt *et al.*,[174] who reported data on a large population with a type I ECG ($n = 212$) with the longest follow-up (40 months on average) so far. They observed only one episode of VF out of a total of 123 asymptomatic individuals (0.8%).

So, according to these two European groups, implantation of an ICD in asymptomatic subjects, highly recommended by Brugada *et al.*, would be not justified.

Whether inducibility of VT/VF during EPS may aid in risk stratification in this subgroup of Brugada syndrome patients is still unresolved.[175–177a]

A recently published meta-analysis on the prognosis in Brugada syndrome, including more than 1500 patients, showed that a history of syncope or SCD, male gender, and the spontaneous appearance of a type I ECG are all associated with an increased risk of arrhythmic events, whereas the presence of an SCN5A mutation or a family history of SCD does not significantly augment the risk of events.[176]

Summary

There has been enormous worldwide interest in Brugada syndrome in the 15 years since its first description. Attempts have been made to recognize ECG parameters, other than J point elevation in V1–V3, that could help in making a correct diagnosis (positioning ECG leads above V1 and V2) or in identifying subjects at high risk (S wave width in V1).

Despite major advances, there are still unresolved issues regarding the epidemiology, unique pathogenesis/arrhythmogenesis, genetic background, and prognosis and treatment of Brugada syndrome. Although it is believed that a history of syncope or SCD and the spontaneous occurrence of a type I ECG represent increased risks for sudden death,[176] many questions about risk stratification and treatment in the large subpopulation of asymptomatic Brugada syndrome patients need to be answered. Aside from economical considerations, ICD implantation does not always represent an ideal treatment for all categories of patients (e.g., children). For these cases and for patients who receive multiple appropriate ICD shocks, quinidine may represent a valid alternative/adjunctive treatment.

Linkage to mutations in the SCN5A gene (in 20–30% of Brugada syndrome patients) has represented the biggest step in understanding the pathogenesis of Brugada syndrome (with reduction in I_{Na} being the common denominator of the mutant proteins) and the recent discovery of a second gene (GPD1L) has confirmed the genetic heterogeneity of this syndrome. For this reason, genetic screening cannot be considered the gold standard in Brugada syndrome; however, it represents a unique instrument to confirm the diagnosis, identify affected family members, and unravel genotype–phenotype relationships in Brugada syndrome, and, as such, is strongly recommended.

Acknowledgments. The author wants to thank A.C. Linnenbank, PhD, and P.G. Postema, MD, (Department of Cardiology, AMC, The Netherlands) for making Figure 32–3 and for helping in the selection and layout of the figures.

References

1. Brugada P, Brugada J. Right bundle branch block, persistent ST segment elevation and sudden cardiac death: A distinct clinical and electrocardiographic syndrome. A multicenter report. *J Am Coll Cardiol* 1992;20(6):1391–1396.
2. Brugada J, Brugada P. Further characterization of the syndrome of right bundle branch block, ST segment elevation, and sudden cardiac death. *J Cardiovasc Electrophysiol* 1997;8(3):325–331.
3. Shimizu W, Matsuo K, Takagi M, *et al.* Body surface distribution and response to drugs of ST

segment elevation in Brugada syndrome: Clinical implication of eighty-seven-lead body surface potential mapping and its application to twelve-lead electrocardiograms. *J Cardiovasc Electrophysiol* 2000;11(4):396–404.
4. Brugada J, Brugada R, Brugada P. Right bundle-branch block and ST-segment elevation in leads V1 through V3: A marker for sudden death in patients without demonstrable structural heart disease. *Circulation* 1998;97(5):457–460.
5. Sangwatanaroj S, Prechawat S, Sunsaneewitayakul B, *et al.* New electrocardiographic leads and the procainamide test for the detection of the Brugada sign in sudden unexplained death syndrome survivors and their relatives. *Eur Heart J* 2001;22(24):2290–2296.
6. Meregalli PG, Wilde AAM, Tan HL. Pathophysiological mechanisms of Brugada syndrome: Depolarization disorder, repolarization disorder or more? *Cardiovasc Res* 2005;67(3):367–378.
7. Antzelevitch C. The Brugada syndrome: Ionic basis and arrhythmia mechanisms. *J Cardiovasc Electrophysiol* 2001;12(2):268–272.
8. Gussak I, Antzelevitch C. Early repolarization syndrome: Clinical characteristics and possible cellular and ionic mechanisms. *J Electrocardiol* 2000;33(4):299–309.
9. Yan GX, Antzelevitch C. Cellular basis for the Brugada syndrome and other mechanisms of arrhythmogenesis associated with ST-segment elevation. *Circulation* 1999;100(15):1660–1666.
10. Nabauer M, Beuckelmann DJ, Uberfuhr P, *et al.* Regional differences in current density and rate-dependent properties of the transient outward current in subepicardial and subendocardial myocytes of human left ventricle. *Circulation* 1996;93(1):168–177.
11. Tukkie R, Sogaard P, Vleugels J, *et al.* Delay in right ventricular activation contributes to Brugada syndrome. *Circulation* 2004;109(10):1272–1277.
12. Ikeda T, Sakurada H, Sakabe K, *et al.* Assessment of noninvasive markers in identifying patients at risk in the Brugada syndrome: Insight into risk stratification. *J Am Coll Cardiol* 2001;37(6):1628–1634.
13. Takami M, Ikeda T, Enjoji Y, *et al.* Relationship between ST-segment morphology and conduction disturbances detected by signal-averaged electrocardiography in Brugada syndrome. *Ann Noninvasive Electrocardiol* 2003;8(1):30–36.
14. Kasanuki H, Ohnishi S, Ohtuka M, *et al.* Idiopathic ventricular fibrillation induced with vagal activity in patients without obvious heart disease. *Circulation* 1997;95(9):2277–2285.
15. Coronel R, Casini S, Koopmann TT, *et al.* Right ventricular fibrosis and conduction delay in a patient with clinical signs of Brugada syndrome: A combined electrophysiological, genetic, histopathologic, and computational study. *Circulation* 2005;112(18):2769–2777.
16. Okazaki O, Yamauchi Y, Kashida M, *et al.* Possible mechanism of ECG features in patients with idiopathic ventricular fibrillation studied by heart model and computer simulation. *J Electrocardiol* 1998;30(Suppl.):98–104.
17. Wilde AA, Antzelevitch C, Borggrefe M, *et al.* Proposed diagnostic criteria for the Brugada syndrome: Consensus report. *Circulation* 2002;106(19):2514–2519.
18. Antzelevitch C, Brugada P, Borggrefe M, *et al.* Brugada syndrome: Report of the second consensus conference: Endorsed by the *Heart Rhythm* Society and the European *Heart Rhythm* Association. *Circulation* 2005;111(5):659–670.
19. Brugada J, Brugada R, Antzelevitch C, *et al.* Long-term follow-up of individuals with the electrocardiographic pattern of right bundle-branch block and ST-segment elevation in precordial leads V1 to V3. *Circulation* 2002;105(1):73–78.
20. Priori SG, Napolitano C, Gasparini M, *et al.* Natural history of Brugada syndrome: Insights for risk stratification and management. *Circulation* 2002;105(11):1342–1347.
21. Chen Q, Kirsch GE, Zhang D, *et al.* Genetic basis and molecular mechanism for idiopathic ventricular fibrillation. *Nature* 1998;392(6673):293–296.
22. Weiss R, Barmada MM, Nguyen T, *et al.* Clinical and molecular heterogeneity in the Brugada syndrome: A novel gene locus on chromosome 3. *Circulation* 2002;105(6):707–713.
23. London B, Sanyal S, Michalec M, *et al.* A mutation in the glycerol-3-phosphate dehydrogenase 1-like gene (GPD1L) causes Brugada syndrome. *Heart Rhythm* 2006;3(1S):S32.
24. Tan HL, Bezzina CR, Smits JP, *et al.* Genetic control of sodium channel function. *Cardiovasc Res* 2003;57(4):961–973.
25. Viskin S, Fish R, Eldar M, *et al.* Prevalence of the Brugada sign in idiopathic ventricular fibrillation and healthy controls. *Heart* 2000;84(1):31–36.
26. Sakabe M, Fujiki A, Tani M, *et al.* Proportion and prognosis of healthy people with coved or saddle-back type ST segment elevation in the right precordial leads during 10 years follow-up. *Eur Heart J* 2003;24(16):1488–1493.

27. Vatta M, Dumaine R, Varghese G, *et al.* Genetic and biophysical basis of sudden unexplained nocturnal death syndrome (SUNDS), a disease allelic to Brugada syndrome. *Hum Mol Genet* 2002;11(3):337–345.
28. Nademanee K, Veerakul G, Nimmannit S, *et al.* Arrhythmogenic marker for the sudden unexplained death syndrome in Thai men. *Circulation* 1997;96(8):2595–2600.
29. Matsuo K, Akahoshi M, Nakashima E, *et al.* The prevalence, incidence and prognostic value of the Brugada-type electrocardiogram: Apopulation-based study of four decades. *J Am Coll Cardiol* 2001;38(3):765–770.
30. Kim JS, Park SY, Min SK, *et al.* Anaesthesia in patients with Brugada syndrome. *Acta Anaesthesiol Scand* 2004;48(8):1058–1061.
31. Teo WS, Kam R, Tan RS, *et al.* The Brugada syndrome in a Chinese population. *Int J Cardiol* 1998;65(3):281–286.
32. Park DW, Nam GB, Rhee KS, *et al.* Clinical characteristics of Brugada syndrome in a Korean population. *Circ J* 2003;67(11):934–939.
33. Priori SG, Napolitano C, Gasparini M, *et al.* Clinical and genetic heterogeneity of right bundle branch block and ST-segment elevation syndrome: A prospective evaluation of 52 families. *Circulation* 2000;102(20):2509–2515.
34. Junttila MJ, Raatikainen MJ, Karjalainen J, *et al.* Prevalence and prognosis of subjects with Brugada-type ECG pattern in a young and middle-aged Finnish population. *Eur Heart J* 2004;25(10):874–878.
35. Alings M, Wilde A. "Brugada" syndrome: Clinical data and suggested pathophysiological mechanism. *Circulation* 1999;99(5):666–673.
36. Sreeram N, Simmers T, Brockmeier K. The Brugada syndrome. Its relevance to paediatric practice. *Z Kardiol* 2004;93(10):784–790.
37. Greer RW, Glancy DL. Prevalence of the Brugada electrocardiographic pattern at the Medical Center of Louisiana in New Orleans. *J LA State Med Soc* 2003;155(5):242–246.
38. Ito H, Yano K, Chen R, *et al.* The prevalence and prognosis of a Brugada-type electrocardiogram in a population of middle-aged Japanese-American men with follow-up of three decades. *Am J Med Sci* 2006;331(1):25–29.
39. Priori SG, Napolitano C, Giordano U, *et al.* Brugada syndrome and sudden cardiac death in children. *Lancet* 2000;355(9206):808–809.
39a. Probst V, Denjoy I, Meregalli PG, *et al.* Clinical aspects and prognosis of Brugada syndrome in children. *Circulation* 2007;115(15):2042–2048.
40. Suzuki H, Torigoe K, Numata O, *et al.* Infan case with a malignant form of Brugada syndrome *J Cardiovasc Electrophysiol* 2000;11(11):1277 1280.
41. Atarashi H, Ogawa S, Harumi K, *et al.* Characteristics of patients with right bundle branch block and ST-segment elevation in right precordia leads. Idiopathic Ventricular Fibrillation Investigators. *Am J Cardiol* 1996;78(5):581–583.
42. Antzelevitch C, Brugada P, Brugada J, *et a* Brugada syndrome: A decade of progress. *Cir Res* 2002;91(12):1114–1118.
43. Hermida JS, Lemoine JL, Aoun FB, *et al.* Prevalence of the Brugada syndrome in an apparentl healthy population. *Am J Cardiol* 2000;86(1) 91–94.
44. Atarashi H, Ogawa S, Harumi K, *et al.* Three-yea follow-up of patients with right bundle branc block and ST segment elevation in the righ precordial leads: Japanese Registry of Brugad Syndrome. Idiopathic Ventricular Fibrillatio Investigators. *J Am Coll Cardiol* 2001;37(7):1916-1920.
45. Morita H, Morita ST, Nagase S, *et al.* Ventricula arrhythmia induced by sodium channel blocke in patients with Brugada syndrome. *J Am Col Cardiol* 2003;42(9):1624–1631.
46. Antzelevitch C, Brugada P, Brugada J, *et al* Brugada syndrome: 1992–2002: A historical perspective. *J Am Coll Cardiol* 2003;41(10):1665-1671.
47. Matsuo K, Kurita T, Inagaki M, *et al.* The circadian pattern of the development of ventricula fibrillation in patients with Brugada syndrome *Eur Heart J* 1999;20(6):465–470.
48. Itoh H, Shimizu M, Ino H, *et al.* Arrhythmias in patients with Brugada-type electrocardiographic findings. *Jpn Circ J* 2001;65(6):483–486.
49. Chalvidan T, Deharo JC, Dieuzaide P, *et al.* Nea fatal electrical storm in a patient equipped with an implantable cardioverter defibrillator fo Brugada syndrome. *Pacing Clin Electrophysio* 2000;23(3):410–412.
50. Brugada P, Brugada J, Brugada R. The Brugada syndrome. *Card Electrophysiol Rev* 2002;6(1–2) 45–48.
51. Bjerregaard P, Gussak I, Kotar SL, *et al.* Recurrent syncope in a patient with prominent J wave *Am Heart J* 1994;127(5):1426–1430.
52. Dubner SJ, Gimeno GM, Elencwajg B, *et al.* Ventricular fibrillation with spontaneous reversion on ambulatory ECG in the absence of heart disease. *Am Heart J* 1983;105(4):691-693.

53. Patt MV, Podrid PJ, Friedman PL, *et al.* Spontaneous reversion of ventricular fibrillation. *Am Heart J* 1988;115(4):919–923.
54. Kontny F, Dale J. Self-terminating idiopathic ventricular fibrillation presenting as syncope: A 40-year follow-up report. *J Intern Med* 1990;227(3): 211–213.
55. Shimada M, Miyazaki T, Miyoshi S, *et al.* Sustained monomorphic ventricular tachycardia in a patient with Brugada syndrome. *Jpn Circ J* 1996; 60(6):364–370.
56. Mok NS, Chan NY. Brugada syndrome presenting with sustained monomorphic ventricular tachycardia. *Int J Cardiol* 2004;97(2):307–309.
57. Ogawa M, Kumagai K, Saku K. Spontaneous right ventricular outflow tract tachycardia in a patient with Brugada syndrome. *J Cardiovasc Electrophysiol* 2001;12(7):838–840.
58. Gang ES, Priori SS, Chen PS. Short coupled premature ventricular contraction initiating ventricular fibrillation in a patient with Brugada syndrome. *J Cardiovasc Electrophysiol* 2004; 15(7):837.
59. Kakishita M, Kurita T, Matsuo K, *et al.* Mode of onset of ventricular fibrillation in patients with Brugada syndrome detected by implantable cardioverter defibrillator therapy. *J Am Coll Cardiol* 2000;36(5):1646–1653.
60. Sanchez-Aquino RM, Peinado R, Peinado A, *et al.* [Recurrent ventricular fibrillation in a patient with Brugada syndrome successfully treated with procainamide]. *Rev Esp Cardiol* 2003;56(11):1134–1136.
61. Chinushi M, Washizuka T, Chinushi Y, *et al.* Induction of ventricular fibrillation in Brugada syndrome by site-specific right ventricular premature depolarization. *Pacing Clin Electrophysiol* 2002;25(11):1649–1651.
62. Haissaguerre M, Extramiana F, Hocini M, *et al.* Mapping and ablation of ventricular fibrillation associated with long-QT and Brugada syndromes. *Circulation* 2003;108(8):925–928.
63. Morita H, Kusano-Fukushima K, Nagase S, *et al.* Atrial fibrillation and atrial vulnerability in patients with Brugada syndrome. *J Am Coll Cardiol* 2002;40(8):1437–1444.
64. Eckardt L, Kirchhof P, Loh P, *et al.* Brugada syndrome and supraventricular tachyarrhythmias: A novel association? *J Cardiovasc Electrophysiol* 2001;12(6):680–685.
65. Antzelevitch C. The Brugada syndrome. *J Cardiovasc Electrophysiol* 1998;9(5):513–516.
66. Matsuo K, Shimizu W, Kurita T, *et al.* Dynamic changes of 12-lead electrocardiograms in a patient with Brugada syndrome. *J Cardiovasc Electrophysiol* 1998;9(5):508–512.
67. Tsunoda Y, Takeishi Y, Nozaki N, *et al.* Presence of intermittent J waves in multiple leads in relation to episode of atrial and ventricular fibrillation. *J Electrocardiol* 2004;37(4):311–314.
68. Fujiki A, Usui M, Nagasawa H, *et al.* ST segment elevation in the right precordial leads induced with class IC antiarrhythmic drugs: Insight into the mechanism of Brugada syndrome. *J Cardiovasc Electrophysiol* 1999;10(2):214–218.
69. Naccarelli GV, Antzelevitch C, Wolbrette DL, *et al.* The Brugada syndrome. *Curr Opin Cardiol* 2002;17(1):19–23.
70. Bordachar P, Reuter S, Garrigue S, *et al.* Incidence, clinical implications and prognosis of atrial arrhythmias in Brugada syndrome. *Eur Heart J* 2004;25(10):879–884.
71. Oto A. Brugada sign: A normal variant or a bad omen? Insights for risk stratification and prognostication. *Eur Heart J* 2004;25(10):810–811.
72. Matsuo K, Akahoshi M, Seto S, *et al.* Disappearance of the Brugada-type electrocardiogram after surgical castration: A role for testosterone and an explanation for the male preponderance. *Pacing Clin Electrophysiol* 2003;26(7Pt. 1):1551–1553.
73. Shimizu W, Matsuo K, Kokubo Y, *et al.* Sex hormone and gender difference–role of testosterone on male predominance in Brugada syndrome. *J Cardiovasc Electrophysiol* 2007;18(4): 415–421.
74. Bidoggia H, Maciel JP, Capalozza N, *et al.* Sex differences on the electrocardiographic pattern of cardiac repolarization: Possible role of testosterone. *Am Heart J* 2000;140(4):678–683.
75. Di Diego JM, Cordeiro JM, Goodrow RJ, *et al.* Ionic and cellular basis for the predominance of the Brugada syndrome phenotype in males. *Circulation* 2002;106(15):2004–2011.
76. Fish JM, Antzelevitch C. Cellular and ionic basis for the sex-related difference in the manifestation of the Brugada syndrome and progressive conduction disease phenotypes. *J Electrocardiol* 2003;36(Suppl.):173–179.
77. Gellens ME, George AL Jr, Chen LQ, *et al.* Primary structure and functional expression of the human cardiac tetrodotoxin-insensitive voltage-dependent sodium channel. *Proc Natl Acad Sci USA* 1992;89(2):554–558.
78. Plummer NW, Meisler MH. Evolution and diversity of mammalian sodium channel genes. *Genomics* 1999;57(2):323–331.
79. Moric E, Herbert E, Trusz-Gluza M, *et al.* The implications of genetic mutations in the sodium

channel gene (SCN5A). *Europace* 2003;5(4):325–334.

80. Balser JR. The cardiac sodium channel: Gating function and molecular pharmacology. *J Mol Cell Cardiol* 2001;33(4):599–613.
81. Bezzina CR, Rook MB, Wilde AA. Cardiac sodium channel and inherited arrhythmia syndromes. *Cardiovasc Res* 2001;49(2):257–271.
82. Tan HL, Bink-Boelkens MT, Bezzina CR, *et al.* A sodium-channel mutation causes isolated cardiac conduction disease. *Nature* 2001;409(6823): 1043–1047.
83. Herfst LJ, Potet F, Bezzina CR, *et al.* Na+ channel mutation leading to loss of function and non-progressive cardiac conduction defects. *J Mol Cell Cardiol* 2003;35(5):549–557.
84. Mohler PJ, Rivolta I, Napolitano C, *et al.* Nav1.5 E1053K mutation causing Brugada syndrome blocks binding to ankyrin-G and expression of Nav1.5 on the surface of cardiomyocytes. *Proc Natl Acad Sci USA* 2004;101(50):17533–17538.
85. Brugada R, Brugada J, Antzelevitch C, *et al.* Sodium channel blockers identify risk for sudden death in patients with ST-segment elevation and right bundle branch block but structurally normal hearts. *Circulation* 2000;101(5):510–515.
86. Smits JP, Eckardt L, Probst V, *et al.* Genotype-phenotype relationship in Brugada syndrome: Electrocardiographic features differentiate SCN5A-related patients from non-SCN5A-related patients. *J Am Coll Cardiol* 2002;40(2):350–356.
87. Probst V, Allouis M, Sacher F, *et al.* Progressive cardiac conduction defect is the prevailing phenotype in carriers of a Brugada syndrome SCN5A mutation. *J Cardiovasc Electrophysiol* 2006;17(3): 270–275.
88. Gussak I, Antzelevitch C, Bjerregaard P, *et al.* The Brugada syndrome: Clinical, electrophysiologic and genetic aspects. *J Am Coll Cardiol* 1999;33(1): 5–15.
89. Shimizu W. The Brugada syndrome–an update. *Intern Med* 2005;44(12):1224–1231.
90. Antzelevitch C, Brugada R. Fever and Brugada syndrome. *Pacing Clin Electrophysiol* 2002;25(11): 1537–1539.
91. Bezzina C, Veldkamp MW, van den Berg MP, *et al.* A single Na(+) channel mutation causing both long-QT and Brugada syndromes. *Circ Res* 1999;85(12):1206–1213.
92. Kyndt F, Probst V, Potet F, *et al.* Novel SCN5A mutation leading either to isolated cardiac conduction defect or Brugada syndrome in a large French family. *Circulation* 2001;104(25):3081–3086.
93. Hirata K, Takagi Y, Nakada M, *et al.* Beat-to-be variation of the ST segment in a patient wit right bundle branch block, persistent ST segmer elevation, and ventricular fibrillation: A cas report. *Angiology* 1998;49(1):87–90.
94. Goethals P, Debruyne P, Saffarian M. Drug induced Brugada syndrome. *Acta Cardiol* 1998;5 (3):157–160.
95. Shimizu W, Antzelevitch C, Suyama K, *et a* Effect of sodium channel blockers on S segment, QRS duration, and corrected Q interval in patients with Brugada syndrome. *Cardiovasc Electrophysiol* 2000;11(12):1320 1329.
96. Miyazaki T, Mitamura H, Miyoshi S, *et al.* Autonomic and antiarrhythmic drug modulation c ST segment elevation in patients with Brugad syndrome. *J Am Coll Cardiol* 1996;27(5) 1061–1070.
97. Sumiyoshi M, Nakata Y, Hisaoka T, *et al.* A cas of idiopathic ventricular fibrillation with incomplete right bundle branch block and persistent S segment elevation. *Jpn Heart J* 1993;34(5):661 666.
98. Plunkett A, Hulse JA, Mishra B, *et al.* Variabl presentation of Brugada syndrome: Lessons fron three generations with syncope. *BMJ* 2003;32 (7398):1078–1079.
99. Santambrogio LG, Mencherini S, Fuardo M, *et a* The surgical patient with Brugada syndrome: four-case clinical experience. *Anesth Analg* 2005 100(5):1263–1266.
100. Cordery R, Lambiase P, Lowe M, *et al.* Brugad syndrome and anesthetic management. *J Cardiothorac Vasc Anesth* 2006;20(3):407–413.
101. Edge CJ, Blackman DJ, Gupta K, *et al.* Genera anaesthesia in a patient with Brugada syndrome *Br J Anaesth* 2002;89(5):788–791.
102. Candiotti KA, Mehta V. Perioperative approac to a patient with Brugada syndrome. *J Clin Anest* 2004;16(7):529–532.
103. Watanabe A, Kusano KF, Morita H, *et a* Low-dose isoproterenol for repetitive ventricula arrhythmia in patients with Brugada syndrome *Eur Heart J* 2006;27(13):1579–1583.
104. Tanaka H, Kinoshita O, Uchikawa S, *et al.* Successful prevention of recurrent ventricular fibrillation by intravenous isoproterenol in a patien with Brugada syndrome. *Pacing Clin Electrophysiol* 2001;24(8Pt. 1):1293–1294.
105. Saura D, Garcia-Alberola A, Carrillo P, *et a* Brugada-like electrocardiographic pattern induced by fever. *Pacing Clin Electrophysiol* 2002 25(5):856–859.

106. Porres JM, Brugada J, Urbistondo V, *et al.* Fever unmasking the Brugada syndrome. *Pacing Clin Electrophysiol* 2002;25(11):1646–1648.
107. Kum LC, Fung JW, Sanderson JE. Brugada syndrome unmasked by febrile illness. *Pacing Clin Electrophysiol* 2002;25(11):1660–1661.
108. Smith J, Hannah A, Birnie DH. Effect of temperature on the Brugada ECG. *Heart* 2003;89(3):272.
109. Dumaine R, Towbin JA, Brugada P, *et al.* Ionic mechanisms responsible for the electrocardiographic phenotype of the Brugada syndrome are temperature dependent. *Circ Res* 1999;85(9):803–809.
110. Kalla H, Yan GX, Marinchak R. Ventricular fibrillation in a patient with prominent J (Osborn) waves and ST segment elevation in the inferior electrocardiographic leads: A Brugada syndrome variant? *J Cardiovasc Electrophysiol* 2000;11(1):95–98.
111. Sahara M, Sagara K, Yamashita T, *et al.* J wave and ST segment elevation in the inferior leads: A latent type of variant Brugada syndrome? *Jpn Heart J* 2002;43(1):55–60.
112. Potet F, Mabo P, Le Coq G, *et al.* Novel Brugada SCN5A mutation leading to ST segment elevation in the inferior or the right precordial leads. *J Cardiovasc Electrophysiol* 2003;14(2):200–203.
113. Hisamatsu K, Morita H, Fukushima KK, *et al.* Evaluation of the usefulness of recording the ECG in the 3rd intercostal space and prevalence of Brugada-type ECG in accordance with recently established electrocardiographic criteria. *Circ J* 2004;68(2):135–138.
114. Hermida JS, Denjoy I, Jarry G, *et al.* Electrocardiographic predictors of Brugada type response during Na channel blockade challenge. *Europace* 2005;7(5):447–453.
115. Bruns HJ, Eckardt L, Vahlhaus C, *et al.* Body surface potential mapping in patients with Brugada syndrome: Right precordial ST segment variations and reverse changes in left precordial leads. *Cardiovasc Res* 2002;54(1):58–66.
116. Meregalli PG, Ruijter JM, Hofman N, *et al.* Diagnostic value of flecainide testing in unmasking SCN5A-related Brugada syndrome. *J Cardiovasc Electrophysiol* 2006;17(8):857–864.
117. Wilde AA, Antzelevitch C, Borggrefe M, *et al.* Proposed diagnostic criteria for the Brugada syndrome. *Eur Heart J* 2002;23(21):1648–1654.
118. Atarashi H, Ogawa S. New ECG criteria for high-risk Brugada syndrome. *Circ J* 2003;67(1):8–10.
119. Tatsumi H, Takagi M, Nakagawa E, *et al.* Risk stratificatuion in patients with Brugada syndrome: Analysis of daily fluctuations in 12-lead electrocardiogram (ECG) and signal-averaged electrocardiogram (SAECG). *J Cardiovasc Electrophysiol* 2006;17:705–711.
120. Ikeda T, Takami M, Sugi K, *et al.* Noninvasive risk stratification of subjects with a Brugada-type electrocardiogram and no history of cardiac arrest. *Ann Noninvasive Electrocardiol* 2005;10(4):396–403.
121. Tada H, Nogami A, Shimizu W, *et al.* ST segment and T wave alternans in a patient with Brugada syndrome. *Pacing Clin Electrophysiol* 2000;23(3):413–415.
122. Nakazato Y, Suzuki T, Yasuda M, *et al.* Manifestation of Brugada syndrome after pacemaker implantation in a patient with sick sinus syndrome. *J Cardiovasc Electrophysiol* 2004;15(11):1328–1330.
123. Martini B, Nava A, Thiene G, *et al.* Ventricular fibrillation without apparent heart disease: Description of six cases. *Am Heart J* 1989;118(6):1203–1209.
124. Morita H, Fukushima-Kusano K, Nagase S, *et al.* Sinus node function in patients with Brugada-type ECG. *Circ J* 2004;68(5):473–476.
125. van den Berg MP, Wilde AA, Viersma TJW, *et al.* Possible bradycardic mode of death and successful pacemaker treatment in a large family with features of long QT syndrome type 3 and Brugada syndrome. *J Cardiovasc Electrophysiol* 2001;12(6):630–636.
126. Aizawa Y, Naitoh N, Washizuka T, *et al.* Electrophysiological findings in idiopathic recurrent ventricular fibrillation: Special reference to mode of induction, drug testing, and long-term outcomes. *Pacing Clin Electrophysiol* 1996;19(6):929–939.
127. Brugada R. Use of intravenous antiarrhythmics to identify concealed Brugada syndrome. *Curr Control Trials Cardiovasc Med* 2000;1(1):45–47.
128. Rolf S, Bruns HJ, Wichter T, *et al.* The ajmaline challenge in Brugada syndrome: Diagnostic impact, safety, and recommended protocol. *Eur Heart J* 2003;24(12):1104–1112.
129. Matana A, Goldner V, Stanic K, *et al.* Unmasking effect of propafenone on the concealed form of the Brugada phenomenon. *Pacing Clin Electrophysiol* 2000;23(3):416–418.
130. Gasparini M, Priori SG, Mantica M, *et al.* Flecainide test in Brugada syndrome: A reproducible but risky tool. *Pacing Clin Electrophysiol* 2003;26(1Pt. 2):338–341.
131. Wolpert C, Echternach C, Veltmann C., *et al.* Intravenous drug challenge using flecainide and

ajmaline in patients with Brugada syndrome. *Heart Rhythm* 2005;2:254–260.

132. Hong K, Brugada J, Oliva A, *et al.* Value of electrocardiographic parameters and ajmaline test in the diagnosis of Brugada syndrome caused by SCN5A mutations. *Circulation* 2004;110(19):3023–3027.
133. Tada H, Aihara N, Ohe T, *et al.* Arrhythmogenic right ventricular cardiomyopathy underlies syndrome of right bundle branch block, ST-segment elevation, and sudden death. *Am J Cardiol* 1998; 81(4):519–522.
134. Corrado D, Nava A, Buja G, *et al.* Familial cardiomyopathy underlies syndrome of right bundle branch block, ST segment elevation and sudden death. *J Am Coll Cardiol* 1996;27(2):443–448.
135. Martini B, Nava A. 1988–2003. Fifteen years after the first Italian description by Nava-Martini-Thiene and colleagues of a new syndrome (different from the Brugada syndrome?) in the Giornale Italiano di Cardiologia: Do we really know everything on this entity? *Ital Heart J* 2004;5(1):53–60.
136. Takagi M, Aihara N, Kuribayashi S, *et al.* Localized right ventricular morphological abnormalities detected by electron-beam computed tomography represent arrhythmogenic substrates in patients with the Brugada syndrome. *Eur Heart J* 2001;22(12):1032–1041.
137. Takagi M, Aihara N, Kuribayashi S, *et al.* Abnormal response to sodium channel blockers in patients with Brugada syndrome: Augmented localised wall motion abnormalities in the right ventricular outflow tract region detected by electron beam computed tomography. *Heart* 2003; 89(2):169–174.
138. Papavassiliu T, Wolpert C, Fluchter S, *et al.* Magnetic resonance imaging findings in patients with Brugada syndrome. *J Cardiovasc Electrophysiol* 2004;15(10):1133–1138.
139. Frustaci A, Priori SG, Pieroni M, *et al.* Cardiac histological substrate in patients with clinical phenotype of Brugada syndrome. *Circulation* 2005;112(24):3680–3687.
140. Royer A, V Veen T, Le Bouter S, *et al.* A mouse model of SCN5A-linked hereditary Lenegre's disease. *Circulation* 2005;111:1738–1746.
141. Bezzina CR, Rook MB, Groenewegen WA, *et al.* Compound heterozygosity for mutations (W156X and R225W) in SCN5A associated with severe cardiac conduction disturbances and degenerative changes in the conduction system. *Circ Res* 2003;92(2):159–168.
142. Andersen HR, Falk E, Nielsen D. Right ventricular infarction. The evolution of ST-segment elevation and Q wave in right chest leads. *J Electrocardiol* 1989;22(3):181–186.
143. Goldberger AL. *Myocardial Infarction: Electrocardiographic Differential Diagnosis*, 4th ed. St Louis, MO: Mosby-Year Book Inc., 1991.
144. Kataoka H. Electrocardiographic patterns of the Brugada syndrome in right ventricular infarction/ischemia. *Am J Cardiol* 2000;86(9):1056.
145. Sasaki T, Niwano S, Kitano Y, *et al.* Two cases of Brugada syndrome associated with spontaneous clinical episodes of coronary vasospasm. *Inter Med* 2006;45(2):77–80.
146. Chinushi M, Kuroe Y, Ito E, *et al.* Vasospastic angina accompanied by Brugada-type electrocardiographic abnormalities. *J Cardiovasc Electrophysiol* 2001;12(1):108–111.
147. Douglas PS, Carmichael KA, Palevsky PM. Extreme hypercalcemia and electrocardiographic changes. *Am J Cardiol* 1984;54(6):674–675.
148. Levine HD, Wanzer SH, Merrill JP. Dialyzable currents of injury in potassium intoxication resembling acute myocardial infarction or pericarditis. *Circulation* 1956;13(1):29–36.
149. Spodick DH, Greene TO, Saperia G. Images in cardiovascular medicine. Acute myocarditis masquerading as acute myocardial infarction. *Circulation* 1995;91(6):1886–1887.
150. Rowlands DJ. *Clinical Electrocardiography*. Philadenphia, PA: J. B. Lippincott Company, 1991.
151. Myers GB. Other QRS-T pattern that may be mistaken for myocardial infarction. IV. Alteration in blood potassium: Myocardial ischemia, subepicardial myocarditis; distortion associated with arrhythmias. *Cirulation* 1950;2:75.
152. Sreeram N, Cheriex EC, Smeets JL, *et al.* Value of the 12-lead electrocardiogram at hospital admission in the diagnosis of pulmonary embolism. *Am J Cardiol* 1994;73(4):298–303.
153. Corrado D, Basso C, Buja G, *et al.* Right bundle branch block, right precordial ST-segment elevation, and sudden death in young people. *Circulation* 2001;103(5):710–717.
154. Priori SG, Napolitano C, Schwartz PJ, *et al.* The elusive link between LQT3 and Brugada syndrome: The role of flecainide challenge. *Circulation* 2000;102(9):945–947.
155. Noda T, Shimizu W, Tanaka K, *et al.* Prominent J wave and ST segment elevation: Serial electrocardiographic changes in accidental hypothermia. *J Cardiovasc Electrophysiol* 2003;14(2):223.
156. Perloff JK, Henze E, Schelbert HR. Alterations in regional myocardial metabolism, perfusion, and wall motion in Duchenne muscular dystrophy

studied by radionuclide imaging. *Circulation* 1984;69(1):33–42.
157. Grauer K. Bizarre ECG in a young adult. *Intern Med Alert* 1997;19:56.
158. Hersch C. Electrocardiographic changes in head injuries. *Circulation* 1961;23:853–860.
159. Abbott JA, Cheitlin MD. The nonspecific camel-hump sign. *JAMA* 1976;235(4):413–414.
160. Tarin N, Farre J, Rubio JM, *et al.* Brugada-like electrocardiographic pattern in a patient with a mediastinal tumor. *Pacing Clin Electrophysiol* 1999;22(8):1264–1266.
161. Shimizu W. Acquired forms of the Brugada syndrome. *J Electrocardiol* 2005;38(4Suppl.):22–25.
162. Fish JM, Antzelevitch C. Role of sodium and calcium channel block in unmasking the Brugada syndrome. *Heart Rhythm* 2004;1(2):210–217.
163. Ortega-Carnicer J, Bertos-Polo J, Gutierrez-Tirado C. Aborted sudden death, transient Brugada pattern, and wide QRS dysrrhythmias after massive cocaine ingestion. *J Electrocardiol* 2001;34(4):345–349.
164. Babaliaros VC, Hurst JW. Tricyclic antidepressants and the Brugada syndrome: An example of Brugada waves appearing after the administration of desipramine. *Clin Cardiol* 2002;25(8):395–398.
165. Rouleau F, Asfar P, Boulet S, *et al.* Transient ST segment elevation in right precordial leads induced by psychotropic drugs: Relationship to the Brugada syndrome. *J Cardiovasc Electrophysiol* 2001;12(1):61–65.
166. Bolognesi R, Tsialtas D, Vasini P, *et al.* Abnormal ventricular repolarization mimicking myocardial infarction after heterocyclic antidepressant overdose. *Am J Cardiol* 1997;79(2):242–245.
167. Goldgran-Toledano D, Sideris G, Kevorkian JP. Overdose of cyclic antidepressants and the Brugada syndrome. *N Engl J Med* 2002;346(20):1591–1592.
168. Chow BJ, Gollob M, Birnie D. Brugada syndrome precipitated by a tricyclic antidepressant. *Heart* 2005;91(5):651.
169. Alings M, Dekker L, Sadee A, *et al.* Quinidine induced electrocardiographic normalization in two patients with Brugada syndrome. *Pacing Clin Electrophysiol* 2001;24(9Pt. 1):1420–1422.
170. Hermida JS, Denjoy I, Clerc J, *et al.* Hydroquinidine therapy in Brugada syndrome. *J Am Coll Cardiol* 2004;43(10):1853–1860.
171. Belhassen B, Glick A, Viskin S. Efficacy of quinidine in high-risk patients with Brugada syndrome. *Circulation* 2004;110(13):1731–1737.
172. Nademanee K, Veerakul G, Mower M, *et al.* Defibrillator versus beta-blockers for unexplained death in Thailand (DEBUT): A randomized clinical trial. *Circulation* 2003;107(17):2221–2226.
173. Brugada J, Brugada R, Brugada P. Determinants of sudden cardiac death in individuals with the electrocardiographic pattern of Brugada syndrome and no previous cardiac arrest. *Circulation* 2003;108(25):3092–3096.
174. Eckardt L, Probst V, Smits JP, *et al.* Long-term prognosis of individuals with right precordial ST-segment-elevation Brugada syndrome. *Circulation* 2005;111(3):257–263.
175. Brugada P, Brugada R, Brugada J. Should patients with an asymptomatic Brugada electrocardiogram undergo pharmacological and electrophysiological testing? *Circulation* 2005;112(2):279–292.
176. Gehi AK, Duong TD, Metz LD, *et al.* Risk stratification of individuals with the Brugada electrocardiogram: A meta-analysis. *J Cardiovasc Electrophysiol* 2006;17:577–583.
177. Priori SG, Napolitano C. Should patients with an asymptomatic Brugada electrocardiogram undergo pharmacological and electrophysiological testing? *Circulation* 2005;112(2):279–292.
177a. Paul M, Gerss J, Schulze-Bahr E, *et al.* Role of programmed ventricular stimulation in patients with Brugada syndrome: a meta-analysis of worldwide published data. *Eur Heart J* 2007;[Epub ahead of print].
178. Phillips N, Priestley M, Denniss AR, *et al.* Brugada-type electrocardiographic pattern induced by epidural bupivacaine. *Anesth Analg* 2003;97(1):264–267.
179. Corrado D, Basso C, Thiene G. Sudden cardiac death in young people with apparently normal heart. *Cardiovasc Res* 2001;50(2):399–408.

33
Brugada Syndrome: Cellular Mechanisms and Approaches to Therapy

Charles Antzelevitch and Sami Viskin

Introduction

Nearly 15 years have passed since Pedro and Josep Brugada introduced the syndrome of ST-segment elevation and right bundle branch block (RBBB) associated with a high incidence of ventricular tachycardia/ventricular fibrillation (VT/VF) as a new clinical entity.[1] Over 16 years have transpired since the introduction of the concept of phase 2 reentry (induced by sodium channel block), the mechanism believed to underlie the development of arrhythmogenesis in this clinical syndrome.[2,3] Thus, the entity, which in 1996 came to be known as the Brugada syndrome,[4,5] evolved in the experimental laboratory and in the clinic along parallel but separate tracks until the late 1990s.[6]

The Brugada syndrome has attracted great interest because of its prevalence and its association with a high risk of sudden death, especially in males as they enter their third and fourth decade of life. A consensus report published in 2002 delineated diagnostic criteria for the syndrome.[7,8] A second consensus conference report published in 2005 focused on risk stratification schemes and approaches to therapy.[9,10] This chapter provides an overview of the genetic, molecular, and cellular aspects of the Brugada syndrome and considers the various approaches to therapy.

Brugada Syndrome

Clinical Characteristics

A brief description of clinical characteristics is included to provide a perspective for our discussion of mechanisms and therapy. This subject is more thoroughly dealt with in Chapter 32 (this volume). The Brugada syndrome is characterized by an ST- segment elevation in the right precordial electrocardiogram (ECG) leads and a high incidence of sudden death. The average age at the time of initial diagnosis or sudden death is 40 ± 22, although the range is wide with youngest patient diagnosed at 2 days of age and the oldest at 84 years.

The ECG manifestations of the Brugada syndrome are often concealed, but can be unmasked by sodium channel blockers, a febrile state, or vagotonic agents.[5,11–13] Three types of repolarization patterns in the right precordial leads are recognized (Table 33–1).[7,8] Type 1 ST-segment elevation is diagnostic of Brugada syndrome and is characterized by a coved ST-segment elevation ≥2 mm (0.2 mV) followed by a negative T wave. Type 2 ST-segment elevation has a saddleback appearance with a high take-off ST-segment elevation of ≥2 mm followed by a trough displaying ≥1 mm ST elevation followed by either a positive or biphasic T wave. Type 3 ST-segment elevation has either a saddleback or coved appearance with an ST-segment elevation of <1 mm. These three patterns may be observed sequentially in the same patient or following the introduction of specific drugs. Type 2 and Type 3 ST-segment elevation should not be considered diagnostic of the Brugada syndrome. A Brugada ECG refers to the manifestation of a Type 1 ST-segment elevation. Brugada syndrome is definitively diagnosed when a Type 1 ST-segment elevation (Brugada ECG) is observed in more than one right-precordial lead (V1–V3), in the presence or absence of a sodium channel blocking agent, and in conjunction with one or more of the following: documented VF, polymor-

ABLE 33–1. Diagnostic criteria for Brugada syndrome.[a]

	ST-segment abnormalities in leads V1–V3		
	Type 1	Type 2	Type3
J point	≥2 mm	≥2 mm	≥2 mm
T wave	Negative	Positive or biphasic	Positive
ST-T configuration	Coved type	Saddleback	Saddleback
ST segment (terminal portion)	Gradually descending	Elevated ≥1 mm	Elevated <1 mm

ource: From Wilde *et al.*,[7] with permission.
From the first consensus document. 1 mm = 0.1 mV. The terminal portion f the ST segment refers to the latter half of the ST segment.

hic ventricular tachycardia, a family history of udden cardiac death (SCD) (<45 years old), coved ype ECGs in family members, inducibility of VT vith programmed electrical stimulation, syncope, r nocturnal agonal respiration.[7–10]

Diagnosis of Brugada syndrome is also conidered positive when a Type 2 (saddleback pattern) or Type 3 ST-segment elevation is observed n more than one right precordial lead under aseline conditions and can be converted to the liagnostic Type 1 pattern that occurs upon expoure to a sodium channel blocker (ST-segment levation should be ≥2 mm). One or more of the linical criteria described above should also be resent. Drug-induced conversion of Type 3 to Type 2 ST-segment elevation is considered inconlusive for diagnosis of Brugada syndrome.

The ECG manifestations of the syndrome are often concealed, but can be unmasked using odium channel blockers. Definitive diagnosis is lifficult when the degree of basal ST-segment levation is relatively small and the specificity of odium channel blockers such as flecainide, ajmaine, procainamide, disopyramide, propafenone, and pilsicainide[12,14,15] to identify patients at risk is uncertain. A comparison of intravenous ajmaline and flecainide in the same cohort of patients revealed that ajmaline is more effective in unmasking the syndrome.[16] Flecainide failed in 7 of 22 cases (32%) unmasked by ajmaline. A greater inhibition of transient outward current (I_{to}) by flecainide renders it less effective than ajmaline. False-positive as well as false-negative responses have been reported with ajmaline, as well.[17,18] Itoh *et al.* demonstrated that a missense mutation in SCN5A, the gene that encodes the α subunit of the sodium channel, although responsible for the disease, prevented ajmaline from unmasking the syndrome, due to loss of the ability of the drug to produce use-dependent inhibition of sodium channel current.[18]

Most cases of Brugada syndrome display right precordial ST-segment elevation, although isolated cases of inferior lead[19,20] or left precordial lead[21] ST-segment elevation have been reported in Brugada-like syndromes, in some cases associated with *SCN5A* mutations. In rare cases, ST-segment elevation is observed in all precordial leads (unpublished observation).

Placement of the right precordial leads in a superior position (up to the second intercostal spaces above normal) can increase the sensitivity of the ECG for detecting the Brugada phenotype in some patients, both in the presence or absence of a drug challenge.[22,23] Studies are underway to ascertain whether the greater sensitivity is at the cost of a lower specificity and whether a Type I ECG in the elevated leads is as predictive of events as a Type I ECG the in the standard leads. A recent report demonstrates that as many as 1.3% of normal Korean males display a Type 2, but not Type 1, ST-segment elevation when the right precordial leads are recorded from a superior position.[24]

A slight prolongation of the QT interval is sometimes associated with the ST-segment elevation.[15,25,26] The QT interval is prolonged more in the right than the left precordial leads, presumably due to a preferential prolongation of action potential duration (APD) in right ventricular (RV) epicardium secondary to accentuation of the action potential notch.[27] A QTc > 460 msec in V2 has been shown to be associated with arrhythmic risk.[28] Depolarization abnormalities including prolongation of P wave duration, PR, and QRS intervals are frequently observed, particularly in patients linked to *SCN5A* mutations.[29] PR prolongation likely reflects HV conduction delay.[25]

In many cases arrhythmia initiation is bradycardia related.[30] This may contribute to the higher incidence of sudden death at night in individuals with the syndrome and may account for the success of pacing in controlling the arrhythmia in isolated cases of the syndrome.[31] Makiyama and co-workers reported that loss-of-function SCN5A mutations resulting in Brugada syndrome are distinguished by profound bradyarrhythmias.[32] Related to this observation is the recent report by Scornik and co-workers[33] demonstrating expression of the cardiac sodium channel gene, SCN5A, in intracardiac ganglia. This interesting finding suggests that loss of function mutations in SCN5A may not only create the substrate for reentry in ventricular myocardium, but may also increase vagal activity in intracardiac ganglia, thus facilitating the development of arrhythmias in patients with the Brugada syndrome.

A polymorphic VT is most commonly associated with the Brugada syndrome. Monomorphic VT is observed infrequently and is generally more prevalent in children and infants.[34–39]

The majority of congenital Brugada syndrome patients are believed to possess a structurally normal heart, consistent with the notion that this is a primary electrical heart disease.[40] While fibrosis and myocarditis may exacerbate or indeed trigger events in patients with the Brugada syndrome, it seems clear that in the vast majority of cases these structural changes are unrelated to arrhythmogenic right ventricular cardiomyopathy/dysplasia (ARVC/D).

Prognosis and Risk Stratification

Risk stratification of patients with the Brugada syndrome has been an issue of lively debate. It is generally accepted that Brugada syndrome patients presenting with aborted sudden death are at high risk for recurrence and that they should be protected by an implantable cardiac defibrillator (ICD). There is also little argument that patients presenting with syncope, particularly when the clinical history suggests an arrhythmic syncope (as opposed to typical vasovagal syncope) and the ECG shows a Type I abnormality, are at high risk. In contrast, risk stratification of asymptomatic patients has met with considerable debate.[41–45] Several invasive and noninvasive parameters have been proposed for identification of patients at risk of sudden death, including the presence of spontaneous Type 1 ST-segment elevation, the characteristics of the S wave,[46] the presence of late potentials,[47] and inducibility of VT/VF using programmed electrical stimulation (PES).[48]

In 1998, Brugada *et al.*[49] reported that over 34-month follow-up period, 27% of previousl asymptomatic patients experienced a first VF o SCD. This figure corresponds to an occurrence c life-threatening events of approximately 10% year. In 2002, with a mean follow-up of 27 ± 2 months, Brugada *et al.*[41] reported that 8% of pre viously asymptomatic patients had become symp tomatic, an occurrence of a life-threatening even of 3.5%/year. In 2005, Brugada *et al.*[43] reporte that 6% of asymptomatic patients displayed a firs event during a mean follow-up of 42 ± 42 month corresponding to an event rate of 1.7%/year. Thi progressive decline in first event rate in previ ously asymptomatic patients most likely reflects reduced severity of phenotypes referred to th Brugada registry in subsequent years. In contras Priori *et al.* in 2002[42] reported that asymptomati patients have a cumulative probability of 14% fo developing a cardiac arrest by age 40 years corresponding to a natural history incidence o cardiac arrest of 0.35%/year. In 2005, they reporte a first event rate of 3% (4/132) over a 31-mont follow-up period, corresponding to an event rat of 1%/year.[44]

The reason behind the disparity in the data gen erated by these two groups is not clearly eviden It was suggested by Brugada *et al.*[43] that the dif ference my be due to the inclusion by Priori an co-workers of patients with Type 2 and 3 ST segment elevation, which is not considered diag nostic of the Brugada syndrome.[7–10] Priori an co-workers argue that exclusion of Type 2 and from the diagnosis of the syndrome can lead t missed diagnosis of the disease.[44] While this i clearly the case, it may be a rare occurrence, an the exclusion appears justified on the basis that i avoids a large number of false-positive diagnoses As a result of the failure to exclude individual with Type 2 and 3 ST-segment elevation, th European registry may contain many individual who do not have the syndrome. However, a recen report by Eckardt and co-workers[45] suggests tha other factors may be involved. They report that 1 out of 123 asymptomatic individuals with a Typ 1 ECG (0.8%) had a first arrhythmic event durin a 40 ± 50-month follow-up. This translates into first event rate of 0.24% per year, considerably les than the other two registries. Thus, as additiona data have become available, it has become clea at the prognosis of asymptomatic patients is ssociated with much less risk than was initially erceived.

The large registry studies agree that Brugada yndrome patients at higher risk for the developent of subsequent events are those presenting ith a spontaneous Type 1 ST-segment elevation r Brugada ECG and/or those with a previous VT/F or SCD.[45] The registries also agree that PES ducibility is greatest among patients with previus VT/VF or syncope. Approximately one-third f asymptomatic patients are inducible. In the tudies by Priori *et al.*[44] and Eckardt *et al.*[45] inducility of VT/VF in asymptomatic patients was ot associated with risk. The lack of association etween inducibility and spontaneous VF in rugada patients was also reported by a number f smaller studies, such as that of Kanada *et al.*[50]

In sharp contrast, Brugada *et al.*[51] found that e risk for developing VT/VF is considerably reater in patients who are inducible during PES, hether or not a Type 1 ST-segment elevation is pontaneously present and whether or not they ere symptomatic. The reason for the marked isparity in the predictive power of PES inducibilty among the different studies is not immediately pparent. The discrepancies may be due to differnces in patient characteristics and the use of multiple testing centers with nonstandardized or oncomparable stimulation protocols.[52] Addiional studies are clearly needed to further define isk stratification strategies for asymptomatic atients.

It is noteworthy that in experimental models of he Brugada syndrome involving the coronaryerfused wedge preparation, polymorphic VT is eadily inducible with a single ventricular extrasimulus, but only when applied on the epicardial urface of the wedge. Inducibility is not possible r much more difficult when extrastimulation is pplied to the endocardial surface. The shorter efractory period of epicardium allows extrastimli direct access to the vulnerable window across he ventricular wall, thus facilitating the induction f reentry. These relationships suggest that PES pplied to the epicardium may provide a more ccurate assessment of risk than the current clinial approach in which stimuli are applied to the ndocardial surface. In support of this hypothesis, arlsson *et al.* reported that a Brugada syndrome patient with recurrent syncope due to polymorphic ventricular tachycardia could not be induced with right ventricular endocardial stimulation. However, epicardial stimulation from a left ventricular site through the coronary sinus led to the development of polymorphic VT.[53]

Gehi *et al.*[54] recently reported the results of a meta-analysis of 30 prospective studies that included 1545 patients with a Brugada ECG to assess predictors of events. The meta-analysis suggested that a history of syncope or SCD, the presence of a spontaneous Type I Brugada ECG, and male gender predict a more malignant natural history. The findings, however, did not support the use of a family history of SCD, the presence of an SCN5A gene mutation, or electrophysiologic study to guide the management of patients with a Brugada ECG. The results of the meta-analysis should be viewed with some reservation in that the study pooled data from prognostic studies that used very different criteria to identify patients with Brugada syndrome. Moreover the six studies that were used to evaluate the role of electrophysiological study in risk stratification of patients were quite heterogeneous. A prospective study termed PRELUDE (PRogrammed ElectricaL stimUlation preDictivE) currently underway in Italy is designed to provide further insight into the ongoing debate.

Genetic Basis

Brugada syndrome shows an autosomal dominant mode of inheritance. The first gene to be linked to the syndrome is SCN5A, the gene that encodes the α subunit of the cardiac sodium channel gene.[55] Figure 33–1 highlights the diversity of SCN5A mutations associated with the Brugada syndrome. Of note, mutations in SCN5A are also responsible for the long QT3 (LQT3) form of the long QT syndrome and cardiac conduction disease. A number of mutations have been reported to cause overlapping syndromes; in some cases all three phenotypes are present.[56] Nearly 100 mutations in SCN5A have been associated with the syndrome in recent years (see Antzelevitch *et al.*[57] for references; also see www.fsm.it/cardmoc).

Only a fraction of these mutations has been studied in expression systems and shown to result in loss of function. A number of mechanisms have

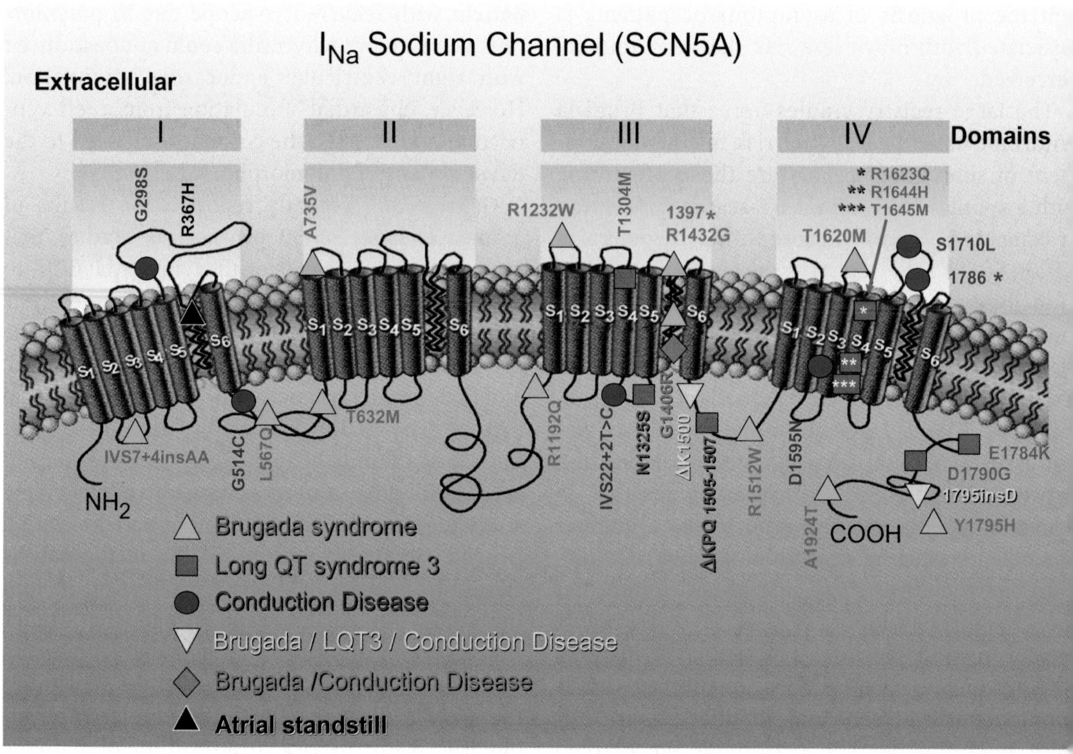

FIGURE 33–1. Schematic of SCN5A, the gene that encodes the α subunit of the sodium channel, illustrating mutations linked to Brugada syndrome, long QT3 syndrome, conduction disease, and atrial standstill. Some mutations are associated with combine phenotypes. (Modified from Antzelevitch C. Brugada syndrom *PACE* 2006;29(10):1130–1159.)

been delineated for the reduction in sodium channel current (I_{Na}), including[58–62] (1) failure of the sodium channel to express, (2) a shift in the voltage and time dependence of sodium channel current (I_{Na}) activation, inactivation, or reactivation, (3) entry of the sodium channel into an intermediate state of inactivation from which it recovers more slowly, or (4) accelerated inactivation of the sodium channel. In *in vitro* expression systems, the premature inactivation of the sodium channel is sometimes observed at physiological temperatures, but not at room temperature.[63] Acceleration of I_{Na} inactivation was still more accentuated at higher than physiological temperatures, suggesting that the syndrome may be unmasked, and that patients with the Brugada syndrome may be at an increased risk during a febrile state.[63] A number of Brugada patients displaying fever-induced polymorphic VT have been identified since the publication of this report.[13,36,64–71]

Mutation in the *SCN5A* gene account fo approximately 18–30% of Brugada syndrom cases. A higher incidence of *SCN5A* mutations ha been reported in familial than in sporadic cases. It is important to recognize that a negative *SCN5* result does not rule this gene out as a cause, sinc the promoter region, cryptic splicing mutations or the presence of gross rearrangements are gen erally not part of a routine investigation. A recen report by Hong *et al.*[72] provided the first report o a dysfunctional sodium channel created by a intronic mutation giving rise to cryptic splice sit activation in SCN5A in a family with the Brugad syndrome. The deletion of fragments of segment 2 and 3 of domain IV of SCN5A caused complet loss of function.

Evidence in support of the hypothesis tha an SCN5A promoter polymorphism common i Asians modulates variability in cardiac conduc tion, and may contribute to the high prevalenc of Brugada syndrome in the Asian population as recently advanced by Bezzina and coorkers.[73] Sequencing of the SCN5A promoter lentified a haplotype variant consisting of six olymorphisms in near-complete linkage disequibrium that occurred at an allele frequency of 2% in Asian subjects and was absent in whites nd blacks. These findings demonstrate that odium channel transcription in the human heart ay vary considerably among individuals and aces and may be associated with variable conducon velocity and arrhythmia susceptibility.

A second locus on chromosome 3, close to but istinct from SCN5A, has been linked to the synrome[74] in a large pedigree in which the syndrome associated with progressive conduction disease, low sensitivity to procainamide, and a relatively ood prognosis. The gene was recently identified s the glycerol-3-phosphate dehydrogenase 1-like ene (GPD1L). In a preliminary report, a mutaon in GPD1L was shown to result in a partial eduction of I_{Na}.[75]

It is generally accepted that identification of pecific mutations may not be very helpful in forulating a diagnosis or providing a prognosis. Mutations have been reported throughout the CN5A gene and no hotspots have been identified. t is not clear whether some mutations are associted with a greater risk of arrhythmic events or udden death. Genetic testing is recommended for upport of the clinical diagnosis, for early detecon of relatives at potential risk, and particularly or the purpose of advancing research and our nderstanding of genotype–phenotype relations.

ellular and Ionic Mechanisms Underlying he Development of the Brugada Phenotype

ransmural Cellular and Ion Channel Distinctions

entricular myocardium is known to be comrised of at least three electrophysiologically and unctionally distinct cell types: epicardial, M, and ndocardial cells.[76,77] These three principal venricular myocardial cell types differ with respect o phase 1 and phase 3 repolarization characteristics. Ventricular epicardial and M, but not endoardial, cells generally display a prominent phase , due to a large 4-aminopyridine (4-AP)-sensitive ransient outward current (I_{to}), giving the action otential a spike and dome or notched configuration. These regional differences in I_{to}, first suggested on the basis of action potential data,[78] have now been directly demonstrated in canine,[79] feline,[80] rabbit,[81] rat,[82] and human[83,84] ventricular myocytes. Differences in the magnitude of the action potential notch and corresponding differences in I_{to} have also been described between right and left ventricular epicardium.[85] Similar interventricular differences in I_{to} have also been described for canine ventricular M cells.[86] This distinction is thought to form the basis for why the Brugada syndrome, a channelopathy-mediated form of sudden death, is a right ventricular disease.

The molecular basis for the transmural distribution of I_{to} has long been a subject of debate. The transmural gradient of I_{to} in dogs has been ascribed to a transmural distribution of (1) the KCND3 gene (Kv4.3), which encodes the α subunit of the I_{to} channel,[87] (2) KChIP2, a β subunit that coassembles with Kv4.3,[88] and (3) IRX5, a transcriptional factor regulating KCND3.[89]

Myocytes isolated from the epicardial region of the left ventricular wall of the rabbit show a higher density of cAMP-activated chloride current when compared to endocardial myocytes.[90] I_{to2}, initially ascribed to a K^+ current, now thought to be primarily due to the calcium-activated chloride current ($I_{Cl(Ca)}$), is also thought to contribute to the action potential notch, but it is not known whether this current differs among the three ventricular myocardial cell types.[91]

Recent studies involving canine ventricular myocytes have shown that calcium current (I_{Ca}) is similar among cells isolated from epicardium, M, and endocardial regions of the left ventricular wall.[92,93] One study, however, reported differences in Ca^{2+} channel properties between epicardial and endocardial canine ventricular cells. In that study, I_{Ca} was found to be larger in endocardial than in epicardial myocytes (3.4 ± 0.2 vs. 2.3 ± 0.1 pA/pF). A low-threshold, rapidly activating and inactivating Ca^{2+} current that resembled the T-type current was also recorded in all endocardial myocytes, but was small or absent in epicardial myocytes. The T-like current was comprised of two components: an Ni^{2+}-sensitive T-type current and a tetrodotoxin-sensitive Ca^{2+} current.[94]

The surface epicardial and endocardial layers are separated by transitional and M cells. M cells are distinguished by the ability of their action potential to prolong disproportionately relative to the action potential of other ventricular myocardial cells in response to a slowing of rate and/or in response to action potential duration (APD)-prolonging agents.[76,95,96] In the dog, the ionic basis for these features of the M cell includes the presence of a smaller slowly activating delayed rectifier current (I_{Ks}),[97] a larger late sodium current (late I_{Na}),[98] and a larger Na–Ca exchange current ($I_{Na\text{-}Ca}$).[99] In the canine heart, the rapidly activating delayed rectifier (I_{Kr}) and inward rectifier (I_{K1}) currents are similar in the three transmural cell types. Transmural and apicobasal differences in the density of I_{Kr} channels have been described in the ferret heart.[100] I_{Kr} message and channel protein are much larger in the ferret epicardium. I_{Ks} is larger in M cells isolated from the right than from the left ventricles of the dog.[86]

Cellular Basis for the Electrocardiographic J Wave

The presence of a prominent action potential notch in epicardium but not endocardium gives rise to a transmural voltage gradient during ventricular activation that manifests as a late delta wave following the QRS or what more commonly is referred to as a J wave[4] or Osborn wave. A distinct J wave is often observed under baseline conditions in the ECG of some animal species, including dogs and baboons. Humans more commonly display a J point elevation rather than a distinct J wave. A prominent J wave in the human ECG is considered pathognomonic of hypothermia[101–103,103] or hypercalcemia.[104,105]

A transmural gradient in the distribution of I_{to} is responsible for the transmural gradient in the magnitude of phase 1 and action potential notch, which in turn gives rise to a voltage gradient across the ventricular wall responsible for the inscription of the J wave or J point elevation in the ECG.[78,79,106] Direct evidence in support of the hypothesis that the J wave is caused by a transmural gradient in the magnitude of the I_{to}-mediated action potential notch derives from experiments conducted in the arterially perfused right ventricular wedge preparation showing a correlation between the amplitude of the epicardial action potential notch and that of the J wave recorded during interventions that alter the appearance of the electrocardiographic J wave, including hypothermia, premature stimulation (restitution), and block of I_{to} by 4-AP.[4]

Transmural activation within the thin wall of the RV is relatively rapid causing the J wave to be buried inside the QRS. Thus, although the action potential notch is most prominent in RV epicardium, RV myocardium would be expected to contribute relatively little to the manifestation of the J wave under normal conditions. These observations are consistent with the manifestation of the J wave in ECG leads in which the mean vector axis is transmurally oriented across the left ventricle and septum. Accordingly, the J wave in the dog is most prominent in leads II, III, aVR, and aVF, and mid to left precordial leads V3 through V6. A similar picture is seen in the human ECG.[105,107] In addition, vectorcardiography indicates that the J wave forms an extra loop that occurs at the junction of the QRS and T loops.[1 It is directed leftward and anteriorly, which explains its prominence in leads associated with the left ventricle.

The first description of the J wave was in the 1920s in animal experiments involving hypercalcemia.[104] The first extensive description and characterization appeared 30 years later by Osborn in a study involving experimental hypothermia in dogs.[109] The appearance of a prominent J wave in the clinic is typically associated with pathophysiological conditions, including hypothermia[101,1 and hypercalcemia.[104,105] The prominent J wave induced by hypothermia is the result of a marked accentuation of the spike-and-dome morphology of the action potential of M and epicardial cells (i.e., an increase in both width and magnitude of the notch). In addition to inducing a more prominent notch, hypothermia produces a slowing of conduction, which permits the epicardial notch to clear the QRS so as to manifest a distinct J wave. Hypercalcemia-induced accentuation of the J wave[104,105,110] may also be explained on the basis of an accentuation of the epicardial action potential notch, possibly as a result of an augmentation of the calcium-activated chloride current and a decrease in I_{Ca}.[111] Accentuation of the action potential notch also underlies the electrocardiographic and arrhythmogenic manifestations of the Brugada syndrome.

Exaggeration of the J Wave as the Basis for ST-Segment Elevation in Brugada Syndrome

Amplification of epicardial and transmural dispersion of repolarization secondary to the presence of genetic defects, pathophysiological factors, and pharmacological influences leads to accentuation of the J wave and eventually to loss of the action potential dome, giving rise to extrasystolic activity in the form of phase 2 reentry. Activation of I_{to} leads to a paradoxical prolongation of APD in canine ventricular tissues,[112] but to abbreviation of ventricular APD in species that normally exhibit brief action potentials (e.g., mouse and rat).[113] Pathophysiological conditions (e.g., ischemia, metabolic inhibition) and some pharmacological interventions (e.g., I_{Na} or I_{Ca} blockers or $I_{K\text{-}ATP}$, I_{to}, I_{Kr}, or I_{Ks} activators) can lead to marked abbreviation of APD in canine and feline[114] ventricular cells where I_{to} is prominent. Under these conditions, canine ventricular epicardium exhibits an all-or-none repolarization as a result of the shift in the balance of currents flowing at the end of phase 1 of the action potential. All-or-none repolarization of the action potential occurs when phase 1 reaches approximately −30 mV. This leads to loss of the action potential dome as the outward currents overwhelm the inward currents. Loss of the dome generally occurs at some epicardial sites but not others, resulting in the development of a marked dispersion of repolarization within the epicardium as well as transmurally, between epicardium and endocardium. Propagation of the action potential dome from the epicardial site at which it is maintained to sites at which it is abolished can cause local reexcitation of the preparation. This mechanism, termed phase 2 reentry, produces extrasystolic beats capable of initiating circus movement reentry[115] (Figure 33–2). Phase 2 reentry has been shown to occur when right ventricular epicardium is exposed to (1) K^+ channel openers such as pinacidil,[116] (2) sodium channel blockers such as flecainide,[3] (3) increased $[Ca^{2+}]_o$,[111] (4) calcium channel blockers such as verapamil, (5) metabolic inhibition,[117] and (6) simulated ischemia.[115]

Exaggerated or otherwise abnormal J waves have long been linked to idiopathic ventricular fibrillation as well as to the Brugada syndrome.[1,19,118–121] The Brugada syndrome is characterized by an exaggerated J wave that manifests as an ST-segment elevation in the right precordial leads.[1] A number of studies have emphasized the similarities between the conditions that predispose to phase 2 reentry and those that attend the appearance of the Brugada syndrome. Loss of the action potential dome in epicardium, but not endocardium, generates a transmural current that manifests on the ECG as an ST-segment elevation, similar to that encountered in patients with the Brugada syndrome.[4,117,122] Evidence in support of a phase 2 reentrant mechanism in humans was recently provided by Thomsen *et al.*[123,124]

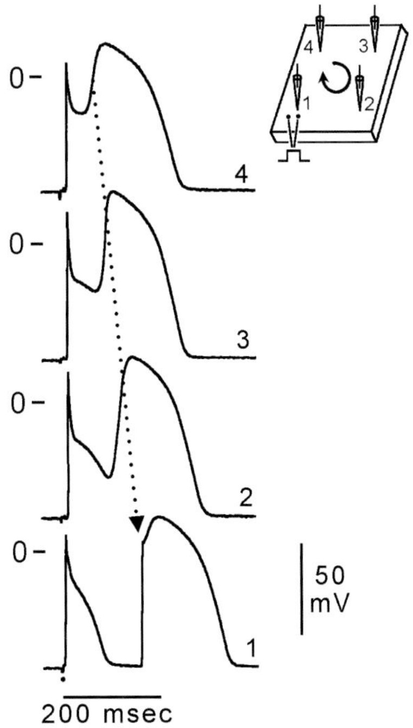

FIGURE 33–2. Phase 2 reentry. Reentrant activity induced by exposure of a canine ventricular epicardial preparation (0.7 cm^2) to simulated ischemia. Microelectrode recordings were obtained from four sites as shown in the schematic (upper right). After 35 min of ischemia, the action potential dome develops normally at site 4, but not at sites 1, 2, or 3. The dome then propagates in a clockwise direction reexciting sites 3, 2, and 1 with progressive delays, thus generating a closely coupled reentrant extrasystole (156 msec) at site 1. In this example of phase 2 reentry, propagation of the dome occurs in a direction opposite to that of phase 0, a mechanism akin to reflection. Basic cycle length (BCL) = 700 msec. (Modified from Lukas and Antzelevitch,[115] with permission.)

Parasympathetic agonists like acetylcholine facilitate loss of the action potential dome[125] by suppressing I_{Ca} and/or augmenting potassium current. β-Adrenergic agonists restore the dome by augmenting I_{Ca}. Sodium channel blockers also facilitate loss of the canine right ventricular action potential dome via a negative shift in the voltage at which phase 1 begins.[2,3] These findings are consistent with accentuation of ST-segment elevation in patients with the Brugada syndrome following vagal maneuvers or Class I antiarrhythmic agents as well as normalization of the ST-segment elevation following β-adrenergic agents and phosphodiesterase III inhibitors.[4,5,126] Loss of the action potential dome is more readily induced in right than in left canine ventricular epicardium[85,117,122] because of the more prominent I_{to}-mediated phase 1 in action potentials in this region of the heart. As previously noted, this distinction is believed to be the basis for why the Brugada syndrome is an RV disease.

Hence, accentuation of the RV epicardial action potential notch underlies the ST-segment elevation. Eventual loss of the dome of the RV epicardial action potential further exaggerates ST-segment elevation. A vulnerable window is created both within epicardium, as well as transmurally, which serves as the substrate for the development of reentry. Phase 2 reentry provides the extrasystole that serves as the trigger that precipitates episodes of VT and fibrillation in the Brugada syndrome. Evidence in support of this hypothesis was recently provided in an arterially perfused canine RV experimental model of the Brugada syndrome (Figure 33–3).[127] The VT and VF generated in these preparations are usually polymorphic, resembling a rapid form of torsade de pointes (TdP). This activity is likely related to the migrating spiral wave shown to generate a pattern resembling a polymorphic VT.[128,129]

In the past, much of the focus has been on the ability of a reduction in sodium channel current to unmask the Brugada syndrome and create an arrhythmogenic substrate. A recent report shows that a combination of I_{Na} and I_{Ca} block is more effective than I_{Na} inhibition alone in precipitating the Brugada syndrome in the arterially perfused wedge preparation (Figure 33–4).[130] High concentrations of terfenadine (5 μM) produce a potent block of I_{Na} and I_{Ca}, leading to accentuation of the epicardial action potential notch following acceleration of the rate from a basic cycle length (BCL) of 800 msec to 400 msec. Accentuation of the notch is due to the effect of the drug to depress phase 0, augment the magnitude of phase 1, and delay the appearance of the second upstroke. With continued rapid pacing, phase 1 becomes more accentuated, until all-or-none repolarization occurs at the end of phase 1 at some epicardial sites but not others, leading to the development of both epicardial (EDR) and transmural (TDR) dispersion of repolarization (Figure 33–4C). Propagation of the dome from the region where it is maintained to the region at which it is lost results in the development of local phase 2 reentry (Figure 33–4D). Figure 33–5 shows the ability of terfenadine-induced phase 2 reentry to generate an extrasystole, couplet, and polymorphic VT/VF. Figure 33–5D illustrates an example of programmed electrical stimulation to initiate VT/VF under similar conditions.

The ST-segment elevation associated with the Brugada syndrome has been attributed to (1) a conduction delay in the RV epicardial free wall in the region of the outflow tract (RVOT)[131] and/or (2) accentuation of the RV epicardial action potential that may lead to loss of the action potential dome.[132] The cellular mechanism thought to be responsible for the development of the Brugada phenotype via hypothesis 2 is schematically illustrated in Figure 33–6.[133,134]

The ST segment is usually isoelectric because of the absence of transmural voltage gradients at the level of the action potential plateau (Figure 33–6A). Accentuation of the RV notch under pathophysiological conditions leads to exaggeration of transmural voltage gradients and thus to accentuation of the J wave or to J point elevation. When epicardial repolarization precedes repolarization of the cells in the M and endocardial regions the T wave remains positive. This results in a saddleback configuration of the repolarization waves (Figure 33–6B). Further accentuation of the notch may be accompanied by a prolongation of the epicardial action potential such that the direction of repolarization across the RV wall and transmural voltage gradients are reversed, leading to the development of a coved-type ST-segment elevation and inversion of the T wave (Figure 33–6C), typically observed in the ECG of Brugada patients. A delay in epicardial activation may also contribute to inversion of the T wave. The downsloping ST-segment elevation observed in the experimen-

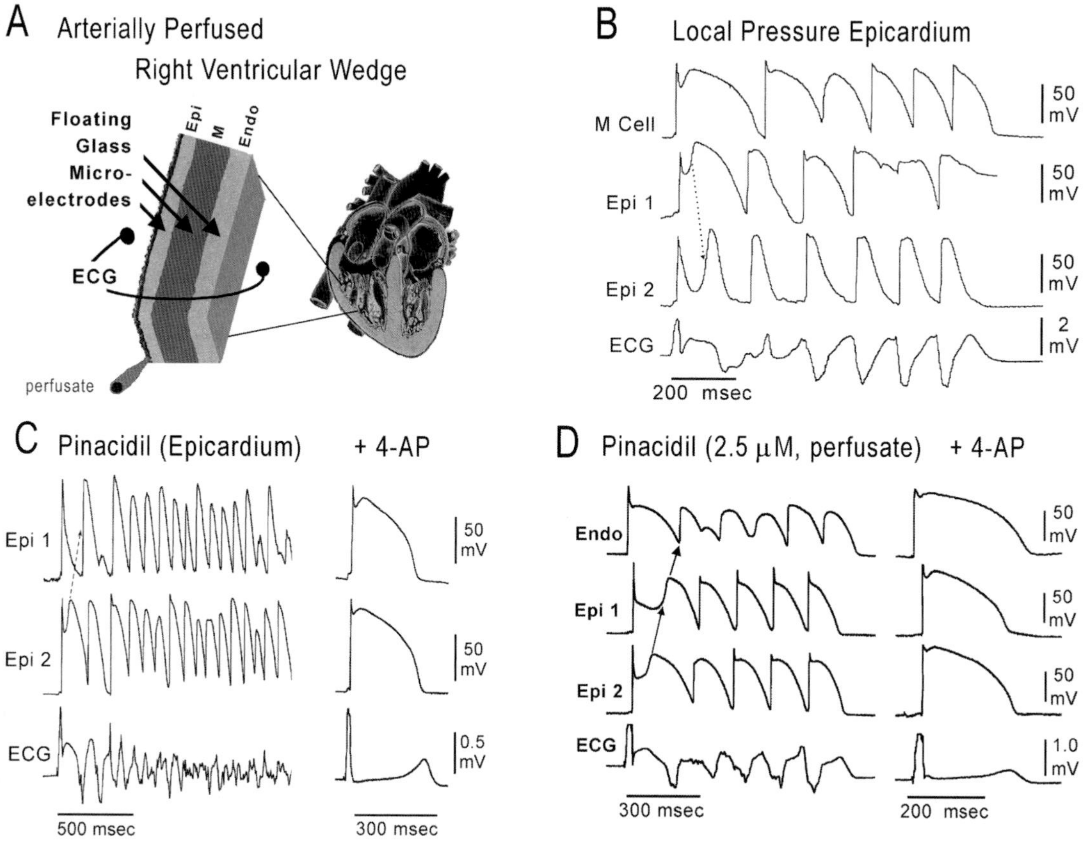

FIGURE 33–3. An ECG and arrhythmias with typical features of the Brugada syndrome recorded from canine coronary-perfused right ventricular wedge preparations. (A) Schematic of arterially perfused right ventricular wedge preparation. (B) Pressure-induced phase 2 reentry and VT. Shown are transmembrane action potentials simultaneously recorded from two epicardial (Epi 1 and Epi 2) and one M region (M) sites, together with a transmural ECG. Local application of pressure near Epi 2 results in loss of the action potential dome at that site but not at the Epi 1 or M sites. The dome at Epi 1 then reexcites Epi 2 giving rise to a phase 2 reentrant extrasystole that triggers a short run of ventricular tachycardia. Note the ST-segment elevation due to loss of the action potential dome in a segment of epicardium. (C) Polymorphic VT/VF induced by local application of the potassium channel opener pinacidil (10 μM) to the epicardial surface of the wedge. Action potentials from two epicardial sites (Epi 1 and Epi 2) and a transmural ECG were simultaneously recorded. Loss of the dome at Epi 1 but not Epi 2 creates a marked dispersion of repolarization, giving rise to a phase 2 reentrant extrasystole. The extrasystolic beat then triggers a long episode of ventricular fibrillation (22 sec). Right panel: Addition of 4-aminopyridine (4-AP, 2 mM), a specific I_{to} blocker, to the perfusate restored the action potential dome at Epi 1, thus reducing dispersion of repolarization and suppressing all arrhythmic activity. BCL = 2000 msec. (D) Phase 2 reentry gives rise to VT following addition of pinacidil (2.5 μM) to the coronary perfusate. Transmembrane action potentials forming two epicardial sites (Epi 1 and Epi 2) and one endocardial site (Endo) as well as a transmural ECG were simultaneously recorded. Right panel: 4-AP (1 mM) markedly reduces the magnitude of the action potential notch in epicardium, thus restoring the action potential dome throughout the preparation and abolishing all arrhythmic activity. (Panel D is from Yan and Antzelevitch,[127] with permission.)

tal wedge models often appears as an R′, suggesting that the appearance of an RBBB morphology in Brugada patients may be due at least in part to early repolarization of RV epicardium, rather than a major impulse conduction block in the right bundle.

Gussak and co-workers pointed out that a majority of RBBB-like morphologies encountered in cases of Brugada syndrome do not fit the criteria for RBBB.[135] Moreover, attempts by Miyazaki and co-workers to record delayed activation of the RV in Brugada patients met with failure.[5]

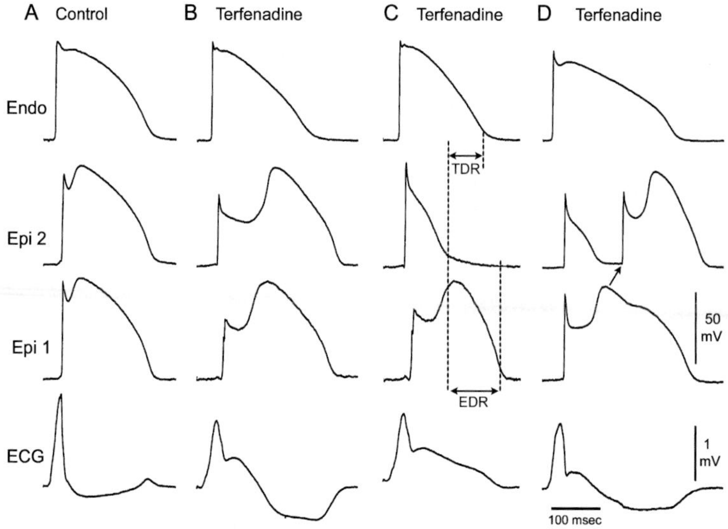

FIGURE 33–4. Terfenadine-induced ST-segment elevation, T wave inversion, transmural and endocardial dispersion of repolarization, and phase 2 reentry. Each panel shows transmembrane action potentials from one endocardial (top) and two epicardial sites together with a transmural ECG recorded from a canine arterially perfused right ventricular wedge preparation. (A) Control (BCL = 400 msec). (B) Terfenadine (5 μM) accentuated the epicardial action potential notch creating a transmural voltage gradient that manifests as an ST-segment elevation or exaggerated J wave in the ECG. The first beat was recorded after changing from BCL 800 msec to BCL 400 msec. (C) Continued pacing at BCL = 400 msec results in all-or-none repolarization at the end of phase 1 at some epicardial sites but not others, creating a local epicardial dispersion of repolarization (EDR) as well as a transmural dispersion of repolarization (TDR). (D) Phase 2 reentry occurs when the epicardial action potential dome propagates from a site where it is maintained to regions where it has been lost. (Modified from Fish and Antzelevitch,[130] with permission.)

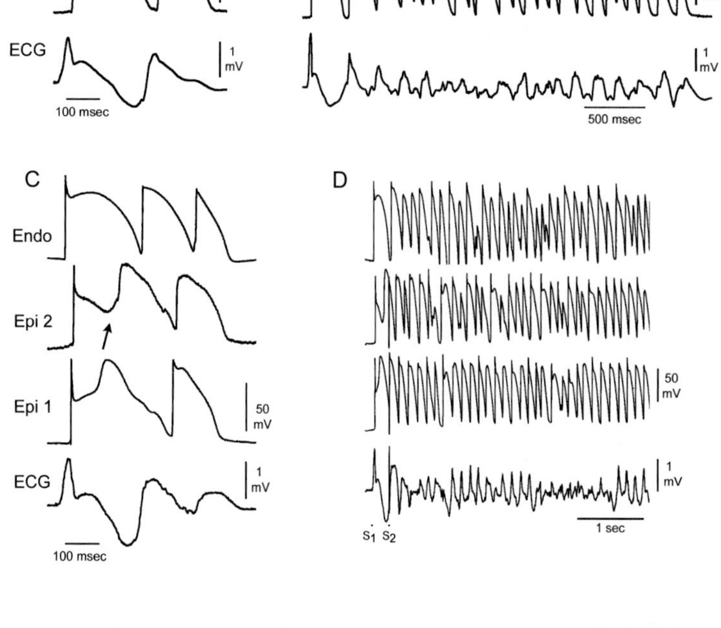

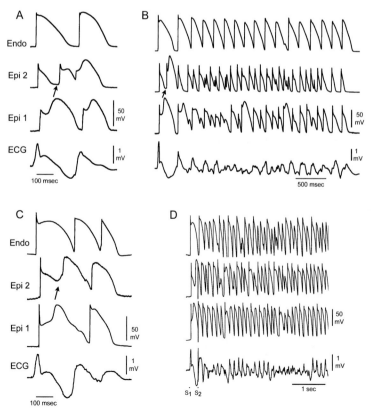

FIGURE 33–5. Spontaneous and programmed electrical stimulation-induced polymorphic VT in RV wedge preparations pretreated with terfenadine (5–10 μM). (A) Phase 2 reentry in epicardium gives rise to a closely coupled extrasystole. (B) Phase 2 reentrant extrasystole triggers a brief episode of polymorphic VT. (C) Phase 2 reentry followed by a single circus movement reentry in epicardium gives rise to a couplet. (D) Extrastimulus (S1 – S2 = 250 msec) applied to epicardium triggers a polymorphic VT. (Modified from Fish and Antzelevitch,[130] with permission.)

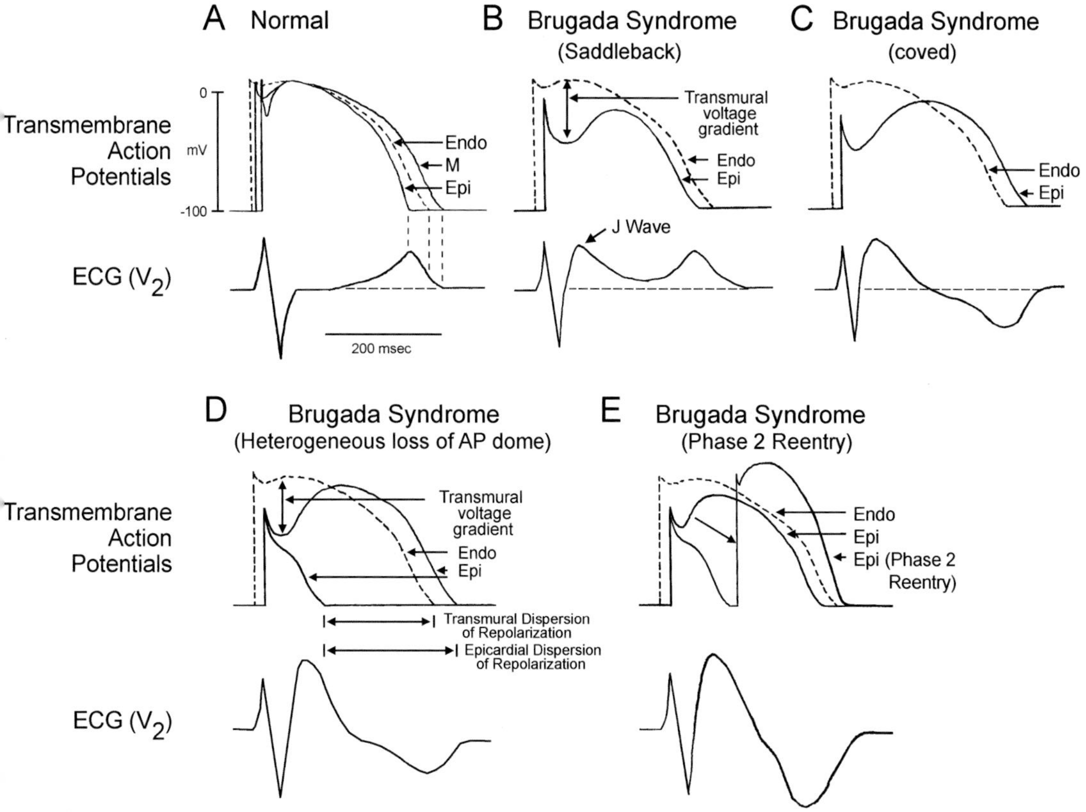

FIGURE 33–6. Schematic representation of right ventricular epicardial action potential changes (A–E) proposed to underlie the electrocardiographic manifestation of the Brugada syndrome. (Modified from Antzelevitch,[133] with permission.)

It is important to point out that although the typical Brugada morphology is present in Figure 33–6B and C, an arrhythmogenic substrate is absent. The arrhythmogenic substrate is thought to develop when a further shift in the balance of current leads to loss of the action potential dome at some epicardial sites but not others (Figure 33–6D). Loss of the action potential dome in epicardium but not endocardium results in the development of a marked transmural dispersion of repolarization and refractoriness, responsible for the development of a vulnerable window during which a premature impulse or extrasystole can induce a reentrant arrhythmia. Conduction of the action potential dome from sites at which it is maintained to sites at which it is lost causes local reexcitation via a phase 2 reentry mechanism, leading to the development of a very closely coupled extrasystole, which captures the vulnerable window across the wall, thus triggering a circus movement reentry in the form of VT/VF (Figure 33–6E).[115,127] The phase 2 reentrant beat fuses with the T wave of the basic response, thus accentuating the negative T wave. This morphology is often observed in the clinic preceding the onset of polymorphic VT.

Studies involving the arterially perfused right ventricular wedge preparation provide evidence in support of these hypotheses.[127] Aiba *et al.*[136] used a high- resolution optical mapping system that allows simultaneous recording of transmembrane action potentials from 256 sites along the transmural surface of the arterially perfused canine RV wedge preparation to demonstrate that a steep repolarization gradient between the region at which the dome is lost and the region at which it is maintained is essential for the development of a closely coupled phase 2 reentrant extrasystole. This study also showed that reentry initially rotates in the epicardium and gradually shifts to a transmural orientation, responsible for nonsustained polymorphic VT or VF.

Kurita *et al.* placed monophasic action potential (MAP) electrodes on the epicardial and endocardial surfaces of the RVOT in patients with the Brugada syndrome and demonstrated an accentuated notch in the epicardial response, thus providing support for this mechanism in humans.[137,138]

The marked accentuation of the epicardial action potential dome and the development of concealed phase 2 reentry suggest that activation forces may extend beyond the QRS in Brugada patients. Indeed, signal averaged ECG (SAECG) recordings have demonstrated late potentials in patients with the Brugada syndrome, especially in the anterior wall of the RVOT.[139–144] The basis for these late potentials, commonly ascribed to delayed conduction within the ventricle, is largely unknown. Endocardial recordings have been unrevealing. Nagase and co-workers[142] introduced a guide wire into the conus branch of the right coronary artery to record signals from the epicardial surface of the anterior wall of the RVOT in patients with the Brugada syndrome. The unipolar recordings displayed delayed potentials, which coincided with late potentials recorded in the SAECG, particularly after administration of Class IC antiarrhythmic agents. It was concluded that recordings from the conus branch of the right coronary artery can identify an "epicardial abnormality" in the RVOT that is accentuated in the presence of IC agents, thus uncovering part of the arrhythmogenic substrate responsible for VT/VF in Brugada syndrome, which may be related to the second upstroke or a concealed phase 2 reentrant beat. Late potentials are often regarded as being representative of delayed activation of the myocardium, but in the case of the Brugada syndrome other possibilities exist as discussed above. The second upstroke of the epicardial action potential, thought to be greatly accentuated in Brugada syndrome,[133] might be capable of generating late potentials when RVOT activation is otherwise normal. Moreover, the occurrence of phase 2 reentry, especially when concealed (i.e., when it fails to trigger transmural reentry), may contribute to the generation of delayed unipolar and late SAECG potentials.

The rate dependence of the ST-segment elevation may be useful in discriminating between these two hypotheses. If the Brugada ECG sign is due to delayed conduction in the RVOT, acceleration of the rate would be expected to further aggravate conduction and thus accentuate the ST-segment elevation and the RBBB morphology of the ECG. If, on the other hand, the Brugada ECG sign is secondary to accentuation of the epicardial action potential notch, at some point leading to loss of the action potential dome, acceleration of the rate would be expected to normalize the ECG, by restoring the action potential dome and reducing the notch. This occurs because the transient outward current, which is at the heart of this mechanism, is slow to recover from inactivation and is less available at faster rates. It should be noted that the presence of sodium channel blockers with strong use-dependent properties may confound the results, since in their presence accentuation of the action potential notch will occur as the stimulation rate is increased.

It is well known that Brugada patients usually display a normalization of their ECG or no change when the heart rate is increased, thus favoring the second hypothesis as the predominant mechanism. Further evidence in support of this hypothesis derives from the recent of observations of Shimizu and co-workers.[145] Using a unipolar catheter introduced into the great cardiac vein, they recorded unipolar activation recovery intervals (ARIs), a measure of local APD, from the epicardial surface of the RVOT in a 53-year-old Brugada patient. The ARIs in the RVOT were observed to abbreviate[146] dramatically whenever the ST segment was elevated in V2 following a pause or the administration of a sodium channel blocker. Additional support for the hypothesis derives from the demonstration by Watanabe and co-workers[147] that quinidine *suppresses* late potentials recorded in a patient with Brugada syndrome. This effect of the drug is presumably due to inhibition of I_{to} leading to diminution of the epicardial action potential notch and normalization of the repolarization heterogeneities. If the late potentials were due to delayed conduction, quinidine-induced I_{Na} inhibition would be expected to accentuate the appearance of the late potentials. Finally, magnetocardiograms recorded from patients with complete RBBB have been shown to generate currents from RVOT to the upper left chest that are opposite from those recorded in patients with Brugada syndrome.[146] Thus, the available data, both basic and clinical, point to

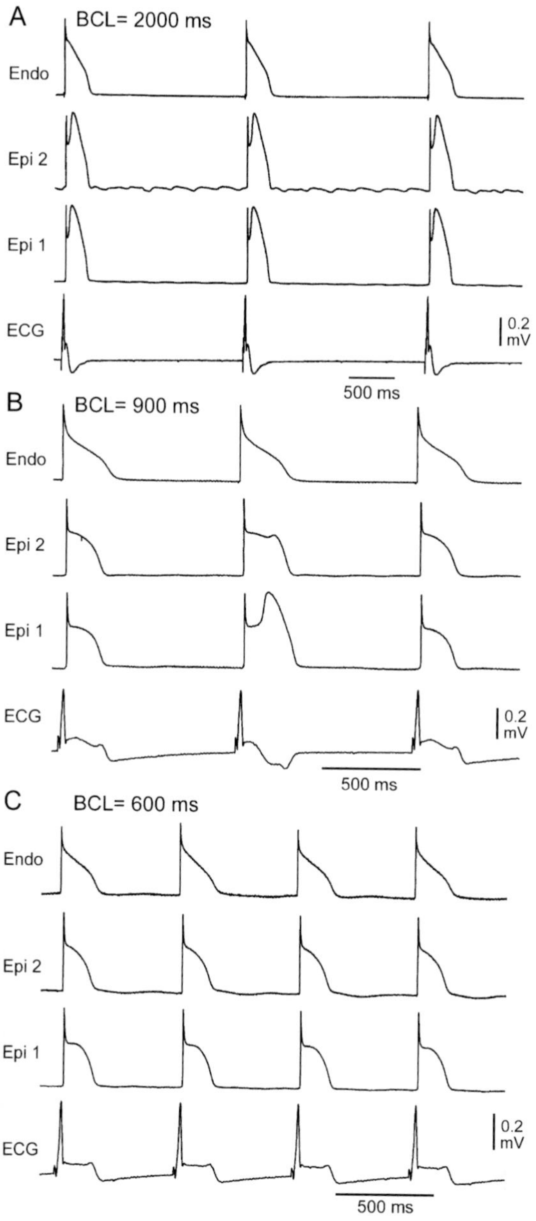

FIGURE 33–7. Verapamil (1 μM)-induced loss of the epicardial action potential dome in alternate beats causes T wave alternans in a canine arterially perfused right ventricular wedge preparation. (A) At a BCL of 2000 msec, endocardial and epicardial action potentials repolarize almost simultaneously, generating little or no T wave on the ECG. (B) Decreasing the cycle length to 900 msec induces heterogeneous loss of the epicardial action potential dome in alternate beats while the endocardial response remains constant, resulting in profound T wave alternans. (C) Decreasing the cycle length to 600 msec leads to homogeneous loss of the action potential dome on all beats, leading to ST-segment elevation but no T wave alternans in the ECG. (Fish and Antzelevitch, unpublished.)

transmural voltage gradients that develop secondary to accentuation of the epicardial notch and loss of the action potential dome as being in large part responsible for the Brugada ECG signature.

These facts notwithstanding, there are likely to be cases in which a conduction defect may predominate. The presence of a prominent S wave displaying rate-dependent boarding was observed in intracavitary unipolar leads.[148]

T Wave Alternans

T wave alternans (TWA) is characterized by beat-to-beat alteration in the amplitude, polarity, and/or morphology of the electrocardiographic T wave. TWA has been reported in patients with the Brugada syndrome and is thought to be associated with an increased risk for development of VT/VF.[149–156] Experimental studies suggest that T wave alternans is due to at least two cellular mechanisms, including (1) loss of the epicardial action potential dome on alternate beats (Figure 33–7) and (2) concealed phase 2 reentry on alternating beats (Figure 33–8).[130,157]

Acquired Forms of Brugada Syndrome and Modulating Factors

The electrocardiographic and arrhythmic manifestations of the Brugada syndrome can be induced and modulated by a large number of agents and factors. The Brugada ECG can be unmasked or modulated by sodium channel blockers, a febrile state, vagotonic agents, α-adrenergic agonists, β-adrenergic blockers, tricyclic or tetracyclic antidepressants, first generation antihistaminics (dimenhydrinate), a combination of glucose and insulin, hyperkalemia, hypokalemia, hypercalcemia, and by alcohol and cocaine toxicity (Figure 33–9)[5,11,12,158–165] These agents may also induce acquired forms of the Brugada syndrome (Table 33–2). Although a definitive list of drugs to avoid in the Brugada syndrome is not yet formulated, the list of agents in Table 33–2 may provide some guidance. One of the more recent additions to this group is lithium. This widely used drug is a blocker of cardiac sodium channels and can unmask patients with the Brugada syndrome.[166]

Myocardial infarction or acute ischemia due to vasospasm involving the RVOT mimics

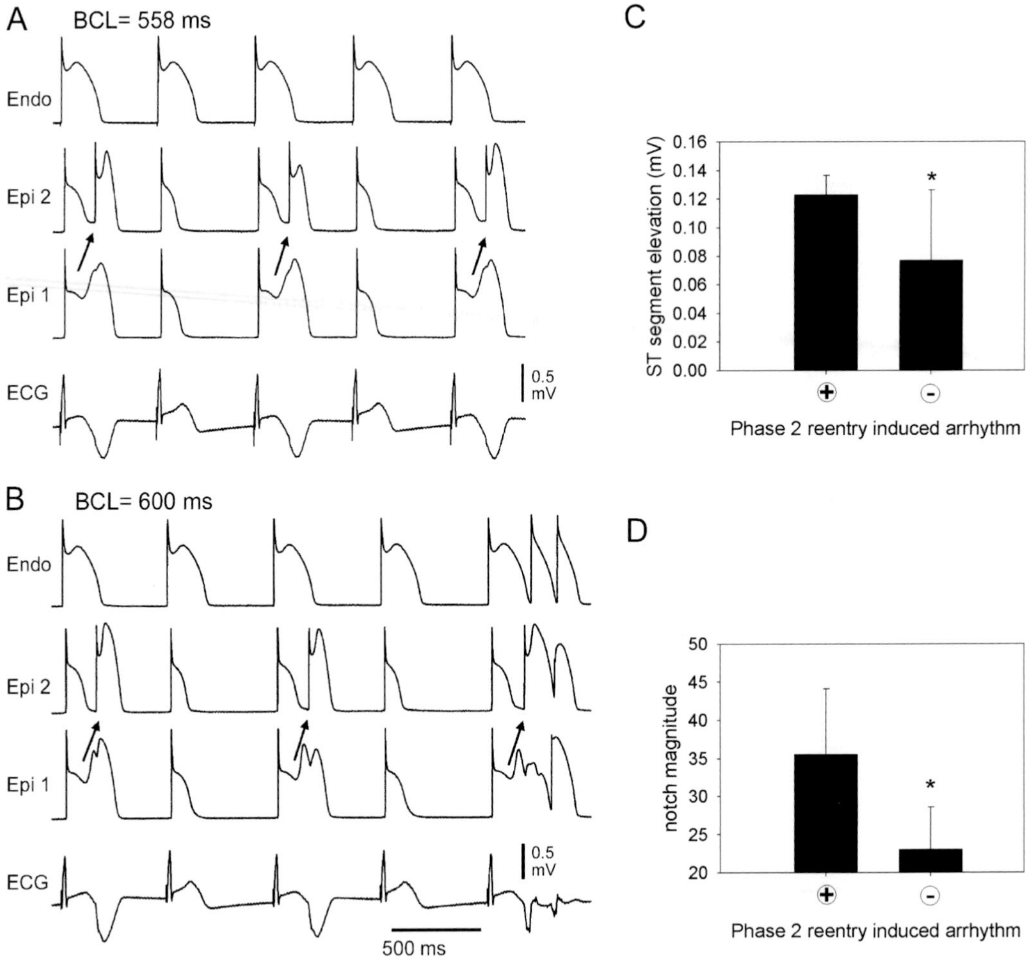

FIGURE 33–8. Verapamil (1 μM)-induced concealed phase 2 reentry in alternate beats leading to T wave alternans in the coronary-perfused right ventricular wedge preparation. (A) T wave alternans occurs as a result of concealed phase 2 reentry. The dome propagates from Epi 1 to Epi 2 on alternating beats while the endocardial response remains constant. The concealed phase 2 reentry results in a negative T wave. BCL = 558 msec. (B) Increasing the cycle length to 600 msec exaggerates the T wave alternans. The phase relationship between Epi 1, Epi 2, and Endo shifts slightly, allowing the previously concealed phase 2 reentry to propagate transmurally, leading to two extrasystoles. (C) The ST-segment elevation, measured 50 msec after the end of the QRS, is greater during alternans secondary to concealed phase 2 reentry compared to alternans due to alternating loss of the epicardial action potential dome [$n = 10$ phase 2 reentry plus (+) and 12 phase 2 reentry minus (–) episodes, $*p = 0.027$]. (D) The size of the epicardial action potential notch magnitude (ph2 amp – ph1 amp/ph2 amp) at BCL = 2000 msec during control was significantly smaller in preparations not displaying phase 2 reentry-induced arrhythmias than in those that did ($n = 5$ for each category, $*p = 0.025$). (Fish and Antzelevitch, unpublished.)

ST-segment elevation similar to that seen in Brugada syndrome. This effect is secondary to the depression of I_{Ca}, inactivation of I_{Na}, and the activation of $I_{K\text{-}ATP}$ during ischemia, and suggests that patients with congenital and possibly acquired forms of Brugada syndrome may be at a higher risk for ischemia-related sudden cardiac death.[167] Although the coexistence of Brugada syndrome and vasospastic angina in the same patient is not rare, Chinushi *et al.* have failed to observe an enhanced susceptibility to VF or a proarrhythmic effect of Ca antagonist in this setting.[168]

Hypokalemia has been suggested to be a contributing factor in the high prevalence of sudden

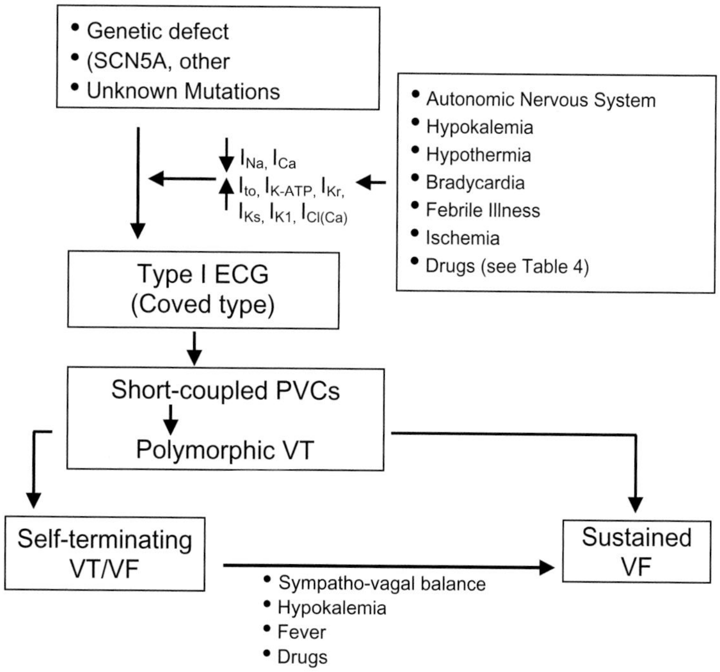

FIGURE 33–9. Factors predisposing to the electrocardiographic and arrhythmic manifestations of the Brugada syndrome. (Modified from Nademanee *et al.*,[206] with permission.)

TABLE 33–2. Drug-induced Brugada-like ECG patterns.

I. Antiarrhythmic drugs
  1. Na^+ channel blockers
     Class IC drugs (flecainide,[12,14,140,207,208] pilsicainide,[145,209] propafenone[210])
     Class IA drugs (ajmaline,[12,211] procainamide,[5,12] disopyramide,[5,8] cibenzoline[150,212])
  2. Ca^{2+} channel blockers
     Verapamil
  3. β Blockers
     Propranolol intoxication[213]

II. Antianginal drugs
  1. Ca^{2+} channel blockers
     Nifedipine, diltiazem
  2. Nitrate
     Isosorbide dinitrate, nitroglycerine[214]
  3. K^+ channel openers
     Nicorandil

III. Psychotropic drugs
  1. Tricyclic antidepressants[215]
     Amitriptyline,[216,217] nortriptyline,[166] desipramine,[158] clomipramine[159]
  2. Tetracyclic antidepressants
     Maprotiline[216]
  3. Phenothiazine
     Perphenazine,[216] cyamemazine
  4. Selective serotonin reuptake inhibitors
     Fluoxetine[217]
  5. Lithium[166]

IV. Other drugs
  1. Histaminic H1 receptor antagonists
     Dimenhydrinate[161]
     Diphenhydramine[218]
  2. Cocaine intoxication[162,219]
  3. Alcohol intoxication

Source: Modified from Antzelevitch *et al.*[62] and Shimizu,[220] with permission.

unexpected nocturnal death syndrome (SUNDS) in the northeastern region of Thailand where potassium deficiency is endemic.[164,169] Serum potassium in the northeastern population is significantly lower than that of the population in Bangkok, which lies in the central part of Thailand where potassium is abundant in the food. A recent case report highlights the ability of hypokalemia to induce VF in a 60-year-old man who had asymptomatic Brugada syndrome without a family history of sudden cardiac death.[164] This patient was initially treated for asthma by steroids, which lowered serum potassium from 3.8 mmol/liter on admission to 3.4 and 2.9 mmol/liter on day 7 and 8 of admission, respectively. Both were associated with unconsciousness. Ventricular fibrillation was documented during the last episode, which reverted spontaneously to sinus rhythm. Hypokalemia may exert these effects by increasing the chemical gradient for K^+ and thus the intensity of I_{to}.

Both VT/VF and sudden death in the Brugada syndrome usually occur at rest and at night. Circadian variation of sympathovagal balance, hormones, and other metabolic factors is likely to contribute to this circadian pattern. Bradycardia, due to altered sympathovagal balance or other factors, may contribute to initiation of arrhythmia.[30,170,171] Abnormal [^{123}I]metaiodobenzylguanidine (MIBG) uptake in 8 (17%) of the 17 Brugada syndrome patients but none in the control group was demonstrated by Wichter *et al.*[172] Segmental reduction of [^{123}I]MIBG in the inferior and the septal left ventricular wall was observed indicating presynaptic sympathetic dysfunction. Of note, imaging of the RV, particularly the RVOT, is difficult with this technique, so that insufficient information is available concerning sympathetic function in the regions known to harbor the arrhythmogenic substrate. Moreover, it remains unclear what role the reduced uptake function plays in the arrhythmogenesis of the Brugada syndrome. If the RVOT is similarly affected, this defect may indeed alter the sympathovagal balance in favor of the development of an arrhythmogenic substrate.[125,127]

The Thai Ministry of Public Health Report (1990) found an association between a large meal on the night of death in SUNDS patients.[169] Consistent with this observation, a recent study by Nogami *et al.* found that glucose and insulin could unmask the Brugada ECG.[163] Another possibility is that sudden death in these patients is due to the increased vagal tone produced by the stomach distention. A recent study by Ikeda *et al.*[173] has shown that a full stomach after a large meal can unmask a Type I ECG, particularly in Brugada syndrome patients at high risk for arrhythmic events, thus suggesting that this technique may be of diagnostic and prognostic value.

Accelerated inactivation of the sodium channel caused by *SCN5A* mutations associated with the Brugada syndrome has been shown to be accentuated at higher temperatures[63] suggesting that a febrile state may unmask the Brugada syndrome. Indeed, several case reports have emerged recently demonstrating that febrile illness could reveal the Brugada ECG and precipitate VF.[13,64,65,174–176] A recent report from Keller *et al.*[177] has identified a missense mutation, F1344S, in SCN5A in a patient with Brugada syndrome and fever-induced VT/VF. Expression of F1344S showed a shift in the voltage dependence of activation, which was further accentuated at high temperatures mimicking fever. Thus fever may also cause a loss of function in I_{Na} by accelerating inactivation as well as producing a shift in the voltage dependence of activation.

Anecdotal data point to hot baths as a possible precipitating factor. Of note, the northeastern part of Thailand, where the Brugada syndrome is most prevalent, is known for its very hot climate. A study is underway to assess whether this extreme climate influences the prognosis of the disease.

Sex-Related Differences in the Manifestation of the Brugada Syndrome

Although the mutation responsible for the Brugada syndrome is equally distributed between the sexes, the clinical phenotype is 8 to 10 times more prevalent in males than in females. The basis for this sex-related distinction has been shown to be due to a more prominent I_{to}-mediated action potential notch in the RV epicardium of males than in females[178] (Figures 33–10 and 33–11). The more prominent I_{to} causes the end of

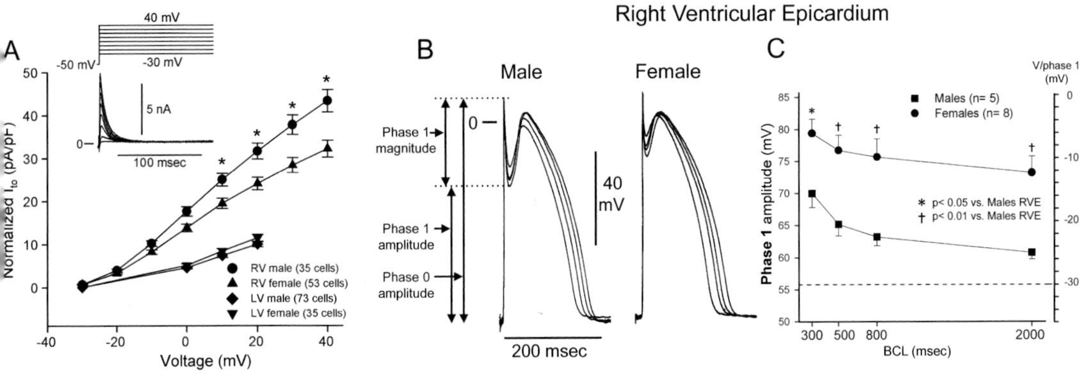

FIGURE 33–10. Sex-based and interventricular differences in I_{to}. (A) Mean I–V relationship for I_{to} recorded from RV epicardial cells isolated from hearts of male and female dogs. Inset: Representative I_{to} current traces and voltage protocol. I_{to} density was significantly greater in male than in female RV epicardial cells. No sex differences were observed in LV. (B) Transmembrane action potentials recorded from isolated canine RV epicardial male and female tissue slices. BCLs = 300, 500, 800, and 2000 msec. (C) Rate dependence of phase 1 amplitude and voltage at the end of phase 1 (V/phase 1, mV) in males (solid squares) versus females (solid circles). (Modified from Di Diego *et al.*,[178] with permission.)

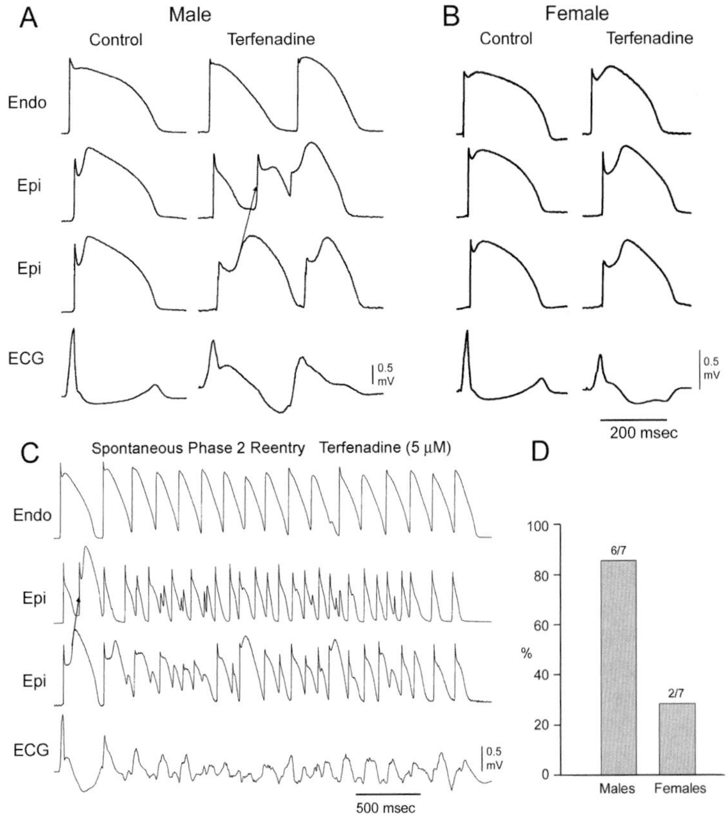

FIGURE 33–11. Terfenadine induces the Brugada phenotype more readily in male than female RV wedge preparations. Each panel shows action potentials recorded from two epicardial sites and one endocardial site, together with a transmural ECG. Control recordings were obtained at a BCL of 2000 msec, whereas terfenadine data were recorded at a BCL of 800 msec after a brief period of pacing at a BCL of 400 msec. (A) Terfenadine (5 μM)-induced, heterogeneous loss of action potential dome, ST-segment elevation, and phase 2 reentry (arrow) in a male RV wedge preparation. (B) Terfenadine fails to induce Brugada phenotype in a female RV wedge preparation. (C) Polymorphic VT triggered by spontaneous phase 2 reentry in a male preparation. (D) Incidence of phase 2 reentry in male (six of seven) versus female (two of seven) RV wedge preparations when perfused with 5 μM terfenadine for up to 2 h. (Modified from Di Diego *et al.*,[178] with permission.)

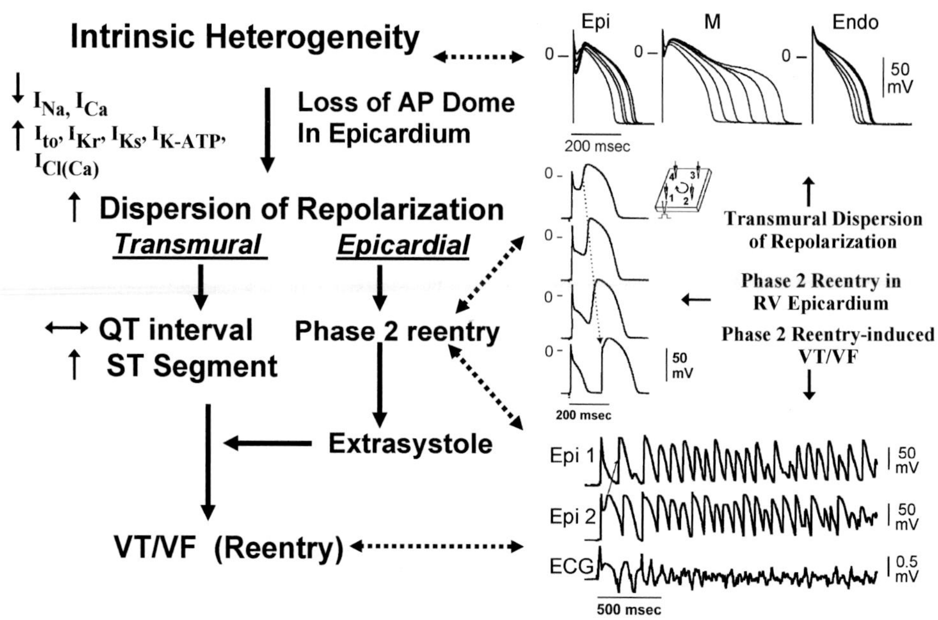

FIGURE 33–12. Proposed mechanism for the Brugada syndrome. A shift in the balance of currents serves to amplify existing heterogeneities by causing loss of the action potential dome at some epicardial, but not endocardial sites. A vulnerable window develops as a result of the dispersion of repolarization and refractoriness within the epicardium as well as across the wall. Epicardial dispersion leads to the development of phase 2 reentry, which provides the extrasystole that captures the vulnerable window and initiates VT/VF via a circus movement reentry mechanism. (Modified from Antzelevitch,[134] with permission.)

phase 1 of the RV epicardial action potential to repolarize to more negative potentials in tissue and arterially perfused wedge preparations from males, facilitating loss of the action potential dome and the development of phase 2 reentry and polymorphic VT.

The proposed cellular mechanism for the Brugada syndrome is summarized in Figure 33–12. Available data support the hypothesis that the Brugada syndrome results from amplification of heterogeneities intrinsic to the early phases of the action potential among the different transmural cell types. This amplification is secondary to a rebalancing of currents active during phase 1, including a decrease in I_{Na} or I_{Ca} or augmentation of any one of a number of outward currents. ST-segment elevation similar to that observed in patients with the Brugada syndrome occurs as a consequence of the accentuation of the action potential notch, eventually leading to loss of the action potential dome in RV epicardium, where I_{to} is most prominent. Loss of the dome gives rise to both a transmural as well as epicardial dispersion of repolarization. The transmural dispersion is responsible for the development of ST-segment elevation and the creation of a vulnerable window across the ventricular wall, whereas the epicardial dispersion is responsible for phase 2 reentry, which provides the extrasystole that captures the vulnerable window, thus precipitating VT/VF. The VT generated is usually polymorphic, resembling a very rapid form of torsade de pointes (TdP).

Approach to Therapy

Device Therapy

The only proven effective therapy for the Brugada syndrome is an ICD (Table 33–3).[179,180] Recommendations for ICD implantation from the Second Consensus Conference [9,10] are presented in Table 33–4 and are summarized as follows.

Table 33–3. Device and pharmacological approach to therapy.

- Devices and ablation
  - ICD[179]
  - ? Ablation or cryosurgery[181]
  - ? Pacemaker[221]
- Pharmacological approach to therapy
  - Ineffective
    - Amiodarone[49]
    - β Blockers[49]
    - Class IC antiarrhythmics
      - Flecainide[14]
      - Propafenone[210]
    - ? Disopyramide[186]
    - Class IA antiarrhythmics
      - Procainamide[12]
  - Effective for treatment of electrical storms
    - β Adrenergic agonists—isoproterenol[5,22]
    - Phosphodiesterase III Inhibitors—cilostazol[126]
    - Quinidine[204]
  - Effective general therapy
    - Quinidine[38,127,184,189,190,192–194,204]
  - Experimental therapy
    - I_{to} Blockers—cardioselective and ion channel specific
      - Quinidine[127]
      - 4-Aminopyridine[127]
      - Tedisamil[197]
      - AVE0118[201]

Symptomatic patients with a Type 1 ST-segment elevation or Brugada ECG (either spontaneously or after sodium channel blockade) who present with aborted sudden death should receive an ICD as a Class I indication without additional need for electrophysiological study (EPS). Similar patients presenting with related symptoms such as syncope, seizure, or nocturnal agonal respiration should also undergo ICD implantation as a Class I indication after vasovagal syncope has been excluded on clinical grounds and noncardiac causes of these symptoms have been carefully ruled out. The Task Force recommended that symptomatic patients undergo EPS only for the assessment of supraventricular arrhythmia.

Asymptomatic patients with a Brugada ECG (spontaneously or after sodium channel block) should undergo EPS if there is a family history of sudden cardiac death suspected to be due to Brugada syndrome. An EPS may be justified when the family history is negative for sudden cardiac death if the Type 1 ST-segment elevation occurs spontaneously. If inducible for ventricular arrhythmia, the patient should receive an ICD. This was recommended as a Class IIa indication for patients presenting with a spontaneous Type I ST-segment elevation and as a Class IIb for patients who display a Type I ST-segment elevation only after sodium block challenge. More recent data have called these recommendations into question and suggest that it might be more appropriate to consider both as Class IIb indications.

Asymptomatic patients who have no family history and who develop a Type 1 ST-segment elevation only after sodium channel blockade should be closely followed-up. As additional data become available, these recommendations will no doubt require further finetuning.

Although arrhythmias and sudden cardiac death generally occur during sleep or at rest and have been associated with slow heart rates, a potential therapeutic role for cardiac pacing remains largely unexplored. Haissaguerre and co-workers[181] reported that focal radiofrequency ablation aimed at eliminating the ventricular premature beats that trigger VT/VF in the Brugada syndrome may be useful in controlling arrhythmogenesis. However, data relative to a cryosurgical approach or the use of ablation therapy are very limited at this point in time.

Pharmacological Approach to Therapy

Although ICD implantation is the mainstay of therapy for the Brugada syndrome, implantation can be challenging in infants and is not an adequate solution for patients residing in regions of the world where an ICD is unaffordable. Also, ICD implantation in "asymptomatic high-risk patients" is not trivial, in particular because the level of risk is still being debated (see the section on Prognosis and Risk Stratification above). In the Antiarrhythmics versus Implantable Defibrillators (AVID) trial, a multicenter study of ICD implantation for patients with heart disease and malignant arrhythmias, the risk for ICD-related complications serious enough to warrant reintervention was 12%.[182] The rate of serious complications from ICD implantation for patients with Brugada syndrome is likely to be higher than the 12% reported for the patients in AVID, who were relatively old (65 ± 11 years) and had a 3-year mortality rate of

TABLE 33–4. Indications for ICD implantation in patients with the Brugada syndrome.[a]

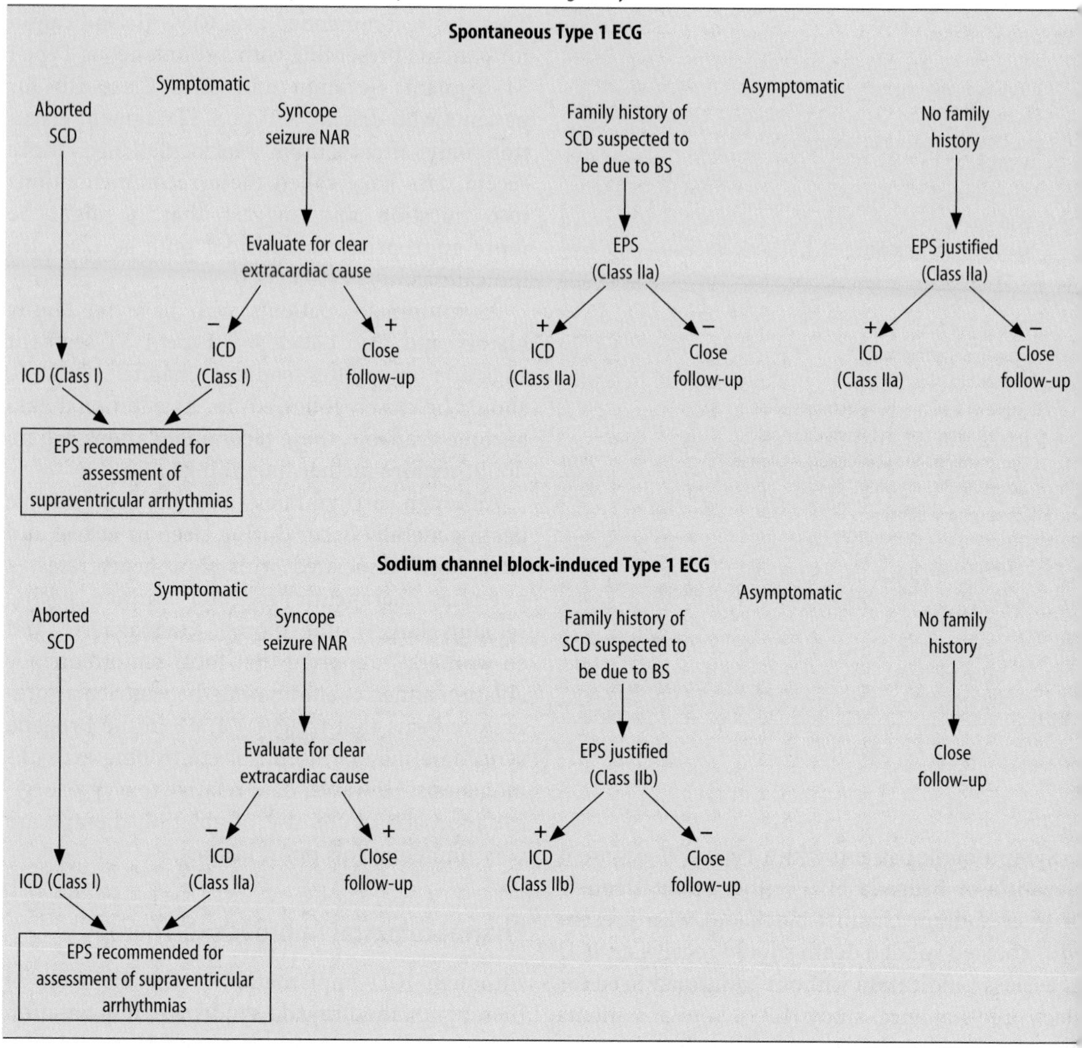

Source: From Antzelevitch *et al.*[9,10] with permission.

[a]Class I: Clear evidence that the procedure or treatment is useful or effective. Class II: Conflicting evidence concerning usefulness or efficacy. Class IIa: Weight of evidence in favor of usefulness or efficacy. Class IIb: Usefulness or efficacy less well established. BS, Brugada syndrome; EPS, electrophysiological study; NAR, nocturnal agonal respiration; SCD, sudden cardiac death.

25%.[183] Patients with Brugada syndrome are younger, have a very low risk for nonarrhythmic cardiac death, and will remain at risk for ICD-related complications for many more years. In particular, the risk for potentially serious complications such as infection or lead-insulation break leading to inappropriate ICD shocks will increase over the years and after repeated ICD replacements. Therefore, although the ICD represents the most effective way for preventing arrhythmic death in Brugada syndrome, pharmacological solutions may be desirable as an alternative to device therapy for selected cases[184] as well as for minimizing the firing of the ICD in patients with frequent events.[9,57,184,185]

The search for a pharmacological treatment has been focused on rebalancing of the ion channel current active during the early phases of the epicardial action potential in the RV so as to reduce the magnitude of the action potential notch and/

or restore the action potential dome. Table 33–3 lists the various pharmacological agents thus far investigated. Antiarrhythmic agents such as amiodarone and β blockers have been shown to be ineffective.[49] Class IC antiarrhythmic drugs, such as flecainide and propafenone, and Class IA agents, such as procainamide, are contraindicated because they unmask the Brugada syndrome and induce arrhythmogenesis. Disopyramide is a Class IA antiarrhythmic that has been demonstrated to normalize ST-segment elevation in some Brugada patients but to unmask the syndrome in others.[186]

The presence of a prominent I_{to} is fundamental to the mechanism underlying the Brugada syndrome. Consequently, the most prudent general approach to therapy, regardless of the ionic or genetic basis for the disease, is to partially inhibit I_{to}. Cardioselective and I_{to}-specific blockers are not currently available. 4-Aminopyridine is an agent that is ion-channel specific at low concentrations, but is not cardioselective in that it inhibits I_{to} in the nervous system. Although it is effective in suppressing arrhythmogenesis in wedge models of the Brugada syndrome[127] (Figure 33–13), it is unlikely to be of clinical benefit because of neurally mediated adverse effects.

Quinidine is an agent currently on the market in the United States and other regions of the world with significant I_{to} blocking properties. Accordingly, we suggested several years ago that this agent may be of therapeutic value in the Brugada syndrome.[187] Quinidine has been shown to be effective in restoring the epicardial action potential dome, thus normalizing the ST segment and preventing phase 2 reentry and polymorphic VT in experimental models of the Brugada syndrome (Figure 33–13).[127,188] Clinical evidence of the effectiveness of quinidine in normalizing ST-segment elevation in patients with the Brugada syndrome has been reported as well (Figure 33–14).[184,189–191] Quinidine has also been reported to be effective in suppressing arrhythmogenesis in an infant too young to receive an ICD.[38]

In a prospective study of 25 Brugada syndrome patients orally administered quinidine bisulfate (1483 ± 240 mg), Belhassen and co-workers[190] evaluated the effectiveness of quinidine in preventing inducible and spontaneous VF. There were 15 symptomatic patients (7 cardiac arrest

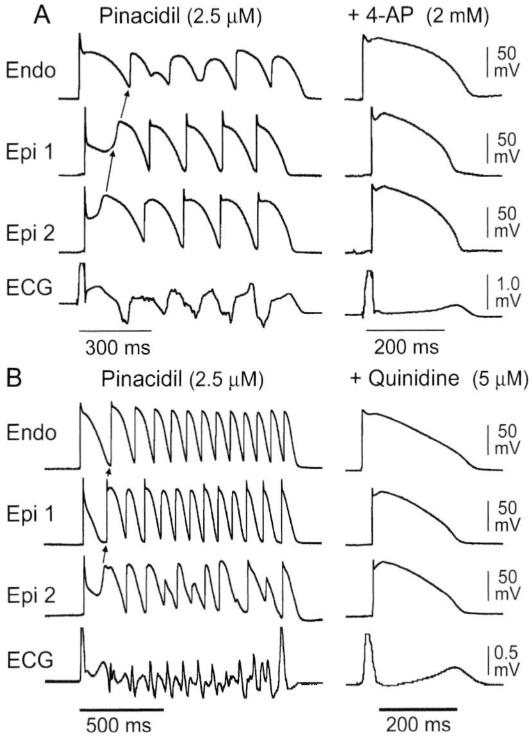

FIGURE 33–13. Effects of I_{to} blockers 4-AP and quinidine on pinacidil-induced phase 2 reentry and VT in the arterially perfused RV wedge preparation. In both examples, 2.5 mM pinacidil produced heterogeneous loss of AP dome in epicardium, resulting in ST-segment elevation, phase 2 reentry, and VT (left); 4-AP (A) and quinidine (B) restored the epicardial AP dome, reduced both transmural and epicardial dispersion of repolarization, normalized the ST segment, and prevented phase 2 reentry and VT in the continued presence of pinacidil. (From Yan and Antzelevitch,[127] with permission.)

survivors and 7 with unexplained syncope) and 10 asymptomatic patients. All 25 patients had inducible VF at baseline electrophysiological study. Quinidine prevented VF induction in 22 of the 25 patients (88%). After a follow-up period of 6 months to 22.2 years, all patients were alive. Of 19 patients treated with oral quinidine (without ICD back-up) for 6 to 219 months (56 ± 67 months), none developed arrhythmic events. Administration of quinidine was associated with a 36% incidence of side effects, principally diarrhea, which resolved after drug discontinuation. It was concluded that quinidine effectively suppresses VF induction as well as spontaneous arrhythmias in patients with Brugada syndrome and may be

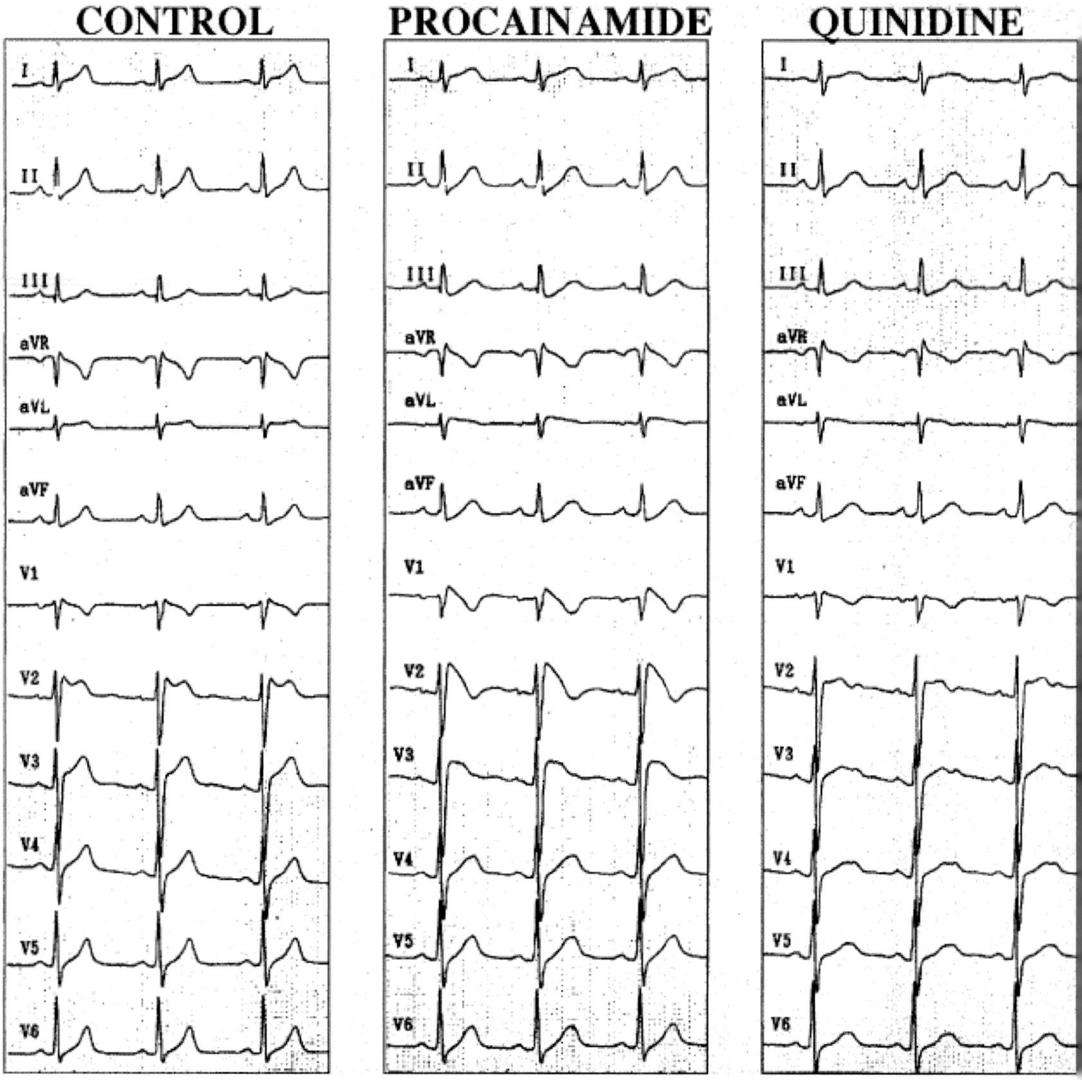

Figure 33–14. Twelve-lead electrocardiogram (ECG) tracings in an asymptomatic 26-year-old man with the Brugada syndrome. Left: Baseline: Type 2 ECG (not diagnostic) displaying a "saddle-back-type" ST-segment elevation is observed in V2. Center: After intravenous administration of 750 mg procainamide, the Type 2 ECG is converted to the diagnostic Type 1 ECG consisting of a "coved-type" ST-segment elevation. Right: A few days after ora[l] administration of quinidine bisulfate (1500 mg/day, serum quini-dine level 2.6 mg/liter), ST-segment elevation is attenuated in the right precordial leads. VF could be induced during control and procainamide infusion, but not after quinidine. (From Belhassen *et al.*,[184] with permission.)

useful as an adjunct to ICD therapy. It was also suggested that EPS-guided quinidine therapy may be used *as an alternative* to ICD in cases in which an ICD is refused or unaffordable as well as when patients who are well informed about the risks and benefits of ICD and EP-guided quinidine therapy prefer medical therapy to device implantation.[191] The results are consistent with those reported by the same group in prior years[184,192] and more recently by other investigators.[193–195] A relatively small recent study by Mizusawa *et al.*[196] also showed that low-dose quinidine (300–600 mg) can prevent electrophysiological induction of VF and has a potential as an adjunctive therapy for Brugada syndrome in patients with frequent implantable cardioverter defibrillator discharges. There is a clear need for a large randomized controlled clinical trial to assess the effectiveness of quinidine, preferably in patients with frequent events who have already received an ICD.

The quest for additional cardioselective and I_{to}-specific blockers is ongoing. Another agent being considered for this purpose is the drug tedisamil, currently being evaluated for the treatment of atrial fibrillation. Tedisamil may be more potent than quinidine because it lacks the inward current blocking actions of quinidine, while potently blocking I_{to}. The effect of tedisamil to suppress phase 2 reentry and VT in a wedge model of the Brugada syndrome is illustrated in Figure 33–15.[197]

Tedisamil and quinidine are both capable of suppressing the substrate and trigger for the Brugada syndrome via their inhibition of I_{to}. Both, however, also block I_{Kr} and thus have the potential to induce an acquired form of the long QT syndrome. Thus these agents may substitute one form of polymorphic VT for another, particularly under conditions that promote TdP, such as bradycardia and hypokalemia. However, the majority of patients with Brugada syndrome are otherwise healthy males, for whom the risk of drug-induced TdP is small.[198] This effect of quinidine is minimized at high plasma levels because at these concentrations quinidine block of I_{Na} counters the effect of I_{Kr} block to increase transmural dispersion of repolarization, the substrate for the development of TdP arrhythmias.[77,199,200] High doses of quinidine (1000–1500 mg/day) are recommended in order to effect I_{to} block without inducing TdP.

Another potential therapeutic candidate is an agent reported to be a relatively selective I_{to} and I_{Kur} blocker, AVE0118.[201] Figure 33–16 shows the ability of AVE0118 to normalize the ECG and suppress phase 2 reentry in a wedge model of the Brugada syndrome. This drug has the advantage that it does not block I_{Kr}, and therefore does not prolong the QT interval or have the potential to induce TdP. The disadvantage of this particular drug is that it undergoes first-pass hepatic metabolism and is therefore not effective with oral administration.

Appropriate clinical trials are needed to establish the effectiveness of all of the above pharmacological agents as well as the potential role of pacemakers in some forms of the disease.

Drugs that increase the calcium current, such as β-adrenergic agents like isoproterenol, are useful as well.[126,127,133] Isoproterenol, sometimes in combination with quinidine, has been shown to be effective in normalizing ST-segment elevation

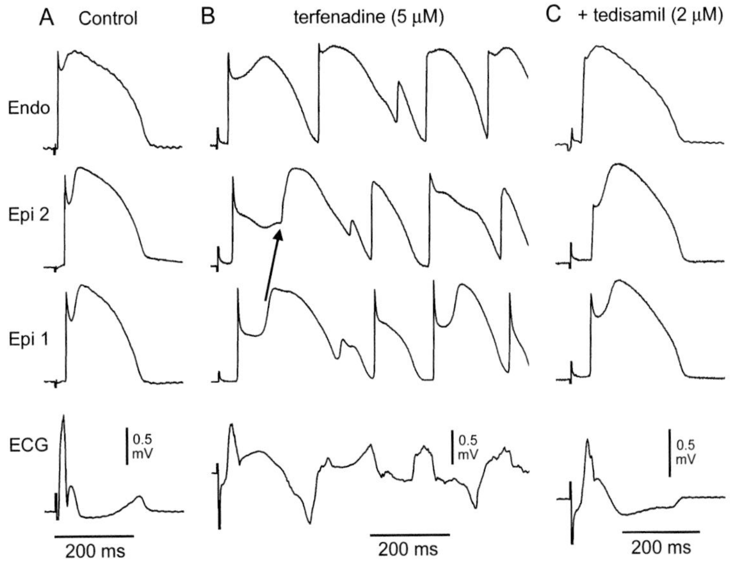

FIGURE 33–15. Effects of I_{to} block with tedisamil to suppress phase 2 reentry induced by terfenadine in an arterially perfused canine RV wedge preparation. (A) Control, BCL = 800 msec. (B) Terfenadine (5 μM) induces ST-segment elevation as a result of heterogeneous loss of the epicardial action potential dome, leading to phase 2 reentry, which triggers an episode of poly VT (BCL = 800 msec). (C) Addition of tedisamil (2 μM) normalizes the ST segment and prevents loss of the epicardial action potential dome and suppresses phase 2 reentry-induced and polymorphic VT (BCL = 800 ms). (From Antzelevitch and Fish,[185] with permission.)

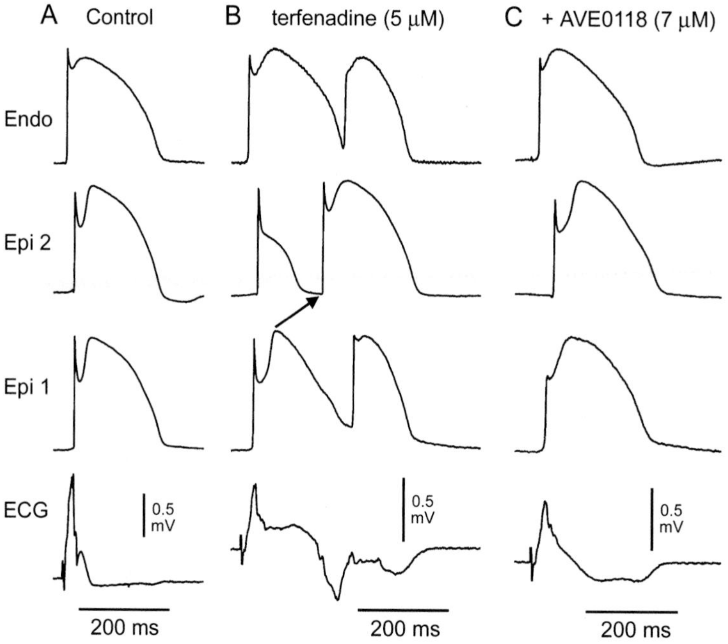

FIGURE 33–16. Effects of I_{to} blockade with AVE0118 to suppress phase 2 reentry induced by terfenadine in an arterially perfused canine RV wedge preparation. (A) Control, BCL = 800 msec. (B) Terfenadine (5 μM) induces ST-segment elevation as a result of heterogeneous loss of the epicardial action potential dome, leading to phase 2 reentry, which triggers a closely coupled extrasystole (BCL = 800 msec). (C) Addition of AVE0118 (7 μM) prevents loss of the epicardial action potential dome and phase 2 reentry-induced arrhythmias (BCL = 800 msec). (From Antzelevitch and Fish,[185] with permission.)

in patients with the Brugada syndrome and in controlling electrical storms, particularly in children.[22,184,189,194,202–204] A new addition to the pharmacological armamentarium is the phosphodiesterase III inhibitor cilostazol,[126] which normalizes the ST segment, most likely by augmenting the calcium current (I_{Ca}) as well as by reducing I_{to} secondary to an increase in heart rate.

Another pharmacological approach is to augment a component of I_{Na} that is active during phase 1 of the epicardial action potential. Dimethyl lithospermate B (dmLSB) is an extract of Danshen, a traditional Chinese herbal remedy, which slows inactivation of I_{Na}, but only during a window of time corresponding to the action potential notch. This leads to increased inward current during the early phases of the action potential. Figure 33–17 shows the effectiveness of dmLSB in eliminating the arrhythmogenic substrate responsible for the Brugada syndrome in three different experimental models of the syndrome.[205] The Brugada syndrome phenotype was created in canine arterially perfused RV wedge preparations using either terfenadine or verapamil to inhibit I_{Na} and I_{Ca}, or pinacidil to activate $I_{K\text{-}ATP}$. Terfenadine, verapamil, and pinacidil each induced all-or-none repolarization at some epicardial sites but not others, leading to ST-segment elevation as well as an increase in both epicardial and transmural dispersions of repolarization from 12.9 ± 9.6 msec to 107.0 ± 54.8 msec and 22.4 ± 8.1 msec to 82.2 ± 37.4 msec, respectively ($p < 0.05$, $n = 9$). Under these conditions, phase 2 reentry developed as the epicardial action potential dome propagated from sites where it was maintained to sites at which it was lost, generating closely coupled extrasystoles and VT/VF. Addition of dmLSB (10 μM) to the coronary perfusate restored the epicardial action potential dome, reduced both epicardial and transmural dispersion of repolarization, and abolished phase 2 reentry-induced extrasystoles and VT/VF in nine of nine preparations. Our data suggest that dmLSB may be a candidate for pharmacological treatment of Brugada syndrome in cases in which an ICD is not feasible or affordable or as an adjunct to ICD use.

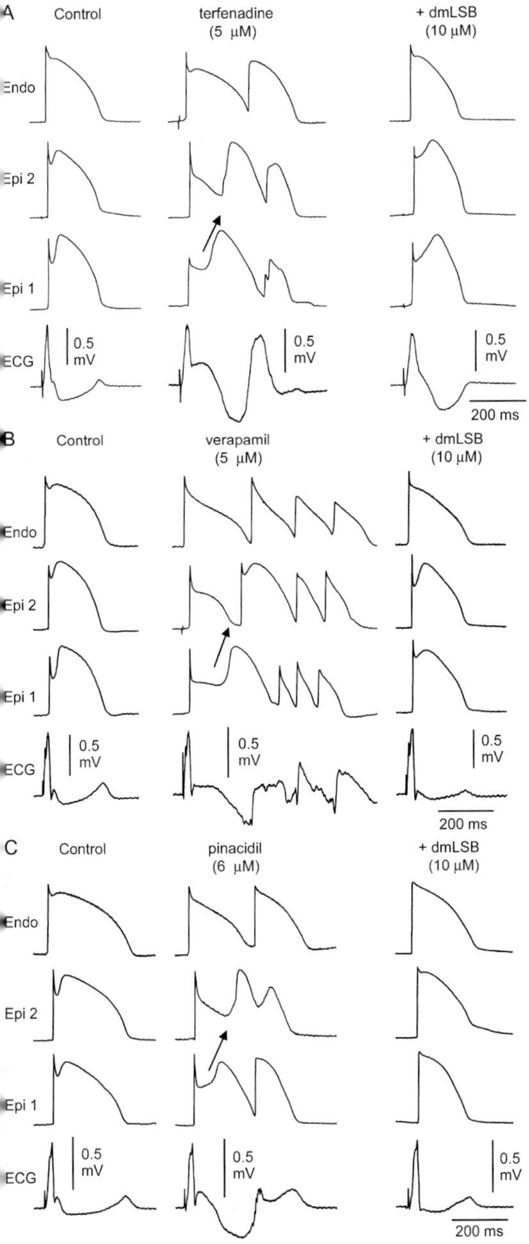

FIGURE 33–17. Effect of dmLSB suppression of the arrhythmogenic substrate of the Brugada syndrome in three experimental models. Phase 2 reentry was induced in three separate models of the Brugada syndrome. Terfenadine (5 μM, A), verapamil (5 μM, B), and pinacidil (6 μM, C) induce heterogeneous loss of the epicardial action potential dome and ST-segment elevation. Phase 2 reentry occurs as the dome is propagated from Epi 1 to Epi 2, triggering either a closely coupled extrasystole or polymorphic ventricular tachycardia. In all three models, addition of dmLSB (10 μM) normalizes the ST segment and abolishes phase 2 reentry and resultant arrhythmias. (From Fish *et al.*,[205] with permission.)

References

1. Brugada P, Brugada J Right bundle branch block, persistent ST segment elevation and sudden cardiac death: A distinct clinical and electrocardiographic syndrome: A multicenter report. *J Am Coll Cardiol* 1992;20:1391–1396.
2. Krishnan SC, Antzelevitch C. Sodium channel block produces opposite electrophysiological effects in canine ventricular epicardium and endocardium. *Circ Res* 1991;69:277–291.
3. Krishnan SC, Antzelevitch C. Flecainide-induced arrhythmia in canine ventricular epicardium. Phase 2 reentry? *Circulation* 1993;87:562–572.
4. Yan GX, Antzelevitch C. Cellular basis for the electrocardiographic J wave. *Circulation* 1996;93:372–379.
5. Miyazaki T, Mitamura H, Miyoshi S, Soejima K, Aizawa Y, Ogawa S. Autonomic and antiarrhythmic drug modulation of ST segment elevation in patients with Brugada syndrome. *J Am Coll Cardiol* 1996;27:1061–1070.
6. Antzelevitch C. The Brugada syndrome. *J Cardiovasc Electrophysiol* 1998;9:513–516.
7. Wilde AA, Antzelevitch C, Borggrefe M, Brugada J, Brugada R, Brugada P, Corrado D, Hauer RN, Kass RS, Nademanee K, Priori SG, Towbin JA. Proposed diagnostic criteria for the Brugada syndrome: Consensus report. *Eur Heart J* 2002;23:1648–1654.
8. Wilde AA, Antzelevitch C, Borggrefe M, Brugada J, Brugada R, Brugada P, Corrado D, Hauer RN, Kass RS, Nademanee K, Priori SG, Towbin JA. Proposed diagnostic criteria for the Brugada syndrome: Consensus report. *Circulation* 2002;106:2514–2519.
9. Antzelevitch C, Brugada P, Borggrefe M, Brugada J, Brugada R, Corrado D, Gussak I, LeMarec H, Nademanee K, Perez Riera AR, Shimizu W, Schulze-Bahr E, Tan H, Wilde A. Brugada Syndrome. Report of the Second Consensus Conference. Endorsed by the Heart Rhythm Society and the European Heart Rhythm Association. *Circulation* 2005;111:659–670.
10. Antzelevitch C, Brugada P, Borggrefe M, Brugada J, Brugada R, Corrado D, Gussak I, LeMarec H, Nademanee K, Perez Riera AR, Shimizu W, Schulze-Bahr E, Tan H, Wilde A. Brugada syndrome: Report of the second consensus conference. *Heart Rhythm* 2005;2:429–440.
11. Brugada P, Brugada J, Brugada R. Arrhythmia induction by antiarrhythmic drugs. *Pacing Clin Electrophysiol* 2000;23:291–292.
12. Brugada R, Brugada J, Antzelevitch C, Kirsch GE, Potenza D, Towbin JA, Brugada P. Sodium channel

blockers identify risk for sudden death in patients with ST-segment elevation and right bundle branch block but structurally normal hearts. *Circulation* 2000;101:510–515.

13. Antzelevitch C, Brugada R. Fever and the Brugada syndrome. *Pacing Clin Electrophysiol* 2002;25: 1537–1539.
14. Shimizu W, Antzelevitch C, Suyama K, Kurita T, Taguchi A, Aihara N, Takaki H, Sunagawa K, Kamakura S. Effect of sodium channel blockers on ST segment, QRS duration, and corrected QT interval in patients with Brugada syndrome. *J Cardiovasc Electrophysiol* 2000;11:1320–1329.
15. Priori SG, Napolitano C, Gasparini M, Pappone C, Della BP, Brignole M, Giordano U, Giovannini T, Menozzi C, Bloise R, Crotti L, Terreni L, Schwartz PJ. Clinical and genetic heterogeneity of right bundle branch block and ST-segment elevation syndrome: A prospective evaluation of 52 families. *Circulation* 2000;102:2509–2515.
16. Wolpert C., Echternach C, Veltmann C, Antzelevitch C, Thomas GP, Sphel S, Streitner F, Kuschyk J, Schimpf R, Haase KK, Borggrefe M. Intravenous drug challenge using flecainide and ajmaline in patients with Brugada syndrome. *Heart Rhythm* 2005;2:254–260.
17. Hong K, Brugada J, Oliva A, Berruezo-Sanchez A, Potenza D, Pollevick GD, Guerchicoff A, Matsuo K, Burashnikov E, Dumaine R, Towbin JA, Nesterenko VV, Brugada P, Antzelevitch C, Brugada R. Value of electrocardiographic parameters and ajmaline test in the diagnosis of Brugada syndrome caused by SCN5A mutations. *Circulation* 2004;110:3023–3027.
18. Itoh H, Shimizu M, Takata S, Mabuchi H, Imoto K. A novel missense mutation in the SCN5A gene associated with Brugada syndrome bidirectionally affecting blocking actions of antiarrhythmic drugs. *J Cardiovasc Electrophysiol* 2005;16:486–493.
19. Kalla H, Yan GX, Marinchak R. Ventricular fibrillation in a patient with prominent J (Osborn) waves and ST segment elevation in the inferior electrocardiographic leads: A Brugada syndrome variant? *J Cardiovasc Electrophysiol* 2000;11:95–98.
20. Ogawa M, Kumagai K, Yamanouchi Y, Saku K. Spontaneous onset of ventricular fibrillation in Brugada syndrome with J wave and ST-segment elevation in the inferior leads. *Heart Rhythm* 2005;2:97–99.
21. Horigome H, Shigeta O, Kuga K, Isobe T, Sakakibara Y, Yamaguchi I, Matsui A. Ventricular fibrillation during anesthesia in association with J waves in the left precordial leads in a child with coarctation of the aorta. *J Electrocardiol* 2003;36: 339–343.
22. Shimizu W, Matsuo K, Takagi M, Tanabe Y, Aiba T, Taguchi A, Suyama K, Kurita T, Aihara N, Kamakura S. Body surface distribution and response to drugs of ST segment elevation in Brugada syndrome: Clinical implication of eighty-seven-lead body surface potential mapping and its application to twelve-lead electrocardiograms. *J Cardiovasc Electrophysiol* 2000;11:396–404.
23. Sangwatanaroj S, Prechawat S, Sunsaneewitayakul B, Sitthisook S, Tosukhowong P, Tungsanga K. New electrocardiographic leads and the procainamide test for the detection of the Brugada sign in sudden unexplained death syndrome survivors and their relatives. *Eur Heart J* 2001;22:2290–2296.
24. Shin SC, Ryu S, Lee JH, Chang BJ, Shin JK, Kim HS, Heo JH, Yang DH, Park HS, Cho Y, Chae SC, Jun JE, Park WH. Prevalence of the Brugada-type ECG recorded from higher intercostal spaces in healthy Korean males. *Circulation J* 2005;69:1064–1067.
25. Alings M, Wilde A. "Brugada" syndrome: Clinical data and suggested pathophysiological mechanism. *Circulation* 1999;99:666–673.
26. Bezzina C, Veldkamp MW, van Den Berg MP, Postma AV, Rook MB, Viersma JW, Van Langen IM, Tan-Sindhunata G, Bink-Boelkens MT, Der Hout AH, Mannens MM, Wilde AA. A single Na(+) channel mutation causing both long-QT and Brugada syndromes. *Circ Res* 1999;85:1206–1213.
27. Pitzalis MV, Anaclerio M, Iacoviello M, Forleo C, Guida P, Troccoli R, Massari F, Mastropasqua F, Sorrentino S, Manghisi A, Rizzon P. QT-interval prolongation in right precordial leads: An additional electrocardiographic hallmark of Brugada syndrome. *J Am Coll Cardiol* 2003;42:1632–1637.
28. Castro HJ, Antzelevitch C, Tornes BF, Dorantes SM, Dorticos BF, Zayas MR, Quinones Perez MA, Fayad RY. Tpeak-Tend and Tpeak-Tend dispersion as risk factors for ventricular tachycardia/ventricular fibrillation in patients with the Brugada syndrome. *J Am Coll Cardiol* 2006;47:1828–1834.
29. Smits JP, Eckardt L, Probst V, Bezzina CR, Schott JJ, Remme CA, Haverkamp W, Breithardt G, Escande D, Schulze-Bahr E, LeMarec H, Wilde AA. Genotype-phenotype relationship in Brugada syndrome: Electrocardiographic features differentiate SCN5A-related patients from non-SCN5A-related patients. *J Am Coll Cardiol* 2002;40: 350–356.
30. Kasanuki H, Ohnishi S, Ohtuka M, Matsuda N, Nirei T, Isogai R, Shoda M, Toyoshima Y, Hosoda

S. Idiopathic ventricular fibrillation induced with vagal activity in patients without obvious heart disease. *Circulation* 1997;95:2277–2285.
31. Proclemer A, Facchin D, Feruglio GA, Nucifora R. Recurrent ventricular fibrillation, right bundle-branch block and persistent ST-segment elevation in V1–V3: A new arrhythmia syndrome? A clinical case report (see comments). *G Ital Cardiol* 1993; 23:1211–1218.
32. Makiyama T, Akao M, Tsuji K, Doi T, Ohno S, Takenaka K, Kobori A, Ninomiya T, Yoshida H, Takano M, Makita N, Yanagisawa F, Higashi Y, Takeyama Y, Kita T, Horie M. High risk for bradyarrhythmic complications in patients with Brugada syndrome caused by SCN5A gene mutations. *J Am Coll Cardiol* 2005;46:2100–2106.
33. Scornik FS, Desai M, Brugada R, Guerchicoff A, Pollevick GD, Antzelevitch C, Perez GJ. Functional expression of "cardiac-type" Na(v)1.5 sodium channel in canine intracardiac ganglia. *Heart Rhythm* 2006;3:842–850.
34. Shimada M, Miyazaki T, Miyoshi S, Soejima K, Hori S, Mitamura H, Ogawa S. Sustained monomorphic ventricular tachycardia in a patient with Brugada syndrome. *Jpn Circ J* 1996;60:364–370.
35. Pinar BE, Garcia-Alberola A, Martinez SJ, Sanchez Munoz JJ, Valdes CM. Spontaneous sustained monomorphic ventricular tachycardia after administration of ajmaline in a patient with Brugada syndrome [see comments]. *Pacing Clin Electrophysiol* 2000;23:407–409.
36. Dinckal MH, Davutoglu V, Akdemir I, Soydinc S, Kirilmaz A, Aksoy M. Incessant monomorphic ventricular tachycardia during febrile illness in a patient with Brugada syndrome: Fatal electrical storm. *Europace* 2003;5:257–261.
37. Mok NS, Chan NY. Brugada syndrome presenting with sustained monomorphic ventricular tachycardia. *Int J Cardiol* 2004;97:307–309.
38. Probst V, Evain S, Gournay V, Marie A, Schott JJ, Boisseau P, Le MH. Monomorphic ventricular tachycardia due to Brugada syndrome successfully treated by hydroquinidine therapy in a 3-year-old child. *J Cardiovasc Electrophysiol* 2006; 17:97–100.
39. Sastry BK, Narasimhan C, Soma RB. Brugada syndrome with monomorphic ventricular tachycardia in a one-year-old child. *Indian Heart J* 2001;53: 203–205.
40. Remme CA, Wever EFD, Wilde AAM, Derksen R, Hauer RNW. Diagnosis and long-term follow-up of Brugada syndrome in patients with idiopathic ventricular fibrillation. *Eur Heart J* 2001;22:400–409.
41. Brugada J, Brugada R, Antzelevitch C, Towbin J, Nademanee K, Brugada P. Long-term follow-up of individuals with the electrocardiographic pattern of right bundle-branch block and ST-segment elevation in precordial leads V(1) to V(3). *Circulation* 2002;105:73–78.
42. Priori SG, Napolitano C, Gasparini M, Pappone C, Della BP, Giordano U, Bloise R, Giustetto C, De Nardis R, Grillo M, Ronchetti E, Faggiano G, Nastoli J. Natural history of Brugada syndrome: Insights for risk stratification and management. *Circulation* 2002;105:1342–1347.
43. Brugada P, Brugada R, Brugada J. Patients with an asymptomatic Brugada electrocardiogram should undergo pharmacological and electrophysical testing. *Circulation* 2005;112:279–285.
44. Priori SG, Napolitano C. Management of patients with Brugada syndrome should not be based on programmed electrical stimulation. *Circulation* 2005;112:285–291.
45. Eckardt L, Probst V, Smits JP, Bahr ES, Wolpert C, Schimpf R, Wichter T, Boisseau P, Heinecke A, Breithardt G, Borggrefe M, LeMarec H, Bocker D, Wilde AA. Long-term prognosis of individuals with right precordial ST-segment-elevation Brugada syndrome. *Circulation* 2005;111:257–263.
46. Atarashi H, Ogawa S, for The Idiopathic Ventricular Fibrillation Investigators. New ECG criteria for high-risk Brugada syndrome. *Circ J* 2003;67:8–10.
47. Morita H, Takenaka-Morita S, Fukushima-Kusano K, Kobayashi M, Nagase S, Kakishita M, Nakamura K, Emori T, Matsubara H, Ohe T. Risk stratification for asymptomatic patients with Brugada syndrome. *Circ J* 2003;67:312–316.
48. Viskin S. Inducible ventricular fibrillation in the Brugada syndrome: Diagnostic and prognostic implications. *J Cardiovasc Electrophysiol* 2003;14: 458–460.
49. Brugada J, Brugada R, Brugada P. Right bundle-branch block and ST-segment elevation in leads V_1 through V_3. A marker for sudden death in patients without demonstrable structural heart disease. *Circulation* 1998;97:457–460.
50. Kanda M, Shimizu W, Matsuo K, Nagaya N, Taguchi A, Suyama K, Kurita T, Aihara N, Kamakura S. Electrophysiologic characteristics and implications of induced ventricular fibrillation in symptomatic patients with Brugada syndrome. *J Am Coll Cardiol* 2002;39:1799–1805.
51. Brugada J, Brugada R, Brugada P. Determinants of sudden cardiac death in individuals with the electrocardiographic pattern of Brugada syndrome and no previous cardiac arrest. *Circulation* 2003; 108:3092–3096.

52. Eckardt L, Kirchhof P, Johna R, Haverkamp W, Breithardt G, Borggrefe M. Wolff-Parkinson-White syndrome associated with Brugada syndrome. *Pacing Clin Electrophysiol* 2001;24:1423–1424.
53. Carlsson J, Erdogan A, Schulte B, Neuzner J, Pitschner HF. Possible role of epicardial left ventricular programmed stimulation in Brugada syndrome. *Pacing Clin Electrophysiol* 2001;24:247–249.
54. Gehi AK, Duong TD, Metz LD, Gomes JA, Mehta D. Risk stratification of individuals with the Brugada electrocardiogram: A meta-analysis. *J Cardiovasc Electrophysiol* 2006;17:577–583.
55. Chen Q, Kirsch GE, Zhang D, Brugada R, Brugada J, Brugada P, Potenza D, Moya A, Borggrefe M, Breithardt G, Ortiz-Lopez R, Wang Z, Antzelevitch C, O'Brien RE, Schultze-Bahr E, Keating MT, Towbin JA, Wang Q. Genetic basis and molecular mechanisms for idiopathic ventricular fibrillation. *Nature* 1998;392:293–296.
56. Grant AO, Carboni MP, Neplioueva V, Starmer CF, Memmi M, Napolitano C, Priori SG. Long QT syndrome, Brugada syndrome, and conduction system disease are linked to a single sodium channel mutation. *J Clin Invest* 2002;110:1201–1209.
57. Antzelevitch C, Brugada P, Brugada J, Brugada R. *The Brugada Syndrome: From Bench to Bedside.* Oxford, UK: Blackwell Futura, 2005.
58. Balser JR. The cardiac sodium channel: Gating function and molecular pharmacology. *J Mol Cell Cardiol* 2001;33:599–613.
59. Schulze-Bahr E, Eckardt L, Breithardt G, Seidl K, Wichter T, Wolpert C, Borggrefe M, Haverkamp W. Sodium channel gene (SCN5A) mutations in 44 index patients with Brugada syndrome: Different incidences in familial and sporadic disease. *Hum Mutat* 2003;21:651–652.
60. Bezzina CR, Wilde AA, Roden DM. The molecular genetics of arrhythmias. *Cardiovasc Res* 2005;67:343–346.
61. Tan HL, Bezzina CR, Smits JP, Verkerk AO, Wilde AA. Genetic control of sodium channel function. *Cardiovasc Res* 2003;57:961–973.
62. Antzelevitch C, Brugada P, Brugada J, Brugada R. The Brugada syndrome. From cell to bedside. *Curr Probl Cardiol* 2005;30:9–54.
63. Dumaine R, Towbin JA, Brugada P, Vatta M, Nesterenko VV, Nesterenko DV, Brugada J, Brugada R, Antzelevitch C. Ionic mechanisms responsible for the electrocardiographic phenotype of the Brugada syndrome are temperature dependent. *Circ Res* 1999;85:803–809.
64. Saura D, Garcia-Alberola A, Carrillo P, Pascual D, Martinez-Sanchez J, Valdes M. Brugada-like electrocardiographic pattern induced by fever. *Pacing Clin Electrophysiol* 2002;25:856–859.
65. Porres JM, Brugada J, Urbistondo V, Garcia F, Reviejo K, Marco P. Fever unmasking the Brugada syndrome. *Pacing Clin Electrophysiol* 2002;25:1646–1648.
66. Mok NS, Priori SG, Napolitano C, Chan NY, Chahine M, Baroudi G. A newly characterized SCN5A mutation underlying Brugada syndrome unmasked by hyperthermia. *J Cardiovasc Electrophysiol* 2003;14:407–411.
67. Ortega-Carnicer J, Benezet J, Ceres F. Fever-induced ST-segment elevation and T-wave alternans in a patient with Brugada syndrome. *Resuscitation* 2003;57:315–317.
68. Patruno N, Pontillo D, Achilli A, Ruggeri G, Critelli G. Electrocardiographic pattern of Brugada syndrome disclosed by a febrile illness: Clinical and therapeutic implications. *Europace* 2003;5:251–255.
69. Peng J, Cui YK, Yuan FH, Yi SD, Chen ZM, Meng SR. [Fever and Brugada syndrome: Report of 21 cases.]. *Di Yi Jun Yi Da Xue Xue Bao* 2005;25:432–434.
70. Dulu A, Pastores SM, McAleer E, Voigt L, Halpern NA. Brugada electrocardiographic pattern in a postoperative patient. *Crit Care Med* 2005;33:1634–1637.
71. Aramaki K, Okumura H, Shimizu M. Chest pain and ST elevation associated with fever in patients with asymptomatic Brugada syndrome. Fever and chest pain in Brugada syndrome. *Int J Cardiol* 2005;103:338–339.
72. Hong K, Guerchicoff A, Pollevick GD, Oliva A, Dumaine R, de Zutter M, Burashnikov E, Wu YS, Brugada J, Brugada P, Brugada R. Cryptic 5′ splice site activation in SCN5A associated with Brugada syndrome. *J Mol Cell Cardiol* 2005;38:555–560.
73. Bezzina CR, Shimizu W, Yang P, Koopmann TT, Tanck MW, Miyamoto Y, Kamakura S, Roden DM, Wilde AA. Common sodium channel promoter haplotype in Asian subjects underlies variability in cardiac conduction. *Circulation* 2006;113:338–344.
74. Weiss R, Barmada MM, Nguyen T, Seibel JS, Cavlovich D, Kornblit CA, Angelilli A, Villanueva F, McNamara DM, London B. Clinical and molecular heterogeneity in the Brugada syndrome. A novel gene locus on chromosome 3. *Circulation* 2002;105:707–713.
75. London B, Sanyal S, Michalec M, Pfahnl AE, Shang LL, Kerchner BS, Lagana S, Aleong RG, Mehdi H,

Gutmann R, Weiss R, Dudley SC. AB16-1: A mutation in the glycerol-3-phosphate dehydrogenase 1-like gene (GPD1L) causes Brugada syndrome. *Heart Rhythm* 2006;3:S32 (abstract).
76. Antzelevitch C, Sicouri S, Litovsky SH, Lukas A, Krishnan SC, Di Diego JM, Gintant GA, Liu DW. Heterogeneity within the ventricular wall. Electrophysiology and pharmacology of epicardial, endocardial, and M cells. *Circ Res* 1991;69:1427–1449.
77. Antzelevitch C, Shimizu W, Yan GX, Sicouri S, Weissenburger J, Nesterenko VV, Burashnikov A, Di Diego JM, Saffitz J, Thomas GP. The M cell: Its contribution to the ECG and to normal and abnormal electrical function of the heart. *J Cardiovasc Electrophysiol* 1999;10:1124–1152.
78. Litovsky SH, Antzelevitch C. Transient outward current prominent in canine ventricular epicardium but not endocardium. *Circ Res* 1988;62:116–126.
79. Liu DW, Gintant GA, Antzelevitch C. Ionic bases for electrophysiological distinctions among epicardial, midmyocardial, and endocardial myocytes from the free wall of the canine left ventricle. *Circ Res* 1993;72:671–687.
80. Furukawa T, Myerburg RJ, Furukawa N, Bassett AL, Kimura S. Differences in transient outward currents of feline endocardial and epicardial myocytes. *Circ Res* 1990;67:1287–1291.
81. Fedida D, Giles WR. Regional variations in action potentials and transient outward current in myocytes isolated from rabbit left ventricle. *J Physiol (Lond)* 1991;442:191–209.
82. Clark RB, Bouchard RA, Salinas-Stefanon E, Sanchez-Chapula J, Giles WR. Heterogeneity of action potential waveforms and potassium currents in rat ventricle. *Cardiovasc Res* 1993;27:1795–1799.
83. Wettwer E, Amos GJ, Posival H, Ravens U. Transient outward current in human ventricular myocytes of subepicardial and subendocardial origin. *Circ Res* 1994;75:473–482.
84. Nabauer M, Beuckelmann DJ, Uberfuhr P, Steinbeck G. Regional differences in current density and rate-dependent properties of the transient outward current in subepicardial and subendocardial myocytes of human left ventricle. *Circulation* 1996;93:168–177.
85. Di Diego JM, Sun ZQ, Antzelevitch C. I_{to} and action potential notch are smaller in left vs. right canine ventricular epicardium. *Am J Physiol Heart Circ Physiol* 1996;271:H548–H561.
86. Volders PG, Sipido KR, Carmeliet E, Spatjens RL, Wellens HJ, Vos MA. Repolarizing K+ currents ITO1 and IKs are larger in right than left canine ventricular midmyocardium. *Circulation* 1999;99:206–210.
87. Zicha S, Xiao L, Stafford S, Cha TJ, Han W, Varro A, Nattel S. Transmural expression of transient outward potassium current subunits in normal and failing canine and human hearts. *J Physiol* 2004;561:735–748.
88. Rosati B, Pan Z, Lypen S, Wang HS, Cohen I, Dixon JE, McKinnon D. Regulation of KChIP2 potassium channel beta subunit gene expression underlies the gradient of transient outward current in canine and human ventricle. *J Physiol* 2001;533:119–125.
89. Costantini DL, Arruda EP, Agarwal P, Kim KH, Zhu Y, Zhu W, Lebel M, Cheng CW, Park CY, Pierce SA, Guerchicoff A, Pollevick GD, Chan TY, Kabir MG, Cheng SH, Husain M, Antzelevitch C, Srivastava D, Gross GJ, Hui CC, Backx PH, Bruneau BG. The homeodomain transcription factor Irx5 establishes the mouse cardiac ventricular repolarization gradient. *Cell* 2005;123:347–358.
90. Takano M, Noma A. Distribution of the isoprenaline-induced chloride current in rabbit heart. *Pflugers Arch* 1992;420:223–226.
91. Zygmunt AC. Intracellular calcium activates chloride current in canine ventricular myocytes. *Am J Physiol Heart Circ Physiol* 1994;267:H1984–H1995.
92. Cordeiro JM, Greene L, Heilmann C, Antzelevitch D, Antzelevitch C. Transmural heterogeneity of calcium activity and mechanical function in the canine left ventricle. *Am J Physiol Heart Circ Physiol* 2004;286:H1471–H1479.
93. Banyasz T, Fulop L, Magyar J, Szentandrassy N, Varro A, Nanasi PP. Endocardial versus epicardial differences in L-type calcium current in canine ventricular myocytes studied by action potential voltage clamp. *Cardiovasc Res* 2003;58:66–75.
94. Wang HS, Cohen IS. Calcium channel heterogeneity in canine left ventricular myocytes. *J Physiol* 2003;547:825–833.
95. Sicouri S, Antzelevitch C. A subpopulation of cells with unique electrophysiological properties in the deep subepicardium of the canine ventricle. The M cell. *Circ Res* 1991;68:1729–1741.
96. Anyukhovsky EP, Sosunov EA, Rosen MR. Regional differences in electrophysiologic properties of epicardium, midmyocardium and endocardium: *In vitro* and *in vivo* correlations. *Circulation* 1996;94:1981–1988.
97. Liu DW, Antzelevitch C. Characteristics of the delayed rectifier current (IKr and IKs) in canine ventricular epicardial, midmyocardial, and endocardial myocytes. *Circ Res* 1995;76:351–365.

98. Zygmunt AC, Eddlestone GT, Thomas GP, Nesterenko VV, Antzelevitch C. Larger late sodium conductance in M cells contributes to electrical heterogeneity in canine ventricle. *Am J Physiol Heart Circ Physiol* 2001;281:H689–H697.
99. Zygmunt AC, Goodrow RJ, Antzelevitch C. I(NaCa) contributes to electrical heterogeneity within the canine ventricle. *Am J Physiol Heart Circ Physiol* 2000;278:H1671–H1678.
100. Brahmajothi MV, Morales MJ, Reimer KA, Strauss HC. Regional localization of ERG, the channel protein responsible for the rapid component of the delayed rectifier, K^+ current in the ferret heart. *Circ Res* 1997;81:128–135.
101. Clements SD, Hurst JW. Diagnostic value of ECG abnormalities observed in subjects accidentally exposed to cold. *Am J Cardiol* 1972;29:729–734.
102. Thompson R, Rich J, Chmelik F, Nelson WL. Evolutionary changes in the electrocardiogram of severe progressive hypothermia. *J Electrocardiol* 1977;10:67–70.
103. RuDusky BM. The electrocardiogram in hypothermia—the J wave and the Brugada syndrome. *Am J Cardiol* 2004;93:671–672.
104. Kraus F. Ueber die wirkung des kalziums auf den kreislauf. *Dtsch Med Wochenschr* 1920;46:201–203.
105. Sridharan MR, Horan LG. Electrocardiographic J wave of hypercalcemia. *Am J Cardiol* 1984;54:672–673.
106. Antzelevitch C, Sicouri S, Lukas A, Nesterenko VV, Liu DW, Di Diego JM. Regional differences in the electrophysiology of ventricular cells: Physiological and clinical implications. In: Zipes DP, Jalife J, Eds. *Cardiac Electrophysiology: From Cell to Bedside,* 2nd ed. Philadelphia, PA: W.B. Saunders Co., 1995:228–245.
107. Eagle K. Images in clinical medicine. Osborn waves of hypothermia. *N Engl J Med* 1994;10:680.
108. Emslie-Smith D, Sladden GE, Stirling GR. The significance of changes in the electrocardiogram in hypothermia. *Br Heart J* 1959;21:343–351.
109. Osborn JJ. Experimental hypothermia: Respiratory and blood pH changes in relation to cardiac function. *Am J Physiol* 1953;175:389–398.
110. Sridharan MR, Johnson JC, Horan LG, Sohl GS, Flowers NC. Monophasic action potentials in hypercalcemic and hypothermic "J" waves—a comparative study. *Am Fed Clin Res* 1983;31:219.
111. Di Diego JM, Antzelevitch C. High $[Ca^{2+}]$-induced electrical heterogeneity and extrasystolic activity in isolated canine ventricular epicardium: Phase 2 reentry. *Circulation* 1994;89:1839–1850.
112. Litovsky SH, Antzelevitch C. Rate dependence of action potential duration and refractoriness in canine ventricular endocardium differs from that of epicardium: Role of the transient outward current. *J Am Coll Cardiol* 1989;14:1053–1066.
113. Kilborn MJ, Fedida D. A study of the developmental changes in outward currents of rat ventricular myocytes. *J Physiol (Lond)* 1990;430:37–60.
114. Furukawa Y, Akahane K, Ogiwara Y, Chiba S. K+-channel blocking and anti-muscarinic effects of a novel piperazine derivative, INO 2628, on the isolated dog atrium. *Eur J Pharm* 1991;193:217–222.
115. Lukas A, Antzelevitch C. Phase 2 reentry as a mechanism of initiation of circus movement reentry in canine epicardium exposed to simulated ischemia. *Cardiovasc Res* 1996;32:593–603.
116. Di Diego JM, Antzelevitch C. Pinacidil-induced electrical heterogeneity and extrasystolic activity in canine ventricular tissues. Does activation of ATP-regulated potassium current promote phase 2 reentry? *Circulation* 1993;88:1177–1189.
117. Antzelevitch C, Sicouri S, Lukas A, Di Diego JM, Nesterenko VV, Liu DW, Roubache JF, Zygmunt AC, Zhang ZQ, Iodice A. Clinical implications of electrical heterogeneity in the heart: The electrophysiology and pharmacology of epicardial, M, and endocardial cells. In: Podrid PJ, Kowey PR, Eds. *Cardiac Arrhythmia: Mechanism, Diagnosis and Management.* Baltimore, MD: William & Wilkins, 1995:88–107.
118. Yan GX, Lankipalli RS, Burke JF, Musco S, Kowey PR. Ventricular repolarization components on the electrocardiogram: Cellular basis and clinical significance. *J Am Coll Cardiol* 2003;42:401–409.
119. Aizawa Y, Tamura M, Chinushi M, Naitoh N, Uchiyama H, Kusano Y, Hosono H, Shibata A. Idiopathic ventricular fibrillation and bradycardia-dependent intraventricular block. *Am Heart J* 1993;126:1473–1474.
120. Aizawa Y, Tamura M, Chinushi M, Niwano S, Kusano Y, Naitoh N, Shibata A, Tohjoh T, Ueda Y, Joho K. An attempt at electrical catheter ablation of the arrhythmogenic area in idiopathic ventricular fibrillation. *Am Heart J* 1992;123:257–260.
121. Bjerregaard P, Gussak I, Kotar Sl, Gessler JE. Recurrent syncope in a patient with prominent J-wave. *Am Heart J* 1994;127:1426–1430.
122. Lukas A, Antzelevitch C. Differences in the electrophysiological response of canine ventricular epicardium and endocardium to ischemia: Role of the transient outward current. *Circulation* 1993;88:2903–2915.
123. Thomsen PE, Joergensen RM, Kanters JK, Jensen TJ, Haarbo J, Hagemann A, Vestergaard A, Saermark K. Phase 2 reentry in man. *Heart Rhythm* 2005;2:797–803.

124. Antzelevitch C. *In vivo* human demonstration of phase 2 reentry. *Heart Rhythm* 2005;2:804–806.
125. Litovsky SH, Antzelevitch C. Differences in the electrophysiological response of canine ventricular subendocardium and subepicardium to acetylcholine and isoproterenol. A direct effect of acetylcholine in ventricular myocardium. *Circ Res* 1990;67:615–627.
126. Tsuchiya T, Ashikaga K, Honda T, Arita M. Prevention of ventricular fibrillation by cilostazol, an oral phosphodiesterase inhibitor, in a patient with Brugada syndrome. *J Cardiovasc Electrophysiol* 2002;13:698–701.
127. Yan GX, Antzelevitch C. Cellular basis for the Brugada syndrome and other mechanisms of arrhythmogenesis associated with ST segment elevation. *Circulation* 1999;100:1660–1666.
128. Pertsov AM, Davidenko JM, Salomonsz R, Baxter WT, Jalife J. Spiral waves of excitation underlie reentrant activity in isolated cardiac muscle. *Circ Res* 1993;72:631–650.
129. Asano Y, Davidenko JM, Baxter WT, Gray RA, Jalife J. Optical mapping of drug-induced polymorphic arrhythmias and torsade de pointes in the isolated rabbit heart. *J Am Coll Cardiol* 1997; 29:831–842.
130. Fish JM, Antzelevitch C. Role of sodium and calcium channel block in unmasking the Brugada syndrome. *Heart Rhythm* 2004;1:210–217.
131. Tukkie R, Sogaard P, Vleugels J, De Groot IK, Wilde AA, Tan HL. Delay in right ventricular activation contributes to Brugada syndrome. *Circulation* 2004;109:1272–1277.
132. Antzelevitch C, Fish J, Di Diego JM. Cellular mechanisms underlying the Brugada syndrome. In: Antzelevitch C, Brugada P, Brugada J, Brugada R, Eds. *The Brugada Syndrome: From Bench to Bedside.* Oxford, UK: Blackwell Futura, 2004:52–77.
133. Antzelevitch C. The Brugada syndrome: Ionic basis and arrhythmia mechanisms. *J Cardiovasc Electrophysiol* 2001;12:268–272.
134. Antzelevitch C. The Brugada syndrome: Diagnostic criteria and cellular mechanisms. *Eur Heart J* 2001;22:356–363.
135. Gussak I, Antzelevitch C, Bjerregaard P, Towbin JA, Chaitman BR. The Brugada syndrome: Clinical, electrophysiologic and genetic aspects. *J Am Coll Cardiol* 1999;33:5–15.
136. Shimizu W, Aiba T, Kamakura S. Mechanisms of disease: Current understanding and future challenges in Brugada syndrome. *Nat Clin Pract Cardiovasc Med* 2005;2:408–414.
137. Antzelevitch C, Brugada P, Brugada J, Brugada R, Shimizu W, Gussak I, Perez Riera AR. Brugada syndrome. A decade of progress. *Circ Res* 2002;91: 1114–1119.
138. Kurita T, Shimizu W, Inagaki M, Suyama K, Taguchi A, Satomi K, Aihara N, Kamakura S, Kobayashi J, Kosakai Y. The electrophysiologic mechanism of ST-segment elevation in Brugada syndrome. *J Am Coll Cardiol* 2002;40:330–334.
139. Futterman LG, Lemberg L. Brugada. *Am J Crit Care* 2001;10:360–364.
140. Fujiki A, Usui M, Nagasawa H, Mizumaki K, Hayashi H, Inoue H. ST segment elevation in the right precordial leads induced with class IC antiarrhythmic drugs: Insight into the mechanism of Brugada syndrome. *J Cardiovasc Electrophysiol* 1999;10:214–218.
141. Antzelevitch C. Late potentials and the Brugada syndrome. *J Am Coll Cardiol* 2002;39:1996–1999.
142. Nagase S, Kusano KF, Morita H, Fujimoto Y, Kakishita M, Nakamura K, Emori T, Matsubara H, Ohe T. Epicardial electrogram of the right ventricular outflow tract in patients with the Brugada syndrome: Using the epicardial lead. *J Am Coll Cardiol* 2002;39:1992–1995.
143. Eckardt L, Bruns HJ, Paul M, Kirchhof P, Schulze-Bahr E, Wichter T, Breithardt G, Borggrefe M, Haverkamp W. Body surface area of ST elevation and the presence of late potentials correlate to the inducibility of ventricular tachyarrhythmias in Brugada syndrome. *J Cardiovasc Electrophysiol* 2002;13:742–749.
144. Ikeda T, Takami M, Sugi K, Mizusawa Y, Sakurada H, Yoshino H. Noninvasive risk stratification of subjects with a Brugada-type electrocardiogram and no history of cardiac arrest. *Ann Noninvasive Electrocardiol* 2005;10:396–403.
145. Shimizu W, Aiba T, Kurita T, Kamakura S. Paradoxic abbreviation of repolarization in epicardium of the right ventricular outflow tract during augmentation of Brugada-type ST segment elevation. *J Cardiovasc Electrophysiol* 2001;12:1418–1421.
146. Kandori A, Shimizu W, Yokokawa M, Noda T, Kamakura S, Miyatake K, Murakami M, Miyashita T, Ogata K, Tsukada K. Identifying patterns of spatial current dispersion that characterise and separate the Brugada syndrome and complete right-bundle branch block. *Med Biol Eng Comput* 2004;42:236–244.
147. Watanabe H, Chinushi M, Osaki A, Okamura K, Izumi D, Komura S, Hosaka Y, Tanabe Y, Furushima H, Washizuka T, Aizawa Y. Elimination of late potentials by quinidine in a patient with Brugada syndrome. *J Electrocardiol* 2006;39: 63–66.

148. Marquez MF, Bisteni A, Medrano G, De Micheli A, Guevara M, Iturralde P, Colin L, Hermosillo G, Cardenas M. Dynamic electrocardiographic changes after aborted sudden death in a patient with Brugada syndrome and rate-dependent right bundle branch block. *J Electrocardiol* 2005;38: 256–259.
149. Nishizaki M, Fujii H, Sakurada H, Kimura A, Hiraoka M. Spontaneous T wave alternans in a patient with Brugada syndrome—responses to intravenous administration of class I antiarrhythmic drug, glucose tolerance test, and atrial pacing. *J Cardiovasc Electrophysiol* 2005;16:217–220.
150. Tada H, Nogami A, Shimizu W, Naito S, Nakatsugawa M, Oshima S, Taniguchi K. ST segment and T wave alternans in a patient with Brugada syndrome. *Pacing Clin Electrophysiol* 2000;23: 413–415.
151. Chinushi M, Washizuka T, Okumura H, Aizawa Y. Intravenous administration of class I antiarrhythmic drugs induced T wave alternans in a patient with Brugada syndrome. *J Cardiovasc Electrophysiol* 2001;12:493–495.
152. Chinushi Y, Chinushi M, Toida T, Aizawa Y. Class I antiarrhythmic drug and coronary vasospasm-induced T wave alternans and ventricular tachyarrhythmia in a patient with Brugada syndrome and vasospastic angina. *J Cardiovasc Electrophysiol* 2002;13:191–194.
153. Takagi M, Doi A, Takeuchi K, Yoshikawa J. Pilsicanide-induced marked T wave alternans and ventricular fibrillation in a patient with Brugada syndrome. *J Cardiovasc Electrophysiol* 2002;13: 837.
154. Ohkubo K, Watanabe I, Okumura Y, Yamada T, Masaki R, Kofune T, Oshikawa N, Kasamaki Y, Saito S, Ozawa Y, Kanmatsuse K. Intravenous administration of class I antiarrhythmic drug induced T wave alternans in an asymptomatic Brugada syndrome patient. *Pacing Clin Electrophysiol* 2003;26:1900–1903.
155. Morita H, Morita ST, Nagase S, Banba K, Nishii N, Tani Y, Watanabe A, Nakamura K, Kusano KF, Emori T, Matsubara H, Hina K, Kita T, Ohe T. Ventricular arrhythmia induced by sodium channel blocker in patients with Brugada syndrome. *J Am Coll Cardiol* 2003;42:1624–1631.
156. Morita H, Nagase S, Kusano K, Ohe T. Spontaneous T wave alternans and premature ventricular contractions during febrile illness in a patient with Brugada syndrome. *J Cardiovasc Electrophysiol* 2002;13:816–818.
157. Morita H, Zipes DP, Lopshire J, Morita ST, Wu J. T wave alternans in an in vitro canine tissue model of Brugada syndrome. *Am J Physiol Heart Circ Physiol* 2006;291:H421–H428.
158. Babaliaros VC, Hurst JW. Tricyclic antidepressants and the Brugada syndrome: An example of Brugada waves appearing after the administration of desipramine. *Clin Cardiol* 2002;25:395–398.
159. Goldgran-Toledano D, Sideris G, Kevorkian JP. Overdose of cyclic antidepressants and the Brugada syndrome. *N Engl J Med* 2002;346:1591–1592.
160. Tada H, Sticherling C, Oral H, Morady F. Brugada syndrome mimicked by tricyclic antidepressant overdose. *J Cardiovasc Electrophysiol* 2001;12 275.
161. Pastor A, Nunez A, Cantale C, Cosio FG. Asymptomatic Brugada syndrome case unmasked during dimenhydrinate infusion. *J Cardiovasc Electrophysiol* 2001;12:1192–1194.
162. Ortega-Carnicer J, Bertos-Polo J, Gutierrez-Tirado C. Aborted sudden death, transient Brugada pattern, and wide QRS dysrrhythmias after massive cocaine ingestion. *J Electrocardiol* 2001;34: 345–349.
163. Nogami A, Nakao M, Kubota S, Sugiyasu A, Doi H, Yokoyama K, Yumoto K, Tamaki T, Kato K, Hosokawa N, Sagai H, Nakamura H, Nitta J, Yamauchi Y, Aonuma K. Enhancement of J-ST-segment elevation by the glucose and insulin test in Brugada syndrome. *Pacing Clin Electrophysiol* 2003;26:332–337.
164. Araki T, Konno T, Itoh H, Ino H, Shimizu M. Brugada syndrome with ventricular tachycardia and fibrillation related to hypokalemia. *Circ J* 2003;67:93–95.
165. Akhtar M, Goldschlager NF. Brugada electrocardiographic pattern due to tricyclic antidepressant overdose. *J Electrocardiol* 2006;39:336–339.
166. Darbar D, Yang T, Churchwell K, Wilde AA, Roden DM. Unmasking of Brugada syndrome by lithium. *Circulation* 2005;112:1527–1531.
167. Noda T, Shimizu W, Taguchi A, Satomi K, Suyama K, Kurita T, Aihara N, Kamakura S. ST-segment elevation and ventricular fibrillation without coronary spasm by intracoronary injection of acetylcholine and/or ergonovine maleate in patients with Brugada syndrome. *J Am Coll Cardiol* 2002; 40:1841–1847.
168. Chinushi M, Furushima H, Tanabe Y, Washizuka T, Aizawaz Y. Similarities between Brugada syndrome and ischemia-induced ST-segment elevation. Clinical correlation and synergy. *J Electrocardiol* 2005;38(Suppl.):18–21.
169. Nimmannit S, Malasit P, Chaovakul V, Susaengrat W, Vasuvattakul S, Nilwarangkur S. Pathogenesis

of sudden unexplained nocturnal death (lai tai) and endemic distal renal tubular acidosis. *Lancet* 1991;338:930–932.

170. Proclemer A, Facchin D, Feruglio GA, Nucifora R. Recurrent ventricular fibrillation, right bundle-branch block and persistent ST segment elevation in V1–V3: A new arrhythmia syndrome? A clinical case report (see comments). *G Ital Cardiol* 1993; 23:1211–1218.
171. Mizumaki K, Fujiki A, Tsuneda T, Sakabe M, Nishida K, Sugao M, Inoue H. Vagal activity modulates spontaneous augmentation of ST elevation in daily life of patients with Brugada syndrome. *J Cardiovasc Electrophysiol* 2004;15:667–673.
172. Wichter T, Matheja P, Eckardt L, Kies P, Schafers K, Schulze-Bahr E, Haverkamp W, Borggrefe M, Schober O, Breithardt G, Schafers M. Cardiac autonomic dysfunction in Brugada syndrome. *Circulation* 2002;105:702–706.
173. Ikeda T, Abe A, Yusa S, Nakamura K, Ishiguro H, Mera H, Yotsukura M, Yoshino H. The full stomach test as a novel diagnostic technique for identifying patients at risk for Brugada syndrome. *J Cardiovasc Electrophysiol* 2006;17:602–607.
174. Gonzalez Rebollo G, Madrid H, Carcia A, Garcia de Casto A, Moro AM. Reccurrent ventricular fibrillation during a febrile illness in a patient with the Brugada syndrome. *Rev Esp Cardiol* 2000;53: 755–757.
175. Madle A, Kratochvil Z, Polivkova A. [The Brugada syndrome]. *Vnitr Lek* 2002;48:255–258.
176. Kum L, Fung JWH, Chan WWL, Chan GK, Chan YS, Sanderson JE. Brugada syndrome unmasked by febrile illness. *Pacing Clin Electrophysiol* 2002;25:1660–1661.
177. Keller DI, Huang H, Zhao J, Frank R, Suarez V, Delacretaz E, Brink M, Osswald S, Schwick N, Chahine M. A novel SCN5A mutation, F1344S, identified in a patient with Brugada syndrome and fever-induced ventricular fibrillation. *Cardiovasc Res* 2006;70:521–529.
178. Di Diego JM, Cordeiro JM, Goodrow RJ, Fish JM, Zygmunt AC, Perez GJ, Scornik FS, Antzelevitch C. Ionic and cellular basis for the predominance of the Brugada syndrome phenotype in males. *Circulation* 2002;106:2004–2011.
179. Brugada J, Brugada R, Brugada P. Pharmacological and device approach to therapy of inherited cardiac diseases associated with cardiac arrhythmias and sudden death. *J Electrocardiol* 2000;33 (Suppl.):41–47.
180. Brugada P, Brugada R, Brugada J, Geelen P. Use of the prophylactic implantable cardioverter defibrillator for patients with normal hearts. *Am J Cardiol* 1999;83:98D-100D.
181. Haissaguerre M, Extramiana F, Hocini M, Cauchemez B, Jais P, Cabrera JA, Farre G, Leenhardt A, Sanders P, Scavee C, Hsu LF, Weerasooriya R, Shah DC, Frank R, Maury P, Delay M, Garrigue S, Clementy J. Mapping and ablation of ventricular fibrillation associated with long-QT and Brugada syndromes. *Circulation* 2003;108:925–928.
182. Kron J, Herre J, Renfroe EG, Rizo-Patron C, Raitt M, Halperin B, Gold M, Goldner B, Wathen M, Wilkoff B, Olarte A, Yao Q. Lead- and device-related complications in the antiarrhythmics versus implantable defibrillators trial. *Am Heart J* 2001;141:92–98.
183. A comparison of antiarrhythmic-drug therapy with implantable defibrillators in patients resuscitated from near-fatal ventricular arrhythmias. The Antiarrhythmics versus Implantable Defibrillators (AVID) Investigators. *N Engl J Med* 1997; 337:1576–1583.
184. Belhassen B, Viskin S, Antzelevitch C. The Brugada syndrome: Is an implantable cardioverter defibrillator the only therapeutic option? *Pacing Clin Electrophysiol* 2002;25:1634–1640.
185. Antzelevitch C, Fish JM. Therapy for the Brugada syndrome. In: Kass R, Clancy CE, Eds. *Handbook of Experimental Pharmacology*. New York: Springer-Verlag, 2006:305–330.
186. Chinushi M, Aizawa Y, Ogawa Y, Shiba M, Takahashi K. Discrepant drug action of disopyramide on ECG abnormalities and induction of ventricular arrhythmias in a patient with Brugada syndrome. *J Electrocardiol* 1997;30:133–136.
187. Antzelevitch C, Brugada P, Brugada J, Brugada R, Nademanee K, Towbin JA. *Clinical Approaches to Tachyarrhythmias. The Brugada Syndrome*. Armonk, NY: Futura Publishing Company, Inc., 1999.
188. Grant AO. Electrophysiological basis and genetics of Brugada syndrome. *J Cardiovasc Electrophysiol* 2005;16(Suppl. 1):S3–S7.
189. Alings M, Dekker L, Sadee A, Wilde A. Quinidine induced electrocardiographic normalization in two patients with Brugada syndrome. *Pacing Clin Electrophysiol* 2001;24:1420–1422.
190. Belhassen B, Viskin S. Pharmacologic approach to therapy of Brugada syndrome: Quinidine as an alternative to ICD therapy? In: Antzelevitch C, Brugada P, Brugada J, Brugada R, Eds. *The Brugada Syndrome: From Bench to Bedside*. Oxford, UK: Blackwell Futura, 2004:202–211.

191. Marquez MF, Rivera J, Hermosillo AG, Iturralde P, Colin L, Moragrega JL, Cardenas M. Arrhythmic storm responsive to quinidine in a patient with Brugada syndrome and vasovagal syncope. *Pacing Clin Electrophysiol* 2005;28:870–873.
192. Belhassen B, Viskin S, Fish R, Glick A, Setbon I, Eldar M. Effects of electrophysiologic-guided therapy with Class IA antiarrhythmic drugs on the long-term outcome of patients with idiopathic ventricular fibrillation with or without the Brugada syndrome. *J Cardiovasc Electrophysiol* 1999;10: 1301–1312.
193. Hermida JS, Denjoy I, Clerc J, Extramiana F, Jarry G, Milliez P, Guicheney P, Di Fusco S, Rey JL, Cauchemez B, Leenhardt A. Hydroquinidine therapy in Brugada syndrome. *J Am Coll Cardiol* 2004;43:1853–1860.
194. Mok NS, Chan NY, Chi-Suen CA. Successful use of quinidine in treatment of electrical storm in Brugada syndrome. *Pacing Clin Electrophysiol* 2004;27:821–823.
195. Marquez MF, Rivera J, Hermosillo AG, Iturralde P, Colin L, Moragrega JL, Cardenas M. Arrhythmic storm responsive to quinidine in a patient with Brugada syndrome and vasovagal syncope. *Pacing Clin Electrophysiol* 2005;28:870–873.
196. Mizusawa Y, Sakurada H, Nishizaki M, Hiraoka M. Effects of low-dose quinidine on ventricular tachyarrhythmias in patients with Brugada syndrome: Low-dose quinidine therapy as an adjunctive treatment. *J Cardiovasc Pharmacol* 2006;47: 359–364.
197. Fish JM, Extramiana F, Antzelevitch C. Tedisamil abolishes the arrhythmogenic substrate responsible for VT/VF in an experimental model of the Brugada syndrome. *Heart Rhythm* 2004;1(1S): S158 (abstract).
198. Zeltser D, Justo D, Halkin A, Prokhorov V, Heller K, Viskin S. Torsade de pointes due to noncardiac drugs: Most patients have easily identifiable risk factors. *Medicine (Baltimore)* 2003;82:282–290.
199. Antzelevitch C, Shimizu W. Cellular mechanisms underlying the long QT syndrome. *Curr Opin Cardiol* 2002;17:43–51.
200. Belardinelli L, Antzelevitch C, Vos MA. Assessing predictors of drug-induced torsade de pointes. *Trends Pharmacol Sci* 2003;24:619–625.
201. Fish JM, Extramiana F, Antzelevitch C. AVE0118, an I_{to} and I_{Kur} blocker, suppresses VT/VF in an experimental model of the Brugada syndrome. *Circulation* 2004;110(17):III-193 (abstract).
202. Suzuki H, Torigoe K, Numata O, Yazaki S. Infant case with a malignant form of Brugada syndrome. *J Cardiovasc Electrophysiol* 2000;11:1277–1280.
203. Tanaka H, Kinoshita O, Uchikawa S, Kasai H, Nakamura M, Izawa A, Yokoseki O, Kitabayashi H, Takahashi W, Yazaki Y, Watanabe N, Imamura H, Kubo K. Successful prevention of recurrent ventricular fibrillation by intravenous isoproterenol in a patient with Brugada syndrome. *Pacing Clin Electrophysiol* 2001;24:1293–1294.
204. Haghjoo M, Arya A, Heidari A, Sadr-Ameli MA. Suppression of electrical storm by oral quinidine in a patient with Brugada syndrome. *J Cardiovasc Electrophysiol* 2005;16:674.
205. Fish JM, Welchons DR, Kim YS, Lee SH, Ho WK, Antzelevitch C. Dimethyl lithospermate B, an extract of danshen, suppresses arrhythmogenesis associated with the Brugada syndrome. *Circulation* 2006;113:1393–1400.
206. Nademanee K, Veerakul G, Schwab M. Predisposing factors in the Brugada syndrome. In Antzelevitch C, Brugada P, Eds. *Brugada Syndrome*. Elmsford, UK: Blackwell Publishing, 2004: 157–165.
207. Krishnan SC, Josephson ME. ST segment elevation induced by class IC antiarrhythmic agents: Underlying electrophysiologic mechanisms and insights into drug-induced proarrhythmia. *J Cardiovasc Electrophysiol* 1998;9:1167–1172.
208. Gasparini M, Priori SG, Mantica M, Napolitano C, Galimberti P, Ceriotti C, Simonini S. Flecainide test in Brugada syndrome: A reproducible but risky tool. *Pacing Clin Electrophysiol* 2003;26:338–341.
209. Takenaka S, Emori T, Koyama S, Morita H, Fukushima K, Ohe T. Asymptomatic form of Brugada syndrome. *Pacing Clin Electrophysiol* 1999;22:1261–1263.
210. Matana A, Goldner V, Stanic K, Mavric Z, Zaputovic L, Matana Z. Unmasking effect of propafenone on the concealed form of the Brugada phenomenon. *Pacing Clin Electrophysiol* 2000;23: 416–418.
211. Rolf S, Bruns HJ, Wichter T, Kirchhof P, Ribbing M, Wasmer K, Paul M, Breithardt G, Haverkamp W, Eckardt L. The ajmaline challenge in Brugada syndrome: Diagnostic impact, safety, and recommended protocol. *Eur Heart J* 2003;24:1104–1112.
212. Sarkozy A, Caenepeel A, Geelen P, Peytchev P, de Zutter M., Brugada P. Cibenzoline induced Brugada ECG pattern. *Europace* 2005;7:537–539.
213. Aouate P, Clerc J, Viard P, Seoud J. Propranolol intoxication revealing a Brugada syndrome. *J Cardiovasc Electrophysiol* 2005;16:348–351.
214. Matsuo K, Shimizu W, Kurita T, Inagaki M, Aihara N, Kamakura S. Dynamic changes of 12-lead electrocardiograms in a patient with Brugada syn

drome. *J Cardiovasc Electrophysiol* 1998;9:508–512.
215. Bigwood B, Galler D, Amir N, Smith W. Brugada syndrome following tricyclic antidepressant overdose. *Anaesth Intensive Care* 2005;33:266–270.
216. Bolognesi R, Tsialtas D, Vasini P, Conti M, Manca C. Abnormal ventricular repolarization mimicking myocardial infarction after heterocyclic antidepressant overdose. *Am J Cardiol* 1997;79:242–245.
217. Rouleau F, Asfar P, Boulet S, Dube L, Dupuis JM, Alquier P, Victor J. Transient ST segment elevation in right precordial leads induced by psychotropic drugs: Relationship to the Brugada syndrome. *J Cardiovasc Electrophysiol* 2001;12:61–65.
218. Lopez-Barbeito B, Lluis M, Delgado V, Jimenez S, az-Infante E, Nogue-Xarau S, Brugada J. Diphenhydramine overdose and Brugada sign. *Pacing Clin Electrophysiol* 2005;28:730–732.
219. Littmann L, Monroe MH, Svenson RH. Brugada-type electrocardiographic pattern induced by cocaine. *Mayo Clin Proc* 2000;75:845–849.
220. Shimizu W. Acquired forms of the Brugada syndrome. *J Electrocardiol* 2005;38(Suppl.):22–25.
221. van Den Berg MP, Wilde AA, Viersma TJW, Brouwer J, Haaksma J, van der Hout AH, Stolte-Dijkstra I, Bezzina TCR, Van Langen IM, Beaufort-Krol GC, Cornel JH, Crijns HJ. Possible bradycardic mode of death and successful pacemaker treatment in a large family with features of long QT syndrome type 3 and Brugada syndrome. *J Cardiovasc Electrophysiol* 2001;12:630–636.

34
Catecholaminergic Polymorphic Ventricular Tachycardia

Nian Liu, Carlo Napolitano, and Silvia G. Priori

Introduction

Catecholaminergic polymorphic ventricular tachycardia (CPVT) is an inherited disease characterized by adrenergically mediated polymorphic ventricular tachycardia (VT) leading to syncope and sudden cardiac death. It was initially described by Coumel *et al.* in 1978.[1] A series of cases were reported by the same group in 1995.[2] The clinical presentation encompasses exercise- or emotion-induced syncopal events and a distinctive pattern of reproducible, stress-related, bidirectional VT in the absence of both structural heart disease and a prolonged QT interval. Since 2001, molecular genetic studies have reveiled that CPVT results from inherited defects of intracellular calcium handling in cardiac myocytes.[3] In this chapter, the current knowledge of CPVT will be reviewed with a focus on the genetics, pathophysiology, and clinical management.

Genetics

The CPVT phenotype most often shows an autosomal dominant pattern of transmission, although sporadic cases seem to be rather frequent and a familial history of juvenile sudden death and stress-induced syncope is present in about 30% of cases.[2] In 1999, Swan *et al.*[4] mapped the disease to chromosome 1q42–q43 in two affected families. In December 2000, Priori *et al.*[3] identified ryanodine receptor (RyR2) mutations in four families with the typical pattern of CPVT and history of sudden cardiac death, thus demonstrating that RyR2 is the gene for autosomal dominant CPVT. These data have been confirmed by Laitinen *et al.* To date, more than 60 RyR2 mutations have been reported (more information is available online at http://www.fsm.it/cardmoc/). All RyR2 mutations identified so far in CPVT are mostly single-base pair substitutions leading to the replacement of highly conserved amino acids. Most RyR2 mutations are localized in the C-terminal region or in the central region; a minority of RyR2 mutations is localized in the other regions of the gene (see Figure 34–1). Interestingly, some investigators[6,] claimed to have identified RyR2 mutations in families diagnosed with an atypical form of right ventricular cardiomyopathy, ARVD2, that combines mild or nearly absent macroscopic structural abnormalities of the right ventricle with typical stress-induced polymorphic VTs. However they could not prove the cosegregation of RyR2 mutations with both catecholaminergic VT and with structural abnormalities of the heart because biopsies were not available for all carriers of RyR2 mutations. As a consequence, at present, whether mutations in RyR2 cause ARVD2 is still debated.

In 2001, Lahat *et al.*[8] described a recessively inherited CPVT phenotype and mapped the disease locus to a 16-megabase interval on chromosome 1p13–21. Subsequently the same group[9] identified a missense mutation in a highly conserved region of the calsequestrin 2 gene (CASQ2) as the potential cause of the autosomal recessive form. To date, the reported CASQ2 mutation gives rise to a pathological clinical phenotype only in homozygous carriers, while heterozygous carriers are usually silent.

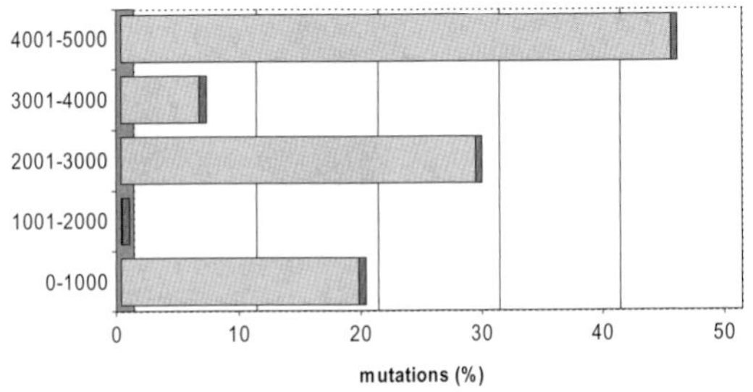

GURE 34–1. Bar graph showing the clustering of mutations in R2. Shown on the *y* axis are the numbers corresponding to the usters of amino acids of the RyR2 protein; on the *x* axis is the ercentage of mutations identified. Bars represent the proportion mutations located in each cluster of amino acids. The N-rminus (amino acid 0–1000), the central region of the protein mino acid 2001–3000), and the C-terminus (amino acid 4001–nd) show the higher percentage of mutations.

We recently reported the first CPVT patient arrier of two distinct CASQ2 mutations, thus emonstrating that the compound heterozygous nutations lead to a catecholaminergic VT henotype.[10]

A disease-causing mutation in RyR2 or CASQ2 an be identified in 50–70% of CPVT patients,[11,12] hus other, yet unknown, CPVT genes are likely to xist.

athophysiology

he hypothesis that arrhythmias in CPVT are initiated by delayed afterdepolarizations (DADs) nd triggered activity had been advanced based n the observation that the bidirectional VT bserved in CPVT patients closely resembles ligitalis-induced arrhythmias.[2] Digitalis-induced ntracellular Ca^{2+} overload leads to the activation f sodium–calcium exchanger that, in turn, genertes a net inward current (the so-called "transient nward" I_{Ti} current). I_{Ti} underlies diastolic nembrane depolarizations, DADs, that may each threshold for sodium current activation nd trigger abnormal beats. This mechanism for rrhythmia initiation is defined as "triggered ctivity." The proof of concept that triggered ctivity is the mechanism for arrhythmias in PVT came because of the availability of the conlitional knockin mouse model carrier of the RyR2 4496C mutation that is equivalent to the R4497C mutations identified in some CPVT families. This transgenic animal model develops typical bidirectional VT upon exposure to caffeine and epinephrine.[13] Recently we[14] studied ventricular myocytes isolated from the heart of $RyR2^{R4496C+/-}$ knockin mouse and demonstrated that DADs are already spontaneously present in $RyR2^{R4496C+/-}$ myocytes in the absence of adrenergic stimulation but not in wild-type myocytes (see Figure 34–2). Upon exposure to β-adrenergic stimulation we observed further enhancement of DADs and the development of multiple triggered action potentials arising from DADs (see Figure 34–3).

RyR2-Related Catecholaminergic Polymorphic Ventricular Tachycardia

The cardiac ryanodine receptor is a tetrameric intracellular Ca^{2+} release channel required for cardiac excitation–contraction coupling. Under normal conditions, RyR2 channels are activated by Ca^{2+} entering the cell through the voltage-dependent L-type Ca^{2+} channels, causing the release of Ca^{2+} from the sarcoplasmic reticulum (SR) into the cytosol, a mechanism known as Ca^{2+}-induced Ca^{2+} release (CICR).[15] Increased cytosolic Ca^{2+} levels activate the contractile apparatus. Ca^{2+} release is terminated when SR luminal Ca^{2+} levels fall below a threshold level, causing a decline in RyR2 activity via a mechanism called luminal Ca^{2+}-dependent deactivation.[16] Multiple accessory proteins exquisitely control the gating of RyR2 channels and the Ca^{2+} fluxes in myocytes.

In vitro studies (lipid bilayer, HEK293 cells, HL1-cardiomyocytes)[17–19] suggest that the RyR2 mutations produce "gain of function" and cause a Ca^{2+} "leakage" from the SR in association with sympathetic (catecholamines) activation. As a consequence, DADs and triggered activity may arise due to cytosolic Ca^{2+} overload.

Despite intensive investigations, the molecular mechanisms by which RyR2 mutations alter the physiological properties of RyR2 in CPVT remain controversial.[20] Wehrens *et al.*[21,22] first proposed that RyR2 mutants reduce the binding affinity of RyR2 for the regulatory protein FKBP12.6. This protein is considered to act as a "stabilizer" of RyR2 that binds to the RyR2 tetramers and reduces the opening probability of the channel. It was suggested that the defective mutation-dependent

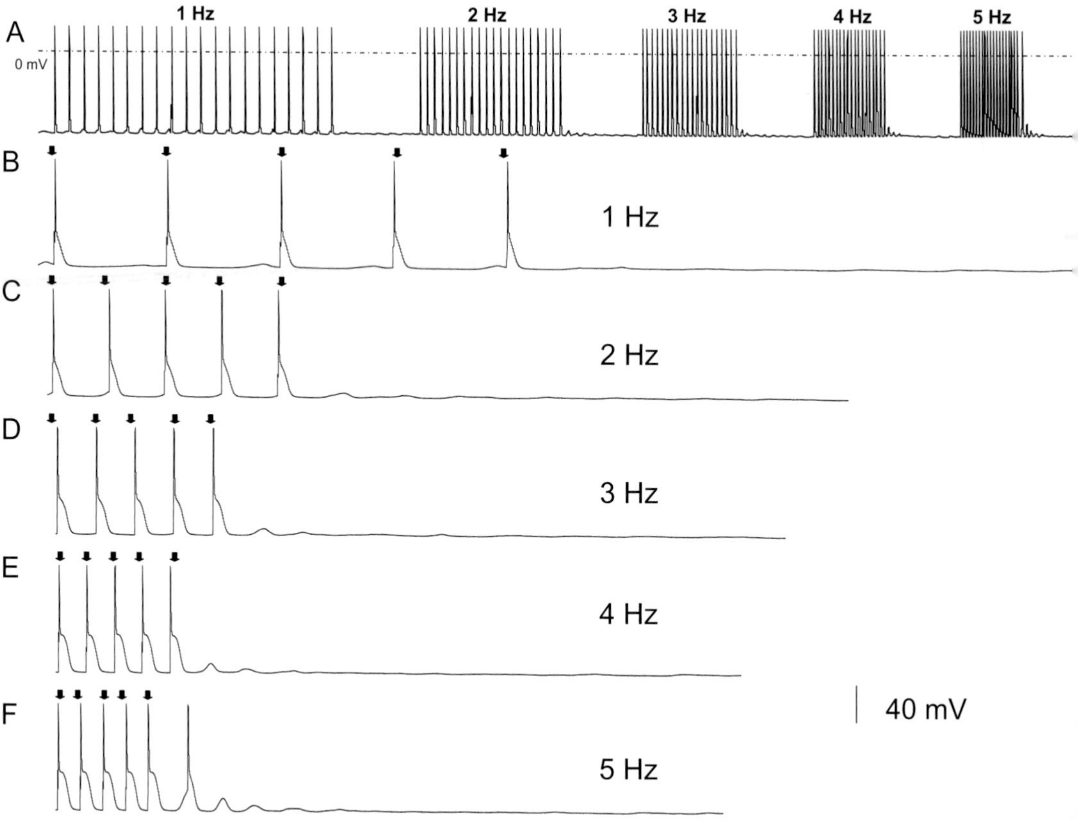

FIGURE 34–2. (A) Action potentials recorded from RyR2$^{R4496C+/-}$ myocytes stimulated at 1–5 Hz are shown: DADs develop when pacing is interrupted. (B–F) The last five driven action potentials at each pacing frequency and DADs and triggered activity developing when pacing is discontinued are shown. Note that the DAD amplitude increases and the DAD coupling interval decreases at faster pacing frequencies. At 5 Hz (F) one triggered beat develops.

RyR2/FKBP12.2 interaction is already present in the resting state. Upon adrenergic stimulation it further deteriorates, since phosphokinase A (PKA) phosphorylates the channel causing even greater dissociation of FKBP12.6 and promoting Ca^{2+} leakage from the SR.

Other investigators questioned the central role of FKBP12.6 in the pathogenesis of CPVT arrhythmias. George *et al.*[18] found that mutant channels had a normal RyR2/FKBP12.6 interaction but an abnormally augmented response to isoproterenol and forskolin. Jiang *et al.*[23] revealed that phosphorylation of RyR2 by PKA did not dissociate FKBP12.6 from RyR2.

It is known that when the SR stored Ca^{2+} content reaches a critical level, spontaneous Ca^{2+} release occurs, a process referred to as store-overload-induced Ca^{2+} release (SOICR). Subsequently, Jiang *et al.*[23] demonstrated that disease-causing RyR2 mutations, by enhancing RyR2 luminal Ca^{2+} activation, reduce the threshold for SOICR, which in turn increases the propensity for triggered arrhythmia.

Recently we[14] demonstrated that K201, a 1,4-benzothiazepine derivative (formerly called JTV-519) that enhances the binding of FKBP12.6 to RyR2,[19] is unable to prevent triggered activity in RyR2$^{R4496C+/-}$ myocytes and ventricular arrhythmias in RyR2$^{R4496C+/-}$ mice, thus suggesting that it is unlikely that the R4496C mutation induces CPVT by interfering with the RyR2/FKBP12.6 complex.

RyR2 is a macromolecular complex that binds several proteins, such as calmodulin, CaM kinase II, FKBP12.6, sorcin, and phosphatases PP1 and PP2A (see Figure 34–4).[24] Accordingly, it is likely

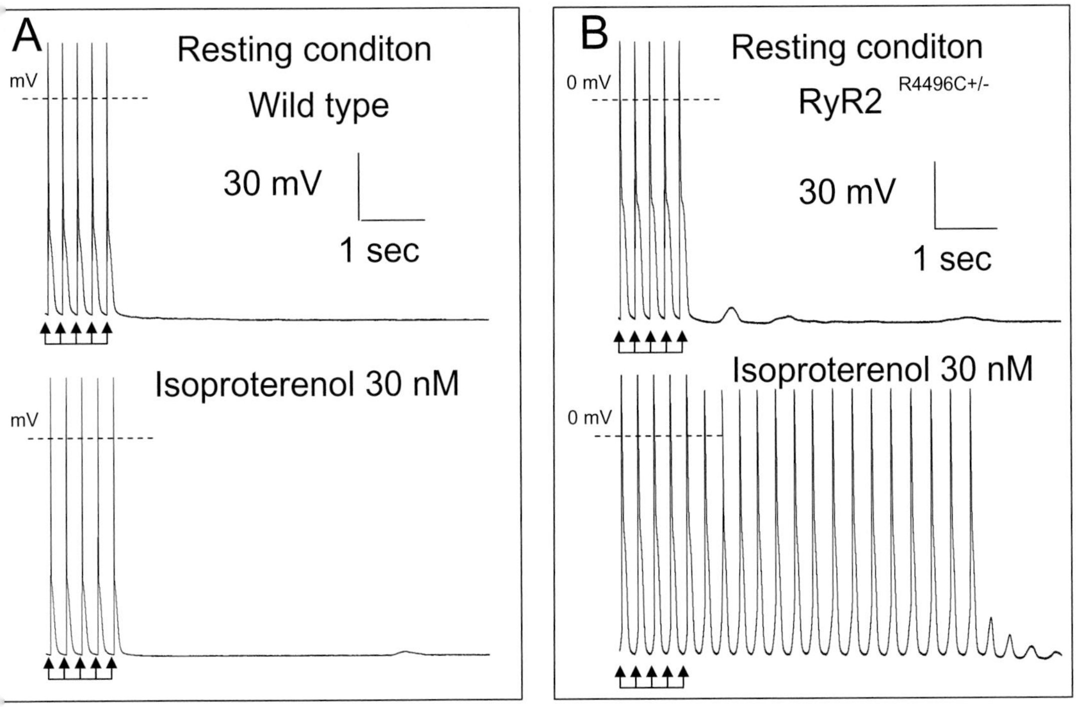

FIGURE 34–3. Action potential recording from a wild-type myocyte (A) and an RyR2$^{R4496C+/-}$ myocyte (B) in the absence (top panel) and in the presence (bottom panel) of isoproterenol (30 nM). Arrows indicate the last five paced action potentials.

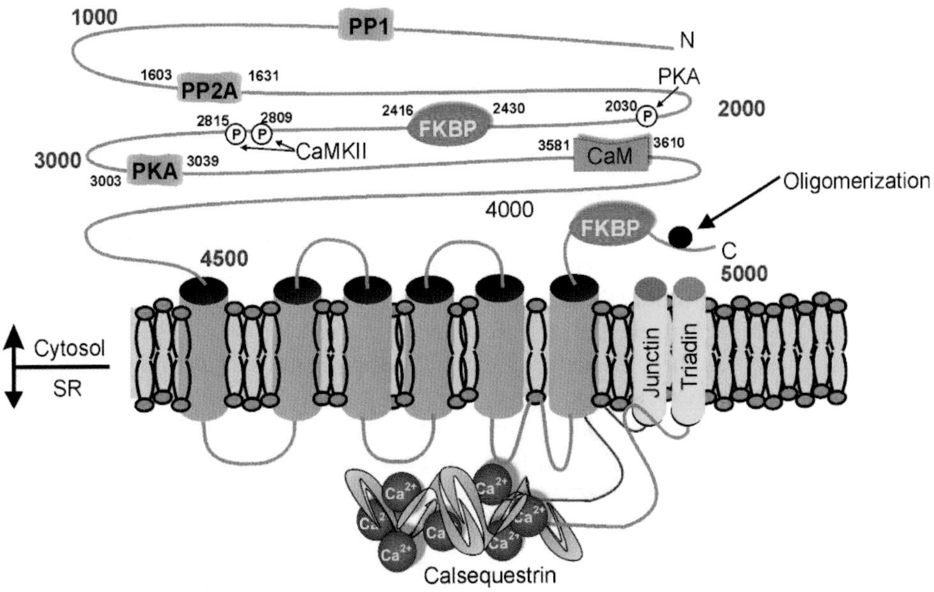

FIGURE 34–4. Schematic showing the predicted structure of the cardiac ryanodine receptor, RyR2, including the sites of interaction with ancillary proteins and the phosphorylation sites. Calsequestrin, junctin, and triadin, proteins interacting with ryanodine receptors in the SR, are also depicted. PP, protein phosphatase; P, phosphorylation sites; CaM, calmodulin; CaMKII, calmodulin-dependent protein kinase II.

that none of these proteins is the sole mediator of the functional consequences of RyR2 mutations. Since mutations linked to the CPVT phenotype are located in physically and functionally distinct regions of the protein,[25] it is likely that the position of each mutation along the RyR2 amino acidic sequence can alter different functional domains. Therefore, it may be hypothesized that all mutations lead to the final common pathway of promoting diastolic calcium leak from RyR2, DADs, and triggered arrhythmias by acting on different molecular targets.

CASQ2-Related Catecholaminergic Polymorphic Ventricular Tachycardia

The CASQ2 protein serves as the major Ca^{2+} reservoir within the SR of cardiac myocytes and is part of a protein complex that contains the ryanodine receptor. The presence of a 50% loss of calsequestrin (in heterozygous carriers) and a normal clinical phenotype suggest that the calsequestrin-related Ca^{2+} buffering process can tolerate quite severe functional impairments. Only two CASQ2 mutations have so far been investigated functionally *in vitro*. Viatchenko-Karpinski *et al.*[26] introduced the CASQ2-D307H mutation (the one reported by Lahat *et al.* in their original study) in adult rat myocytes. This study showed that D307H impairs SR Ca^{2+} storing and reduces the buffering capabilities of Ca^{2+}. Recently the same group of investigators[27] reported that another CASQ2-CPVT mutation (R33Q) disrupts the interaction of CASQ2–RyR2 and impairs luminal Ca^{2+}-dependent RyR2 regulation. These data suggest that CASQ2 and RyR2 are both functionally and physically linked to finely regulate the Ca^{2+} release process from SR. Taken together, the defects of CASQ2 mutations can enhance the responsiveness of RyR2s to luminal Ca^{2+}, which in turn leads to the generation of diastolic spontaneous Ca^{2+} transients, DADs, and triggered action potentials.

Finally, it is interesting to observe that basic science investigations suggest that both the dominant and the recessive CPVT variants share the same final pathway for the onset of arrhythmias: DADs and triggered activity.

Clinical Management

Clinical Manifestations

Syncope, triggered by exercise or emotional stres is often the first manifestation of CPVT.[2,] Approximately 30% of patients present with family history of stress-related syncope, seizur or sudden death. Most events occur in the first o second decade of life.

In the series of cases reported by Leenhard *et al.*,[2] the mean age at first event was 7.8 ± 4 year similar to our results (8 ± 2 years).[11] Usually CPV diagnosis is established after an average delay o 2 years from the first syncope, because thes events are often attributed to vasovagal events o to neurological factors. Increasing evidence show that sudden cardiac death can be the first mani festation of the disease.[11,12] Recently Tester *et al.* reported mutations in RyR2 underlying sudde infant death syndrome.

Electrocardiogram

The resting ECG of CPVT patients is usuall normal with the exception of prominent U wave and mild sinus bradycardia in some patient which is especially abnormal for children of thi age.[2,29] There is normal QTc, normal atrioven tricular conduction, and no evidence of a Brugada like pattern.

Exercise or acute emotional stress is the typica trigger of CPVT-related arrhythmias. The ven tricular rhythm disturbances during exercis stress testing appear quite constantly at heart rat of 110–130 beats per minute.[2,11] The complexit and frequency of ventricular arrhythmia progres sively worsen with an increase in workload, fro isolated premature beats to bigeminy and to ven tricular tachyarrhythmia (see Figure 34–5). Whe the exercise stops, arrhythmias gradually dis appear. The most typical ventricular tachycardi observed in CPVT patients presents an alternat ing QRS axis morphology with a rotation of 18 degrees on a beat-to-beat basis, the so-called bidi rectional ventricular tachycardia. It is importan to acknowledge that supraventricular arrhyth mias and tachycardia are also part of the CPV phenotype. In light of the role of triggered activit

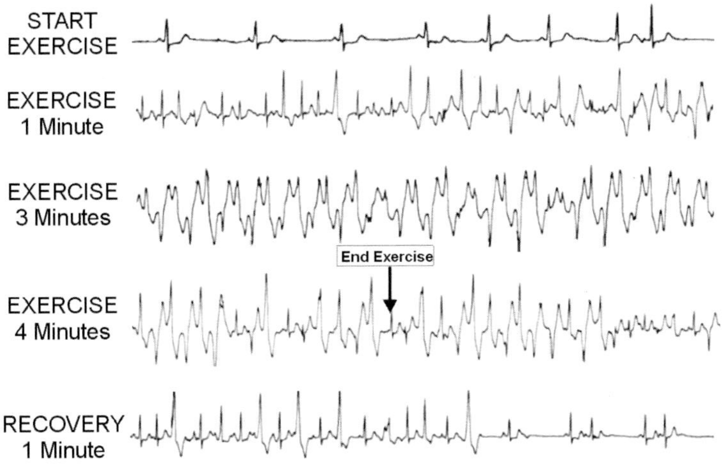

IGURE 34–5. Exercise stress test in a atient with polymorphic VT and RyR2 utation. Ventricular arrhythmias are bserved with a progressive worsening uring exercise. Typical bidirectional VT evelops after 3 min of exercise with a inus heart rate of approximately 120 bpm. rrhythmias rapidly recede during ecovery.

s a mechanism for arrhythmias in CPVT, it is nteresting to note that fast supraventricular tachcardia may act as a trigger for the development f DADs and triggered activity in the ventricle.

enotype–Phenotype Correlation

n 2002, Priori *et al.*[11] reported the clinical characterization of a large cohort of CPVT patients. he clinical phenotype of the 30 probands and of 18 family members was evaluated. Genotype–henotype analysis showed patients with nongnotyped CPVT were predominantly females and ecame symptomatic later in life (20 ± 12 years); atients with RyR2 CPVT became symptomatic arlier (8 ± 2 years), and males were at higher risk f cardiac events. In 2004, we[12] presented an pdate of the clinical profile of our population of PVT patients and reported data on 102 CPVT atients from 60 families suggesting that RyR2 nutations can be identified in approximately 70% f patients and that they have a mean penetrance f 80%. CPVT is a malignant disease: 20% of atients in our series died suddenly at a median ge of 16 years and SCD was the first manifestaion of the disease in 10% of the cases. Because pproximately 20% of RyR2 mutation carriers nay have no phenotype (incomplete penetrate) nd sudden cardiac death can be the first clinical resentation in CPVT, early genetic evaluation is ery important for all family members of CPVT robands.[7,12]

To date, a limited number of CASQ2 genotyped patients has been reported. The autosomal recessive inheritance is typical of the CASQ2-related CPVT. In our experience[12] only 7% (4 out of 60) of CPVT probands harbor CASQ2 mutations, suggesting that this is a relatively uncommon variant of CPVT.[30] The genotype–phenotype correlation in CASQ2-related CPVT awaits more clinical and genetic data.

Diagnosis

Exercise or emotion-induced syncope in a patient with a normal electrocardiogram (normal QT interval) and without structural abnormalities should always suggest the possibility of CPVT. An exercise stress test is the most important tool for diagnosis since the bidirectional or polymorphic VT may be reproducibly elicited during physical activity in most of the patients. Furthermore, even in patients showing polymorphic (and not bidirectional) VT, the progressive worsening of arrhythmias with exercise is to be considered as diagnostic for CPVT. Holter recordings can also be extremely useful, especially in young children for whom it might be difficult to reach a high heart rate during a treadmill test.

Interestingly, the bidirectional pattern of VT may appear in patients with Andersen syndrome.[31] This disease is a variant of the long QT syndrome (also called LQT7) caused by loss of function mutations of the *KCNJ2* gene encoding for the cardiac inward rectifier potassium current. The reasons for this apparent "phenocopy arrhythmia" are still unclear, but differential diagnosis between the two conditions should be considered.

Invasive eletrophysiological testing with programmed electrical stimulation is of no value (either diagnostic or prognostic) in CPVT as patients are largely not inducible with programmed electrical stimulation. Ventricular arrhythmia may be induced by isoproterenol infusion, but the predictive value of inducibility for risk stratification has never been demosntrated.[11,32]

Treatment

Since the catecholamine-dependent onset of ventricular tachycardia the rational treatment of CPVT is that of chronic administration of β-adrenergic blockers.

Acute intravenous administration of propranolol is the treatment of choice for the acute termination of CPVT-related arrhythmias.[33]

Chronic treatment with β-adrenergic blockers can prevent recurrent syncope in some patients. Nadolol at a daily dose of 1–2.5 mg/kg/day is the drug used at our center. Individual tolerability of the drug should be always considered. In our experience, some patients may be treated with up to 3.5–4 mg/kg/day of nadolol without clinically relevant side effects and increased protection from arrhythmic events. However, it is important to be aware that some patients still develop repetitive ventricular arrhythmias during exercise stress test even with maximal tolerated dose of β-blocking agents (see below).

Leenhardt *et al.*[2] reported that a complete efficiency of nadolol, a long acting drug, in CPVT patients: three syncope and two sudden deaths occurred in their series at follow-up, probably due to treatment noncompliance. On the other hand, Priori *et al.*[11] reported that β-adrenergic blockers provided only incomplete protection from recurrence of sustained ventricular tachycardia and ventricular fibrillation; 18 of 39 patients with CPVT treated with β-adrenergic blockers still developed cardiac arrhythmias. Bauce *et al.*[7] observed that 35% (9 out of 26) of CPVT patients treated with β-adrenergic blockers presented with effort-induced polymorphic ventricular arrhythmia, while no patient on β-adrenergic blocker therapy had syncopal episodes or died suddenly during follow-up. Sumitomo *et al.*[32] reported that β-adrenergic blockers completely controlled CPVT in only 31% cases; 4 out of 21 patients treated with β-adrenergic blockers died suddenly.

Overall, agreement exists on the fact that β-blockers reduce the occurrence of cardiac events, postpone the induction of VTs during exercise stress testing, and slow the rate of VT; however incomplete protection from sudden cardiac death has been reported. This suggests that the implant of an implantable cardioverter defibrillator (ICD) should be considered for primary prevention of cardiac arrest in CPVT patients in whom severe ventricular arrhythmias (sustained VT or rapid VT) are still observed while on β-blocker therapy. In our study, 50% of patients with an ICD had received an appropriate shock to terminate ventricular tachyarrhythmia within 2 years of follow-up.[11]

Reports of arrhythmic storms leading to sudden cardiac death in CPVT patients implanted with the ICD stress the importance of ensuring that even when an ICD is provided, the maximally tolerated doses of β-adrenergic blockers should be recommended.

Verapamil, a Ca^{2+} channel antagonist, has been shown to directly inhibit the function of the ryanodine receptor.[34] Since CPVT mutant RyR2 proteins cause a "gain of function" and uncontrolled calcium release from SR, verapamil may theoretically be an alternative option for treatment. In 2003, Sumitomo *et al.*[32] reported that acute administration of verapamil did not completely suppress CPVT; however, the endurance time was prolonged and the number of CPVT episodes decreased; all three patients treated with verapamil survived during the follow-up period. Subsequently, Swan *et al.*[35] also observed that intravenous administration of verapamil could significantly decrease the prevalence of ventricular arrhythmia in all patients with CPVT during an exercise stress test and significantly increase the threshold heart rate at which the arrhythmia appeared. Thus, verapamil may be at least partially effective in CPVT, but the limited data available do not suggest that it be recommended as an alternative to β-blockers. Verapamil may provide further protection when used in combination with β-blockers. The limited experience with amiodar ne, mexiletine, and magnesium produced unavorable results.[2,32,35]

References

1. Coumel P, Fidelle J, Lucet V, *et al.* Catecholamine-induced severe ventricular arrhythmias with Adams-Stokes syndrome in children: Report of four cases. *Br Heart J* 1978;40(Suppl.):28–37.
2. Leenhardt A, Lucte V, Denjoy I, *et al.* Catecholaminergic polymorphic ventricular tachycardia in children. A 7-year follow-up of 21 patients. *Circulation* 1995;91:1512–1519.
3. Priori SG, Napolitano C, Tiso N, *et al.* Mutations in the cardiac ryanodine receptor gene (hRyR2) underlie catecholaminergic polymorphic ventricular tachycardia. *Circulation* 2001;103:196–200.
4. Swan H, Piippo K, Viitasalo M, *et al.* Arrhythmic disorder mapped to chromosome 1q42–q43 causes malignant polymorphic ventricular tachycardia in structurally normal hearts. *J Am Coll Cardiol* 1999; 34:2035–2042.
5. Laitinen PJ, Brown KM, Piippo K, *et al.* Mutations of the cardiac ryanodine receptor (RyR2) gene in familial polymorphic ventricular tachycardia. *Circulation* 2001;103:485–490.
6. Tiso N, Stephan DA, Nava A, *et al.* Identification of mutations in the cardiac ryanodine receptor gene in families affected with arrhythmogenic right ventricular cardiomyopathy type 2 (ARVD2). *Hum Mol Genet* 2001;10:189–194.
7. Bauce B, Rampazzo A, Basso C, *et al.* Screening for ryanodine receptor type 2 mutations in families with effort-induced polymorphic ventricular arrhythmias and sudden death: Early diagnosis of asymptomatic carriers. *J Am Coll Cardiol* 2002;40: 341–349.
8. Lahat H, Eldar M, Levy-Nissenbaum E, *et al.* Autosomal recessive catecholamine- or exercise-induced polymorphic ventricular tachycardia: Clinical features and assignment of the disease gene to chromosome 1p13-21. *Circulation* 2001;103:2822–2827.
9. Lahat H, Pras E, Olender T, *et al.* A missense mutation in a highly conserved region of CASQ2 is associated with autosomal recessive catecholamine-induced polymorphic ventricular tachycardia in Bedouin families from Israel. *Am J Hum Genet* 2001;69:1378–1384.
10. Raffaele di Barletta M, Viatchenko-Karpinski S, Nori A, *et al.* Clinical phenotype and functional characterization of CASQ2 mutations associated with catecholaminergic polymorphic ventricular tachycardia. *Circulation* 2006;114(10):1012–1019.
11. Priori SG, Napolitano C, Memmi M, *et al.* Clinical and molecular characterization of patients with catecholaminergic polymorphic ventricular tachycardia. *Circulation* 2002;106:69–74.
12. Cerrone M, Colombi B, Bloise R, *et al.* Clinical and molecular characterization of a large cohort of patients affected with catecholaminergic polymorphic ventricular tachycardia. *Circulation* 2004;110 (Suppl. II):552.
13. Cerrone M, Colombi B, Santoro M *et al.* Bidirectional ventricular tachycardia and fibrillation elicited in a knock-in mouse model carrier of a mutation in the cardiac ryanodine receptor (RyR2). *Circ Res* 2005;96:e77–e82.
14. Liu N, Colombi B, Memmi M, *et al.* Arrhythmogenesis in catecholaminergic polymorphic ventricular tachycardia: Insights from a RyR2 R4496C knock-in mouse model. *Circ Res* 2006;99: 292–298.
15. Fabiato A. Time and calcium dependence of activation and inactivation of calcium-induced release of calcium from the sarcoplasmic reticulum of a skinned canine cardiac Purkinje cell. *J Gen Physiol* 1985;85:247–289.
16. Terentyev D, Viatchenko-Karpinski S, Valdivia HH, *et al.* Luminal Ca^{2+} controls termination and refractory behavior of Ca^{2+}-induced Ca^{2+} release in cardiac myocytes. *Circ Res* 2002;91:414–420.
17. Jiang D, Xiao B, Zhang L, *et al.* Enhanced basal activity of a cardiac Ca2+ release channel (ryanodine receptor) mutant associated with ventricular tachycardia and sudden death. *Circ Res* 2002;91:218–225.
18. George CH, Higgs GV, Lai FA. Ryanodine receptor mutations associated with stress-induced ventricular tachycardia mediate increased calcium release in stimulated cardiomyocytes. *Circ Res* 2003;93: 531–540.
19. Lehnart SE, Wehrens XH, Laitinen PJ, *et al.* Sudden death in familial polymorphic ventricular tachycardia associated with calcium release channel (ryanodine receptor) leak. *Circulation* 2004;109:3208–3214.
20. Priori SG, Napolitano C. Intracellular calcium handling dysfunction and arrhythmogenesis: A new challenge for the electrophysiologist. *Circ Res* 2005; 97:1077–1079.
21. Wehrens XH, Lehnart SE, Huang F, *et al.* FKBP12.6 deficiency and defective calcium release channel (ryanodine receptor) function linked to exercise-induced sudden cardiac death. *Cell* 2003;113:829–840.
22. Wehrens XH, Lehnart SE, Reiken SR, Deng SX, Vest JA, Cervantes D, Coromilas J, Landry DW, Marks

AR. Protection from cardiac arrhythmia through ryanodine receptor–stabilizing protein calstabin2. *Science* 2004;304:292–296.
23. Jiang D, Wang R, Xiao B, *et al.* Enhanced store overload-induced Ca2+ release and channel sensitivity to luminal Ca^{2+} activation are common defects of RyR2 mutations linked to ventricular tachycardia and sudden death. *Circ Res* 2005;97:1173–1181.
24. Bers DM. Macromolecular complexes regulating cardiac ryanodine receptor function. *J Mol Cell Cardiol* 2004;37:417–429.
25. Thomas NL, Lai FA, George CH. Differential Ca2+ sensitivity of RyR2 mutations reveals distinct mechanisms of channel dysfunction in sudden cardiac death. *Biochem Biophys Res Commun* 2005;331:231–238.
26. Viatchenko-Karpinski S, Terentyev D, Györke I, *et al.* Abnormal calcium signaling and sudden cardiac death associated with mutation of calsequestrin. *Circ Res* 2004;94:471–477.
27. Terentyev D, Nori A, Santoro M, Viatchenko-Karpinski S, *et al.* Abnormal interactions of calsequestrin with the ryanodine receptor calcium release channel complex linked to exercise-induced sudden cardiac death. *Circ Res* 2006;98:1151–1158.
28. Tester D, Carturan E, Dura M, *et al.* Molecular and functional characterization of novel RyR2-encoded cardiac ryanodine receptor/calcium release channel mutations in sudden infant death syndrome. *Heart Rhythm* 2006;3(Issue 1S):S67.
29. Postma AV, Denjoy I, Kamblock J, *et al.* Catecho laminergic polymorphic ventricular tachycardia RYR2 mutations, bradycardia, and follow up of th patients. *J Med Genet* 2005;42:863–870.
30. Lahat H, Pras E, Eldar M. RYR2 and CASQ2 muta tions in patients suffering from catecholaminergi polymorphic ventricular tachycardia. *Circulatio* 2003;107:e29; author reply e29.
31. Zhang L, Benson DW, Tristani-Firouzi M, *et a* Electrocardiographic features in Andersen-Tawi syndrome patients with KCNJ2 mutations: Charac teristic T-U-wave patterns predict the KCNJ2 geno type. *Circulation* 2005;111:2720–2726.
32. Sumitomo N, Harada K, Nagashima M, *et a* Catecholaminergic polymorphic ventricular tachy cardia: Electrocardiographic characteristics an optimal therapeutic strategies to prevent sudde death. *Heart* 2003;89:66–70.
33. De Rosa G, Delogu AB, Piastra M, *et al.* Catecho laminergic polymorphic ventricular tachycardia Successful emergency treatment with intravenou propranolol. *Pediatr Emerg Care* 2004;20:175–177
34. Valdivia HH, Valdivia C, Ma J, *et al.* Direct binding of verapamil to the ryanodine receptor channel o sarcoplasmic reticulum. *Biophys J* 1990;58:471–481
35. Swan H, Laitinen P, Kontula K, *et al.* Calcium channel antagonism reduces exercise-induce ventricular arrhythmias in catecholaminergi polymorphic ventricular tachycardia patients wit RyR2 mutations. *J Cardiovasc Electrophysiol* 2005 16:162–166.

35
Andersen–Tawil and Timothy Syndromes

Martin Tristani-Firouzi and Tania Ferrer

Introduction

This chapter summarizes two relatively new ion channelopathies, Andersen–Tawil and Timothy syndromes. Both disorders are pleiotropic in nature, with multiple clinical manifestations outside the cardiovascular system. While both Andersen–Tawil and Timothy syndromes are disorders of ventricular repolarization, their unique clinical phenotype distinguishes them from the traditional forms of long QT syndrome (LQTS). The degree of QT prolongation in each disorder is directly related to the contribution of the disordered ion channel to the various phases of the cardiac action potential. This chapter discusses the most recent genetic, cellular, and clinical data underlying these unique ion channelopathies.

Andersen–Tawil Syndrome

In 1971, Andersen reported a series of patients with periodic skeletal muscle paralysis, ventricular ectopy, and dysmorphic features, the triad of clinical manifestations known as Andersen's syndrome.[1] Prolongation of the QT interval was incorporated as an important cardiac manifestation in subsequent larger studies of this disorder.[2] The syndrome was renamed Andersen–Tawil syndrome (ATS) in recognition of the exceptional contributions of the clinical neurologist Dr. Rabi Tawil. Within the cardiovascular field, this disorder remained obscure until mutations in the K^+ channel gene *KCNJ2* were identified as a cause of ATS.[3] *KCNJ2* encodes the inward rectifier K^+ channel Kir2.1, a component of the inward rectifier current I_{K1}. I_{K1} provides substantial repolarizing current during the most terminal repolarization phase of the cardiac action potential and is the primary conductance controlling the diastolic membrane potential.[4]

Clinical Manifestations of Andersen–Tawil Syndrome

The clinical features of ATS represent a spectrum of phenotypic manifestations encompassing the skeletal muscle and cardiac systems, in addition to craniofacial and skeletal anomalies (Figure 35–1). A major obstacle in the clinical diagnosis of ATS is the high degree of phenotypic variability and nonpenetrance. The full triad of clinical features (ventricular arrhythmias, periodic paralysis, and characteristic dysmorphic features) is present in 58–78% of mutation-positive patients,[5] while between 32% and 81% manifest involvement of two of the three organ systems.[3,5,6] Nonpenetrance ranges from 6% to 20% of mutation-positive individuals.[5,6] In an interesting report, a large ATS family presented with sex-specific clinical manifestations. In this kindred, females manifested ventricular arrhythmias, while affected males had periodic paralysis. None of 41 mutation carriers expressed the complete triad of ATS features.[6] These sex-specific clinical findings, however, appear to be specific for this particular family in that the same mutation was reported in other individuals who manifested the typical ATS triad.[7]

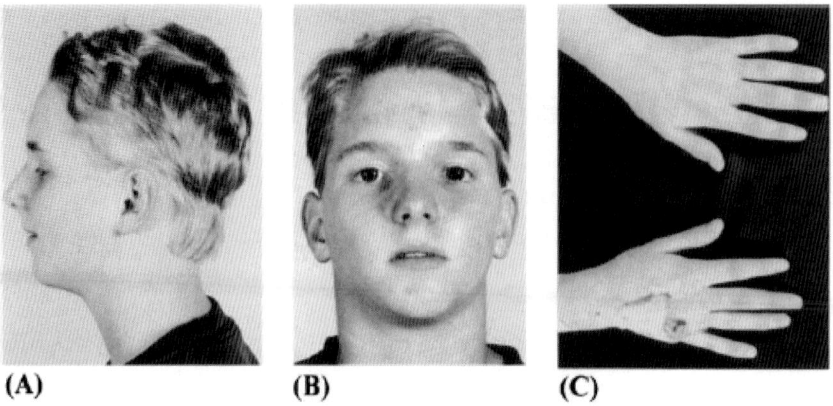

FIGURE 35–1. Typical dysmorphic features in an ATS subject. Note the low set ears, hypertelorism (wide interpupillary distance), micrognathia (small jaw) (A and B), and clinodactyly of the fifth digits (C). (From Plaster *et al.*,[3] © 2001 Elsevier. Reprinted with permission.)

Recently, the ATS phenotype was expanded to include several consistent craniofacial features, dental and skeletal anomalies that were observed in all members of a small cohort, irrespective of cardiac or neuromuscular findings.[8] These new findings help to establish the clinical diagnosis when cardiac or skeletal muscle findings are absent.

Andersen–Tawil syndrome is an autosomal dominant or sporadic disorder of ventricular repolarization manifested by mild QTc interval prolongation, but marked prolongation of the QUc interval.[5,9] Prominent U waves are commonly described. Zhang and colleagues recently reported distinct electrocardiographic (ECG) findings unique to ATS that included prolongation of the T wave downslope, a wide T-U junction, and high amplitude, broad U waves (Figure 35–2).[9] Arrhythmias in ATS patients include frequent premature ventricular contractions (PVCs), bigeminy, and polymorphic ventricular tachycardia (VT).[5] Typically, VT is nonsustained and bidirectional in nature with heart rates in the 130–150 range. The degree of ventricular ectopy is quite variable between subjects, but up to 50% of all beats may be ventricular in origin.[8] While tachycardia burden is often high in ATS subjects,[10] degeneration into lethal ventricular arrhythmias is relatively uncommon.[11] For example, torsade de pointes was documented in only 3 of 96 *KCNJ2* mutation-positive individuals.[9]

The frequent ventricular ectopy typical of ATS is notoriously difficult to suppress with pharma-

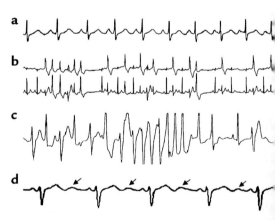

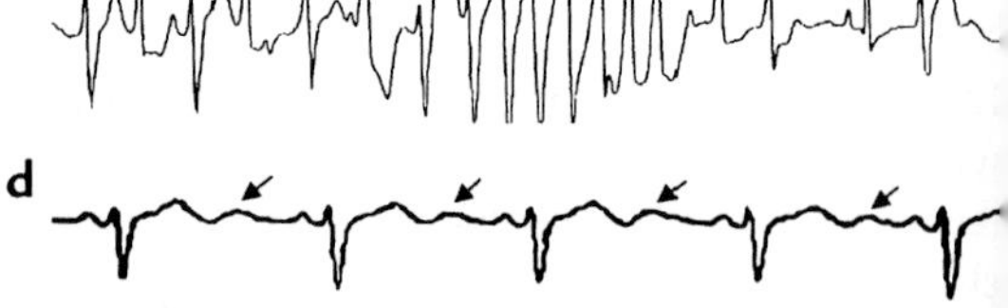

FIGURE 35–2. Representative ECGs from ATS subjects. (a) An ECG demonstrating prolongation of the QT interval. (b) ECG traces demonstrating a short run of nonsustained polymorphic VT followed by bigeminy. (c) Bidirectional VT (note alternating QRS axis polarity) degenerating into a brief run of polymorphic VT. (d) An ECG trace demonstrating a prominent U wave (indicated by arrows) (From Tristani-Firouzi *et al.*,[5] © 2002 by the American Society for Clinical Investigation. Reprinted with permission.)

cological therapy.[10,12] Given that many patients with frequent ventricular ectopy are entirely asymptomatic, therapy may not be indicated in most patients. However, identifying the subset of ATS patients at risk for life-threatening arrhythmias remains a daunting task,[10,12] primarily due to the paucity of data in the literature. In light of the absence of known criteria, any patient with runs of rapid polymorphic VT or symptoms such as syncope should be considered a candidate for placement of an implantable cardioverter defibrillator (ICD).

The Molecular Correlate of I_{K1}

The inward rectifier potassium current I_{K1} is the major determinant of the resting membrane potential in the heart and participates in the most terminal phase of action potential repolarization.[4] I_{K1} is conducted by homotetrameric and/or heterotetrameric channels formed by coassembly of the Kir2.x subfamily of proteins (Kir2.1, Kir2.2, and Kir2.3). Message and protein expression studies indicate that Kir2.1 is the most abundant subfamily member in ventricular tissue.[13,14] The finding that mutations in *KNCJ2* cause human disease (but not the genes enconding Kir2.2 and 2.3) further underscores the pivotal role of Kir2.1 as a primary component of I_{K1}.

The Cellular Basis of Andersen–Tawil Syndrome

Nearly all the *KCNJ2* mutations described to date cause dominant-negative suppression of Kir2.1 channel function. A minority of mutations alter channel assembly and trafficking, with resultant accumulation of subunits within the endoplasmic reticulum and Golgi apparatus.[15] Most mutant subunits coassemble with wild-type subunits and traffic appropriately to the cell surface, but fail to function normally. The mechanism underlying this abnormal function is an altered sensitivity of the mutant channel to the membrane-delimited second messenger phosphatidylinositol 4,5-bisphosphate (PIP_2), an essential activator of most inward rectifier K^+ channels.[16] Nearly one-half of all reported *KCNJ2* mutations occur at residues known to be important for PIP_2–channel interaction, supporting the idea that reduced PIP_2 binding is critical to the pathogenesis of ATS.[7] Recently, the effects of ATS mutations were studied at the atomic level by crystallizing the N-terminal and C-terminal cytoplasmic domains of Kir2.1 (Figure 35–3).

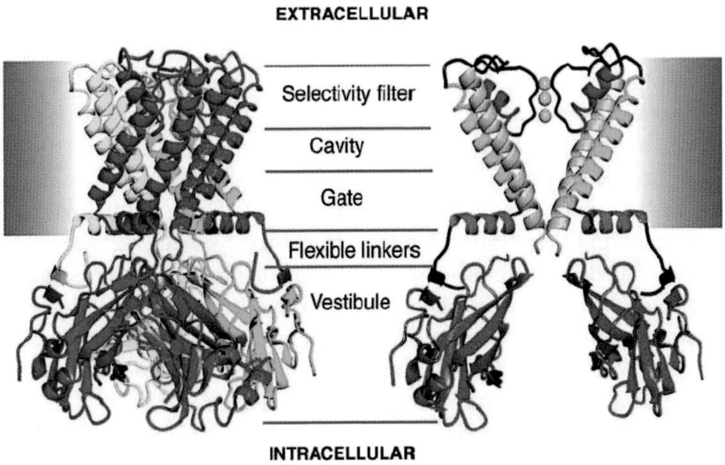

FIGURE 35–3. Crystal structure of a related inward rectifier channel, KirBac1.1. The left panel shows all four subunits, while the right panel eliminates two subunits for clarity. The majority of ATS mutations are located on the N-terminal slide helix and the C-terminal cytoplasmic domain. (From Kuo *et al.*,[29] © 2003 AAAS. Reprinted with permission.)

Arg-218 and Glu-303 in the C-terminus form charged and polar interactions with neighboring residues Thr-309 and Arg-312.[17,18] ATS mutations at Arg-218 and Glu-303 destabilize these interactions and likely render the channel insensitive to the activating effects of PIP_2.[17,18] To date, there is no clear genotype–phenotype relationship in ATS. No single mutation described to date has a higher likelihood of unstable arrhythmias.

How does reduced Kir2.1 channel function lead to susceptibility to arrhythmia? Selective I_{K1} blockade in feline Purkinje fibers results in action potential prolongation and an increased frequency of spontaneous action potentials.[19] In an elegant *in vivo* study, gene transfer of a Kir2.1 dominant-negative construct resulted in QT prolongation in adenoviral-transfected guinea pigs as well as spontaneous action potentials in isolated ventricular myocytes.[20] Both studies support the idea that a reduction in I_{K1} leads to the generation of spontaneous ventricular activity. The cellular consequences of reduced I_{K1} have been studied using *in silico* approaches. Reductions in I_{K1} initially cause mild prolongation of the most terminal foot of the cardiac action potential.[21] Greater reductions in I_{K1} result in the generation of spontaneous action potentials that are triggered by the Na^+/Ca^{2+} exchanger.[5,21,22] This is unlike the traditional forms of LQTS whereby prolongation of the plateau phase results in L-type Ca^{2+}-triggered early afterdepolarizations. Computer simulations of reduced I_{K1} in virtual left ventricular tissue reveal an increase in action potential duration across the ventricular wall, without an increase in transmural dispersion of repolarization.[21] Thus, the low frequency of torsade de pointes arrhythmia in ATS patients may be a consequence of the lack of transmural dispersion of repolarization in the setting of reduced I_{K1}, despite the fact that action potential duration is prolonged. The *in silico* data are consistent with data from the isolated canine wedge preparation using $BaCl_2$ as a model of ATS.[23] Interestingly, the contribution of I_{Kr} to phase 3 repolarization increased dramatically in the setting of computer-simulated I_{K1} reductions.[21] The consequences of this observation are that patients with ATS may be particularly susceptible to changes in I_{Kr} (such as hERG channel blockers or decreased $[K^+]_o$) given the baseline reduced repolarization reserve and the dependence upon I_{Kr} as a substitute for reduced I_{K1}.

Timothy Syndrome

The first case of what we now call Timothy syndrome (TS) was described in 1992 in a German report of an infant with 2 : 1 atrioventricular block, prolonged QT interval, syndactyly, and subsequent sudden death.[24] The association between severe LQT and syndactyly was further defined in a small cohort of three patients, two of whom died of ventricular fibrillation.[25] Mutations in the known LQTS genes were excluded in this population as well as mutations in the coding sequence of the cardiac L-type calcium channel Cav1.2. Subsequently, novel alternatively spliced Cav1.2 isoforms were described and a mutation in a splice variant was identified in a cohort of TS patients.[26]

Clinical Manifestations of Timothy Syndrome

Timothy syndrome is a rare, primarily sporadic disorder that affects the development of multiple organ systems. Although originally described as severe LQT and syndactyly, the ascertainment of additional subjects revealed a more complex clinical constellation, including congenital heart disease, developmental delay (including autism), abnormal dentition, and facial dysmorphic features (Figure 35–4).[26] One hundred percent of TS subjects display QT prolongation, syndactyly, baldness at birth, and small teeth.[26] The majority of subjects display 2:1 atrioventricular block in the neonatal period as a consequence of severe LQT. As the sinus rate slows down with advancing age, 1:1 atrioventricular conduction ensues. Consistent with the severe degree of QT prolongation, these individuals are at high risk for sudden cardiac death. The pleiotropic manifestations of this disease are a consequence of the wide expression pattern of the alternatively spliced variant of Cav1.2, including heart, brain, gastrointestinal system, lungs, immune system, and smooth muscle.[26] Two cases of atypical TS were recently

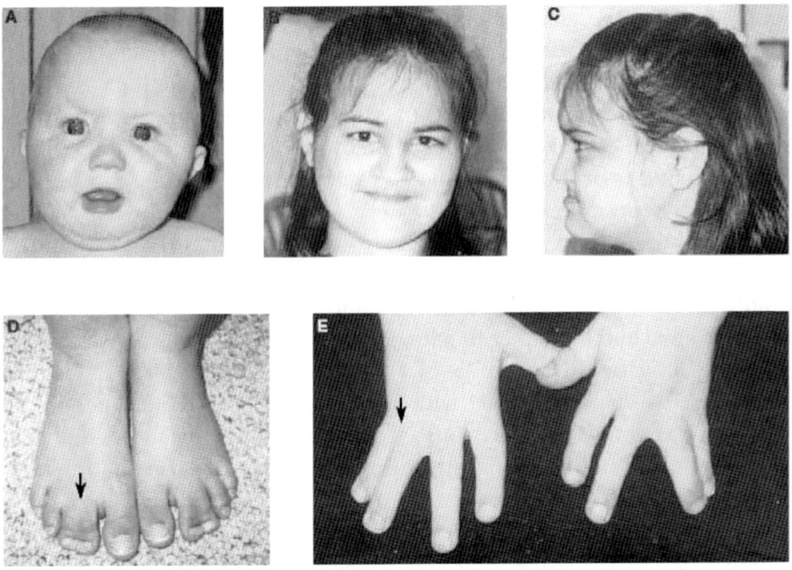

FIGURE 35–4. Typical dysmorphic features in TS subjects. (A–C) The TS individuals exhibited dysmorphic facial features including round face, flat nasal bridge, receding upper jaw, and thin upper lip. (D and E) Webbing of the toes and fingers (syndactyly). (From Splawski *et al.*,[26] © 2004 Elsevier. Reprinted with permission.)

described (TS2) notable for the absence of the cardinal feature of syndactyly. As discussed below, mutations in the primary Cav1.2 transcript were identified in this subset of patients.[27]

Molecular and Cellular Basis of Timothy Syndrome

A remarkable feature of TS is its molecular homogeneity; all of the original cases occurred as the result of the identical, *de novo* missense mutation in exon 8A (G406R), an alternatively spliced variant of Cav1.2. In the heart, approximately 23% of calcium channels are encoded by the exon 8A variant, with 77% encoded by exon 8.[26] In the heterozygote state, only 11.5% of Cav1.2 channels carry the G406R mutation; however, this causes sufficient calcium channel dysfunction to produce severe QT prolongation. The *de novo* predilection for the G406R exon 8A mutation is likely related to the high incidence of infant mortality, making its inheritance rare. In TS2, which is characterized by the absence of syndactyly, two mutations in the dominant splice variant exon 8 were identified, G402S and G406R.[27] All TS mutations are localized to the most terminal portion of the S6 transmembrane domain in Domain I.

L-type calcium channels display two forms of inactivation: a calcium-dependent and voltage-dependent inactivation. Expression of TS mutant Cav1.2 channels in heterologous expression systems revealed that mutant channels displayed near complete loss of voltage-dependent inactivation, while maintaining calcium-dependent inactivation.[26,27] Computer simulations of the effect of reduced Cav1.2 voltage-dependent inactivation in the heterozygous state revealed marked action potential duration prolongation and the development of delayed afterdepolarizations (DADs).[26,27] Thus, the cellular basis of arrhythmia in TS is reduced Cav1.2 inactivation, leading to a sustained inward calcium current during the plateau phase of the cardiac action potential, marked action potential prolongation, and subsequent QT prolongation. The sustained inward calcium current leads to secondary DADs, ventricular arrhythmias, and sudden death.

The molecular mechanisms underlying voltage- and calcium-dependent inactivation in L-type Ca^{2+} channels are not completely understood;

however, distinct regions of the channel appear to differentially regulate each process (Figure 35–5). The cytoplasmic linker between domain I and II (I–II linker) likely represents an important structural determinant of voltage-dependent inactivation. The I–II linker is proposed to function as a "lid" or inactivating blocking particle that occludes the inner mouth of the channel pore. The TS mutation G406R is located in the S6 C-terminal region of Domain I and likely influences the ability of the adjacent I–II linker to participate in channel inactivation (Figure 35–6). Substitution of the glycine at position 406 with charged, polar, or hydrophobic residues also impairs channel inactivation, implying that glycine is an absolute requirement for voltage-dependent inactivation.[27] Glycine is a flexible amino acid and functions as a hinge in other ion channels. G406 may function as a hinge that allows proper bending of the intracellular inactivation gate.

Although mutant Cav1.2 channels do not inactivate, they remain sensitive to L-type calcium channel blockers with potencies in nanomolar concentrations.[26] This would suggest that calcium channel blockers may prove to be useful therapeutic strategies for TS. Indeed, in a recent case report, Jacobs and colleagues describe a TS patient in whom verapamil successfully reduced the incidence of ventricular arrhythmias.[28]

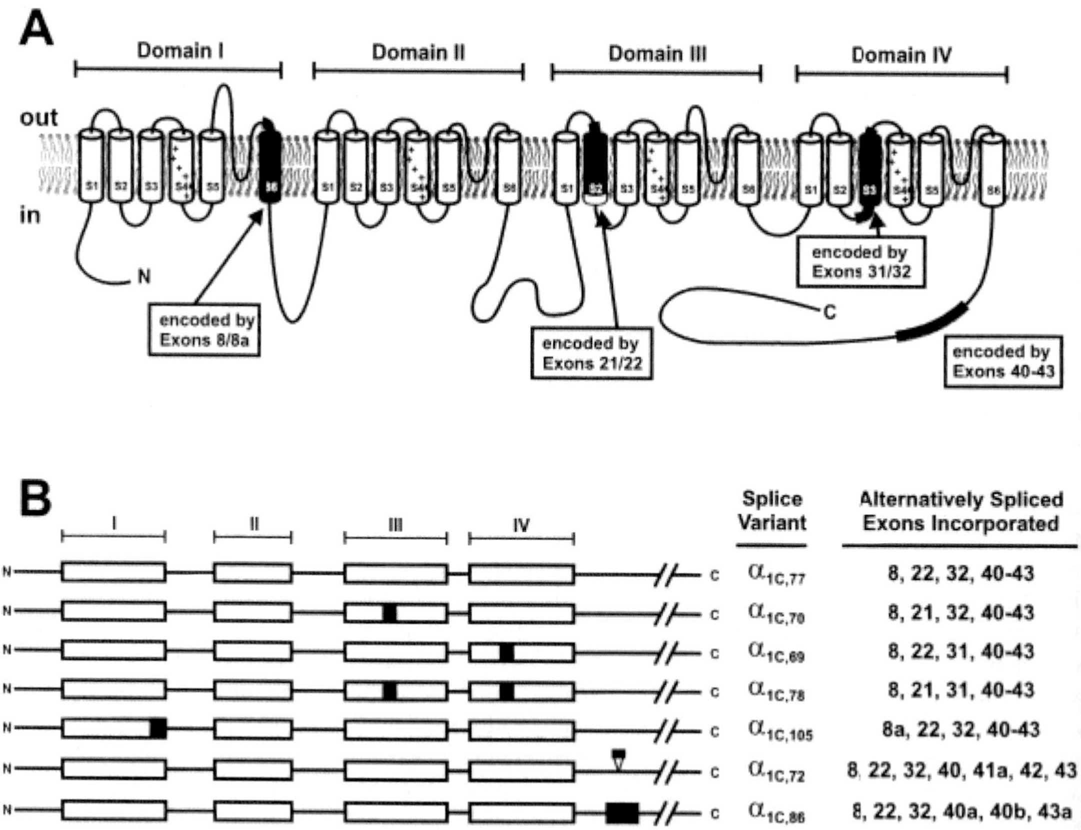

FIGURE 35–5. Schematic representation of the L-type calcium α_{1C} subunit and its isoforms. (A) The human α_{1C} subunit is characterized by four homologous domains (I–IV), each containing six transmembrane segments (S1–S6). Segments encoded by alternatively spliced exons are indicated. (B) The cDNA constructs with alternatively spliced exons are schematically presented, with the respective exon combinations indicated in the right column. Exons 8 and 8a, 21 and 22, as well as 31 and 32 are pairs of mutually exclusive homologous exons. (From Zuhlke *et al.*,[30] © 1998 Elsevier. Reprinted with permission.)

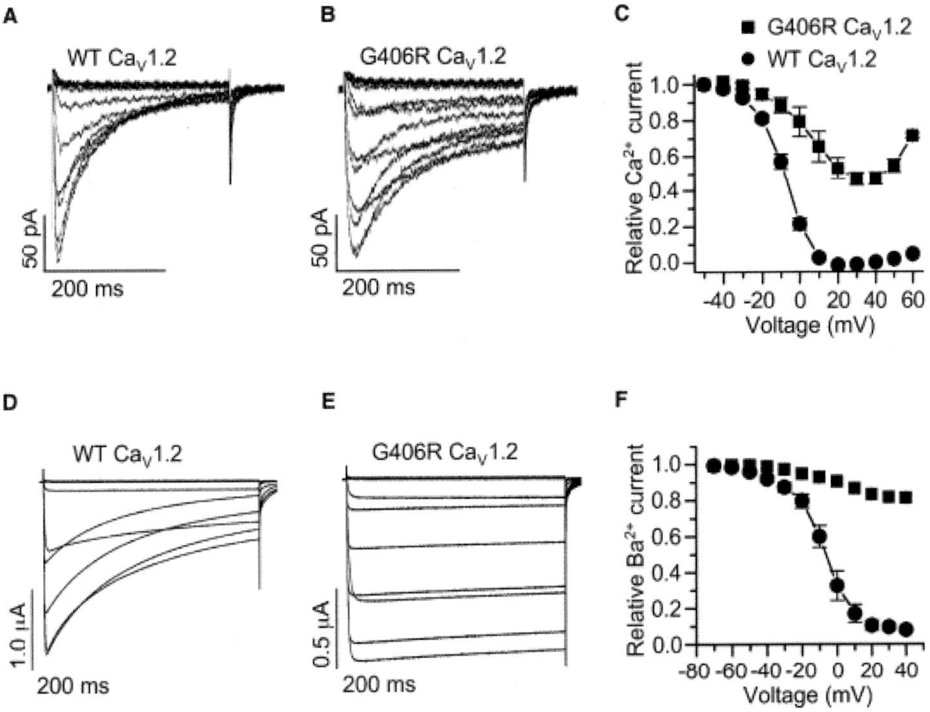

FIGURE 35–6. Timothy syndrome mutation reduces Cav1.2 channel inactivation. Wild-type (A) and G406R (B) Cav1.2 channel currents are recorded from CHO cells in response to voltage pulses applied in 10 mV increments from −40 to +60 mV. Note that both wild-type and mutant channels display decreased current with time, consistent with intact calcium-dependent inactivation. (C) Voltage dependence of Ca^{2+} current inactivation. (D and E) Wild-type (A) and G406R (B) Cav1.2 channel currents recorded with the voltage protocol described above but using Ba^{2+} as the charge carrier to abolish calcium-dependent inactivation. Note that the mutant current does not decline, consistent with voltage-dependent inactivation. (F) Voltage dependence of Ba^{2+} current inactivation. (From Splawski *et al.*,[26] © 2004 Elsevier. Reprinted with permission.)

Summary

The identification of the molecular bases of ATS and TS has advanced our understanding of the fundamental biophysical properties of Kir2.1 and Cav1.2 channels, respectively. Discerning the cellular mechanisms of these disorders has provided additional insight into the clinical manifestations of each disorder. Kir2.1 channels provide repolarizing current during the most terminal phase of the cardiac action potential. Reduced Kir2.1 channel function causes mild prolongation of action potential duration, resulting in mild QT prolongation. Disrupted Cav1.2 inactivation results in sustained inward calcium current during the plateau phase, causing marked action potential prolongation and, secondarily, marked QT prolongation. Thus, the degree of QT prolongation in each disorder is directly related to the contribution of the disordered ion channel to the various phases of the cardiac action potential. The identification of the molecular basis of TS also allowed tailoring of treatment strategies. The sensitivity of mutant Cav1.2 channels to traditional calcium channel blockers paved the way for a limited trial of verapamil to control ventricular arrhythmias. An activator of Kir2.1 channels remains to be discovered; however, such an agent could prove beneficial in the treatment of ATS.

References

1. Andersen ED, Krasilnikoff PA, Overvad H. Intermittent muscular weakness, extrasystoles, and multiple developmental anomalies. A new syndrome? *Acta Paediatr Scand* 1971;60(5):559–564.
2. Sansone V, Griggs RC, Meola G, *et al.* Andersen's syndrome: A distinct periodic paralysis. *Ann Neurol* 1997;42:305–312.
3. Plaster NM, Tawil R, Tristani-Firouzi M, *et al.* Mutations in Kir2.1 cause the developmental and episodic electrical phenotypes of Andersen's syndrome. *Cell* 2001;105(4):511–519.
4. Sanguinetti MC, Tristani-Firouzi M. Delayed and inward rectifier potassium channels. In: Zipes DP, Jalife J, Eds. *Cardiac Electrophysiology From Cell to Bedside*, 3rd ed. Philadelphia, PA: W.B. Saunders Co., 2000:Chapter 9.
5. Tristani-Firouzi M, Jensen JL, Donaldson MR, *et al.* Functional and clinical characterization of KCNJ2 mutations associated with LQT7 (Andersen syndrome). *J Clin Invest* 2002;110(3):381–388.
6. Andelfinger G, Tapper AR, Welch RC, Vanoye CG, George AL Jr, Benson DW. KCNJ2 mutation results in Andersen syndrome with sex-specific cardiac and skeletal muscle phenotypes. *Am J Hum Genet* 2002;71(3):663–668.
7. Donaldson MR, Jensen JL, Tristani-Firouzi M, *et al.* PIP(2) binding residues of Kir2.1 are common targets of mutations causing Andersen syndrome. *Neurology* 2003;60(11):1811–1816.
8. Yoon G, Oberoi S, Tristani-Firouzi M, *et al.* Andersen-Tawil syndrome: Prospective cohort analysis and expansion of the phenotype. *Am J Med Genet A* 2006;140(4):312–321.
9. Zhang L, Benson DW, Tristani-Firouzi M, *et al.* Electrocardiographic features in Andersen-Tawil syndrome patients with KCNJ2 mutations: Characteristic T-U-wave patterns predict the KCNJ2 genotype. *Circulation* 2005;111(21):2720–2726.
10. Chun TU, Epstein MR, Dick M 2nd, *et al.* Polymorphic ventricular tachycardia and KCNJ2 mutations. *Heart Rhythm* 2004;1(2):235–241.
11. Venance SL, Cannon SC, Fialho D, *et al.* The primary periodic paralyses: Diagnosis, pathogenesis and treatment. *Brain* 2006;129(Pt. 1):8–17.
12. Tristani-Firouzi M. Polymorphic ventricular tachycardia associated with mutations in KCNJ2. *Heart Rhythm* 2004;1(2):242–243.
13. Wang Z, Yue L, White M, Pelletier G, Nattel S. Differential distribution of inward rectifier potassium channel transcripts in human atrium versus ventricle. *Circulation* 1998;98(22):2422–2428.
14. Zobel C, Cho HC, Nguyen TT, *et al.* Molecular dis section of the inward rectifier potassium curren (IK1) in rabbit cardiomyocytes: Evidence for heter omeric co-assembly of Kir2.1 and Kir2.2. *J Physic* 2003;550(Pt. 2):365–372.
15. Bendahhou S, Donaldson MR, Plaster NM Tristani-Firouzi M, Fu YH, Ptacek LJ. Defectiv potassium channel Kir2.1 trafficking underlie Andersen-Tawil syndrome. *J Biol Chem* 2003;27 (51):51779–51785.
16. Lopes CM, Zhang H, Rohacs T, Jin T, Yang J, Logo thetis DE. Alterations in conserved Kir channel PIP2 interactions underlie channelopathies. *Neuro* 2002;34(6):933–944.
17. Pegan S, Arrabit C, Slesinger PA, Choe S. Andersen' syndrome mutation effects on the structure an assembly of the cytoplasmic domains of Kir2.1 *Biochemistry* 2006;45(28):8599–8606.
18. Pegan S, Arrabit C, Zhou W, *et al.* Cytoplasmi domain structures of Kir2.1 and Kir3.1 show site for modulating gating and rectification. *Nat Neurosci* 2005;8(3):279–287.
19. Sanchez-Chapula JA, Salinas-Stefanon E, Torres Jacome J, Benavides-Haro DE, Navarro-Polanc RA. Blockade of currents by the antimalarial dru chloroquine in feline ventricular myocytes. *J Pharmacol Exp Ther* 2001;297(1):437–445.
20. Miake J, Marban E, Nuss HB. Biological pacemake created by gene transfer. *Nature* 2002;419(6903) 132–133.
21. Seemann G, Sachse FB, Weiss DL, Ptáček LP Tristani-Firouzi M. Modeling of IK1 mutation in human left ventricular myocytes and tissue *Am J Physiol Heart Circ Physiol* 2006:292(1):H549-559.
22. Silva J, Rudy Y. Mechanism of pacemaking ir I(K1)-downregulated myocytes. *Circ Res* 2003;92(3) 261–263.
23. Tsuboi M, Antzelevitch C. Cellular basis for electro cardiographic and arrhythmic manifestations o Andersen-Tawil syndrome (LQT7). *Heart Rhythm* 2006;3(3):328–335.
24. Reichenbach H, Meister EM, Theile H. [The heart-hand syndrome. A new variant of disorders of hear conduction and syndactylia including osseou changes in hands and feet]. *Kinderarztl Prax* 1992 60(2):54–56.
25. Marks ML, Whisler SL, Clericuzio C, Keating M. A new form of long QT syndrome associated with syndactyly. *J Am Coll Cardiol* 1995;25(1):59–64.
26. Splawski I, Timothy KW, Sharpe LM, *et al.* Ca(V)1.2 calcium channel dysfunction causes a multisystem disorder including arrhythmia and autism. *Cell* 2004;119(1):19–31.

27. Splawski I, Timothy KW, Decher N, *et al.* Severe arrhythmia disorder caused by cardiac L-type calcium channel mutations. *Proc Natl Acad Sci USA* 2005;102(23):8089–8096; discussion 8086–8088.
28. Jacobs A, Knight BP, McDonald KT, Burke MC. Verapamil decreases ventricular tachyarrhythmias in a patient with Timothy syndrome (LQT8). *Heart Rhythm* 2006;3(8):967–970.
29. Kuo A, Gulbis JM, Antcliff JF, Rahman T, Lowe ED, Zimmer J, Cuthbertson J, Ashcroft FM, Ezaki T, Doyle DA. Crystal structure of the potassium channel KirBac1.1 in the closed state. *Science* 2003; 300(5627):1922–1926.
30. Zuhlke RD, Bouron A, Soldatov NM, Reuter H. Ca2+ channel sensitivity towards the blocker isradipine is affected by alternative splicing of the human alpha1C subunit gene. *FEBS Lett* 1998;427(2):220–224.

36
Short QT Syndrome

Preben Bjerregaard and Ihor Gussak

Introduction

A prolonged QT interval has long been known to be a harbinger of life-threatening ventricular arrhythmias, and long QT syndrome is recognized as a hereditary condition with an increased risk of sudden cardiac death.[1] A short QT interval, on the other hand, was not considered arrhythmogenic and was seen mostly in relation to hypercalcemia.[2] This way of thinking changed after the first description in 2000 of a sporadic case of short QT interval and sudden cardiac death and of a family with short QT interval and paroxysmal atrial fibrillation (AF).[3]

In 2003, families with short QT interval and sudden cardiac death were described.[4] Despite being very rare, with only nine families and five sporadic cases identified so far, there has been great interest in the genetic and cellular electrophysiological characteristics, which can explain the high risk of atrial as well as ventricular fibrillation (VF) often seen as the initial presentation of the disease.

Definition and Terminology

By definition, any clinical syndrome is a combination of signs and symptoms that occur together and characterize a particular abnormality. In this context, short QT syndrome (SQTS) is best defined as a new inheritable, primary electrical heart disease that is characterized by a short QT interval (Figure 36–1) and paroxysmal atrial and/or ventricular tachyarrhythmias resulting from an accelerated cardiac (atrial and ventricular) repolarization due to congenital (genetically heterogeneous) cardiac channelopathies. It requires exclusion of patients with secondary short QT interval, and without documentation of associated arrhythmogenic complications in the patient or the patient's family a short QT interval is only an electrocardiogram (ECG) abnormality. Unexplained sudden cardiac death (SCD) in a family with members having SQTS is also considered a manifestation of SQTS.

Even though there is some debate about the upper limit of normal for the QT interval, a corrected QT interval >450 msec in males and >460 msec in females is generally considered prolonged. Numbers for the lower limit of normal are seldom given. Based upon data from the study by Rautaharju *et al.*,[5] we previously suggested that a *short QT interval* is <350 msec (two standard deviations below the mean predicted value) and an *abnormally short QT interval* is <320 msec (<80% of the mean predicted value), below which SQTS should be strongly considered.[6] In all published articles about SQTS to date, where the diagnosis was based upon an ECG in a symptomatic patient, the QT interval at a normal heart rate was ≤320 msec, but recent data (see later) suggest that some patients with SQTS may present with QT intervals longer than that. The QT interval is traditionally corrected for heart rate, but in patients with SQTS there are only minimal changes in the QT interval with a change in heart rate. Therefore, if the usual correction for heart rate is applied to the QT interval, in particular at fast heart rates, a diagnosis of SQTS may be missed. Corrected by Bazett's formula, at a heart rate of 130–140 beats/min, the corrected QT intervals in our patients were all >350 msec. To make a diagnosis of SQTS, the heart rate has to be <130 beats/min, and

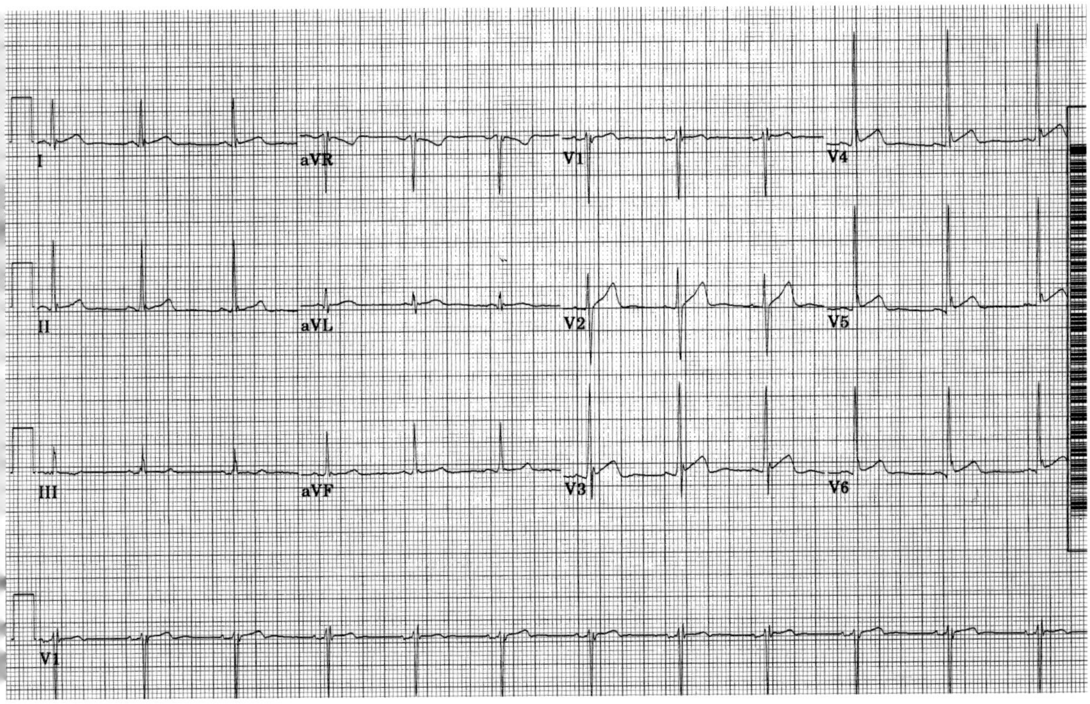

FIGURE 36–1. Twelve-lead ECG from a patient with SQTS based on a short QT interval and paroxysmal atrial fibrillation. The ECG shows sinus rhythm at a heart rate of 75 beats/min. The QT interval is 240 msec.

preferably <100 beats/min. This is particularly important to remember when dealing with children, whose heart rates are often fast, even at rest, and SQTS has been documented as the cause behind aborted SCD in an 8-month-old child and the likely cause for SCD in a 3-month-old child. Recently SQTS was diagnosed in a newborn with bradycardia *in utero* due to atrial fibrillation with a slow ventricular response.[7]

The first indication of the prognostic significance of a relatively short QT interval was from a study in 1993 by Algra *et al.*[8] Out of 6693 patients who underwent 24 h Holter monitoring and who were followed for 2 years, patients with a QTc <400 msec. had a 2.4-fold increase in sudden death rate compared to patients with a QTc of 400–440 msec. This was even more than patients with a QTc >440 msec, who had a 2.3-fold increase. Algra *et al.*[8] argued strongly that their finding could be a true pathophysiological phenomenon with a relative short QT interval possibly leading to life threatening arrhythmias.

Evidence that shortening of the QT interval may play a role in the occurrence of idiopathic ventricular tachycardia (VT) was provided by Fei and Camm in 1995.[9] Twenty-four hour Holter monitoring was used to detect 60 episodes of monomorphic repetitive VT in 10 patients. Analysis of three consecutive QT intervals immediately before the onset of VT found these QT intervals significantly shorter than the intervals measured 40 min before at the same heart rates (342 ± 34 vs. 353 ± 35 msec, $p < 0.001$). Of the 60 episodes, the QT intervals were shortened in 45 (75%) compared to the intervals 40 min earlier. The shortening was explained by sudden parasympathetic withdrawal leading to sympathetic predominance and thereby QT shortening. The shortening was considered to play an important role in the pathogenesis of idiopathic VF.

In 1999 we presented a case of paradoxic shortening of the QT interval to 216 msec during severe transient bradycardia in a child with recurrent cardiac arrest and discussed *deceleration-dependent shortening of the QT interval* as a trigger of arrhythmic events.[10] We proposed activation of Ik_{Ach} due to an unusually high vagal discharge to the heart as a possible mechanism responsible for both slowing of the heart rate and shortening of the QT interval.

Visken *et al.*[11] compared ECGs of 28 patients with *idiopathic VF* (17 men and 11 women, aged 31 ±17 years) to those of 270 age- and gender-matched healthy controls. They found that the QTc of males with idiopathic VF was shorter than the QTc of healthy males (371 ± 22 msec vs. 385 ± 19 msec, $p = 0.034$), and 35% of the male patients had QTc <360 msec (range 326—350 msec) compared to only 10% of male controls (345–360 msec). However, no such differences were found among women. They suggested that QTc intervals shorter than 360 msec might entail some arrhythmic risk.

Based upon there own observations Maury *et al.*[12] also suggested that the lower limit for the QT interval in patients with SQTS should be higher than the 300 msec seen in previously published cases. They presented a 15-year-old male with aborted SCD and QT interval ranging from 245 to 310 msec. Repeated ECGs in the patient's two brothers displayed QT intervals ≤300 msec in one sibling and 320 msec in the other. QT intervals in his mother varied between 300 and 320 msec. Ventricular arrhythmias could be induced during EP study only in the brother with the longest QT intervals, and he received a prophylactic ICD. As shown in Table 36–1, we have seen similar slightly

TABLE 36–1. Sporadic cases and families with short QT syndrome.

Reference	Age (years)	Gender	Short QT interval	SCD	Aborted SCD	AF[a]	QT	HR	QTc
Gussak *et al.*[3]	37	Female	Yes	Yes			266	52	248
	84	Male	Yes			Yes			
	51	Female	Yes			Yes	260	74	289
	21	Male				Yes	272	58	267
	17	Female	Yes			Yes	280	69	300
Gaita *et al.*[4]	35	Male	Yes			Yes	280	52	261
	31	Female	Yes				220	96	278
	6	Male	Yes		Yes (8 months)		260	92	322
	3 months			Yes					
	39	Male		Yes					
	49	Female		Yes					
	?	Female		Yes					
	39	Female		Yes					
	67	Female	Yes			Yes	270	72	324
	15	Male	Yes				260	80	300
	40	Female	Yes				240	75	268
	45	Female		Yes					
	62	Female	Yes	Yes		Yes	310	85	369
	26	Male		Yes					
Brugada *et al.*[14]	51	Male	Yes		Yes				288
	50	Male	Yes						293
Priori *et al.*[16]	5	Female	Yes						315
	35	Male	Yes						320
Anttonen *et al.*[17]	19	Male	Yes				280		313
	55	Male	Yes				310		307
	79	Male	Yes		Yes		280		
Riera *et al.*[18]	27	Yes				Yes	320		315
Maury *et al.*[12]	15	Male	Yes		Yes		283		340
	?	Male	Yes				<300		310–335
	?	Male	Yes				320		330–335
	?	Female	Yes				300–320		365
Kirilmaz *et al.*[19]	20	Male	Yes			Yes	300	54	<340
Hong *et al.*[7]	Newborn	Female	Yes			Yes	280		
Bjerregaard (unpublished observations)	13	Male	Yes		Yes		300	65	325
	15	Female	Yes				310	73	377
	38	Female	Yes				335	59	332
	56	Female	Yes				324	68	345
	21	Male	Yes		Yes		299	70	322
	60	Male	Yes				340	54	323
	25	Female	Yes				330	81	383

[a]SCD, sudden cardiac death; AF, atrial fibrillation.

longer QT intervals in family members of patients with SQTS among the two previously unpublished U.S. families; until more data become available, we would also consider that such patients have SQTS.[13–18] To this point, however, no genetic defect has been found in any of the cases with a QT interval greater than 300 msec labeled as SQTS.

It has been stated repeatedly that patients with SQTS show very little change in QT interval with a change in heart rate, and the question has been raised whether the QT/RR slope would be helpful in making the diagnosis of SQTS in questionable cases with QT intervals in the 310–350 msec range. The faster the heart rate, the more the QT interval in these patients will look normal. The QT/RR slope in normal subjects is generally from 0.12 to 0.17. In a study by Fujiki *et al.*[19] of patients with idiopathic VF in the setting of a normal QT, the average 24-h QT/RR slope was 0.09 compared to 0.14 in normal subjects. The calculated mean QT interval in these patients was 384 msec at 60 beats/min. Preliminary data from our study of 10 patients from four U.S. families including two studies of families not previously published (Table 36–1) have shown a similar result, suggesting that a QT/RR ratio <0.1 might be a way to distinguish between patients with short QT interval at risk for arrhythmic events and normal subjects with a QT interval at the lower level of normal.

Before making the diagnosis of SQTS it is important to exclude patients with *secondary short QT interval.* There are only few causes for a short QT interval, and it is a rare occurrence in normal clinical practice. It is well known, however, that hypercalcemia[2] can shorten the QT interval as well as hyperkalemia and hyperthermia. It is seen in acidosis and can occur immediately following ventricular fibrillation terminated spontaneously[20] or by a DC shock, most likely as a consequence of a high intracellular calcium level. Administration of acetylcholine and catecholamine will often shorten the QT interval out of proportion to the increase in heart rate, and early repolarization (Figure 36–2) is often accompanied by shortening of the QT interval.

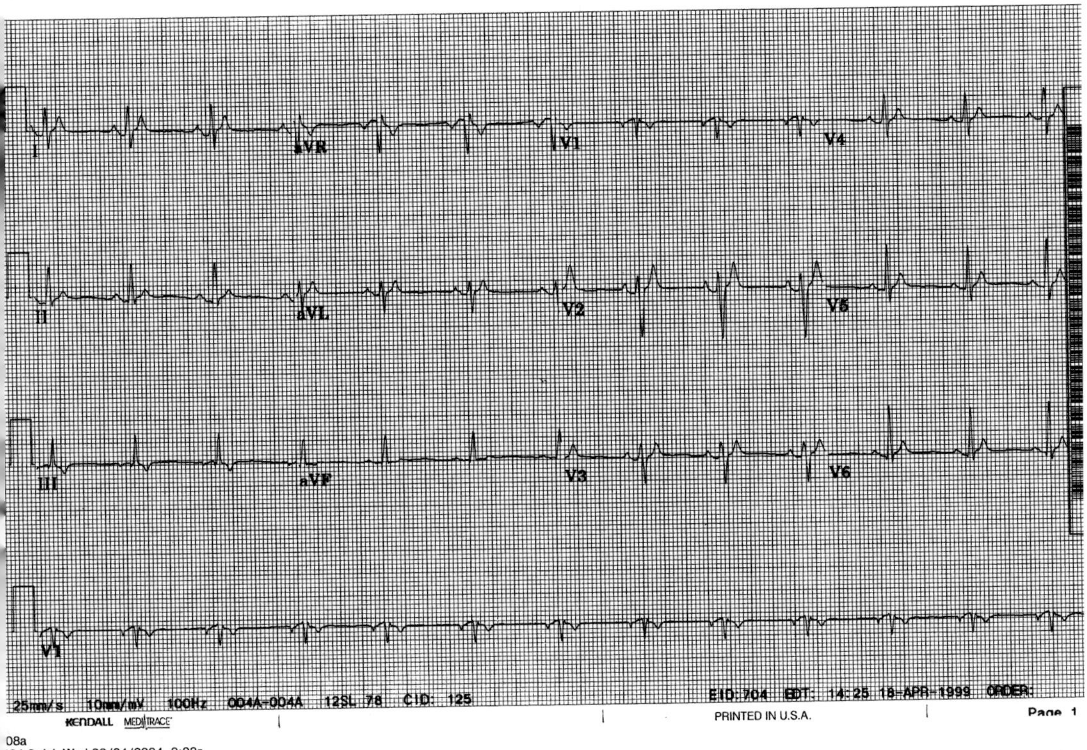

08a
304.8 dpi, Wed 08/04/2004, 9:22a

Figure 36–2. Twelve-lead ECG from an asymptomatic African-American male. The ECG shows sinus rhythm at a heart rate of 70 beats/min and early repolarization. The QT interval is most likely secondary to early repolarization.

History and Incidence

In February 1999, a 17-year-old white female developed atrial fibrillation with fast ventricular response while undergoing laparoscopic cholecystectomy. Her ECG showed an unusually short QT interval (225 msec), which was not explained by hypercalcemia. Further cardiac examination including Doppler echocardiography was normal. She had no history of palpitations, syncope, or dizziness and her family history was negative for SCD. Her only sibling (a 21-year-old brother) and her 51-year-old mother also had short QT intervals in their ECGs (240 and 230 msec, respectively), while her father's ECG was normal. It was later discovered that her maternal grandfather (born in 1914 and an immigrant from Italy) had a long-standing history of chronic AF and a similar short QT interval (245 msec).

This family and a 37-year-old Spanish woman, who suddenly died a few days after an ECG revealed a QT interval of 266 msec, formed the basis for the first description of SQTS.[3]

In addition to the four families with SQTS living in the United States, there are case reports from Italy, Germany, France, The Netherlands, Finland, Turkey, and Brazil (Table 36–1). Including the two unpublished studies of families from the United States, information is available about nine families and five sporadic cases of SQTS, with a total number of 41 patients with SQTS worldwide. Thirty-four patients have been diagnosed by short QT interval in the ECG and seven have been diagnosed by a combination of sudden cardiac death and a family history of SQTS.

Genetics, Etiology, and Mechanism

In the first two families from Europe with SQTS reported in 2004 by Gaita *et al.*,[4] two different missense mutations (C1764A and C1764G) were found to result in the same amino acid change (N588K) in the S5-P loop region of the cardiac I_{Kr} channel KCNH2 (human ether-à-go-go-related gene, hERG).[13] It was followed within the same year by a case report from France and the Netherlands of a 70-year-old male with idiopathic VF and a short QT interval in whom analysis of candidate genes identified a mutation (V307L) in the KCNQ1 gene encoding the I_{Ks} channel KvLQT1.[1] Another mutation (V141M) in the *KCNQ1* gene leading to SQTS was recently discovered in a newborn with bradycardia *in utero* secondary to atrial fibrillation with a slow ventricular response.[7] In 2005 a third genetic mutation was found in an Italian family with SQTS.[15] The defect was found in the gene encoding for the inwardly rectifying Kir2.1 (I_{K1}) channel. The affected members had a G514A substitution in the KCNJ2 gene resulting in a change from aspartic acid to aspargine at position 172. Meanwhile in 2005 the genetic mutation in the first reported family with SQTS from the United States initially published in 2000 had been determined.[21] It turned out to be the same as previously shown in the European family from Germany [missense mutation (C1764G) resulting in an amino acid change (N588K) in KCNH2]. A genetic mutation has been found in a total of 13 patients from five families with SQTS, but almost as many in other families with SQTS have undergone genetic screening without finding any mutation, which suggests that other genetic defects may be involved.

The three different mutations identified to date in patients with SQTS have all been investigated *in vitro*.[22] They all affect potassium channels leading to a gain in function with either a large increase in potassium current with failure to rectify at physiological membrane potentials, a shift in activation toward an earlier phase of the action potential, or an increased current accelerating the final phase of repolarization. The net effect is an abbreviation of the action potential and refractoriness. Shortening of refractoriness is one of the key elements in the reentry mechanism behind many tachyarrhythmias and is likely the main reason for the increased propensity to AF and VF seen in SQTS; however, it is also possible that the abbreviation of the action potential may affect different cells differently, leading to dispersion of refractoriness as an additional arrhythmogenic factor.[23] As pointed out by Cerrone *et al.*,[24] it is likely that the mechanisms that lead to electrical instability and eventually result in VF in patients carrying mutations in hERG or KvLQT1 would be different from those resulting from gain-of-function substitutions in Kir2.1. In the only patient monitored so far during the onset of spontaneous VF, where the SQTS was linked to mutations in hERG, the arrhythmia occurred during sleep following a premature beat with a very short coupling interval.[25]

Within the past year several cellular electrophysiological studies and computer models have focused upon the etiology behind arrhythmias in patients with SQTS.

Cordeiro *et al.*[26] measured the characteristics of hERG current generated by wild-type KCNH2 and the N588K mutant channel expressed in mammalian TSA201 cells. They found that the ventricular action potentials were preferentially reduced in SQTS, while the Purkinje fiber action potentials remained unchanged. This would lead to a shortening of the refractory period in the ventricles, but not in the Purkinje fibers. They suggested that the longer action potentials in the Purkinje fibers might reexcite the repolarized endocardial layer of the ventricles and thereby create tacharrhythmias. This may also explain the wider than usual separation between T and U waves seen in SQTS patients.

McPate *et al.*[27] examined at physiological temperature the importance of the S5-P linker for hERG channel function. They demonstrated that N588K–hERG contributes increased repolarizing current earlier in the ventricular action potential due to a ~+60 mV shift in voltage dependence of I_{hERG} inactivation. This explains the accelerated repolarization and short QT interval in some SQTS patients.

Weiss *et al.*[28] have been able to create a computer model of human cardiomyocytes that incorporates modifications in I_{Kr} as seen in some SQTS patients. They found a heterogeneous abbreviation of the action potential duration leading to a decreased dispersion of repolarization in heterogeneous tissue. Repolarization was homogenized and the final repolarization was shifted to epicardial sites.

Finally Tanabe *et al.*[29] have been able to create a model based upon fetal rat cardiomyocytes with overexpression of Kv1.5 leading to shortening of the action potential. They have suggested that this model can be used to study the arrhythmogenic substrate of SQTS.

Electrophysiological Findings

Atrial and ventricular-programmed electrical stimulation studies have been performed in eight patients with short QT interval.[4,15] In one patient the shortest coupling interval applied was 180 msec, with the ventricular effective refractory period (ERP) shorter than that, and no arrhythmias were induced. In the remaining seven patients, ERP was determined in both atria and ventricles. In five of these patients, ERP was found to be between 120 and 160 msec, while AF was induced in two patients. Atrioventricular (AV) node ERP was determined in two patients and was found to be 210 and 440 msec. Ventricular ERP was remarkably short and consistent in all seven patients (130–140 msec). Ventricular fibrillation was inducted in five patients and a monomorph VT (CI 150 msec) in one patient. A finding in patients with SQTS, which is quite rare in patients undergoing electrophysiological studies in general, was the induction of VF by catheter positioning in the right ventricle prior to programmed stimulation. It occurred in two patients (a 35-year-old male and a 31-year-old female) in the study by Gaita *et al.*[4] and in the 17-year-old girl from our first family.[3] Two of these patients had paroxysmal AF starting as a teenager, but none of them had experienced episodes of spontaneous ventricular tachyarrhythmias; this is, therefore, another indication of how little it takes for VF to occur in patients with SQTS.

Clinical Manifestations and Clinical Course

Out of the 14 probands with SQTS, 10 presented with either SCD or aborted SCD. Two presented as AF (one *in utero*) and one as a short QT interval in a routine ECG evaluation of a 5-year-old Italian girl. In one case the presentation was not mentioned.

In 1997, Brugada and Ardiaca observed the case of a patient who died a few days after an ECG revealed a QT interval of 266 msec (J. Brugada and A. Ardiaca, personal communication), but it was an article by Gaita *et al.*[4] that brought attention to the high incidence of SCD in members of two families with short QT interval. Both families were later found to have a hERG gene mutation. In one of the families, which was Italian, six members had died suddenly. Of those six, one had documented short QT interval. Two living members also were known to have short QT interval. In the other family, which was German, three members had died suddenly, one with documented short QT interval in an ECG taken prior to death. Two members of that family with short QT interval were alive. At the present time there are reports of 16 individuals with short QT interval who have either died suddenly or have been resuscitated with defibrillation following sudden collapse (Table 36–1). This places the short QT interval as one of the high risks for SCD, similar to other channelopathies such as Brugada syndrome and long QT syndrome. In addition, an episode of aborted SCD in an 8-month-old baby with short QT interval suggests that it may be one of the possible explanations for sudden death in infants.

In the first family with SQTS, the development of AF at a very early age led to the detection of a short QT interval. This patient was only 17 years old when she presented with recurrent AF, and her brother was 25 years old, when an asymptomatic episode of AF was detected by his implantable cardioverter defibrillator (ICD). Their mother at the age of 55 also had paroxysmal AF and their maternal grandfather had persistent AF for many years prior to his death at age 85. Four more patients with short QT intervals have been reported to have a history of AF (ages 27, 35, 62, and 67 years old), bringing the total number of reported cases to 8 out of 28 (29%) for whom such information is available.

Syncope and palpitations have been some of the other symptoms reported by patients with SQTS, but there are no studies in which such symptoms have been correlated with any arrhythmia.

Left anterior hemiblock has been observed in two asymptomatic subjects and right bundle branch block (RBBB) in two other, including the 25-year-old sister of a patient with SQTS and aborted SCD (Figure 36–3). Her QT interval at a heart rate of 54 beats/min was 340 msec, and she eventually received an ICD without further diagnostic testing. The occurrence of a conduction disturbance in 4 out of 37 young adults is more than expected, and suggests that it may be another consequence of the underlying channellopathy. The patients with left anterior hemiblock have a hERG mutation, whereas the mutation in patients with RBBB is unknown.

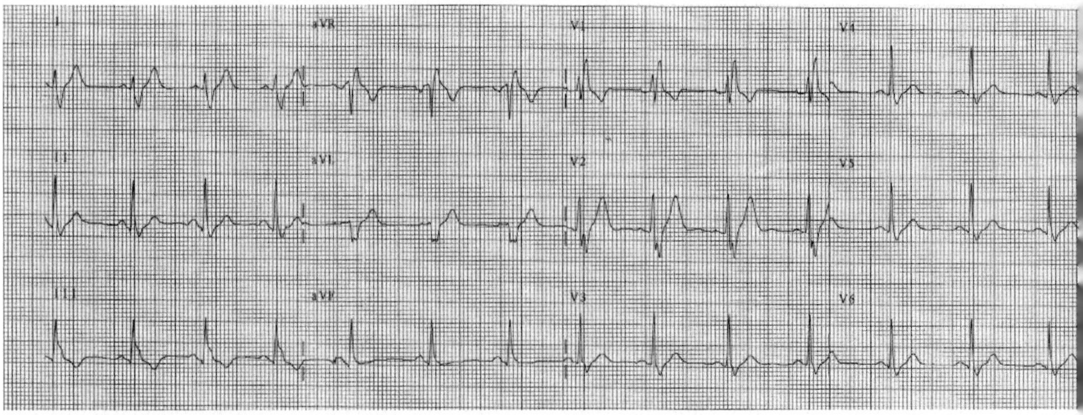

FIGURE 36–3. Twelve-lead ECG from an asymptomatic female with SQTS based on a short QT interval and a sibling with an aborted SCD due to SQTS. The ECG shows sinus rhythm at a heart rate of 81 beats/min, RBBB, and R axis deviation. The QT interval varies between different leads from 320 msec to 360 msec. Twenty-four-hour Holter monitoring showed a QT/RR slope of 0.1 both during the day and during the night, suggesting minimal variability in QT interval with changes in heart rate. The person had an ICD implanted for primary prevention of SCD.

Treatment

Antiarrhythmic therapy in patients with SQTS has mainly been necessary for paroxysmal AF and as primary prophylaxis against SCD. In patients with frequent shocks from an ICD or in whom an ICD is not implanted, medical therapy is needed as prophylaxis against VF. Due to the unknown risk of sudden cardiac death an ICD is currently offered to everyone with SQTS, but occasionally it is turned down or may be difficult to implement, as for instance in small children. Due to the low number of cases of SQTS, no controlled clinical trial of antiarrhythmic drugs has yet been done, and clinical experience is limited. Gaita *et al.*[30] tested the effect of several antiarrhythmic drugs (flecainide, sotalol, ibutilide, and hydroquinidine) on the OT interval in seven patients with SQTS. Flecainide caused a slight prolongation of the QT interval, primarily due to prolongation of the QRS complex, whereas sotalol and ibutilide had no effect on the QT interval. Hydroquinidine caused QT prolongation, with an increase in QT intervals from 263 ± 12 msec to 362 ± 25 msec and a normalization of rate adaptation of the QT interval; in addition, VF was no longer inducible. We have used propafenone in two patients with paroxysmal AF without recurrence of the arrhythmia for over 2 years. Propafenone had no prolonging effect on the QT interval.

Although abnormalities in three different potassium channels, (KCNH2, KCNQ1 and KCNJ2) have been recognized, it is only in 13 patients from five different families and is likely the main reason why molecular-target-based strategies for the management of the short QT syndrome have not yet been successfully developed. Clinical testing of such an approach would not be feasible. Since acceleration of repolarization due to gain-of-function mutations in cardiac potassium channels appears to be a common theme in the short QT syndrome, pharmacological blockade of potassium channels could serve as the basis for the development of antiarrhythmic strategy. Triggers and modulating factors that destabilize the underlying substrate of altered repolarization also form potential targets for drug development.[31]

Concluding Remarks

Short QT syndrome is the latest among a group of electrical diseases of the heart, easily diagnosed by an ECG, but likely missed quite often because of lack of knowledge about its existence and the difficulties many physicians still have in measuring the QT interval correctly and interpreting an abnormal interval. Despite a rather low number of patients with SQTS, it is remarkable how much interest there has been in many laboratories both in Europe and the United States in studying the mechanism by which a short QT interval is generated, and how it can lead to arrhythmias. The similarities with long QT syndrome have likely been a fascination to many.

Based upon the most recent cases of family members of aborted SCD victims with QT intervals between 320 and 350 msec, SQTS should be considered a possibility in anyone with a QT interval <350 msec and no evidence of secondary QT interval shortening. Any patient with AF at a young age or aborted SCD has to have the QT interval thoroughly scrutinized, and likewise members of families of victims of SCD. When a patient with SQTS is diagnosed with the disease it is very important that other family members are examined by electrocardiography. If it is difficult to obtain an ECG at a normal heart rate preferably close to 60 beats/min, a 24-h Holter monitor should be requested and the QT interval measured at different heart rates. A short QT interval combined with minimal variability in QT interval with changes in heart rate supports a diagnosis of SQTS.

SQTS is a very malignant disease, and anyone with that diagnosis should have an ICD implanted until a reliable medical alternative becomes available or we find ways to risk stratify these patients.

References

1. Ackerman MJ. The long QT ayndrome: Ion channel diseases of the heart. *Mayo Clin Proc* 1998;73:250–259.
2. Nierenberg DW, Ransil BJ. Q-aTc interval as a clinical indicator of hypercalcemia. *Am J Cardiol* 1979; 44:243–248.

3. Gussak I, Brugada P, Brugada J, Wright RS, Kopecky SL, Chaitman BR, Bjerregaard P. Idiopathic short QT interval: A new clinical syndrome? *Cardiology* 2000;94:99–102.
4. Gaita F, Giustetto C, Bianchi F, Wolpert C, Schrimpf R, Riccardi R, Grossi S, Richiardi E, Borggrefe M. Short QT syndrome. A familial cause of sudden death. *Circulation* 2003;108:965–970.
5. Rautaharju PM, Zhou SH, Wong S, Calhoun HP, Berenson GS, Prineas R, Davignon A. Sex differences in the evolution of the electrocardiographic QT interval with age. *Can J Cardiol* 1992;8:690–695.
6. Gussak I, Brugada P, Brugada J, Antzelevich C, Osbakken M, Bjerregaard, P. ECG phenomenon of idiopathic and paradoxical short QT intervals. *Card Electrophysiol Rev* 2002;6:49–53.
7. Hong K, Piper DR, Diaz-Valdecantos A, Brugada J, Oliva A, Burashnikov E, Santas-de Soto J, Grueso-Montero J, Diaz-Enfante E, Brugada P, Sachse F, Sanguinetti MC, Brugada R. De novo *KCNQ1* mutation responsible for atrial fibrillation and short QT syndrome in utero. *Cardiovas Res* 2005;68:433–440.
8. Algra A, Tijssen JG, Roelandt JR, Pool J, Lubsen J. QT interval variables from 24-hour electrocardiography and the two year risk of sudden death. *Br Heart J* 1993;70(1):43–48.
9. Fei L, Camm AJ. Shortening of the QT interval immediately preceding the onset of idiopathic spontaneous ventricular tachycardia. *Am Heart J* 1995;130(4):915–917.
10. Gussak I, Liebl N, Nouri S, Bjerregaard P, Zimmerman F, Chaitman BR. Deceleration-dependent shortening of the QT interval: A new electrocardiographic phenomenon? *Clin Cardiol* 1999;22:124–126.
11. Viskin S, Zeltser D, Ish-Shalom M, Katz A, Glikson M, Justo D, Tekes-Manova D, Belhassen B. Is idiopathic ventricular fibrillation a short QT syndrome? Comparison of QT intervals of patients with idiopathic ventricular fibrillation and healthy controls. *Heart Rhythm* 2004;1(5):587–591.
12. Maury P, Hollington L, Duparc A, Brugada R. Short QT syndrome: Should we push the frontier forward? *Heart Rhythm* 2005;2:1135–1137.
13. Brugada R, Hong K, Dumaine R, Cordeiro J, Gaita F, Borggrefe M, Menendez TM, Brugada J, Pollevick GD, Wolpert C, Burachnikov E, Matsuo K, Wu YS, Guerchicoff A, Bianchi F, Giustetto C, Schrimpf R, Brugada P, Antzelevich C. Sudden death associated with short-QT syndrome linked to mutations in HERG. *Circulation* 2004,109:30–35.
14. Bellocq C, van Ginneken ACG, Bezzina CR, Alders M, Escande D, Mannens MM, Baro I, Wilde AA. Mutation in the *KCNQ1* gene leading to the short QT-interval syndrome. *Circulation* 2004;109:2394–2397.
15. Priori SG, Pandit SV, Rivolta I, Berenfeld O, Ronchetti E, Dhamoon A, Napolitano C, Anumonwo J, Raffaele di Bartella M, Gudapakkam S, Bosi G, Stramba-Badiale M, Jalife J. A novel form of short QT syndrome (SQT3) is caused by a mutation in the KCNJ2 gene. *Circ Res* 2005;96:800–807.
16. Anttonen O, Kokkonen L, Huikuri H. Short QT syndrome as a cause of sudden cardiac death. *Duodecim* 2004;120(24):2915–2918.
17. Riera ARP, Ferreira C, Dubner SJ, Schapachnik E, Soares JD, Francis J. Brief review of the recently described short QT syndrome and other cardiac channelopathies. *Ann Noninvasive Electrocardiol* 2005;10(3):371–377.
18. Kirilmaz A, Ulusoy RE, Kardesoglu E, Ozmen N, Demiralp E. Short QT interval syndrome: A case report. *J Electrocardiol* 2005;38:371–374.
19. Fujiki A, Sugao M, Nishida K,Sakabe M, Tsuneda T, Mizumaki K, Inoue H. Repolarization abnormality in idioathic ventricular fibrillation: Assessment using 24-hour QT-RR and QaT-RR relationships. *J Cardiovasc Electrophysiol* 2004;15:59–63.
20. Kontny F, Dale J. Self-terminating ventricular fibrillation presenting as syncope: A 40-year follow-up report. *J Int Med* 1990;227:211–213.
21. Hong K, Bjerregaard P, Gussak I, Brugada R. Short QT syndrome and atrial fibrillation caused by mutation in KCNH2. *J Cardiovasc Electrophysiol* 2005;16:394–396.
22. Wolpert C, Schimpf R, Veltman C, Giustetto C, Gaita F, Borggrefe M. Clinical characteristics and treatment of short QT syndrome. *Expert Rev Cardiovasc Ther* 2005;3(4):611–617.
23. Extramiana F, Antzelevitch C. Amplified transmural dispersion of repolarization as the basis for arrhythmogenesis in a canine ventricular-wedge model of short-QT syndrome. *Circulation* 2004;110:3661–3666.
24. Cerrone M, Noujaim S, Jalife J. The short QT syndrome in a paradigm to understand the role of potassium channels in ventricular fibrillation. *J Int Med* 2006;259:24–38.
25. Schimpf R, Bauersfeld U, Gaita F, Wolpert C. Short QT syndrome: Successful prevention of sudden cardiac death in an adolescent by implantable cardioverter-defibrillator treatment for primary prophylaxis. *Heart Rhythm* 2005;2:416–417.
26. Cordeiro JM, Brugada R, Wu YS, Hong K, Dumaine R. Modulation of I_{Kr} inactivation by mutation N588K in KCNH2: A link to arrhythmogenesis in short QT syndrome. *Cardiovasc Res* 2005;67:498–509.

27. McPate MJ, Duncan RS, Milnes JT, Witchel HJ, Hancox JC. The N588K-HERG K^+ channel mutation in the "short QT syndrome": Mechanism of gain-in-function determined at 37 °C. *Biochem Biophys Res Commun* 2005;334:441–449.
28. Weiss DL, Seeman G, Sachse FB, Dossel O. Modelling of short QT syndrome in a heterogeneous model of the human ventricular wall. *Eurpace* 2005;7:S105–S117.
29. Tanabe Y, Hatada K, Naito N, Aizawa Y, Chinushi M, Nawa H, Aizawa Y. Over-expression of Kv1.5 in rat cardiomyocytes extremely shortens the duration of the action potential and causes rapid excitation. *Biochem Biophys Res Commun* 2006:345:1116–1121.
30. Gaita F, Giustetto C, Bianchi F, Schrimpf R, Haissaguerre M, Calo L, Brugada R, Antzelevitch C, Borggrefe M, Wolpert C. Short QT syndrome: Pharmacological treatment. *J Am Coll Cardiol* 2004;43: 1494–1499.
31. Bjerregaard P, Jahangir A, Gussak I. Targeted therapy for short QT syndrome. *Expert Opin Ther Targets* 2006;10(3):393–400.

37
Progressive Cardiac Conduction Disease

Jean-Jacques Schott, Flavien Charpentier, and Hervé Le Marec

Introduction

Cardiac conduction defect (CCD) is a serious and potentially life-threatening disorder.[1] It belongs to a group of pathologies with an alteration of cardiac conduction through the atrioventricular (AV) node, the His-Purkinje system with right or left bundle branch block, and widening of QRS complexes. CCD can lead to complete AV block and cause syncope and sudden death.[1,2] Originally CCD was considered a structural disease of the heart with anatomic changes in the conduction system underlying abnormal impulse propagation. In a substantial number of cases, however, conduction disturbances are found to occur in the absence of anatomical abnormalities. In these cases functional rather then structural alterations appear to underlie conduction disturbances. These functional defects are called "primary electrical disease of the heart."[3–6] The pathophysiological mechanisms underlying CCD are diverse, but the most frequent form of CCD is a degenerative form also called Lenègre–Lev disease[7,8] (idiopathic bilateral bundle branch fibrosis). Today Lenègre–Lev disease represents a major cause of pacemaker implantation in the world.

Familial clustering has been noted and published pedigrees show autosomal dominant inheritance with either early or late onset of AV conduction disease.

This chapter aims to briefly review the history of CCD and to focus on the recent molecular advances in isolated progressive cardiac conduction defect.

First Description of Cardiac Conduction Defect

Morgagni[9] was probably the first to associate recurrent fainting episodes in a man with a simultaneous observed slow pulse rate. In the nineteenth century Adams[10] and Stokes[11] made similar observations. The first known report of an Adams–Stokes attack combined with electrocardiographic (ECG) recordings came from van den Heuvel,[12] who described a case of congenital heart block. Lenègre[7] and Lev[8] combined ECG, clinical observations, and detailed post mortem studies of the heart and proved their direct relationship in the 1960s. The names of Lenègre and Lev became synonymous with progressive cardiac conduction defect (PCCD). Lenègre–Lev disease is characterized by progressive alteration of cardiac conduction through the His-Purkinje system with right or left bundle branch block (RBBB or LBBB) and widening of QRS complexes, leading to complete AV block and causing syncope and sudden death.[13–15] In both diseases a sclerodegenerative process causes fibrosis of the His-Purkinje system. The severity and extent of the fibrotic lesions differ in the descriptions of Lev and Lenègre. For Lenègre, histological studies identified diffuse fibrotic degeneration of the common trunk, the proximal and distal portions of the right and left branches, and the His bundle; the sinus node and the AV node remained unaffected. For Lev the sclerodegenerative abnormalities affect the specialized conduction system and the fibrous skeleton of the heart.[13–15]

Therefore PCCD is considered as a primary degenerative disease or an exaggerated aging process with sclerosis affecting only the conduction tissue even if an inherited component is involved.

Cardiac Conduction Defect a Genetic Disease?

Morquio[16] and Osler[17] are credited with the earliest reports of a familial disturbance in cardiac conduction. Although most reports of congenital heart block have concerned affected siblings (most of which may represent cases of congenital complete heart block due to circulating autoantibodies in the mother with lupus), two or more generations have been affected often enough to prove dominant inheritance.[18–20] In the family reported by Gazes *et al.*,[21] conduction disturbances occurred in three generations. In most of the affected persons the heart block was of second degree with episodes of third-degree (complete) AV block.

Identification of the First Locus for Cardiac Conduction Defect

Combrink *et al.*[22] described a South African large family in which the mother had RBBB and died at the age of 35 years from a Stokes–Adams attack. Of her four children, three had RBBB. The mother's parents both died suddenly in their 30 s. One of her brothers was suspected of having a cardiac conduction disturbance and another had dextrocardia; three other siblings were apparently normal. Follow-up of this kindred revealed RBBB in one of seven grandchildren. Steenkamp[23] described a South African family in which 6 of the 17 studied members showed rhythm or conduction disturbance. Brink and Torrington[24] suggested that the disorder, referred as type I progressive familial heart block (PFHB), is prevalent in South Africa and is the same disorder reported by Combrink *et al.*[22] and Steenkamp.[25] Type I heart block in their description tends to have the pattern of an RBBB and/or left anterior hemiblock, manifesting clinically when complete heart block supervenes with syncopal episodes or sudden death. In two studies, van der Merwe *et al.*[26,27] provided follow-up information on the kindred reported by Brink and Torrington[24] and documented progression of the disorder. They also reported a second type of CCD (PFHB type II) in which the onset of complete heart block is associated with narrow complexes. Electrocardiographic changes were bundle branch disease and AV nodal disease with an AV block and an idionodal escape rhythm.

In 1978, Stephan[28] described a large Lebanese family. Among the 209 patients included in the study, 31 were diagnosed with conduction defects and 3 were implanted with a pacemaker.[28] Within the family, conduction defects were mostly RBBB (12 patients), incomplete RBBB (7 patients), RBBB with left axis deviation (6 patients), RBBB with right axis deviation (4 patients), and complete AV block (2 patients).

In 1997 Stephan *et al.* reported a follow-up of a family spanning five generations composed of 47 patients with major CCD and 36 patients with minor CCD.[29] Conduction defects in this family were diagnosed early in life and were progressive in 5–15% of the patients, evolving to complete AV block.

Interestingly, in 1995, the Lebanese and South African families reported previously were both genetically mapped on chromosome 19q13.2–13.3,[30,31] representing the first locus for type I PFHB. The penetrance of the disease appears variable in the Lebanese families, whereas it was almost complete in the South African family. As of 2006, the disease-causing gene had not yet been identified.

Identification of the First Gene for Progressive Cardiac Conduction Defect

In 1999, our team described a large family with PCCD[32] (Figure 37–1A). Molecular genetics excluded the chromosome 19 locus and linkage analysis mapped the disease locus on chromosome 3 near the *SCN5A* gene encoding the cardiac-specific sodium channel Nav1.5. *SCN5A* was considered as a candidate gene and direct sequencing of affected members identified a splice donor site mutation in exon 22 of the *SCN5A* gene (IVS.22+2T->C) in 25 affected members.[32]

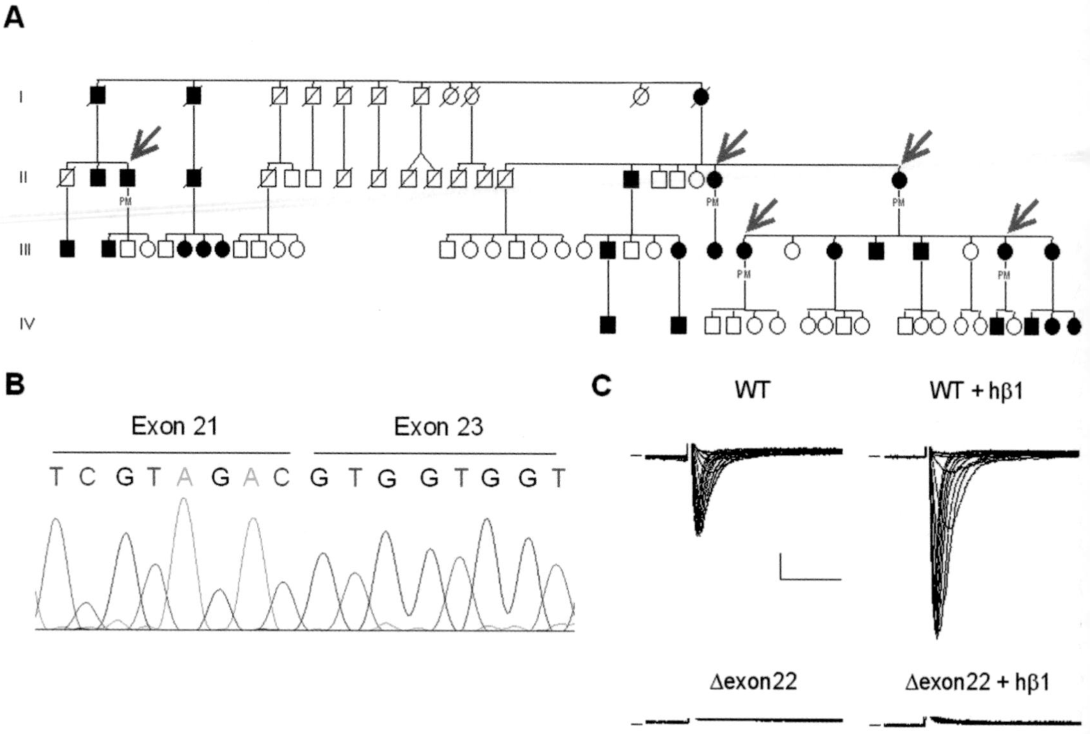

Figure 37–1. (A) Pedigree of the four-generation family with progressive cardiac conduction defect. Filled symbols: patients carrying the mutation or obligate carriers; open symbols: non-carriers. PM, patients with a pacemaker. (B) Sequence analysis of the splice product confirms exon 22 skipping in the mutant allele. (C) Functional experiments of the mutated gene product. Whole-cell patch-clamp recordings of wild-type *SCN5A* (top panel) and delta exon 22-*SCN5A* (bottom panel) in the absence or presence of the β_1 regulatory subunit. Holding potential, −100 mV. Depolarizing steps from −60 mV to +30 mV in 10-mV increments. Vertical bar = 0.5 nA. Horizontal bar = 5 msec.

Phenotypic Description of the Family

Familial and clinical investigation of this Lenègre pedigree started after the identification of a member with RBBB and syncope, a brother with RBBB, and a sister with complete AV block and syncope. Among the 65 family members included in the study, 15 had clinical and ECG abnormalities.[33] Familial investigation found all types of CCD in the family (Figure 37–2): RBBB was present in five, left bundle branch block (LBBB) in two, left anterior or posterior hemiblock in three, and long PR interval (more than 210 msec) in eight members. None had a structural heart disease. Five members had a pacemaker implanted because of syncope or complete AV block. A typical example of progressive development of a conduction defect in the same patient is shown in Figure 37–3. Electrocardiograms recorded in 1982, 1998, and 2000 show a progressive increase in QRS duration (QRS: 130, 140, and 172 msec).

Long-term follow-up of several affected members demonstrated that their conduction defects increased in severity with age. The age of the patients who participated to the study ranged from 15 to 81 years. We plotted conduction parameters in relation to age (see Figure 37–5A). Whatever the age, averaged and filtered P wave, PR, and QRS duration were longer in affected than in unaffected patients. There was a shift in the regression line for P wave and PR duration toward higher values in affected patients, whereas the slopes, expressed in milliseconds per year, were comparable in the two groups. In contrast, the QRS duration evolved differently in relation to

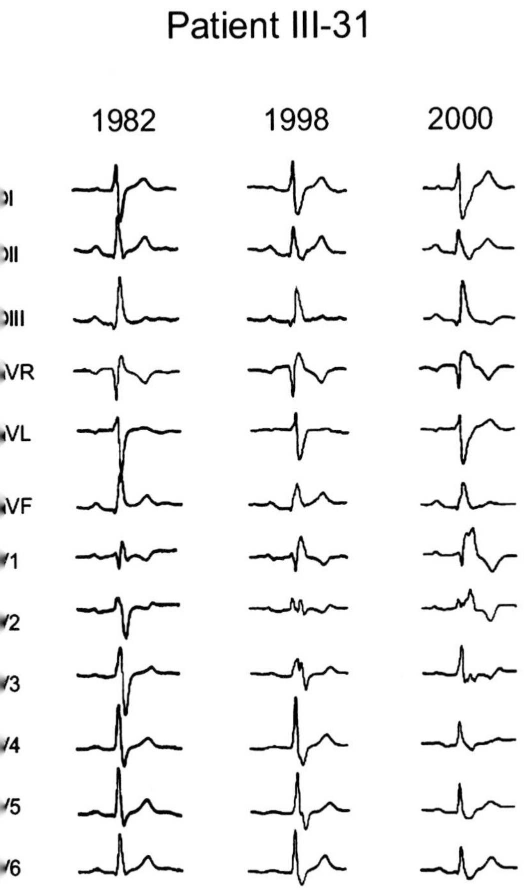

FIGURE 37–2. Serial electrocardiograms performed in patient III-31 showing progressive development of a conduction defect. Electrocardiograms recorded in 1982, 1998, and 2000 show a progressive increase in QRS duration (QRS: 130, 140, and 172 msec).

age between the two groups. There was a more pronounced QRS lengthening with age in affected than in unaffected patients. In addition, an age-dependent variability in the QRS duration was evidenced in the affected group.

These data demonstrate that conduction was already abnormal early in life in the absence of specific conduction defects, which are never observed before the age of 40 years. In the family, young affected patients have ECG parameters considered within "normal limits." Using the presence of selective conduction defects as a selective criteria, penetrance is complete only late during aging.

Pathophysiology of Progressive Cardiac Conduction Defect

Functional Consequences of the *SCN5A* Splice Mutation

The abnormal transcript is predicted to an in-frame skipping of exon 22 and an impaired gene product missing the voltage-sensitive DIIIS4 segment.[33] *In vitro* exon-trapping experiments of the mutated *SCN5A* IVS.22+2T→C gene confirmed skipping of exon 22 (Figure 37–1B).

Wild-type and exon 22-deleted Nav1.5 channels were expressed in COS-7 cells. Illustrative current traces show that Lenègre disease results from a loss-of-function mutation[33] (Figure 37–1C). Immunostaining in cells transfected with exon 22-deleted *SCN5A* suggests that the protein is correctly processed to the cell membrane.

Altogether, in this family, a supposed 50% reduction in sodium current is tolerated to some extent. The effect of the mutation becomes evident only later in age, when conduction in the heart becomes impaired because of the naturally occurring aging process. Interestingly the normal aging process usually involves sclerosis, although evidence is emerging (as described in the following section) that sclerosis is enhanced in carriers of loss-of-function *SCN5A* mutations.

An *Scn5a*$^{+/-}$ Mouse Model Mimics Lenègre Disease

The model used is the *Scn5a*-deficient mouse created by Andrew Grace's group at the University of Cambridge. In this model, exon 2 of the *SCN5A* gene was replaced with a splice acceptor (SA)-*Gfp*-PGK-neomycin cassette.

In the first phenotypic characterization of the *Scn5a* knockout mouse model, it was shown that disruption of the *scn5a gene* causes intrauterine lethality in homozygotes with severe defects in ventricular morphogenesis, whereas heterozygotes show normal survival. Whole cell patch-clamp analyses of isolated ventricular myocytes from 8- to 10-week-old heterozygote (*Scn5a*$^{+/-}$) mice demonstrated that the cardiac sodium current is reduced by about 50% as compared to wild-type mice. It was also shown that *Scn5a*$^{+/-}$ mice have several cardiac electrical defects including impaired AV conduction and delayed intramyocardial conduction (see Figure 37–5A).

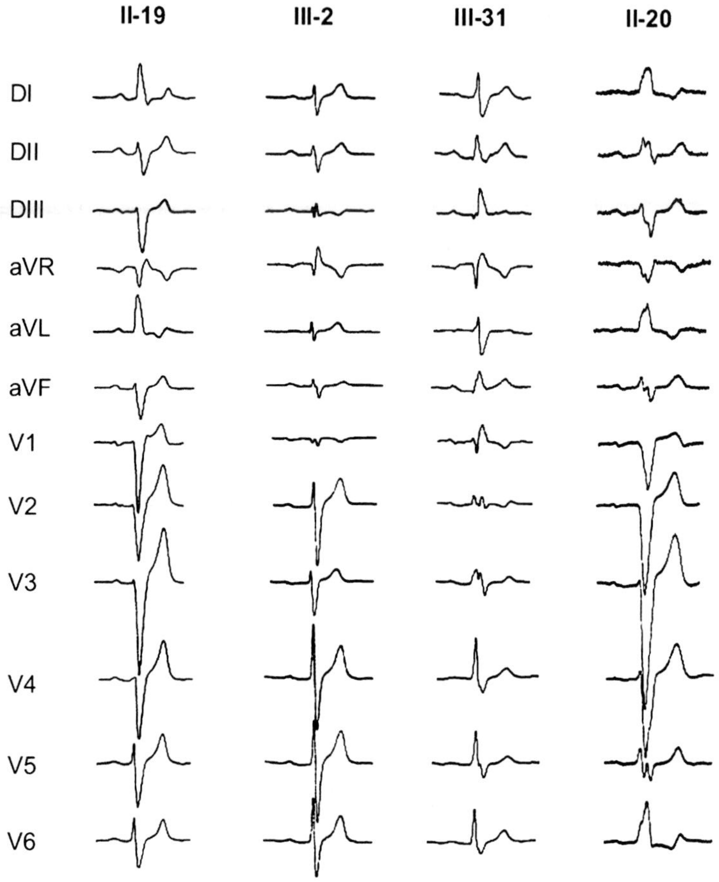

FIGURE 37–3. Examples of electrocardiogram patterns in affected members. Patient II-19 was a 70-year-old woman with parietal block and left-axis deviation [heart rate (HR), 64 beats/min; P, 144 msec; PR, 215 msec; QRS, 160 msec]. A pacemaker was implanted because of several episodes of syncope. Patient III-2 was a 49-year-old man with a parietal block and undetermined axis (HR, 54 beats/min; P, 150 msec; PR, 244 msec; QRS, 128 msec). Patient III-31 was a 48-year-old woman with right bundle branc block (HR, 64 beats/min; P, 153 msec; PR, 205 msec; QRS, 172 msec Sudden widening of QRS complexes and the occurrence of 2-1 A block during exercise led to pacemaker implantation. Patient II-2 was a 78-year-old woman with left bundle branch block (HR, 5 beats/min; P, 157 msec; PR, 248 msec; QRS, 196 msec). A pace maker was implanted after two episodes of syncope.

This first characterization suggests that *Scn5a*$^{+/-}$ mice could be a model for human cardiac pathologies linked to slow conduction. Since that first study, *Scn5a*$^{+/-}$ mice have been further characterized.[34,35] Based on ECG studies performed on *Scn5a*$^{+/-}$ and wild-type mice ranging in age from 4 to 71 weeks, it was shown that (1) the phenotype of *Scn5a*$^{+/-}$ mice worsens with age (Figure 37–4B), with the appearance of bundle branch blocks and a deviation of the cardiac axis; and (2) the phenotype of *Scn5a*$^{+/-}$ mice is highly variable, for instance, the QRS interval can vary from 15 mse (a normal value) to 35 msec (Figure 37–2B). Al these features are also found in human hereditar PCCD, suggesting that *Scn5a*$^{+/-}$ mice represent good model for hereditary Lenègre disease due t mutations in the *SCN5A* gene.[35]

Activation mapping performed in Langendorff perfused hearts showed that in young *Scn5a*$^{+/}$ mice, conduction velocity was affected only in th right ventricle. In old mice (50–75 weeks), righ ventricular conduction defects were furthe

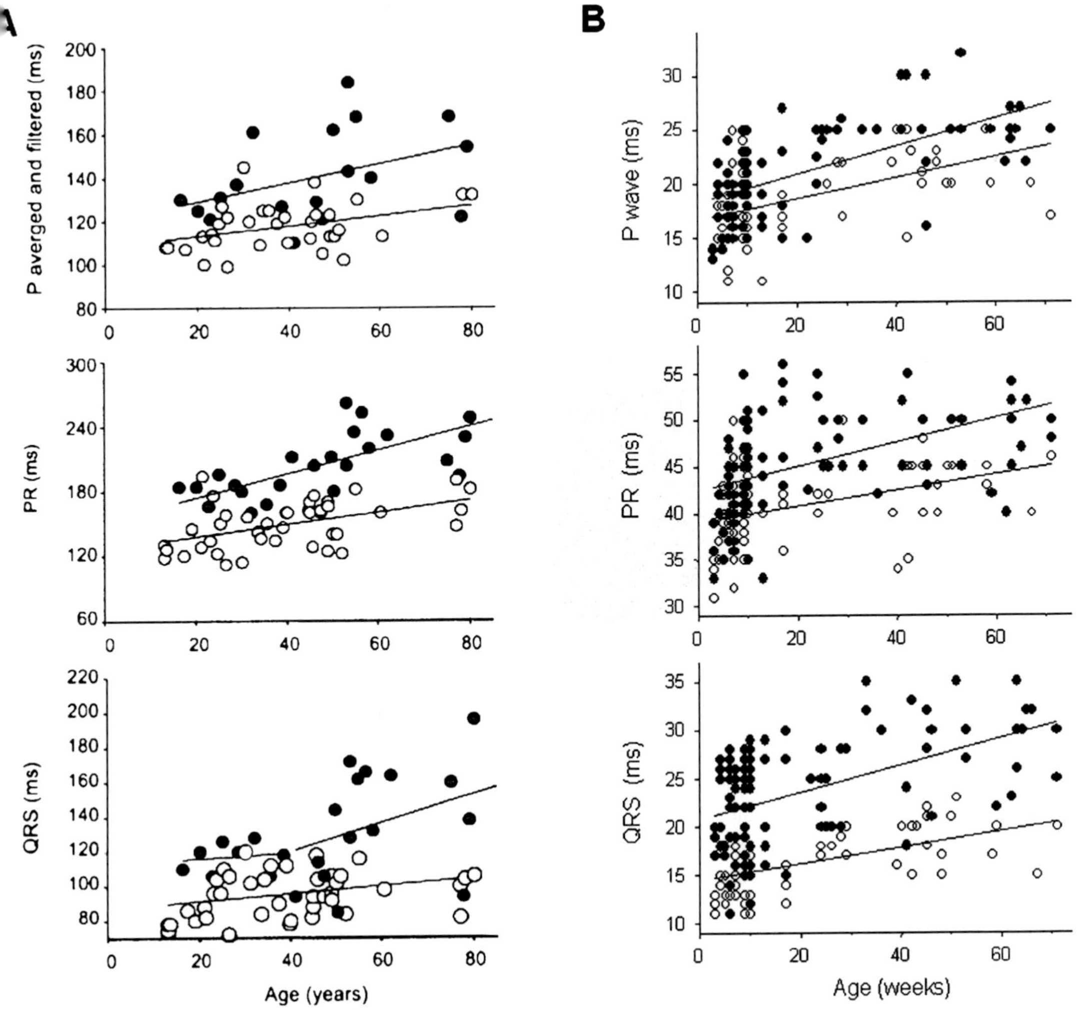

GURE 37–4. Evolution with aging of conduction parameters in umans and in an scn5a$^{+/-}$ knockout mouse model. (A) Evolution ith aging of conduction parameters in affected (filled symbols) nd unaffected subjects (open symbols). Top panel: Averaged and tered P wave duration. Middle panel: PR duration. Bottom panel: RS duration. In the top and middle panels, data were fitted with linear regression analysis. In the bottom panel, assessment of the residuals showed that the linear model was poorly adapted to fit the relationship between QRS duration and aging in affected members. The variance was significantly different before and after the age of 40 (ratio variance test; $p < 0.001$) and was indicative of a threshold effect of age. (B) Effects of age on P wave duration, PR interval duration, and QRS interval duration in wild-type (open symbols) and Scn5a$^{+/-}$ (filled symbols) mice.

ncreased and were associated with an alteration f conduction velocity in the left ventricle. urthermore, 50- to 75-week-old *Scn5a*$^{+/-}$ mice are haracterized by extensive ventricular fibrosis nd a redistribution of connexin43 expression Figure 37–5B). Finally, a downregulation of connexin40 atrial expression was also observed. These studies show that in the mouse model the disease seems to result from both a primary decrease in Na^+ current and secondary progressive fibrosis and remodeling of connexin expression with aging.

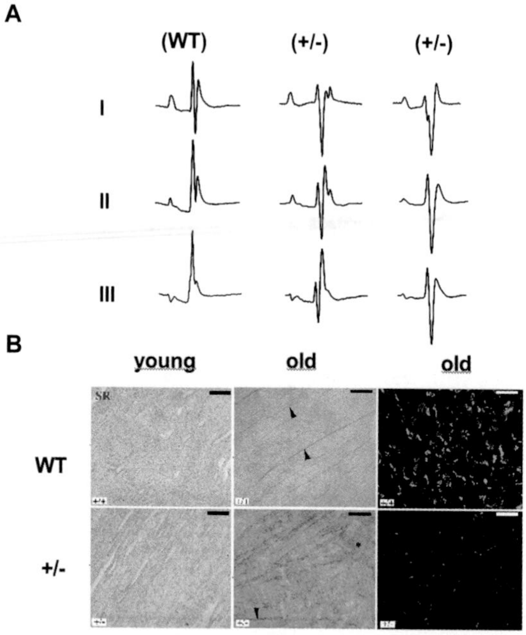

FIGURE 37–5. Surface ECG recordings and histology of wild-type and Scn5A$^{+/-}$ mice. (A) Surface ECGs in wild-type (WT) and Scn5a$^{+/-}$ mice. Representative ECG recordings (leads I, II, and III) in a WT and two different Scn5a$^{+/-}$ mice. (B) Ventricular fibrosis and expression of connexin43. Ventricular fibrosis (in red) in young mice (left) is almost absent in WT mice, which leaves the expression pattern of Cx43 unaffected. Fibrosis in old WT animals is increased in the interstitium between the muscle fibers, whereas locally massive fibrosis is observed in Scn5A$^{+/-}$ old animals. Fibrosis is accompanied by a downregulation and redistribution of Cx43 in old Scn5A$^{+/-}$ mice, whereas Cx43 in old WT hearts appears unaffected. Bar = 50 μm in panels showing Cx43 and 100 μm in those showing Sirius red.

Other Familial Forms of Cardiac Conduction Defects Linked to *SCN5A* Mutations

Since its first description in 1999, over a dozen reports have identified new *SCN5A* mutations causing PCCD or nonprogressive CCD, sometimes associated with dilated cardiomyopathy or arrhythmias (Figure 37–6).

In 1999, together with the first description of the Lenègre disease *SCN5A*-causing mutation, a second *SCN5A*-5280 del G frame shift mutation[32,36] was described in a Dutch family with nonprogressive conduction defect. The proband presented after birth with an asymptomatic first-degree A block associated with RBBB (PR interval and QR duration: 200 and 120 msec, respectively). Thre brothers were asymptomatic, one of whom ha RBBB (QRS duration: 110 msec). The asympto matic mother had an unspecified conductio defect (QRS duration: 120 msec).

In 2001, Tan *et al.*[37] provided a functional char acterization of an *SCN5A* mutation that causes sustained, isolated conduction defect with patho logical slowing of the cardiac rhythm. ECG find ings reported bradycardia, AV nodal escape and a broad P wave, long PR, and wide QRS By analyzing the *SCN5A* coding region, they re ported an *SCN5A*-G514C mutation in five affecte family members. Biophysical characterization c the mutant channel showed abnormal voltage dependent "gating" behavior.

In 2002, Wang *et al.*[38] described two new *SCN5* mutations that resulted in AV conduction bloc and that presented during childhood. Molecula genetic studies revealed a first *SCN5A*-G298 mutation in a proband with progressive AV bloc (QRS = 135 msec at age 9 and QRS = 133 msec a age 20). A second *SCN5A*-D1595N mutation wa identified in a proband with complete heart bloc at the age of 12 years. The functional consequence of the two mutations are impaired fast inactiva tion but not sustained noninactivating current The mutations reduce sodium current density an enhance slow inactivation components.

In 2003, Bezzina *et al.*[39] described a family i which the proband was born in severe distres with irregular wide complex tachycardia. An olde sister died at 1 year of age from severe conductio disease with similarly widened QRS complexes Mutational analysis in the proband demonstrate compound heterozygosity for a nonsense *SCN5A* W156X mutation, inherited from the father, an an *SCN5A*-R225W missense mutation, inherite from the mother. Expression studies showed tha the W156X mutation is a loss-of-function muta tion, whereas the R225W mutation leads to a severe reduction in current density and is als associated with gating changes. Histologica examination of the heart from the deceased siblin revealed changes consistent with a dilated type o cardiomyopathy and severe degenerative abnor malities of the specialized conduction system These morphological changes may have occurre

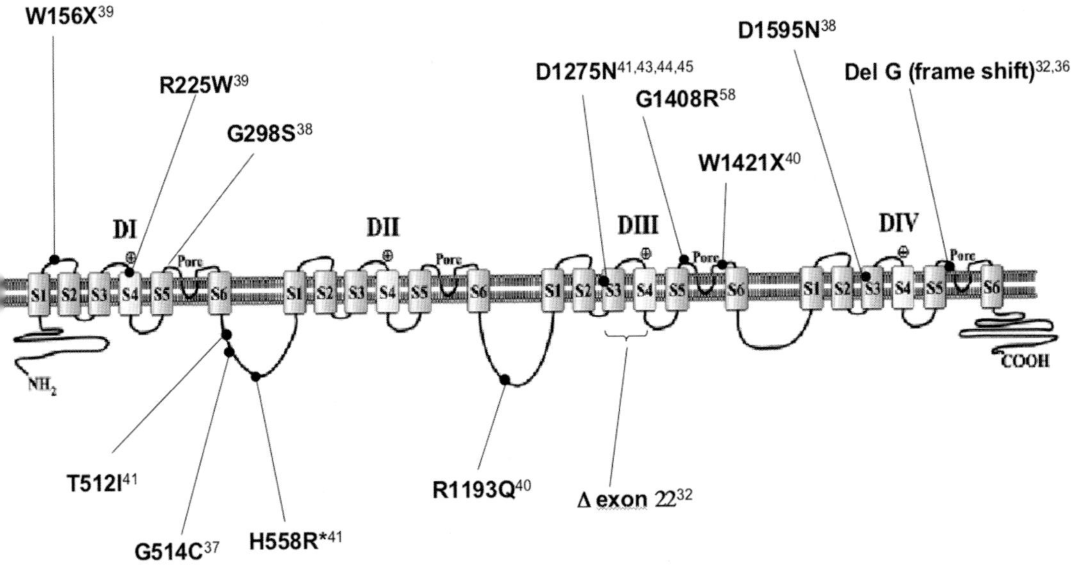

IGURE 37–6. *SCN5A* diagram with location of previously identified *SCN5A* mutations resulting in conduction system disease (*common olymorphism).

econdary to the sodium channel abnormality nd contributed to the severity of the disorder in his individual.

In 2006, Niu *et al.*[40] described a novel *SCN5A*-V1421X mutation in a four-generation family vith cardiac conduction abnormalities and several ases of sudden death. Most family members who arry this W1421X mutation have developed najor clinical manifestations. However, in a 73-ear-old grandfather, who carried the *SCN5A*-V1421X mutation, a second *SCN5A*-R1193Q ariant was identified. This patient has remained ealthy and presents only minor ECG abnormalities, whereas most of his siblings, who carried a ingle mutation (W1421X), had died early or had najor disease manifestations. This observation uggests that the R1193Q mutation has a complenentary role in alleviating the deleterious effects onferred by W1421X in the function of the *SCN5A* gene. This report provides a good example f the mechanism of penetrance of genetic lisorders.

The work of Viswanathan *et al.*[41] provides a econd illustration of phenotypic modulation by n *SCN5A* polymorphism. They identified a noel mutation, *SCN5A*-T512I, in a 2-year-old boy liagnosed with second-degree AV conduction lock. The T512I mutation, when heterologously expressed, causes hyperpolarizing shifts in activation and inactivation, and enhances slow inactivation. However, the common *SCN5A*-H558R polymorphism also found in this child had no effect on the wild-type sodium current but attenuated the gating effects caused by the T512I mutation. The polymorphism entirely restored the voltage-dependent activation and inactivation voltage shifts caused by the T512I mutation, and partially restored the kinetic features of slow inactivation. This mutation and the H558R polymorphism were both found in the same allele of the child with isolated conduction disease, suggesting a direct functional association between a polymorphism and a mutation in the same gene.

Four reports identified the same *SCN5A*-D1275N mutation associated with CCD and various cardiac arrhythmias or structural cardiomyopathies.

In 2003, Groenewegen *et al.*[42] described an *SCN5A*-D1275N mutation cosegregating with two connexin40 genotypes [(−44 (G→A) and +71 (A→G)] in familial atrial standstill (AS). *SCN5A*-D1275N channels show only a small depolarizing shift in activation compared with wild-type channels. It was proposed that although the functional effect of each genetic change is relatively benign, the combined effect of genetic changes eventually progresses to total atrial standstill. More recently, an *SCN5A*-L212P mutation associated with the same connexin40 polymorphism combination was reported in another atrial standstill family.[43]

In 2004, McNair WP *et al.*[44] described a large family diagnosed with CCD associated with sinus node dysfunction, arrhythmia, and right and occasionally left ventricular dilatation and dysfunction. Screening family members for mutations identified an *SCN5A*-D1275N defect. This finding expands the clinical spectrum of disorders of the cardiac sodium channel to cardiac dilation and dysfunction and supports the hypothesis that genes encoding ion channels can be implicated in dilated cardiomyopathies.

In 2005, Olson *et al.*[45] described an *SCN5A*-D1275N mutation associated with susceptibility to heart failure and atrial fibrillation.

In 2006, Laitinen-Forsblom *et al.*[46] described five family members with atrial arrhythmias and intracardiac conduction defects. Interestingly, left ventricle dilatation was also seen in one individual and three individuals had a slightly enlarged right ventricle. Premature death due to stroke occurred in one subject, and two other members had suffered from stroke at a young age. Direct sequencing disclosed a *SCN5A*-D1275N mutation. This alteration was present not only in all affected individuals, but also in two young individuals lacking clinical symptoms.

Conduction Defects in Other Syndromes

Besides isolated PCCD, many diseases such as dilated or restrictive cardiomyopathies are associated with CCD.[47,48] Mutations in the *NKX2-5* gene (cardiac-specific homeo box) have been reported in association with septal defects[49] as well as with a much wider clinical spectrum including ventricular septal defects and tetralogy of Fallot.[50] Mutations in the *LMNA A/C* gene encoding lamin were found to be causally involved in Emery–Dreiffus muscular dystrophy[51] as well as in families with dilated cardiomyopathies and severe CCD without skeletal muscle involvement.[51–53] Finally, mutations in the *PRKAG2* gene encoding a noncatalytic, gamma-2 subunit of an AMP-activated protein kinase were found in patients with Wolf–Parkinson–White syndrome, a disease characterized by ventricular preexcitation, atrial fibrillation, and CCD.[54]

Lenègre Disease and Brugada Syndrome: An Overlap Syndrome?

Brugada syndrome (BS) is a genetically inherited arrhythmogenic disorder characterized by an ECG pattern of ST segment elevation in the right precordial leads and an increased risk of sudden cardiac death resulting from episodes of polymorphic ventricular tachyarrhythmias and fibrillation.[55] Loss-of-function mutations in the *SCN5A* gene account for about 20% of BS.[56]

An intriguing overlap exists between Lenègre disease and BS: (1) decreased availability of the sodium channel accounts for both clinical entities; (2) we have previously described a family in which the same G1408R *SCN5A* mutation leads to BS or Lenègre disease depending on the familial branches;[57] and (3) in preceding work, we and others have shown that BS *SCN5A*-linked probands have an impaired cardiac conduction when compared to BS patients not related to *SCN5A*. Finally, sodium channel blockers have been shown to induce a more pronounced QRS widening in Brugada patients.[58,59]

We characterized a cardiac conduction defect in relation to aging in a cohort of 78 individuals carrying an *SCN5A* mutation associated with BS in their pedigree.[60] In this population, the penetrance of the spontaneous Brugada syndrome phenotype is low (36%), whereas the penetrance of conduction defects is high (76%), consistent with the recent report by Hong *et al.*[61] *SCN5A* BS-type mutation carriers exhibit various degrees of cardiac conduction defects. This phenotype is similar to that of hereditary Lenègre disease. As in Lenègre disease, we found various types of conduction defects in *SCN5A* BS-type mutation carriers, although with clear predominance of RBBB and parietal block. When conduction parameters were plotted in relation to age, PR and QRS interval durations were longer in gene carriers than in noncarriers regardless of age. The interaction between age and PR interval is not significant, whereas the interaction between age and QRS interval is highly significant, showing a progressive alteration of intraventricular conduction (Figure 37–7).

IGURE 37–7. Evolution with aging of onduction parameters in affected (solid mbols) and unaffected (open symbols) ubjects. (A) PR interval. (B) QRS duration. egardless of age, PR and QRS duration as longer in mutated patients. The interction between age and PR interval was ot significant, whereas the interaction etween age and QRS interval reached gnificance ($p = 0.0057$), showing a proressive alteration of the intraventricular onduction with age.

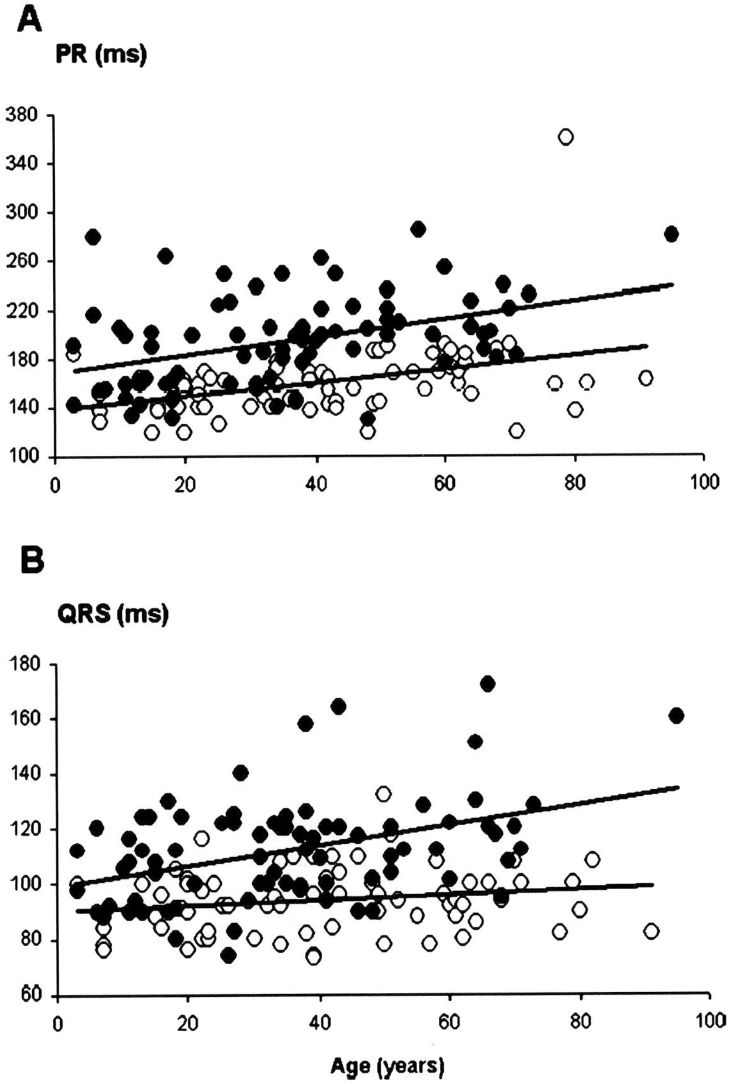

In this study, the conduction defects worsen vith age in the *SCN5A* BS-type mutation carriers egardless of their BS phenotype and lead in five ases of pacemaker implantation. Thus, the conluction phenotype of BS-type and Lenègre-type *SCN5A* mutation carriers is indistinguishable. This positive correlation between the age and the progression of the conduction defect was found at a single time point, and only a follow-up of patients for a long period of time could definitively prove the progressive evolution of the conluction defects with aging. Longitudinal follow-up as been achieved in the *Scn5aA*$^{+/-}$ mouse and firmly demonstrates slow progression of the conduction defect with aging.

Nevertheless, Lenègre disease and Brugada syndrome remain distinct entities with a different arrhythmic risk. Indeed, with programmed electrical stimulation, we were unable to provoke VF or ventricular tachycardia in gene carriers without a BS phenotype, whereas 33% of the investigated patients with the Brugada phenotype experienced polymorphic ventricular tachycardia or ventricular fibrillation. These observations, despite an overlap of Lenègre and BS, further support the concept that Lenègre disease differs from BS not only because of the absence of ST-segment elevation, but also because the risk for life-threatening ventricular arrhythmias remains a major characteristic of BS.

Conclusions

Progressive CCD, also called Lenègre–Lev disease, is a frequently occurring disease with an expected increasing prevalence given the general aging of the population. It is a heritable heterogeneous condition of mostly unknown origin. It is likely that the most common form of PCCD has a mutifactorial origin, combining environmental and genetic factors. However, in some cases, familial PCCD with a monogenetic origin has been described. Today, a single gene encoding the cardiac-specific sodium channel *SCN5A* has been identified. Since its original description in 1999, many *SCN5A* mutations leading to either progressive or nonprogressive CCD have been reported. Genotype–phenotype studies reveal that in addition to variable penetrance, generally described in almost all monogenic diseases, *SCN5A* mutation carriers exhibit a wide phenotypic spectrum, associating structural cardiomyopathies and arrhythmias. The study of an scn5a-haploinsufficiency mouse model mimicking Lenègre's disease provides a unique opportunity to understand the underlying pathophysiological bases of Lenègre disease. It already appears that the disease-causing mechanism due to a single channel defect is a consequence of a complex remodeling process and not just a slowing of the propagation of the electrical impulse through the conduction system. Increased fibrosis in *Scn5A* heterozygous mice reconciles the original description of Lenègre and Lev in which a combination of aging and fibrosis explains the progressive alteration in conduction velocity.

Today pacemaker implantation constitutes the only therapeutic treatment used to prevent sudden death in PCCD. It is conceivable that in the near future, once the precise pathophysiological mechanism of PCCD is identified, less invasive approaches will become available improving patient management.

References

1. Michaelsson M, Jonzon A, Riesenfeld T. Isolated congenital complete atrioventricular block in adult life. A prospective study. *Circulation* 1995;92(3): 442–449.
2. Balmer C, Fasnacht M, Rahn M, *et al.* Long-term follow up of children with congenital complete atrioventricular block and the impact of pacemaker therapy. *Europace* 2002;4(4):345–349.
3. Tan HL, Bezzina CR, Smits JP, Verkerk AO, Wilde AA. Genetic control of sodium channel function. *Cardiovasc Res* 2003;57(4):961–973.
4. Roden DM, Balser JR, George AL Jr, *et al.* Cardiac ion channels. *Annu Rev Physiol* 2002;64:431–475.
5. Roden DM, George AL Jr. Structure and function of cardiac sodium and potassium channels. *Am J Physiol* 1997;273(2 Pt 2):H511–525.
6. Benson DW. Genetics of atrioventricular conduction disease in humans. *Anat Rec A Discov Mol Cell Evol Biol* 2004;280(2):934–939 (review).
7. Lenegre J. The pathology of complete atrioventricular block. *Prog Cardiovasc Dis* 1964;6:317–323.
8. Lev M, Kinare SG, Pick A. The pathogenesis of complete atrioventricular block. *Prog Cardiovasc Dis*1964;6:317–326.
9. Morgagni GB. De sedibus, et causis morborum per anatomen indagatis libri quinque. 2 volumes. In 1. Venetis, typ. Remondiniana 1761.
10. Adams R. Cases of disease of the heart, accompanied with pathological observation. *Dublin Hosp Rep* 1827;4:353–453.
11. Stokes W. Observations on some cases of permanently slow pulse. *Q J Med Sci* 1846;2:73–85.
12. van den Heuvel GCJ. Die ziekte van Stokres-Adams en een geval van aangeborne hart blok. Groningen, 1908.
13. Lev M, Kinare SG, Pick A. The pathogenesis of atrioventricular block in coronary disease. *Circulation* 197;42:409–425.
14. Bharati S, Lev M, Dhingra RC, *et al.* Electrophysiologic and pathologic correlations in two cases of chronic second degree atrioventricular block with left bundle branch block. *Circulation* 1975;52(2): 221–229.
15. Lev M, Cuadros H, Paul MH. Interruption of the atrioventricular bundle with congenital atrioventricular block. *Circulation* 1971;43(5):703–710.
16. Morquio L. Sur une maladie infantile et familiale caracterisee par des modifications permanentes du pouls, des attaques syncopales et epileptiformes et la mort subite. *Arch Med Enfants* 1901;4:467–475.

7. Osler W. On the so-called Stokes-Adams disease. *Lancet* II 1903;516–524.
8. Fulton ZMK, Judson, CF, Norris GW. Congenital heart block occurring in a father and two children, one an infant. *Am J Med Sci* 1910;140:339–348.
9. Wallgren A, Winblad S. Congenital heart-block. *Acta Paediatr* 1937;20:175–204.
0. Wendkos MH. Familial congenital complete A-V heart blocks. *Am Heart J* 1947;34:138–142.
1. Gazes PC, Culler RM, Taber E, *et al.* Congenital familial cardiac conduction defects. *Circulation* 1965;32:32–34.
2. Combrink JMD, Davis WH, Snyman HW. Familial bundle branch block. *Am Heart J* 1962;64:397–400.
3. Steenkamp WF. Familial trifascicular block. *Am Heart J* 1972;84:758–760.
4. Brink AJ, Torrington M. Progressive familial heart block—two types. *S Afr Med J* 1977;52:53–59.
5. Steenkamp WF. Familial trifascicular block. *Am Heart J* 1972;84(6):758–760.
6. Van der Merwe PL, Weymar HW, Torrington M, Brink AJ. Progressive familial heart block. Part II. Clinical and ECG confirmation of progression–report on 4 cases. *S Afr Med J* 1986;70(6):356–357.
7. Van der Merwe PL, Weymar HW, Torrington M, Brink AJ. Progressive familial heart block (type I). A follow-up study after 10 years. *S Afr Med J* 1988;73:275–276.
8. Stephan E. Hereditary bundle branch system defect: Survey of a family with four affected generations. *Am Heart J* 1978;95:89–95.
9. Stephan E, de Meeus A, Bouvagnet P. Hereditary bundle branch defect: Right bundle branch blocks of different causes have different morphologic characteristics. *Am Heart J* 1997;133:249–256.
0. Brink PA, Ferreira A, Moolman JC, *et al.* Gene for progressive familial heart block type I maps to chromosome 19q13. *Circulation* 1995;91:1633–1640.
1. de Meeus A, Stephan E, Debrus S, Jean MK, Loiselet J, Weissenbach J, Demaille J, Bouvagnet P. An isolated cardiac conduction disease maps to chromosome 19q.*Circ Res* 1995;77(4):735–740.
2. Schott JJ, Alshinawi C, Kyndt F, *et al.* Cardiac conduction defects associate with mutations in *SCN5A*. *Nat Genet* 1999;23:20–21.
3. Probst V, Kyndt F, Potet F, *et al.* Haploinsufficiency in combination with aging causes SCN5A-linked hereditary Lenegre disease. *J Am Coll Cardiol* 2003; 41(4):643–652.
4. Van Veen TA, Stein M, Royer A, *et al.* Impaired impulse propagation in Scn5a-knockout mice: Combined contribution of excitability, connexin expression, and tissue architecture in relation to aging. *Circulation* 2005;112(13):1927–1935.
35. Royer A, van Veen TA, Le Bouter S, *et al.* Mouse model of SCN5A-linked hereditary Lenegre's disease: Age-related conduction slowing and myocardial fibrosis.*Circulation* 2005;111(14):1738–1746.
36. Herfst LJ, Potet F, Bezzina CR, *et al.* Na+ channel mutation leading to loss of function and non-progressive cardiac conduction defects. *J Mol Cell Cardiol* 2003;35(5):549–557.
37. Tan HL, Bink-Boelkens MT, Bezzina CR, *et al.* A sodium-channel mutation causes isolated cardiac conduction disease. *Nature* 2001;409:1043–1047.
38. Wang DW, Viswanathan PC, Balser JR, *et al.* Clinical, genetic, and biophysical characterization of *SCN5A* mutations associated with atrioventricular conduction block. *Circulation* 2002;105:341–346.
39. Bezzina CR, Rook MB, Groenewegen WA, *et al.* Compound heterozygosity for mutations (W156X and R225W) in *SCN5A* associated with severe cardiac conduction disturbances and degenerative changes in the conduction system. *Circ Res* 2003; 92:159–168.
40. Niu DM, Hwang B, Hwang HW, *et al.* A common SCN5A polymorphism attenuates a severe cardiac phenotype caused by a non-sense SCN5A mutation in a Chinese family with an inherited cardiac conduction defect. *J Med Genet* 2006;43(10):817–821.
41. Viswanathan PC, Benson DW, Balser JR. A common SCN5A polymorphism modulates the biophysical effects of an SCN5A mutation. *J Clin Invest* 2003; 111(3):341–346.
42. Groenewegen WA, Firouzi M, Bezzina CR, *et al.* A cardiac sodium channel mutation cosegregates with a rare connexin40 genotype in familial atrial standstill. *Circ Res* 2003;92(1):14–22.
43. Makita N, Sasaki K, Groenewegen WA, *et al.* Congenital atrial standstill associated with coinheritance of a novel SCN5A mutation and connexin 40 polymorphisms. *Heart Rhythm* 2005;2(10):1128–1134.
44. McNair WP, Ku L, Taylor MR, *et al.* SCN5A mutation associated with dilated cardiomyopathy, conduction disorder, and arrhythmia. *Circulation* 2004;110(15):2163–2167.
45. Olson TM, Michels VV, Ballew JD, *et al.* Sodium channel mutations and susceptibility to heart failure and atrial fibrillation. *JAMA* 2005;293(4): 447–454.
46. Laitinen-Forsblom PJ, Makynen P, Makynen H, *et al.* SCN5A mutation associated with cardiac

conduction defect and atrial arrhythmias. *J Cardiovasc Electrophysiol* 2006;17(5):480–485.

47. Hanson EL, Jakobs PM, Keegan H, *et al.* Cardiac troponin T lysine 210 deletion in a family with dilated cardiomyopathy. *J Card Fail* 2002;8:28–32.
48. Oropeza ES, Cadena CN. New phenotype of familial dilated cardiomyopathy and conduction disorders. *Am Heart J* 2003;145:317–323.
49. Schott JJ, Benson DW, Basson CT, *et al.* Congenital heart disease caused by mutations in the transcription factor *NKX2.5*. *Science* 1998;281:108–111.
50. McElhinney DB, Geiger E, Blinder J, Benson DW, Goldmuntz E. NKX2.5 mutations in patients with congenital heart disease. *J Am Coll Cardiol* 2003; 42(9):1650–1655.
51. Kanada M, Demirtas M, Guzel R, *et al.* Cardiomyopathy and atrioventricular block in Emery-Dreifuss muscular dystrophy–a case report. *Angiology* 2002;53:109–112.
52. Graber HL, Unverferth DV, Baker PB, *et al.* Evolution of a hereditary cardiac conduction and muscle disorder: A study involving a family with six generations affected. *Circulation* 1986;74:21–35.
53. Ohkubo R, Nakagawa M, Higuchi I, *et al.* Familial skeletal myopathy with atrioventricular block. *Intern Med* 1999;38:856–860.
54. Gollob MH, Green MS, Tang AS, *et al.* Identification of a gene responsible for familial Wolff-Parkinson-White syndrome. *N Engl J Med* 2001;344(24):1823–1831.
55. Brugada P, Brugada J. Right bundle branch block, persistent ST segment elevation and sudden cardiac death: A distinct clinical and electrocardiographi syndrome. A multicenter report. *J Am Coll Cardi* 1992;20:1391–1396.
56. Priori SG, Napolitano C, Gasparini M, *et al.* Clinic and genetic heterogeneity of right bundle branc block and ST-segment elevation syndrome: prospective evaluation of 52 families. *Circulatio* 2000;102:2509–2515.
57. Kyndt F, Probst V, Potet F, *et al.* Novel *SCN5* mutation leading either to isolated cardiac conduc tion defect or Brugada syndrome in a large Frenc family. *Circulation* 2001;104:3081–3086.
58. Smits JP, Eckardt L, Probst V, *et al.* Genotype phenotype relationship in Brugada syndrom Electrocardiographic features differentiate SCN5A related patients from non-SCN5A-related patient *J Am Coll Cardiol* 2002;40:350–356.
59. Shimizu W, Antzelevitch C, Suyama K, *et al.* Effec of sodium channel blockers on ST segment, QR duration, and corrected QT interval in patient with Brugada syndrome. *J Cardiovasc Electrophys iol* 2000;11:1320–1329.
60. Probst V, Allouis M, Sacher F, *et al.* Progressiv cardiac conduction defect is the prevailing pheno type in carriers of a Brugada syndrome SCN5 mutation. *J Cardiovasc Electrophysiol* 2006;17(3 270–275.
61. Hong K, Brugada J, Oliva A, Berruezo-Sanchez A *et al.* Value of electrocardiographic parameters an ajmaline test in the diagnosis of Brugada syndrom caused by SCN5A mutations. *Circulation* 2004;11 3023–3027.

38

Familial Atrial Fibrillation and Standstill

Bas A. Schoonderwoerd, J. Peter van Tintelen, Ans C.P. Wiesfeld, and Isabelle C. van Gelder

Introduction

Atrial fibrillation (AF), the most common arrhythmia, is associated with an unfavorable prognosis.[1,2] The majority of patients have AF in association with underlying (cardiac) diseases.[3] In 15–30% of the patients, however, a known etiology is absent.[4,5] This condition is called lone AF. Some of these patients have a positive family history for AF and may have a genetic cause or predisposition.[6] Atrial fibrillation as an inherited disease was first reported in 1943.[7] Darbar *et al.*[8] observed that familial AF is more common than previously recognized. Of the 914 patients with AF, 36% had lone AF. A positive family history for AF was present in 15% of these lone AF patients (5% of all AF patients).[8,9]

The prognosis for AF patients is determined by the associated cardiovascular disease as well as by arrhythmia-related events. Identifying patients with genetic defects predisposing to AF may therefore have important implications. Identification of the genes that play a role in the initiation of the arrhythmia may provide new insights into the development of the disease and improve our understanding of the disease and may provide new therapeutic options. Also, early recognition of patients at risk may, eventually, reduce morbidity and mortality.[1,3]

Atrial fibrillation is also related to other monogenic (cardiac) diseases including dilated cardiomyopathy,[10–13] hypertrophic cardiomyopathy,[14] skeletal myopathies,[15,16] long QT syndromes,[17,18] short QT syndromes,[19–21] Brugada syndrome,[22] familial amyloidosis,[23] congenital cardiac abnormalities,[24] and preexcitation syndromes.[25] In some of these conditions, AF will occur secondary to left ventricular dysfunction rather than to primary atrial disease.[26] These associations will not be discussed in this chapter.

We will focus on genetic defects that cause familial forms of lone AF. We will discuss polymorphisms that have been associated with the occurrence of AF in the setting of underlying disease, such as hypertension and coronary artery disease, as well as the genetic aspects of atrial standstill.

Atrial Fibrillation Without Structural Heart Disease

The incidence of lone AF depends on the type of AF (paroxysmal versus persistent) and how rigorously the patient has been evaluated. Depending on its mechanism of initiation, lone AF may be divided into vagally induced AF, adrenergically induced AF, or a combination of both types. Although never systematically investigated, most patients seem to suffer from a combination of both types of AF.

Monogenic Forms of Lone Atrial Fibrillation

Although a hereditary form of AF had been recognized as early as 1943,[7] Brugada *et al.* in 1997 were the first to identify linkage to a locus on chromosome 10q22–q24 for familial AF in three different Spanish families.[27] In these families, AF segregated as an autosomal dominant disease with high penetrance. In a three-generation family, 10 of the 26 living family members were affected. The mean age was 18 years and nine had permanent AF, with seven of them being asymptomatic. In two of them an increase in the left ventricular diameters, with left ventricular ejection fractions of 51% and 54%, respectively, was observed. All others had no echocardiographic abnormalities. One patient died suddenly at the age of 36 years. In the other two families, all nine affected persons had permanent AF and were asymptomatic without any echocardiographic abnormality (Table 38–1). The causative gene has not yet been identified. Sequencing several candidate genes including genes encoding α- and β-adrenergic receptors and G-protein receptor kinase in or in the vicinity of the locus identified did not reveal any mutations, and these can therefore be excluded as causative genes. Darbar *et al.*,[8] however, could not confirm linkage to chromosome 10q22–q24 in three other families with familial paroxysmal AF and rapid ventricular response and in one AF family with a slow ventricular response (Tab 38–1). In contrast to the other three families, A in the latter family was often asymptomatic. Eventually, 4 of the 10 patients of this family develope a junctional rhythm, and 5 of the 10 patients lef ventricular enlargement with a low-normal lef ventricular ejection fraction. The latter findin suggests that the phenotype of the fourth A family is characterized by an additional cardiomyopathy and atrial conduction disease. Linkag with the AF-associated 3p22–p25 region and th LMNA gene, associated with familial AF, conduction system disease and dilated cardiomyopath was excluded.[8,13,28] Nevertheless, clinicians shoul be aware of the development of conduction disturbances or a cardiomyopathy in (young) patient with familial AF and a slow ventricular respons It also highlights the importance of adequatel describing the phenotype in studies searchin for genes underlying arrhythmias, e.g., AF. Th second family in the study by Darbar *et al.* is completely different from the first one with a differen

TABLE 38–1. Monogenic forms of lone AF.[a]

Gene/chromosome	MOI	Fam	Type AF	Age	Race	HR	(A)symp	TCM	QTc (msec)	Mechanism
I. No locus and gene identified										
FAF 1–3[8]	AD	3	PAF	38–51	?	High	Symp	$n = 2$	Normal	?
FAF 4[8]	AD	1	PAF	37	?	Slow	Asymp	No	Too long in 2	?
II. Locus identified										
10q22–q24[27]										
FAF 1	AD	1	CAF (PAF)	18	White	na	Asymp	No	na	?
FAF 2–3	AD	2	CAF	2–46	White	na	Asymp	No	na	?
6q14–q16[29]	AD	1	PAF, CAF	21–72	White	na	na	No[b]	na	?
5p13[37c]	AR	1	CAF	Young	Chin	High	Symp	Some	Normal	?
III. Gene identified										
KCNQ1[31]	AD	1	CAF	>5	Chin	na	na	na	50% long	I_{Ks} ↑
KCNE2[35]	AD	2	PAF	>40	Chin	118–138	Symp	No	Normal	I_{Ks} ↑
KCNJ2[38]	AD	1	PAF,CAF	50–58	Chin	63–118	Symp	No	Normal	I_{K1} ↑
KCNA5[40]	AD	1	PAF	30–40	?	na	Symp	No	na	I_{Kur} ↓
SCN5A[41d]	AD	1	PAF/AFL	12–20	White	na	Symp	No	Normal	Excitability ↓
GJA5[43]	?	1[e]	PAF	41	?	na	Symp	na	na	Dispersed conduction

[a]AD, autosomal dominant; AF, atrial fibrillation; AFL, atrial flutter; (A)symp, (a)symptomatic; CAF, chronic/permanent AF; Chin, Chinese; FAF, familial A Fam, number of families; HR, heart rate; MOI, mode of inheritance; na, not available; PAF, paroxysmal AF; TCM, tachycardia-induced cardiomyopathy; unknown.

[b]One patient had a reversible tachycardiomyopathy and one carrier had peripartum cardiomyopathy but no AF.

[c]Multiple sudden deaths occurred at a very young age.

[d]Three carriers suffered from stroke.

[e]No families but subjects.

clinical outcome. This suggests at least two distinct mechanisms (and possible associated genes) involved in AF in these families.

In a large family with autosomal dominantly inherited lone AF, eight individuals with AF were identified.[29] In this family, AF started as paroxysmal AF in younger individuals and became permanent in older family members. The age of onset was variable, ranging from young to elderly family members. The left ventricular function was normal except for one individual who had a left ventricular ejection fraction of 40% while in AF with a rapid ventricular response (Table 38–1). Remarkably, two other individuals in this family had a history of peripartum cardiomyopathy but no AF. The disease locus was mapped to chromosome 6q14–q16, but the causative gene has not yet been identified. Both the locus found by Brugada *et al.*[27] and this locus[29] overlap with known loci for familial autosomal dominant dilated cardiomyopathy on chromosomes 10q21–23 and 6q12–q16, respectively.[10,11,30] The exact relationship between AF and cardiomyopathy in this family remains to be investigated. Moreover, four of the affected women have had 17 pregnancies without signs of cardiomyopathy being reported in the article.

In 2003 Chen *et al.*[31] published data on a large Chinese family with autosomal dominantly inherited lone AF (Table 38–1). Atrial fibrillation was permanent in all patients. The causative mutation (S140G) was located in the KCNQ1 gene on chromosome 11p15.5. The KCNQ1 gene encodes the pore-forming α subunit of the cardiac I_{Ks} potassium channel (KCNQ1/ KCNE1) and the KCNQ1/ KCNE2, KCNQ1/ KCNE3, KCNQ1/ KCNE4,[32] and KCNQ1/KCNE5 potassium channels.[33] Functional analysis of this mutation revealed a gain-of-function effect on the KCNQ1/KCNE1 and the KCNQ1/KCNE2 currents, thereby reducing the action potential duration and the effective refractory period in atrial myocytes, which in turn may set the stage for initiation and maintenance of AF. Although I_{Ks} and KCNQ1/KCNE2 are also expressed in the ventricle, the QT interval in the affected AF individuals was prolonged rather than shortened (in 9 of 16 patients the QT interval was between 460 and 530 msec). The clinical importance of this mutation may be limited, since it could not be confirmed in either six additional Chinese families and 19 sporadic idiopathic AF patients or in an unselected group of 141 AF patients in the United States (largely of Northern European descent).[34]

The same group[35] also identified a mutation (R27C) of the KCNE2 gene in two Chinese families with lone AF (Table 38–1). The KCNE gene family encodes small proteins that function as β subunits of several voltage-gated cation channels.[36] KCNE2 is the β subunit of the KCNQ1–KCNE2 channel, which produces a background potassium current. The age at diagnosis was higher than observed in the family with the KCNQ1 mutation, between 40 and 60 years. Most patients had symptomatic paroxysmal AF and also frequent premature atrial complexes. The left atrial size and left ventricular ejection fraction were within normal limits. Functional analyses also revealed a gain-of-function effect resulting in both inward and outward KCNQ1–KCNE2 potassium currents leading to a shortening of the action potential duration, which again may trigger and perpetuate AF.

Oberti *et al.*[37] identified a locus on chromosome 5p13 in autosomal recessively inherited neonatal AF. The affected children showed a rapidly progressive disease: AF with early onset at the fetal stage, neonatal sudden death, ventricular arrhythmias, and cardiomyopathy (Table 38–1). The heterozygous parents, all without AF, could be identified by a broad P wave on the electrocardiogram (ECG). Whether this disease is caused primarily by AF or, more likely, by an underlying cardiomyopathy remains to be determined.

Xia *et al.*[38] studied 30 unrelated Chinese kindreds with familial AF (Table 38–1). They identified one family in which a missense mutation (V93I) in the KCNJ2 gene, encoding the Kir2.1 potassium channel, was present in all affected family members. These subjects had no underlying heart disease and a normal QT interval. The Kir2.1 channel is responsible for the I_{K1} inward rectifier current. Expression of this mutant in COS-7 and human embryonic kidney cells resulted in a shortening of the action potential duration and effective refractory period caused by a gain in function of Kir2.1. The investigators analyzed this gene in another 154 patients with lone AF, but no mutations were detected.[38] Additionally, they studied the KCNQ1, KCNH2, SCN5A, ANK-B, and KCNE1–5 genes in the 30 families, which did not reveal additional mutations. However, it is not clear whether the population studied overlaps the previously described population.[35] In 96 American patients with familiar AF no mutations in the KCNJ2 gene could be identified.[39]

In another family with lone AF, Olson *et al.*[40] identified a mutation in the KCNA5 gene (Table 38–1). This gene encodes for the atrial-specific Kv1.5, potassium channel responsible for the ultrarapid delayed rectifier current (I_{Kur}). A heterozygous nonsense mutation (1123G>T) in exon 4 of KCNA5, resulting in a premature stop codon at residue 375 (E375X), was found. This mutation results in I_{Kur} loss of function by a dominant-negative effect on Kv1.5. Thus, the atrial action potential is prolonged and early afterdepolarizations may develop. The E375X mutation was not found in 540 unrelated control subjects.

In addition to changes in atrial action potential duration, such as caused by the above-mentioned mutations in atrial potassium channels, alterations in atrial conduction may lead to predisposition to AF. Laitinen-Forsblom *et al.*[41] identified a mutation in the SCN5A gene in a large Finnish family with cardiac conduction defects and atrial arrhythmias (Table 38–1). Six of 44 family members were affected, of whom five had a pacemaker implanted due to conduction defects and/or bradycardia before the age of 20. Five of these six subjects suffered from various atrial arrhythmias including paroxysmal AF and atrial flutter. Three suffered from stroke between the age of 20 and 30. None had symptoms before their teens. All six affected individuals had a normal left ventricular ejection fraction, although the left ventricle and right ventricle were enlarged in one and three individuals, respectively. A mutation (D1275N) in the SCN5A gene was found in the six affected individuals as well as in two young asymptomatic family members. One of these two carriers had an abnormally wide QRS complex (116 msec). The other was only 12 years old at the time of analysis. The D1275N mutation has also been reported in a family with atrial standstill[42] (see below) and in different families with dilated cardiomyopathy.[13,28] Although atrial standstill due to the D1275N mutation has been demonstrated to occur only in combination with polymorphisms in the promotor and untranslated region of the connexin40 gene,[42] it is currently unknown why this mutation expresses these different phenotypes and whether the phenotype described in the Finnish family may be considered to be true lone AF.

Gollob *et al.*[43] sequenced the GJA5 gene encoding connexin40 in cardiac tissue and lymphocytes in 15 unrelated patients with lone atrial fibrillation (Table 38–1). In three patients a novel heterozygous missense mutation was identified in cardiac tissue alone (somatic mutation). However, in one patient the mutation (286G>T) was present in both cardiac tissue and lymphocytes (germ-line mutation). This indicates that somatic mutations may underlie AF, but inheritable germ-line GJA5 mutations can occur. Analysis of the expression of the mutant proteins revealed impaired intracellular transport or reduced intercellular electrical coupling, which may result in anisotropic atrial conduction, promoting reentry. These results indicate that in some patients lone AF may have a genetic basis confined to the diseased myocardial tissue.

Genetic Aspects of Atrial Fibrillation in Acquired Structural Heart Disease

Atrial fibrillation predominantly occurs in the setting of structural (heart) diseases, in particular hypertension, coronary artery disease, and heart failure. A familial occurrence in these patients is uncertain yet conceivable. However, genetic differences may also contribute to this more common form of AF, since in the setting of heart failure some will suffer from AF repeatedly, while others never will. This is also suggested by recent data. Fox *et al.* demonstrated that parental AF not only increases the risk for offspring AF in lone AF, but also in the more common forms of AF in the setting of structural diseases.[6] In a cohort study within the Framingham Heart Study, they found that 681 of 2243 persons (30%) had at least one parent with documented AF. During follow-up, 70 of these 681 persons (10%) developed AF. If AF was present in at least one parent, the risk of offspring AF increased by 1.85 (95% confidence interval 1.12–3.06, $p = 0.02$) when compared to the absence of parental AF. As expected, the results were stronger if only younger parents and offspring (<75 years) without a previous myocardial infarction, heart failure, or valvular disease were assessed (odds ratio 3.17, 95% confidence interval 1.71–5.86, $p<0.001$). The polymorphisms described below have been associated with the more common forms of AF, i.e., AF occurring in the presence of risk factors for AF.

Polymorphisms Associated with Atrial Fibrillation in the Presence of Precipitating Factors

Lai *et al.* performed a case–control study in 108 consecutive nonfamilial AF patients from Taiwan with any underlying disease but they excluded patients with hyperthyroidism.[44] The mean age was 63 years and a history of hypertension was present in 52% of the patients. More than 80% of the patients had permanent AF (Table 38–2). Matching was performed regarding sex, age, left ventricular dysfunction, and valvular disease. An association between the KCNE1 (encoding the minK β subunit of the I_{Ks} potassium channel) 38G allele and AF was observed. The odds ratios for AF in patients with one and two KCNE1 38G alleles were 2.16 (95% confidence interval 0.81–5.74) and 3.58 (95% confidence interval 1.38–9.27), respectively, compared to patients without the KCNE1 38G allele. Recently, the functional role of this polymorphism has been demonstrated.[45]

Fatini *et al.*[46] also found an association between the presence of the 38G minK allele and nonvalvular atrial fibrillation in 331 white patients. Additionally, they studied several polymorphisms in the endothelial nitric oxide synthase (eNOS) gene including the G894T nucleotide exchange in exon 7, a T/C exchange in the promoter region (–T786C), and the eNOS 4a/4b polymorphism. Only eNOS –T786C was significantly more prevalent in patients with AF when compared to healthy volunteers. Surprisingly, the combined presence of minK 38G and eNOS –786C resulted in a stronger predisposition for AF than the minK variant alone (Table 38–2).

Firouzi *et al.* reported evidence that a connexin40 gene promotor polymorphism (–44AA genotype) is linked to enhanced atrial vulnerability as measured by an increased coefficient of spatial dispersion of refractoriness and an increased risk of AF (Table 38–2).[47] They investigated the coefficient of dispersion, defined as the standard deviation of all local mean fibrillatory intervals expressed as a percentage of the overall mean fibrillatory interval, in 30 unrelated adults. On the basis of previous work, they defined a coefficient of dispersion of a value >3 to be associated with enhanced spatial dispersion of atrial refractoriness. These patients had no structural heart disease and underwent an electrophysiological study because of the presence of an accessory pathway ($n = 27$) or atrioventricular nodal reentrant tachycardias ($n = 3$). Of these subjects, 14 had prior documented sporadic episodes of AF, whereas 16 had no history of AF. The AF patients suffered a mean of one (range one to five) previous episode of AF with a median duration of 1 h (range 15 min to 3 h). The AF free interval before the study was 148 days (range 9–365 days). The prevalence of the minor Cx40 allele (–44A)

Table 38–2. Polymorphisms associated with AF in patients with concomitant underlying heart disease.[a]

Gene/chromosome	Number of subjects	Type AF	Age	Race	HR	(A)symp	UHD	Mechanism
38G KCNE1[44]	108	CAF	63	Chin	na	na	Yes	$I_{Ks}\downarrow$
38G KCNE1 ± –786T > C eNOS[46]	331	CAF	73	White	na	na	Yes	$I_{Ks}\downarrow$
–44AA Connexin40[47]	30	PAF	33	White	na	Symp	WPW	Possible
M235T, G-217A and G-6A angiotensinogen[49]	250	CAF	68	Chin	na	Symp	Yes	Possible
C825T GNB3 G-protein β3[51]	227	PAF, CAF	58	?	na	na	59% hypertension	Possible ($I_{K,Ach}$)
97T KCNE5[52]	158	CAF, PAF	66	White	na	na	na	Possible (I_{Ks})
–174G/C interleukin-6[53]	110	Post op AF	61	?	na	na	Yes	Inflammation?

[a]AF, atrial fibrillation; (A)symp, (a)symptomatic; CAF, chronic/permanent AF; Chin, Chinese; na, not available; HR, heart rate; PAF, paroxysmal AF; Post op AF, postoperative AF; UHD, underlying heart disease; WPW, Wolff–Parkinson–White syndrome; ?, unknown.

and −44AA genotype was significantly higher in subjects with increased dispersion ($n = 13$) compared to patients with a normal coefficient of dispersion ($n = 17$, $p = 0.00046$ and $p = 0.025$, odds ratio 6.7 and 7.4, respectively). Subjects with the −44AA genotype had a significantly higher coefficient of dispersion than those with the −44GG genotype. Finally, all subjects with an increased dispersion had a history of AF compared with only one subject with a normal coefficient of dispersion. The mechanism is at present unknown. It may be surmised that an abnormal gap junction distribution may cause abnormal conduction with increased anisotropy. By creating a substrate, this may result in an increased propensity for AF.

In a case–control study Yamashita *et al.*[48] could not demonstrate a significant association between angiotensin-converting enzyme gene insertion/deletion polymorphisms and AF.

Tsai *et al.*[49] investigated several gene polymorphisms of the renin–angiotensin system in 250 patients with nonfamilial AF in the setting of underlying heart diseases and 250 matched controls. They observed, comparable to the data of Yamashita *et al.*, no association between the angiotensin-converting enzyme gene insertion/deletion polymorphism and nonfamilial structural AF. The same was found for the investigated polymorphism of the angiotensin II receptor gene. However, the angiotensinogen M235T, G-217A, and G-6A polymorphisms were associated with AF. The odds ratios for AF were 2.5 (95% confidence interval 1.7–3.3) with the M235/M235 plus M235/T235 genotype, 3.3 (95% confidence interval 1.3–10.0) with the G-6/G-6 genotype, and 2.0 (95% confidence interval 1.3–2.5) with the G-217/G-217 genotype, respectively. Furthermore, these data might explain why drugs affecting the renin–angiotensin system may have beneficial effects on the prevention of AF.[50]

Schreieck *et al.*[51] determined the genotype of the C825T polymorphism in the G-protein β3 subunit gene (GNB3) in 291 patients with AF and 292 controls. This polymorphism is a risk factor for hypertension. In this study, 59% of AF patients and 62% of controls suffered from hypertension. Patients with coronary artery disease, valvular heart disease, or cardiomyopathy were excluded. The TT genotype was significantly less present in the AF group when compared to the control group (5.8% vs. 12.0%) and was associated with a 51% decrease in the unadjusted risk for the occurrence of AF (OR, 0.49; 95% CI, 0.28–0.85; $p = 0.01$). The presence of the CC and CT genotypes was not statistically different between both groups.

Ravn *et al.*[52] investigated the 97T polymorphism of the KCNE5 gene. This gene is located on the X-chromosome and encodes an inhibitory β subunit, MiRP4, of the repolarizing cardiac potassium channel KCNQ1. When compared to 158 patients with AF, a greater proportion of the 96 healthy control subjects was carrier of the 97T allele (15.2% vs. 29.2%). The OR for AF if a patient did not have a copy of the 97T allele was 2.17 (95% CI 0.89–5.28) in men and 1.94 (95% CI 0.80–4.75) in women. Because the gene is located on the X-chromosome, the protection of the 97T polymorphism may explain gender-related differences in AF. The exact mechanism by which this gene influences atrial electrophysiology has not been investigated.

Gaudino *et al.*[53] assessed the role of the −174G/C interleukin-6 polymorphism in 110 patients undergoing coronary artery bypass surgery. This polymorphism has been previously associated with postoperative interleukin-6 levels. In the postoperative period, 26 patients developed AF. Analysis of the polymorphism demonstrated a significant prevalence of the GG genotype in patients with AF (34% vs. 10%). This resulted in an OR of 3.25 (95% CI 1.23–8.62). These results show a possible role of an inflammatory component in the development of postoperative AF.

Atrial Standstill

Atrial standstill is a rare arrhythmia characterized by the total absence of electrical and mechanical activity in the atria. On the electrocardiogram, P waves are absent and usually a junctional escape rhythm is present. Also intraatrial electrograms are absent and the atria are inexcitable by electrical stimulation. On the echocardiogram, the atrial wall does not contract and the mitral A-wave is missing.

Atrial standstill may be complete or partial. In the latter, electrical silence exists in one part of the atria together with a rapid atrial rate in another part of the atria at the same time.[54,55] Atrial standstill may be transient as well as permanent, depending on the underlying condition. The treatment consists of VVI pacemaker implantation in combination with anticoagulation, since atrial standstill is associated with an increased risk of thromboembolic complications.

Atrial standstill may be due to different nonheritable causes including digitalis or quinidine intoxication, hyperkalemia, myocardial ischemia or infarction, cardiac surgery, myocarditis, diabetes, and hypothermia.[56] Atrial standstill is associated with a number of inheritable disorders. Familial forms in the absence of underlying (cardiac) disease (isolated familial atrial standstill) have also been described.

Atrial Standstill in Inheritable (Cardiac) Disorders

Atrial standstill occurs in up to 45% of patients with Emery–Dreifuss muscular dystrophy.[57] This disease can be inherited as an X-linked recessive, autosomal dominant, or autosomal recessive disorder. The X-linked form is caused by mutations in the gene encoding emerin, whereas the autosomal forms are caused by mutations in the gene encoding lamin A/C. The disease is characterized by progressive skeletal muscle wasting with contractures. Cardiac involvement may include the development of cardiomyopathy and AV conduction abnormalities. Both AF and atrial flutter, often anticipating atrial standstill, may occur. Atrial standstill has also been described in patients suffering from autosomal recessive spinal muscular atrophy type 3 (Kugelberg–Welander syndrome).[58]

Fazelifar *et al.*[59] described two Iranian siblings, one male aged 34 years and one female aged 44 years, who were evaluated because of frequent syncope. Both had atrial standstill on the 12-lead ECG with a broad QRS escape rhythm, mildly enlarged ventricles and atria on echocardiography, and a left ventricular ejection fraction between 30% and 40%. There were no signs of amyloidosis or muscular disease. The male developed syncope due to self-terminating polymorphic ventricular tachycardia. The family history disclosed two sudden deaths in a brother and a nephew at the ages of 34 and 21 years, respectively. The nephew previously had a pacemaker implanted because of symptomatic bradycardia. Although no genetic analysis was performed, an autosomal inheritance of this form of dilated cardiomyopathy in combination with atrial standstill is likely.

A case of father and son with Ebstein's anomaly and atrial standstill has been reported[60] as well as a single case with this combination.[61]

Takehara *et al.* reported a case of atrial standstill in a patient with Brugada syndrome (Table 38–3).[62] This 37-year-old Japanese woman suffered from recurrent syncope. Her ECG demonstrated coved-type ST elevation compatible with Brugada syndrome. During admission she suffered from episodes of ventricular fibrillation that were preceded by a long pause due to atrial standstill. Atrial standstill could also be provoked by administration of procainamide. A mutation in exon 9 of the SCN5A gene leading to amino acid substitution R367H was found in the patient as well as in her son. Her son's ECG, however, demonstrated a saddleback ST elevation. The family history was negative for sudden cardiac death.

TABLE 38–3. Mutations associated with familial atrial standstill.[a]

Gene and mutation	Number of Families (subjects)	Age	Race	UHD
Homozygous Cx40 −44G > A; +71A > G together with SCN5A–D1275N[42]	1(4)	22–33	White	No
Heterozygous Cx40 − 44G > A; +71A > G together with SCN5A–L212P[68]	1(1)	3	Jpn	No
SCN5A–R367H[62]	1(2)	37	Jpn	Brugada

[a]Cx40, connexin40; Jpn, Japanese; UHD, underlying heart disease.

Isolated Familial Atrial Standstill

Familial forms of atrial standstill are extremely rare. A number of families have been described in the past decades.[63–67]

In 2003 a Dutch family with a progressive form of atrial standstill was reported.[42] In this family atrial standstill was present in four individuals (Table 38–3). Symptoms of dizziness and syncope started in their early 20 s, progressing in the years thereafter and prompting medical evaluation by

30–40 years of age. On an invasive electrophysiological study, the atria could either be partially stimulated or not stimulated. Genetic analysis revealed a mutation in the cardiac sodium channel gene SCN5A (D1275N) in all three living affected individuals and five unaffected family members. Additionally, two gap junction protein connexin40-related polymorphisms (–44G>A and +71A>G) were found in all affected patients and five other healthy relatives. Eight relatives were *homozygous* for both polymorphisms, of whom three were affected with atrial standstill. Therefore, only the combination of the SNCA5 mutation and the rare Cx40 genotype led to atrial standstill in this family. Remarkably, AF was present in only one individual in this family, aged 68 years, after myocardial infarction, although AF has been described in D1275N carriers.[41] Functional measurements of D1275N sodium channels revealed a shift of the voltage dependence of activation toward more depolarized voltages, resulting in decreased excitability. The combination of the rare Cx40 genotypes was demonstrated to cause a reduction in Cx40 expression *in vitro*.

Two years later, Makita *et al.*[68] reported a Japanese boy presenting with sick sinus syndrome in combination with paroxysmal AF at the age of 3 years (Table 38-3). When he was 11 years old, total atrial standstill was present. No underlying (cardiac) disease was present. Genetic screening revealed a mutation in exon 6 of the SCN5A gene leading to substitution of proline for leucine at position 212 (L212P). His father, although asymptomatic, was also found to be the carrier of this mutation. Additionally, a *heterozygous* Cx40 polymorphism (–44GA/+71AG) was found in the boy and in his asymptomatic mother and maternal grandmother.

In conclusion, a genetic defect in SCN5A seems to underlie familial atrial standstill, but in itself does not lead to the severe phenotype. Coinheritance of connexin40 polymorphisms modifies the clinical expression of the arrhythmia.

Conclusions

Familial AF is clinically and genetically heterogeneous and seems more common than previously suspected. Proper identification of the phenotype of patients with AF is of utmost importance. Different phenotypes may point to distinct mechanisms and genes underlying familial AF. Genetic heterogeneity and a relatively low yield of genetic testing until now hamper extensive genetic evaluation in clinical practice. The observations in patients with nonfamilial AF in the presence of underlying heart disease suggest some form of genetic control in the pathogenesis of this more common form of AF.

Obviously, the data are promising and may help to clarify why some people develop AF while others never do. Atrial standstill is an extremely rare arrhythmia and is usually caused by a reversible condition. Furthermore, it may be associated with a variety of inheritable diseases with distinct phenotypes. Cases of isolated familial atrial standstill have been described.

References

1. Benjamin EJ, Wolf PA, D'Agostino RB, Silbershatz H, Kannel WB, Levy D. Impact of atrial fibrillation on the risk of death: The Framingham Heart Study. *Circulation* 1998;98:946–952.
2. Dries DL, Exner DV, Gersh BJ, Domanski MJ, Waclawiw MA, Stevenson LW. Atrial fibrillation is associated with an increased risk for mortality and heart failure progression in patients with asymptomatic and symptomatic left ventricular systolic dysfunction: A retrospective analysis of the SOLVD trials. Studies of Left Ventricular Dysfunction. *J Am Coll Cardiol* 1998;32:695–703.
3. Fuster V, Ryden LE, Cannom DS, *et al.* ACC/AHA/ESC 2006 Guidelines for the Management of Patients with Atrial Fibrillation: A report of the American College of Cardiology/American Heart Association Task Force on Practice Guidelines and the European Society of Cardiology Committee for Practice Guidelines (Writing Committee to Revise the 2001 Guidelines for the Management of Patients with Atrial Fibrillation): Developed in collaboration with the European Heart Rhythm Association and the Heart Rhythm Society. *Circulation* 2006;114: e257–e354.
4. Murgatroyd FD, Camm AJ. Atrial arrhythmias. *Lancet* 1993;341:1317–1322.
5. Levy S, Maarek M, Coumel P, *et al.* Characterization of different subsets of atrial fibrillation in general practice in France: The ALFA study. The College of French Cardiologists. *Circulation* 1999; 99:3028–3035.

6. Fox CS, Parise H, D'Agostino RB Sr, *et al.* Parental atrial fibrillation as a risk factor for atrial fibrillation in offspring. *JAMA* 2004;291:2851–2855.
7. Wolf L. Familial auricular atrial fibrillation. *N Engl J Med* 1943;229:396–397.
8. Darbar D, Herron KJ, Ballew JD, *et al.* Familial atrial fibrillation is a genetically heterogeneous disorder. *J Am Coll Cardiol* 2003;41:2185–2192.
9. Kopecky SL, Gersh BJ, McGoon MD, *et al.* The natural history of lone atrial fibrillation. A population-based study over three decades. *N Engl J Med* 1987;317:669–674.
10. Bowles KR, Gajarski R, Porter P, *et al.* Gene mapping of familial autosomal dominant dilated cardiomyopathy to chromosome 10q21-23. *J Clin Invest* 1996;98:1355–1360.
11. Bowles KR, Abraham SE, Brugada R, *et al.* Construction of a high-resolution physical map of the chromosome 10q22-q23 dilated cardiomyopathy locus and analysis of candidate genes. *Genomics* 2000;67:109–127.
12. Sebillon P, Bouchier C, Bidot LD, *et al.* Expanding the phenotype of LMNA mutations in dilated cardiomyopathy and functional consequences of these mutations. *J Med Genet* 2003;40:560–567.
13. Olson TM, Michels VV, Ballew JD, *et al.* Sodium channel mutations and susceptibility to heart failure and atrial fibrillation. *JAMA* 2005;293:447–454.
14. Gruver EJ, Fatkin D, Dodds GA, *et al.* Familial hypertrophic cardiomyopathy and atrial fibrillation caused by Arg663His beta-cardiac myosin heavy chain mutation. *Am J Cardiol* 1999;83:13H–18H.
15. Ohkubo R, Nakagawa M, Higuchi I, *et al.* Familial skeletal myopathy with atrioventricular block. *Intern Med* 1999;38:856–860.
16. Sakata K, Shimizu M, Ino H, *et al.* High incidence of sudden cardiac death with conduction disturbances and atrial cardiomyopathy caused by a nonsense mutation in the STA gene. *Circulation* 2005;111:3352–3358.
17. Schott JJ, Charpentier F, Peltier S, *et al.* Mapping of a gene for long QT syndrome to chromosome 4q25-27. *Am J Hum Genet* 1995;57:1114–1122.
18. Mohler PJ, Schott JJ, Gramolini AO, *et al.* Ankyrin-B mutation causes type 4 long-QT cardiac arrhythmia and sudden cardiac death. *Nature* 2003;421:634–639.
19. Hong K, Piper DR, az-Valdecantos A, *et al.* De novo KCNQ1 mutation responsible for atrial fibrillation and short QT syndrome in utero. *Cardiovasc Res* 2005;68:433–440.
20. Hong K, Bjerregaard P, Gussak I, Brugada R. Short QT syndrome and atrial fibrillation caused by mutation in KCNH2. *J Cardiovasc Electrophysiol* 2005;16:394–396.
21. Giustetto C, Di MF, Wolpert C, *et al.* Short QT syndrome: Clinical findings and diagnostic-therapeutic implications. *Eur Heart J* 2006;27:2440–2447.
22. Morita H, Kusano-Fukushima K, Nagase S, *et al.* Atrial fibrillation and atrial vulnerability in patients with Brugada syndrome. *J Am Coll Cardiol* 2002;40:1437–1444.
23. Gillmore JD, Booth DR, Pepys MB, Hawkins PN. Hereditary cardiac amyloidosis associated with the transthyretin Ile122 mutation in a white man. *Heart* 1999;82:e2.
24. Gutierrez-Roelens I, Roy LD, Ovaert C, *et al.* A novel CSX/NKX2-5 mutation causes autosomal-dominant AV block: Are atrial fibrillation and syncopes part of the phenotype? *Eur J Hum Genet* 2006;14(12):1313–1316.
25. Gollob MH, Seger JJ, Gollob TN, *et al.* Novel PRKAG2 mutation responsible for the genetic syndrome of ventricular preexcitation and conduction system disease with childhood onset and absence of cardiac hypertrophy. *Circulation* 2001;104:3030–3033.
26. Schoonderwoerd BA, Van Gelder IC, Van Veldhuisen DJ, Van Den Berg MP, Crijns HJ. Electrical and structural remodeling: Role in the genesis and maintenance of atrial fibrillation. *Prog Cardiovasc Dis* 2005;48:153–168.
27. Brugada R, Tapscott T, Czernuszewicz GZ, *et al.* Identification of a genetic locus for familial atrial fibrillation. *N Engl J Med* 1997;336:905–911.
28. McNair WP, Ku L, Taylor MR, *et al.* SCN5A mutation associated with dilated cardiomyopathy, conduction disorder, and arrhythmia. *Circulation* 2004;110:2163–2167.
29. Ellinor PT, Shin JT, Moore RK, Yoerger DM, MacRae CA. Locus for atrial fibrillation maps to chromosome 6q14-16. *Circulation* 2003;107:2880–2883.
30. Sylvius N, Tesson F, Gayet C, *et al.* A new locus for autosomal dominant dilated cardiomyopathy identified on chromosome 6q12-q16. *Am J Hum Genet* 2001;68:241–246.
31. Chen YH, Xu SJ, Bendahhou S, *et al.* KCNQ1 gain-of-function mutation in familial atrial fibrillation. *Science* 2003;299:251–254.
32. Grunnet M, Jespersen T, Rasmussen HB, *et al.* KCNE4 is an inhibitory subunit to the KCNQ1 channel. *J Physiol* 2002;542:119–130.
33. Angelo K, Jespersen T, Grunnet M, Nielsen MS, Klaerke DA, Olesen SP. KCNE5 induces time- and voltage-dependent modulation of the KCNQ1 current. *Biophys J* 2002;83:1997–2006.

34. Ellinor PT, Moore RK, Patton KK, Ruskin JN, Pollak MR, MacRae CA. Mutations in the long QT gene, KCNQ1, are an uncommon cause of atrial fibrillation. *Heart* 2004;90:1487–1488.
35. Yang Y, Xia M, Jin Q, *et al.* Identification of a KCNE2 gain-of-function mutation in patients with familial atrial fibrillation. *Am J Hum Genet* 2004; 75:899–905.
36. Jiang M, Zhang M, Tang DG, *et al.* KCNE2 protein is expressed in ventricles of different species, and changes in its expression contribute to electrical remodeling in diseased hearts. *Circulation* 2004;109: 1783–1788.
37. Oberti C, Wang L, Li L, *et al.* Genome-wide linkage scan identifies a novel genetic locus on chromosome 5p13 for neonatal atrial fibrillation associated with sudden death and variable cardiomyopathy. *Circulation* 2004;110:3753–3759.
38. Xia M, Jin Q, Bendahhou S, *et al.* A Kir2.1 gain-of-function mutation underlies familial atrial fibrillation. *Biochem Biophys Res Commun* 2005; 332:1012–1019.
39. Ellinor PT, Petrov-Kondratov VI, Zakharova E, Nam EG, MacRae CA. Potassium channel gene mutations rarely cause atrial fibrillation. *BMC Med Genet* 2006;7:70.
40. Olson TM, Alekseev AE, Liu XK, *et al.* Kv1.5 channelopathy due to KCNA5 loss-of-function mutation causes atrial fibrillation. *Hum Mol Genet* 2006; 15:2185–2191.
41. Laitinen-Forsblom PJ, Makynen P, Makynen H, *et al.* SCN5A mutation associated with cardiac conduction defect and atrial arrhythmias. *J Cardiovasc Electrophysiol* 2006;17:480–485.
42. Groenewegen WA, Firouzi M, Bezzina CR, *et al.* A cardiac sodium channel mutation cosegregates with a rare connexin40 genotype in familial atrial standstill. *Circ Res* 2003;92:14–22.
43. Gollob MH, Jones DL, Krahn AD, *et al.* Somatic mutations in the connexin 40 gene (GJA5) in atrial fibrillation. *N Engl J Med* 2006;354:2677–2688.
44. Lai LP, Su MJ, Yeh HM, *et al.* Association of the human minK gene 38G allele with atrial fibrillation: Evidence of possible genetic control on the pathogenesis of atrial fibrillation. *Am Heart J* 2002;144: 485–490.
45. Ehrlich JR, Zicha S, Coutu P, Hebert TE, Nattel S. Atrial fibrillation-associated minK38G/S polymorphism modulates delayed rectifier current and membrane localization. *Cardiovasc Res* 2005;67: 520–528.
46. Fatini C, Sticchi E, Genuardi M, *et al.* Analysis of minK and eNOS genes as candidate loci for predisposition to non-valvular atrial fibrillation. *Eur Heart J* 2006;27:1712–1718.
47. Firouzi M, Ramanna H, Kok B, *et al.* Association of human connexin40 gene polymorphisms with atrial vulnerability as a risk factor for idiopathic atrial fibrillation. *Circ Res* 2004;95:e29–e33.
48. Yamashita T, Hayami N, Ajiki K, *et al.* Is ACE gene polymorphism associated with lone atrial fibrillation? *Jpn Heart J* 1997;38:637–641.
49. Tsai CT, Lai LP, Lin JL, *et al.* Renin-angiotensin system gene polymorphisms and atrial fibrillation. *Circulation* 2004;109:1640–1646.
50. Madrid AH, Bueno MG, Rebollo JM, *et al.* Use of irbesartan to maintain sinus rhythm in patients with long-lasting persistent atrial fibrillation: A prospective and randomized study. *Circulation* 2002;106:331–336.
51. Schreieck J, Dostal S, von BN, *et al.* C825T polymorphism of the G-protein beta3 subunit gene and atrial fibrillation: Association of the TT genotype with a reduced risk for atrial fibrillation. *Am Heart J* 2004;148:545–550.
52. Ravn LS, Hofman-Bang J, Dixen U, *et al.* Relation of 97T polymorphism in KCNE5 to risk of atrial fibrillation. *Am J Cardiol* 2005;96:405–407.
53. Gaudino M, Andreotti F, Zamparelli R, *et al.* The −174G/C interleukin-6 polymorphism influences postoperative interleukin-6 levels and postoperative atrial fibrillation. Is atrial fibrillation an inflammatory complication? *Circulation* 2003;108(Suppl. 1):II195–199.
54. Effendy FN, Bolognesi R, Bianchi G, Visioli O. Alternation of partial and total atrial standstill. *J Electrocardiol* 1979;12:121–127.
55. Talwar KK, Dev V, Chopra P, Dave TH, Radhakrishnan S. Persistent atrial standstill—clinical, electrophysiological, and morphological study. *Pacing Clin Electrophysiol* 1991;14:1274–1280.
56. Ruff P, Leier CV, Schaal SF. Temporary atrial standstill. *Am Heart J* 1979;98:413–420.
57. Boriani G, Gallina M, Merlini L, *et al.* Clinical relevance of atrial fibrillation/flutter, stroke, pacemaker implant, and heart failure in Emery-Dreifuss muscular dystrophy: A long-term longitudinal study. *Stroke* 2003;34:901–908.
58. Liu YB, Chen WJ, Lee YT. Atrial standstill in a case of Kugelberg-Welander syndrome with cardiac involvement: An electrophysiologic study. *Int J Cardiol* 1999;70:207–210.
59. Fazelifar AF, Arya A, Haghjoo M, Sadr-Ameli MA. Familial atrial standstill in association with dilated cardiomyopathy. *Pacing Clin Electrophysiol* 2005; 28:1005–1008.
60. Pierard LA, Henrard L, Demoulin JC. Persistent atrial standstill in familial Ebstein's anomaly. *Br Heart J* 1985;53:594–597.

1. Carballal J, Asensio E, Hernandez R, *et al.* Ebstein's anomaly, atrial paralysis and atrio-ventricular block: An uncommon association. *Europace* 2002; 4:451–454.

2. Takehara N, Makita N, Kawabe J, *et al.* A cardiac sodium channel mutation identified in Brugada syndrome associated with atrial standstill. *J Intern Med* 2004;255:137–142.

3. Harrison WH Jr, Derrick JR. Atrial standstill: A review, and presentation of two new cases of familial and unusual nature with reference to epicardial pacing in one. *Angiology* 1969;20:610–617.

4. Ward DE, Ho SY, Shinebourne EA. Familial atrial standstill and inexcitability in childhood. *Am J Cardiol* 1984;53:965–967.

65. Shah MK, Subramanyan R, Tharakan J, Venkitachalam CG, Balakrishnan KG. Familial total atrial standstill. *Am Heart J* 1992;123:1379–1382.

66. Balaji S, Till J, Shinebourne EA. Familial atrial standstill with coexistent atrial flutter. *Pacing Clin Electrophysiol* 1998;21:1841–1842.

67. Disertori M, Guarnerio M, Vergara G, *et al.* Familial endemic persistent atrial standstill in a small mountain community: Review of eight cases. *Eur Heart J* 1983;4:354–361.

68. Makita N, Sasaki K, Groenewegen WA, *et al.* Congenital atrial standstill associated with coinheritance of a novel SCN5A mutation and connexin 40 polymorphisms. *Heart Rhythm* 2005;2: 1128–1134.

39
Idiopathic Ventricular Fibrillation

Sami Viskin and Bernard Belhassen

Introduction

Idiopathic ventricular fibrillation (VF) is an uncommon disease of unknown etiology that manifests as syncope or cardiac arrest caused by rapid polymorphic ventricular tachycardia (VT) or VF in the absence of organic heart disease or identifiable channelopathy. Because the term "idiopathic" means "absence of identifiable etiology," idiopathic VF is essentially a diagnosis by exclusion. However, typical clinical and electrophysiological characteristics present in some patients often allows for a straightforward positive diagnosis.

History

In 1929, Dock published what probably represents the first description of idiopathic VF.[1] This case report describes a 36-year-old male with clusters of syncope caused by documented VF that terminated spontaneously. Organic heart disease was appropriately excluded with the technologies then available. Similar case reports followed, and in 1987 Belhassen published the first series of idiopathic VF,[2] emphasizing the importance of electrophysiological evaluation with programmed ventricular stimulation and the high efficacy of quinidine in preventing inducible and spontaneous VF.[2]

In 1990, we published the first systematic review on idiopathic VF,[3] including data on 54 cases published by then. The typical characteristics of idiopathic VF, including the onset of symptoms during early adulthood in both genders, the relatively high incidence of arrhythmic storms (with clusters of VF episodes), the high inducibility rate of VF with programmed ventricular stimulation and the excellent response to quinidine therapy were first summarized in that review.

The mode of onset of spontaneous arrhythmias in idiopathic VF, namely, the triggering of rapid polymorphic VT/VF by single ventricular extrasystoles with very short (R-on-T) coupling intervals, already evident from the initial reports, was described by Leenhardt and Coumel[4] as "short-coupled variant of torsade de pointes" and was finally described in detail by us in 1997.[5] Six years later, Haissaguerre demonstrated that the short-coupled extrasystoles triggering VF in this disease are very-early ectopic beats originating from Purkinje fibers.[6]

The differential diagnosis of idiopathic VF also evolved in recent years. When we wrote the first review on this topic in 1990,[3] the differential diagnosis included (in addition to subtle forms of organic heart disease) the following arrhythmia disorders: the long QT syndrome (described in 1957),[7–9] the catecholamine-sensitive polymorphic VT (CPVT) (described in 1995),[10] and the syndrome of nocturnal sudden death of South East Asia (known since 1960).[11] However, in 1992, the Brugada brothers described patients with otherwise idiopathic VF who had a peculiar electrocardiogram showing right bundle branch block with persistent ST-segment elevation in the right precordial leads.[12] It soon became evident that >20% of patients thought until then to have idiopathic VF had what we now call "Brugada syndrome."[13] Moreover, in 1997 it became clear that the "syndrome of unexplained nocturnal sudden death in South East Asia" was in fact, an "endemic" manifestation of Brugada syndrome in Asia.[14] More recently, patients with the congenital short QT syndrome (first described in 2000)[15,16] proved to have inducible[15] and spontaneous[17] ventricular arrhythmias indistinguishable from those of idiopathic VF patients. In fact, we recently proposed that idiopathic VF may very well be a "*short QT syndrome with not very short QT intervals*" (QTc intervals in the range of 340–360 msec).[18] Detailed descriptions of the above-mentioned disorders appear in Chapters 35–38 of this volume.

Etiology

Almost 80 years after the original description of idiopathic VF,[1] the etiology of this disorder remains a mystery. Several lines of evidence suggest that idiopathic VF is a channelopathy. First, the spontaneous and inducible ventricular arrhythmias of idiopathic VF are remarkably similar to those observed in the Brugada syndrome and the short QT syndromes, two well-described channelopathies involving hereditary malfunction of sodium channels (Brugada syndrome)[19] or potassium channels (short QT syndromes).[20–22] Second, patients with Brugada syndrome may have a diagnostic electrocardiogram (with ST-segment elevation in the right precordial leads) some time, but may have normal or near-normal electrocardiograms at other times, making distinction of patients with idiopathic VF and Brugada syndrome challenging. In fact, a diagnosis of idiopathic VF is not considered definite until a "Brugada syndrome with near normal electrocardiogram" is excluded by performing a drug challenge with a sodium channel blocker. This is because slow intravenous injection of a sodium channel blocker (such as ajmaline,[23–25] flecainide,[25–27] disopyramide,[28] or procainamide[29]) will worsen any inborn malfunction of sodium channels, augmenting the ST-segment elevation in up to 40% of patients with Brugada syndrome who have a normal electrocardiogram.[19,25,30] As mentioned above, male patients with idiopathic VF have borderline-short QT intervals,[18] suggesting that the short QT syndrome and idiopathic VF represent a continuum.[18] On the other hand, the fact that only a minority of patients with idiopathic VF report a familial history of sudden death[3,31,32] is a strong argument against the role of genetic channelopathies in this disease.

Haissaguerre *et al.* recently proposed that idiopathic VF represents a "focal VF" triggered by ectopic beats originating from Purkinje fibers.[33] These Purkinje extrasystoles are so premature that they fall on the vulnerable period of the surrounding ventricular tissue, initiating reentrant VF. The very early Purkinje ectopic beats have been demonstrated by intracardiac recordings,[33] but the reason for this very premature focal activity remains to be determined.

Clinical Manifestations

Patients with idiopathic VF present with either syncope or cardiac arrest in early adulthood. The mean age at presentation in several series has been 35–45 years and the majority are older than 20 years and younger than 65 years old at the time of presentation.[31,34] Two-thirds of the patients are males.[31,34]

The arrhythmias provoking syncope (Figure 39–1) and those causing cardiac arrest are similar in terms of mode of onset, ventricular rate, and polymorphic morphology. It is not clear why some events of polymorphic VT terminate spontaneously (causing syncope) while others deteriorate to fine VF (causing cardiac arrest) (Figure 39–1B and C). However, the proportion of patients presenting with cardiac arrest (as opposed to syncope) is much higher in idiopathic VF than in other channelopathies causing polymorphic ventricular tachyarrhythmias like the long QT syndrome (LQTS) or CPVT.[35] In other words, arrhythmias in idiopathic VF occur rarely, but once they occur they are generally sustained. As a rule, syncope and cardiac arrest in idiopathic VF are *not* related to effort or emotional stress.[3,31,32] Sleep-related arrhythmias, which are common in sodium channelopathies (Brugada syndrome and LQTS of the LQT3 type), are rare in idiopathic VF.[13,32] Finally, about 25% of patients with idiopathic VF present with arrhythmic storms, that is, with clusters of VF episodes recurring within

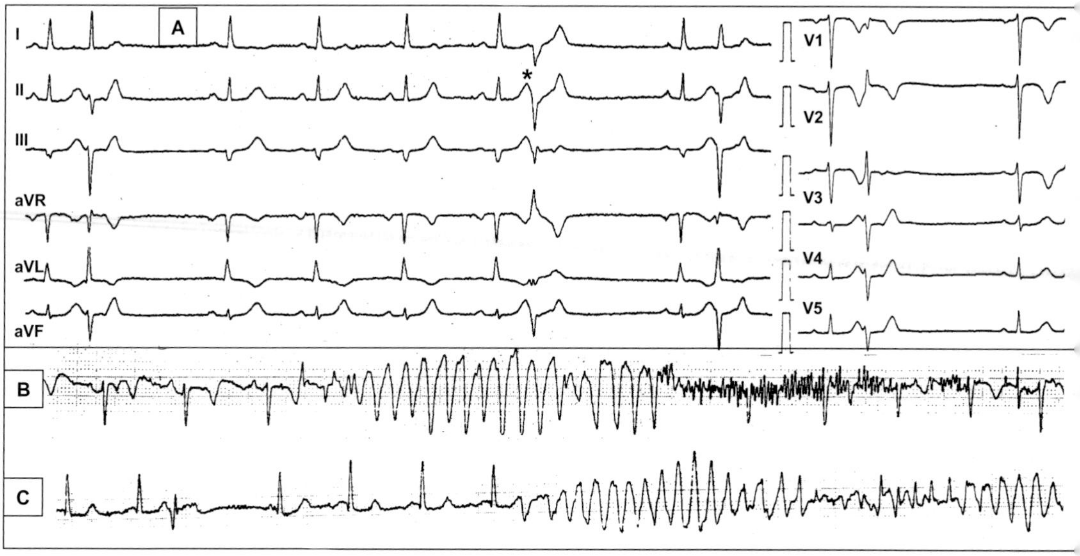

FIGURE 39–1. Typical example of idiopathic VF. This 54 year old female was referred for neurological consultation because of "recurrent seizures." Her baseline electrocardiogram shows sinus rhythm with normal PR, QRS, and QT intervals (A). However, there are several ventricular extrasystoles with varying coupling intervals, including short-coupled extrasystoles falling on the peak of the preceding T wave (*). Because of the short-coupled extrasystoles the patient was admitted to the Cardiology Department (instead of the Neurology Department). Soon thereafter, a self-terminating episode of rapid polymorphic ventricular tachycardia was recorded during one of her "seizures" (B). Ventricular fibrillation requiring defibrillation was also recorded shortly thereafter (C). The patient was diagnosed with "idiopathic ventricular fibrillation" and has been free of ventricular arrhythmias during treatment with quinidine for more than 9 years.

24–48 h.[3,31] Some of these VF clusters have been triggered by fever.[36]

Electrocardiogram

By definition, the electrocardiogram (ECG) of patients with idiopathic VF is normal during sinus rhythm. Japanese investigators report that patients with idiopathic VF often have J-point elevation in the inferior leads,[37] but it remains to be demonstrated that such a finding is more common in idiopathic VF than among healthy controls. Male patients with idiopathic VF have a disproportionably high prevalence of "relatively short QT" (see below).[18] The T_{peak}–T_{end} interval (the interval from the summit to the end of the T wave), which is a marker of the ventricular dispersion of repolarization and arrhythmic risk in the LQTSs[38,39] and Brugada syndrome,[40] is normal in idiopathic VF.[18]

Ventricular extrasystoles occur only rarely in patients with idiopathic VF, but when they do, they have varying coupling intervals with some extrasystoles closely coupled to the preceding complex (mean coupling interval = 302 ± 52 msec in our series,[5] 297 ± 41 msec in the series of Haissaguerre *et al.*,[32] and 300 ± 35 msec in the series of Champagne *et al.*[34]). Because of the short coupling interval, the extrasystoles fall on the summit or the descending limb of the T wave (Figures 39–1 and 39–2). In our series,[5] all VF episodes started by ventricular extrasystoles falling within 40 msec (with the majority falling within 20 msec) of the peak of the T wave. There appears to be an inverse relationship between the coupling interval of the extrasystoles and the risk for malignant arrhythmias with longer bursts of polymorphic VT triggered by extrasystoles with shorter coupling intervals.[32] In contrast to the polymorphic ventricular arrhythmias recorded in the LQTS,[41,42] the QT and QTc of the sinus complexes immediately before the onset of arrhythmias are normal (QT = 357 ± 41 msec and QTc = 397 ± 56 msec)[5,34]

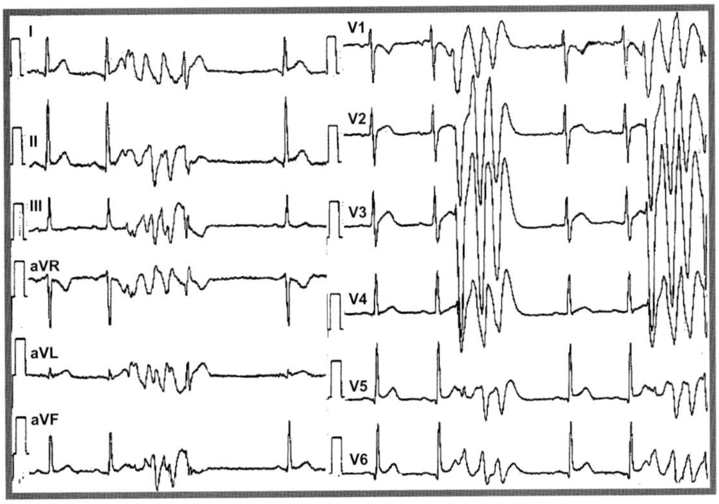

GURE 39–2. Typical mode of onset of idi- ɔathic VF. Note the very short coupling terval of the extrasystoles initiating the ɔlymorphic ventricular tachycardia. Also ɔte that despite the polymorphic mor- hology of the arrhythmia, when more ıan a VT episode is recorded (as in the recordial leads), the first, second and third ɔmplexes of the tachycardias are remark- ɔly similar.

nd arrhythmias are (as a rule) *not* pause lependent.[3,31,32,34]

Aorphology of Extrasystoles

n early reports showing the onset of idiopathic 'F,[1,3,43] an ECG pattern similar to the first short- oupled ventricular extrasystole was observed, ıamely, a left bundle branch block pattern and eft axis (Figure 39–2). However, later reports,[32,33] howed that extrasystoles with other patterns do xist, suggesting various possible sites of origin. nterestingly, when multiple episodes of polymor- hic VT are noted with 6-lead or 12-lead record- ngs, the morphology of the initiating beats of all hese episodes is similar. This applies not only to he first complex, but to the second and third omplexes of the polymorphic arrhythmias as vell (Figure 39–2). The last observation supports he notion that idiopathic VF has a focal origin see below).[32,33]

Electrophysiologic Data

Patients with idiopathic VF have normal A–H and I–V intervals, and their ventricular refractory eriods are within normal limits.[2,44] This is in con- rast to patients with Brugada syndrome, who often have a prolonged H–V interval[12] and patients vith short QT syndrome (SQTS), who invariably ıave short refractory periods in the atrium and he ventricle.[15,45,46]

The ventricular arrhythmias induced by programmed ventricular stimulation are invariably of polymorphic morphology, namely polymorphic VT or VF (Figure 39–3). Induction of monomorphic VT excludes the diagnosis of idiopathic VF. This is at variance with patients with Brugada syndrome who also have primarily VF,[47] but rarely have monomorphic VT.[48–53]

The inducibility rate is a function of the protocol used during programmed ventricular stimulation. Many electrophysiologists are reluctant to shorten the coupling interval of the delivered ventricular extrastimuli beyond a "nominal" value of 200 msec. This is because the risk of "accidentally" inducing VF in healthy individuals also increases as the coupling intervals of the second and third extrastimuli are shortened below 200 msec.[54–56] Indeed, in small studies performed 20 years ago, 6% of healthy individuals *without* documented or suspected spontaneous ventricular arrhythmias had inducible VF when the coupling intervals were limited only by ventricular refractoriness.[54–56] Moreover, an additional 40% of the last group of healthy controls had inducible nonsustained polymorphic VT, which led to premature discontinuation of the pacing protocol.[54–56] Therefore, *at least* 6% of healthy individuals will have inducible VF if aggressive protocols of extrastimulation (with double and triple extrastimulation with coupling intervals shorter than 200 msec) are used.[54–56] On the other hand, in our experience, as many as *80% of patients with idiopathic VF* have inducible VF

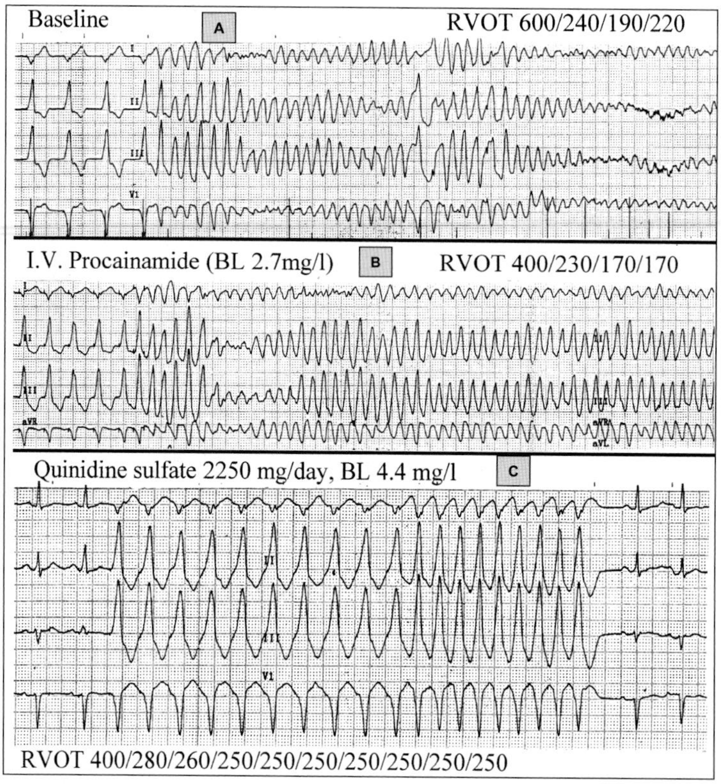

FIGURE 39–3. Typical results of an electrophysiological study in idiopathic VF. (A) At the baseline study, VF is induced by triple ventricular extrastimulation with short coupling intervals from the right ventricular outflow tract. Basic ventricular pacing at 100 beats/min (cycle length 600 msec) is followed by three extrastimuli 240, 190, and 220 msec apart; this initiates a VF that required direct current shock for termination. (B) After intravenous administration of 1000 mg of procainamide, the protocol of extrastimulation is repeated and VF is induced again. Note that despite of therapeutic levels of procainamide the effective refractory period is sufficientl short to allow ventricular capture of the ventricle with short cou pling intervals (230, 170, and 170 msec for the first, second, an third extrastimuli, respectively). (C) After 5 days of oral therap with quinidine it is no longer possible to capture the ventricle wit short coupling intervals. No ventricular arrhythmias could b induced despite a maximally aggressive protocol of extrastimula tion, including nine extrastimuli. This survivor of cardiac arrest ha been free of arrhythmias for >5 years on quinidine therapy.

with aggressive protocols of extrastimulation consisting of double and triple ventricular extrastimulation at two right ventricular pacing sites and using repetition of extrastimulation at the shortest coupling interval that captures the ventricle.[44,57] This very high inducibility rate suggests that the induction of VF, with aggressive protocols of extrastimulation, is a valid endpoint of programmed ventricular stimulation that then may be used for guiding antiarrhythmic therapy with quinidine in patients with idiopathic VF (Figure 39–3) (see the section on "Prognosis and Therapy of Idiopathic Ventricular Fibrillation" below).

Recently, Haissaguerre *et al.* performed endocardial recordings in patients with idiopathic VF at a time when they had frequent spontaneous ventricular extrasystoles and/or bursts of poly morphic VT.[32,33] The investigators were able t locate the site of origin of these ventricula arrhythmias in 27 patients. Successful localizatio of the site of origin of the ventricular arrhythmia was guided by very early endocardial recording and confirmed by abolition of ventricular arrhythmias following radiofrequency ablation of th firing focus. Purkinje potentials were recorded a the site of origin of ventricular arrhythmias in 2 (85%) out these 27 patients (in the left ventricula septum in 10 patients, the anterior right ventricl in 9 patients, and in both locations in 4). Th Purkinje potentials preceded the local myocardia activation by 11 ± 5 sec during sinus rhythm an by 10 ± 150 msec during spontaneous ventricula ectopy.[32] Based on these endocardial recordings, it seems that the arrhythmias in idiopathic VF have a focal origin, and that the triggering focus is within the Purkinje fibers in the majority of patients. Of note, the firing focus was not within the Purkinje network in only four (15%) patients, and in all these patients the arrhythmias originated in the right ventricular outflow tract (RVOT). Noda and Shimizu recently observed a large series of patients with polymorphic VT/VF originating in the RVOT.[58] Their observations are discussed in the section on "Differential Diagnosis" of idiopathic VF below.

Diagnosis

Diagnosing idiopathic VF in a cardiac arrest survivor is straightforward when the onset of spontaneous polymorphic VT/VF is recorded (usually during an arrhythmic storm) and this shows initiation of polymorphic VT/VF by very short coupled ventricular extrasystoles[3,31,42] (Figures 39–1 and 39–2). This is because the only three other conditions that lead to such a characteristic mode of VF initiation (myocardial ischemia,[59,60] Brugada syndrome,[61] and short QT syndrome)[17] can be identified with appropriate testing.

More often, however, patients are admitted after resuscitation from cardiac arrest and have documented VF, but recordings of the onset of arrhythmia are not available. In such cases, the diagnosis of idiopathic VF is established by excluding all identifiable causes and is further supported by the inducibility of VF with programmed ventricular stimulation. A discussion of all potential causes of sudden death is beyond the scope of this chapter, but a practical approach is presented in Figure 39–4.

The diagnosis of idiopathic VF most be considered in patients presenting with syncope without documented arrhythmias. Having said that, it

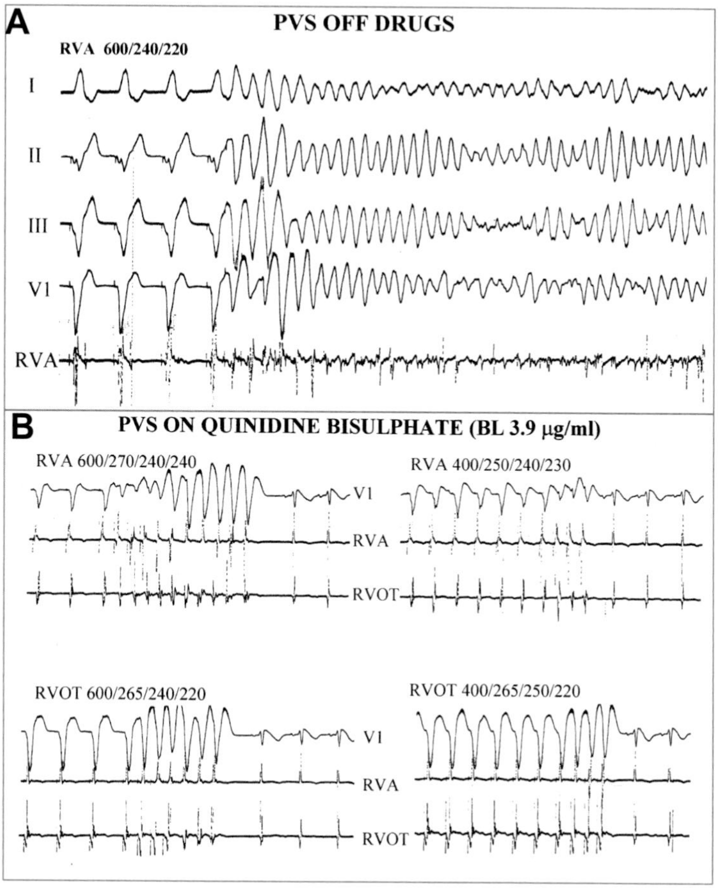

FIGURE 39–4. Easy induction of VF with double ventricular extrastimulation in the absence of drugs in a patient with idiopathic VF. In the same patient after treatment with quinidine no arrhythmias could be induced despite a very aggressive protocol including repetition of double and triple ventricular extrastimulation at the shortest coupling intervals that capture the ventricle. PVS, programmed ventricular stimulation.

most be emphasized that in the overwhelming majority of patients presenting with syncope in the absence of heart disease, a diagnosis of vasovagal syncope (rather than arrhythmic syncope) will be evident from the clinical history. Also, the majority of patients with syncope that does *not* appear to be of vasovagal origin also have ECG or echocardiographic abnormalities that will suggest an underlying diagnosis. Therefore, only very rarely a patient presents with syncope in whom the history is sufficiently worrisome to suggest an arrhythmic origin yet all noninvasive studies [including drug challenges to exclude Brugada syndrome,[25,30] LQTS,[62–65] and Wolff–Parkinson–White syndrome (WPW)][66] are negative. In such cases, an electrophysiological evaluation can be performed to exclude intra-His block as the cause of syncope. However, recommending the performance of programmed ventricular stimulation to a patient with syncope who has no evidence of heart disease and no documented arrhythmias (particularly closed-coupled ventricular extrasystoles) is problematic. This is because in the absence of organic heart disease, inducible ventricular arrhythmias (if any) are likely to be of polymorphic morphology. Understanding the significance of inducible VF in the absence of documented spontaneous arrhythmias is difficult, because such arrhythmias may be induced in at least 6% of healthy individuals.[54–56] Therefore, programmed ventricular stimulation should be performed only when both physician and patient are prepared to accept the induction of VF as a "positive" response.

Differential Diagnosis

Subtle Forms of Organic Heart Disease

Excluding all forms of organic heart disease is essential before the diagnosis of idiopathic VF can be considered. However, it should be noted that some forms of organic heart disease may cause malignant ventricular arrhythmias at a time when the anatomic abnormalities are minimal and difficult to detect by imaging modalities. For example, patients with hypertrophic cardiomyopathy due to troponin-T mutations may be at risk for arrhythmic death at a time when left ventricular hypertrophy is still mild.[67,68] Similarly, right ventricular dysplasia is sometimes identified as the underlying cause of sudden death only during forensic examination and despite a negative extensive diagnostic workup.[69] Of note, subtle anatomic abnormalities, like mitral valve prolapse without hemodynamic significance, should not necessarily be accepted as the cause of cardiac arrest. On the other hand, signs of severe left ventricular dysfunction after resuscitation should not necessarily be used to exclude the diagnosis of idiopathic VF because prolonged resuscitation may result in transient electrocardiographic and ECG abnormalities that are indistinguishable from those seen in patients with dilated cardiomyopathy.[70] If such abnormalities resolve, the diagnosis of idiopathic VF should obviously be considered.

Wolff–Parkinson–White Syndrome

Patients with atrioventricular (AV) accessory pathways may have minimal or no ventricular preexcitation (i.e., may have narrow QRS complexes) if they also have fast conduction along the AV node or if their accessory pathways are located on the left lateral wall (far from the sinus node). Yet these pathways may have short refractory periods. Such patients may develop atrial fibrillation with rapid ventricular rates that may deteriorate to VF. If the preexcited atrial fibrillation is not recorded and the patient is found in VF, the near-normal ECG during sinus rhythm may lead to a wrong diagnosis of "idiopathic VF" because all imaging tests will be normal. The wrong diagnosis of idiopathic VF may gain further support from electrophysiological studies if *atrial* stimulation is not performed prior to ventricular pacing, because programmed ventricular stimulation is likely to induce VF in patients with WPW syndrome.[71] Therefore, excluding accessory pathways, either with adenosine injection as a bedside test or with atrial pacing during electrophysiological studies, is a mandatory step in the workup of VF survivors even when the ECG is judged to be "normal." Of note, rare cases of cardiac arrest caused by very rapid supraventricular tachyarrhythmias in patients without WPW syndrome have also been described.[72]

Catecholamine-Sensitive Polymorphic Ventricular Tachycardia

Physicians maydecide to skip exercise testing in cardiac arrest survivors reasoning that coronary angiography will eventually reveal any significant coronary lesion. We have encountered patients with CPVT who were erroneously diagnosed with "idiopathic VF" only because exercise stress testing was not performed. Since all other tests, including electrophysiological studies, are invariably normal in this disease, an exercise stress test is mandatory in cardiac arrest survivors. Although the majority of patients with CPVT have a pathognomonic response to exercise (exercise-induced atrial fibrillation followed my multifocal ventricular extrasystoles, bidirectional VT, and polymorphic VT), it was recently recognized that some patients with genetically proven CPVT have only single ventricular extrasystoles that look like typical "benign RVOT extrasystoles" during maximal exercise.[73] Such patients may be wrongly diagnosed as having "idiopathic VF."

Long QT Syndrome

The QTc intervals of the healthy population, as well as the QTc of patients with LQTS have a normal distribution and there is considerable overlapping between the QTc of both populations. Importantly, 12% of patients with genetically proven LQTS have "normal" QT when the latter is defined as QTc < 440 msec.[74] Identifying patients with LQTS who have borderline QT is especially challenging in the LQT1 genotype because the T wave morphology, which is frequently abnormal in LQT2 and LQT3, is most often normal in LQT1. Fortunately, the epinephrine challenge test is especially effective in unraveling abnormal QT responses in LQT1.[62–64,75]

Short QT Syndrome

The newly described SQTS[15,16] is caused by genetic mutations involving the same potassium channels that cause the LQTS but with an opposite effect.[20,22,30,76–78] In other words, in the SQTS there is excessive outflow of potassium currents, shortening the duration of the action potential and the effective ventricular refractory period. Distinguishing idiopathic VF from SQTS is not easy. Although the original cases of SQTS had extremely short QT intervals (QTc shorter than 300 msec),[15,16] more recently described cases of genetically proven SQTS have QTc intervals of 320 msec.[22] Also, we recently showed that "relatively short" QT intervals (QTc < 360 msec) are frequently observed in healthy males but are statistically more common in males with idiopathic VF.[18] Moreover, patients with idiopathic VF have normal QT intervals at normal heart rates, but their QT fails to lengthen as their heart rate slows down, leading to abnormally short QTc values during bradycardia.[79–81] Finally, patients with SQTS and patients with idiopathic VF share the following clinical characteristics. (1) Both patient groups have similar spontaneous[5,17] and inducible[3,46] ventricular arrhythmias, (2) both patient groups appear to respond especially well to quinidine therapy,[2,44,45,82] and (3) both patient groups are at risk for inappropriate implantable cardioverter defibrillator (ICD) shocks because of intracardiac T wave oversensing.[83,84] Patients with SQTS may be misdiagnosed as "idiopathic VF" if the QT interval is measured only during relatively rapid heart rates. This is because the main problem in the SQTS is failure of appropriate QT lengthening during bradycardia.[46]

Brugada Syndrome

We estimated that one out of five patients originally diagnosed as "idiopathic VF" in fact have Brugada syndrome[13] and very similar numbers were reported by others.[85] Moreover, if all patients with idiopathic VF undergo systematic testing with repeated ECGs (placing the right precordial electrodes at higher positions)[86] and with a pharmacological challenge test using sodium channel blockers to unravel subtle sodium channel malfunctions, as many as 40% with idiopathic VF could be diagnosed as having Brugada syndrome.[19]

Short-Coupled Variant of Right Ventricular Outflow Tachycardia

The RVOT is the site of origin of the most common type of VT occurring in patients *without* organic heart disease.[31] This RVOT-VT has a distinctive morphology (QRS complexes with a left bundle branch block pattern and tall R waves in the inferior leads) and, in general, does not lead to hemodynamic decompensation. Therefore, RVOT-VT is considered a benign arrhythmia.[31] However, our group[87] and the group of Noda and Shimizu[58] recently described patients with otherwise typical "benign RVOT ectopy" who went on to develop spontaneous VF or polymorphic VT.[88] It is not clear if patients with idiopathic VF and patients with this newly described form of "polymorphic VT from the RVOT"[58,87,89] represent different aspects of one disease or two distinct disorders.[88] However, several characteristics differ among both groups. (1) Otherwise typical *monomorphic* RVOT-VT is *also* seen in patients with malignant polymorphic RVOT-VT,[58,87] but is never seen in idiopathic VF.[3,31,32] (2) Only 5% of patients with "malignant polymorphic VT" have inducible VF by programmed ventricular stimulation, whereas the majority of patients with idiopathic VF have inducible VF.[44] (3) The coupling interval of the ventricular extrasystoles initiating the malignant ventricular arrhythmias is invariably very short in idiopathic VF,[5,32] but is longer, varying from "relatively short"[87] to "normal,"[58] in the "polymorphic RVOT-VT." The last observation is consistent with the results of intracardiac mapping performed by Haissaguerre *et al.*[32] In that series, idiopathic VF originated from Purkinje fibers in 86% of the patients and from the RVOT in the remaining 14%. Again, the coupling interval of the extrasystoles initiating VF was *longer* for arrhythmias originating in the RVOT than for arrhythmias triggered by Purkinje fibers (355 ± 30 msec vs. 280 ± 26 msec, $p < 0.01$).

Prognosis and Therapy of Idiopathic Ventricular Fibrillation

The rate of recurrence of malignant ventricular arrhythmias in idiopathic VF, in the absence of therapy, is unacceptably high. At a mean follow-up of 6 years, more than 40% of patients have recurrent VF and the risk is higher for those with normal ECGs (that is, after excluding those with possible Brugada syndrome).[90] In a recent series of patients with "truly idiopathic VF" (that is, excluding not only those with a Brugada-type ECG at baseline but also those who developed ST-segment elevation when challenged with sodium channel blockers), the risk for recurrent VF was 39% at 3.4 ± 2.3 years.[34] Therefore, once a diagnosis of idiopathic VF is made, some form of therapy is mandatory. Therapy may include ICD implantation, drug therapy with quinidine, radiofrequency ablation of the triggering focus, or combinations of the above.

Drug Therapy with Quinidine

The first patients with idiopathic VF described in the literature, back in 1929[1] and 1949,[91] were treated with quinidine after multiple episodes of spontaneous polymorphic VT and VF were clearly documented. Both patients had an excellent response.[1,91] In fact, a second publication reporting the long-term follow-up of the patient initially reported in 1949 established that this patient eventually died of cancer at old age, without ever experiencing a recurrence of arrhythmia while on quinidine therapy for 40 years.[92] In 1987, Belhassen pioneered the therapy of idiopathic VF with electrophysiological-guided quinidine after observing that VF is easily inducible at the baseline state but is no longer inducible after quinidine therapy.[2] Of note, one of the patients included in that original report[43] recently completed 25 uneventful years of electrophysiological-guided therapy with amiodarone and quinidine after experiencing arrhythmic storms of VF in the absence of therapy and recurrent arrhythmic syncope on amiodarone alone.[93]

In 1990, when we first reviewed the topic of idiopathic VF,[3] we found that the recurrence rate of cardiac arrest was high during therapy with other antiarrhythmic drugs (including amiodarone, β blockers, or verapamil).[3] The high rate of recurrence of arrhythmia with verapamil is worth noting because that drug was empirically proposed by Leenhardt and Coumel to treat the "short-coupled variant of torsade de pointes,"[4] an entity that probably represents idiopathic VF. In contrast, we found that there was no recurrence rate with quinidine.[3] Therefore, when the ICD became commercially available, *we continued to recommend quinidine as the sole therapy for appropriately selected patients with idiopathic VF, including patients resuscitated from spontaneous ardiac arrest.*[94] Our criteria for quinidine therapy n VF survivors include all of the following: (1) iagnosis of idiopathic VF with or without rugada syndrome, (2) inducible VF in the bsence of drugs with programmed ventricular timulation (Figure 39–5), (3) no inducible rrhythmias during oral quinidine therapy despite very aggressive protocol of ventricular stimula-ion (Figure 39–5),[44,57] (4) informed consent by a atient who is well aware of the risks and benefits f ICD and quinidine therapy for this disease,[94] nd (5) repeated assertion of drug compliance uring long-term follow-up (compliance is ssessed with quinidine serum levels and quini-ine effect on the QT interval).

Our results using such an approach were published in 1999.[44] These results are shown in Figure 39–6 and may be summarized as follows. Of 34 patients with idiopathic VF (all after resuscitation from cardiac arrest), 26 (80%) had inducible VF at baseline electrophysiological study and all but one of them were rendered noninducible with quinidine. Side effects from quinidine led to discontinuation of quinidine therapy in 14% of our patients. Nevertheless, 23 patients (two out of three patients from the original cohort of cardiac arrest survivors) remained on quinidine therapy (without ICD backup); all are alive and all have been completely free of arrhythmic symptoms for more than 10 years. Relatively early in our experience,

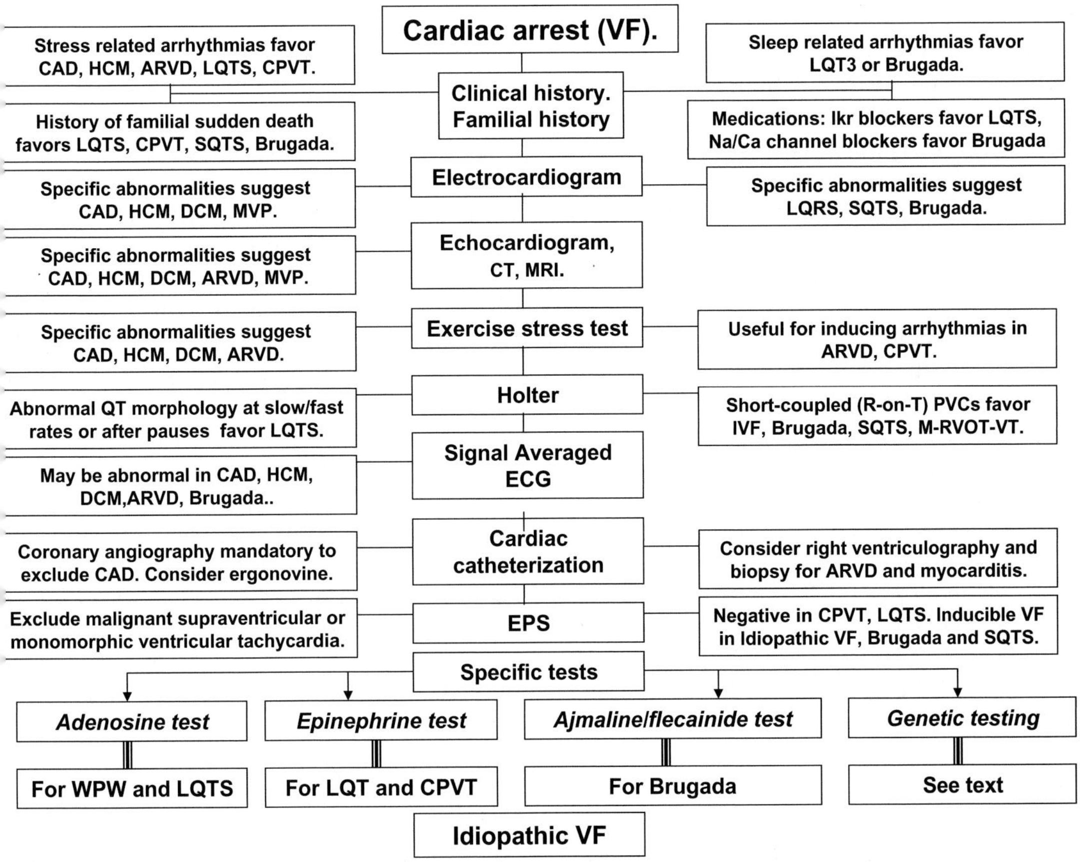

FIGURE 39–5. Proposed basic algorithm to diagnose idiopathic VF. CAD, coronary artery disease; HCM and DCM, hypertrophic and dilated cardiomyopathy, respectively; ARVD, arrhythmogenic right ventricular dysplasia/cardiomyopathy; LQTS, long QT syndrome; CPVT, catecholaminergic polymorphic ventricular tachycardia; LQT3, long QT syndrome of LQT3 genotype; SQTS, short QT syndrome; MVP, mitral valve prolapse; CT, computerized tomography; MRI, magnetic resonance imaging; M-RVOT-VT, malignant form of idiopathic ventricular tachycardia originating from the right ventricular outflow tract; WPW, Wolff–Parkinson–White syndrome.

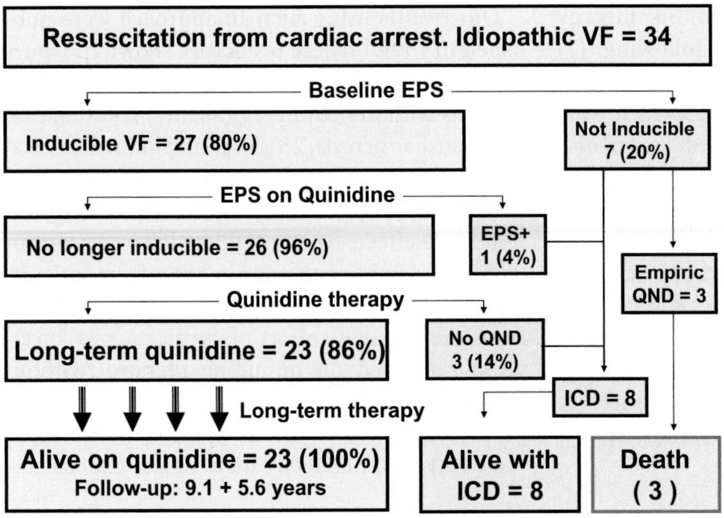

FIGURE 39–6. Our experience with quinidine therapy as published in 1999.[44] VF, ventricular fibrillation; EPS, electrophysiological study with programmed ventricular stimulation; EPS+, positive electrophysiological study, i.e., inducible VF with programmed ventricular stimulation; QND, quinidine; ICD, implantable cardioverter defibrillator.

three patients who had negative electrophysiological studies in the absence of drugs received empiric quinidine. All these patients died 4–8 years after the original VF episode. These three patients discontinued follow-up long before they died. Therefore, we do not know if the fatalities were due to poor compliance or due to drug failure and whether such failure was related to the fact that quinidine therapy for these particular patients was empiric and not guided by electrophysiological studies (since these three patients were noninducible at baseline). Nevertheless, we no longer recommend empiric use of quinidine for noninducible patients, a subgroup of patients for whom ICD implantation is mandatory. However, we have successfully used quinidine to control arrhythmic storms of ventricular fibrillations in patients who originally received an ICD either because of noninducibility in the baseline EPS or because of (the extremely rare) persistence of inducibility while on quinidine therapy. The excellent response of VF storms in idiopathic VF with Brugada syndrome has also been repeatedly reported.[95–97] Of note, the fatalities that occurred 4–8 years after the first VF event clearly demonstrate that patients with idiopathic VF remain at risk for fatal recurrence of arrhythmia even after long asymptomatic periods. Thus, long asymptomatic periods after the first VF episode should not be interpreted as resolution of an unidentified "myocarditis" and cannot be taken as a "good prognostic sign."

Radiofrequency Ablation

Catheter-based radiofrequency ablation of the triggering focus is now an accepted mode of therapy for *atrial* fibrillation. Haissaguerre[32,33] and others[58,98,99] have used the same concept to treat idiopathic VF. This form of therapy has been used primarily to treat patients with implanted ICDs who are receiving multiple ICD shocks because of arrhythmic storms. The first successful ablation was reported by Aizawa *et al.* in 1992,[98] whereas relatively large series have been reported by Haissaguerre *et al.*[32,33] and by Noda *et al.*[58] These differ in the site of origin of the targeted arrhythmias: Noda *et al.* targeted polymorphic VT originating from the right ventricular outflow tract.[58] In contrast, 85% of the polymorphic ventricular arrhythmias ablated by Haissaguerre *et al.* were mapped to the Purkinje system in the right or left ventricle, whereas the site of origin of the VF was in the right ventricular outflow tract in only four (15%) patients.[32] An acute successful abolition was achieved in all cases; 24 patients (89%) had no recurrence of VF without drugs during follow-up. Such favorable results certainly encourage adopting such a curative option for treating patients with idiopathic VF. However, this is a therapy that can be considered only for the rare patients with repetitive ventricular arrhythmias. In our 27-year experience dealing with 35 patients with idiopathic VF, only three could have been candidates for ch a mode of therapy in our institution.[2] Also, nce the etiology of idiopathic VF is unknown, it impossible to state at this point that this is a cal disease.

nplantable Cardioverter efibrillator Implantation

here is no doubt that ICD offers the most effecve therapy for preventing arrhythmic death in liopathic VF. Indeed, ICD implantation is condered "the only" effective therapy for idiopathic F by most investigators. However, when comaring ICD implantation with quinidine therapy r radiofrequency ablation for idiopathic VF, it is ecessary to also take into consideration the otential adverse events of all these interventions.

In Antiarrhythmics versus Implantable Defiillators (AVID), a large multicenter study of ICD nplantation for malignant ventricular arrhythnias in patients with organic heart disease,[100] the isk of adverse events, serious enough to warrant eintervention was 12%.[101] Since only experienced lectrophysiologists from prestigious centers parcipated in AVID, this 12% complication rate is kely to be a moderate estimate. Moreover, the ate of complications from ICD implantation in liopathic VF could likely be higher than the 12% eported in AVID. This is because patients in VID were relatively old (mean age 65 ± 11 ears)[100] and had a 3-year mortality rate of 25% espite the ICD related to their underlying organic eart disease.[100] In contrast, patients with idioathic VF are significantly younger and have n extremely low risk of nonarrhythmic cardiac eath. Therefore, idiopathic VF patients will renain at risk for ICD-related complications for nany more years. In particular, the risk of potenially serious complications such as infection or a reak in lead insulation leading to inappropriate CD shocks will increase over the years and after epeated ICD replacements.

eferences

1. Dock W. Transitory ventricular fibrillation as a cause of syncope and its prevention by quinidine sulfate. *Am Heart J* 1929;4:709–714.
2. Belhassen B, Shapira I, Shoshani D, Paredes A, Miller H, Laniado S. Idiopathic ventricular fibrillation: Inducibility and beneficial effects of class I antiarrhythmic agents. *Circulation* 1987;75:809–816.
3. Viskin S, Belhassen B. Idiopathic ventricular fibrillation. *Am Heart J* 1990;120:661–671.
4. Leenhardt A, Glaser E, Burguera M, Nurnberg M, Maison-Blanche P, Coumel P. Short-coupled variant of torsade de pointes. A new electrocardiographic entity in the spectrum of idiopathic ventricular tachyarrhythmias. *Circulation* 1994;89:206–215.
5. Viskin S, Lesh M, Eldar M, *et al.* Mode of onset of malignant ventricular arrhythmias in idiopathic ventricular fibrillation. *J Cardiovasc Electrophysiol* 1997;8:1115–1120.
6. Haissaguerre M, Extramiana F, Hocini M, *et al.* Mapping and ablation of ventricular fibrillation associated with long-QT and Brugada syndromes. *Circulation* 2003;108:925–928.
7. Jervell A, Lange-Nielsen F. Congenital deaf-mutism, functional heart disease with prolongation of the Q-T interval and sudden death. *Am Heart J* 1957;54:59–68.
8. Romano C, Gemme G, Pongiglione R. Aritmie cardiache rare dell'eta pediatrica. *Clin Pediatr* 1963;45:656–683.
9. Ward OC. A new familial cardiac syndrome in children. *J Irish Med Assoc* 1964;54:103–106.
10. Leenhardt A, Lucet V, Denjoy I, Grau F, Ngoc D, Coumel P. Catecholaminergic polymorphic ventricular tachycardia in children. A 7-year follow-up of 21 patients. *Circulation* 1995;91:1512–1519.
11. Aponte G. The enigma of "Bangungut." *Ann Intern Med* 1960;52:1258–1263.
12. Brugada P, Brugada J. Right bundle branch block, persistent ST segment elevation and sudden cardiac death: A distinct clinical and electrocardiographic syndrome. A multicenter report. *J Am Coll Cardiol* 1992;20:1391–1396.
13. Viskin S, Fish R, Eldar M, *et al.* Prevalence of the Brugada sign in idiopathic ventricular fibrillation and healthy controls. *Heart* 2000;84:31–36.
14. Nademanee K, Veerakul G, Nimmannit S, *et al.* Arrhythmogenic marker for the sudden unexpected death syndrome in Thai men. *Circulation* 1997;96:2595–2600.
15. Gaita F, Giustetto C, Bianchi F, *et al.* Short QT syndrome: A familial cause of sudden death. *Circulation* 2003;108:965–970.
16. Gussak I, Brugada P, Brugada J, *et al.* Idiopathic short QT interval: A new clinical syndrome? Cardiology 2000;94:99–102.
17. Schimpf R, Bauersfeld U, Gaita F, Wolpert C. Short QT syndrome: Successful prevention of sudden

cardiac death in an adolescent by implantable cardioverter-defibrillator treatment for primary prophylaxis. *Heart Rhythm* 2005;2:416–417.

18. Viskin S, Zeltser D, Ish-Shalom M, *et al.* Is idiopathic ventricular fibrillation a short QT syndrome? Comparison of QT intervals of patients with idiopathic ventricular fibrillation and healthy controls. *Heart Rhythm* 2004;1:587–591.
19. Chen Q, Kirsch GE, Zhang D, *et al.* Genetic basis and molecular mechanism for idiopathic ventricular fibrillation. *Nature* 1998;392:293–296.
20. Bellocq C, van Ginneken AC, Bezzina CR, *et al.* Mutation in the KCNQ1 gene leading to the short QT-interval syndrome. *Circulation* 2004;109: 2394–2397.
21. Brugada R, Hong K, Dumaine R, *et al.* Sudden death associated with short-QT syndrome linked to mutations in HERG. *Circulation* 2004;109: 30–35.
22. Priori SG, Pandit SV, Rivolta I, *et al.* A novel form of short QT syndrome (SQT3) is caused by a mutation in the KCNJ2 gene. *Circ Res* 2005;96: 800–807.
23. Hong K, Brugada J, Oliva A, *et al.* Value of electrocardiographic parameters and ajmaline test in the diagnosis of Brugada syndrome caused by SCN5A mutations. *Circulation* 2004;110: 3023–3027.
24. Rolf S, Bruns HJ, Wichter T, *et al.* The ajmaline challenge in Brugada syndrome: Diagnostic impact, safety, and recommended protocol. *Eur Heart J* 2003;24:1104–1112.
25. Wolpert C, Echternach C, Veltmann C, *et al.* Intravenous drug challenge using flecainide and ajmaline in patients with Brugada syndrome. *Heart Rhythm* 2005;2:254–260.
26. Meregalli PG, Ruijter JM, Hofman N, Bezzina CR, Wilde AA, Tan HL. Diagnostic value of flecainide testing in unmasking SCN5A-related Brugada syndrome. *J Cardiovasc Electrophysiol* 2006;17(8): 857–864.
27. Priori SG, Napolitano C, Schwartz PJ, Bloise R, Crotti L, Ronchetti E. The elusive link between LQT3 and Brugada syndrome: The role of flecainide challenge. *Circulation* 2000;102:945–947.
28. Chinushi M, Aizawa Y, Ogawa Y, Shiba M, Takahashi K. Discrepant drug action of disopyramide on ECG abnormalities and induction of ventricular arrhythmias in a patient with Brugada syndrome. *J Electrocardiol* 1997;30:133–136.
29. Sangwatanaroj S, Prechawat S, Sunsaneewitayakul B, Sitthisook S, Tosukhowong P, Tungsanga K. New electrocardiographic leads and the procainamide test for the detection of the Brugada sign in sudden unexplained death syndrome survivor and their relatives. *Eur Heart J* 2001;2 2290–2296.
30. Hong K, Bjerregaard P, Gussak I, Brugada R. Sho QT syndrome and atrial fibrillation caused b mutation in KCNH2. *J Cardiovasc Electrophysi* 2005;16:394–396.
31. Belhassen B, Viskin S. Idiopathic ventricular tach ycardia and fibrillation. *J Cardiovasc Electrophys iol* 1993;4:356–368.
32. Haissaguerre M, Shoda M, Jais P, *et al.* Mappin and ablation of idiopathic ventricular fibrillatior *Circulation* 2002;106:962–967.
33. Haissaguerre M, Shah DC, Jais P, *et al.* Role c Purkinje conducting system in triggering of idic pathic ventricular fibrillation. *Lancet* 2002;35 677–678.
34. Champagne J, Geelen P, Philippon F, Brugada Recurrent cardiac events in patients with idio pathic ventricular fibrillation, excluding patient with the Brugada syndrome. *BMC Med* 2005; 1–6.
35. Viskin S, Belhassen B. Polymorphic ventricula tachyarrhythmias in the absence of organic hear disease. Classification, differential diagnosis an implications for therapy. *Prog Cardiovasc Di* 1998;41:17–34.
36. Pasquie JL, Sanders P, Hocini M, *et al.* Fever as precipitant of idiopathic ventricular fibrillation i patients with normal hearts. *J Cardiovasc Electro physiol* 2004;15:1271–1276.
37. Takagi M, Aihara N, Takaki H, *et al.* Clinical char acteristics of patients with spontaneous or induc ible ventricular fibrillation without apparent hear disease presenting with J wave and ST segmen elevation in inferior leads. *J Cardiovasc Electro physiol* 2000;11:844–848.
38. Shimizu W, Horie M, Ohno S, *et al.* Mutation site specific differences in arrhythmic risk and sensi tivity to sympathetic stimulation in the LQT form of congenital long QT syndrome: Multicente study in Japan. *J Am Coll Cardiol* 2004;44 117–125.
39. Yan GX, Antzelevitch C. Cellular basis for th normal T wave and the electrocardiographic man ifestations of the long-QT syndrome. *Circulatio* 1998;98:1928–1936.
40. Castro Hevia J, Antzelevitch C, Tornes Barzaga F *et al.* Tpeak-Tend and Tpeak-Tend dispersion a risk factors for ventricular tachycardia/ventricu lar fibrillation in patients with the Brugada syn drome. *J Am Coll Cardiol* 2006;47:1828–1834.
41. Noda T, Shimizu W, Satomi K, *et al.* Classificatio and mechanism of torsade de pointes initiation i

patients with congenital long QT syndrome. *Eur Heart J* 2004;25:2149–2154.
42. Viskin S, Alla SR, Barron HV, *et al.* Mode of onset of torsade de pointes in congenital long QT syndrome. *J Am Coll Cardiol* 1996;28:1262–1268.
43. Belhassen B, Pelleg A, Miller HI, Laniado S. Serial electrophysiological studies in a young patient with recurrent ventricular fibrillation. *Pacing Clin Electrophysiol* 1981;4:92–99.
44. Belhassen B, Viskin S, Fish R, Glick A, Setbon I, Eldar M. Effects of electrophysiologic-guided therapy with Class IA antiarrhythmic drugs on the long-term outcome of patients with idiopathic ventricular fibrillation with or without the Brugada syndrome. *J Cardiovasc Electrophysiol* 1999;10: 1301–1312.
45. Gaita F, Giustetto C, Bianchi F, *et al.* Short QT syndrome: Pharmacological treatment. *J Am Coll Cardiol* 2004;43:1494–1499.
46. Gussak I, Bjerregaard P. Short QT syndrome–5 years of progress. *J Electrocardiol* 2005;38:375–377.
47. Brugada P, Geelen P, Brugada R, Mont L, Brugada J. Prognostic value of electrophysiologic investigations in Brugada syndrome. *J Cardiovasc Electrophysiol* 2001;12:1004–1007.
48. Boersma LV, Jaarsma W, Jessurun ER, Van Hemel NH, Wever EF. Brugada syndrome: A case report of monomorphic ventricular tachycardia. *Pacing Clin Electrophysiol* 2001;24:112–115.
49. Dinckal MH, Davutoglu V, Akdemir I, Soydinc S, Kirilmaz A, Aksoy M. Incessant monomorphic ventricular tachycardia during febrile illness in a patient with Brugada syndrome: Fatal electrical storm. *Europace* 2003;5:257–261.
50. Mok NS, Chan NY. Brugada syndrome presenting with sustained monomorphic ventricular tachycardia. *Int J Cardiol* 2004;97:307–309.
51. Sastry BK, Narasimhan C, Soma Raju B. Brugada syndrome with monomorphic ventricular tachycardia in a one-year-old child. *Indian Heart J* 2001;53:203–205.
52. Shimada M, Miyazaki T, Miyoshi S, *et al.* Sustained monomorphic ventricular tachycardia in a patient with Brugada syndrome. *Jpn Circ J* 1996;60: 364–370.
53. Viskin S, Belhassen B. Clinical problem solving: When you only live twice. *N Engl J Med* 1995;332: 1221–1225.
54. Brugada P, Green M, Abdollah H, Wellens HJ. Significance of ventricular arrhythmias initiated by programmed ventricular stimulation: The importance of the type of ventricular arrhythmia induced and the number of premature stimuli required. *Circulation* 1984;69:87–92.
55. Morady F, DiCarlo L, Baerman J, de Buitleir M. Comparison of coupling intervals that induce clinical and nonclinical forms of ventricular tachycardia during programmed stimulation. *Am J Cardiol* 1986;57:1269–1273.
56. Stevenson WG, Brugada P, Waldecker B, Zehender M, Wellens HJ. Can potentially significant polymorphic ventricular arrhythmias initiated by programmed stimulation be distinguished from those that are nonspecific? *Am Heart J* 1986;111: 1073–1080.
57. Belhassen B, Shapira I, Sheps D, Laniado S. Programmed ventricular stimulation using up to two extrastimuli and repetition of double extrastimulation for induction of ventricular tachycardia: A new highly sensitive and specific protocol. *Am J Cardiol* 1990;65:615–622.
58. Noda T, Shimizu W, Taguchi A, *et al.* Malignant entity of idiopathic ventricular fibrillation and polymorphic ventricular tachycardia initiated by premature extrasystoles originating from the right ventricular outflow tract. *J Am Coll Cardiol* 2005; 46:1288–1294.
59. Myerburg R, Kessler K, Mallon S, *et al.* Life-threatening ventricular arrhythmias in patients with silent myocardial ischemia due to coronary-artery spasm. *N Engl J Med* 1992;326:1451–1455.
60. Wolfe CL, Nibley C, Bhandari A, Chatterjee K, Scheinman M. Polymorphous ventricular tachycardia associated with acute myocardial infarction. *Circulation* 1991;84:1543–1551.
61. Kakishita M, Kurita T, Matsuo K, *et al.* Mode of onset of ventricular fibrillation in patients with Brugada syndrome detected by implantable cardioverter defibrillator therapy. *J Am Coll Cardiol* 2000;36:1646–1653.
62. Ackerman MJ, Khositseth A, Tester DJ, Hejlik JB, Shen WK, Porter CB. Epinephrine-induced QT interval prolongation: A gene-specific paradoxical response in congenital long QT syndrome. *Mayo Clin Proc* 2002;77:413–421.
63. Shimizu W, Noda T, Takaki H, *et al.* Epinephrine unmasks latent mutation carriers with LQT1 form of congenital long-QT syndrome. *J Am Coll Cardiol* 2003;41:633–642.
64. Viskin S. Drug challenge with epinephrine or isoproterenol for diagnosing a long QT syndrome: Should we try this at home? *J Cardiovasc Electrophysiol* 2005;16:285–287.
65. Viskin S, Rosso R, Rogowski O, *et al.* Provocation of sudden heart rate oscillation with adenosine exposes abnormal QT responses in patients with long QT syndrome: A bedside test for diagnosing long QT syndrome. *Eur Heart J* 2006;27:469–475.

66. Garratt CJ, Antoniou A, Griffith MJ, Ward DE, Camm AJ. Use of intravenous adenosine in sinus rhythm as a diagnostic test for latent preexcitation. *Am J Cardiol* 1990;65:868–873.
67. Varnava A, Baboonian C, Davison F, *et al.* A new mutation of the cardiac troponin T gene causing familial hypertrophic cardiomyopathy without left ventricular hypertrophy. *Heart* 1999;82:621–624.
68. Varnava AM, Elliott PM, Baboonian C, Davison F, Davies MJ, McKenna WJ. Hypertrophic cardiomyopathy: Histopathological features of sudden death in cardiac troponin T disease. *Circulation* 2001;104:1380–1384.
69. Fontaine G, Fornes P, Hebert JL. Ventricular tachycardia in arrhythmogenic right ventricular cardiomyopathies. In: Zipes DP, Jalife J, Eds. *Cardiac Electrophysiology: From Cell to Bedside*, 3rd ed. Philadelphia, PA: W.B. Saunders, 2003.
70. Deantonio HJ, Kaul S, Lerman BB. Reversible myocardial depression in survivors of cardiac arrest. *Pacing Clin Electrophysiol* 1990;13:982–985.
71. Brembilla-Perrot B, Terrier de la Chaise A, Isaaz K, Marcon F, Cherrier F, Pernot C. Inducible multiform ventricular tachycardia in Wolff-Parkinson-White syndrome. *Br Heart J* 1987;58:89–95.
72. Wang Y, Griffin J, Lesh M, Cohen T, Chien W, Scheinman M. Patients with supraventricular tachycardia presenting with aborted sudden death: Incidence, mechanism and long-term follow-up. *J Am Coll Cardiol* 1991;18:1720–1721.
73. Tester DJ, Kopplin LJ, Will ML, Ackerman MJ. Spectrum and prevalence of cardiac ryanodine receptor (RyR2) mutations in a cohort of unrelated patients referred explicitly for long QT syndrome genetic testing. *Heart Rhythm* 2005;2:1099–1105.
74. Vincent GM, Timothy KW, Leppert M, Keating M. The spectrum of symptoms and QT intervals in carriers of the gene for the long QT syndrome. *N Engl J Med* 1992;327:846–852.
75. Shimizu W, Noda T, Takaki H, *et al.* Diagnostic value of epinephrine test for genotyping LQT1, LQT2, and LQT3 forms of congenital long QT syndrome. *Heart Rhythm* 2004;3:273–286.
76. Borggrefe M, Wolpert C, Antzelevitch C, *et al.* Short QT syndrome. Genotype-phenotype correlations. *J Electrocardiol* 2005;38:75–80.
77. Hong K, Piper DR, Diaz-Valdecantos A, *et al.* De novo KCNQ1 mutation responsible for atrial fibrillation and short QT syndrome in utero. *Cardiovasc Res* 2005;68:433–440.
78. McPate MJ, Duncan RS, Milnes JT, Witchel HJ, Hancox JC. The N588K-HERG K+ channel mutation in the "short QT syndrome": Mechanis of gain-in-function determined at 37 degrees *Biochem Biophys Res Commun* 2005;334:441–44
79. Fujiki A, Sugao M, Nishida K, *et al.* Repolarizatio abnormality in idiopathic ventricular fibrillatio Assessment using 24-hour QT-RR and QaT-R relationships. *J Cardiovasc Electrophysiol* 2004;1 59–63.
80. Sugao M, Fujiki A, Nishida K, *et al.* Repolarizatio dynamics in patients with idiopathic ventricul fibrillation: Pharmacological therapy with bepri and disopyramide. *J Cardiovasc Pharmacol* 200 45:545–549.
81. Sugao M, Fujiki A, Sakabe M, *et al.* New quant tative methods for evaluation of dynamic chang in QT interval on 24 hour Holter ECG recor ings: QT interval in idiopathic ventricular fibri lation and long QT syndrome. *Heart* 2006;9 201–207.
82. Wolpert C, Schimpf R, Giustetto C, *et al.* Furthe insights into the effect of quinidine in short Q syndrome caused by a mutation in HERG. *J Ca diovasc Electrophysiol* 2005;16:54–58.
83. Schimpf R, Wolpert C, Bianchi F, *et al.* Congenit short QT syndrome and implantable cardiovert defibrillator treatment: Inherent risk for inappr priate shock delivery. *J Cardiovasc Electrophysi* 2003;14:1273–1277.
84. Strohmer B, Schernthaner C, Pichler M. T-wav oversensing by an implantable cardioverter def brillator after successful ablation of idiopath ventricular fibrillation. *Pacing Clin Electrophysi* 2006;29:431–435.
85. Remme CA, Wever EF, Wilde AA, Derksen R Hauer RN. Diagnosis and long-term follow-up c the Brugada syndrome in patients with idiopath ventricular fibrillation. *Eur Heart J* 2001;2 400–409.
86. Shimizu W, Matsuo K, Takagi M, *et al.* Bod surface distribution and response to drugs of S segment elevation in Brugada syndrome: Clinic implication of eighty-seven-lead body surfac potential mapping and its application to twelve lead electrocardiograms. *J Cardiovasc Electro physiol* 2000;11:396–404.
87. Viskin S, Rosso R, Rogowski O, Belhassen B. Th short-coupled variant of right ventricular outflo ventricular tachycardia. A not-so-benign form o benign ventricular tachycardia. *J Cardiovasc Elec trophysiol* 2005;16:912–916.
88. Viskin S, Antzelevitch C. The cardiologists' wors nightmare: Sudden death from "benign" ventricu lar arrhythmias. *J Am Coll Cardiol* 2005;46:1295 1297.

89. Ashida K, Kaji Y, Sasaki Y. Abolition of torsade de pointes after radiofrequency catheter ablation at right ventricular outflow tract. *Int J Cardiol* 1997; 59:171–175.
90. Wever EF, Robles de Medina EO. Sudden death in patients without structural heart disease. *J Am Coll Cardiol* 2004;43:1137–1144.
91. Moe T. Morgagni-Adams-Stokes attacks caused by transient recurrent ventricular fibrillation in a patient without apparent heart disease. *Am Heart J* 1949;37:811–818.
92. Konty F, Dale J. Self-terminating idiopathic ventricular fibrillation presenting as syncope: A 40-year follow-up report. *J Intern Med* 1990;227: 211–213.
93. Belhassen B. A 25-year control of idiopathic ventricular fibrillation with electrophysiologic-guided antiarrhythmic drug therapy. *Heart Rhythm* 2004; 1:352–354.
94. Belhassen B, Viskin S. Management of idiopathic ventricular fibrillation: Implantable defibrillators? Antiarrhythmic drugs? *Ann Noninvasive Electrocardiol* 1998;3:125–128.
95. Haghjoo M, Arya A, Heidari A, Sadr-Ameli MA. Suppression of electrical storm by oral quinidine in a patient with Brugada syndrome. *J Cardiovasc Electrophysiol* 2005;16:674.
96. Marquez MF, Rivera J, Hermosillo AG, *et al.* Arrhythmic storm responsive to quinidine in a patient with Brugada syndrome and vasovagal syncope. *Pacing Clin Electrophysiol* 2005;28: 870–873.
97. Mok NS, Chan NY, Chiu AC. Successful use of quinidine in treatment of electrical storm in Brugada syndrome. *Pacing Clin Electrophysiol* 2004;27:821–823.
98. Aizawa Y, Tamura M, Chinushi M, *et al.* An attempt at electrical catheter ablation of the arrhythmogenic area in idiopathic ventricular fibrillation. *Am Heart J* 1992;123:257–260.
99. Kusano KF, Yamamoto M, Emori T, Morita H, Ohe T. Successful catheter ablation in a patient with polymorphic ventricular tachycardia. *J Cardiovasc Electrophysiol* 2000;11:682–685.
100. The Antiarrhythmic Versus Implantable Defibrillators (AVID) Investigators. A comparison of antiarrhythmic-drug therapy with implantable defibrillators in patients resuscitated from near-fatal ventricular arrhythmias. *N Engl J Med* 1997; 337:1576–1583.
101. Kron J, Herre J, Renfroe EG, *et al.* Lead- and device-related complications in the antiarrhythmics versus implantable defibrillators trial. *Am Heart J* 2001;141:92–98.

Part IV
Secondary Hereditary Electrical Diseases and Clinical Syndromes

Cardiac Remodeling

Jeffrey E. Saffitz

The chapters in this section are focused on mechanisms responsible for lethal arrhythmias in patients with underlying diseases of heart muscle. Alterations in the structure of the heart are a common theme in these conditions. The pertinent structural derangements may affect all or most of the heart, as in the dilated and hypertrophic cardiomyopathies. They may occur regionally, as in arrhythmogenic right ventricular cardiomyopathy, or they may entail highly localized, even microscopic, abnormalities in cardiac anatomy, such as those responsible for the preexcitation syndromes. In each case, however, the structural derangement itself appears to play a critical role in arrhythmogenesis. Indeed, efforts to elucidate mechanisms of arrhythmias that arise in the cardiomyopathies challenge us to explain not only the interplay between anatomic and functional substrates of arrhythmias, but also how altered function, both contractile and electrophysiological, can contribute to the development of altered tissue structure. Thus, the concept of *cardiac remodeling* in all of its complexities and subtleties, in forward and reverse directions, and as both a cause and an effect of cardiac pathophysiology, is fundamental to understanding arrhythmogenesis in the cardiomyopathies.

Structural changes that are thought to play an important role in arrhythmogenesis in the cardiomyopathies arise from diverse genetic, inflammatory, toxic, or metabolic injuries to cardiac myocytes. The arrhythmogenic potential in the cardiomyopathies is thought, therefore, to emerge from the development of anatomic substrates. But while there is considerable evidence to support this mechanistic progression, the precise roles of altered structure and the complex relationships between altered structure and altered function in arrhythmogenesis in the cardiomyopathies have been difficult to isolate and identify. At the same time, there is abundant evidence that altered function can promote altered structure, which, in turn, leads to a further deterioration in function in a complex reciprocating fashion. This aspect of cardiac remodeling has been recognized in many settings, which have served to deepen our understanding of the pathobiological processes underlying sudden death in heart muscle disease.

Perhaps the purest example of an arrhythmia causing heart muscle damage is pacing-induced heart disease. Widely employed as a means of inducing heart failure in experimental animals, this entity may have a clinical counterpart in patients in whom tachyarrhythmias may contribute to the progression or exacerbation of heart failure. A more clinically relevant counterpart to pacing-induced ventricular failure in experimental animals is tachycardia-induced electrical remodeling of the atria. Prolonged rapid atrial pacing reduces the atrial refractory period and diminishes or reverses the normal rate adaptation of the refractory period. In fact, these observations first gave rise to the concept of "electrical remodeling," which has since been explored in much greater detail in a variety of experimental and clinical settings. Significant reductions in the densities of the L-type voltage-gated Ca^{2+} current, the transient outward K^+ current, and the ultrarapid delayed rectifier K^+ current develop in atrial myocytes in patients with long-standing atrial fibrillation. These changes, referred to in isolation as electrical remodeling, go hand-in-hand with contractile derangements likely related to a reduction in the Ca^{2+} inward current. Importantly, however, rapid atrial pacing and persistent atrial fibrillation can also cause changes in the structure of atrial myocytes that bear a striking resemblance to those seen in hibernating ventricular myocytes including an increase in cell size, perinuclear accumulation of glycogen, and central loss of sarcomeres associated with fragmentation of the sarcoplasmic reticulum.[1] The extent to which these structural alterations further contribute to the ongoing atrial fibrillation is difficult to identify, but it should be stressed that many of these changes are potentially reversible.

A similar type of remodeling occurs in ventricular myocytes in the setting of hypertrophy and heart failure. Prolongation of action potential duration is a consistent feature in these conditions. Normal ventricles exhibit a transmural gradient in the kinetics of action potential repolarization related, at least in part, to transmural differences in the expression of ion channel proteins including the transient outward K^+ current. In heart failure, preferential conduction from subendocardial to subepicardial myocytes is lost, and the resultant abnormality in transmural dispersion of repolarization likely contributes to ventricular tachycardia by promoting phase 2 reentry. Here again, the time course and the cause–effect relationships between electrical remodeling and structural remodeling are difficult to elucidate, but the yin-yang of "altered structure begets altered function begets altered structure" appears to be a recurrent theme in various heart diseases associated with important atrial and ventricular arrhythmias. And recently, conventional thinking about electrical/contractile functions has been broadened to include other fundamental biological processes such as the role of metabolic derangements in electrical remodeling. For example, the transient outward K^+ current may be modulated by oxidoreductase systems and receptor tyrosine kinases that control the intracellular redox state and glucose metabolism.[2] These observations provide new insights linking altered expression and function of critical ion channel proteins in disparate diseases through identification of common pathogenic pathways.

Additional insights into the fascinating relationship between altered contractile function and lethal arrhythmias may come from the application of cardiac resynchronization therapy in the management of heart failure. A significant proportion of patients with systolic heart failure exhibits prolonged QRS duration, typically manifested as left bundle branch block. The resultant left ventricular dyssynchrony impairs ventricular filling, promotes mitral regurgitation, and reduces left ventricular contractility. The extent to which this dyssynchrony also alters expression and/or function of ion channels and other gene products critical in cardiac electrophysiology has not been explored in detail, but emerging evidence implicates such a relationship.[3] Attempts to restore the normal temporal/spatial pattern of electrical activation of the failing ventricle with resynchronization therapy may, therefore, reverse pathophysiologically relevant aspects of electrical remodeling and, perhaps, even some types of structural remodeling.

Finally, identification of genetic mutations responsible for the "channelopathies" has also broadened our understanding of the links between electrical remodeling and structural remodeling in the heart. While the long QT and Brugada syndromes are considered "primary electrical" diseases arising in myocardium that is otherwise structurally and functionally normal, some patients with the electrocardiographic features of these syndromes may also have structural heart disease, raising the possibility that the electrophysiological abnormality may promote structural changes. This notion is supported by observations of age-dependent myocardial fibrosis and progressive slowing of atrial and ventricular conduction in mice with a single null allele for *SCN5A*.[4] Additional insights have come from recognition that mutations in proteins conventionally thought to fulfill structural roles may contribute to the pathogenesis of lethal arrhythmias. For example, identification of ankyrin B mutations in the long QT syndrome has focused attention on the critical importance of chaperones and scaffolding proteins responsible for the trafficking and assembly of ion channel proteins and a variety of accessory and regulatory proteins into macromolecular complexes. A similar relationship may apply in the case of desmosomal protein mutations implicated in arrhythmogenic right ventricular cardiomyopathy. Here, a common theme is emerging that mutations in proteins responsible for intercellular adhesion can give rise to highly arrhythmogenic substrates in which remodeling of gap junctions may play a role.[5]

Realization of a fundamental molecular understanding of mechanisms of arrhythmia remains a major challenge. We are far from the goal of effective mechanism-based therapy. Nevertheless, the vigorous application of contemporary tools of cellular and molecular biology has vastly expanded our understanding of the myriad factors that underlie the development of anatomic and functional substrates, and has led to an increasingly sophisticated understanding of how they interact with acute triggering mechanisms to determine whether a lethal arrhythmia will arise. Further progress can certainly be anticipated.

References

1. Allessie M, Ausma J, Schotten M. Electrical and structural remodeling during atrial fibrillation. *Cardiovasc Res* 2002;54:230–246.
2. Li X, Li S, Xu Z, *et al.* Redox control of K+ channel remodeling in rat ventricle. *J Mol Cell Cardiol* 2006; 40:339–349.
3. Spragg DD, Leclercq, Loghmani M, *et al.* Regional alterations in protein expression in the dyssynchronous failing heart. *Circulation* 2003;108:929–932.
4. Royer A, van Veen TA, Le Bouter S, *et al.* Mouse model of SCN5A-linked hereditary Lenegre's disease: Age-related conduction slowing and myocardial fibrosis. *Circulation* 2005;111:1738–1746.
5. Saffitz JE. Adhesion molecules: Why they are important to the electrophysiologist. *J Cardiovasc Electrophysiol* 2006;17:225–229.

40
Arrhythmogenic Malignancies in Hypertrophic Cardiomyopathy

Shaji C. Menon, J. Martijn Bos, Steve R. Ommen, and Michael J. Ackerman

Introduction

Cardiomyopathies are diseases of the myocardium associated with cardiac dysfunction. According to the World Health Organization (WHO) classification, cardiomyopathies are classified either as primary or secondary cardiomyopathies. Based on morphological and functional criteria, heritable cardiomyopathies are classified into four primary categories including hypertrophic cardiomyopathy (HCM), dilated cardiomyopathy (DCM), arrhythmogenic right ventricular cardiomyopathy (ARVC), and restrictive cardiomyopathy (RCM). More recently, left ventricular noncompaction (LVNC) syndrome has been added. Secondary cardiomyopathies include, for example, ischemic and hypertensive cardiomyopathy. This chapter focuses solely on HCM, with particular attention to its arrhythmogenic features.

Definition

Hypertrophic cardiomyopathy is a primary myocardial disease associated with increased cardiac mass and, typically, asymmetric but diffuse or segmental left (and occasionally right) ventricular hypertrophy.[1] Genetically, HCM is a heterogeneous disease with mutations identified in at least 23 HCM-susceptibility genes, permitting a genomics-based classification of HCM into myofilament-HCM, Z-disc-HCM, energetic/storage disease (metabolic)-HCM, and mitochondrial-HCM (Table 40–1).

Nomenclature

Hypertrophic cardiomyopathy is encompassed by a confusing nomenclature that includes numerous alternative disease labels such as hypertrophic obstructive cardiomyopathy (HOCM), familial hypertrophic cardiomyopathy (FHC), and idiopathic hypertrophic subaortic stenosis (IHSS). Since left ventricular outflow tract obstruction (LVOTO) is not a prerequisite for the disease process, we will refer to the entity of unexplained cardiac hypertrophy as HCM throughout this chapter.[2] Approximately 25–50% of patients with HCM do not have obstructive disease.

Epidemiology of Hypertrophic Cardiomyopathy and Sudden Cardiac Death

Hypertrophic cardiomyopathy is one of the most common heritable cardiovascular diseases with a prevalence of 0.2% (1:500) in the adult general population across multiple ethnicities based on echocardiographic screening.[2–4] An estimated 500,000 people in the United States have HCM. In developed countries, sudden cardiac death (SCD) causes more deaths than any other medical condition. In the United States, for example, nearly 1000 people die suddenly every day and over 300,000 SCDs occur each year.[5] The majority of these deaths stem from coronary artery disease involving the middle aged or elderly. However, SCD in the young occurs, and among young

TABLE 40–1. Summary of hypertrophic cardiomyopathy (HCM) susceptibility genes.

	Gene	Locus	Protein	Frequency (%)
Myofilament HCM				
Giant filament	*TTN*	2q24.3	Titin	<1
Thick filament	*MYH7*	14q11.2–q12	β-Myosin heavy chain	15–25
	MYH6	14q11.2–q12	α-Myosin heavy chain	<1
	MYL2	12q23–q24.3	Ventricular regulatory myosin light chain	<2
	MYL3	3p21.2–p21.3	Ventricular essential myosin light chain	<1
Intermediate filament	*MYBPC3*	11p11.2	Cardiac myosin-binding protein C	15–25
Thin filament	*TNNT2*	1q32	Cardiac troponin T	<5
	TNNI3	19p13.4	Cardiac troponin I	<5
	TPM1	15q22.1	α-Tropomyosin	<5
	ACTC	15q14	α-Cardiac actin	<1
Z-disc HCM				
	CSRP3	11p15.1	Muscle LIM protein	<1
	TCAP	17q12–q21.1	Telethonin	<1
	VCL	10q22.1–q23	Vinculin/metavinculin	<1
	ZASP/LBD3	10q22.2–q23.3	Z-band alternatively spliced PDZ-motif protein/LIM binding domain 3	1–5
	ACTN2	1q42–q43	α-Actinin 2	<1
Calcium-handling HCM				
	RyR2	1q42.1–q43	Cardiac ryanodine receptor	<1
	JPH2	20q12	Junctophilin-2	<1
	PLN	6q22.1	Phospholamban	<1
Storage disease HCM				
	PRKAG2	7q35–q36.36	AMP-activated protein kinase	<1
	LAMP2	Xq24	Lysosome-associated membrane protein 2	<1
	GLA	Xq22	α-Galactosidase A	<1
Mitochondrial HCM				
	FRDA	9q13	Frataxin	<1
Miscellaneous				
	CAV3	3p25	Caveolin-3	<1

individuals heritable cardiomyopathies such as HCM and ARVC represent the most common identifiable causes.[5]

In a population-based study of sudden death in young individuals from Australia encompassing >90% of all sudden deaths, >50% were of cardiac origin.[6] Hypertrophic cardiomyopathy is one of the most common causes of SCD in people under 30 years of age in the United States. Hypertrophic cardiomyopathy is the most common cause of SCDs occurring on the athletic field (36%), with no warning signs in almost 50% of these patients.[5] The majority of competition-related SCDs involves males and these occur during or immediately following exertion (90%).[5] Notably, in Italy, the most common cause of youthful SCD is ARVC, followed by HCM, a difference that might be attributed to genetic predisposition for ARVC or possibly to the increased primary prevention for HCM due to screening efforts.[5,7] It is now recognized that in HCM, the overall annual incidence of SCD is ~1%/year, and many individuals with HCM are destined to a lifelong asymptomatic state.[1,8,9] In contrast, the highest risk subset of HCM exhibits a 5–10%/year risk of SCD, and here HCM is truly an arrhythmogenic malignancy.[10]

This chapter focuses on the current understanding of the molecular pathogenic mechanisms and arrhythmias of HCM, SCD risk stratification, clinical management, athletics in HCM, and screening for HCM.

Pathology/Pathophysiology/Pathogenetics of Hypertrophic Cardiomyopathy

The histopathology in HCM is characterized by unexplained, markedly enlarged, and bizarre shaped myocytes, myocyte disorientation (myofibrillar disarray), and premature death of hypertrophic muscle cells and its replacement with fibroblasts and extracellular matrix (replacement fibrosis).[2,4] The areas of myocyte disarray vary from focal to extensive involvement of myocardium.

Molecular Basis of Hypertrophic Cardiomyopathy and Yield of Genetic Testing

Hypertrophic cardiomyopathy is generally considered a "disease of the sarcomere" or more accurately a "disease of the myofilament," with hundreds of mutations identified in the thick, intermediate, and thin cardiac myofilaments that comprise the cardiac sarcomere. However, mutations in proteins of the cardiac Z-disc, proteins involved in calcium handling, and glycogen storage diseases have also been implicated in the pathogenesis of HCM (Table 40–1). Hypertrophic cardiomyopathy has an autosomal dominant mode of inheritance, although autosomal recessive forms and spontaneous germline mutations have also been identified. A familial history of HCM is present in 33–50% of all index cases.[4]

Among various ethnically diverse cohorts of patients with HCM, MYH7, MYBPC3, and TNNT2 are cited as the three most common HCM-associated genes accounting for, respectively, 15–25%, 15–25%, and <5% of all HCM cases (Table 40–1).[11–14] Derived from the largest published cohort of unrelated patients with HCM, the Mayo Clinic series reported that nearly 40% of patients with clinical HCM had an identifiable mutation localizing to one of eight myofilament-encoding genes that comprise the commercially available HCM genetic test, with the two most common genetic subtypes being MYBPC3- and MYH7-HCM.[11–14]

Nonsarcomeric protein missense mutations involving the gamma-2-regulatory subunit of AMP-activated protein kinase encoded by PRKAG2 and the lysosome-associated membrane protein 2 encoded by LAMP2 have been associated with HCM.[15] PRKAG2-HCM is associated with minimal hypertrophy, conduction system defects, and glycogen accumulation in myocytes in the absence of characteristic myocyte disarray. These patients show ventricular preexcitation and progressive conduction disease with heart block.[16] Mutations in LAMP2 lead to the glycogen storage disease of Danon's syndrome showing HCM with massive hypertrophy and preexcitation on a surface electrocardiogram (ECG).[3,4] Genetic testing for PRKG2- and LAMP2-HCM is available clinically.[1] Besides the aforementioned primary HCM-causing genetic substrates, the variability in expression of these causal genes may be modulated by single nucleotide polymorphisms (SNPs) located in the coding or regulatory region of other genes not to mention other acquired factors.[18,19]

The yield of genetic testing ranges from about 30% to 70% depending on the series of patients with HCM examined. The yield of genetic testing is higher with positive family history, severe hypertrophy, young age at diagnosis, and presence of an internal cardioverter defibrillator (ICD).[13,14] Moreover, the yield was most dependent and in multivariate analyses exclusively dependent upon the manifest septal morphology.[20] Again, for the eight myofilament-encoding genes that constitute the clinically available HCM genetic test, the yield ranged from only 8% for sigmoidal contour-HCM to nearly 80% for reverse septal curvature-HCM (Figure 40–1).[20] These two anatomical/morphological subtypes represent the two most common clinical subsets of HCM, suggesting a possible role for echo-guided genetic testing.

Arrhythmias and Arrhythmogenic Mechanisms in Hypertrophic Cardiomyopathy

The various mechanisms and types of arrhythmias in HCM include (1) reentrant tachycardia, (2) focal automaticity, (3) bradyarrhythmias, and (4) supraventricular or ventricular tachyarrhythmias. Hypertrophic cardiomyopathy is characterized by myocardium consisting of areas of fibrosis, disruption of cellular architecture, and hypertro

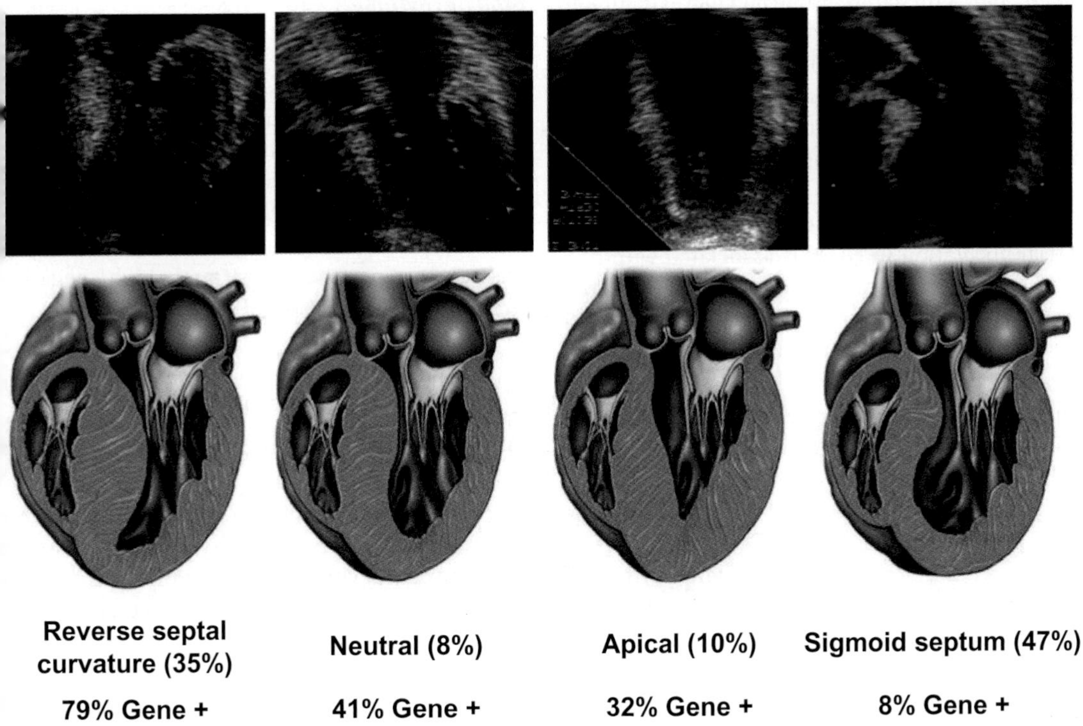

FIGURE 40–1. Hypertrophic cardiomyopathy septal morphology subtypes and yield of myofilament (Panel A and Panel B) genetic testing. Starting with the highest yield, the morphological subtype classification from left to right is reverse curve-, neutral-, apical-, and sigmoidal septal contour-HCM based on standard echocardiography long-axis views taken at end diastole. The percentage following the contour type indicates the relative frequency of that particular morphological subtype seen at the Mayo Clinic. The percentage at the bottom of each panel indicates the yield of the commercially available genetic test for each particular HCM morphology. Gene +, presence of myofilament mutation (positive Panel A/B test).

phied/dysplastic myocytes, creating an inhomogeneous and unstable, proarrhythmic electrical milieu.[21,22] Regional inhomogeneity in action potential durations (APDs) and enhanced spatial and temporal dispersion of APDs form the basis for reentry.[18] Alteration in gap junctions, transmural and transseptal dispersion of repolarization, cell-to-cell coupling, and intracellular calcium homeostasis lead to dyshomogeneity of APDs. Defective repolarization predisposes to delayed and early afterdepolarization, a source of extrasystole.[18,22] Small afterpotentials with low amplitude and high frequency in the ventricle represent a local abnormality of impulse propagation and can lead to reentrant arrhythmia.[18]

Patients with atrial enlargement due to valvular pathology or abnormal loading conditions are prone to supraventricular arrhythmias, especially atrial fibrillation (AF). In some patients supraventricular tachyarrhythmias could trigger ventricular tachyarrhythmias. Associated conditions such as electrolyte imbalance secondary to diuretic treatment and QT interval prolongation, and proarrhythmic properties of antiarrhythmic drugs may precipitate these arrhythmias. The underlying pathophysiological abnormality leading to SCD ranges from supraventricular tachycardia, sinus arrest, ventricular tachycardia, myocardial ischemia, and acute hemodynamic changes caused by physical or emotional stress.

Atrial Fibrillation

Atrial fibrillation is the most common arrhythmia observed in HCM.[2] Ultimately, paroxysmal or chronic AF occurs in 20–25% of patients with

HCM, and is linked to left atrial enlargement and increasing age.[2,23,24] Older patients with chronic high left ventricular (LV) end diastolic pressures and diastolic dysfunction are prone to chronic sustained AF secondary to a dilating left atrium.[23] Young patients with significant outflow tract obstruction and dilated left atrium also have a greater propensity to develop paroxysmal AF. Atrial fibrillation in HCM is associated with progressive heart failure, stroke, and disease progression.[23] Due to the increased risk of systemic thromboembolization, the threshold for initiation of anticoagulant therapy (i.e., coumadin) should be low, such as after one or two episodes of paroxysmal AF. In some patients supraventricular tachyarrhythmias could trigger ventricular arrhythmias;[25] however, there is currently insufficient evidence linking AF to SCD in HCM. Nevertheless, AF is independently associated with heart failure-related death and occurrence of fatal and nonfatal stroke. Amiodarone is the drug of choice for prevention of paroxysmal AF, whereas chronic AF can be treated with rate control medications, β-blockers, and verapamil.[2] There is no consensus regarding the various modalities for treatment of AF (i.e., radiofrequency ablation, the surgical MAZE procedure, or implantable atrial defibrillators).[24]

Other Supraventricular Tachycardias

Other arrhythmias include supraventricular tachycardia, AV block, and sinus bradycardia. Wolf–Parkinson–White (WPW) syndrome can also be seen in HCM. In fact, the presence of WPW in HCM should prompt the consideration for glycogen storage-HCM mediated by mutations in PRKAG2.[16]

Ventricular Arrhythmias

Ventricular arrhythmias are an important clinical feature in adults with HCM. In a study of 178 adults with HCM, 90% had ventricular arrhythmias, including premature ventricular depolarizations (88%), ventricular couplets (42%), nonsustained bursts of ventricular tachycardia (NSVT) (31%), and supraventricular tachycardia (SVT) (37%) recorded by routine ambulatory (Holter) 24-h ECG monitoring.[26]

Bradyarrhythmias

Bradycardia may cause syncope and sudden death. Sudden death is less frequently due to bradycardia. Bradycardia was found to be more common in patient with hypertrophy involving the mid-low part of the ventricular septum. Some patients with bradyarrhythmias may require back-up pacing. Routine ambulatory monitoring has a low positive (9%) and high negative predictive value (95%) for SCD.[26]

Clinical Presentation of Hypertrophic Cardiomyopathy

The clinical presentation of HCM is often underscored by extreme variability ranging from an asymptomatic course to that of severe heart failure, arrhythmias, and premature and/or sudden cardiac death. The age of presentation varies from infancy to 90 years, with the majority of patients presenting during adolescence and young adulthood.[2,3] Twenty-five percent of patients achieve a normal life span (75 years or more).[27,28] Most patients with HCM are asymptomatic or only mildly symptomatic, and the first manifestation may be sudden death.[2] Hypertrophic cardiomyopathy occurs equally in men and women, but may be underdiagnosed in women, minorities, and underprivileged populations.[27,29] Variable expressivity and age-dependent penetrance have been described in patients with HCM mutations. MYBPC3-HCM, for example, has been associated with delayed onset of hypertrophy.[3,30] However, in one large series, there was no difference in age at diagnosis between MYBPC3-HCM and MYH7-HCM.[11] Rarely, infants and young children may present with heart failure, and these patients have a poor prognosis.[3,31] Sudden cardiac death can be the tragic sentinel event for HCM in children, adolescents, and young adults.

Symptomatic patients may present with exertional dyspnea, chest pain, and syncope/presyncope. Physical findings of dynamic systolic ejection murmur with characteristic response to bedside maneuvers and bifid pulse are classic signs indicating LVOTO and obstructive HCM Progression to "end-stage" disease with systolic dysfunction and heart failure occurs in approximately 5% of patients.[32,33] Other serious life threatening complications including embolic stroke and arrhythmias, which can occur as a consequence of HCM.[27]

Periodically, all patients with HCM should undergo examination with meticulous recording of personal and family history, two-dimensional echocardiography and/or cardiac magnetic resonance (CMR), 12-lead ECG and 24–48 h ambulatory Holter electrocardiogram, and exercise stress testing (for evaluation of exercise tolerance, blood pressure, and ventricular tachyarrhythmias).[27]

Diagnosis of Hypertrophic Cardiomyopathy

Conventional two-dimensional echocardiography is the diagnostic modality of choice for the clinical diagnosis of HCM.[27] Cardiac magnetic resonance is being utilized increasingly to aid in the diagnosis of HCM, particularly among patients with suboptimal echocardiographic images. Cardiac magnetic resonance with delayed gadolinium hyperenhancement may also indicate the presence and degree of intramyocardial fibrosis.[34,35] Hypertrophic cardiomyopathy is characterized by unexplained and usually asymmetric, diffuse, or segmental hypertrophy associated with a nondilated and hyperdynamic LV independent of the presence or absence of LVOTO. Echocardiography can provide details of location, degree of hypertrophy, mitral valve and subvalvular apparatus position and function, and assessment of systolic and diastolic cardiac function.[1]

Hypertrophic cardiomyopathy can be subdivided into at least four anatomical, morphological variants based on the shape of the septal myocardium: sigmoidal septal contour, reverse septal curvature, apical-HCM hypertrophy, and neutral septal contour (Figure 40–1).[20,36] A left ventricular wall thickness (LVWT) ≤12 mm is typically regarded as normal in adults. An LVWT measuring 13–15 mm is generally classified as borderline LVH while a measurement ≥15 mm is the absolute cutoff generally accepted for the clinical diagnosis of HCM in an adult (in children, it is two or more standard deviations from the mean relative to body surface, i.e., a *Z*-score of two or more).[27] However, it should be appreciated that cutoff values will result inevitably in misclassifications. For example, patients can have LVWT well in the normal range but have genetically proven HCM (so-called nonpenetrance or "not yet expressivity," while athletes without any genetic perturbations may nonetheless exceed this 15-mm cutoff value.

Sudden Cardiac Death Risk Stratification in Hypertrophic Cardiomyopathy

Hypertrophic cardiomyopathy accounts for over half of all cases of sudden cardiac death in young individuals below 25 years of age. Overall, the annual mortality is <1%, but reaches 5–10%/year for the highest risk subset.[27] High-risk HCM constitutes a small part of the total HCM population. Sudden cardiac death is more frequent in adolescents and young adults (<35 years old), and could be the first presenting symptom.

No single clinical, morphological, genetic, or electrophysiological (EP) factor has emerged as a single reliable predictor of sudden death risk in HCM (Figure 40–2). Clearly, the patients at highest risk of sudden death are those already experiencing and surviving an out-of-hospital cardiac arrest (OHCA), ventricular fibrillation (VF), and sustained VF.[8,9,27] To the established minor risk factors belong an abnormal blood pressure response during exercise, extreme hypertrophy, family history of SCD, nonsustained ventricular tachycardia (NSVT) on Holter monitoring, and unexplained (especially when during exercise) syncope. In addition, gadolinium-derived measurements of fibrosis by CMR, genetic substrate, and LVOTO likely represent disease modifiers. SCD risk stratification based solely on the genetic test result should not be performed.[37,38]

Established Minor Risk Factors

Abnormal Blood Pressure Response to Exercise

An abnormal blood pressure response to exercise is defined as hypotension or failed blood pressure increase (<20 mm Hg) with exercise. A

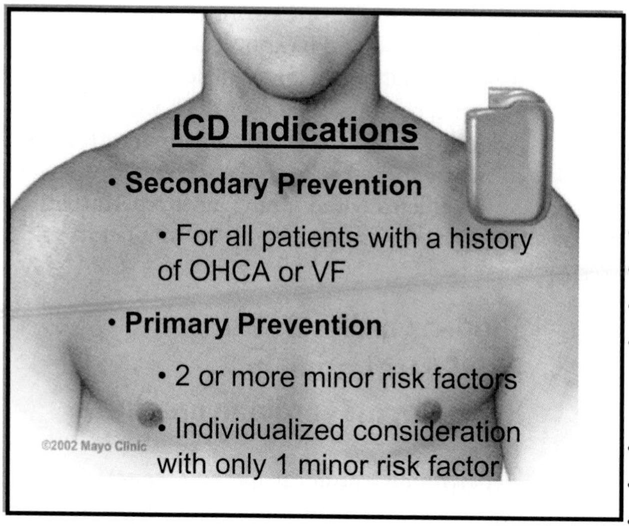
ICD Indications
• Secondary Prevention
• For all patients with a history of OHCA or VF
• Primary Prevention
• 2 or more minor risk factors
• Individualized consideration with only 1 minor risk factor
©2002 Mayo Clinic
Major Risk Factors
• Out of Hospital Cardiac Arrest (OHCA)
• Ventricular Fibrillation (VF)
Minor Risk Factors
• Abnormal Blood Pressure Response during Exercise
• Extreme Hypertrophy (≥ 30 mm)
• Family History of Sudden Cardiac Death
• Non-Sustained Ventricular Tachycardia
• Unexplained Syncope (especially exercise-induced)
Possible Modifiers
• Delayed Gadolinium Hyper-Enhancement on CMR
• Genetic Test Result
• Left Ventricular Outflow Tract Obstruction

FIGURE 40–2. Summary of ICD indications and the major, minor, and possible modifying factors in sudden death risk stratification in HCM.

hypotensive blood pressure response during exercise occurred in over 20% of a community-based patient cohort with HCM, and was associated with a higher incidence of cardiovascular mortality and SCD (odds ratio of 4.5) in patients <50 years old.[39]

Extreme Hypertrophy

In one study, the risk of sudden death was directly related to septal wall thickness. Hypertrophy of 30 mm or more is associated with a 2%/year mortality (recall that the overall annual mortality for the disease is around 0.5–1%) in contrast to an extremely low yearly mortality associated with a wall thickness less than 20 mm.[40] There is a direct and continuous relationship between maximal LV thickness and risk of SCD.[10,41] However, it is possible to have a predisposition for SCD despite minimal hypertrophy.[41] Some investigators have reported that massive hypertrophy is a higher risk factor for sudden death in young patients <30 years, but not in middle-aged and older patients.[10,40,42,43] In patients over 60 years old with massive hypertrophy, higher mortality is secondary to heart failure, AF, and stroke. In addition, the majority of patients with HCM experiencing SCD will not exhibit this echo marker of badness and will die suddenly despite a wall thickness <30 mm.

Family History of Sudden Death

A family history of two or more cases of SCD is a clear indication for ICD. In addition, most view a single sudden death as indicative of a positive family history despite the fact that the published risk factor requires at least two deaths. In the case of a single incidence of SCD in a family, the decision to implant an ICD should be based on other associated risk factors and should be discussed with the patient.

Nonsustained Ventricular Tachycardia

Especially in young patients, NSVT may be a risk factor for SCD.[25] In a study of 531 patients followed for 70 ± 40 months, 20% of patients showed NSVT. The incidence of NSVT had a direct correlation with LV wall thickness and LA diameter. The annual mortality was approximately 4%/year when NSVT was recorded compared to ~1% when it was absent.[25]

Unexplained Syncope

Syncope in HCM can be caused by neurally mediated responses leading to cardioinhibition and/or vasodepression.[33,44] In young patients with HCM, syncope with exertion or at rest should be considered a risk factor for sudden death.[24,45] A dual chamber ICD may be better in neurally mediated syncope due to its role in maintaining a normal heart rate and atrial contribution to LV.[33]

Other Potential Testing for Sudden Cardiac Death Risk Stratification

There is no single ECG test, clinical marker, or biomarker for risk stratification and identification of an SCD substrate. Various proposed tests for recognition of substrates for SCD include EP study, signal-averaged ECG, microvolt T wave alternans, QT dispersion, ejection fraction, number of ventricular premature beats, heart rate variability, and baroreceptor sensitivity.[25] These tests and a clinical history should be repeated periodically to restratify the risk as the disease progresses.

Gadolinium Hyperenhancement by Cardiac Magnetic Resonance

Delayed gadolinium hyperenhancement by CMR is a marker of irreversible myocardial injury. Myocardial hyperenhancement in HCM may indicate areas of replacement fibrosis. In a cohort of 42 patients myocardial hyperenhancement was found in 79%. The extent of hyperenhancement was greater in patients with progressive disease (28.5% vs. 8.7%, $p < 0.001$) and in patients with two or more risk factors for SCD (15.7% vs. 8.6%, $p = 0.02$).[35]

Genetic Testing for Sudden Cardiac Death Risk

The role of genetic testing in SCD risk stratification for HCM is controversial. One study showed a higher incidence of ECG abnormalities with mutations in troponin I (99%), troponin T (88%), and myosin-binding protein C (83%) as compared to 79% in other patients.[46] ST-T wave abnormalities were more frequently observed in patient with troponin T mutation (81%) compared to 55% and 66% with troponin I and myosin-binding protein C, respectively.[47] The ECG might have a significant role in screening of family members of HCM patients, athletes, and military recruits.[27] Electrocardiographic changes may precede phenotypic manifestation on echocardiography, especially in young children, providing invaluable clinical clues.[30,47–49] P wave duration (>134.5 msec) and P wave dispersion (>52.5 msec), markers of intaatrial and interatrial conduction time, have a sensitivity of 90%+ and specificity of 80%+ in predicting AF and LA enlargement.[50] Electrocardiographic late potentials have low sensitivity and prevalence in the detection of subclinical VT.

Initial genotype–phenotype correlative studies suggested the possibility of specific genotype–phenotype correlations, particularly specific mutations being associated with a "malignant" or "benign" natural history and SCD risk. Some experts consider that HCM precipitated by mutations in troponin T and I, tropomyosin, and particular missense mutations (R403Q, R453C, and R719W, for example) in the β-myosin heavy chain is associated with increased risk of sudden death.[51] However, this association was not seen in other studies, and the frequency of specific so-called "malignant mutations" in HCM cohorts is very low (1%).[38] In the current era, the genetic test result should not be used as a principal determinant of SCD risk.[11–14] Each HCM-associated mutation provides the fundamental pathogenetic substrate, but the degree of penetrance and expressivity varies based on gene modifiers, epigenetic factors, and environmental triggers.[14] At present, it is difficult to prognosticate based upon the genetic mutation. A decision to place an ICD should not be based on the patient's HCM-causing mutation.[14] Clinical genetic testing for HCM comprising the eight most common HCM-associated myofilament genes is now commercially available.[17]

Left Ventricular Outflow Tract Obstruction

Left ventricular outflow tract obstruction is a predictor of death due to adverse cardiovascular events.[9] The risk of progression to New York Heart Association (NYHA) class III or IV or death specifically from heart failure or stroke was also greater among patients with obstruction.[52] There are some reports of symptomatic patients with severe LVOTO being an independent risk factor for SCD/ICD in HCM (relative risk, 2.0).[52] A recent study, however, showed that with an increasing number of risk factors, there was a significant trend toward increased mortality in patients with or without LVOTO.

Electrocardiographic Findings in Hypertrophic Cardiomyopathy

Traditionally, 12-lead electrocardiography has played a significant role in the screening and evaluation of family members and athletes for HCM.[53] The 12-lead ECG is abnormal in 75–95% of patients who have HCM.[2,41] The ECG in HCM is nonspecific, however, and does not predict clinical status, magnitude of hypertrophy, and degree of left ventricular outflow tract (LVOT) obstruction. The ECG may show high voltage, nonspecific ST and T wave changes, abnormal Q waves, left atrial enlargement, diminished R waves in left precordial leads, left ventricular hypertrophy (LVH), and in a few patients right ventricular hypertrophy (RVH).[47] QT dispersion and QT interval prolongation may be seen. Longer QRS duration and prolonged QT interval are common findings in HCM. In adults, a weak correlation can be demonstrated between ECG voltages and the magnitude of LVH assessed by echocardiography.[53] The various voltage criteria (Romhilt–Ester score, Cornell voltage score, LV strain pattern, sum of R and S waves in 12 leads, and sum of S wave in lead V1 or V2 and R wave in V6 or V5) have a weak correlation (correlation coefficients of 0.2–0.3) with LV hypertrophy.[53] In one study, Rohmilt–Ester voltage criteria and 12-lead ECG criteria were found to be 23% sensitive in the diagnosis of prehypertrophic carrier states.[48] It seems that inclusion of ST-T wave changes in ECG criteria increases the sensitivity. The relationship of voltage criteria with severity of hypertrophy and SCD risk is not very strong.[53,54] Less than 50% of patients with massive hypertrophy have ECG abnormalities.[53]

Echocardiography for Sudden Cardiac Death Risk

Apart from the value of echocardiography in identifying the SCD substrates, degree of hypertrophy and LVOTO and Doppler myocardial imaging-derived intra-left ventricular electromechanical asynchrony and delay have high sensitivity and specificity in identifying patients with HCM and a subset with a higher risk for SCD. An intraventricular conduction delay >30 msec identifies patients with HCM and >45 msec is associated with NSVT on Holter monitoring and with a higher risk for SCD.[55] Intraventricular conduction delay also helps to differentiate true HCM and athlete's heart. Maximal left atrial volume is also a sensitive indicator predicting susceptibility for paroxysmal AF.

Signal-Averaged Electrocardiogram

A signal-averaged ECG (SECG) is helpful in reducing the extraneous noise from a spectral ECG. The traditional method of analysis, time domain analysis, called high-pass filtering, helps in reducing the large amplitude; low frequency noise signals and help in detecting QRS duration and aberrations in terminal QRS (late potentials).[25] An SECG, although abnormal in HCM, is not useful in risk stratification.[25,56]

QT Interval Variability

Time domain and spectral analysis-derived QT interval variability is increased in patients with HCM compared to normal subjects. These repolarization abnormalities can predispose to syncope and SCD.[57] QT dispersion has not proven to be useful in SCD risk stratification.[56]

T Wave Alternans

T wave alternans (TWA), reflecting a beat-to-beat fluctuation in T waves associated with dispersion of repolarization, may predict the extent of disarray on biopsy and risk for ventricular arrhythmias.[25,58] However, assessment of microscopic TWA has not been utilized routinely in the evaluation of HCM.

Heart Rate Variability

Heart rate variability (HRV) indicates the modulation of the sinus node by the autonomic nervous system. Fast Fourier analysis of a 3- to 5-min ECG derived high-frequency (HF) fluctuation (index of vagal activity) and low-frequency (LF) fluctuation (sympathetic activity). Heart rate variability is decreased in patients with HCM. An LF:HF ratio of <1.2 predicted a higher risk of SCD (80% positive and 90% negative predictive value).[25] In studies in adults, low HRV has been correlated with increased risk of SCD in cardiomyopathy.[25]

Role of Electrophysiology Studies

Electrical instability is a common factor in SCD. Ventricular tachycardia induced in EP studies (i.e., programmed ventricular stimulation) has been associated with a higher risk of sudden death in one study, but not in other studies.[59] During EP study VT can be induced in less than one-third of patients with HCM and seems to be a nonspecific EP response.[44] This has low positive and negative predictive value in risk stratification.[25,27,60] Electrophysiological study may be of value in patients with unexplained syncope.[27] However, there is no role for an EP study in the evaluation of a patient with imaging (echocardiography or CMR)-positive HCM.

Myocardial Bridging

Myocardial bridging of the epicardial coronary artery is not a risk factor for SCD, but surgical resection of myocardial bridges may relieve clinical signs and symptoms of ischemia.[4,61]

Clinical Management of Hypertrophic Cardiomyopathy

The Impact of Symptomatic Therapies on Sudden Cardiac Death Risk

The Role and Impact of Pharmacological Therapy

Negative Inotropic Therapy

β Blockers. β Blockers due to their negative inotropic effects are the traditional mainstay of HCM therapy. β Blockers are used in symptomatic patients with or without obstruction to control heart failure and anginal chest pain. The dose–response relationship of these medications varies significantly from patient to patient. Commonly used β blockers include propranolol, atenolol, metoprolol, and nadolol.[24,62]

Calcium-Blocker Therapy. The calcium channel antagonist verapamil is another drug used in HCM for its negative inotropic effect. It should be avoided in infants and used with caution in patients with heart failure and/or significant obstruction.[27]

Disopyramide. Disopyramide is a negative inotrope and type 1-A antiarrhythmic agent. It may help some patients with obstruction. It decreases cardiac output in nonobstructive HCM and is used primarily in patients not responding to β blocker and/or calcium channel blocker therapy. There are no data that indicate that these medications alter the risk of sudden death.[27]

Drugs to Be Used with Caution in Hypertrophic Cardiomyopathy. Angiotensin-converting enzymes inhibitors (ACE inhibitors), angiotensin II blockers, nifedipine, and other afterload reducing agents should be used with caution, as afterload reduction may worsen LVOTO.[8,24] β-Adrenergic agents such as dopamine, dobutamine, or epinephrine, agents with increased inotropic activity, may worsen LVOTO.[27]

Antiarrhythmic Drug Therapy

Amiodarone. Medical treatment strategies with β blockers, quinidine, procainamide, and amiodarone have shown variable and conflicting results in the reduction of SCD risk.[9] To be sure, the possible protective effect is dwarfed by the safety profile and efficacy of ICD in long-term primary and secondary prevention of SCD.[9] In the current era, medical therapy does not play a principal role in primary or secondary prevention of SCD.[4,63]

The Role and Impact of Nonpharmacological Therapy

Septal Myectomy Surgery

Ventricular septal myectomy remains the gold standard for treating drug refractory obstructive HCM.[24,64,65] Surgery is usually indicated in patients with a peak instantaneous LVOT Doppler gradient of 50 mm Hg or higher under rest or provocation and/or severely symptomatic patients (NYHA class 3 or 4).[24,27,65] This profile represents approximately 5% of patients with HCM.[66] More extensive, extended septal myectomy involving the anterolateral papillary muscle and mitral valvuloplasty may be needed in patients with abnormal papillary muscle apparatus and mitral valve abnormalities.[67] The surgical mortality is <1% in most major centers.[2,65] Long-term survival after surgical myectomy is equal to that observed in the general population.[67] Surgery provides long-term improvement in LVOT gradient, mitral valve regurgitation, and symptomatic improvement.[2,65,67]

Septal Ablation

In the alcohol septal ablation technique ethanol (95% alcohol 1–3 ml) is injected in specific septal branches of the left anterior descending artery producing a controlled septal infarction; this often provides dramatic symptomatic improvement in some patients.[27,56] The criteria for patient selection for alcohol septal ablation are similar to myectomy with the following caveat: the impact of alcohol septal ablation on SCD risk is unknown. Scarring associated with alcohol septal ablation may create a permanent arrhythmogenic substrate.[27] Complications include complete atrioventricular block requiring permanent pacemakers (5–10% of patients), large myocardial infarction, acute mitral valve regurgitation, VF, and death (2–4%).[8,24,64] Alcohol septal ablation is not suitable for patients with LVOTO secondary to an abnormal mitral valve apparatus and an unusual location of hypertrophy away from the area supplied by the septal perforator. Given the unknown future risks of alcohol septal ablation, it is not recommended in children or young adults.[27]

Dual-Chamber Pacing

There has been a great deal of debate surrounding the use of pacing as a means of relieving ventricular obstruction. Some studies have shown a beneficial effect, while others demonstrated a significant placebo effect.[27] The average decrease in the LVOTO gradient with pacing ranged from a modest 25% to 40% and varied substantially.[27] There is evidence to suggest that appropriately used dual chamber pacing may decrease the LVOT gradient and provide symptomatic relief.[68] Thus, there may be a limited role of dual chamber pacing for a select group of patients, for example, patients with advanced age (>65 years) and with higher surgical mortality. There is no evidence to suggest any change in SCD risk or disease progression.[33]

MAZE Procedures

A surgical Maze procedure combined with myectomy may be a feasible therapeutic option in HCM with LVOTO and AF. There are small case series reporting low operative mortality and morbidity and a high likelihood of patients remaining in sinus rhythm postprocedure.[69] Larger studies with longer follow-up are needed to better define the risks and benefits of the surgical MAZE procedure in HCM.

Internal Cardioverter Defibrillator and Hypertrophic Cardiomyopathy

Functions of the Internal Cardioverter Defibrillator

The ICD plays an important role in primary and secondary prevention of SCD. In many young patients, the ICD prolongs life substantially and provides the potential for near-normal life expectancy. In a multicenter study of ICDs in patients with HCM, the device intervened appropriately, terminating ventricular tachycardia/ventricular fibrillation (VT/VF) at a rate of 5% per year for those patients implanted as primary prevention and 11% per year for secondary prevention, over an average follow-up of 3 years.[4] The three main functions of the ICD are detection of arrhythmia, delivery of appropriate electrical therapy, and storage of diagnostic information, including ECGs and details of treated episodes. In addition, ICDs provide antibradycardia pacing. In patients with sinus node dysfunction, supraventricular tachyarrhythmias precipitating VT/VF, and paroxysmal or sustained AF, a dual-chamber ICD is preferred.[33]

Single- or Dual-Chamber System

In general, a single-chamber ICD is indicated for primary/secondary prevention of SCD. Dual-chamber devices are utilized if pacing is needed or anticipated or if the patient also has paroxysmal AF.

Complication of Internal Cardioverter Defibrillator Use

There are several potential complications of ICD therapy, particularly in young patients with long-term ICD use. These risks include (1) perforation, (2) high pacing thresholds, (3) inadequate sensing or pacing, (4) contraindication for magnetic resonance imaging, (5) infection, (6) thrombosis, (7) valvular regurgitation, (8) unwarranted shock therapy, and (9) multiple battery changes.[33] Malfunction of a transvenous ICD lead, fracture, and erosion can occur at an estimated frequency of 4–7%/year.[33,70] This is an important issue to be considered in young patients with HCM. Given the primary prevention rate of 5%/year, families and patients must be informed that patients are as likely to experience a complication from the ICD as they will experience a potentially life-saving, VF-terminating therapy when the device is implanted as primary prevention.

Contradictions for Internal Cardioverter Defibrillator Therapy

1. Wolff–Parkinson–White syndrome patients presenting with VF secondary to AF should undergo catheter or surgical ablation if their accessory pathways are amenable to such treatment.
2. New York Heart Association Class IV drug-refractory congestive heart failure patients who are not candidates for cardiac transplantation or who have a life expectancy not exceeding 6 months are not candidates for a device.
3. Patients with incessant VT or VF not responsive to antitachycardia pacing or pharmacological therapy are not suitable candidates for a device.
4. A history of psychiatric disorders, including uncontrolled depression and substance abuse, that interferes with the meticulous care and follow-up needed by these patients is a relative contraindication to device therapy.
5. Syncope of undetermined cause in a patient without inducible ventricular tachyarrhythmias is a contraindication indication for ICD therapy.

Summary of Internal Cardioverter Defibrillator Indications in Hypertrophic Cardiomyopathy (Figure 40–2)

Secondary Prevention (Aborted Cardiac Arrest)

In general, secondary prevention ICD therapy is indicated for all patients with a history of out of hospital cardiac arrest, aborted cardiac arrest, VF, or sustained VT.[27]

Primary Prevention

Primary prevention ICD therapy is generally advised if two minor risk factors are present. Here, the relative risk for SCD is 2-fold greater than the annual mortality attributed to HCM. Debate continues as to whether ICDs are indicated if only a single minor risk factor is present.[24,27]

Low-Risk Group. Asymptomatic patients with hypertrophy less than 20 mm, no family history of sudden death, an LVOTO gradient <30 mm, normal atrial size, normal blood pressure response to exercise, and absence of NSVT on Holter have a low risk of sudden death and a life expectancy similar to the general population.[27] There is no evidence that in low-risk individuals standard pharmacological therapy may change the course of disease.[27,44,62]

One-Risk Factor Group. In contrast to European experts, experts from the United States strongly advocate ICD implantation in the presence of a single minor risk factor.[28,63,71] The clinical decision for ICD implantation in patients with a single risk factor should be based on the strength of the risk factor, the individual risk profile, and the level of risk acceptable to the patient and family and should be made only after a detailed discussion about the pro and cons of ICD factors.

Two or More Risk Factors Group. There is consensus on the use of ICD for primary prevention of SCD in patients with multiple risk factors (two or more minor risk factors).[24]

The Interaction between Athletics and Hypertrophic Cardiomyopathy

One of the important diagnostic challenges is distinguishing between HCM and the "athlete's heart." Caution should be exercised in the diagnosis of "athlete's heart," as even among very elite competitive athletes, only a small portion will develop LVH. Differentiating features include an absence of family history of HCM and genetic mutation, some degree of LV dilation in addition to their hypertrophy, an absence of SAM, female gender, a normal diastolic filling pattern, the absence of abnormal ECG findings, above-normal oxygen consumption, and an LV wall thickness rarely exceeding 15 mm.[2,72] If necessary, a period of deconditioning may help distinguish between the two entities as deconditioning typically produces a regression of hypertrophy in the "athlete's heart."

Sports Participation and Screening

Intense physical exertion can potentially trigger SCD in individuals with HCM. According to the 2005 Bethesda Conference #36 recommendations, athletes with HCM should be excluded from participation in contact and most organized competitive sports, with the possible exception of low-intensity, class IA sports (golf, bowling, cricket, billiards, and riflery).[73] According to these expert opinion guidelines, the presence of an ICD does not alter these recommendations.[73]

Athletes with a Family History of Hypertrophic Cardiomyopathy

Athletes with a family history of HCM should undergo a detailed cardiac evaluation including ECG, ambulatory (Holter) 24-h ECG monitoring, exercise testing, echocardiogram, and genetic testing for disease screening and risk stratification before they are cleared for sports.

Athletes with a Hypertrophic Cardiomyopathy Mutation, But Normal Echocardiogram

Athletes with an HCM mutation and a normal echocardiogram diagnosed by family screening should undergo a comprehensive clinical evaluation similar to patients with known HCM before they are cleared for sports. Currently, there are no data on the usefulness of drug therapy in preventing or delaying symptoms or hypertrophy. Although SCD has been reported among patients with troponin T mutations, for example, and minimal hypertrophy, overall there are few data on SCD risk in asymptomatic HCM carriers with a normal echocardiogram (i.e., genotype positive/phenotype negative). Although current recommendations advise restricting such a patient from competitive sports, this is not based on extensive data and is viewed by some as being too restrictive.[27] On the other hand, if all parameters including HCM mutation analysis are normal, then restriction from competitive athletic activities is not recommended.[27]

Family Screening in Hypertrophic Cardiomyopathy

Nongenetic Screening Recommendations in Hypertrophic Cardiomyopathy

All first- and second-degree relatives of an index case of HCM should be screened with an ECG and echocardiogram. In general, annual screening is recommended for adolescents and young adults (age 12–25 years) and athletes.[56] Before age 12 and after age 25, some periodicity of screening is advised (every 3–5 years), although yearly evaluations are probably most prudent if the individual is an athlete or has symptoms, or if a family history suggests early onset disease.

Screening guidelines:

1. A thorough family history and physical examination.[56]
2. Two-dimensional echocardiography.[27,56]
3. Twelve-lead ECG. [27,56]
4. DNA testing (optional) is now more widely available; costs are covered by medical insurance and have decreased. Mutation analysis may alter the need for lifelong echocardiographic surveillance making it cost effective.

Role of Genetic Testing in Family Screening and Hypertrophic Cardiomyopathy

If the HCM-causing mutation is known, first-degree relatives should have confirmatory genetic testing in addition to a screening ECG and echo. Depending on the established familial versus sporadic pattern, confirmatory genetic testing should proceed in concentric circles of relatedness. For example, if the HCM-associated mutation is established in the patient's father, then the patient's paternal grandparents should be tested, and if necessary, then the paternal aunts and uncles, and so forth.

Genetic testing will play a key role in the screening and identification of at-risk family members, even with preclinical HCM, and guide proper surveillance of those harboring an HCM-predisposing genetic substrate. In the future, perhaps, predisease interventions with antifibrotic and myocardial remodeling agents such as aldactone, ACE inhibitors, angiotensin receptor blockers, calcium channel blockers, and/or 3-hydroxy-3-methylglutaryl coenzyme A (HMG-CoA) inhibitors may favorably alter the natural history of HCM.[14]

References

1. Yetman AT, McCrindle BW. Management of pediatric hypertrophic cardiomyopathy. *Curr Opin Cardiol* 2005;20:80–83.
2. Poliac LC, Barron ME, Maron BJ. Hypertrophic cardiomyopathy. *Anesthesiology* 2006;104:183–192.
3. Maron BJ, Seidman JG, Seidman CE. Proposal for contemporary screening strategies in families with hypertrophic cardiomyopathy. *J Am Coll Cardiol* 2004;44:2125–2132.
4. Franz WM, Muller OJ, Katus HA. Cardiomyopathies: From genetics to the prospect of treatment. *Lancet* 2001;358:1627–1637.
5. Ellsworth EG, Ackerman MJ. The changing face of sudden cardiac death in the young. *Heart Rhythm* 2005;2:1283–1285.
6. Puranik R, Chow CK, Duflou JA, Kilborn MJ, McGuire MA. Sudden death in the young. *Heart Rhythm* 2005;2:1277–1282.
7. Corrado D, Basso C, Thiene G. Sudden cardiac death in young people with apparently normal heart. *Cardiovasc Res* 2001;50:399–408.
8. Roberts R, Sigwart U. Current concepts of the pathogenesis and treatment of hypertrophic cardiomyopathy. *Circulation* 2005;112:293–296.
9. Klein GJ, Krahn AD, Skanes AC, Yee R, Gula LJ. Primary prophylaxis of sudden death in hypertrophic cardiomyopathy, arrhythmogenic right ventricular cardiomyopathy, and dilated cardiomyopathy. *J Cardiovasc Electrophysiol* 2005;16(Suppl. 1):S28–34.
10. Elliott PM, Gimeno Blanes JR, Mahon NG, Poloniecki JD, McKenna WJ. Relation between severity of left-ventricular hypertrophy and prognosis in patients with hypertrophic cardiomyopathy. *Lancet* 2001;357:420–424.
11. Van Driest SL, Vasile VC, Ommen SR, Will ML, Gersh BJ, Nishimura RA, Tajik AJ, Ackerman MJ. Myosin binding protein C mutations and compound herterozygosity in hypertrophic cardiomyopathy. *J Am Coll Cardiol* 2004;44:1903–1910.
12. Van Driest SL, Ommen SR, Tajik AJ, Gersh BJ, Ackerman MJ. Yield of genetic testing in hypertrophic cardiomyopathy. *Mayo Clinic Proc* 2005;80: 739–744.
13. Van Driest SL, Ommen SR, Tajik AJ, Gersh BJ, Ackerman MJ. Sarcomeric genotyping in hypertrophic cardiomyopathy. *Mayo Clin Proc* 2005;80:463–469.
14. Ackerman MJ. Genetic testing for risk stratification in hypertrophic cardiomyopathy and long QT syndrome: Fact or fiction? *Curr Opin Cardiol* 2005;20: 175–181.
15. Arad M, Maron BJ, Gorham JM, Johnson WH Jr, Saul JP, Perez-Atayde AR, Spirito P, Wright GB, Kanter RJ, Seidman CE, Seidman JG. Glycogen storage diseases presenting as hypertrophic cardiomyopathy. *N Engl J Med* 2005;352:362–372.
16. Arad M, Perez-Atayde AR, Moskowitz IP, Berul CI, Seidman JG, Seidman CE. Genetic studies link glycogen storage to mechanism of familial WPW. Keystone Symposia on Molecular Biology of Cardiac Disease. Keystone, CO, March 7–12, 2004.
17. Harvard Medical School–Partners Heathcare Center for Genetics and Genomics. Laboratory for Molecular Medicine: Tests. Avalaible at http://www.hpcgg.org/LMM/tests.jsp.
18. Antzelevitch C. Molecular genetics of arrhythmias and cardiovascular conditions associated with arrhythmias. *J Cardiovasc Electrophysiol* 2003;14: 1259–1272.
19. Perkins MJ, Van Driest SL, Ellsworth EG, Will ML, Gersh BJ, Ommen SR, Ackerman MJ. Gene-specific modifying effects of pro-LVH polymorphisms involving the renin-angiotensin-aldosterone system among 389 unrelated patients with hypertrophic cardiomyopathy. *Eur Heart J* 2005;26:2457–2462.
20. Binder J, Ommen SR, Gersh BJ, Van Driest SL, Tajik AJ, Nishimura RA, Ackerman MJ. Echocardiography-guided genetic testing in hypertrophic cardiomyopathy: Septal morphological features predict the presence of myofilament mutations. *Mayo Clin Proc* 2006;81:459–467.
21. Wolf CM, Moskowitz IP, Arno S, Branco DM, Semsarian C, Bernstein SA, Peterson M, Maida M, Morley GE, Fishman G, Berul CI, Seidman CE, Seidman JG. Somatic events modify hypertrophic cardiomyopathy pathology and link hypertrophy to arrhythmia. *Proc Natl Acad Sci USA* 2005;102: 18123–18128.
22. Tomaselli GF, Marban E. Electrophysiological remodeling in hypertrophy and heart failure. *Cardiovasc Res* 1999;42:270–283.

23. Olivotto I, Cecchi F, Casey SA, Dolara A, Traverse JH, Maron BJ. Impact of atrial fibrillation on the clinical course of hypertrophic cardiomyopathy. *Circulation* 2001;104:2517–2524.
24. Spirito P, Autore C. Management of hypertrophic cardiomyopathy. *BMJ* 2006;332:1251–1255.
25. Attari M, Dhala A. Role of invasive and noninvasive testing in risk stratification of sudden cardiac death in children and young adults: An electrophysiologic perspective. *Pediatr Clin North Am* 2004;51:1355–1378.
26. Adabag AS, Casey SA, Kuskowski MA, Zenovich AG, Maron BJ. Spectrum and prognostic significance of arrhythmias on ambulatory Holter electrocardiogram in hypertrophic cardiomyopathy. *J Am Coll Cardiol* 2005;45:697–704.
27. Maron BJ, McKenna WJ, Danielson GK, Kappenberger LJ, Kuhn HJ, Seidman CE, Shah PM, Spencer WH, 3rd, Spirito P, Ten Cate FJ, Wigle ED. American College of Cardiology/European Society of Cardiology clinical expert consensus document on hypertrophic cardiomyopathy. A report of the American College of Cardiology Foundation Task Force on Clinical Expert Consensus Documents and the European Society of Cardiology Committee for Practice Guidelines. *J Am Coll Cardiol* 2003;42:1687–1713.
28. Maron BJ. Hypertrophic cardiomyopathy: A systematic review. *J Am Med Assoc* 2002;287:1308–1320.
29. Maron BJ, Carney KP, Lever HM, Lewis JF, Barac I, Casey SA, Sherrid MV. Relationship of race to sudden cardiac death in competitive athletes with hypertrophic cardiomyopathy. *J Am Coll Cardiol* 2003;41:974–980.
30. Seidman JG, Seidman C. The genetic basis for cardiomyopathy: From mutation identification to mechanistic paradigms. *Cell* 2001;104:557–567.
31. Maron BJ, Tajik AJ, Ruttenberg HD, Graham TP, Atwood GF, Victorica BE, Lie JT, Roberts WC. Hypertrophic cardiomyopathy in infants: Clinical features and natural history. *Circulation* 1982;65:7–17.
32. Spirito P, Maron BJ, Bonow RO, Epstein SE. Occurrence and significance of progressive left ventricular wall thinning and relative cavity dilatation in hypertrophic cardiomyopathy. *Am J Cardiol* 1987;60:123–129.
33. Boriani G, Maron BJ, Shen WK, Spirito P. Prevention of sudden death in hypertrophic cardiomyopathy: But which defibrillator for which patient? *Circulation* 2004;110:e438–442.
34. Debl K, Djavidani B, Buchner S, Lipke C, Nitz W, Feuerbach S, Riegger G, Luchner A. Delayed hyper-enhancement: Frequent finding in magnetic resonance imaging of left ventricular hypertrophy due to aortic stenosis and hypertrophic cardiomyopathy. *Heart* 2006;92(10):1447–1451.
35. Moon JC, McKenna WJ, McCrohon JA, Elliott PM, Smith GC, Pennell DJ. Toward clinical risk assessment in hypertrophic cardiomyopathy with gadolinium cardiovascular magnetic resonance. *J Am Coll Cardiol* 2003;41:1561–1567.
36. Lever HM, Karam RF, Currie PJ, Healy BP. Hypertrophic cardiomyopathy in the elderly. Distinctions from the young based on cardiac shape. *Circulation* 1989;79:580–589.
37. Van Driest SV, Ackerman MJ, Ommen SR, Shakur R, Will ML, Nishimura RA, Tajik AJ, Gersh BJ. Prevalence and severity of "benign" mutations in the beta myosin heavy chain, cardiac troponin-T, and alpha tropomyosin genes in hypertrophic cardiomyopathy. *Circulation* 2002;106:3085–3090.
38. Ackerman MJ, Van Driest SV, Ommen SR, Will ML, Nishimura RA, Tajik AJ, Gersh BJ. Prevalence and age-dependence of malignant mutations in the beta-myosin heavy chain and troponin T gene in hypertrophic cardiomyopathy: A comprehensive outpatient perspective. *J Am Coll Cardiol* 2002;39:2042–2048.
39. Olivotto I, Maron BJ, Montereggi A, Mazzuoli F, Dolara A, Cecchi F. Prognostic value of systemic blood pressure response during exercise in a community-based patient population with hypertrophic cardiomyopathy. *J Am Coll Cardiol* 1999;33:2044–2051.
40. Spirito P, Bellone P, Harris KM, Bernabo P, Bruzzi P, Maron BJ. Magnitude of left ventricular hypertrophy and risk of sudden death in hypertrophic cardiomyopathy. *N Engl J Med* 2000;342:1778–1785.
41. Maron BJ. Hypertrophic cardiomyopathy in childhood. *Pediatr Clin North Am* 2004;51:1305–1346.
42. Sorajja P, Nishimura RA, Ommen SR, Ackerman MJ, Tajik AJ, Gersh BJ. Use of echocardiography in patients with hypertrophic cardiomyopathy: Clinical implications of massive hypertrophy. *J Am Soc Echocardiogr* 2006;19:788–795.
43. Maron BJ. The electrocardiogram as a diagnostic tool for hypertrophic cardiomyopathy: Revisited. *Ann Noninvasive Electrocardiol* 2001;6:277–279.
44. Spirito P, Seidman CE, McKenna WJ, Maron BJ. The management of hypertrophic cardiomyopathy. *N Engl J Med* 1997;336:775–785.
45. Maron BJ MW, Danielson GK, Kappenberger LJ, Kuhn HJ, Seidman CE, Shah PM, Spencer WH 3rd, Spirito P, Ten Cate FJ, Wigle ED; Task Force on Clinical Expert Consensus Documents. American

College of Cardiology; Committee for Practice Guidelines. European Society of Cardiology. American College of Cardiology/European Society of Cardiology clinical expert consensus document on hypertrophic cardiomyopathy. A report of the American College of Cardiology Foundation Task Force on Clinical Expert Consensus Documents and the European Society of Cardiology Committee for Practice Guidelines. *J Am Coll Cardiol* 2003;42:1687.
46. Konno T SM, Ino H, Fujino N, Hayashi K, Uchiyama K, Kaneda T, Inoue M, Masuda E, Mabuchi H. Phenotypic differences between electrocardiographic and echocardiographic determination of hypertrophic cardiomyopathy in genetically affected subjects. *J Intern Med* 2005; 258:216–224.
47. Konno T, Shimizu M, Ino H, Fujino N, Hayashi K, Uchiyama K, Kaneda T, Inoue M, Masuda E, Mabuchi H. Phenotypic differences between electrocardiographic and echocardiographic determination of hypertrophic cardiomyopathy in genetically affected subjects. *J Intern Med* 2005; 258:216–224.
48. Konno T, Shimizu M, Ino H, Fujino N, Hayashi K, Uchiyama K, Kaneda T, Inoue M, Fujita T, Masuta E, Funada A, Mabuchi H. Differences in diagnostic value of four electrocardiographic voltage criteria for hypertrophic cardiomyopathy in a genotyped population. *Am J Cardiol* 2005;96:1308–1312.
49. Maron BJ, Spirito P, Wesley Y, Arce J. Development and progression of left ventricular hypertrophy in children with hypertrophic cardiomyopathy. *N Engl J Med* 1986;315:610–614.
50. Ozdemir O, Soylu M, Demir AD, Topaloglu S, Alyan O, Turhan H, Bicer A, Kutuk E. P-wave durations as a predictor for atrial fibrillation development in patients with hypertrophic cardiomyopathy. *Int J Cardiol* 2004;94:163–166.
51. Franz WM MO, Katus HA. Cardiomyopathies: From genetics to the prospect of treatment. *Lancet* 2001;358:1627–1637.
52. Maron MS, Olivotto I, Betocchi S, Casey SA, Lesser JR, Losi MA, Cecchi F, Maron BJ. Effect of left ventricular outflow tract obstruction on clinical outcome in hypertrophic cardiomyopathy. *N Engl J Med* 2003;348:295–303.
53. Montgomery JV, Harris KM, Casey SA, Zenovich AG, Maron BJ. Relation of electrocardiographic patterns to phenotypic expression and clinical outcome in hypertrophic cardiomyopathy. *Am J Cardiol* 2005;96:270–275.
54. Ostman-Smith I, Wettrell G, Keeton B, Riesenfeld T, Holmgren D, Ergander U. Echocardiographic and electrocardiographic identification of those children with hypertrophic cardiomyopathy who should be considered at high-risk of dying suddenly. *Cardiol Young* 2005;15:632–642.
55. D'Andrea A, Caso P, Severino S, Scotto di Uccio F, Vigorito F, Ascione L, Scherillo M, Calabro R. Association between intraventricular myocardial systolic dyssynchrony and ventricular arrhythmias in patients with hypertrophic cardiomyopathy. *Echocardiography* 2005;22:571–578.
56. Maron BJ, Towbin JA, Thiene G, Antzelevitch C, Corrado D, Arnett D, Moss AJ, Seidman CE, Young JB. Contemporary definitions and classification of the cardiomyopathies: An American Heart Association Scientific Statement from the Council on Clinical Cardiology, Heart Failure and Transplantation Committee; Quality of Care and Outcomes Research and Functional Genomics and Translational Biology Interdisciplinary Working Groups; and Council on Epidemiology and Prevention. *Circulation* 2006;113:1807–1816.
57. Cuomo S, Marciano F, Migaux ML, Finizio F, Pezzella E, Losi MA, Betocchi S. Abnormal QT interval variability in patients with hypertrophic cardiomyopathy: Can syncope be predicted? *J Electrocardiol* 2004;37:113–119.
58. Kuroda N, Ohnishi Y, Yoshida A, Kimura A, Yokoyama M. Clinical significance of T-wave alternans in hypertrophic cardiomyopathy. *Circ J* 2002; 66:457–462.
59. Zhu DW, Sun H, Hill R, Roberts R. The value of electrophysiology study and prophylactic implantation of cardioverter defibrillator in patients with hypertrophic cardiomyopathy. *Pacing Clin Electrophysiol* 1998;21:299–302.
60. Fananapazir L, Chang AC, Epstein SE, McAreavey D. Prognostic determinants in hypertrophic cardiomyopathy. Prospective evaluation of a therapeutic strategy based on clinical, Holter, hemodynamic, and electrophysiological findings. *Circulation* 1992; 86:730–740.
61. Mohiddin SA, Begley D, Shih J, Fananapazir L. Myocardial bridging does not predict sudden death in children with hypertrophic cardiomyopathy but is associated with more severe cardiac disease. *J Am Coll Cardiol* 2000;36:2270–2278.
62. Elliott P, McKenna WJ. Hypertrophic cardiomyopathy. *Lancet* 2004;363:1881–1891.
63. Maron BJ. Contemporary considerations for risk stratification, sudden death and prevention in hypertrophic cardiomyopathy. *Heart* 2003;89:977–978.
64. Nishimura RA, Holmes DR Jr. Clinical practice. Hypertrophic obstructive cardiomyopathy. *N Engl J Med* 2004;350:1320–1327.

65. Maron BJ, Dearani JA, Ommen SR, Maron MS, Schaff HV, Gersh BJ, Nishimura RA. The case for surgery in obstructive hypertrophic cardiomyopathy. *J Am Coll Cardiol* 2004;44:2044–2053.
66. Elliott PMW. Hypertrophic cardiomyopathy. *Lancet* 2004;363:1881–1891.
67. Ommen SR, Maron BJ, Olivotto I, Maron MS, Cecchi F, Betocchi S, Gersh BJ, Ackerman MJ, McCully RB, Dearani JA, Schaff HV, Danielson GK, Tajik AJ, Nishimura RA. Long-term effects of surgical septal myectomy on survival in patients with obstructive hypertrophic cardiomyopathy. *J Am Coll Cardiol* 2005;46:470–476.
68. Maron BJ, Nishimura RA, McKenna WJ, Rakowski H, Josephson ME, Kieval RS. Assessment of permanent dual-chamber pacing as a treatment for drug-refractory symptomatic patients with obstructive hypertrophic cardiomyopathy. A randomized, double-blind, crossover study (M-PATHY). *Circulation* 1999;99:2927–2933.
69. Chen MS, McCarthy PM, Lever HM, Smedira NG, Lytle BL. Effectiveness of atrial fibrillation surgery in patients with hypertrophic cardiomyopathy. *Am J Cardiol* 2004;93:373–375.
70. DiMarco JP. Implantable cardioverter-defibrillators. *N Engl J Med* 2003;349:1836–1847.
71. Maron BJ, Estes NAM, Maron MS, Almquist AK, Link MS, Udelson JE. Primary prevention of sudden death as a novel treatment strategy in hypertrophic cardiomyopathy. *Circulation* 2003;107:2872–2875.
72. Maron BJ, Pelliccia A, Spirito P. Cardiac disease in young trained athletes. Insights into methods for distinguishing athlete's heart from structural heart disease, with particular emphasis on hypertrophic cardiomyopathy. *Circulation* 1995;91:1596–1601.
73. Maron BJ, Chaitman BR, Ackerman MJ, Bayes de Luna A, Corrado D, Crosson JE, Deal BJ, Driscoll DJ, Estes NA 3rd, Araujo CG, Liang DH, Mitten MJ, Myerburg RJ, Pelliccia A, Thompson PD, Towbin JA, Van Camp SP. Recommendations for physical activity and recreational sports participation for young patients with genetic cardiovascular diseases. *Circulation* 2004;109:2807–2816.

41
Sudden Death in Dilated Cardiomyopathy and Skeletal Myopathies

Jop H. van Berlo and Yigal M. Pinto

Introduction

It is obvious to assume that diseases that affect skeletal muscle also affect the heart. Indeed, different myopathies share common cardiac abnormalities. While many different skeletal myopathies can be recognized, only a few different types of cardiomyopathies can be clinically distinguished. This suggests that different skeletal myopathies cause actually quite similar cardiac abnormalities. The reason for this is not clear. It might indicate that the underlying defects in skelatal myopathies all induce common pathways in the heart despite their underlying different pathobiological mechanisms. This probably reflects the very different capacities of skeletal muscle and cardiac muscle. A very important difference between cardiac and skeletal muscle is that unlike the heart, skeletal muscle can be electrically activated only by neurons. Another important difference is the existence of a specialized conduction system within the heart. A third important difference is the type of fibers that make up the contractile elements. The skeletal muscles are all composed of a mixture of fast and slow fibers. Fast fibers contain large amounts of glycolytic enzymes, have an extensive sarcoplasmic reticulum, and have less blood supply and are therefore ideal for fast contraction with great strength of contraction. Slow fibers contain large amounts of mitochondria, have a more extended blood supply, and contain myoglobin for oxygen storage, which makes these fibers red. The heart is built up of striated muscle fibers, similar to skeletal muscle, but consists of single cardiac myocytes that can pass through electrical signals via the intercalated disc.

Despite these differences, there are also many obvious similarities. This is emphasized by the fact that indeed many skeletal myopathies also show cardiac involvement. However, the extent of this cardiac involvement depends not only on the type of skeletal myopathy, but also on other, so far unrecognized factors. Therefore, whenever the heart could be involved in a skeletal myopathy, cardio logical consultation is advisable. Most often cardiac involvement is evidenced by conduction system disease, cardiac arrhythmias, and/or heart failure or ultimately sudden cardiac death. The goal of this chapter is not to exhaustively describe dilated cardiomyopathy or the neurological diseases, but to give an overview of the most frequent cardiac complications of skeletal myopathies. Furthermore, the risk of sudden death is discussed for each skeletal myopathy and for dilated cardiomyopathy.

Dilated Cardiomyopathy

Older studies have shown that dilated cardiomyopathy (DCM) has an incidence of around 20/100,000 per year with a prevalence of 38/100,000 per year.[1] In recent years, the 5-year mortality rate has dropped from 70% to approximately 20%.[2–4] The cause of DCM is typically unknown, however, with a thorough medical history and physical examination focused on possible causes of DCM combined with endomyocardial biopsies, in almost 50% of patients a diagnosis could be reached in a tertiary referral clinic.[5] Most studies that look at DCM and risk of sudden death did not specify the cause of DCM, but usually indicated that it was nonischemic. For the purpose of this chapter, we will focus on nonischemic DCM in general, and only briefly comment on specific forms of DCM, e.g., hereditary DCM or myocarditis.

In ischemic DCM, mortality is mainly determined by arrhythmic causes (sudden death), progressive heart failure, or noncardiac causes of death. In DCM (nonischemic) the cause of death is not always clear. Most patients die due to progressive heart failure. Nevertheless, sudden death is also a major problem in DCM and accounts for approximately 30% of all deaths.[6] However, the arrhythmic origin of these sudden deaths is not always well established, and other causes such as bradyarrhythmias, pulmonary or systemic embolization, or pulseless electrical activity account for up to 50% of sudden deaths in some reports.[7–10] Whether the treatment to prevent sudden death in ischemic heart failure should differ from the treatment in nonischemic DCM has not yet been tested in prospective randomized clinical trials. Most studies have reported similar survival rates for DCM and ischemic heart failure with current treatment regimes. Irrespective of these remarks, a number of randomized clinical trials have been performed that addressed the problem of sudden death in DCM, albeit not always specifically DCM.

Risk of Sudden Death in Dilated Cardiomyopathy

Sudden death in the general population accounts for 20% of all deaths.[11] When looking at autopsy studies that identified the cause of sudden death, above the age of 30 years, the main cause of sudden death is atherosclerosis. Below the age of 30 years, DCM could be identified as the cause of sudden death in 5–12% of cases.[12,13] Hypertrophic cardiomyopathy was as often found to be the cause of sudden death as DCM in these two studies.

A number of studies have focused on prevention of sudden death in DCM, both secondary and primary. Although prospective cohort studies are important to identify risk factors for SD to justify implantable cardioverter defibrillator (ICD) implantation in subgroups of DCM patients, we will focus on the more general randomized clinical trials with ICDs in DCM. Recently, a meta-analysis was performed that included all randomized clinical trials that included DCM patients.[14] This meta-analysis included three secondary prevention trials and five primary prevention trials. Obviously it is beyond debate that ICD therapy has a role in secondary prevention to treat malignant ventricular arrhythmias. Three trials have assessed the role of ICD therapy for secondary prevention in patients with DCM and compared ICD implantation to antiarrhythmic drug therapy.[15–17] Although the Antiarrhymics versus Implantable Defibrillators (AVID)[15] study showed a statistically significant survival benefit of ICD over amiodarone in the entire study population, in the nonischemic DCM subgroup improved survival with ICD therapy failed to reach statistical significance, which is remarkable for a secondary prevention strategy. The other trials failed to reach statistical significance. Probably, the power to find a difference was too low in the entire study population to begin with, due to low mortality rates. When analyzing the nonischemic subgroup from these studies, the power to detect a difference in treatment is even less. Another explanation could be the relatively high proportion of crossovers in the studies or the proportion of non-arrhythmic sudden deaths in DCM. The survival benefit, however, was 31% for secondary prevention of sudden death.

Primary prevention of sudden death in (nonischemic) DCM was tested in five randomized clinical trials.[18–22] Most of these trials were unable to show a statistically significant survival benefit for ICD implantation, although the ICD was usually associated with improved survival. In a meta-analysis of all these trials, the combined trials with only the DCM patients clearly showed a significant reduction in mortality of 31%.[14] This reduction in mortality was not dependent on one single trial. Therefore, the meta-analysis concluded that ICDs for primary prevention may reduce all-cause mortality in nonischemic DCM patients. However, the mortality rates in the control groups were relatively low, which resulted in a low absolute benefit of ICD implantation. Based on the combined mortality rates of these trials and an estimated risk reduction of all-cause mortality by the ICD of 31%, a number needed to treat (NNT) of 25 to prevent one death in 2 years was calculated.[14] In patients with a reduced ejection fraction after myocardial infarction the NNT is approximately 18.[23] Not withstanding the relevance of ICD therapy in this group, these numbers also indicate that in nonischemic DCM, the combination of improved diagnosis and therapy with lowered mortality rates, and the combination of various forms of morbidity and mortality preclude a major impact of ICD therapy so that a substantial number of ICDs need to be implanted to prevent death. This further emphasizes the urgent need to better identify patients who are at increased risk for sudden death.

Risk Factors for Sudden Death in Dilated Cardiomyopathy

To identify subgroups at increased risk for sudden death, many prospective studies have been performed. QT dispersion, electrophysiology testing, signal-averaged electrocardiograms (ECGs), heart rate variability, and baroreflex sensitivity to predict sudden death in DCM have yielded opposing results.[24–26] The factors that have consistently been associated with sudden death in DCM are depressed ejection fraction, severity of heart failure according to New York Heart Association (NYHA) class, and presence of nonsustained ventricular tachycardias (VTs).[27] The use of microvolt T wave alternans is still under debate. Three studies have found a positive relation with T wave alternans, although one excluded all undetermined cases in the analysis, and one study could not find any relation.[28–31] Therefore a prospective study was performed in patients with a reduced ejection fraction but without sustained ventricular tachycardias.[32] This study included over 500 patients with heart failure, both ischemic and nonischemic, and performed microvolt T wave alternans (MTWA) testing in all patients. They found an association for both positive and indeterminate MTWA tests and sudden death (2.4% events in negative MTWA and 17.8% and 12.3% for indeterminate and positive MTWA, respectively).[32,33] Another factor that is often associated with sudden death in DCM is lack of β blocker therapy.[24,32] The above shows that there are still no precise measures to predict the chance of sudden death in DCM.

Whether myocarditis is an important risk factor for sudden death is not entirely clear. It is known that patients with fulminant myocarditis often suffer from severe ventricular tachyarrhythmias. In autopsy studies of sudden death victims, the proportion of patients that show signs of myocarditis varies greatly from 5% to 40%.[12,13,34–36] However, whether these patients all suffered from a clinically relevant myocarditis is not known; neither is it known whether the myocarditis was causally related to the sudden death event.[37] There are no studies that report the frequency of myocarditis on autopsy of noncardiac deaths, such as car accident victims. Nevertheless, myocarditis could be an important risk factor for sudden death and prospective follow-up of patients with proven myocarditis could provide insight in the risk of sudden death in clinically relevant myocarditis. Another risk factor for sudden death is DCM caused by Chagas disease. Within this subgroup of DCM, arrhythmias are more the rule than the exception.[38,39] When these patients are treated with an ICD implantation for secondary prevention, more than 90% of patients show appropriate device therapy within 1 year of ICD implantation.[40]

Finally, some forms of genetic DCM carry an increased risk of sudden death. Whether the increased risk is due to a certain gene that is mutated, or due to specific mutations within one gene, environmental factors, genetic modifiers, or still unidentified factors is not known. One example of probable environmental or genetic modulatory factors comes from a paper that described two families with DCM that was mapped to chromosome 10q25–26.[41] Although the causal gene mutation has not yet been identified, both families showed linkage to this locus. Surprisingly, only one family showed a phenotype of sudden cardiac death, while within the other family all patients died due to congestive heart failure. DCM causing gene mutations that are associated with sudden death include, for example, troponin T, delta sarcoglycan, desmin, and lamin A/C. The risk of sudden death varies among these different genes. The risk of sudden death in lamin A/C gene mutations was reported to be exceptionally high (45%).[42] Therefore, a prospective primary prevention trial was performed in 19 patients with a lamin A/C gene mutation, who were all in need of a pacemaker, but received ICD implantation with pacing capacities.[43] After almost 3 years of follow-up of 19 included patients, 42% of patients underwent appropriate ICD shock, while none of the patients died during this period. This is the first report of a primary prevention sudden death trial in DCM patients based on gene mutation.

In conclusion, the risk of sudden death in DCM patients is very high and selected patients might benefit from ICD implantation for primary prevention of sudden death. The difficulty is to predict which patient benefits most from ICD implantation. Factors that are associated with arrhythmic events in DCM patients include low ejection fraction, nonsustained VT on Holter examination, lack of β blocker use, a positive or indeterminate MTWA test, and possibly a lamin A/C mutation as cause of DCM.

Skeletal Myopathies

Duchenne Muscular Dystrophy

General

Duchenne muscular dystrophy (DMD) was first described by Edward Meryon in 1851.[44] The characteristic clinical features are progressive proximal muscle weakness with typical pseudohypertrophy of the calves.[45] Serum creatine kinase levels are usually elevated. The progressive nature of the disease is shown by the fact that most patients are wheelchair bound by the age of 12 years. The disease is caused by mutations in the dystrophin gene that is located on the X-chromosome. Therefore only boys are affected with full-blown muscular dystrophy. Ten to 15% of female carriers do show signs of muscular weakness and enlarged calves are quite frequent.[45] These women are called manifesting carriers. Mental retardation is a frequent finding in DMD; 20–30% of patients have a full scale intelligence quotient below 75.[46,47] Smooth muscle may also be involved and could lead to gastric dilation or acute intestinal obstruction eventually resulting in death.

In different studies an incidence rate of 20–30 per 100,000 live male births has been reported.[48–50] The prevalence rate varies between 1:18,496 and 1:31,646.

Cardiac Involvement

The heart is usually involved in DMD. Up to 95% of boys have signs of cardiac disease at the end of their lives. The ECG shows typical features, tall right precordial R waves, deep limb lead, and left precordial Q waves.[51] Further cardiac abnormalities include inappropriate sinus tachycardia, atrial flutter, both atrial and ventricular premature beats, and paroxysmal ventricular tachycardia. Conduction system disease evidenced by right or left bundle branch block can also occur. Left and/or right ventricular dilation and systolic dysfunction are frequent findings in DMD.[52–54] Due to improved respiratory support with use of tracheostoma, more patients survive to develop these echocardiographic abnormalities at the end of their life. An additional problem in DMD is the deformed chest, which can make conventional echocardiography challenging or impossible. Overt heart failure, however, is quite infrequent, probably due to patient immobility. Again, due to improved survival from respiratory failure, the incidence of heart failure in DMD patients has increased in the past decades.[55] Before the development of global cardiomyopathy with severely depressed systolic function, many patients already show regional wall motion abnormalities.

Cause of Death

The usual cause of death in DMD used to be respiratory failure. However, with improved treatment with steroids and respiratory support with ambulatory ventilators, cardiac causes of death have become more frequent.[56] Up to 40% of deaths are thought to be due to cardiac causes based on autopsy findings.[57] Heart failure is a quite frequent finding in the final stage of DMD and probably end-stage heart failure is a common cause of death.[55] As might be expected, patients with DMD often die suddenly. The cause of this sudden death, however, is not always known. One study evaluated the use of 24-h Holter registration to predict sudden death.[56] None of the patients had symptomatic arrhythmias, but one showed sustained VT on this relatively short Holter monitoring. During a 3-year follow-up, 15 of 45 patients died. The risk of dying during follow-up was 50% if patients showed complex ventricular ectopy on Holter monitoring (multiform VPB or VPB couplets), while it was only 8% in patients without complex ventricular ectopy. Although suggestive, this still does not establish that these patients died due to tachyarrhythmias. Adding to the suggestion of ventricular arrhythmia is another study that also found that ectopic activity and depressed systolic function are associated with an increased chance of death,[58] yet definite evidence that ventricular tachyarrhythmias cause sudden death is still lacking.

Becker Muscular Dystrophy

General

Becker muscular dystrophy (BMD) is the less severe variant of Duchenne muscular dystrophy. The two diseases are allelic, so BMD is also caused by mutations in dystrophin. In general, DMD is caused by frameshift mutations, while in BMD the reading frame remains intact. The result is a total absence of dystrophin at the sarcolemma in DMD, while dystrophin protein levels are reduced only in BMD. Similar muscle groups are affected, but the disease usually presents only after the age of 12 years.[45] Some patients have no symptoms until later in life. Patients can become wheelchair bound; the age at which this occurs varies from adolescence onward. Possible future treatments for Duchenne muscular dystrophy involve exon skipping techniques that are estimated to function in about 60% of DMD patients.[59,60] The result of exon skipping would be a return to the restoration of the normal reading frame, but with a mutated protein. Protein levels would thereby be increased and DMD patients would develop a Becker type of muscular dystrophy. The first trials in patients are currently being performed. If this therapy becomes widely applied, this would have a major impact on the prevalence of BMD.

Cardiac Involvement

Cardiac involvement is as frequent as in DMD; some patients may present with cardiac abnormalities before the development of a skeletal muscular phenotype, or even with pure cardiac disease without muscular weakness.[61] Electrocardiographic abnormalities are frequent with the usually small R waves and/or Q waves in lateral leads (90%), prominent R waves in right precordial leads (47%), and prominent Q waves in inferior leads (37%). These ECG changes are comparable to changes with DMD, with the difference that the most common finding in DMD is tall R waves in right precordial leads (88%).[62] Echocardiographic abnormalities range from wall motion abnormalities to right and/or left ventricular dilation to hypertrophic cardiomyopathy.[61–63] Systolic function may be depressed. However, despite this high frequency of abnormalities on cardiac examination, most patients are without complaints until late in the disease.[61] Fourteen years of median follow-up of 27 BMD patients showed progressive disease, both in terms of muscular disease and cardiac disease, in 24.[64] Only five patients were without cardiac abnormalities after this follow-up period. Five patients died during follow-up, of whom four died due to heart failure.

Cause of Death

Due to the milder muscular involvement in BMD, patients are more likely to be limited by cardiac complaints. Second, the cause of death in BMD patients is therefore more often cardiac than respiratory related. Heart failure was the leading cause of death in the previously mentioned study of Hoogerwaard *et al.*[64] Sudden death has been reported in BMD in up to 30% of cases.[65] This emphasizes that defects in dystrophin have severe cardiac consequences, and that such cardiac consequences are less prominent in DMD simply because of the much more extensive skeletal myopathy in DMD. The exact cause of death is usually hard to establish and could be either heart failure, respiratory failure, or arrhyrhmias. Although sustained VTs are usually not seen on 24-h Holter monitoring, arrhythmic sudden death cannot be excluded. One study found QT-interval dispersion as a predictor of sudden death in BMD.[65] This dispersion of ventricular repolarization is also seen in dilated cardiomyopathy, where sudden cardiac death is often encountered.[25,66] Cardiovascular health supervision with a proactive approach is advocated in BMD and DMD patients by the American Academy of Pediatrics.[67] This way we might be able to delay deterioration of cardiac function in BMD patients. Furthermore, it is important to obtain insight into the mechanism of sudden death in BMD patients. If the cause is tachyarrhythmic, these patients might benefit from prophylactic ICD implantation.

Female Carriers of Duchenne Muscular Dystrophy and Becker Muscular Dystrophy Gene Mutations

Female carriers of a DMD or BMD mutation can develop muscular weakness and cardiac disease.[68] The incidence of carriers with symptoms varies between 2.5 and 22%.[69–72] Most studies only report on either muscle weakness or cardiac involvement. A large survey by Hoogerwaard *et al.* investigated 127 proven carriers with a mean age of 37 years for the presence of both muscular complaints and cardiac abnormalities.[73] They found myalgia, cramps, or muscle weakness in 20 of 84 (24%) DMD carriers and in 8 of 43 (19%) BMD carriers. Cardiac abnormalities were present in 23 of 84 (27%) DMD carriers and in 7 of 43 (16%) BMD carriers. However, dilated cardiomyopathy was far less prevalent, with 7 of 84 (8%) DMD carriers and 0 of 43 BMD carriers. The significance of left ventricular dilation in 23 carriers is not known; furthermore it is not known if this should be interpreted as the initial stage of dilated cardiomyopathy. Sudden death has been described in carriers of DMD and BMD. This might be suggestive of arrhythmia with asymptomatic dilated cardiomyopathy. However, the frequency of sudden death in carriers of DMD or BMD is not established.

Myotonic Dystrophy

General

Myotonic dystrophy (MD) is a rather frequent autosomal dominant disease with an incidence of 1 in 8000 births and a worldwide estimated prevalence of 2.1 to 14.3/100,000 inhabitants.[74] Myotonic dystrophy is a multisystem disease, as it affects many other systems besides the musculature. Clinically, myotonic dystrophy is divided into three subtypes: congenital, classical, and mild or minimal. Congenital MD is the most severe subtype with neonatal hypotonia, motor and mental retardation, and facial diplegia. Respiratory difficulties are common in neonates and are often fatal (~10%). If newborns survive this period most turn out to have mental retardation (60–70%).[75] Eventually these children develop myotonia and the characteristics of classical myotonic dystrophy.

In the classical form a diagnosis is made by the presence of progressive distal and bulbar dystrophy in the presence of myotonia, delayed relaxation after muscle contraction. Typically signs become evident in middle life, but symptoms may start in the second decade. Progression of muscle weakness is usually slow, while the myotonia is stable. This is often accompanied by frontal balding and/or cataract, but other organs may also be involved. Mild cases present after the age of 50 years and may only show cataract; therefore the diagnosis can be difficult in mild MD. The cause is an instable region on chromosome 19 in type 1 and on chromosome 3 in type 2. Due to genomic instability, during mitosis and meiosis the number of cytosine–thymine–guanine (CTG) (type 1) or CCTG (type 2) repeats can increase or in rare cases decrease. Due to an increase in the number of repeats during meiosis classic anticipation is seen, so that the disease becomes more severe in later generations.

Cardiac Involvement

Cardiac features are rather common in myotonic dystrophy.[76] At biopsies or at postmortem examination, unspecific findings such as interstitial fibrosis, myocyte hypertrophy, and fatty infiltration can be seen. Occasionally lymphocyte infiltration, focal myocarditis, or myofiber disarray can be seen. Typically, during life, cardiac involvement is evidenced by conduction system disease, supraventricular arrhythmias, or ventricular arrhythmias.[77–80] Conduction system disease can affect any part of the conduction system, but the His-Purkinje system is most often involved.[81] The main concern is the development of complete heart block.[82] Usually the conduction system disease is slowly progressive; a pacemaker may become necessary in up to 15% of patients. However, some cases of rapid progression have been reported and cannot be predicted. Less often there are left ventricular dysfunction and heart failure or ischemic heart disease. Mitral valve rolapse has been reported in 25–40% of patients nd is thought to be related to papillary muscle lysfunction. Mitral valve prolapse is not associ- ted with arrhythmias.[76]

Cause of Death

Life expectancy is also reduced in patients with he less severe adult-onset myotonic dystrophy. Median survival for male patients was 59 years nd 60 years for females in one longitudinal study of 180 patients after 45 years of follow-up.[83] The usual cause of death in myotonic dystrophy is (aspiration) pneumonia, sudden death, or post-operative death.[83] Sudden death can be due to bradyarrhythmias as well as to tachyarrhythmias. The rate of sudden death in myotonic dystrophy varies between 2% and 30%. Some studies found an association between CTG size and progression of conduction system disease, cardiac arrhythmias, and sudden cardiac death.[84] However, others failed to show such an association.[85] One prospective study implanted pacemakers in 49 patients with HV >70 msec.[79] After a mean follow-up of 54 months in patients with a mean age of 46 years, 10 patients had died. Four patients died suddenly, but arrhythmias could be excluded in two of those. The cause of death could not be established in only two deaths. Four patients died due to chronic or acute-on-chronic respiratory failure; one suffered from massive pulmonary embolism and one patient died due to an embolic cerebrovascular accident. This analysis suggests that the usual cause of death in myotonic dystrophy is respiratory failure. Sudden death does occur, but is not necessarily due to bradyarrhythmias or tachyarrhytmias. Although tachyarrhythmias and also ventricular tachyarrhythmias are frequently seen in myotonic dystrophy, whether patients die due to tachyarrhythmias is less certain. Prophylactic pacemaker implantation in patients with HV >70 msec was unable to prevent the 40% sudden death rate in one study.[79]

Patients with congenital myotonic dystrophy can develop severe myocardial involvement and are at higher risk of tachyarrhythmic death. There might be an association between exercise and tachyarrhythmias in these patients. One study reported tachyarrhythmias in 40% of younger patients with congenital myotonic dystrophy and showed ventricular fibrillation in 2 out of 11 patients (18%).[80] In myotonic dystrophy type 2 a recent report retrospectively identified four cases of sudden death out of a total population of 297 patients from 120 families.[86] Due to lack of data on total follow-up and lack of mortality numbers, the rate of sudden death in MD2 could not be established. Whether these patients died due to bradyarrhythmias or tachyarrhythmias is not certain, but three of them showed signs of dilated cardiomyopathy at the time of death. At postmortem examination of the heart, fibrosis of the conduction system was found in two patients.

Emery–Dreifuss Muscular Dystrophy

General

Emery–Dreifuss muscular dystrophy (EDMD) is a rather uncommon type of muscular dystrophy.[45] Inheritance patterns can be X-linked, autosomal dominant, or rarely autosomal recessive. The most frequent type is X-linked and is caused by mutations in the gene Emerin. This is a nuclear envelope protein. The autosomal dominant and recessive forms are caused by mutations in the gene LMNA. LMNA encodes two nuclear envelope proteins, lamin A and C. For both the X-linked and the autosomal type of EDMD the molecular pathobiology is unknown. Key features of EDMD are tendon contractures at a young age (4–7 years), mainly of the elbows, Achilles tendons, and posterior neck msucles. These contractures usually proceed to humeroperoneal muscular dystrophy. The muscular dystrophy is hardly progressive and respiratory failure or pneumonia due to muscular weakness usually does not occur.

Cardiac Involvement

Cardiac involvement is usual in EDMD. This starts with conduction system disease (CSD) and/or atrial arrhythmias at a young age.[42] The CSD starts with mild first-degree atrioventricular (AV) block and/or sinus bradycardia or atrial fibrillation with slow ventricular response. Evidence of cardiac disease is usually present by age 30 years. Usually the CSD is progressive and necessitates pacemaker implantation in almost 50% of the patients. Dilated cardiomyopathy and heart failure are more often seen in the autosomal disease, but are not uncommon in the X-linked form.[87] In the autosomal dominant form heart failure can be seen without muscular involvement. If heart failure is present it is often severe and progressive. In retrospective studies of heart transplantation patients with idiopathic dilated cardiomyopathy, 9% were found to have a lamin A/C gene mutation.[88] Another study found that 33% of patients undergoing heart transplantation for familial cardiomyopathy carried a lamin A/C gene mutation.[89]

Cause of Death

Although the muscular dystrophy is considered benign by neurologists, the cardiac consequences of the disease are not. There seems to be a difference between cause of death in X-linked and autosomal dominant EDMD. In X-linked EDMD sudden death has been frequently reported. However, there are few cases of sudden death when a pacemaker was implanted. Therefore, it seems that patients with X-linked EDMD are especially at risk of bradyarrhythmias and complete heart block.[90] Before the description of autosomal EDMD and its causative gene, female carriers of EDMD had been described and sudden death had been reported in these women.[91] Now autosomal EDMD is recognized as a separate disease entity, so that in retrospect, it could be questioned whether these families could have suffered from autosomal EDMD. Patients with autosomal dominant EDMD are at risk of both bradyarrhythmias and tachyarrhythmias. The risk of dying suddenly does not depend on pacemaker implantation.[42] Therefore, a prospective trial was performed on 19 patients with lamin A/C gene mutations with or without muscular involvement.[43] These patients all received an ICD with pacing capacities and were followed for 3 years. After this period eight had experienced ICD shock, with six for ventricular fibrillation. This indicates that patients with lamin A/C mutations, which can cause EDMD, are at high risk of sudden death despite pacemaker implantation, and therefore an ICD should be considered.

Limb-Girdle Muscular Dystrophy

General

Limb-girdle muscular dystrophy (LGMD) mainly affects the proximal limb-girdle musculature.[92] It is a genetically heterogeneous disease with at least six autosomal dominant and 10 autosomal recessive types. Muscular weakness usually presents itself in the second or third decade with a mild progression compared to DMD. Due to the very heterogeneous nature of this type of muscular dystrophy, the exact clinical presentation and the differences between the limb-girdle muscular dystrophies will not be discussed here. Nevertheless, it is very important that an accurate diagnosis is made by a specialized neurologist, because the prevalence of severe complications is very different for the different types of LGMD. The types of LGMD that show cardiac involvement are LGMD1B caused by mutations in lamin A/C, LGMD1D with an unknown genetic defect, LGMD2C-F caused by mutations in the sarcoglycans, and LGMD2I caused by mutations in Fukutin-related protein.

Cardiac Involvement

In LGMD1B the heart is usually involved.[93] The type of cardiac involvement mimics that of autosomal dominant EDMD, but may be less severe. In LGMD1B the conduction system disease is also affected with first- to third-degree AV block. Eventually patients may develop heart failure, but this is less common compared to EDMD. LGMD1D has been described in only one family.[94] This family combined dilated cardiomyopathy with conduction system disease with LGMD, very much like mutations in lamin A/C do. Nevertheless, only one family with this type of LGMD has been described and the gene defect is not known. Because the phenotype resembles the phenotype of lamin A/C gene mutations so closely, it could be hypothesized that a lamin A/C-associated mechanism like a binding protein could be involved in this disease. Similar to mutations in lamin A/C, the cardiac involvement in LGMD1D starts with low-grade AV block that progresses to high-grade AV block; heart failure usually begins later than the conduction system disease. LGMD2C-F can show cardiac involvement quite frequently.[95,96] Usually this is restricted to ECG abnormalities that show Q-waves or an increased QT/PQ ratio, which could point to a prepreclinical cardiomyopathy in skeletal muscle disease.[96] In some patients, however, severe congestive heart failure may develop necessitating cardiac ansplantation. Finally, some patients show ven-icular ectopic activity and may show ventricular chycardias on 24-h Holter monitoring. LGMD2I ten shows cardiac involvement. A retrospective ulticenter study found cardiac involvement 39% of 38 patients, while another six showed ossible cardiac involvement with only ECG normalities.[97] Congestive heart failure can evelop independently of muscular severity of the isease, with a severe course necessitating cardiac ansplantation.

use of Death

he muscular phenotype in LGMD can be quite riable. In the case of LGMD2C-F it can be Duch-ne-like with confinement to a wheelchair by the ge of 16 years. However, other cases with less vere muscular involvement have also been escribed. Therefore the cause of death can be redominantly from respiratory failure in case of vere muscular involvement, but it can also be ue to congestive heart failure if there is severe rdiac involvement. Sudden cardiac death has een described, especially in the autosomal domi-ant types of LGMD,[93,94] where the muscular isease is usually less severe. In the case of GMD1B the cause of sudden death could very ell be tachyarrhythmias.[42] In the case of LGMD1D ost sudden deaths were preceded by a period of ongestive heart failure.

esmin-Related Myopathy

eneral

esmin-related myopathies have been known to ause skeletal myopathies, dilated cardiomyopa-hies, and a combination of the two.[98] Both the keletal muscular phenotype and the cardiac henotype may vary significantly depending on e specific gene mutation. There seems to be a elation between phenotype and type of mutation, e it dominant, recessive, or *de novo*. Desmin yopathies can be caused by mutations in desmin, ut also in desmin-related proteins, such as αB-rystallin. The most typical finding in desmin-elated myopathies is the accumulation of protein ggregates that stain positive for desmin immu-ostaining. Muscular weakness usually starts dis-lly and progresses proximally and may become eneralized. The age of onset differs significantly, ranging from patients who are already affected before the age of 10 years to patients with only slight muscular weakness at the age of 50 years.[99]

Cardiac Involvement

The heart is often involved in desmin-related myopathies.[100,101] In some patients the heart is more severely affected, while in others the muscular phenotype is more prominent. If cardiac involvement is present, it usually starts with conduction system disease, often requiring pacemaker implantation later in the disease course. This can be so severe that before the age of 10 years a pacemaker was implanted in three out of four siblings with a desmin mutation.[102] Later during the disease course dilated cardiomyopathy or restrictive cardiomyopathy can develop.[103] In both cases patients suffer from congestive heart failure. Finally, arrhythmias are also quite frequently reported in desmin-related myopathies sometimes necessitating ICD implantation.[104] If patients with pure cardiomyopathy without muscular involvement are screened for desmin mutations, usually no mutation is found, suggesting that isolated cardiac disease due to desmin mutations is rare.[105]

Cause of Death

Desmin-related myopaties are typically progressive, both for the muscular and the cardiac phenotypes. Depending on the rate of progression patients therefore either die from respiratory insufficiency or from cardiac disease.[100,101] In the case of cardiac disease this can be death due to heart failure, although sudden death has also been described. The sudden death in desmin-related myopathy could very well be tachyarrhythmic in origin, as nonsustained VTs have been described as well as ICD discharges on VTs.[104,106] What is certain is that the life span is limited in desmin-related myopathy.

Congenital Muscular Dystrophies

General

The group of congenital muscular dystrophies (CMD) is a very heterogeneous group of disorders, all showing at least muscular weakness before the age of 6 months.[107] The rate of progression is very different and the number of other organ systems involved also varies. Due to its heterogeneity we will discuss only the most relevant ones in this chapter. Mutations in collagen VI can cause Bethlem myopathy or Ullrich muscular dystrophy depending on the presence of dominant or recessive mutations, respectively.[108] Only in Bethlem myopathy has a cardiac phenotype been described, but only in a few cases.[109] Fukuyama is the second most common form of muscular dystrophy in Japan and is caused by mutations in fukutin. In other parts of the world this type of muscular dystrophy is rarely seen. Patients show generalized muscle weakness and hypotonia in combination with brain malformations. Finally, congenital muscular dystrophy 1c (MDC1C) is caused by mutations in the fukutin-related protein. MDC1C is a severe muscular dystrophy with hypotonia after birth, muscle hypertrophy, severe weakness, and inability to achieve ambulation without help. A milder form of muscular dystrophy that is also caused by mutations in the fukutin-related protein is LGMD1I.

Cardiac Involvement

One study examined 27 patients with Bethlem myopathy, but found cardiac involvement in only one patient in the form of asymmetrical cardiac hypertrophy.[109] A later study examining 121 patients from 61 families, however, identified cardiac involvement in about 10% of cases, although the cardiac involvement was usually mild.[110] One patient showed a nonsustained VT on 24-h Holter monitoring. Cardiac abnormalities in Ullrich muscular dystrophy have not been described, but the neurological disorder is more severe than Bethlem myopathy with hypotonia and multiple contractures at birth or in the neonatal period. Fukuyama congenital muscular dystrophy rarely had cardiac involvement. Nevertheless, on autopsy of a 17-year-old male Japanese patient severe myocardial fibrosis was found.[111] A recent report systematically investigated 34 patients with Fukuyama congenital muscular dystrophy (FMDC) and found an age-dependent cardiac involvement. Above the age of 15 years more than 80% of the patients showed depressed ventricular function.[112] In MDC1C cardiac involvement has also been reported.[113]

Cause of Death

The cause of death in congenital muscular dystr phies is usually respiratory insufficiency. In FMI some patients died due to heart failure and o patient was reported to have died suddenly the age of 17 years. The heart is often fibrotic FMDC on autopsy. Patients with MDC1C usua die from respiratory insufficiency.[113] Patients wi Bethlem myopathy usually do not die from cardi causes. Sudden death is rarely reported in co genital muscular dystrophies.

Facioscapulohumeral Muscular Dystrophy

General

Facioscapulohumeral muscular dystrophy (FSHI derives its name from the muscle groups that a first affected—facial and shoulder girdle.[45] It is t third most common muscular dystrophy, aft Duchenne and myotonic dystrophy. Clinical sig are highly variable and may appear from infan to late life, but typically start in the second decad There may be a congenital defect of certain musc groups, e.g., the pectoral muscle. The disea can be inherited over several generations. Son patients may show progression in muscle wastir and weakness, but others do not show progre sion. Disease severity also varies considerab even within families. This disease is caused by deletion of a tandem repeat element on chrom some 4q35.

Cardiac Involvement

The heart is usually not involved in th disease.[114] However, anecdotal reports are avai able in the literature of atrial paralysis i patients with FSHD. Cardiomyopathy or hea failure has never been described. Atrial arrhyt mias seem to occur ranging from paroxysm atrial fibrillation to sustained supraventricul tachycardias.[115]

Cause of Death

Life span is not limited in FSHD and sudde cardiac death has not been described in thes patients.

onclusions

any skeletal myopathies have at least minor ardiac involvement. In particular, the most revalent forms of muscular dystrophy, i.e., DMD nd myotonic dystrophy, do show major cardiac nvolvement during the later phases of the disease. e think it is very important to screen patients ith muscular dystrophies for cardiac abnoralities. At this moment there are no guidelines uggesting, for example, a regular cardiological heckup every 3 years. Therefore, we propose that ese patients should be referred to specialized linics where both neurological and cardiological xpertise regarding muscular dystrophies can be ombined. This would make it possible to detect arly cardiac involvement and hopefully prevent apid deterioration. As a result, life span, which is lready limited in most muscular dystrophies, ould become somewhat longer. If the promising ew therapies for DMD successfully change the isease to a kind of BMD, cardiological expertise ecomes more important in muscular dystrophies. Whether prophylactic defibrillators should e considered depends entirely on the underlying yopathy and individual patient risk factors, so hat general recommendations cannot be given. uture studies might show a more prominent role or prophylactic defibrillators in preventing udden death in skeletal myopathies.

eferences

1. Codd MB, Sugrue DD, Gersh BJ, Melton LJ 3rd. Epidemiology of idiopathic dilated and hypertrophic cardiomyopathy. A population-based study in Olmsted County, Minnesota, 1975–1984. *Circulation* 1989;80:564–572.
2. Fuster V, Gersh BJ, Giuliani ER, Tajik AJ, Brandenburg RO, Frye RL. The natural history of idiopathic dilated cardiomyopathy. *Am J Cardiol* 1981;47:525–531.
3. Di Lenarda A, Secoli G, Perkan A, Gregori D, Lardieri G, Pinamonti B, Sinagra G, Zecchin M, Camerini F. Changing mortality in dilated cardiomyopathy. The Heart Muscle Disease Study Group. *Br Heart J* 1994;72:S46–51.
4. Dec GW, Fuster V. Idiopathic dilated cardiomyopathy. *N Engl J Med* 1994;331:1564–1575.
5. Felker GM, Hu W, Hare JM, Hruban RH, Baughman KL, Kasper EK. The spectrum of dilated cardiomyopathy. The Johns Hopkins experience with 1,278 patients. *Medicine (Baltimore)* 1999;78:270–283.
6. Carson PA, O'Connor CM, Miller AB, Anderson S, Belkin R, Neuberg GW, Wertheimer JH, Frid D, Cropp A, Packer M. Circadian rhythm and sudden death in heart failure: Results from Prospective Randomized Amlodipine Survival Trial. *J Am Coll Cardiol* 2000;36:541–546.
7. Priori SG, Aliot E, Blomstrom-Lundqvist C, Bossaert L, Breithardt G, Brugada P, Camm AJ, Cappato R, Cobbe SM, Di Mario C, Maron BJ, McKenna WJ, Pedersen AK, Ravens U, Schwartz PJ, Trusz-Gluza M, Vardas P, Wellens HJ, Zipes DP. Task Force on Sudden Cardiac Death of the European Society of Cardiology. *Eur Heart J* 2001; 22:1374–1450.
8. Luu M, Stevenson WG, Stevenson LW, Baron K, Walden J. Diverse mechanisms of unexpected cardiac arrest in advanced heart failure. *Circulation* 1989;80:1675–1680.
9. Tamburro P, Wilber D. Sudden death in idiopathic dilated cardiomyopathy. *Am Heart J* 1992;124:1035–1045.
10. Kelly P, Coats A. Variation in mode of sudden cardiac death in patients with dilated cardiomyopathy. *Eur Heart J* 1997;18:879–880.
11. de Vreede-Swagemakers JJ, Gorgels AP, Dubois-Arbouw WI, van Ree JW, Daemen MJ, Houben LG, Wellens HJ Out-of-hospital cardiac arrest in the 1990's: A population-based study in the Maastricht area on incidence, characteristics and survival. *J Am Coll Cardiol* 1997;30:1500–1505.
12. Wisten A, Forsberg H, Krantz P, Messner T. Sudden cardiac death in 15–35-year olds in Sweden during 1992–1999. *J Intern Med* 2002;252:529–536.
13. Puranik R, Chow CK, Duflou JA, Kilborn MJ, McGuire MA. Sudden death in the young. *Heart Rhythm* 2005;2:1277–1282.
14. Desai AS, Fang JC, Maisel WH, Baughman KL. Implantable defibrillators for the prevention of mortality in patients with nonischemic cardiomyopathy: A meta-analysis of randomized controlled trials. *JAMA* 2004;292:2874–2879.
15. The Antiarrhythmics versus Implantable Defibrillators (AVID) Investigators. A comparison of antiarrhythmic-drug therapy with implantable defibrillators in patients resuscitated from near-fatal ventricular arrhythmias. *N Engl J Med* 1997;337:1576–1583.
16. Connolly SJ, Gent M, Roberts RS, Dorian P, Roy D, Sheldon RS, Mitchell LB, Green MS, Klein GJ, O'Brien B. Canadian implantable defibrillator

study (CIDS): A randomized trial of the implantable cardioverter defibrillator against amiodarone. *Circulation* 2000;101:1297–1302.
17. Kuck KH, Cappato R, Siebels J, Ruppel R. Randomized comparison of antiarrhythmic drug therapy with implantable defibrillators in patients resuscitated from cardiac arrest: The Cardiac Arrest Study Hamburg (CASH). *Circulation* 2000; 102:748–754.
18. Bansch D, Antz M, Boczor S, Volkmer M, Tebbenjohanns J, Seidl K, Block M, Gietzen F, Berger J, Kuck KH. Primary prevention of sudden cardiac death in idiopathic dilated cardiomyopathy: The Cardiomyopathy Trial (CAT). *Circulation* 2002; 105:1453–1458.
19. Strickberger SA, Hummel JD, Bartlett TG, Frumin HI, Schuger CD, Beau SL, Bitar C, Morady F. Amiodarone versus implantable cardioverter-defibrillator: Randomized trial in patients with nonischemic dilated cardiomyopathy and asymptomatic nonsustained ventricular tachycardia–AMIOVIRT. *J Am Coll Cardiol* 2003;41:1707–1712.
20. Bristow MR, Saxon LA, Boehmer J, Krueger S, Kass DA, De Marco T, Carson P, DiCarlo L, DeMets D, White BG, DeVries DW, Feldman AM. Cardiac-resynchronization therapy with or without an implantable defibrillator in advanced chronic heart failure. *N Engl J Med* 2004;350:2140–2150.
21. Kadish A, Dyer A, Daubert JP, Quigg R, Estes NA, Anderson KP, Calkins H, Hoch D, Goldberger J, Shalaby A, Sanders WE, Schaechter A, Levine JH. Prophylactic defibrillator implantation in patients with nonischemic dilated cardiomyopathy. *N Engl J Med* 2004;350:2151–2158.
22. Bardy GH, Lee KL, Mark DB, Poole JE, Packer DL, Boineau R, Domanski M, Troutman C, Anderson J, Johnson G, McNulty SE, Clapp-Channing N, Davidson-Ray LD, Fraulo ES, Fishbein DP, Luceri RM, Ip JH. Amiodarone or an implantable cardioverter-defibrillator for congestive heart failure. *N Engl J Med* 2005;352:225–237.
23. Moss AJ, Zareba W, Hall WJ, Klein H, Wilber DJ, Cannom DS, Daubert JP, Higgins SL, Brown MW, Andrews ML. Prophylactic implantation of a defibrillator in patients with myocardial infarction and reduced ejection fraction. *N Engl J Med* 2002; 346:877–883.
24. Rankovic V, Karha J, Passman R, Kadish AH, Goldberger JJ. Predictors of appropriate implantable cardioverter-defibrillator therapy in patients with idiopathic dilated cardiomyopathy. *Am J Cardiol* 2002;89:1072–1076.
25. Grimm W, Steder U, Menz V, Hoffman J, Maisch B. QT dispersion and arrhythmic events in idiopathic dilated cardiomyopathy. *Am J Cardi*[illegible] 1996;78:458–461.
26. Becker R, Haass M, Ick D, Krueger C, Bauer A, Senges-Becker JC, Voss F, Hilbel T, Niroomand F, Katus HA, Schoels W. Role of nonsustained ventricular tachycardia and programmed ventricular stimulation for risk stratification in patients with idiopathic dilated cardiomyopathy. *Basic Re*[illegible] *Cardiol* 2003;98:259–266.
27. Grimm W, Hoffmann JJ, Muller HH, Maisch B. Implantable defibrillator event rates in patients with idiopathic dilated cardiomyopathy, nonsustained ventricular tachycardia on Holter and left ventricular ejection fraction below 30%. *J A*[illegible] *Coll Cardiol* 2002;39:780–787.
28. Klingenheben T, Zabel M, D'Agostino RB, Cohe[illegible] RJ, Hohnloser SH. Predictive value of T-wav[illegible] alternans for arrhythmic events in patients wit[illegible] congestive heart failure. *Lancet* 2000;356:651 652.
29. Kitamura H, Ohnishi Y, Okajima K, Ishida A, Galeano E, Adachi K, Yokoyama M. Onset hear[illegible] rate of microvolt-level T-wave alternans provide[illegible] clinical and prognostic value in nonischemi[illegible] dilated cardiomyopathy. *J Am Coll Cardiol* 200[illegible] 39:295–300.
30. Hohnloser SH, Klingenheben T, Bloomfield D, Dabbous O, Cohen RJ. Usefulness of microvo[illegible] T-wave alternans for prediction of ventricula[illegible] tachyarrhythmic events in patients with dilate[illegible] cardiomyopathy: Results from a prospective ob[illegible] servational study. *J Am Coll Cardiol* 2003;41:2220 2224.
31. Grimm W, Christ M, Bach J, Muller HH, Maisc[illegible] B. Noninvasive arrhythmia risk stratification i[illegible] idiopathic dilated cardiomyopathy: Results o[illegible] the Marburg Cardiomyopathy Study. *Circulatio*[illegible] 2003;108:2883–2891.
32. Bloomfield DM, Bigger JT, Steinman RC, Namerov[illegible] PB, Parides MK, Curtis AB, Kaufman ES, Davidenko JM, Shinn TS, Fontaine JM. Microvo[illegible] T-wave alternans and the risk of death or sus[illegible] tained ventricular arrhythmias in patients wit[illegible] left ventricular dysfunction. *J Am Coll Cardi*[illegible] 2006;47:456–463.
33. Kaufman ES, Bloomfield DM, Steinman RC, Namerow PB, Costantini O, Cohen RJ, Bigger JT Jr. "Indeterminate" microvolt T-wave alternan[illegible] tests predict high risk of death or sustained ven[illegible] tricular arrhythmias in patients with left ventri[illegible] cular dysfunction. *J Am Coll Cardiol* 2006;48 1399–1404.
34. Phillips M, Robinowitz M, Higgins JR, Boran KJ, Reed T, Virmani R. Sudden cardiac death in Ai[illegible]

Force recruits. A 20-year review. *JAMA* 1986;256:2696–2699.
35. Lecomte D, Fornes P, Fouret P, Nicolas G. Isolated myocardial fibrosis as a cause of sudden cardiac death and its possible relation to myocarditis. *J Forensic Sci* 1993;38:617–621.
36. Liberthson RR. Sudden death from cardiac causes in children and young adults. *N Engl J Med* 1996;334:1039–1044.
37. Fontaine G, Fornes P, Fontaliran F. Myocarditis as a cause of sudden death. *Circulation* 2001;103:e12; author reply e12.
38. Rabinovich R, Muratore C, Iglesias R, Gonzalez M, Daru V, Valentino M, Liprandi AS, Luceri R. Time to first shock in implantable cardioverter defibrillator (ICD) patients with Chagas cardiomyopathy. *Pacing Clin Electrophysiol* 1999;22:202–205.
39. Martinelli Filho M, De Siqueira SF, Moreira H, Fagundes A, Pedrosa A, Nishioka SD, Costa R, Scanavacca M, D'Avila A, Sosa E. Probability of occurrence of life-threatening ventricular arrhythmias in Chagas' disease versus non-Chagas' disease. *Pacing Clin Electrophysiol* 2000;23:1944–1946.
40. Cardinalli-Neto A, Greco OT, Bestetti RB. Automatic implantable cardioverter-defibrillators in Chagas' heart disease patients with malignant ventricular arrhythmias. *Pacing Clin Electrophysiol* 2006;29:467–470.
41. Ellinor PT, Sasse-Klaassen S, Probst S, Gerull B, Shin JT, Toeppel A, Heuser A, Michely B, Yoerger DM, Song BS, Pilz B, Krings G, Coplin B, Lange PE, Dec GW, Hennies HC, Thierfelder L, MacRae CA. A novel locus for dilated cardiomyopathy, diffuse myocardial fibrosis, and sudden death on chromosome 10q25–26. *J Am Coll Cardiol* 2006; 48:106–111.
42. van Berlo JH, de Voogt WG, van der Kooi AJ, van Tintelen JP, Bonne G, Yaou RB, Duboc D, Rossenbacker T, Heidbuchel H, de Visser M, Crijns HJ, Pinto YM. Meta-analysis of clinical characteristics of 299 carriers of LMNA gene mutations: Do lamin A/C mutations portend a high risk of sudden death? *J Mol Med* 2005;83:79–83.
43. Meune C, Van Berlo JH, Anselme F, Bonne G, Pinto YM, Duboc D. Primary prevention of sudden death in patients with lamin A/C gene mutations. *N Engl J Med* 2006;354:209–210.
44. Meryon E. On fatty degeneration of the voluntary muscles. *Lancet* 1851;2:588–589.
45. Emery AE. The muscular dystrophies. *Lancet* 2002;359:687–695.
46. Zellweger H, Niedermeyer E. Central nervous system manifestations in childhood muscular dystrophy (CMD). I. Psychometric and electroencephalographic findings. *Ann Paediatr* 1965;205: 25–42.
47. Bresolin N, Castelli E, Comi GP, Felisari G, Bardoni A, Perani D, Grassi F, Turconi A, Mazzucchelli F, Gallotti D, *et al.* Cognitive impairment in Duchenne muscular dystrophy. *Neuromuscul Disord* 1994;4:359–369.
48. Nigro G, Comi LI, Limongelli FM, Giugliano MA, Politano L, Petretta V, Passamano L, Stefanelli S. Prospective study of X-linked progressive muscular dystrophy in Campania. *Muscle Nerve* 1983;6: 253–262.
49. Mostacciuolo ML, Lombardi A, Cambissa V, Danieli GA, Angelini C. Population data on benign and severe forms of X-linked muscular dystrophy. *Hum Genet* 1987;75:217–220.
50. van Essen AJ, Busch HF, te Meerman GJ, ten Kate LP. Birth and population prevalence of Duchenne muscular dystrophy in The Netherlands. *Hum Genet* 1992;88:258–266.
51. Perloff JK, Roberts WC, de Leon AC Jr, O'Doherty D. The distinctive electrocardiogram of Duchenne's progressive muscular dystrophy. An electrocardiographic-pathologic correlative study. *Am J Med* 1967;42:179–188.
52. de Kermadec JM, Becane HM, Chenard A, Tertrain F, Weiss Y. Prevalence of left ventricular systolic dysfunction in Duchenne muscular dystrophy: An echocardiographic study. *Am Heart J* 1994;127:618–623.
53. Melacini P, Vianello A, Villanova C, Fanin M, Miorin M, Angelini C, Dalla Volta S. Cardiac and respiratory involvement in advanced stage Duchenne muscular dystrophy. *Neuromuscul Disord* 1996;6:367–376.
54. Parker AE, Robb SA, Chambers J, Davidson AC, Evans K, O'Dowd J, Williams AJ, Howard RS. Analysis of an adult Duchenne muscular dystrophy population. *QJM* 2005;98:729–736.
55. Jefferies JL, Eidem BW, Belmont JW, Craigen WJ, Ware SM, Fernbach SD, Neish SR, Smith EO, Towbin JA. Genetic predictors and remodeling of dilated cardiomyopathy in muscular dystrophy. *Circulation* 2005;112:2799–2804.
56. Chenard AA, Becane HM, Tertrain F, de Kermadec JM, Weiss YA. Ventricular arrhythmia in Duchenne muscular dystrophy: Prevalence, significance and prognosis. *Neuromuscul Disord* 1993;3:201–206.
57. Mukoyama M, Kondo K, Hizawa K, Nishitani H. Life spans of Duchenne muscular dystrophy patients in the hospital care program in Japan. *J Neurol Sci* 1987;81:155–158.

58. Corrado G, Lissoni A, Beretta S, Terenghi L, Tadeo G, Foglia-Manzillo G, Tagliagambe LM, Spata M, Santarone M. Prognostic value of electrocardiograms, ventricular late potentials, ventricular arrhythmias, and left ventricular systolic dysfunction in patients with Duchenne muscular dystrophy. *Am J Cardiol* 2002;89:838–841.
59. Aartsma-Rus A, Janson AA, Kaman WE, Bremmer-Bout M, van Ommen GJ, den Dunnen JT, van Deutekom JC. Antisense-induced multiexon skipping for Duchenne muscular dystrophy makes more sense. *Am J Hum Genet* 2004;74:83–92.
60. Alter J, Lou F, Rabinowitz A, Yin H, Rosenfeld J, Wilton SD, Partridge TA, Lu QL. Systemic delivery of morpholino oligonucleotide restores dystrophin expression bodywide and improves dystrophic pathology. *Nat Med* 2006;12:175–177.
61. Melacini P, Fanin M, Danieli GA, Villanova C, Martinello F, Miorin M, Freda MP, Miorelli M, Mostacciuolo ML, Fasoli G, Angelini C, Dalla Volta S. Myocardial involvement is very frequent among patients affected with subclinical Becker's muscular dystrophy. *Circulation* 1996;94:3168–3175.
62. Saito M, Kawai H, Akaike M, Adachi K, Nishida Y, Saito S. Cardiac dysfunction with Becker muscular dystrophy. *Am Heart J* 1996;132:642–647.
63. Kirchmann C, Kececioglu D, Korinthenberg R, Dittrich S. Echocardiographic and electrocardiographic findings of cardiomyopathy in Duchenne and Becker-Kiener muscular dystrophies. *Pediatr Cardiol* 2005;26:66–72.
64. Hoogerwaard EM, de Voogt WG, Wilde AA, van der Wouw PA, Bakker E, van Ommen GJ, de Visser M. Evolution of cardiac abnormalities in Becker muscular dystrophy over a 13-year period. *J Neurol* 1997;244:657–663.
65. Nigro G, Politano L, Santangelo L, Petretta VR, Passamano L, Panico F, De Luca F, Montefusco A, Comi LI. Is the value of QT dispersion a valid method to foresee the risk of sudden death? A study in Becker patients. *Heart* 2002;87:156–157.
66. Zaidi M, Robert A, Fesler R, Derwael C, Brohet C. Dispersion of ventricular repolarization in dilated cardiomyopathy. *Eur Heart J* 1997;18:1129–1134.
67. Cardiovascular health supervision for individuals affected by Duchenne or Becker muscular dystrophy. *Pediatrics* 2005;116:1569–1573.
68. Mirabella M, Servidei S, Manfredi G, Ricci E, Frustaci A, Bertini E, Rana M, Tonali P. Cardiomyopathy may be the only clinical manifestation in female carriers of Duchenne muscular dystrophy. *Neurology* 1993;43:2342–2345.
69. Moser H, Emery AE. The manifesting carrier i Duchenne muscular dystrophy. *Clin Genet* 1974; 271–284.
70. Norman A, Harper P. A survey of manifesting ca riers of Duchenne and Becker muscular dystroph in Wales. *Clin Genet* 1989;36:31–37.
71. Hoogerwaard EM, Bakker E, Ippel PF, Oosterwi JC, Majoor-Krakauer DF, Leschot NJ, Van Esse AJ, Brunner HG, van der Wouw PA, Wilde AA, d Visser M. Signs and symptoms of Duchenne mus cular dystrophy and Becker muscular dystroph among carriers in The Netherlands: A coho study. *Lancet* 1999;353:2116–2119.
72. Grain L, Cortina-Borja M, Forfar C, Hilton-Jone D, Hopkin J, Burch M. Cardiac abnormalities an skeletal muscle weakness in carriers of Duchenn and Becker muscular dystrophies and control *Neuromuscul Disord* 2001;11:186–191.
73. Hoogerwaard EM, van der Wouw PA, Wilde A Bakker E, Ippel PF, Oosterwijk JC, Majoo Krakauer DF, van Essen AJ, Leschot NJ, de Visse M. Cardiac involvement in carriers of Duchenn and Becker muscular dystrophy. *Neuromusc Disord* 1999;9:347–351.
74. Mathieu J, Allard P, Potvin L, Prevost C, Begin I A 10-year study of mortality in a cohort c patients with myotonic dystrophy. *Neurolog* 1999;52:1658–1662.
75. Roig M, Balliu PR, Navarro C, Brugera R, Losad M. Presentation, clinical course, and outcome c the congenital form of myotonic dystroph *Pediatr Neurol* 1994;11:208–213.
76. Phillips MF, Harper PS. Cardiac disease in myot onic dystrophy. *Cardiovasc Res* 1997;33:13–22.
77. Merino JL, Carmona JR, Fernandez-Lozano Peinado R, Basterra N, Sobrino JA. Mechanisms c sustained ventricular tachycardia in myoton dystrophy: Implications for catheter ablatio *Circulation* 1998;98:541–546.
78. Lazarus A, Varin J, Ounnoughene Z, Radvanyi F Junien C, Coste J, Laforet P, Eymard B, Becan HM, Weber S, Duboc D. Relationships amon electrophysiological findings and clinical statu heart function, and extent of DNA mutation i myotonic dystrophy. *Circulation* 1999;99:1041 1046.
79. Lazarus A, Varin J, Babuty D, Anselme F, Coste Duboc D. Long-term follow-up of arrhythmias i patients with myotonic dystrophy treated b pacing: A multicenter diagnostic pacemaker stud *J Am Coll Cardiol* 2002;40:1645–1652.
80. Bassez G, Lazarus A, Desguerre I, Varin J, Lafor P, Becane HM, Meune C, Arne-Bes M

Ounnoughene Z, Radvanyi H, Eymard B, Duboc D. Severe cardiac arrhythmias in young patients with myotonic dystrophy type 1. *Neurology* 2004; 63:1939–1941.

81. Pelargonio G, Dello Russo A, Sanna T, De Martino G, Bellocci F. Myotonic dystrophy and the heart. *Heart* 2002;88:665–670.
82. Bushby K, Muntoni F, Bourke JP. 107th ENMC International Workshop: The management of cardiac involvement in muscular dystrophy and myotonic dystrophy. 7–9 June, 2002, Naarden, the Netherlands. *Neuromuscul Disord* 2003;13:166–172.
83. de Die-Smulders CE, Howeler CJ, Thijs C, Mirandolle JF, Anten HB, Smeets HJ, Chandler KE, Geraedts JP. Age and causes of death in adult-onset myotonic dystrophy. *Brain* 1998;121 (Pt. 8):1557–1563.
84. Clarke NR, Kelion AD, Nixon J, Hilton-Jones D, Forfar JC. Does cytosine-thymine-guanine (CTG) expansion size predict cardiac events and electrocardiographic progression in myotonic dystrophy? *Heart* 2001;86:411–416.
85. Sabovic M, Medica I, Logar N, Mandic E, Zidar J, Peterlin B. Relation of CTG expansion and clinical variables to electrocardiogram conduction abnormalities and sudden death in patients with myotonic dystrophy. *Neuromuscul Disord* 2003;13: 822–826.
86. Schoser BG, Ricker K, Schneider-Gold C, Hengstenberg C, Durre J, Bultmann B, Kress W, Day JW, Ranum LP. Sudden cardiac death in myotonic dystrophy type 2. *Neurology* 2004;63: 2402–2404.
87. Bonne G, Yaou RB, Beroud C, Boriani G, Brown S, de Visser M, Duboc D, Ellis J, Hausmanowa-Petrusewicz I, Lattanzi G, Merlini L, Morris G, Muntoni F, Opolski G, Pinto YM, Sangiuolo F, Toniolo D, Trembath R, van Berlo JH, van der Kooi AJ, Wehnert M. 108th ENMC International Workshop, 3rd Workshop of the MYO-CLUSTER project: EUROMEN, 7th International Emery-Dreifuss Muscular Dystrophy (EDMD) Workshop, 13–15 September 2002, Naarden, The Netherlands. *Neuromuscul Disord* 2003;13:508–515.
88. Karkkainen S, Reissell E, Helio T, Kaartinen M, Tuomainen P, Toivonen L, Kuusisto J, Kupari M, Nieminen MS, Laakso M, Peuhkurinen K. Novel mutations in the lamin A/C gene in heart transplant recipients with end stage dilated cardiomyopathy. *Heart* 2006;92:524–526.
89. Pethig K, Genschel J, Peters T, Wilhelmi M, Flemming P, Lochs H, Haverich A, Schmidt HH. LMNA mutations in cardiac transplant recipients. *Cardiology* 2005;103:57–62.
90. Emery AE. X-linked muscular dystrophy with early contractures and cardiomyopathy (Emery-Dreifuss type). *Clin Genet* 1987;32:360–367.
91. Fishbein MC, Siegel RJ, Thompson CE, Hopkins LC. Sudden death of a carrier of X-linked Emery-Dreifuss muscular dystrophy. *Ann Intern Med* 1993;119:900–905.
92. Laval SH, Bushby KM. Limb-girdle muscular dystrophies–from genetics to molecular pathology. *Neuropathol Appl Neurobiol* 2004;30:91–105.
93. van der Kooi AJ, Ledderhof TM, de Voogt WG, Res CJ, Bouwsma G, Troost D, Busch HF, Becker AE, de Visser M. A newly recognized autosomal dominant limb girdle muscular dystrophy with cardiac involvement. *Ann Neurol* 1996;39:636–642.
94. Messina DN, Speer MC, Pericak-Vance MA, McNally EM. Linkage of familial dilated cardiomyopathy with conduction defect and muscular dystrophy to chromosome 6q23. *Am J Hum Genet* 1997;61:909–917.
95. Ginjaar HB, van der Kooi AJ, Ceelie H, Kneppers AL, van Meegen M, Barth PG, Busch HF, Wokke JH, Anderson LV, Bonnemann CG, Jeanpierre M, Bolhuis PA, Moorman AF, de Visser M, Bakker E, Ommen GJ Sarcoglycanopathies in Dutch patients with autosomal recessive limb girdle muscular dystrophy. *J Neurol* 2000;247:524–529.
96. Politano L, Nigro V, Passamano L, Petretta V, Comi LI, Papparella S, Nigro G, Rambaldi PF, Raia P, Pini A, Mora M, Giugliano MA, Esposito MG. Evaluation of cardiac and respiratory involvement in sarcoglycanopathies. *Neuromuscul Disord* 2001; 11:178–185.
97. Poppe M, Bourke J, Eagle M, Frosk P, Wrogemann K, Greenberg C, Muntoni F, Voit T, Straub V, Hilton-Jones D, Shirodaria C, Bushby K. Cardiac and respiratory failure in limb-girdle muscular dystrophy 2I. *Ann Neurol* 2004;56:738–741.
98. Goldfarb LG, Vicart P, Goebel HH, Dalakas MC. Desmin myopathy. *Brain* 2004;127:723–734.
99. Olive M, Goldfarb L, Moreno D, Laforet E, Dagvadorj A, Sambuughin N, Martinez-Matos JA, Martinez F, Alio J, Farrero E, Vicart P, Ferrer I. Desmin-related myopathy: Clinical, electrophysiological, radiological, neuropathological and genetic studies. *J Neurol Sci* 2004;219:125–137.
100. Goebel HH, Fardeau M. Familial desmin-related myopathies and cardiomyopathies–from myopathology to molecular and clinical genetics. 36th European Neuromuscular Center (ENMC)-

Sponsored International Workshop. 20–22 October, 1995, Naarden, The Netherlands. *Neuromuscul Disord* 1996;6:383–388.

101. Goebel H, Fardeau M. 121st ENMC International Workshop on Desmin and Protein Aggregate Myopathies. 7–9 November 2003, Naarden, The Netherlands. *Neuromuscul Disord* 2004;14:767–773.

102. Goldfarb LG, Park KY, Cervenakova L, Gorokhova S, Lee HS, Vasconcelos O, Nagle JW, Semino-Mora C, Sivakumar K, Dalakas MC. Missense mutations in desmin associated with familial cardiac and skeletal myopathy. *Nat Genet* 1998; 19:402–403.

103. Pruszczyk P, Kostera-Pruszczyk A, Shatunov A, Goudeau B, Draminska A, Takeda K, Sambuughin N, Vicart P, Strelkov SV, Goldfarb LG, Kaminska A. Restrictive cardiomyopathy with atrioventricular conduction block resulting from a desmin mutation. *Int J Cardiol* 2007;117(2):244–253.

104. Dagvadorj A, Olive M, Urtizberea JA, Halle M, Shatunov A, Bonnemann C, Park KY, Goebel HH, Ferrer I, Vicart P, Dalakas MC, Goldfarb LG. A series of West European patients with severe cardiac and skeletal myopathy associated with a de novo R406W mutation in desmin. *J Neurol* 2004;251:143–149.

105. Tesson F, Sylvius N, Pilotto A, Dubosq-Bidot L, Peuchmaurd M, Bouchier C, Benaiche A, Mangin L, Charron P, Gavazzi A, Tavazzi L, Arbustini E, Komajda M. Epidemiology of desmin and cardiac actin gene mutations in a european population of dilated cardiomyopathy. *Eur Heart J* 2000;21: 1872–1876.

106. Luethje LG, Boennemann C, Goldfarb L, Goebel HH, Halle M. Prophylactic implantable cardioverter defibrillator placement in a sporadic desmin related myopathy and cardiomyopathy. *Pacing Clin Electrophysiol* 2004;27:559–560.

107. Guglieri M, Magri F, Comi GP. Molecular etiopathogenesis of limb girdle muscular and congenital muscular dystrophies: Boundaries and contiguities. *Clin Chim Acta* 2005;361:54–79.

108. Lampe AK, Bushby KM. Collagen VI relate muscle disorders. *J Med Genet* 2005;42:673–685.

109. de Visser M, de Voogt WG, la Riviere GV. Th heart in Becker muscular dystrophy, facioscapu lohumeral dystrophy, and Bethlem myopath *Muscle Nerve* 1992;15:591–596.

110. Pepe G, Bertini E, Bonaldo P, Bushby K, Giusti de Visser M, Guicheney P, Lattanzi G, Merlini Muntoni F, Nishino I, Nonaka I, Yaou R Sabatelli P, Sewry C, Topaloglu H, van der Kooi Bethlem myopathy (BETHLEM) and Ullrich scle roatonic muscular dystrophy: 100th ENMC inte national workshop, 23–24 November 200 Naarden, The Netherlands. *Neuromuscul Disor* 2002;12:984–993.

111. Miura K, Shirasawa H. Congenital muscular dys trophy of the Fukuyama type (FCMD) with sever myocardial fibrosis. A case report with postmor tem angiography. *Acta Pathol Jpn* 1987;37:1823 1835.

112. Nakanishi T, Sakauchi M, Kaneda Y, Tomimats H, Saito K, Nakazawa M, Osawa M. Cardia involvement in Fukuyama-type congenital mus cular dystrophy. *Pediatrics* 2006;117:e1187–1192.

113. Brockington M, Blake DJ, Prandini P, Brown SC Torelli S, Benson MA, Ponting CP, Estournet I Romero NB, Mercuri E, Voit T, Sewry CA Guicheney P, Muntoni F. Mutations in the fukutin related protein gene (FKRP) cause a form c congenital muscular dystrophy with secondar laminin alpha2 deficiency and abnormal glyco sylation of alpha-dystroglycan. *Am J Hum Gene* 2001;69:1198–1209.

114. Galetta F, Franzoni F, Sposito R, Plantinga Y Femia FR, Galluzzi F, Rocchi A, Santoro G, Sicili ano G. Subclinical cardiac involvement in patient with facioscapulohumeral muscular dystroph *Neuromuscul Disord* 2005;15:403–408.

115. Trevisan CP, Pastorello E, Armani M, Angelini C Nante G, Tomelleri G, Tonin P, Mongini T Palmucci L, Galluzzi G, Tupler RG, Barchitta A Facioscapulohumeral muscular dystrophy an occurrence of heart arrhythmia. *Eur Neurol* 2006 56:1–5.

42 Ventricular Arrhythmias in Right Ventricular Dysplasia/Cardiomyopathy

Hugh Calkins and Frank I. Marcus

Introduction

Arrhythmogenic right ventricular dysplasia/cardiomyopathy (ARVD/C) is a genetic cardiomyopathy characterized by ventricular arrhythmias and structural abnormalities of the right ventricle (RV). In ARVD/C there is progressive replacement of right ventricular myocardium with fatty and fibrous tissue. The precise prevalence of ARVD/C has been estimated to vary between 1 in 1000 and 1 in 5000 of the general population. The purpose of this chapter is to review the current understanding of ARVD/C and its management. Particular attention will be focused on some of the recent advances in the understanding of the genetic basis of ARVD/C and how this information provides insight into the mechanism of ventricular arrhythmias that can cause sudden death.

Clinical Presentation and Natural History

Most commonly patients with ARVD/C come to clinical attention because of ventricular arrhythmias. The ventricular arrhythmias, which originate in the right ventricle, may be asymptomatic and detected by routine electrocardiogram (ECG), or they may cause palpitations due to premature ventricular beats or nonsustained ventricular tachycardia (VT). Presyncope or syncope may occur due to transient or sustained VT. Sudden cardiac death (SCD) may be triggered by rapid VT that degenerates into ventricular fibrillation (VF). It has been estimated that ARVD/C accounts for approximately 3–10% of SCD in individuals under the age of 65 years. Exercise has been identified as a common precipitant of arrhythmias that occur in ARVD/C.[1–3]

We recently reported the presentation, clinical features, survival, and natural history of ARVD/C in a cohort of 100 patients from the United States.[4] The median age at presentation was 26 years. The most common presenting symptoms were palpitations, syncope, and SCD in 27%, 26%, and 23% of patients, respectively. It is possible that the patients who died suddenly could have had some symptoms prior to death that were not reported to others including family members. Among those who were diagnosed while living (n = 69), the median time between first presentation and diagnosis was 1 year (range, 0–37 years). During a median follow-up of 6 years, implantable cardioverter defibrillators (ICD) were implanted in 47 patients, 29 of whom received an appropriate ICD discharge, including 3 patients who received the ICD for primary prevention. At follow-up, 66 patients were alive, of whom 44 had an ICD implanted, 5 developed signs of heart failure, 2 had a heart transplant, and 18 were on antiarrhythmia drug therapy. Thirty-four patients died either at presentation (n = 23) or during follow-up (n = 11), and one had an ICD implanted. On Kaplan–Meier analysis, the median survival time in the entire population was 60 years. The results of this study extended the findings of prior studies and led to the following observations. First, ARVD/C patients usually present between the second and fifth decades of life either with symptoms of palpitations or syncope associated with VT or with SCD. Second, our data suggest that diagnosis is often delayed. Third, once diagnosed and treated with an ICD, mortality is low. Finally, we observed a wide variation in presentation and course of ARVD/C patients, which may be explained in part by the genetic heterogeneity of the disease.

Diagnosis of Arrhythmogenic Right Ventricular Dysplasia/Cardiomyopathy

The diagnosis of ARVD/C is based on the criteria of the Task Force of the Working Group of Myocardial and Pericardial Disease of the European Society of Cardiology and of the Scientific Council on Cardiomyopathies of the International Society and Federation of Cardiology. These criteria are shown in Table 42–1. Specific cardiac tests that are recommended in all patients suspected of having ARVD/C include an electrocardiogram (ECG), a signal-averaged ECG (SAECG), a Holter monitor, and an echocardiogram. Analysis of right ventricular (RV) size and function can also be obtained by cardiac magnetic resonance imaging (MRI) and/or computed tomography (CT). If the results of the noninvasive tests point toward a diagnosis of ARVD/C, invasive testing including RV angiography, endomyocardial biopsy, and electrophysiology testing is recommended to establish the diagnosis and help provide further information to guide treatment.

Electrocardiographic Evaluation

Electrocardiographic abnormalities are detected in more than 90% of ARVC patients.[4,5] The typical ECG features of ARVD/C are demonstrated by the ECG shown in Figure 42–1, which was obtained from a 37-year-male who presented with sustained VT and was diagnosed with ARVD/C. The ECG features include the presence of precordial T wave inversions beyond V2, an epsilon wave in V1–V3,

Table 42–1. Diagnostic criteria[a] for ARVD/C.[b]

	Major criteria	Minor criteria
Structural or functional abnormalities	1. Severe dilation and reduction of RVEF with mild or no LV involvement 2. Localized RV aneurysm (akinetic or dyskinetic areas with diastolic bulging) 3. Severe segmental dilation of the RV	1. Mild global RV dilation and/or EF reduction with normal LV 2. Mild segmental dilation of the RV 3. Regional RV hypokinesis
Tissue characterization	Infiltration of RV by fat with presence of surviving strands of cardiomyocytes	
ECG depolarization/ conduction abnormalities	1. Localized QRS complex duration >110 msec in V1, V2, or V3 2. Epsilon wave in V1, V2 or V3	Late potentials in SAECG
ECG repolarization abnormalities		Inverted T waves in right precordial leads (V2–V3 above age 12 years in absence of RBBB)
Arrhythmias		1. LBBB VT (sustained or nonsustained) on ECG, Holter, or ETT 2. Frequent PVCs (>1000/24 h on Holter)
Family history	Family history of ARVD confirmed by biopsy or autopsy	1. Family history of premature sudden death (<35 years) due to suspected ARVD 2. Family history of clinical diagnosis based on present criteria

[a] The criteria state that an individual must have two major, or one major plus two minor, or four minor criteria from different categories to meet the diagnosis of ARVD/C.

[b] ARVD/C, arrhythmogenic right ventricular dysplasia/cardiomyopathy; RVEF, right ventricular ejection fraction; EF, ejection fraction; RV/LV, right ventricular/left ventricular; ECG, electrocardiogram; RBBB, LBBB, right and left bundle branch blocks; SAECG, signal-averaged ECG; ETT, exercise treadmill test; PVC, premature ventricular contraction.

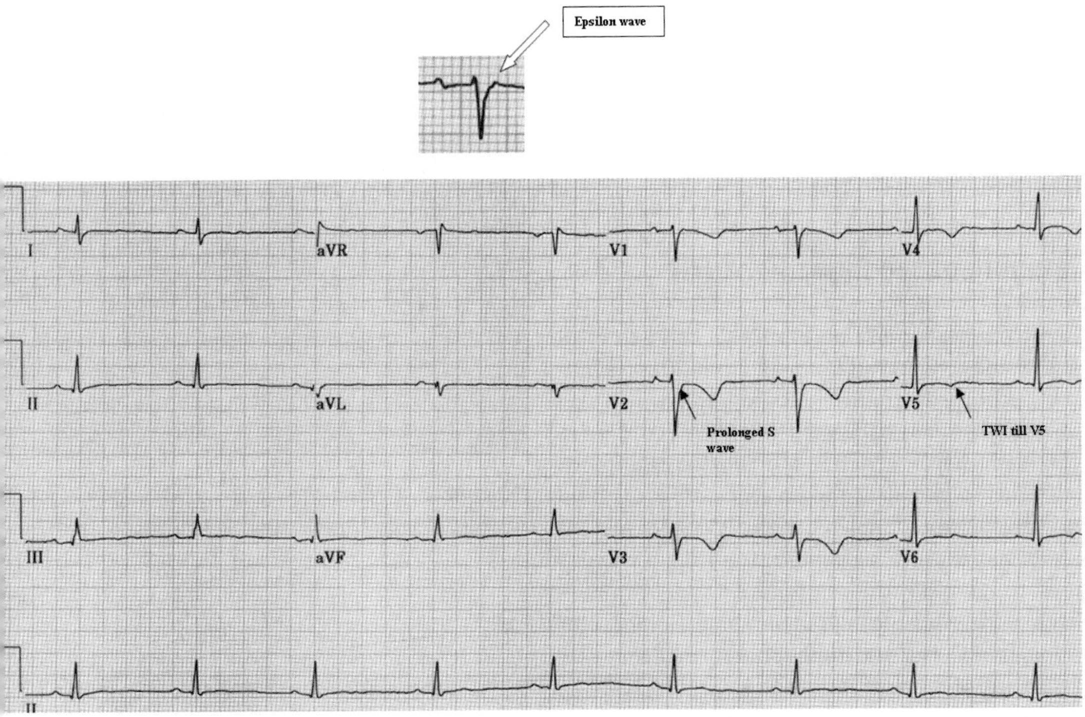

FIGURE 42–1. Typical electrocardiogram from a patient with ARVD/C. The T waves are inverted in V1–V5. The S wave is prolonged in V1–V3 and there is a suggestion of an epsilon wave in V1 that is better seen in the enlargement of a QRS complex above the 12-lead ECG.

and a widened QRS complex in leads V1 to V3 (parietal block).

T wave inversion (TWI) in leads V1–V3 is a well-established ECG feature of ARVD/C, and in the absence of a right bundle branch block (RBBB) is considered a minor diagnostic criterion. The juvenile pattern of TWI in leads V1–V3 or beyond is a normal variant in children under 12 years of age. It is present in 1–3% of a healthy population 19–45 years of age. It is seen in 87% of patients with ARVD/C. T wave inversion beyond V1 in a patient in the above age group who has no apparent heart disease but has ventricular arrhythmias of left bundle branch block (LBBB) morphology should raise the suspicion of ARVD/C.[6]

Another typical ECG feature of ARVD/C is the "epsilon wave," which is a "postexcitation" electrical potential of small amplitude that occurs in the ST segment after the end of the QRS complex. Epsilon waves, which are seen in 33% of ARVD/C patients, are considered a major diagnostic criterion for ARVD/C.[5] Slowed electrical conduction in the right ventricle as a result of ARVD/C may also cause localized widening of QRS complex (≥110 msec) in the right precordial leads, which is seen in 64% of the patients. Prolonged S wave upstroke in V1 through V3 ≥55 msec (Figure 42–1) is the most prevalent ECG feature and is seen in 95% of the patients. A prolonged S wave in V1–V3 of ≥70 msec and QRS dispersion ≥40 msec were each found to be predictors of inducible VT at electrophysiology study.[5]

Late potentials on SAECG recordings are considered a minor criterion for the diagnosis of ARVD/C. The Task Force on SAECG defines an SAECG as abnormal when two or more of the following are present: (1) the duration of the signal-averaged, high-frequency filtered QRS complex (fQRS) is ≥114 msec, (2) the duration of the low-amplitude signal of <40 μV in the terminal portion of the filtered QRS complex (LAS40) is ≥38 msec, and (3) the root mean square voltage of the terminal 40 msec of the filtered QRS complex (RMS40) is <20 μV. The results of several recent studies have shown that the probability of an abnormal SAECG as defined by these criteria is related to the extent of structural disease of the RV.[7,8] An abnormal SAECG has been reported to predict inducibility on electrophysiological testing as well as ICD therapy.[9]

Imaging of the Right Ventricle

Right ventricular size and function can be evaluated using a variety of imaging modalities including echocardiography, angiography, cardiac magnetic resonance (CMR), and CT. According to the Task Force criteria, a major criterion for ARVD/C is defined as the presence of severe dilation and/or functional loss of the RV. A less severe abnormality of RV size and/or function is considered to be minor criteria for ARVD/C. Although each of the available imaging modalities for evaluation of RV size and function can detect severe structural abnormalities of the RV, the diagnostic accuracy of these tests is less certain when used for the evaluation of patients with mild disease. Right ventricular angiography has historically been regarded as the best imaging test for the diagnosis of ARVD/C and has been shown to be highly specific (90%). Compared to RV angiography, echocardiography is noninvasive and represents the first-line imaging approach in evaluating patients with suspected ARVD/C or in screening family members.[10,11] Limitations of echocardiography include the fact that it is subject to obtaining adequate views and that it does not allow for a quantitative evaluation of global RV size and function. Newer echo modalities such as three-dimensional echocardiography and strain and tissue Doppler echocardiography may overcome some of these limitations.[12,13] Cardiac magnetic resonance is an attractive imaging method because it is noninvasive and has the unique ability to characterize tissue, specifically by differentiating fat from muscle.[14–16] It also allows for a highly accurate and quantitative evaluation of RV size and function (Figure 42–2). The newer gadolinium-enhanced MR imaging can localize the fibrosis in the RV myocardium.[17,18] Despite these many advantages, the role of CMR in ARVD/C is limited by the fact that an ICD is generally considered to be a contraindication to performing a CMR. Although we recently defined the extent of interactions between ICDs and CMR, and have shown the feasibility of performing CMR in ICD patients, these results must be considered preliminary. An additional disadvantage is that the results of CMR are highly impacted by the specific protocol with which it is performed, the presence of artifacts caused by ventricular premature beats, and the experience of the physician interpreting these results. It is our experience that CMR is a common cause of "overdiagnosis" of ARVD/C.[19,20] Physicians should be hesitant to diagnose ARVD/C when the only abnormalities are limited to those seen on CMR. In our experience, an abnormality detected with MRI will rarely be the sole abnormality detected in a patient with ARVD/C. It is also important to recognize that the presence of "fat" in the RV myocardium may be normal and should not be considered diagnostic of ARVD/C.[21]

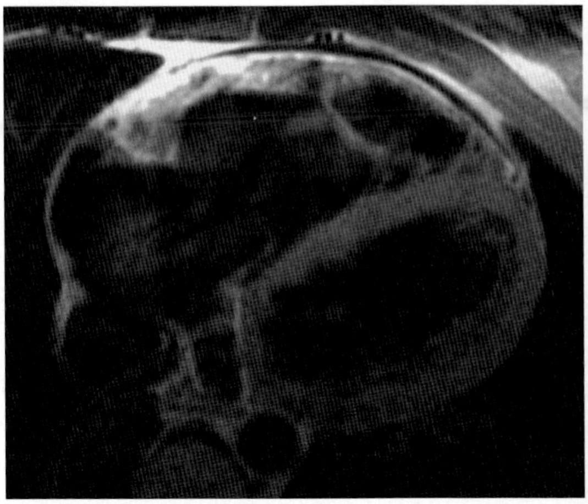

FIGURE 42–2. A cardiac MRI showing an enlarged RV with high signal (fat) is the anterior basal free wall.

Myocardial Biopsy

Performance of an endomyocardial biopsy is recommended for all patients suspected of having ARVD/C. This technique is most sensitive when performed on the free wall at a site adjacent to regional RV dysfunction or thinning. It is important to recognize that ARVD/C can be a patchy disease and that definitive pathological evidence for the diagnosis by myocardiac biopsy will be obtained in approximately one-third of affected individuals. However, when the biopsy shows myocyte loss with fibrosis and fatty infiltration along with surviving strands of myocytes, the diagnosis of ARVD/C is clearly established. An endomyocardial biopsy is also useful in identifying other conditions such as sarcoidosis and myocarditis, which can be confused with ARVD/C.[22]

Differential Diagnosis

Although it is not difficult to diagnose an overt case of ARVD/C, differentiation of ARVD/C at its early stages from idiopathic ventricular tachycardia (IVT), a usually benign and nonfamilial arrhythmic condition that also presents with VT with an LBBB morphology, remains a clinical challenge.[23,24] A typical RV outflow tract IVT is shown in Figure 42–3. The major differences in the two conditions are highlighted in Table 42–2. It is extremely important to determine if the patient has IVT or ARVD/C for two reasons. First, IVT is a benign condition that is not associated with a risk of sudden death and therefore is not an indication for placement of an ICD. In contrast, when the diagnosis of ARVD/C is established. there needs to be serious consideration for ICD implantation because of the risk of SCD. Second, ARVD/C is frequently hereditary whereas IVT is not. As a result, when a diagnosis of ARVD/C is made, screening of all first-degree family members over the age of 10–12 years is recommended.

Krahn *et al.* recently reported that QRS characteristics of VT are different in patients with ARVD/C as compared to those with idiopathic VT, presumably because of altered ventricular conduction through abnormal myocardium.[25] They reported that an algorithm combining lead I QRS duration for sensitivity and axis for specificity is useful in differentiating the two tachycardia substrates. A lead I QRS duration ≥120 msec had a sensitivity of 100%, specificity of 46%, positive predictive value of 61%, and negative predictive value of 100% for ARVD/C. The addition of a mean QRS axis <30 degrees (R < S in lead III) to the above criterion increased specificity for ARVD/C to 100%.[25]

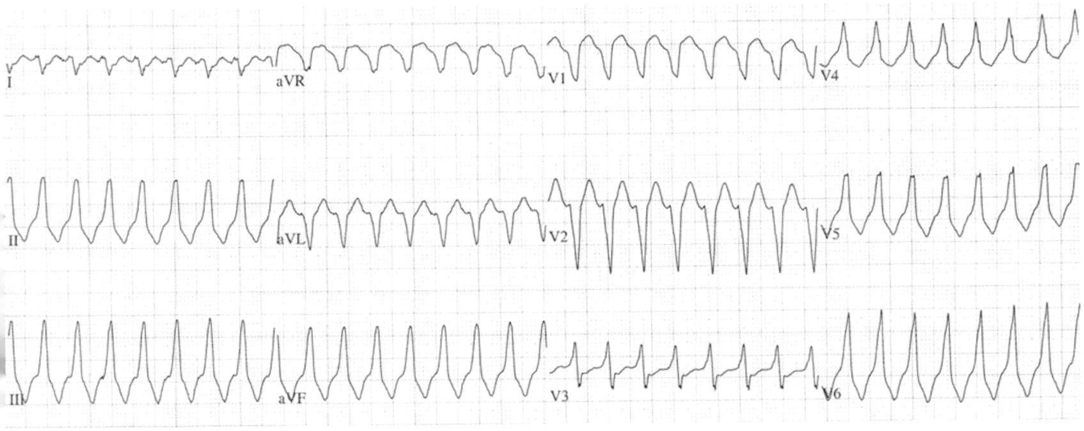

FIGURE 42–3. A 12-lead ECG during VT from a patient with idiopathic VT. Note the inferior QRS axis and the negative QRS in leads AVL. There features indicate that the origin of the VT is from the RV outflow tract.

TABLE 42–2. Differentiation between idiopathic VT and ARVD/C.[a]

	Idiopathic VT	ARVD/C
Clinical features		
Family history of arrhythmias or sudden cardiac death	No	Frequently yes
	Morphology of ventricular arrhythmias	
Arrhythmias	LBBB; +II, III, AVF, −AVL	May be the same, but frequently morphology of ventricular arrhythmias from base of RV LBBB; −II, III, +AVL
	PVCs, nonsustained VT, or sustained VT at rest or with exercise	PVCs, nonsustained VT, or sustained VT at rest or with exercise
Sudden cardiac death	Rare	1% per year
Electrocardiographic features		
T wave morphology	T wave upright V2–V5	T wave inverted V1, V2, V3
Parietal block	QRS duration <110 msec in V1, V2, or V3	QRS duration >110 msec
Epsilon wave V1–V3	Absent	Present in 30%
Prolonged S-wave upstroke	Rarely seen	Present in 95%
Signal averaged ECG	Normal	Usually abnormal
Imaging features		
Echocardiogram	Normal	Increased RV size and/or wall motion abnormalities
RV ventriculogram	Usually normal	Usually abnormal wall motion abnormalities
MRI	Usually normal	Increased signal intensity of RV free wall; wall motion abnormalities with CINE MRI
Treatment		
Response to therapy	Acute: Vagal maneuvers Adenosine, β blockers, verapamil	
	Chronic: β Blockers or verapamil ± class 1 antiarrhythmic drugs	Sotalol Amiodarone ± β blockers
RF ablation	Usually curative	May be curative; can modify substrate to permit AA drugs to be effective; arrhythmias of different morphology tend to recur

[a]VT, ventricular tachycardia; ARVD/C, arrhythmogenic right ventricular dysplasia/cardiomyopathy; LBBB, left bundle branch block; RV, right ventricle; PVC, premature ventricular contraction; ECG, electrocardiogram; MRI, magnetic resonance imaging; AA, antiarrhythmic.

Histopathology and Etiology

The most striking pathological feature of ARVD is the diffuse or segmental replacement of mid-mural or external layers of the RV myocardium and, to a much lesser extent, left ventricular myocardium by fatty tissue and fibrosis. Patchy acute myocarditis with myocyte death and inflammatory infiltrates is also present in nearly two-thirds of the cases. The RV myocardial replacement by fibrofatty tissue has been related to four basic mechanisms: (1) apoptosis or programmed cell death, (2) inflammation, (3) myocardial dystrophy, which might reflect a genetically determined atrophy, and (4) a genetically determined abnormality of the cell-to-cell adhesion (desmosomal) proteins and loss of gap junctions. It is currently unknown whether different mechanisms are present in different patients or whether this is a uniform disease in various stages of evolution.

Genetics

Arrhythmogenic right ventricular dysplasia/cardiomyopathy is a heritable condition, typically with an autosomal dominant pattern of inheritance and variable penetrance. Most studies have reported a familial pattern of disease in approximately one-third of probands.[4] To date, 11 different genetic variants of ARVD/C have been mapped; these are summarized in Table 42–3. Mutations including plakoglobin (JUP), desmoplakin (DSP), the cardiac ryanodine receptor (RyR2), plakophilin-2 (PKP-2), and desmoglein-2 have been reported in ARVD/C.[26–30] The cardiac RyR2 gene offers potential insight into a cause of

TABLE 42–3. Gene defects associated with ARVD/C.[a]

Genetic variant	Inheritance	Chromosome	Gene	Comment
ARVD1	AD	14q24.3	$TGFB_3$	Characterized by progressive degeneration of RV myocardium Causes cytokine-stimulating fibrosis and modulates cell adhesion
ARVD2	AD	1q42–q43	Cardiac ryanodine receptor	Identification of four different mutations in different families Associated with catecholaminergic polymorphic VT Whether ARVD2 and CPMT are different diseases due to different mutations of the RyR2 gene still remains unsettled
ARVD3	AD	14q11–q12	—	—
ARVD4	AD	2q32.1–q32.3	—	Associated with localized LV involvement
ARVD5	AD	3p23	—	Seen in ARVD/C cases in Newfoundland
ARVD6	AD	10p12–14	—	Early onset, high penetrance
ARVD7	AD	10q22	—	Associated with myofibrillar myopathy
ARVD8	AD/AR	6p23–p24	Desmoplakin	Associated with palmoplantar keratoderma and woolly hair
ARVD9 (Naxos)	AR	17q21	Plakoglobin	Associated with palmoplantar keratoderma and woolly hair (Naxos disease)
ARVD10	AD	12p11	Plakophilin-2	Most common genetic defect in familial cases
ARVD11	AD		Desmoglein-2	Component of desmosome

[a]ARVD/C, arrhythmogenic right ventricular dysplasia/cardiomyopathy; AD, autosomal dominant; AR, autosomal recessive; $TGFB_3$, tumor growth factor β_3; RV, right ventricle; VT, ventricular tachycardia; RyR2, ryanodine receptor.

adrenergically mediated ventricular arrhythmias. The RyR2 induces calcium release from the sarcoplasmic reticulum into the cytosol and may be responsible for catecholamine-induced VT. Whether ARVD/C 2 and catecholaminergic polymorphic VT are different diseases or are due to different mutations of the RyR2 gene still remains unsettled. There is also a question as to whether tumor growth factor (TGF)-β is indeed a gene responsible for one variant of ARVD/C. The Naxos variant of ARVD/C is inherited in an autosomal recessive manner and is characterized by the presence of woolly hair and palmoplantar keratoderma usually seen in early infancy, whereas cardiac abnormalities are observed by adolescence. However, the Naxos variant does not represent the usual ARVD/C. In Newfoundland there is a high prevalence of ARVD/C. There are 11 currently separate families with numbers of individuals within those pedigrees ranging from 50 to 1500 over nine generations. The gene loci is linked to chromosome 3p23.[30] Survival analysis shows that 50% of men with this variant of ARVD/C die by the age of 40 years.

Recently, it has been found that ARVD/C due to an abnormality in PKP-2, an essential armadillo-repeat protein of the cardiac desmosome, is a common cause of familial ARVD/C. The disruption of desmosomal function by PKP-2 mutations leads to death of cardiomyocytes and fibrofatty replacement under mechanical stress, thus providing a potential explanation for the frequent occurrence of ventricular tachyarrhythmias and sudden death during exercise. The PKP-2 mutation is present in 30–50% of ARVD/C patients, whereas other mutations are reported less frequently.[27,28] In probands with familial disease, it is present in 70%. Another newly identified genetic cause of ARVD/C is a mutation in desmoglein-2, which is another desmosomal junction protein.[29] Based on the results of these recent studies, it is now evident that in most patients with familial ARVD/C, the genetic abnormality involves one of the desmosomal proteins. This observation helps explain many of the clinical features of this disease, including its delayed onset and higher prevalence in athletes and its predisposition to affect the RV.

Identification of a gene abnormality in a family member does not provide definitive information regarding risk. The presence of an abnormal gene does not indicate the phenotypic expression, which can be variable. For example, family members with plakophilin 2 have been identified who are in middle age or are the parents of an affected proband. These family members have the gene abnormality but no evidence of the disease. Genetic analysis should be of clinical value in identifying those offspring who need to be followed most intensively for the development of ARVD/C. For example, assuming a PKP-2 mutation is identified in a proband with ARVD/C, it would be of potential clinical value to screen the offspring for this mutation. While the absence of this mutation does not totally exclude the risk of development of ARVD/C, it is much less likely to develop. In contrast, if the offspring does carry the PKP-2 mutation more intensive periodic screening for identification of early ARVD/C (i.e., biannual noninvasive testing after puberty) and/or restriction of athletic activity may be warranted.

Management and Use of Implantable Defibrillators

Once the diagnosis of ARVD has been established the main therapeutic decision is whether to implant an ICD for prevention of sudden death.[31–34] ARVD/C patients who are at the highest risk for arrhythmic death include those patients with a history of having been resuscitated from sudden cardiac death, patients with syncope, those who are very young, and those who have marked RV involvement. The presence of left ventricular involvement is also a risk factor. Risk stratification based on any of the above characteristics singularly or in combination is statistically documented. However, the application of these risk factors to the decision to implant an ICD can only be used as a guide. The risk of SCD is low if these risk factors are not present, but it is not zero.

We recently reported our experience with ICDs in 67 patients with definite or probable ARVD/C.[31] Over a mean follow-up of 4.4 ± 2.9 years, 40 (73%) of 55 patients who met Task Force Criteria for ARVD/C and 4 (33%) of 12 patients with probable ARVD/C had appropriate ICD therapies for VT/VF ($p = 0.027$). The mean time to ICD therapy was 1.1 ± 1.4 years. Eleven of 28 patients (39%) who received an ICD in the absence of a prior episode of sustained VT or VF and 33 of 35 patients who received an ICD for secondary prevention (85%) experienced appropriate ICD therapies ($p = 0.001$). Electrophysiological testing did not predict appropriate ICD interventions in patients who received an ICD for primary prevention. Fourteen patients (21%) received ICD therapy for life-threatening (VT/VF > 240 bpm) arrhythmias. There was no difference in the incidence of life-threatening arrhythmias in the primary and secondary prevention groups.

Based on these findings we conclude that patients who meet task force criteria for ARVD are at high risk for SCD and should undergo ICD placement for primary and secondary prevention, regardless of electrophysiological testing results. Further research is needed to identify a low-risk subset of patients who may not require ICD placement. It is our current policy to recommend ICD implantation in patients who meet the strict diagnostic criteria for ARVD/C.

In addition to placement of an ICD, we also recommend that patients with ARVD/C avoid competitive athletics in an attempt to slow the progression of the disease. In addition, we advise that patients with definite or probable ARVD/C avoid activities such as long distance biking or running and long distance swimming and/or weight training and that activity be limited to low-intensity activities such as walking or golf.

There are few data available concerning the use of pharmacological agents in the treatment of patients with ARVD/C for the prevention of SCD. Symptomatic ventricular arrhythmias are treated initially with β blocker therapy. If this is inadequate to control the patient's symptoms or to prevent recurrent VT, membrane-active antiarrhythmic agents such as sotalol[35] and/or amiodarone should be considered. Further research is needed to determine if other commonly used treatments for heart failure such as angiotensin-converting enzyme inhibitors are of value for the treatment of patients with ARVD/C.

Because of the progressive nature of ARVD/C and the result of small clinical studies, catheter ablation is not considered a curative procedure.[35,36] However, with the use of computerized mapping systems and anatomically based ablation strategies, catheter ablation may play a role in decreasing the frequency of sustained ventricular arrhythmias and/or ICD therapies. It is important to note that VT storm, per se, is not an indication for catheter ablation in most ARVD/C patients because the VT generally can be well controlled with antiarrhythmic therapy.[37]

Cardiac transplantation is considered in patients with progressive heart failure and intractable recurrent ventricular arrhythmias.[38] In our experience, few patients with ARVD/C require cardiac transplantation.[4]

Unanswered Questions

There are many unanswered questions regarding the diagnosis and treatment of ARVD/C. For example, it remains uncertain how best to exclude the diagnosis of ARVD/C in patients with a mild form of disease including relatives of affected individuals. Further research is needed to better define which patients suspected of having ARVD/C require ICD implantation to prevent SCD. Further work is also needed to identify other genes that cause ARVD/C. This information will greatly facilitate diagnosis of the disease and would also allow for genotype/phenotype correlations.[39] In addition, the identification of the specific genetic defects may ultimately have specific therapeutic implications for gene therapy. The ongoing Multidisciplinary Study of Right Ventricular Dysplasia, which is a multicenter, collaborative study to investigate the cardiac, clinical, and genetic aspects of ARVD/C funded by a grant from the National Institutes of Health and the National Heart Lung and Blood Institute, should provide information to aid in the diagnosis and treatment of these patients. A larger term follow-up of these patients with ARVD/C and their family members will address important questions regarding the course, prognosis, and appropriate treatment for the individual patient with ARVD/C.[39,40] More information concerning this registry is available at www.arvd.com and www.arvd.org.

References

1. Corrado D, Basso C, Rizzoli G, Schiavon M, *et al.* Does sports activity enhance the risk of sudden death in adolescents and young adults? *J Am Coll Cardiol* 2003;42:1959–1963.
2. Hulot JS, Jouven X, Empana JP, *et al.* Natural history and risk stratification of arrhythmogenic right ventricular dysplasia/cardiomyopathy. *Circulation* 2004;110:1879–1884.
3. Tabib A, Loire R, Chalabreysse L, *et al.* Circumstances of death and gross and microscopic observations in a series of 200 cases of sudden death associated with arrhythmogenic right ventricular cardiomyopathy and/or dysplasia. *Circulation* 2003; 108:3000–3005.
4. Dalal D, Nasir K, Bomma C, *et al.* Arrhythmogenic right ventricular dysplasia: A United States experience. *Circulation* 2005;112:3823–3832.
5. Nasir K, Bomma C, Tandri H, *et al.* Electrocardiographic features of arrhythmogenic right ventricular dysplasia/cardiomyopathy according to disease severity: A need to broaden diagnostic criteria. *Circulation* 2004;110:1527–1534.
6. Marcus FI. Prevalence of T-wave inversion beyond V(1) in young normal individuals and usefulness for the diagnosis of arrhythmogenic right ventricular cardiomyopathy/dysplasia. *Am J Cardiol* 2005; 95:1070–1071.
7. Nasir K, Rutberg J, Tandri H, *et al.* Utility of SAECG in arrhythmogenic right ventricle dysplasia. *Ann Noninvasive Electrocardiol* 2003;8:112–120.
8. Nasir K, Bomma C, Khan FA, *et al.* Utility of a combined signal-averaged electrocardiogram and QT dispersion algorithm in identifying arrhythmogenic right ventricular dysplasia in patients with tachycardia of right ventricular origin. *Am J Cardiol* 2003;92:105–109.
9. Nasir K, Tandri H, Rutberg J, *et al.* Filtered QRS duration on signal-averaged electrocardiography predicts inducibility of ventricular tachycardia in arrhythmogenic right ventricle dysplasia. *Pacing Clin Electrophysiol* 2003;26:1955–1960.
10. Yoerger DM, Marcus F, Sherrill D, *et al.* Echocardiographic findings in patients meeting task force criteria for arrhythmogenic right ventricular dysplasia: New insights from the multidisciplinary study of right ventricular dysplasia. *J Am Coll Cardiol* 2005;45:860–865.
11. Prakasa KR, Dalal D, Wang J, *et al.* Feasibility and variability of three dimensional echocardiography in arrhythmogenic right ventricular dysplasia/cardiomyopathy. *Am J Cardiol* 2006;97:703–709.
12. Donal E, Raud-Raynier P. Transthoracic tissue Doppler study of right ventricular regional

function in a patient with an arrhythmogenic right ventricular cardiomyopathy. *Heart* 2004;90:980.
13. Lopez-Fernandez T, Garcia-Fernandez MA, *et al.* Usefulness of contrast echocardiography in arrhythmogenic right ventricular dysplasia. *J Am Soc Echocardiogr* 2004;17:391–393.
14. Tandri H, Calkins H, Nasir K, *et al.* Magnetic resonance imaging findings in patients meeting task force criteria for arrhythmogenic right ventricular dysplasia. *J Cardiovasc Electrophysiol* 2003;14:476–482.
15. Tandri H, Friedrich MG, Calkins H, *et al.* MRI of arrhythmogenic right ventricular cardiomyopathy/dysplasia. *J Cardiovasc Magn Reson* 2004;6:557–563.
16. Bluemke DA, Krupinski EA, Ovitt T, *et al.* MR imaging of arrhythmogenic right ventricular cardiomyopathy: Morphologic findings and interobserver reliability. *Cardiology* 2003;99:153–162.
17. Tandri H, Saranathan M, Rodriguez ER, *et al.* Noninvasive detection of myocardial fibrosis in arrhythmogenic right ventricular cardiomyopathy using delayed-enhancement magnetic resonance imaging. *J Am Coll Cardiol* 2005;45:98–103.
18. Tandri H, Bomma C, Calkins H, *et al.* Magnetic resonance and computed tomography imaging of arrhythmogenic right ventricular dysplasia. *J Magn Reson Imaging* 2004;19:848–858.
19. Tandri H, Calkins H, Marcus FI. Controversial role of magnetic resonance imaging in the diagnosis of arrhythmogenic right ventricular dysplasia. *Am J Cardiol* 2003;92:649.
20. Bomma C, Rutberg J, Tandri H, *et al.* Misdiagnosis of arrhythmogenic right ventricular dysplasia/cardiomyopathy. *J Cardiovasc Electrophysiol* 2004;15:300–306.
21. Macedo R, Prakasa K, Tucker A, *et al.* MRI findings in patients with fat dissociation syndrome of the right ventricle. Submitted.
22. Shiraishi J, Tatsumi T, Shimoo K, *et al.* Cardiac sarcoidosis mimicking right ventricular dysplasia. *Circ J* 2003;67:169–171.
23. O'Donnell D, Cox D, Bourke J, *et al.* Clinical and electrophysiological differences between patients with arrhythmogenic right ventricular dysplasia and right ventricular outflow tract tachycardia. *Eur Heart J* 2003;24:801–810.
24. Tandri H, Bluemke DA, Ferrari VA, *et al.* Findings on magnetic resonance imaging of idiopathic right ventricular outflow tachycardia. *Am J Cardiol* 2004;94:1441–1445.
25. Ainsworth CD, Skanes AC, Klein GJ, *et al.* Differentiating arrhythmogenic right ventricular cardiomyopathy from right ventricular outflow tract ventricular tachycardia using multilead QRS duration and axis. *Heart Rhythm* 2006;4:416–423.
26. Ahmad F. The molecular genetics of arrhythmogenic right ventricular dysplasia-cardiomyopathy. *Clin Invest Med* 2003;26:167–178.
27. Gerull B, Heuser A, Wichter T, *et al.* Mutations in the desmosomal protein plakophilin-2 are common in arrhythmogenic right ventricular cardiomyopathy. *Nat Genet* 2004;36:1162–1164.
28. Dalal D, Molin LH, Piccini J, *et al.* Clinical features of arrhythmogenic right ventricular dysplasia/cardiomyopathy associated with mutations in plakophilin-2. *Circulation* 2006;113:1641–1649.
29. Awad MM, Dalal D, Cho E, *et al.* DSG2 mutations contribute to arrhythmogenic right ventricular dysplasia/cardiomyopathy. *Am J Hum Genet* 2006;79:136–142.
30. Hodgkinson KA, Parfrey PS, Bassett AS, *et al.* The impact of implantable cardioverter-defibrillator therapy on survival in autosomal-dominant arrhythmogenic right ventricular cardiomyopathy (ARVD5). *J Am Coll Cardiol* 2005;45:400–408.
31. Piccini JP, Dalal D, Roguin A, *et al.* Predictors of appropriate implantable defibrillator therapies in patients with arrhythmogenic right ventricular dysplasia. *Heart Rhythm* 2005;2:1188–1194.
32. Wichter T, Paul M, Wollmann C, *et al.* Implantable cardioverter/defibrillator therapy in arrhythmogenic right ventricular cardiomyopathy: Single-center experience of long-term follow-up and complications in 60 patients. *Circulation* 2004;109:1503–1508.
33. Corrado D, Leoni L, Link msec, *et al.* Implantable cardioverter-defibrillator therapy for prevention of sudden death in patients with arrhythmogenic right ventricular cardiomyopathy/dysplasia. *Circulation* 2003;108:3084–3091.
34. Roguin A, Bomma CS, Nasir K, *et al.* Implantable cardioverter-defibrillators in patients with arrhythmogenic right ventricular dysplasia/cardiomyopathy. *J Am Coll Cardiol* 2004;43:1843–1852.
35. Hiroi Y, Fujiu K, Komatsu S, *et al.* Carvedilol therapy improved left ventricular function in a patient with arrhythmogenic right ventricular cardiomyopathy. *Jpn Heart J* 2004;45:169–177.
36. Zou J, Cao K, Yang B, *et al.* Dynamic substrate mapping and ablation of ventricular tachycardias in right ventricular dysplasia. *J Interv Card Electrophysiol* 2004;11:37–45.
37. Reithmann C, Hahnefeld A, Remp T, *et al.* Electroanatomic mapping of endocardial right ventricular activation as a guide for catheter ablation in patients with arrhythmogenic right ventricular dysplasia. *Pacing Clin Electrophysiol* 2003;26:1308–1316.

38. Lacroix D, Lions C, Klug D, *et al.* Arrhythmogenic right ventricular dysplasia: Catheter ablation, MRI, and heart transplantation. *J Cardiovasc Electrophysiol* 2005;16:235–236.
39. Wichter T, Breithardt G. Implantable cardioverter-defibrillator therapy in arrhythmogenic right ventricular cardiomyopathy: A role for genotyping in decision-making? *J Am Coll Cardiol* 2005;45:409–411.
40. Marcus F, Towbin JA, Zareba W, *et al.* Arrhythmogenic right ventricular dysplasia/cardiomyopathy (ARVD/C): A multidisciplinary study: Design and protocol. *Circulation* 2003;107:2975–2978.

43 The Wolff–Parkinson–White Syndrome and the Risk of Sudden Death

Michael H. Gollob, Rafeeq Samie, David H. Birnie, Martin S. Green, and Robert M. Gow

History

In 1930, Drs. Wolff, Parkinson, and White described a series of patients with the electrocardiographic (ECG) features of a short PR interval and "bundle branch block" QRS pattern, who also had frequent paroxysms of supraventricular tachycardia.[1] The condition would soon bear their name and be termed the Wolff–Parkinson–White (WPW) syndrome. The ECG description would be refined, and the widened QRS described as a slurred upstroke or delta wave and, alternatively, was noted to represent ventricular preexcitation.

Some 15 years following their original clinical description, the anatomic basis for a short PR interval and delta wave was identified through histological examination of hearts from deceased patients with WPW. Wood *et al.*[2] and Ohnell[3] both described the existence of accessory muscular connections (accessory pathways) between atrial and ventricular myocardium. However, debate continued over the role of these observations in relation to the physiological mechanism of ventricular preexcitation and supraventricular tachycardia in the WPW syndrome.[4,5]

The physiological basis of WPW and the mechanism of tachycardia were firmly established by the seminal work of Drs. Durrer and Wellens.[6,7] Through the technique of programmed electrical stimulation and intracardiac catheters recording atrial and ventricular signals, they demonstrated the inducibility of reciprocating tachycardia utilizing the normal atrioventricular (AV) conduction axis and an accessory conducting circuit (the accessory pathway) in WPW patients. The reciprocating or "reentry" mechanism of tachycardia was consistent with the initial hypothesis of tachycardia mechanisms proposed by Ralph Mines in 1914.[8] These landmark studies set the stage for curative therapy, first by an open-heart surgical procedure.[9] In 1984, Morady and Scheinman developed the technique of catheter ablation.[10] The use of this method for eradicating accessory pathway tissue responsible for WPW became routine with the use of radiofrequency energy, and provided a safe, minimally invasive procedure for the cure of WPW.[11–13] The latest advance in the history of this fascinating syndrome has been the identification of a genetic cause for a familial form of WPW,[14] providing the opportunity to now understand the molecular basis and embryological development of the substrate for WPW, the accessory AV connection.

Since the pioneering work of these leaders in the arrhythmia field, much has been learned about variations that exist in the physiology and anatomic basis of the WPW syndrome (Figure 43–1). In addition, it is now recognized that the arrhythmias associated with WPW may present more than just a symptomatic nuisance, and lead to sudden cardiac death in a minority of patients.

Unusual Variations of Accessory Atrioventricular Connections in Wolff–Parkinson–White Syndrome

Many variations of accessory AV connections exist. These variations may be related to unusual accessory pathway anatomic locations, distal

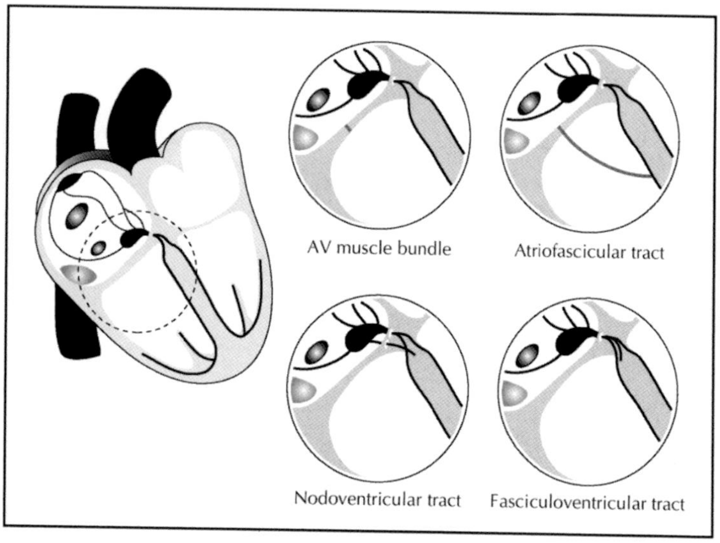

FIGURE 43–1. Graphic illustration of the anatomic variants for ventricular preexcitation. The most common AV accessory connection is a muscle bundle crossing the AV annulus, giving rise to the accessory pathway responsible for most cases of WPW. Variant AV connections may exist, including the atriofascicular pathway that connects the atrial musculature into the distal right bundle branch. True Mahaim fibers, nodoventricular and fasciculoventricular tracts, arise from the normal AV conduction axis and insert into the summit of the interventricular septum.

connections to portions of the conduction system rather than ventricular myocardium, or unusual conduction properties of the accessory connections.

Some of these variations may be present in patients at risk for sudden arrhythmic death, and in some cases these variations may confuse the diagnosis or management. In general, sudden arrhythmic death associated with WPW syndrome is thought to be mainly due to preexcited atrial fibrillation (AF) or flutter with extremely rapid AV conduction over the accessory pathway, and subsequent degeneration to ventricular fibrillation or flutter (VF).[15] Since these accessory pathways must be capable of rapid antegrade conduction, it has been assumed that manifest preexcitation must be a marker of those with a risk for arrhythmic death. However, in occasional patients the preexcitation may not be manifest during sinus rhythm despite the ability of the accessory pathway to sustain rapid antegrade conduction (The Wolff in Sheep's Clothing). This phenomenon is usually related to either accessory pathway location or decremental conduction within the pathway.

The Wolff in Sheep's Clothing

Manifest preexcitation during sinus rhythm occurs when activation from the atria reaches the ventricle via the accessory pathway before the competitive activation via the AV node and His-Purkinje system. However, when accessory pathway conduction is slow (such as is seen with decremental accessory pathways) or when conduction via the AV node is more rapid, ventricular preexcitation on the 12-lead ECG may be minimal during sinus rhythm despite the ability to sustain rapid tachycardia (Figure 43–2). Thus, the degree of preexcitation observed on resting ECG is not a predictor of the risk of malignant arrhythmias.

Unusual Accessory Atrioventricular Pathway Locations

Several unusual accessory pathway locations have been described. These include ventricular insertions in the RV outflow tract[16] and atrial insertions at the RA appendage.[17] In addition, accessory connections may terminate in portions of the specialized conduction system. Typically these are atriofascicular accessory pathways with distal termination in the distal ramifications of the right bundle branch and most often exhibit decremental AV node-like conduction properties.[18–20] There may also be situations where the accessory pathway may serve as the only connection to the right bundle branch, thus serving as a dual conduction system.[21] Atriofascicular accessory connections are potentially troublesome since the ECG during sinus rhythm shows little or no

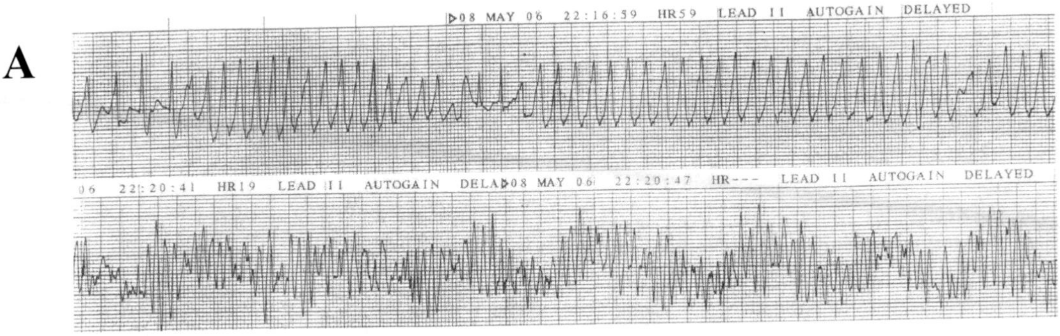

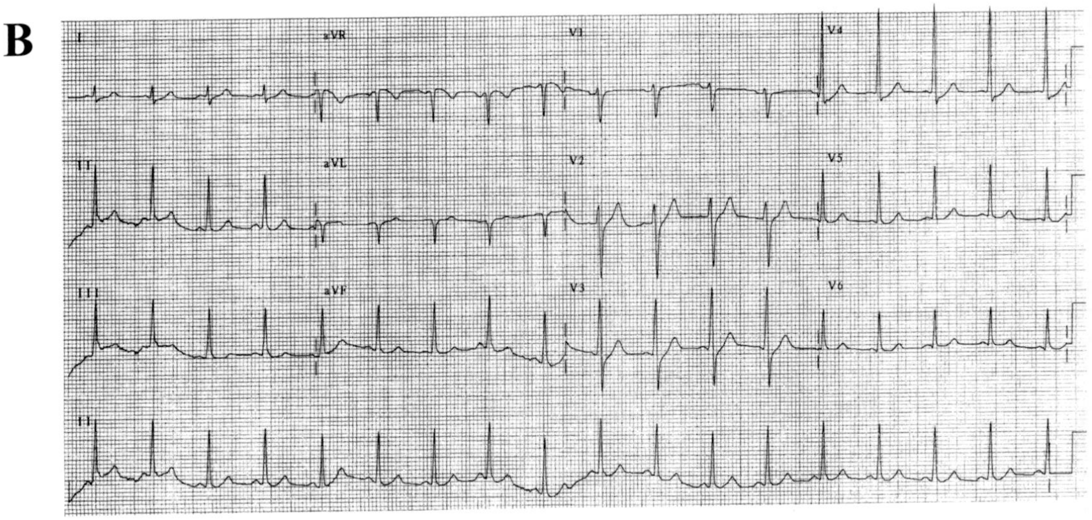

Figure 43–2. (A) A monitor lead from a 27-year-old man who presented to the emergency department with rapid palpitation. The top strip shows preexcited AF. The bottom strip was recorded about 3–4 min later after degeneration to VF. (B) This shows the 12-lead ECG from the same patient recorded after successful defibrillation. Note the absence of manifest preexcitation despite the fact that the accessory pathway was capable of rapid AV conduction. The accessory pathway was successfully ablated on the lateral mitral annulus.

evidence of preexcitation. Once again, the absence of manifest preexcitation does not preclude rapid and potentially life-threatening tachycardia that uses the accessory pathway in the antegrade direction (Figure 43–3). Although there may be clues in the sinus rhythm ECG to the presence of these pathways, these are not universally present.[22] In view of the often normal appearing resting ECG, regular, wide-complex, antedromic tachycardia mediated through these accessory connections is frequently incorrectly diagnosed as ventricular tachycardia by the nonarrhythmia specialist.

Unusual accessory AV connections have also been described in the coronary sinus musculature.[23] In these cases, the latticework array of coronary sinus musculature may connect to the left ventricle via the middle cardiac vein or other posterior coronary vein. In addition, accessory pathways may be associated with a diverticulum at the mouth of the coronary sinus.[24] A characteristic ECG pattern of ventricular preexcitation with QS complexes of the inferior leads is a clue to this unusual connection (Figure 43–4).

Other unusual accessory AV connections exist but are rarely seen to participate in tachycardia. These include fasciculoventricular connections, which represent fibers originating from the His or bundle branch fascicles and connecting to the

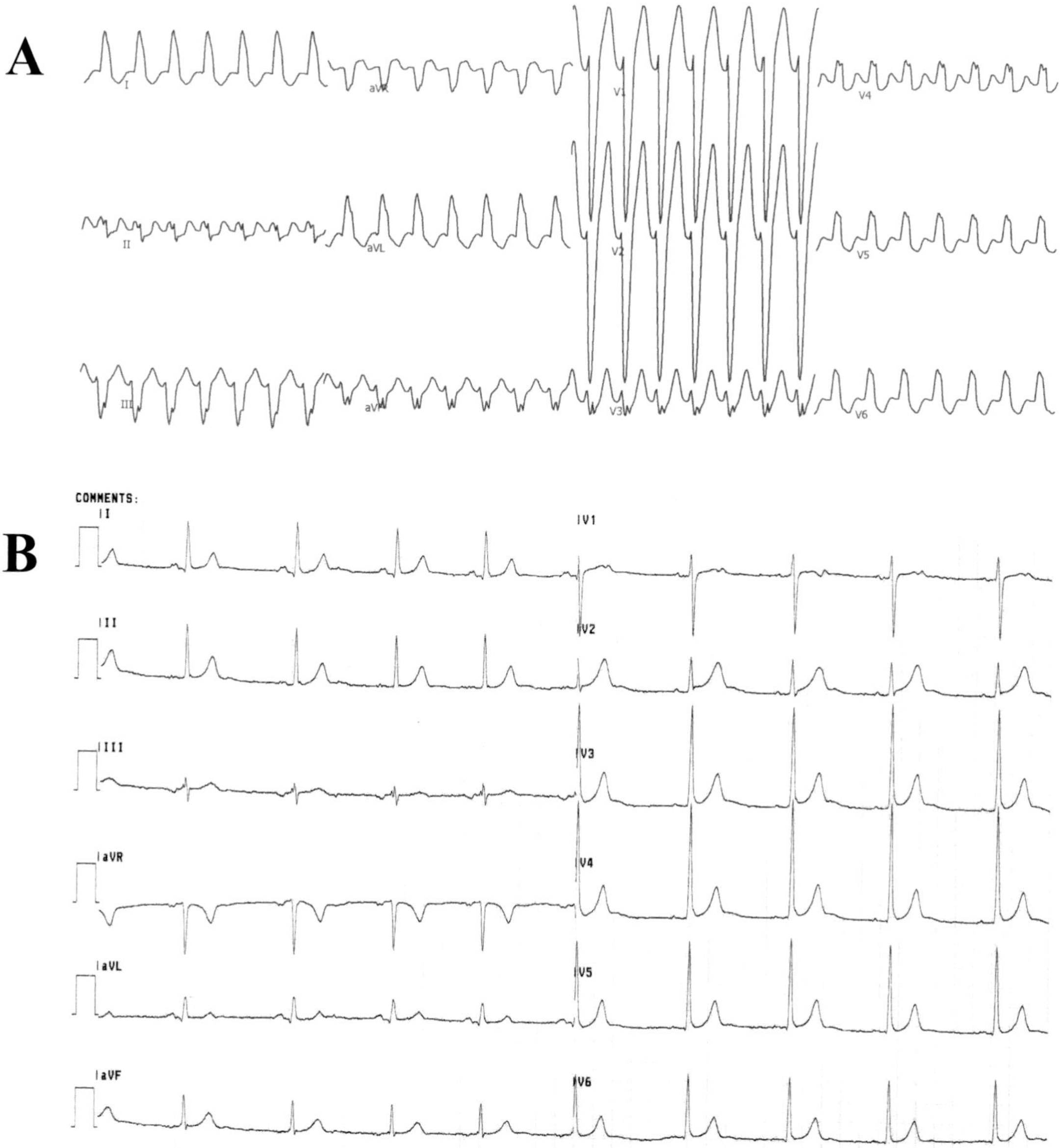

Figure 43–3. (A) A wide QRS tachycardia induced in the electrophysiology laboratory. The tachycardia has left bundle branch block-like morphology with left axis deviation. This was shown to be an antidromic tachycardia using a right anterior atriofascicular accessory pathway in the antegrade direction and the AV node retrogradely. (B) This is the 12-lead ECG from the same patient showing no evident preexcitation. The accessory pathway had decremental conduction properties such that the normal sequence of ventricular activation was preserved. The atriofascicular accessory pathway was successfully ablated in the right anterior region in close proximity to the AV node.

summit of the interventricular septum, as originally described by the pathologist Ivan Mahaim.[25] These accessory connections do not participate in reentrant tachycardia, but may have antegrade conduction and produce some degree of ventricular preexcitation on ECG. Occasionally, these connections may coexist with other arrhythmic substrates.[26–28]

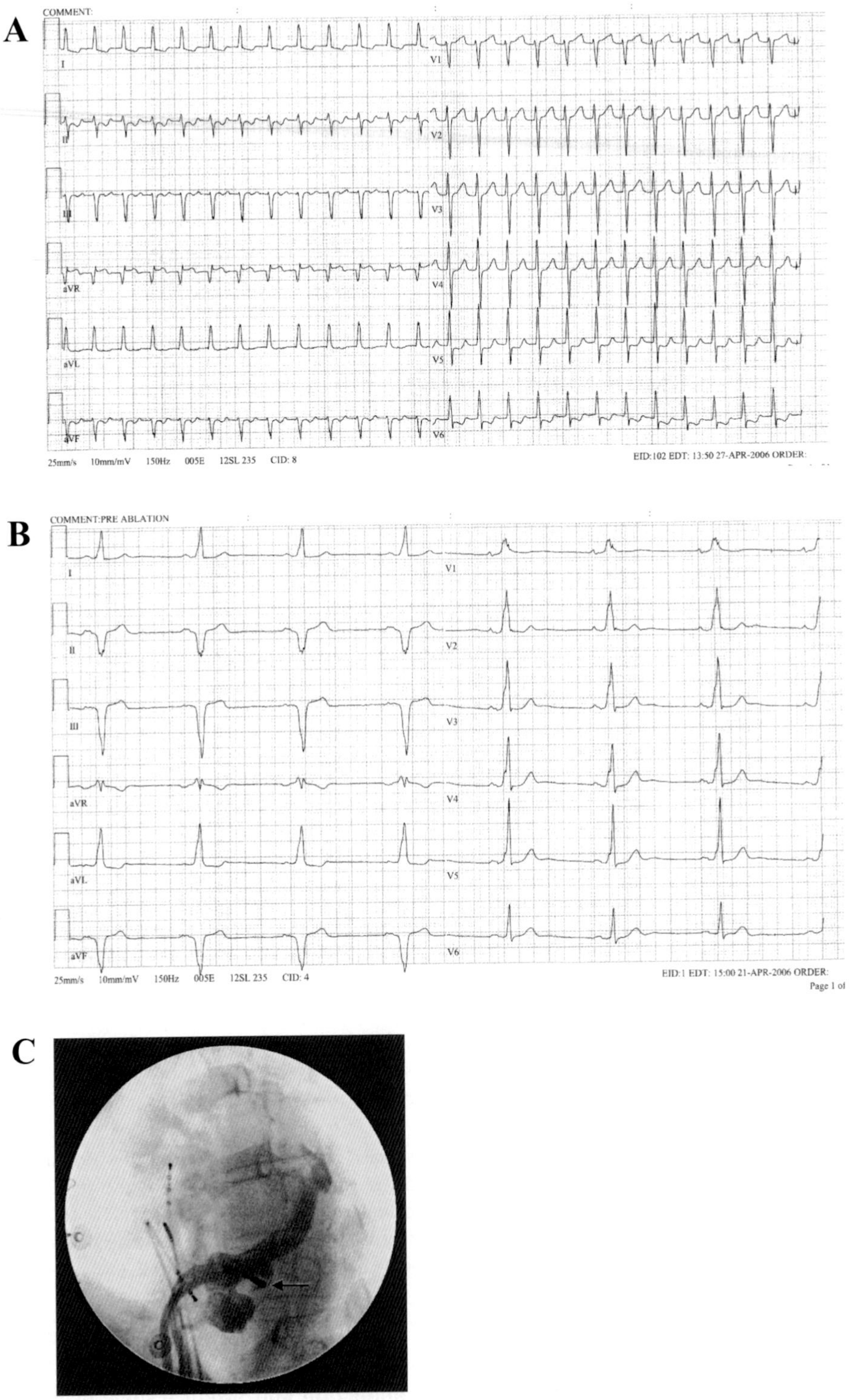

FIGURE 43–4. (A) A rapid, narrow complex tachycardia in a patient proven to have a coronary sinus-mediated accessory AV connection inserting into the posterior left ventricle. (B) Characteristic ECG features of a coronary sinus connection, with negative delta waves and QS complexes in all three inferior leads. (C) Coronary sinus angiography reveals two diverticuli branches. The accessory connection was mapped within the smaller diverticulum, and radiofrequency ablation from with the diverticulum (arrow) successfully eradicated conduction of the accessory connection.

Wolff–Parkinson–White and Congenital Heart Disease

It is recognized that accessory pathways occur more frequently in patients with congenital heart disease than in the general population. A prevalence of between 2.7 and 8.6 per 1000 has been found. More specifically, accessory pathways and the WPW syndrome occur more frequently in some forms of congenital heart disease than others. Ebstein's anomaly of the tricuspid valve is the most common anomaly associated with WPW (10–30%), followed by the various forms of single ventricle, atrial septal defects, and congenitally corrected transposition (L-TGV) among others. The WPW pattern on the ECG is seen in between 4% and 26% of patients with Ebstein's anomaly. Importantly, multiple pathways are found in about 50% of patients, and the pathways are predominantly right sided. Rarely, an accessory pathway may be created during surgical anastomosis of atrial tissue to the ventricular myocardium in the Bjork modification of the Fontan operation.[29]

Uncontrolled arrhythmias causing death in patients with WPW have been described following cardiac surgery to correct congenital abnormalities. Consequently, it has been recommended that accessory pathways be ablated prior to surgery if vascular or cardiac chamber access may be restricted following surgery [Class IIA recommendation, North American Society for Pacing and Electrophysiology (NASPE) position statement].[30]

In general, studies examining sudden death in patients with congenital heart disease have not identified WPW as a significant risk factor. For example, in a population-based prospective study over 45,857 patient years none of the 41 patients that died was reported as having associated WPW.[31] Similarly, in patients with Ebstein's anomaly who died suddenly, WPW was not noted as a predisposing factor.[32] It would seem reasonable, however, to be concerned about a potential risk in patients whose underlying congenital heart disease makes them particularly prone to having atrial tachycardia and AF if they are also found to have WPW. Such patient groups clearly include those with previous Mustard operation, Senning operation, Ebstein's anomaly, and Fontan operations; however, individual patients with a wide range of previously operated congenital heart disease may be at risk for atrial arrhythmias.

Genetics and Wolff–Parkinson–White

A familial occurrence of WPW was described as early as 1959.[33] In 1987, Vidaillet *et al.* reported that a family history of WPW was apparent in 3.4% of patients, and noted a higher incidence of multiple accessory pathways.[34] These observations provided the impetus to identify genes responsible for WPW.

To date, only a single gene has been reported to be responsible for a familial form of WPW.[14] First reported in 1986, a large French-Canadian family demonstrated an autosomal dominant mode of inheritance with a high degree of disease penetrance and variable clinical expressivity.[35] The predominant clinical phenotype observed in approximately 50% of patients was that of the classic ventricular preexcitation pattern of WPW (Figure 43-5). Electrocardiographic variants of preexcitation are commonly observed, including a short PR interval without a delta wave. Clearly distinguishing this familial form of WPW from the more common sporadic variety is the coexistence of cardiac hypertrophy in 30–50% of patients.[14,36] In addition, progressive cardiac conduction system disease, including sinus node dysfunction, is common. Development of paroxysmal and eventual chronic AF is seen in 80% of patients by the sixth decade of life.[37] Electrophysiological studies in affected individuals of the French-Canadian family have identified typical accessory pathways that are responsible for preexcitation and participate in reentry arrhythmias. These observations are consistent with the electrophysiological (EP) findings of other investigators who have assessed unrelated families with the identical genetic syndrome.[38,39] Fasciculoventricular tracts (Figure 43-1), in the absence of typical accessory pathways, have also been observed at EP study in some affected members of the Canadian family. This finding is consistent with the observation of a short PR interval and no delta wave on resting ECG and the presence of preexcited atrial tachycardia in some patients (Figure 43-6).

The disease-causing gene was identified as PRKAG2, a gene coding for the gamma-2

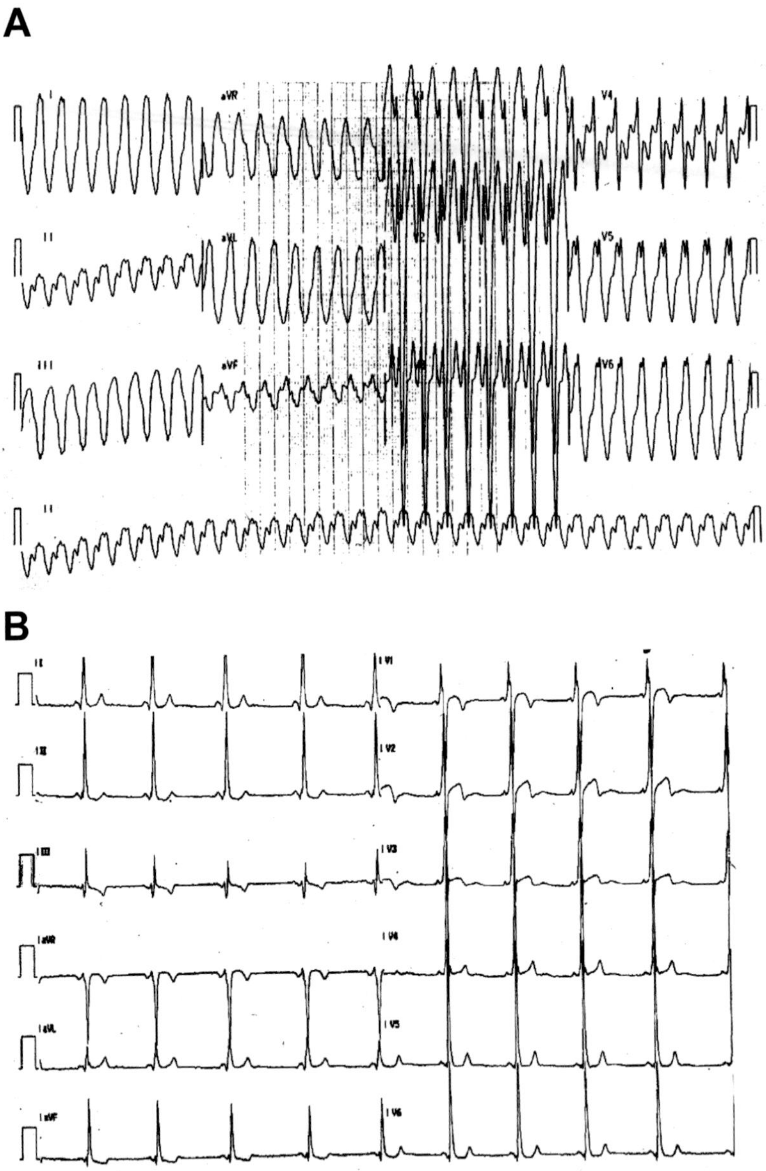

FIGURE 43–5. (A) Presenting 12-lead ECG of a 20-year-old male proven to harbor a PRKAG2 mutation (Arg-302-Gln) responsible for familial WPW. This patient had frequent episodes of presyncope. An electrophysiological study identified the mechanism of this tachycardia as antedromic AVRT utilizing a right free-wall accessory pathway. Following ablation of the right-sided pathway, ventricular preexcitation persisted and a left-sided accessory pathway was evident. (B) A resting ECG of the same patient following cardioversion. A classic pattern of WPW is evident.

regulatory subunit of AMP-activated protein kinase (AMPK). AMP-activated protein kinase is known to have a critical role in the preservation of cellular "energy homeostasis" in the heart by regulating key lipid and glucose metabolic pathways. Thus, it was originally hypothesized that the pathological basis of the cardiac hypertrophy seen in this genetic syndrome in humans may be secondary to abnormal glycogen storage in the heart.[37] This was confirmed by the development of transgenic mice models with cardiac expression of human PRKAG2 mutant genes.[40,41] These mice were found to have a glycogen storage disease of the heart, which has now also been confirmed in affected humans.[42,43] In addition, these mice developed the classic ECG features of WPW, including the inducibility of atrioventricular reentrant tachycardia (AVRT) and accessory pathway block with normalization of the ECG during procainamide infusion.[41]

Although the link between accumulation of cellular glycogen and accessory pathways remains to be elucidated, the present hypothesis considers the effect of excessive glycogen on normal heart

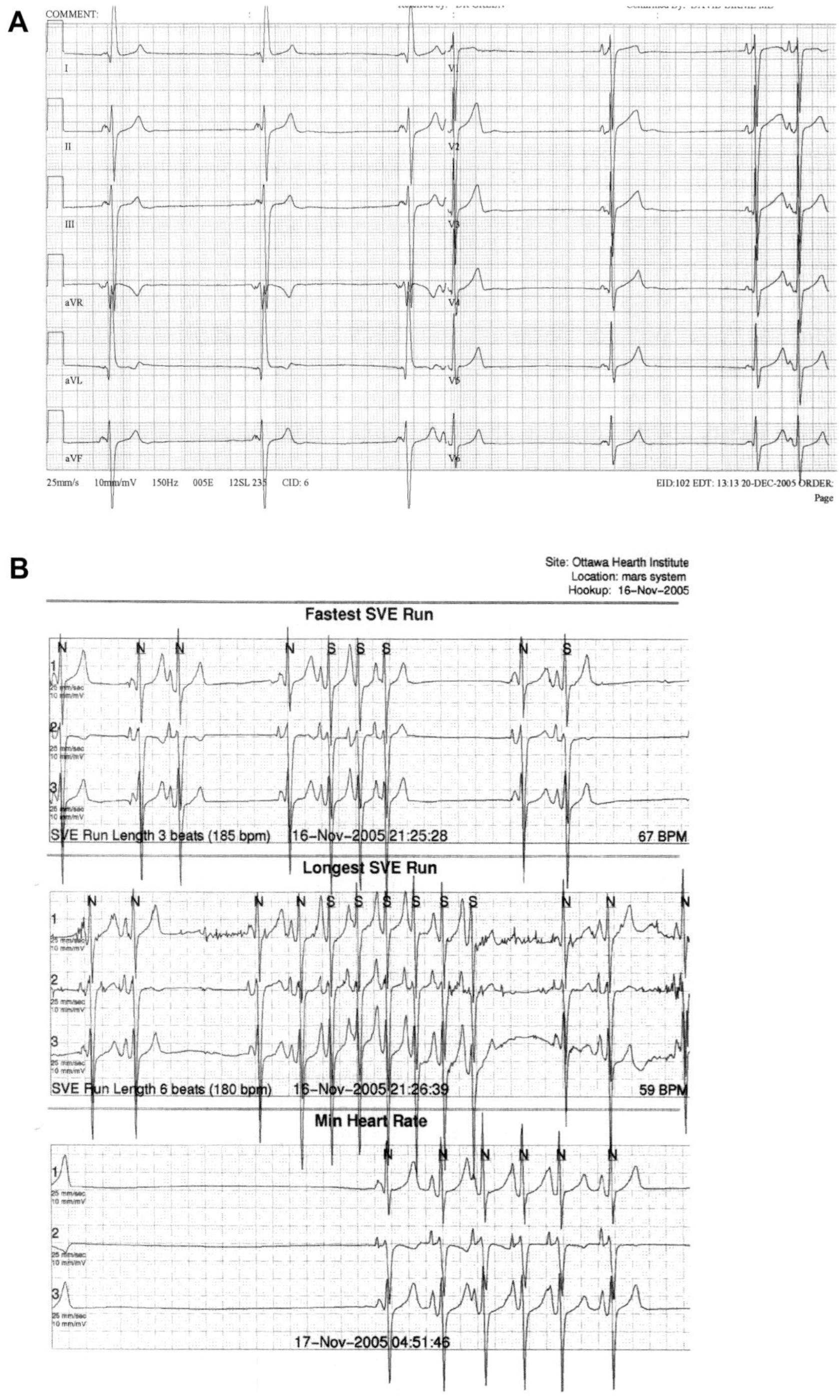

IGURE 43–6. (A) A resting 12-lead ECG in a 26-year-old female ousin of the patient illustrated in Figure 43–5, proven to have the ame PRKAG2 mutation. This patient had severe sinus bradycardia nd a short PR interval without a delta wave. Electrophysiological study showed no evidence of a typical accessory pathway. However, characteristics of a fasciculoventricular pathway were seen. (B) Frequent atrial tachycardias with significant pauses upon termination eventually resulted in permanent pacemaker placement.

development.[44] During early cardiac development, the heart exists as a tubular structure with muscular continuity between atrial and ventricular myocardium.[45] Atrioventricular septation occurs between 7 and 12 weeks of fetal life, with myocardial continuity between atrial and ventricular myocardium now occurring primarily via the developed normal conduction axis.[45] However, it has been well established by histological study that remnants of AV muscle continuity outside of the normal conduction axis are still observed in normal neonatal hearts.[45] The observed accessory fibers connecting atrial and ventricular myocardium in neonatal hearts are described as thin in nature and would therefore not be expected to have the "cable" capacity to conduct a depolarizing electrical wavefront from atrial to ventricular tissue. In this respect, these accessory fibers may be considered quiescent or subclinical and are a normal finding in newborn hearts. The effect of glycogen accumulation may be postulated to promote conduction through these otherwise quiescent accessory fibers. First, the enlargement of these accessory fibers due to glycogen accumulation may improve their "cable" capacity and ability to conduct a depolarizing wavefront. This concept is consistent with the histological finding of abnormally enlarged accessory fibers giving rise to WPW in a patient with glycogen storage disease due to Pompe disease.[46] The effect of increased glycogen in myocytes may further alter electrical properties by other mechanisms. The relationship between decreased cellular pH due to glycogen accumulation and the effect on myocyte conduction properties is unknown. However, given the known sensitivity of ion channel gating and current to intracellular pH,[47,48] a change in kinetics favoring conduction would not be unexpected. The hypothesis presented to account for the presence of WPW in the PRKAG2 cardiac syndrome suggests that this phenotype is secondary to the effects of glycogen on naturally occurring, quiescent, accessory fibers. In this regard, implicating a specific, independent function of AMPK as a direct cause of the WPW phenotype in this genetic syndrome is not necessary. The progression to conduction disease and left ventricular dysfunction in a significant number of affected patients by their fourth decade of life likely reflects a myopathic effect from the long-term cellular glycogen excess.

Wolff–Parkinson–White and the Risk of Sudden Cardiac Death

The Risk of Sudden Cardiac Death in Wolff–Parkinson–White Patients followed Prospectively

In most long-term, population-based follow-u studies, the risk of sudden cardiac death in WP has been reported to be very low. In 1993, Munge *et al.* reported on the natural history of 11 patients with WPW in a population-based stud in Olmsted County, Minnesota.[49] They reporte two cases of premature SCD over an averag patient follow-up of 12 years, suggesting a 1.9 risk of SCD over a 12 year follow-up (0.15%/yea risk) (18). Fitzsimmons *et al.* obtained follow-u on 238 consecutive military aviators with WP over an average of 21.8 years and found tha SCD occurred in only 1 of 228 patients (0.4%).[5] However, limitations in accurately determinin the rate of SCD in both studies arises from th consistent finding of patients lost to follow-up. I the Olmsted County cohort, six patients could n be located for follow-up. Assuming the worse cas scenario of sudden death in these cases, the esti mated range of SCD rate from this cohort woul be a 0.15%/year to 0.58%/year risk (SCD in two t eight of 113 patients over 12 years). Similarly, i the study of Fitzsimmons *et al.*, follow-up on 1 patients could not be ascertained, raising the pos sible range of SCD risk from 0.4% to 4.6% ove a 21.8-year follow-up.

As the above studies suggested a very low ris of sudden cardiac death, the recommendation b most "experts" and professional bodies has bee that WPW patients who are asymptomatic shoul not be considered for potential curative therap via catheter ablation. These recommendation have been challenged by more a recent study b Pappone *et al.*[51] In a follow-up study of 162 WP patients over an average of 3.1 years, they reporte sudden cardiac arrest in three patients, indicatin a 0.61%/year risk of SCD. Furthermore, previou EP studies in these asymptomatic patients ha induced preexcited AF, suggesting the EP stud may have risk stratified these previously asymp tomatic patients for catheter ablation to reduc the risk of cardiac arrest.

Sudden Cardiac Death in the Young and the Incidence of Wolff–Parkinson–White

In early autopsy series assessing the cause of SCD in previously healthy, young patient cohorts, WPW as an etiology has routinely not been reported.[52,53] Similarly, in these early retrospective studies, genetic electrical diseases of the heart such as long QT syndrome (LQTS) or catecholaminergic polymorphic ventricular tachycardia (CPVT), for example, were never reported. The absence of these diagnostic possibilities reflects the limitations of routine autopsy procedures. Pathologists do no routinely assess for histological evidence of accessory pathways responsible for WPW. Such an assessment would require thousands of sections across both AV annuli and an extraordinary time commitment for review. Thus, the possibility of WPW in a structurally normal heart is not addressed as a possibility in the sudden death of a young patient. As well, molecular autopsy in the form of genetic testing is not a standard procedure, excluding the ability to rule out genetic diseases such as LQTS or CPVT. In a unique study, Topaz *et al.* clinically evaluated 22 consecutive young survivors of sudden cardiac death, providing the opportunity to assess for both gross structural and nonstructural causes for cardiac arrest.[54] The most common identifiable causes were dilated cardiomyopathy and WPW, each considered responsible for three cases (13.3%). In two of three WPW patients, AF was induced during EP study. Long QT syndrome and the most commonly attributed cause of SCD in the young, hypertrophic cardiomyopathy, were each found in one case. These data are supported by a study from Basso and colleagues who retrieved prior ECGs on 93 patients aged <35 years who experienced sudden cardiac death. Ten patients (10.5%) had ECG documented ventricular preexcitation, and detailed histological examination of their hearts confirmed the presence of accessory pathways.[55] Importantly, 40% of these patients were asymptomatic prior to their sudden death.

Risk Stratification for Sudden Cardiac Death in Wolff–Parkinson–White

The objective of risk stratifying patients for the risk of sudden death in WPW is motivated by the tragedy of losing an otherwise healthy, young individual to a condition that is most often curable. Unfortunately, significant limitations exist in the development of a protocol with a high predictive accuracy in determining risk. These limitations arise due to the relatively low incidence of sudden death in WPW cohorts and the relatively small number of survivors of sudden death that have been subsequently evaluated. Nevertheless, a number of noninvasive and invasive electrophysiological observations have been proposed to be associated with either a higher or lower estimated risk. These observed variables traditionally endeavor to predict whether or not an accessory pathway is capable of sustaining rapid conduction to the ventricle during AF.

Noninvasive observations such as the presence of intermittent preexcitation on resting ECG have been suggested to predict a low risk of sudden death and to represent a longer ERP of the accessory pathway. Similarly, the apparent block of accessory pathway conduction and loss of preexcitation during exercise have been used to conclude that some WPW patients are at low risk of SCD.[56,57] However, Critelli *et al.* have demonstrated that such patients may still be capable of sustaining AF with rapid ventricular responses despite this observation.[58] Further, Sharma *et al.* described two of six patients with WPW who survived SCD but yet demonstrated loss of preexcitation on exercise treadmill.[59] Thus, robust data supporting noninvasive markers to predict a high or low risk of SCD in WPW do not currently exist.

Invasive EP testing has also been proposed to stratify for the risk of SCD in patients with WPW. The antegrade ERP of the accessory pathway, the shortest preexcited RR interval (SPRR) during AF, and the inducibility of AVRT or AF have all been used to stratify the risk of SCD. The most consistent observation in WPW patients who have survived SCD or who underwent EP study prior to SCD is the ability to induce AF during EP study and the observation of an SPRR of <250 msec.[51,59,60] In 25 patients studied by Klein *et al.*, 24 patients had inducible AF and all had an observed SPRR of 250 msec or less.[60] In three patients subsequently found to develop SCD studied by Pappone *et al.*, all had prior inducibility of AF and a SPRR of <250 msec.[51] Although the sensitivity of an SPRR of <250 mec during AF is high, the specificity is not, as many patients without SCD have been noted to meet this criteria within these studies. In addition, a further study by Sharma *et al.* noted two of nine WPW survivors of SCD who had relatively high SPRR during AF (396 msec and 295 msec),[59] highlighting the lack of complete reassurance that may be provided to young patients. Other EP measures that have been considered for risk stratifying include the accessory pathway antegrade ERP, the shortest preexcited RR interval during atrial pacing, the presence of multiple pathways, or pathway location. Bromberg and colleagues reported a cohort of 60 children with WPW who underwent invasive EP assessment, including 10 with documented VF or asystole.[61] Again, only the SPRR during AF significantly differed between high-risk and low-risk groups. No difference existed in the accessory pathway antegrade refractory period, the shortest preexcited RR interval during atrial pacing, the presence of multiple pathways, or pathway location. Interestingly, clinical history also did not differentiate the high risk patients.

Despite the limitations in the interpretation of EP data, transesophageal EP studies are used as part of the clinical management strategies in children by 50% of practicing pediatric electrophysiologists.[62] However, there are very few data that indicate the information that is provided is useful for risk stratification using standard markers. Physiological parameters that can be measured by transesophageal study (the antegrade accessory pathway refractory period and the shortest RR interval during atrial burst pacing) may not distinguish high-risk pediatric patients from those who are low risk.[61] As well, it has been shown that there is poor agreement between the intervals measured at invasive EP with those measured by the transesophageal route.[63]

Overall, the traditionally accepted indicator for increased risk of sudden death in WPW is an observed SPRR during AF of <250 msec. However, exceptions to this rule exist (Sharma). Conversely, the inability to induce AF during EP study using an aggressive pacing protocol may identify a lower risk population. The small number of studies and patients evaluated preclude definitive risk stratification recommendations.

Clinical Management of Wolff–Parkinson–White

Pharmacological Therapy

Chronic antiarrhythmic drug therapy is one option in the management of patients with symptomatic WPW. However, there are no randomized studies comparing drug therapy with radiofrequency ablation. Similarly, no evidence exists that drug therapy reduces the risk of SCD, although it is presumed that such therapy will minimize the risk of developing AF. Furthermore, it should be clearly discussed with patients that drug therapy is an arrhythmia reduction strategy and is not a cure for the condition. There are some data from the EP laboratory and observational studies about a number of anti-arrhythmic drugs. A summary of guidelines of drug therapy for WPW is shown in Table 43–1.[64] Of critical importance is the avoidance of drugs exerting a predominant AV nodal blocking effect in patients with manifest preexcitation. Drugs such as digoxin and verapamil preferentially block AV nodal conduction without a significant effect on accessory pathway conduction, increasing the risk of rapid conduction of atrial activity via the accessory pathway in the presence of AF, with subsequent degeneration to VF.

Table 43–1. Guidelines for drug therapy for WPW.[a]

Arrhythmia	Recommendation	Classification	Level of evidence
WPW syndrome (preexcitation and symptomatic arrhythmias), well tolerated	Flecainide, propafenone	IIa	C
	Sotalol, amiodarone, β blockers	IIa	C
	Verapamil, diltiazem, digoxin	III	C
Single or infrequent AVRT episode(s) (no preexcitation)	No therapy	I	C
	Vagal maneuvers	I	B
	Pill-in-the-pocket-verapamil	I	B
	Diltiazem, β blockers	IIb	B
	Sotalol, amiodarone, flecainide, propafenone, digoxin	III	C
Preexcitation, asymptomatic	No therapy	I	C

[a]WPW, Wolff–Parkinson–White; AVRT, atrioventricular reentrant tachycardia.

Class IC Antiarrhythmic Drugs

Propafenone and flecainide have been shown to block accessory pathway conduction and render supraventricular tachycardia (SVT) to be noninducible during EP procedures.[65,66] In addition, both propafenone and flecainide have been studied in small, randomized control studies comparing these Class IC agents with placebo in patients with paroxysmal, narrow complex SVT.[67,68] In these studies it is likely that some patients had accessory pathway-mediated tachycardia. The results consistently demonstrated that both drug agents are generally better than placebo; however, even on active therapy up to 25% of patients had recurrent SVT within 2 months,[4] indicating the limitations of drug therapy in patient management.

Class II Antiarrhythmic Drugs

There are no studies looking at the efficiency of β blockers for WPW; however, despite this paucity of data recent consensus guidelines have given β blockers a Class IIa recommendation.[64]

Class III Antiarrhythmic Drugs

Intravenous sotalol has been assessed for an ability to render SVT noninducible in the EP laboratory and has proven to be highly successful,[69] suggesting oral sotalol may be efficacious in management of arrhythmia. Anecdotal reports suggest moderate efficacy of chronic amiodarone in reducing the burden of arrhythmia in WPW[70]; however, in view of the relative toxicity of this drug it is seldom recommended for long-term management of arrhythmia in young patients.

Ablation for Wolff–Parkinson–White

In the current era, catheter ablation for the cure of WPW is usually performed as a day case procedure and under local anesthetic. Venous access is primarily via the femoral vein with some operators also using the internal jugular vein or a subclavian vein. Access for left-sided accessory pathways is achieved either by a retrograde aortic approach using femoral artery access or transseptally from the right to left atrium. The accessory pathway is localized by mapping the site of earliest ventricular activation during sinus rhythm or atrial pacing and/or mapping the earliest atrial activation during ventricular pacing. A successful ablation is seen by loss of delta waves during radiofrequency application.

Indications for ablation of WPW are detailed in Table 43–2.[30,64] Current guidelines consider that the risks of the actual ablation procedure may outweigh the potential benefits. In 2002, the NASPE, now the Heart Rhythm Society, developed a position statement for the use of radiofrequency catheter ablation in children with arrhythmias.[30] Class 1 indications for ablation were (1) a history of aborted sudden death and (2) syncope in a patient with WPW where there is a

Table 43–2. Recommendations for catheter ablation for WPW in adults.[a]

Arrhythmia	Recommendation	Classification	Level of evidence
WPW syndrome (preexcitation and symptomatic arrhythmias), well tolerated	Catheter ablation	I	B
WPW syndrome (with AF and rapid-conduction or poorly tolerated ARVT)	Catheter ablation	I	B
AVRT, poorly tolerated (no preexcitation)	Catheter ablation	I	B
Preexcitation, asymptomatic	Do nothing	I	C
	Catheter ablation	IIa	B

[a]WPW, Wolff–Parkinson–White; AF, atriofibrillation; AVRT, atrioventricular reentrant tachycardia.

short preexcited RR interval during AF (<250 msec) or an antegrade effective refractory period of the accessory pathway <250 msec at EP testing. Asymptomatic WPW was considered to be a Class II indication in children older than 5 years and there was agreement that ablation should not be performed in the asymptomatic child with WPW who is younger than 5 years of age (i.e., a Class III recommendation). Despite these recommendations, a survey of practicing pediatric electrophysiologists showed that 84% use EP studies to risk stratify asymptomatic children with some stratifying patients as young as 1 year of age.[62]

Invasive risk stratification or empiric catheter ablation in an informed patient with asymptomatic WPW remains controversial, but appears to be supported by the recent data of Pappone *et al.*[51] The major potential benefit is the elimination of the small risk of sudden cardiac death associated with WPW. In the case of asymptomatic WPW, the pros and cons of the procedure should be discussed very carefully with the patient/family and a decision should be individualized based on the wishes of an informed patient. Some high-risk occupations (pilots, bus drivers, military personnel) have mandatory requirements for ablation of asymptomatic WPW. However, these requirements are also controversial and vary from jurisdiction to jurisdiction.

In most experienced hands the acute success rate for ablation of WPW is in the range of 95%. The rates are higher in left-sided accessory pathways. There is a small recurrence rate of 1–2% and recurrences usually occur within minutes or hours of the procedure. Most complications associated with the procedure are minor and relate to venous or arterial access. Significant complications of heart block, cardiac tamponade, pneumothorax, myocardial infarction, venous and arterial embolism, vascular injury, and death have been reported. In a European study published in 1993 the complication rate was 4.4% with three deaths in 2222 patients (0.14%).[71] These data were accumulated in the early era of catheter ablation. In 2002, it was reported that the complication rate from ablation procedures in the United States had decreased from 4.2% in the early experience to 3.0% in more recent years,[72] suggesting the knowledge gained through the early experience has resulted in a reduction of complication risk.

References

1. Wolff L, Parkinson J, White PD. Bundle branch block with short PR interval in healthy young people prone to paroxysmal tachycardia. *Am Heart J* 1930;5:686–704.
2. Wood FC, WolferthCC, Geckeler GD. Histologic demonstration of accessory muscular connections between auricle and ventricle in a case of short P-R interval and prolonged QRS. *Am Heart J* 1943;25: 454–462.
3. Ohnell RF. Pre-excitation, cardiac abnormality, pathophysiological, patho-anatomical and clinical studies of excitatory spread phenomenon bearing upon the problem of the WPW (Wolff, Parkinson, and White) electrocardiogram and paroxysmal tachycardia. *Acta Med Scand* 1944;152:1–167.
4. Prinzmetal M. *Accelerated Conduction: The Wolff-Parkinson-White Syndrome and Related Conditions*. New York: Grune & Stratton, 1952.
5. Sodi-Pallares D, Cisneros F, Medrano GA, *et al.* Electrocardiographic diagnosis of myocardial infarction in the presence of bundle branch block (right and left), ventricular premature beats and Wolff-Parkinson-White syndrome. *Prog Cardiovasc Dis* 1963;6:107–136.
6. Durrer D, Schoo L, Schuilenburg RM, *et al.* The role of premature beats in the initiation and the termination of supraventricular tachycardia in the Wolff-Parkinson-White syndrome. *Circulation* 1967;36:644–662.
7. Wellens HJ, Schuilenburg RM, Durrer D. Electrical stimulation of the heart in patients with Wolff-Parkinson-White syndrome, type A. *Circulation* 1971;43:99–114.
8. Mines GR. On circulating excitations in heart muscles and their possible relationship to tachycardia and fibrillation. *Proc Trans R Soc Can* 1914; 8:43–52.
9. Cobb FR, Blumenschein SD, Sealy WC, *et al.* Successful surgical interruption of the bundle of Kent in a patient with Wolff-Parkinson-White syndrome. *Circulation* 1968;38:1018–1029.
10. Morady F, Scheinmann MM. Transvenous catheter ablation of a posteroseptal accessory pathway in a patient with the Wolff-Parkinson-White syndrome. *N Engl J Med* 1984;310:705–707.
11. Jackman WM, Wang XZ, Friday KJ, *et al.* Catheter ablation of accessory atrioventricular pathways (Wolff-Parkinson-White syndrome) by radiofrequency current. *N Engl J Med* 1991;334:1605–1611.
12. Calkins H, Sousa J, el Atassi R, *et al.* Diagnosis and cure of the Wolff-Parkinson-White syndrome or paroxysmal supraventricular tachycardias during a

single electrophysiologic test. *N Engl J Med* 1991; 324:1612–1618.
13. Kuck KH, Schluter M, Geiger M, *et al.* Radiofrequency current catheter ablation of accessory atrioventricular pathways. *Lancet* 1991;337:1557–1561.
14. Gollob MH, Green MS, Tang AS, *et al.* Identification of a gene responsible for familial Wolff-Parkinson-White syndrome. *N Engl J Med* 2001; 344:1823–1831.
15. Dreifus LS, Haiat R, Watanabe Y, *et al.* Ventricular fibrillation–a possible mechanism of sudden death in patients with Wolff-Parkinson-White syndrome. *Circulation* 1971;43:520–527.
16. Petrellis B, Skanes AC, Klein GJ, Gollob MH, Krahn AD, Yee R. An unusual accessory pathway: Anteroseptal to ventricular outflow region connection. *J Cardiovasc Electrophysiol* 2005;16(5):546–551.
17. Shah MJ, Garabedian H, Garoutte MC, Cecchin F. Catheter ablation of a right atrial appendage to the right ventricle connection in a neonate. *Pacing Clin Electrophysiol* 2001;24(9Pt. 1):1427–1429.
18. Tchou P, Lehmann MH, Jazayeri M, Akhtar M. Atriofascicular connection or a nodoventricular Mahaim fiber? Electrophysiologic elucidation of the pathway and associated reentrant circuit. *Circulation* 1988;77:837–848.
19. Klein GJ, Guiraudon GM, Kerr CR, *et al.* "Nodoventricular" accessory pathway: Evidence for a distinct accessory atrioventricular pathway with atrioventricular node-like properties. *J Am Coll Cardiol* 1988;11:1035–1040.
20. McClelland JH, Wang X, Beckman KJ, *et al.* Radiofrequency catheter ablation of right atriofascicular (Mahaim) accessory pathways guided by accessory pathway activation potentials. *Circulation* 1994;89:2655–2666.
21. Lau EW, Green MS, Birnie DH, Lemery R, Tang ASL. Preexcitation masking underlying aberrant conduction: An atriofascicular accessory pathway functioning as an ectopic right bundle branch. *Heart Rhythm* 2004;1(4):497–499.
22. Sternick EB, Timmermans C, Sosa E, *et al.* The electrocardiogram during sinus rhythm and tachycardia in patients with Mahaim fibers. *J Am Coll Cardiol* 2004;44(8):1626–1635.
23. Sun Y, Arruda M, Otomo K, *et al.* Coronary sinus-ventricular accessory connections producing posteroseptal and left posterior accessory pathways: Incidence and electrophysiological identification. *Circulation* 2002;106:1362–1367.
24. Guiraudon GM, Guiraudon CM, Klein GJ, *et al.* The coronary sinus diverticulum: A pathologic entity associated with Wolff-Parkinson-White syndrome. *Am J Cardiol* 1988;62:733–735.
25. Mahaim I, Benatt A. Nouvelles recherches sur les connexions superieures de la branche gauche du faisceau de His-Tawara avec la cloison interventriculaire. *Cardiologia* 1937;1:61–73.
26. Gallagher JJ, Smith WM, Kasell JH, *et al.* Role of Mahaim fibers in cardiac arrhythmias in man. *Circulation* 1981;64:176–189.
27. Sternick EB, Gerken LM, Vrandecic MO, Wellens HJJ. Fasciculoventricular pathways: Clinical and electrophysiologic characteristics of a variant of preexcitation. *J Cardiovasc Electrophysiol* 2003;14 (10):1057–1063.
28. Oh S, Choi YS, Choi EK, *et al.* Electrocardiographic characteristics of fasciculoventricular pathways. *Pacing Clin Electrophysiol* 2005;28:25–28.
29. Razzouk AJ, Gow R, Finley J, Murphy D, Williams WG. Surgically created Wolff-Parkinson-White syndrome after Fontan operation. *Ann Thorac Surg* 1992;54:974–977.
30. Friedman RA, Walsh EP, Silka MJ, *et al.* NASPE Expert Consensus Conference: Radiofrequency catheter ablation in children with and without congenital heart disease. Report of the writing committee. North American Society of Pacing and Electrophysiology. *Pacing Clin Electrophysiol* 2002;25:1000–1017.
31. Silka MJ, Hardy BG, Menashe VD, Morris CD. A population-based prospective evaluation of risk of sudden cardiac death after operation for common congenital heart defects. *J Am Coll Cardiol* 1998;32: 245–251.
32. Oh JK, Holmes DR Jr, Hayes DL, Porter CB, Danielson GK. Cardiac arrhythmias in patients with surgical repair of Ebstein's anomaly. *J Am Coll Cardiol* 1985;6:1351–1357.
33. Harnischfeger WW. Hereditary occurrence of the pre-excitation (Wolff-Parkinson-White) syndrome with re-entry mechanism and concealed conduction. *Circulation* 1959;19:28–40.
34. Vidaillwt HJ Jr, Pressley JC, Henke E, *et al.* Familial occurrence of accessory atrioventricular pathways (preexcitation syndrome). *N Engl J Med* 1987;317: 65–69.
35. Cherry JM, Green MS. Familial cardiomyopathy: A new autosomal dominant form [abstract]. *Clin Invest Med* 1986;9:B31.
36. Gollob MH, Seger JJ, Gollob TN, *et al.* Novel PRKAG2 mutation responsible for the genetic syndrome of ventricular preexcitation and conduction system disease with childhood onset and absence of cardiac hypertrophy. *Circulation* 2001;104:3030–3033.
37. Gollob MH, Green MS, Tang AS, Roberts R. PRKAG2 cardiac syndrome: Familial ventricular

preexcitation, conduction system disease, and cardiac hypertrophy. *Curr Opin Cardiol* 2002;17: 229–234.
38. MacRae CA, Ghasia N, Kass S, *et al.* Familial hypertrophic cardiomyopathy with Wolff-Parkinson-White syndrome maps to a locus on chromosome 7q3. *J Clin Invest* 1995;96:1216–1220.
39. Sinha SC, Nair M, Gambhir DS, *et al.* Genetically transmitted ventricular pre-excitation in a family with hypertrophic cardiomyopathy. *Indian Heart J* 2000;52:76–78.
40. Arad M, Moskowitz IP, Patel, *et al.* Transgenic mice overexpressing mutant PRKAG2 define the cause of Wolff-Parkinson-White syndrome in glycogen storage cardiomyopathy. *Circulation* 2003;107:2850–2856.
41. Sidhu JS, Rajawat YS, Rami TG, *et al.* Transgenic mouse model of ventricular preexcitation and atrioventricular reentrant tachycardia induced by an AMP-activated protein kinase loss-of-function mutation responsible for Wolff-Parkinson-White syndrome. *Circulation* 2005;111:21–29.
42. Gollob MH, Green MS, Veinot JP. Altered AMP-activated protein kinase activity and pathologic cardiac disease. *Heart Metab* 2006;32:28–31.
43. Burwinkel B, Scott JW, Buhrer C, *et al.* Fatal congenital heart glycogenosis caused by a recurrent activating R531Q mutation in the gamma-2 subunit of AMP-activated protein kinase (PRKAG2), not by phosphorylase kinase deficiency. *Am J Hum Genet* 2005;76:1034–1049.
44. Gollob MH. Glyocogen storage disease as a unifying mechanism of disease in the PRKAG2 cardiac syndrome. *Biochem Soc Trans* 2003;31:228–231.
45. Wessels A, Markman MWM, Vermeulen JLM, *et al.* The development of the atrioventricular junction in the human heart. *Circulation Res* 1996;78:110–117.
46. Bulkley BH, Hutchins GM. Pompe's disease presenting as hypertrophic myocardiopathy with Wolff-Parkinson-White syndrome. *Am Heart J* 1978;96:246–252.
47. Komukai K, Brette F, Orchard CH. Electrophysiological response of rat ventricular myocytes to acidosis. *Am J Physiol Heart Circ Physiol* 2002;283: H715–724.
48. Padanilam BJ, Lu T, Hoshi T, *et al.* Molecular determinants of intracellular pH modulation of human Kv1.4 N-type inactivation. *Mol Pharmacol* 2002;62: 127–134.
49. Munger TM, Packer DL, Hammill SC, *et al.* A population study of the natural history of Wolff-Parkinson-White syndrome in Olmsted County, Minnesota, 1953–1989. *Circulation* 1993;87:866–873.
50. Fitzsimmons PJ, McWhirter PD, Peterson DW, *et al.* The natural history of Wolff-Parkinson-White syndrome in 228 military aviators: A long term follow-up of 22 years. *Am Heart J* 2001;142:530–536.
51. Pappone C, Santtinelli V, Rosanio S, *et al.* Usefulness of invasive electrophysiology testing to stratify the risk of arrhythmic events in asymptomatic patients with Wolff-Parkinson-White pattern: Results from a large prospective long-term follow up study. *J Am Coll Cardiol* 2003;41:239–244.
52. Maron BJ, Roberts WC, McAllistair HA, *et al.* Sudden death in young athletes. *Circulation* 1980; 62:218–229.
53. Maron BJ, Epstein SE, Roberts WC. Causes of sudden death in competitive athletes. *J Am Coll Cardiol* 1986;7:204–214.
54. Topaz O, Perin E, Cox M, *et al.* Young adult survivors of sudden cardiac death: Analysis of invasive evaluation of 22 subjects. *Am Heart J* 1989;118: 281–287.
55. Basso C, Corrado D, Rossi L, *et al.* Ventricular preexcitation in children and young adults: Atrial myocarditis as a possible trigger of sudden death. *Circulation* 2001;103:269–275.
56. Strasberg B, Ashley WW, Wyndham CRC, *et al.* Treadmill exercise testing in the Wolff-Parkinson-White syndrome. *Am J Cardiol* 1980;45:742–748.
57. Levy S, Brooustet JP, Clementy J, *et al.* Value of noninvasive techniques in the Wolff-Parkinson-White syndrome with particular reference to exercise testing. In: Levy S, Scheinmann M, Eds. *Cardiac Arrhythmia from Diagnosis to Therapy*. Mt. Kisco, NY: Futura, 1984:301–312.
58. Critelli G, Grassi G, Perticone F, *et al.* Transesophageal pacing for prognostic evaluation of preexcitation syndromes and assessment of protective therapy. *Am J Cardiol* 1983;51:513–518.
59. Sharma AD, Yee R, Guiraudon G, Klein GJ. Sensitivity and specificity of invasive and non-invasive testing for risk of sudden death in Wolff-Parkinson-White syndrome. *J Am Coll Cardiol* 1987;10:373–381.
60. Klein GJ, Bashore TM, Sellers TD, *et al.* Ventricular fibrillation in the Wolff-Parkinson-White syndrome. *N Engl J Med* 1979;301:1080–1085.
61. Bromberg BI, Lindsay BD, Cain ME, Cox JL. Impact of clinical history and electrophysiologic characterization of accessory pathways on management strategies to reduce sudden death among children with Wolff-Parkinson-White syndrome. *J Am Coll Cardiol* 1996;27:690–695.

62. Campbell RM, Strieper MJ, Frias PA, *et al.* Survey of current practice of pediatric electrophysiologists for asymptomatic Wolff-Parkinson-White syndrome. *Pediatrics* 2003;111:e245–e247.
63. Nanthakumar K, Bergfeldt L, Darpo B. Assessment of accessory pathway and atrial refractoriness by transoesophageal and intracardiac atrial stimulation: An analysis of methodological agreement. *Europace* 1999;1:55–62.
64. Blomstrom-Lundqvist C, Scheinman MM, Aliot EM, *et al.* ACC/AHA/ESC guidelines for the management of patients with supraventricular arrhythmias–executive summary. A report of the American College of Cardiology/American Heart Association Task Force on Practice Guidelines and the European Society of Cardiology Committee for Practice Guidelines (writing committee to develop guidelines for the management of patients with supraventricular arrhythmias) developed in collaboration with NASPE-Heart Rhythm Society. *J Am Coll Cardiol* 2003;42:1493–1531.
65. Manolis AS, Katsaros C, Cokkinos DV. Electrophysiological and electropharmacological studies in pre-excitation syndromes: Results with propafenone therapy and isoproterenol infusion testing. *Eur Heart J* 1992;13:1489–1495.
66. Helmy I, Scheinman MM, Herre JM, *et al.* Electrophysiologic effects of isoproterenol in patients with atrioventricular reentrant tachycardia treated with flecainide. *J Am Coll Cardiol* 1990;16:1649–1655.
67. Henthorn RW, Waldo AL, Anderson JL, *et al.* Flecainide acetate prevents recurrence of symptomatic paroxysmal supraventricular tachycardia. The Flecainide Supraventricular Tachycardia Study Group. *Circulation* 1991;83:119–125.
68. UK Propafenone PSVT Study Group. A randomized, placebo-controlled trial of propafenone in the prophylaxis of paroxysmal supraventricular tachycardia and paroxysmal atrial fibrillation. *Circulation* 1995;92:2550–2557.
69. Kunze KP, Schluter M, Kuck KH. Sotalol in patients with Wolff-Parkinson-White syndrome. *Circulation* 1987;75:1050–1057.
70. Tuzcu Em, Gilbo J, Masterson M, Maloney JD. The usefulness of amiodarone in management of refractory supraventricular tachyarrhythmias. *Clev Clin J Med* 1989;56:238–242.
71. Hindricks G. The Multicentre European Radiofrequency Survey (MERFS): Complications of radiofrequency catheter ablation of arrhythmias. The Multicentre European Radiofrequency Survey (MERFS) investigators of the Working Group on Arrhythmias of the European Society of Cardiology. *Eur Heart J* 1993;14:1644–1653.
72. Kugler JD, Danford DA, Houston KS, *et al.* Pediatric radiofrequency catheter ablation registry success, fluoroscopy time, and complication rates for supraventricular tachycardias: Comparison of early and recent eras. *J Cardiovasc Electrophysiol* 2002;13:336–341.

Part V
Iatrogenic (Drug-Induced) Cardiac Channelopathies and Sudden Cardiac Death

Drug-Induced Enhanced Risk for Sudden Cardiac Death in Clinical Practice, Clinical Research, and Drug Development

Joel Morganroth

Introduction

Primum non nocere ("first, do no harm") is one of the fundamental precepts in medicine. It means that possible harm must be considered before "bringing any forth by a healer" to the human body or mind ("iatrogenesis"). Based on numerous iatrogenic studies, it appears that the use of some of the common current medicines arguably could cause more harm than good in many patients.[1] The extent of serious and fatal adverse drug reactions is largely underestimated and is of an important magnitude. Lazarou *et al.* in their meta-analysis of 39 prospective U.S. studies on adverse drug reactions in hospitalized patients revealed that the incidence of serious and fatal adverse drug reactions was 6.7% and 0.32%, respectively. Based on this, iatrogenic drug-induced death is between the fourth and sixth leading cause of death in the United States.[2]

Since 2002, U.S. and Canadian regulators have signaled that convincing assessment of both short- and long-term cardiac safety should be increasingly emphasized before acceptance of new drugs for marketing.[3] The focus has been on defining the effect of new drugs on cardiac repolarization as determined by the surface 12-lead electrocardiogram (ECG), a common safety measurement used in most if not all clinical trials to detect drug-induced cardiac adverse effects.[4] It is widely acknowledged that unwanted prolongation of cardiac repolarization as determined by prolongation of the QTc interval on the ECG is the commonest cause for delays in the drug development process and removal of drugs from the market. Noncardiac drugs that prolong cardiac repolarization have come from many different therapeutic groups and from many different related and unrelated chemical structures. Some examples include the antihistamine terfenadine, the antibiotic grepafloxacin, the antispasmodic terodiline, the calcium channel blocker lidoflazine, the atypical antipsychotic sertindole, the opioid levomethadyl, and the gastric prokinetic agent cisapride.[5]

While the primary focus should be on cardiac repolarization, other data from the ECG should be obtained with as much care and scrutiny. Proarrhythmic-induced ventricular arrhythmias, alteration of sinoatrioventricular conduction, and damage to myocardial cell integrity are important ECG findings.

Regulatory Focus on Cardiac Safety

While it is clear that the QTc interval duration on the ECG may not be highly correlated with the risk for torsade de pointes (TdP), prolongation of the QTc interval is relied upon by drug developers and regulatory authorities as the best predictor of a new drug's cardiac safety risk. This is likely to be the case even if new parameters for detecting cardiac repolarization disturbance are proposed, since those new factors will need to be compared to the ECG QT interval and outcome data on risk for TdP after marketing. A sponsor is unlikely to include a new parameter in clinical trials since discordant findings will not be interpretable and will raise concern without resolution. While European and Canadian ECG guidances were available in 1997 and 2001 but did not capture as much attention from industry,[6,7] the increasing number of marketed products that were withdrawn after unexpected effects on cardiac repolarization were discovered culminated in the U. S.-Canadian Guidance in 2002, which has attracted widespread serious interest among clinical researchers. This concept paper was subjected to the International Committee on Harmonization (ICH) process, which in May 2005 culminated in acceptance of the Step-IV E14 Guidance for Implementation.[8] E14 was also accompanied by an ICH guidance on preclinical cardiac safety assessment (S7B) also reaching Step-IV.[9]

The enhanced regulatory focus on cardiac safety in the past few years should encourage clinical researchers to avoid the pitfalls that probably resulted in lack of premarket identification of the cardiac liability of many drugs. Many of these problems stem from the high rate of spontaneous variability in QTc duration, which requires careful attention to trial design, statistical power, ECG processing methods, and the like to define the actual ECG effect(s) of a drug.[10] In using ECGs in clinical research, it is necessary to avoid analyzing the ECG by having each investigative site fill out a case report form with its attendant variation in quality and consistency. Sites usually use the automated ECG algorithms to determine QT interval duration, which for abnormal ECGs in particular are often inaccurate, rather than using a centralized digital manual method. Hence, as emphasized in the Food and Drug Administration (FDA)-Canadian Concept paper, ECGs in clinical research should be obtained and processed digitally using a validated central ECG laboratory. A single ECG has often been used to establish the baseline, which proves unreliable because of the high degree of spontaneous change in QT duration. Since the ECG data analysis is focused on change from baseline to define the drug effect, an adequate baseline value must be established. This can be accomplished by using as few as three ECGs taken a few minutes apart.

In March 2002, the Cardio-Renal Division of the FDA developed the concept of defining a drug's effect from a single dedicated clinical research trial. General details of this trial first appeared in the FDA-Health Canada paper and were finally defined as a regulatory requirement in the E14 document.

The need to understand precisely the ECG QTc effects of drugs applies to all new bioactive agents as well as any marketed drugs that are brought back for new indications. Drugs that cannot be given to healthy volunteers in the clinical dose range used in patients (e.g., atypical antipsychotic drugs) or at all (e.g., cytotoxic agents) require the use of other approaches to define adequate assessment of cardiac safety.

The principles of the Thorough ECG Trial's (TET) design, the analysis of the resultant data, the required control groups, and the regulatory interpretation of its results are evolving. The following recommendations stem from my extensive experience with over 50 such trials since 2002.

The Thorough Electrocardiographic Trial

A TET should be conducted when there is a clear understanding of the drug's pharmacokinetic profile, metabolism, and nature of metabolites (if any) and a good estimate of a clinically effective dose. The trial should certainly be conducted before launching a very costly Phase III program where large numbers of patients will be exposed. In determining the design of the TET, the new drug must be given in a manner that reflects the extent of exposure of the parent compound and its metabolites that will occur in clinical use. If the pharmacokinetics of a drug following a single dose and at steady state following multiple doses is essentially identical, then a single-dose trial can be conducted. From a clinical point of view, it might seem more meaningful to conduct the TET in the target population or older apparently healthy people. This approach, however, will produce a less robust and perhaps flawed TET since patients have multiple degrees of disease intensity, comorbidities, and concomitant medications, which prohibit the balancing of these factors between the treatment and control groups. Since the effect of drugs on cardiac intervals will occur in healthy as well as abnormal hearts or other clinical conditions, it is more effective to select a homogeneous disease and drug-free group of healthy volunteers (men and women from age 18–45 years) as the study population. However, to mimic the new drug's interaction with any effect modifiers that might be present in the target population (e.g., heart disease, metabolic abnormalities, concomitant drug metabolic inhibitors, or abnormal metabolism), a supratherapeutic dose treatment arm in the healthy volunteers must be employed. It is anticipated that this supratherapeutic dose given to healthy volunteers will mimic the worst-case effects (except for a frank overdose) of the drug in the target population, allowing the TET to be conducted in a small number of healthy volunteers.

The selection of the supratherapeutic dose should be modeled based on the known pharmacological properties of the drug and how the extent of exposure will change under various conditions in the patient population. Alternatively, the magnitude of this supratherapeutic dose can be the maximum tolerated dose in healthy volunteers. As a rough guideline, the minimal clinical dose compared to the supratherapeutic dose is often but not always at least three to five times the usual clinical dose, and for certain agents such as antihistamines or antibiotics it may be much greater. It is critical that all treatment arms in the TET (especially the positive control group) are subjected to the same experimental conditions. The positive control should not be used out of the randomization sequence. All subjects in the trial should have pharmacokinetic blood samples drawn (even if not measured in the control groups to induce the same autonomic tone changes) as an example of keeping the trial's conditions uniform across all treatment groups. For the results of the TET to be most predictive, it is important that all sources of variability in QT intervals have been controlled. To reduce the degree of spontaneous QT variability, attention must be given to sample size, number of ECG measurements at baseline and on treatment, accuracy of the ECG interval durations (centrally validated and consistent manual determinations), homogeneity of the study population (healthy volunteers half of whom are usually females), controls for environmental stresses (activity, food, diurnal effects, time effects, etc.), and using the most suitable means of correcting for the effect of heart rate on QT duration, which is the individually corrected QT interval (QTcI).[11]

To adequately evaluate at baseline and on treatment the effects of the parent and metabolites of a drug as well as time and food effects, ECG and blood samples should be taken at a minimum of 12–16 time points over a day (a number similar to most pharmacokinetic studies). At each of these time points multiple ECGs should be taken to improve a point's precision and to allow for computation of a QTcI exponent.

The choice of whether the TET is conducted using a crossover or parallel design depends on the pharmacokinetics of the new drug and its clinical use. For a crossover design the baselines should be collected before each treatment arm of the crossover.

In the TET an important analysis is the change from baseline in the placebo group to evaluate the control of spontaneous variability, which provides information on how well the trial was conducted. The placebo change from baseline for QTc duration should be within 10 msec of 0. Critical to defining the integrity of the trial is the result of the positive control, which provides assay sensitivity; moxifloxacin has proven to be a reliable and safe agent to produce a 5–10 msec time averaged change in QTc duration. If the placebo and positive control groups show study validity, then the analysis of the two different doses of the test agent will define whether the new agent does or does not affect cardiac repolarization (and other ECG intervals and morphology). Inadequate acquisition or measurement of ECG data may lead to an incorrect assessment of the drug's ECG effects and therefore attention to proper centralized ECG laboratory methods and digital processes are required.[12] New methods of recording the 10–20,000 ECGs that comprise a TET have been validated and used in the majority of these trials to date.[13]

The sample size of the TET is defined by the need to have enough power to detect a 5 msec (±5 msec) QTc effect (change from baseline) with a power of 80% and an α of 0.05. A key determination of sample size is the variance of the QTc, which is in large part determined by the number of ECGs employed in a subject and generally is between 8 msec and 12 msec. Using three ECGs at 12 time points usually requires a sample size of about 60 subjects per treatment (for a parallel trial 60 × 4 or 240 different subjects are recruited, whereas in a crossover trial 60 subjects are recruited and studied four times). If more ECGs per time point are extracted (four or five) then the sample size can be reduced to about 40. As defined in the regulatory E14 guidance, the primary statistical analysis is based on a central tendency determination on the time-matched analysis of QTcI at steady state. The time-matched analysis is based upon the primary endpoint "change from baseline placebo corrected" (the so-called double delta analysis) and is calculated for each of the separate time points. Two-sided 90% confidence intervals (CI) are calculated for each postbaseline time point based upon the pairwise comparison derived from the analysis-of-covariance model with gender and treatment group as factors. If the upper bound exceeds 10 msec then the test drug is declared positive (effects cardiac repolarization). An outlier or categorical analysis is an exploratory analysis. As noted in the regulatory guidances, the general consensus of the relationship of the magnitude of the central tendency QTc result and risk of TdP is as follows: (1) 0–5 msec, imparts no risk of TdP; and (2) if the effect is over 20 msec, the risk is considered quite high for TdP.

Most would say that a 5–10 msec effect for a drug is of minimal concern, but this depends on the risk–benefit ratio of the particular drug. An effect between 10 msec and 20 msec is uncertain.

The decision for approval in reference to cardiac risk of the new drug's effect on the ECG (especially QTc duration-cardiac repolarization) depends on the total data available. The TET is the most important part of the total risk assessment. The TET must be viewed in the context of ECG data in the Phase II–III target population, where it is necessary to look carefully for the presence of unexpected outliers since the TET still cannot be considered 100.0% definitive.

References

1. Leape LL. Error in medicine. *JAMA* 1994;272(23): 1851–1857.
2. Lazarou J, Pomeranz BH, Corey PN. Incidence of adverse drug reactions in hospitalized patients: A meta-analysis of prospective studies. *JAMA* 1998; 279(15):1200–1205.
3. Food and Drug Administration and Health Canada. The clinical evaluation of QT/QTc interval prolongation and proarrhythmic potential for non-antiarrhythmic drugs. Preliminary Concept paper, November 15, 2002: http://www.fda.gov/cder/workshop.htm#upcoming.
4. Morganroth J. Focus on issues in measuring and interpreting changes in the QTc interval duration. *Eur Heart J Suppl* 2001;3(Suppl. K):K105–K111.
5. Morganroth J, Gussak I, Eds. *Cardiac Safety of Noncardiac Drugs*. Totowa, NJ: Humana Press, 2005.
6. Committee for Proprietary Medicinal Products (CPMP). Points to consider: The assessment of the potential for QT interval prolongation by non-cardiovascular medicinal products. The European Agency for the Evaluation of Medicinal Products, 17 December 1997.
7. Health Canada Draft Guidance. Assessment of the QT prolongation potential of non-antiarrhythmic drugs. http://www.hc-sh.gc.ca/hpb-dgps/therapeut/htmleng/guidmain.html. Accessed March 15, 2001.
8. ICH E14 guideline (clinical testing for effect on QT interval). http://www.ich.org/cache/compo/276-254-1.html http://www.emea.eu.int/htms/human/ich/efficacy/ichdraft.htm.
9. ICH S7B guideline (nonclinical testing for effect on ventricular repolarization). http://www.ich.org/cache/compo/276-254-1.html_http://www.emea.eu.int/htms/human/ich/safety/ichdraft.htm.
10. Morganroth J, Brozovich FV, McDonald JT, Jacobs RA. Variability of the QT measurement in healthy men: With implications for selection of an abnormal QT value to predict drug toxicity and proarrhythmia. *Am J Cardiol* 1991;67:774–776.
11. Malik M, Färbom P, Batchvarov V, *et al.* Relation between QT and RR intervals is highly individual among healthy subjects: Implications for heart rate correction of the QT interval. *Heart* 2002;87:220–228.
12. Haverkamp W, Breithardt G, Camm AJ, *et al.* The potential for QT prolongation and proarrhythmia by non-antiarrhythmic drugs: Clinical and regulatory implications. Report on a Policy Conference of the European Society of Cardiology. *Cardiovasc Res* 2000;47:219–233.
13. Sarapa N, Morganroth J, Couderc J-P, Francom SF, Darpo B, Fleishaker JC, McEnroe JD, Chen WT, Zareba W, Moss AJ. Drug-induced QT prolongation in the electrocardiogram: Assessment by different recording and measurement methods. *Ann Noninvasive Electrocardiol* 2004;9:48–57.

44 Pharmacogenomics in Drug Development and Clinical Research

Richard Judson

Introduction

Pharmacogenomics research typically aims to find genetic variants that affect the pharmacokinetics or the pharmacodynamics of a drug. Pharmacokinetic-related genetic variants can cause loss of function for a metabolic enzyme that can in turn decrease the rate at which a drug is metabolized. This increases the amount of drug delivered to the active site, as well as the half-life of the drug in the system. Pharmacodynamic variants can change the binding properties of a receptor to which a drug is targeted, and can therefore affect activity. Alternatively, a variant can simply alter the level of expression of some protein, which can lead to an indirect effect on drug action. Variants can cause *cis* effects, meaning that a variant in the gene has a direct effect on the gene's expression level. Alternatively, the effect can be *trans*, meaning that variation in the gene affects expression levels for other genes. Genes causing such *trans* effects can be far removed from pathways directly involved in drug action.

The aims of pharmacogenomic research in the cardiac safety area are 3-fold: (1) to understand variability in safety that is related to genetic factors, (2) to develop tools to help evaluate the safety of compounds early in clinical trials, and (3) to develop tests to keep susceptible patients off inappropriate drugs, or at safe doses. In almost all therapeutic areas, there is large variability in both safety and response, and this variability is driven in part by genetics.

The goals of this chapter are to review the current knowledge of the genetic factors that affect the risk of drug-induced torsade de pointes (TdP) and to describe possible avenues for further research. The range of possible genetic risk factors is large, so that we are far from being able to screen all patients for genetic risk prior to drug prescription. However, a more modest goal seems to be in reach: that of being able to understand the cause for outliers in clinical trials (excessive QT prolongation or TdP). It may then be possible to quantify the risk of observing significant problems with a drug once it goes into larger clinical trials and onto the market.

Currently, there are about 50 drugs on the market that carry some risk of drug-induced TdP that results from drug-induced QT prolongation. The incidence of TdP ranges from very low (on the order of 1 out of 100,000 users of cisapride)[1] to relatively high (e.g., sotalol, which shows a rate of a few percent).[2–4] Drugs that cause QT prolongation span many classes and indications, but there are some common risk factors. Almost all QT-prolonging drugs block the hERG potassium ion channel.[5] Women are at higher risk than men. Hypokalemia and the use of diuretics increase risk. In addition to these and other "phenotypic" risk factors, there are known "pharmacogenomic" risk factors. We will use the term pharmacogenomic loosely, to mean instances where we can directly relate clinical risk to an underlying genetic mechanism.

The best understood classes of pharmacogenomic risks of TdP involve drug metabolism (pharmacokinetics) and the interaction of drugs, directly or indirectly, with cardiac ion channels (pharmacodynamics).[6] Many QT-prolonging drugs are metabolized by the cytochrome P450 class of enzymes. Some individuals inherit defective versions of these enzymes, which can cause them to be poor metabolizers. Most metabolic enzymes can also be inhibited by other drugs, which can cause patients on multiple medications to receive higher than desired effective concentrations of the drug. On the pharmacodynamic side, certain individuals have genetic defects that alter the ability of their cardiac potassium and sodium ion channels to conduct. This can lead to the familial long QT syndrome (LQTS). The addition of a human ether-à-go-go-related gene (hERG) blocker can be a second hit that will decrease the conductivity of their I_{Kr} channel to the point that significant QT prolongation is seen, which in turn increases the risk of TdP. Although it is known that mild prolongation of the QT interval is not a always good surrogate for risk of TdP,[7] we will discuss both QT prolongation and TdP risk together.

Cisapride offers an example in which both pharmacodynamic and pharmacokinetic genetic risk factors were seen to be important enough to make their way into the label.[8] A family history of LQTS was added as a contraindication, based on evidence that the drug could be the critical "second hit" for individuals who had deleterious mutations in the cardiac ion channel genes. At the same time, the ingestion of grapefruit juice was contraindicated. Cisapride is primarily metabolized by CYP3A4, which is inhibited by grapefruit juice. Taking the two together would greatly increase the effective concentration of the drug. This drug was removed from active marketing due to 341 reports of patients with cardiac events and 80 deaths associated with drug-induced arrhythmias.[8] In these reports, 37% of patients also took other CYP3A4-inhibiting medications; 10% had heart ischemia with previous reports of arrhythmias, 5% had electrolyte imbalance, 5% were simultaneously on a second proarrhythmic drug, and 3% suffered a cisapride overdose. In summary, about 60% of patients with events had obvious risk factors, and many of these were pharmacogenomic in nature, which could explain the cause of their drug-induced arrhythmia. Therefore, there is significant evidence that genetic factors (pharmacokinetic CYP3A4 inhibition or LQTS) played a major role in putting individuals at risk for drug-induced arrhythmias while taking cisapride.

Genetics of Cardiac Repolarization

The genetics of LQTS are dealt with more comprehensively elsewhere, so here we simply provide a brief summary that will be required for further discussion of drug-induced QT prolongation (DI-LQT).

Approximately 75% of congenital LQTS is caused by mutations in currently recognized cardiac channel mutations. Over 400 LQTS-associated mutations have been reported to date across several ion channel genes, including KCNQ1 (LQT1), KCNH2 (LQT2), SCN5A (LQT3), KCNE1 (LQT5), and KCNE2 (LQT6). Notably, KCNH2 directly intersects with both congenital (LQT2) and DI-LQT. Long QT syndrome mutations can have relatively low penetrance (as low as 25%[9]), so that even among siblings who both carry the same LQTS-associated mutation, one may have marked QT prolongation while the other will have a normal baseline QT interval. These "asymptomatic" LQTS carriers may become symptomatic when exposed to a QT-prolonging drug, even at moderate dosage. Long QT syndrome is relatively uncommon with an estimated incidence around 1 in 3000.

The QT interval is the "outer" manifestation of the underlying cardiac action potential (AP) (Figure 44–1). The first phase of the AP is due to

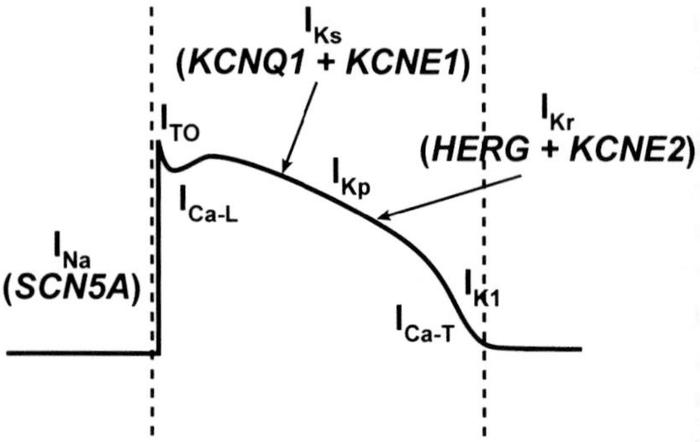

FIGURE 44–1. A schematic of the cardiac action potential indicating the currents and intervals during which proteins coded for by key ion channel genes act.

the opening of the *SCN5A*-encoded sodium channel, which causes rapid depolarization of the cell. Several potassium currents, including I_{Ks} (produced by the combination of *KCNQ1* and *KCNE1*) and I_{Kr} [produced by the channel composed of the protein products of *KCNH2* (commonly called hERG) and *KCNE2*] open in a synchronized manner to allow the cell to repolarize. Generally, LQTS-causing mutations involving potassium channels (causing syndromes labeled LQT1, LQT2, LQT5, and LQT6) cause a loss of function (i.e., decreased repolarization current), whereas LQT3-associated *SCN5A* mutations cause a gain of function (i.e., increased/sustained depolarization current resulting in QT prolongation, as additional time is required for repolarizing forces to counterbalance). In both settings, time to full repolarization is increased, which manifests itself by an increased QT interval. If the potassium channels cannot conduct sufficient current to fully repolarize the cell well before the next depolarization step, synchronization of the cells may fail and an arrhythmia can occur.

Overview of Pharmacogenetics

In the ideal pharmacogenetics study, levels of protein and existence of protein variants with clinical outcome would be correlated. This is usually impractical, often because the tissue of interest (e.g., the heart) is inaccessible. The easiest surrogates to use are DNA variants that can be detected from blood samples. DNA sequence variations range in size from single nucleotide polymorphisms (SNPs) up to whole chromosome deletions and duplications. Single nucleotide polymorphisms are positions in the genome where one letter in the genetic code differs between at least two people. RNA and protein expression (and hence related phenotypes) are loosely tied to the underlying genetic sequence, although noise in expression can cause significant phenotypic differences in even clonal individuals such as twins.[10] This chapter focuses on inborn DNA variation and its effect on clinical outcomes, in particular QT prolongation and TdP.

There are about 15 million SNPs in the human population, or about 1 every 200 base pairs in our genome. For most of these, one of the alleles is rare, so that most people will be homozygous for the common allele. The majority of SNPs are nonfunctional. They do not cause any change in RNA or protein expression and have no effect on the structure or function of any expressed protein. However, silent SNPs can still be useful for tracking nearby functional variants. Most of the functional SNPs have minimal phenotypic effects, which are overwhelmed by environmental and dietary factors. Of the remaining functional variants, there is a gradation of level of effect, ranging from measurable but weak to almost 100% predictive of disease. Into this latter category fall the so-called monogenic disorders such as LQTS.

Figure 44–2 illustrates the distribution of SNPs across functional categories. What is potentially

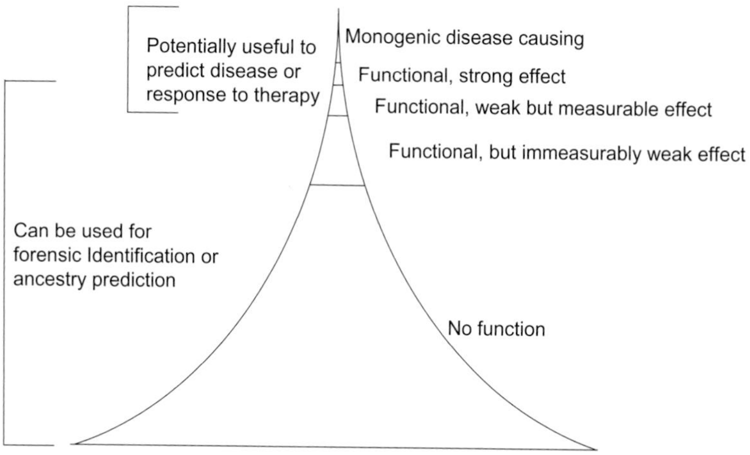

FIGURE 44–2. A schematic of the relative distribution of genetic variants between different functional classes.

unique about an individual's genome are the 15 million variable sites. However, referring to the figure, one can see that only a small fraction of those could have any medical relevance. Currently, of that small potential set, there are only a handful (potentially 100s) of SNPs of proven functional relevance, outside of those responsible for rare monogenic diseases.

Types of Genetic Scans: Candidate Gene Versus Whole Genome

Three types of genetic markers are used in pharmacogenetic studies: known markers, markers in candidate genes, and genome-wide sets of markers. The first category is self-explanatory. A series of known, validated markers (e.g., SNPs that define CYP2D6 activity) are measured and directly used as covariates in an association analysis, or as inclusion/exclusion criteria in a clinical study.

In the candidate gene approach, genes are selected that may be associated with a phenotype; it is then necessary to measure markers in these genes in a patient cohort and to look for correlations with the phenotype. The set of genes may include the target of the drug, ADME genes, or genes in pathways associated with upstream and downstream processes of the drug or the disease. Often, it is necessary to focus on known SNPs found in exons, splice regions, and putative promoter regions. Typically, 5–10 SNPs per gene are required. If the relevant SNPs are expected to be rare (e.g., when looking for predictors of a rare side effect), it is better to resequence the genes in DNA samples from patients.

Genome-wide approaches are quickly becoming practical to apply. These techniques measure a set of SNPs spread across all of the chromosomes, spaced closely enough to use the linkage disequilibrium (LD) properties of the genome. Linkage disequilibrium is a measure of the correlation between nearby markers.[11] In general, LD drops off with distance. Commercially available genome-wide approaches measure markers as densely as one SNP every 2 kb or so, for a total of about 1.5 million. Affymetrix has a 500,000 SNP chip that is widely available, and Parallele has a 200,000 chip focused on genes. Costs to perform a whole genome scan are decreasing, but at present are in the range of $2000–$4000 per clinical subject. Because of the extreme number of tests being performed in a whole genome scan, there is minimal power to rule out false-positive findings. The whole-genome approach should then be viewed as a screen to find candidate regions that can be further evaluated in follow-on studies.

Ethnicity Considerations

Many markers are correlated with an individual's ethnicity or continental ancestry (Africa, Asia, and Europe). This fact is of practical importance because if the phenotype being studied is also correlated with ethnicity, spurious, confounding associations between irrelevant genetic markers and the phenotype will be found. To manage this, ethnicity must be used as a covariate in genetic association analyses. Either self-reported ethnicity or more sophisticated methods such as genomic control can be used.[12] This approach measures a set of genetic markers that is correlated with ethnicity but that is known to be uncorrelated with the phenotype. Each individual's genetic background can then be quantified in an unbiased way.

Association Analysis

The goal of a pharmacogenetic study is to find an association between a genetic variant and a clinical variable. Pharmacogenetic association analyses are in many ways similar to analyses carried out using standard clinical or demographic measures as independent variables. However, there are three special situations to note. The first is the issue of multiple comparisons. Candidate gene and whole-genome studies measure hundreds to hundreds of thousands of markers for each patient. The number of independent variables is then often far greater than the number of subjects, requiring the use of a multiple test correction. Standard correction methods (e.g., Bonferroni based on the total set of markers) are usually too conservative because they incorrectly assume that all tests are independent. This is not the case because of the correlation between nearby SNPs due to LD. A better correction approach uses permutation testing, which properly accounts for correlations between markers.[13–15]

A second property of most genetic markers is that they are diploid—each person can have zero, one, or two copies of the marker. Because of this, dominant, recessive, and additive models should be simultaneously considered. An extension of this occurs when multi-SNP haplotypes are used as part of the analysis strategy. In this case, a locus can have many different haplotypes, all of which need to be tested.[16–18] There is a special situation that occurs in genes such as the cardiac ion channels responsible for LQTS. These genes contain many mutations (hundreds at latest count), any one of which can cause LQTS. So, although there is an association in a population between the gene and the disease, there is little power to detect an association between any specific marker and disease. Instead, a model must be used in which it is not the presence of a given marker that determines risk, but the presence of any one of many variants that is the input. An extension to this is to use the number of variants (common or rare) and to calculate a genetic load as an independent variable in a risk model.

We finish this section with a few comments on the science of genetic testing that emphasize the complexity of the field and our imperfect current understanding of it. First, much of what is known is derived from association studies that look for statistical correlations between (potentially many) genetic variants and some clinical measurement. Such a study can easily find false-positive results, i.e., associations that occur by chance. To be validated, a finding must be reproduced in one or more other studies. Often, even after a finding has been reproduced, it may take many years before the underlying mechanistic explanation for the association is worked out. Also, it is often the case that an association may be reproduced in some populations but will fail to replicate in others. This phenomenon reinforces the fact that genetic variants interact with other factors (including other genes) that differ from population to population. Working out these interactions is especially difficult.

The Food and Drug Administration (FDA) has introduced the concept of a validated biomarker, which (in this context) is a genetic variant, and its associated phenotypic consequence that are backed up by significant experimental evidence and (often) mechanistic understanding. There are relatively few validated biomarkers and they are mainly confined to drug metabolism and cancer markers.

Finally, it needs to be emphasized again that it is rare to find a single gene controlling a trait. Notwithstanding the popular news accounts of the discovery of "the gene for . . . ," almost all measurable traits are affected by multiple genes. Variants in each of these genes play a complicated, interacting role in determining a particular individual's outcome.

Genetics of Drug-Induced QT Prolongation

We next turn to the pharmacogenetics of DI-LQT.[19] Little prospective, systematic work has been done to characterize how genetic variation affects a person's risk of drug-induced QT prolongation or TdP, but we focus on the genetic pathways that are most likely to play a role in this effect. However, it will require careful examination of clinical trial populations to confirm the connection between genetic variation and DI-LQT. We include a proposal to help make this connection.

Moss and Schwartz originally proposed that some instances of drug-induced TdP were actually a manifestation of LQTS that was uncovered only when a patient was treated with a QT-prolonging drug.[20] Roden in turn proposed the concept of "repolarization reserve"[7,21] to bring together the mechanics of repolarization and the understanding of how multiple hits may be required to cause TdP. Under ordinary conditions, cardiac cells have an excess capacity to repolarize. Cells contain more copies of each ion channel than the absolute minimum needed, and there are multiple pathways for ions to enter and exit the cell. This leads to a reserve of repolarization capacity. Numerous factors can cause a decrease in this capacity. At some point the reserve is exhausted and the next additional factor will cause the QT interval to increase. Incomplete penetrance in families that carry even severe LQTS mutations is further evidence that multiple factors are needed to cause TdP.[9,22] Most drugs that cause QT prolongation do so by blocking the KCNH2-encoded hERG potassium channels. For these drugs, ion channel function is measurably affected in all patients, but only a small minority experience TdP. The molecular genetic factors that cause some individuals to be especially susceptible to these drugs are beginning to be understood.

Pharmacokinetic Aspects of Drug-Induced QT Prolongation

Pharmacokinetic factors drive the effective concentration of a drug at its site of action. Although there is conflicting evidence that the risk of TdP is dependent on dose, it must be true that the degree of hERG block will increase with the local drug concentration at the hERG channel. The basic pharmacogenomic risk factor is obvious: if a patient's ability to metabolize the drug is compromised, then the effective concentration at the target is increased, as is the risk for TdP. Metabolism can be compromised by (1) inborn defects in metabolic enzymes, (2) reduced expression of the enzymes due to a condition such as disease or advanced age, or (3) inhibition of the enzyme by another drug. A significant fraction of the reported events that led to the withdrawal of cisapride could be explained by these factors.[8,23]

Figure 44–3A illustrates the effect of changing levels of metabolism. Notionally, the degree of channel block will increase with increasing drug concentration. Due to the exhaustion of the repolarization reserve, there is a nonlinear relationship between drug concentration and change in QT, especially at high concentrations. When the parent drug is active, an individual who is an extensive metabolizer (EM) should see a modest concentration of drug in the heart, and a correspondingly modest QT effect. Poor metabolizers (PMs) or patients taking concomitant drugs that inhibit the relevant metabolizing enzyme will show higher local concentrations. Consistent with this paradigm, dose is a risk factor for QT prolongation by certain drugs, including terfenadine,[24] cisapride,[8] and sotalol.[4] To help illustrate the complementary roles of pharmacokinetics and pharmacodynamics, we refer to the drug concentration axis as the PK axis in this figure.

Many QT-prolonging drugs are metabolized by CYP2D6 or CYP3A4. CYP2D6 has a series of alleles that knock out the function of the gene making it possible to genotype individuals and classify them as having 0, 1, or 2 (and sometimes more) active copies of the gene. The results can be used to individualize the dosage of CYP2D6-metabolized drugs.[25] This is especially valuable in situations in which the patient is on multiple drugs that are substrates for this enzyme. Those with zero copies are classified as PMs. (Note that it is possible for one or both of the parent drug and the metabolite to have hERG-blocking activity. The particular situation will govern how genetic variation information should be used.)

CYP3A4 does not have any knockout alleles as seen in CYP2D6, but still shows variable meta-

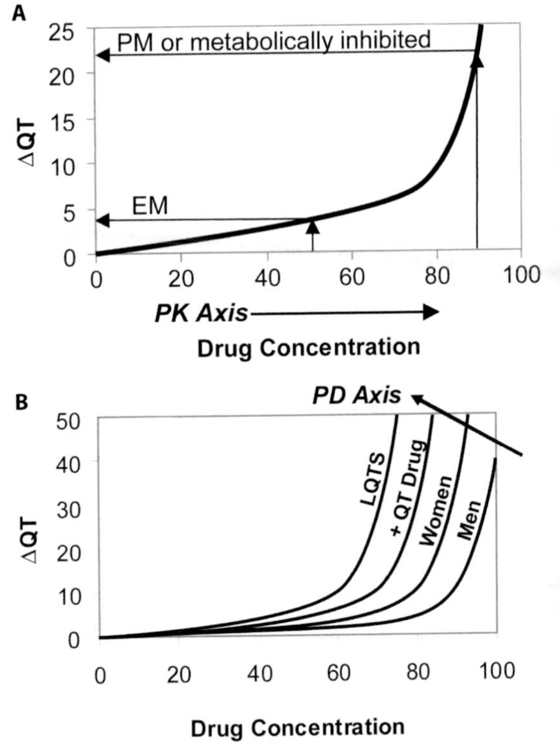

FIGURE 44–3. (A) Illustration of the effect of drug concentration on the expected change in the QT interval. EM, extensive metabolizer; PK, pharmacokinetic; PM, poor metabolizer. (From Judson, *et al.*[89] Reproduced with permission from Adis Data Information BV.) (B) Illustration of the effect of various pharmacodynamic variables on the expected change in QT interval. Women have higher sensitivity than men. The addition of a QT-prolonging drug (+QT Drug) will further increase the sensitivity and the presence of a long QT syndrome (LQTS)-susceptibility cardiac channel mutation/polymorphism (clinical or subclinical) will increase the sensitivity even more. PD, pharmacodynamic. (From Judson, *et al.*[89] Reproduced with permission from Adis Data Information BV.)

bolic efficiency, likely due to alterations in levels of expression. Although specific polymorphisms have been correlated with CYP3A4 activity, the degree of predictivity is usually too low for practical use. Changes in expression can be induced, or can be caused by inhibition by other molecules.[26] A secondary PK effect is seen in elderly patients, in whom total hepatic metabolism is reduced due to a combination of reduced liver mass and decline in blood flow through the liver.

Both CYP2D6 and CYP3A4 can be inhibited by a variety of other drugs as well as by common foods.[27] Although this cause of adverse drug–drug or drug–food interaction is well understood, there are many case reports of incidents in which a patient experienced TdP while simultaneously taking an hERG-blocking drug and a corresponding enzyme inhibitor.[28–31]

In summary, drug metabolism plays a key role in the risk of developing QT prolongation and TdP.[32] If the local concentration of a channel-blocking drug is sufficiently high, QT prolongation will occur. This can arise if the original dose is too high or if the patient cannot adequately metabolize the drug. The latter can occur if the patient is genetically programmed to be a PM or if the patient is taking a concomitant metabolic inhibitor.

Pharmacokinetics covers not only drug metabolism, but also the entire ADME process—administration, distribution, metabolism, and excretion. Genetic differences likely affect how these drugs are processed in the other ADME steps. Currently, however, little is known about how other ADME pathways affect the potential for drug-induced TdP.

Pharmacodynamic Aspects of Drug-Induced QT Prolongation

Genetics also affect the pharmacodynamics of QT-prolonging drugs. The best characterized effect is seen in LQTS. Patients with LQTS have an elevated risk of TdP because of their inherited reduction in repolarization reserve.[22,33–36] Many LQTS variants cause a decrease in function (equivalent to partial blocking) so that normal drug blocking can have increased effect. It has been estimated that between 56% and 71% of patients who experience TdP may have prolonged baseline QT intervals.[37] Several variants in KCNE2, KCNQ1, and SCN5A that are associated with drug-induced TdP have been shown to decrease baseline current, implying that they are LQTS variants that lead to TdP upon drug challenge.[33,34,38–41] The majority of LQTS mutations cause a loss of function in potassium channels, leading to a decrease in the effective repolarization current, and hence the repolarization reserve. This can then lead to an enhanced effect of an hERG-blocking drug. Many LQTS mutations have been functionally characterized *in vitro* (for examples, see Table 44–1). Variants can affect the expression of the channels, the formation of multimeric channels, the current, or the opening/closing dynamics. Additionally, variants that do not cause LQTS may increase drug binding, which can increase the degree of channel block. There are subclinical variants that manifest their effect only in the presence of an additional stress such as a drug challenge. Finally, variants in regulatory pathways likely affect drug response.

Several case studies have shown that LQTS mutations are associated with TdP. Table 44–1 lists a sample of variants in the ion channel genes that have been reported to cause TdP, or have been otherwise functionally characterized. Each variant is classified into one or more of five categories: L, causes LQTS; D, causes TdP; B, the site is demonstrated to be important for drug binding *in vitro*; F, functionally characterized *in vivo*; C, common, i.e., is seen in a reference population of healthy individuals. A more extensive compilation of variants associated with LQTS, Brugada, and TdP is given at the following web site: http://www.fsm.it/cardmoc/.

Functional studies have shown that altering certain residues in the hERG channel can affect dru-binding characteristics. Although there are currently no reported naturally occurring variants at the functionally characterized binding positions, such mutations would change the effect of hERG-blocking drugs *in vivo*.[42–45]

LQTS-associated mutations can compromise the expression of channels and their incorporation into working multiunit channels.[21] Decreased gene expression will have effects similar to those due to loss-of-function variants. Ion channel expression decreases in patients with ischemic heart disease, which is one risk factor for sensitivity to QT-prolonging drugs.[46] Variants also affect

TABLE 44–1. Sample of variants that are characterized as being associated with functional changes in key cardiac ion channel genes.[a]

Gene	Site or variant	Class	Drug	Functional effect	Clinical effect	Minor allele frequency (AA : CA : AS : HL)	Reference
KCNH2	P347S	D,C	Cisapride Clarithromycin		TdP	0.0 : 0.0025 : 0.0 : 0.0	73, 74
KCNH2	N470D	L,B	E4031, astemizole, cisapride	Trafficking deficient, rescued *in vitro* by E4031, astemizole, cisapride	LQTS		44
KCNH2	D540K	B	MK-499	Increase speed of channel opening and decreases drug block			43
KCNH2	G601S	L,B	E4031, astemizole, cisapride	Trafficking deficient, rescued *in vitro* by E4031, astemizole, cisapride	LQTS		44, 75
KCNH2	S620T	B	Dofetilide	Critical for high-affinity binding			76
KCNH2	T623	B	MK-499	Critical for high-affinity binding			42
KCNH2	V625	B	MK-499	Critical for high-affinity binding			42
KCNH2	S631A	B	Dofetilide	Critical for high-affinity binding			45
KCNH2	G648	B	MK-499	Critical for high-affinity binding			42
KCNH2	Y652	B	MK-499, terfenadine, cisapride	Critical for high-affinity binding			42, 77
KCNH2	F656V	B	Dofetilide, quinidine, MK-499, terfenadine, cisapride	Necessary but not sufficient for binding			42, 45, 77
KCNH2	R784W	D	Amiodarone		TdP		33
KCNH2	K897T	F,C		Changes activation and deactivation parameters	Increased baseline QTc, potential TdP	0.0041 : 0.166 : 0.038 : 0.034	56, 73, 74
KCNE2	T8A	L,D,F,C	TMP/SMX, quinidine, amiodarone	Slight decrease in baseline current; similar or increased drug block relative to WT	TdP, QTP, LQTS(?)	0.0 : 0.0055 : 0.0 : 0.0	38, 39, 73,
KCNE2	Q9E	D,F,C	Erythromycin	Clarithromycin shows increased block relative to WT	TdP	0.015 : 0.0 : 0.0 : 0.0	38, 74
KCNE2	M54T	L,D,F	Procainamide	Decrease in baseline current; drug block similar to WT	TdP, LQTS		38, 39
KCNE2	I57T	L,D,F	Oxatomide	Decrease in baseline current	TdP, LQTS		38, 39
KCNE2	A116V	D,F	Quinidine, sulfamethoxazole	Decrease in baseline current	TdP		39
KCNQ1	R259C	L,F		Reduced current relative to WT	Hypokalemia-induced TdP, LQTS		40, 78
KCNQ1	T312	L,B	Novel I_{Ks} blockers	Drug binding site	LQTS		79–81
KCNQ1	Y315C	L,D,F	Cisapride	No current in mutant channel	TdP, LQTS		34, 35, 40,
KCNQ1	I337	B	Novel I_{Ks} blockers	Drug binding site			83
KCNQ1	F339	B	Novel I_{Ks} blockers	Drug binding site	LQTS		83, 84
KCNQ1	F340	B	Novel I_{Ks} blockers	Drug binding site	LQTS		83
KCNQ1	A344	B	Novel I_{Ks} blockers	Drug binding site	LQTS		34, 83
KCNQ1	R555C	L,D	Terfenadine, disopyramide, meflaquine, diuretics		TdP, LQTS		34
KCNQ1	R583C	L,D,F	Dofetilide	Reduced current	TdP, LQTS		33, 85
KCNQ1	G589D	L,F		Site required for binding of complex involved in β-adrenergic modulation	LQTS		64, 65
KCNQ1	Residues 588–616	F		Leucine zipper motif in C-terminus β-adrenergic modulation			64

E 44–1. *Continued*

ne	Site or variant	Class	Drug	Functional effect	Clinical effect	Minor allele frequency (AA:CA:AS:HL)	Reference
NE1	G38S	L,D,C			Potential TdP, LQTS	0.18:0.22:0.082:0.24	73, 74
NE1	Residues 39–43	B	Stilbene, fenamate	Drug interaction site			86
NE1	D76N	L,F	Stilbene, fenamate	Decreased baseline current, activity rescued by drug	LQTS		86
NE1	D85N	D,C	Sotalol, quinidine		TdP	0.0035:0.0055:0.0035:0.0	73
N5A	H558R	D,C			Potential TdP	0.29:0.20:0.092:0.23	73, 74
N5A	G615E	D,F	Quinidine	No effect seen *in vitro* relative to WT	TdP		33
N5A	L618F	D,F	Quinidine	No effect seen *in vitro* relative to WT	TdP		33
N5A	S1102Y	L,F,C		Small change in current	LQTS (weak)	0.063:0.0:0.0:0.0	60
N5A	F1250L	D,F	Sotalol	No effect seen *in vitro* relative to WT	TdP		33
N5A	D1790G	L,F	Flecainide	Decreased current relative to WT with drug	LQTS, unusual flecainide block		87, 88
N5A	Y1795C	L,F	Flecainide	Decreased current relative to WT with drug	LQTS, unusual flecainide block		87
N5A	Y1795H	L,F	Flecainide	Decreased current relative to WT with drug	BrS, unusual flecainide block		87
N5A	L1825P	C	Cisapride	Decreased current relative to WT; drug has no effect on current of mutant or WT	TdP		41

1 of these variants has been classified into one or more of five categories: L, causes LQTS; D, causes TdP; B, the site is demonstrated to be important for drug .ng *in vitro*; F, functionally characterized *in vitro*; C, common, i.e., seen in a reference population of healthy individuals. TdP, torsade de pointes; LQTS, long QT rome; TMP/SMX, trimethoprim/sulfamethoxazole; WT, wild-type.

the transport of the immature protein to the cell membrane.[47,48] In fact, most LQT2-associated mutations are trafficking defective.[49] Regulatory variants also likely affect the expression of mRNA for the LQTS-related genes.

The spatial distribution of ion channels throughout the myocardium is another factor that affects the risk of TdP.[46,50–53] KCNQ1 expression levels are lower in the Purkinje fibers and M cells than in other layers of the myocardium, so that the repolarization reserve in these layers is smaller.[54] The fact that two drugs cause the same degree of QT prolongation but are discordant in their "torsadogenic" potential is likely attributable to spatial heterogeneities in the cardiac channel expression and environment.[21,51–53,55]

Most of the ion channel variants responsible for LQTS are rare mutants. A few common variants in these genes have functional effects *in vitro*, or cause elevated risk for LQTS or for DI-LQT and TdP. These are termed subclinical LQTS polymorphisms. Such polymorphisms have a clinical impact only when combined with other risk factors. Polymorphic variants that have been implicated in either LQTS or drug-induced QT prolongation include KCNE2:T8A,[38,39] KCNE2:Q9E,[38] hERG:K897T,[56–58] hERG:R1047L,[59] SCN5A:S1103Y,[60] and KCNE1:D85N.[61,62] Relevant information on these variants is given in Table 44–1.

Pharmacodynamic effects have been associated with the β-adrenergic pathway that modulates the dynamics of the ion channel proteins. An association links a 2-SNP haplotype in the β_2-adrenergic receptor with risk for TdP.[63] Several intermediate molecules participate in this signaling pathway. The result is the phosphorylation and inactivation of KCNQ1. A key protein in this chain is ACAP9 (yotiao), which interacts with residues 588–616 of the KCNQ1 protein.[64] At least one LQTS-causing mutation has been discovered in this region.[64,65] Variants in other genes in this pathway may also affect ion channel dynamics.

Genes involved in sex hormone regulation may also affect the QT interval.[66,67] The baseline QTc of women is higher than that of men.[68] The QTc effect of ibutilide is correlated with the phase of the menstrual cycle.[67] Estradiol and progesterone may play a role in regulating the QT interval, so genetic factors that alter their levels could be involved in QT-associated risk.[67] This would help explain why the postpartum period is an especially arrhythmogenic period among women with congenital LQTS, particularly LQT2.[69,70] Sex hormones play a role in altering the levels of expression of cardiac potassium channels in an animal model.[71] A contradictory fact is that in one study, the baseline QTc interval did not track with the menstrual cycle phase.[72]

In summary, there are multiple genetic risk factors that may predispose an individual to increased risk for drug-induced QT prolongation. The effects of these are schematically illustrated in Figure 44–3B to contrast with the previously discussed pharmacokinetic effects. These include the following:

1. Poor metabolizer genotype or phenotype.
2. Presence of a mutation in a proven LQTS-causing gene.
3. Presence of a mutation or polymorphism in one of the suspected LQTS-related genes, including the ryanodine and ankyrin receptors, cardiac calcium channels, and cardiac potassium channels other than those currently associated with LQTS.
4. Presence of a subclinical LQT polymorphism that is not by itself sufficient to cause symptoms but may predispose an individual when combined with an additional stressor.
5. Polymorphisms in genes in the β-adrenergic and sex hormone pathways.
6. Decreased repolarization reserve due to spatial heterogeneity and/or decreased expression of ion channel proteins. This could be due to polymorphisms in genes responsible for drug transport in the myocardium.
7. Female gender.

Outlook

We conclude by briefly listing some open questions that are relevant to research into drug-induced QT prolongation. Each of these questions suggests open avenues for research in this area.

- *How much of the variability in the baseline QT interval is explained by genetics?* An understanding of how genetic variability drives baseline QT will also help us understand drug response variability. A key study would measure baseline QT intervals in healthy volunteers over a range of ages and then perform an association analysis, using genes in the pathways discussed. Variants that significantly affect baseline should be considered in subsequent studies for risk of drug-induced QT prolongation.
- *How much variability in drug-induced QT prolongation is genetic?* To answer this question, it is necessary to run association studies for drugs in each relevant class. Genes in the pathways already discussed are good candidates. These studies would be worthwhile only for drugs with significant QT effect, but that still meet significant medical needs.
- *Which genes/polymorphisms contribute?* We already know that variation in the LQTS-associated and drug metabolism genes are risk factors, and that genes in the β-adrenergic and hormonal pathways likely contribute to risk. Other cardiac ion channels and ion channel-related genes are candidates. For drug response, candidates would include genes involved in drug transport across different layers of the myocardium.
- *What are the genetic determinants of other ECG parameters (e.g., T wave morphology, QT interval dispersion)?* The QT interval is the main target of analysis in TQT studies, but it has been proposed that other ECG parameters may help predict the risk of arrhythmias. It would be worthwhile to subject these to the same genetic analysis as the QT interval.
- *What combination of genetics and clinical parameters best predicts significant predisposition to drug-induced QT prolongation and arrhythmia?* Genetics plays some role in risk for TdP, but so do other clinical parameters such as age and electrolyte status. Algorithms could be developed that merge genetic and phenotypic parameters to determine risk for TdP in patients taking QT-prolonging drugs. The test would have to be highly sensitive, specific, and cost effective, in light of the risk–benefit tradeoffs for the use of particular drug.

References

1. Barbey JT, Lazzara R, Zipes DP. Spontaneous adverse event reports of serious ventricular arrhythmias, QT prolongation, syncope, and sudden death in patients treated with cisapride. *J Cardiovasc Pharmacol Ther* 2002;7(2):65–76.
2. Haverkamp W, Martinez-Rubio A, Hief C, *et al.* Efficacy and safety of d,l-sotalol in patients with ventricular tachycardia and in survivors of cardiac arrest. *J Am Coll Cardiol* 1997;30(2):487–495.
3. Lehmann MH, Hardy S, Archibald D, quart B, MacNeil DJ. Sex difference in risk of torsade de pointes with d,l-sotalol. *Circulation* 1996;94(10): 2535–2541.
4. Hohnloser SH. Proarrhythmia with class III antiarrhythmic drugs: Types, risks, and management. *Am J Cardiol* 1997;80(8A):82G-89G.
5. Fermini B, Fossa AA. The impact of drug-induced QT interval prolongation on drug discovery and development. *Nat Rev Drug Discov* 2003;2(6):439–447.
6. Shah RR. Pharmacogenetic aspects of drug-induced torsade de pointes: Potential tool for improving clinical drug development and prescribing. *Drug Saf* 2004;27(3):145–172.
7. Roden DM. Drug-induced prolongation of the QT interval. *N Engl J Med* 2004;350(10):1013–1022.
8. Wysowski DK, Corken A, Gallo-Torres H, Talarico L, Rodriguez EM. Postmarketing reports of QT prolongation and ventricular arrhythmia in association with cisapride and Food and Drug Administration regulatory actions. *Am J Gastroenterol* 2001;96(6):1698–1703.
9. Priori SG, Napolitano C, Schwartz PJ. Low penetrance in the long-QT syndrome: Clinical impact. *Circulation* 1999;99(4):529–533.
10. Raser JM, O'Shea EK. Noise in gene expression: Origins, consequences, and control. *Science* 2005; 309(5743):2010–2013.
11. Devlin B, Risch N. A comparison of linkage disequilibrium measures for fine-scale mapping. *Genomics* 1995;29(2):311–322.
12. Marchini J, Cardon LR, Phillips MS, Donnelly P. The effects of human population structure on large genetic association studies. *Nat Genet* 2004;36(5): 512–517.
13. Pitman EJG. Significance tests which may be applied to samples from any populations. *J R Stat Soc Ser B* 1937;4:119–130.
14. Brown CC, Fears TR. Exact significance levels for multiple binomial testing with application to carcinogenicity screens. *Biometrics* 1981;37:763–774.
15. Heyse J, Rom D. Adjusting for multiplicity of statistical tests in the analysis of carcinogenicity studies. *Biometric J* 1988;30:883–896.
16. Drysdale CM, McGraw DW, Stack CB, *et al.* Complex promoter and coding region beta 2-adrenergic receptor haplotypes alter receptor expression and predict in vivo responsiveness. *Proc Natl Acad Sci USA* 2000;97(19):10483–10488.
17. Judson R, Stephens JC, Windemuth A. The predictive power of haplotypes in clinical response. *Pharmacogenomics* 2000;1(1):15–26.
18. Stephens JC, Schneider JA, Tanguay DA, *et al.* Haplotype variation and linkage disequilibrium in 313 human genes. *Science* 2001;293(5529):489–493.
19. Roden DM, Viswanathan PC. Genetics of acquired long QT syndrome. *J Clin Invest* 2005;115(8):2025–2032.
20. Moss AJ, Schwartz PJ. Delayed repolarization (QT or QTU prolongation) and malignant ventricular arrhythmias. *Mod Concepts Cardiovasc Dis* 1982; 51(3):85–90.
21. Roden DM. Taking the "idio" out of "idiosyncratic": Predicting torsades de pointes. *Pacing Clin Electrophysiol* 1998;21(5):1029–1034.
22. Priori SG, Napolitano C. Genetic defects of cardiac ion channels. The hidden substrate for torsades de pointes. *Cardiovasc Drugs Ther* 2002;16(2):89–92.
23. Judson R, Moss A. Pharmacogenomics in drug development: When and how to apply. In: Morganroth J, Gussak I, Eds. *Cardiac Safety of Non-Cardiac Drugs: Practical Guidelines for Clinical Research and Drug Development.* Totowa, NJ: Humana Press, 2005:83–103.
24. Monahan BP, Ferguson CL, Killeavy ES, Lloyd BK, Troy J, Cantilena LR Jr. Torsades de pointes occurring in association with terfenadine use. *JAMA* 1990;264(21):2788–2790.
25. Kirchheiner J, Brosen K, Dahl ML, *et al.* CYP2D6 and CYP2C19 genotype-based dose recommendations for antidepressants: A first step towards subpopulation-specific dosages. *Acta Psychiatr Scand* 2001;104(3):173–192.
26. Thummel KE, Wilkinson GR. In vitro and in vivo drug interactions involving human CYP3A. *Annu Rev Pharmacol Toxicol* 1998;38:389–430.
27. Fujita K. Food-drug interactions via human cytochrome P450 3A (CYP3A). *Drug Metabol Drug Interact* 2004;20(4):195–217.
28. Carlson AM, Morris LS. Coprescription of terfenadine and erythromycin or ketaconazole: An assessment of potential harm. *J Am Pharm Assoc (Wash)* 1996;NS36(4):263–269.
29. Thompson D, Oster G. Use of terfenadine and contraindicated drugs. *JAMA* 1996;275(17):1339–1341.

30. Curtis LH, Ostbye T, Sendersky V, *et al.* Prescription of QT-prolonging drugs in a cohort of about 5 million outpatients. *Am J Med* 2003;114(2):135–141.
31. Roe CM, Odell KW, Henderson RR. Concomitant use of antipsychotics and drugs that may prolong the QT interval. *J Clin Psychopharmacol* 2003;23(2):197–200.
32. Priori SG. Exploring the hidden danger of noncardiac drugs. *J Cardiovasc Electrophysiol* 1998;9(10):1114–1116.
33. Yang P, Kanki H, Drolet B, *et al.* Allelic variants in long-QT disease genes in patients with drug-associated torsades de pointes. *Circulation* 2002;105(16):1943–1948.
34. Donger C, Denjoy I, Berthet M, *et al.* KVLQT1 C-terminal missense mutation causes a forme fruste long-QT syndrome. *Circulation* 1997;96(9):2778–2781.
35. Napolitano C, Schwartz PJ, Brown AM, *et al.* Evidence for a cardiac ion channel mutation underlying drug-induced QT prolongation and life-threatening arrhythmias. *J Cardiovasc Electrophysiol* 2000;11(6):691–696.
36. Roden DM, Woosley RL, Primm RK. Incidence and clinical features of the quinidine-associated long QT syndrome: Implications for patient care. *Am Heart J* 1986;111(6):1088–1093.
37. Zehender M, Hohnloser S, Just H. QT-interval prolonging drugs: Mechanisms and clinical relevance of their arrhythmogenic hazards. *Cardiovasc Drugs Ther* 1991;5(2):515–530.
38. Abbott GW, Sesti F, Splawski I, *et al.* MiRP1 forms IKr potassium channels with HERG and is associated with cardiac arrhythmia. *Cell* 1999;97(2):175–187.
39. Sesti F, Abbott GW, Wei J, *et al.* A common polymorphism associated with antibiotic-induced cardiac arrhythmia. *Proc Natl Acad Sci USA* 2000;97(19):10613–10618.
40. Jongbloed R, Marcelis C, Velter C, Doevendans P, Geraedts J, Smeets H. DHPLC analysis of potassium ion channel genes in congenital long QT syndrome. *Hum Mutat* 2002;20(5):382–391.
41. Makita N, Horie M, Nakamura T, *et al.* Drug-induced long-QT syndrome associated with a subclinical SCN5A mutation. *Circulation* 2002;106(10):1269–1274.
42. Mitcheson JS, Chen J, Lin M, Culberson C, Sanguinetti MC. A structural basis for drug-induced long QT syndrome. *Proc Natl Acad Sci USA* 2000;97(22):12329–12333.
43. Mitcheson JS, Chen J, Sanguinetti MC. Trapping of a methanesulfonanilide by closure of the HERG potassium channel activation gate. *J Gen Physiol* 2000;115(3):229–240.
44. Ficker E, Obejero-Paz CA, Zhao S, Brown AM. The binding site for channel blockers that rescue misprocessed human long QT syndrome type 2 ether-a-gogo-related gene (HERG) mutations. *J Biol Chem* 2002;277(7):4989–4998.
45. Lees-Miller JP, Duan Y, Teng GQ, Duff HJ. Molecular determinant of high-affinity dofetilide binding to HERG1 expressed in Xenopus oocytes: Involvement of S6 sites. *Mol Pharmacol* 2000;57(2):367–374.
46. Haverkamp W, Breithardt G, Camm AJ, *et al.* The potential for QT prolongation and pro-arrhythmia by non-anti-arrhythmic drugs: Clinical and regulatory implications. Report on a Policy Conference of the European Society of Cardiology. *Cardiovasc Res* 2000;47(2):219–233.
47. Roti EC, Myers CD, Ayers RA, *et al.* Interaction with GM130 during HERG ion channel trafficking. Disruption by type 2 congenital long QT syndrome mutations. Human ether-a-go-go-related gene. *J Biol Chem* 2002;277(49):47779–47785.
48. Valdivia CR, Tester DJ, Rok BA, *et al.* A trafficking defective, Brugada syndrome-causing SCN5A mutation rescued by drugs. *Cardiovasc Res* 2004;62(1):53–62.
49. Anderson CL, Delisle BP, Anson BD, *et al.* Most LQT2 mutations reduce Kv11.1 (hERG) current by a class 2 (trafficking-deficient) mechanism. *Circulation* 2006;113(3):365–373.
50. El Sherif N, Caref EB, Yin H, Restivo M. The electrophysiological mechanism of ventricular arrhythmias in the long QT syndrome. Tridimensional mapping of activation and recovery patterns. *Circ Res* 1996;79(3):474–492.
51. Akar FG, Yan GX, Antzelevitch C, Rosenbaum DS. Unique topographical distribution of M cells underlies reentrant mechanism of torsade de pointes in the long-QT syndrome. *Circulation* 2002;105(10):1247–1253.
52. Shimizu W, McMahon B, Antzelevitch C. Sodium pentobarbital reduces transmural dispersion of repolarization and prevents torsades de pointes in models of acquired and congenital long QT syndrome. *J Cardiovasc Electrophysiol* 1999;10(2):154–164.
53. Keating MT, Sanguinetti MC. Molecular and cellular mechanisms of cardiac arrhythmias. *Cell* 2001;104(4):569–580.
54. Liu DW, Antzelevitch C. Characteristics of the delayed rectifier current (IKr and IKs) in canine ventricular epicardial, midmyocardial, and endocardial myocytes. A weaker IKs contributes to the

longer action potential of the M cell. *Circ Res* 1995;76(3):351–365.
55. Houltz B, Darpo B, Edvardsson N, *et al.* Electrocardiographic and clinical predictors of torsades de pointes induced by almokalant infusion in patients with chronic atrial fibrillation or flutter: A prospective study. *Pacing Clin Electrophysiol* 1998;21(5): 1044–1057.
56. Bezzina CR, Verkerk AO, Busjahn A, *et al.* A common polymorphism in KCNH2 (HERG) hastens cardiac repolarization. *Cardiovasc Res* 2003;59(1):27–36.
57. Crotti L, Lundquist M, Roden DM, George AL Jr, Schwartz PJ. Common KCNH2 polymorphism (K897T) as a genetic modifier of congenital long QT syndrome. *Heart Rhythm* 2005;Abstract Suppl.: P1–P19.
58. Kannankeril PJ, Norris K, Gillani M, George AL Jr, Roden DM. A common polymorphism in KCNH2 (HERG) eliminates gender differences in drug-induced QT prolongation. *Heart Rhythm* 2005; Abstract Suppl.:P2–P34.
59. Sun Z, Milos PM, Thompson JF, *et al.* Role of a KCNH2 polymorphism (R1047 L) in dofetilide-induced torsades de pointes. *J Mol Cell Cardiol* 2004;37(5):1031–1039.
60. Splawski I, Timothy KW, Tateyama M, *et al.* Variant of SCN5A sodium channel implicated in risk of cardiac arrhythmia. *Science* 2002;297(5585):1333–1336.
61. George AL Jr, Roden DM. Method for screening for susceptibility to drug-induced cardiac arrhythmia. U.S. patent US 6,458,542 B1; 2002.
62. Westenskow P, Splawski I, Timothy KW, Keating MT, Sanguinetti MC. Compound mutations. A common cause of severe long-QT syndrome. *Circulation* 2004;109(15):1834–1841.
63. Kanki H, Yang P, Xie HG, Kim RB, George AL Jr, Roden DM. Polymorphisms in beta-adrenergic receptor genes in the acquired long QT syndrome. *J Cardiovasc Electrophysiol* 2002;13(3):252–256.
64. Marx SO, Kurokawa J, Reiken S, *et al.* Requirement of a macromolecular signaling complex for beta adrenergic receptor modulation of the KCNQ1-KCNE1 potassium channel. *Science* 2002;295(5554): 496–499.
65. Piippo K, Swan H, Pasternack M, *et al.* A founder mutation of the potassium channel KCNQ1 in long QT syndrome: Implications for estimation of disease prevalence and molecular diagnostics. *J Am Coll Cardiol* 2001;37(2):562–568.
66. Hara M, Danilo P Jr, Rosen MR. Effects of gonadal steroids on ventricular repolarization and on the response to E4031. *J Pharmacol Exp Ther* 1998;285 (3):1068–1072.
67. Rodriguez I, Kilborn MJ, Liu XK, Pezzullo JC, Woosley RL. Drug-induced QT prolongation in women during the menstrual cycle. *JAMA* 2001;285 (10):1322–1326.
68. Stramba-Badiale M, Locati EH, Martinelli A, Courville J, Schwartz PJ. Gender and the relationship between ventricular repolarization and cardiac cycle length during 24-h Holter recordings. *Eur Heart J* 1997;18(6):1000–1006.
69. Rashba EJ, Zareba W, Moss AJ, *et al.* Influence of pregnancy on the risk for cardiac events in patients with hereditary long QT syndrome. LQTS Investigators. *Circulation* 1998;97(5):451–456.
70. Khositseth A, Tester DJ, Will ML, Bell CM, Ackerman MJ. Identification of a common genetic substrate underlying postpartum cardiac events in congenital long QT syndrome. *Heart Rhythm* 2004; 1(1):60–64.
71. Drici MD, Burklow TR, Haridasse V, Glazer RI, Woosley RL. Sex hormones prolong the QT interval and downregulate potassium channel expression in the rabbit heart. *Circulation* 1996;94(6):1471–1474.
72. Burke JH, Goldberger JJ, Ehlert FA, Kruse JT, Parker MA, Kadish AH. Gender differences in heart rate before and after autonomic blockade: Evidence against an intrinsic gender effect. *Am J Med* 1996; 100(5):537–543.
73. Paulussen AD, Gilissen RA, Armstrong M, *et al.* Genetic variations of KCNQ1, KCNH2, SCN5A, KCNE1, and KCNE2 in drug-induced long QT syndrome patients. *J Mol Med* 2004;82(3):182–188.
74. Ackerman MJ, Tester DJ, Jones GS, Will ML, Burrow CR, Curran ME. Ethnic differences in cardiac potassium channel variants: Implications for genetic susceptibility to sudden cardiac death and genetic testing for congenital long QT syndrome. *Mayo Clin Proc* 2003;78(12):1479–1487.
75. Swan H, Viitasalo M, Piippo K, Laitinen P, Kontula K, Toivonen L. Sinus node function and ventricular repolarization during exercise stress test in long QT syndrome patients with KvLQT1 and HERG potassium channel defects. *J Am Coll Cardiol* 1999;34(3): 823–829.
76. Ficker E, Jarolimek W, Kiehn J, Baumann A, Brown AM. Molecular determinants of dofetilide block of HERG K+ channels. *Circ Res* 1998;82(3):386–395.
77. Chen J, Seebohm G, Sanguinetti MC. Position of aromatic residues in the S6 domain, not inactivation, dictates cisapride sensitivity of HERG and eag potassium channels. *Proc Natl Acad Sci USA* 2002; 99(19):12461–12466.
78. Kubota T, Shimizu W, Kamakura S, Horie M. Hypokalemia-induced long QT syndrome with an

underlying novel missense mutation in S4-S5 linker of KCNQ1. *J Cardiovasc Electrophysiol* 2000;11(9): 1048–1054.
79. Seebohm G, Scherer CR, Busch AE, Lerche C. Identification of specific pore residues mediating KCNQ1 inactivation. A novel mechanism for long QT syndrome. *J Biol Chem* 2001;276(17):13600–13605.
80. Wang Q, Curran ME, Splawski I, *et al.* Positional cloning of a novel potassium channel gene: KVLQT1 mutations cause cardiac arrhythmias. *Nat Genet* 1996;12(1):17–23.
81. Shalaby FY, Levesque PC, Yang WP, *et al.* Dominant-negative KvLQT1 mutations underlie the LQT1 form of long QT syndrome. *Circulation* 1997;96(6): 1733–1736.
82. Splawski I, Shen J, Timothy KW, Vincent GM, Lehmann MH, Keating MT. Genomic structure of three long QT syndrome genes: KVLQT1, HERG, and KCNE1. *Genomics* 1998;51(1):86–97.
83. Seebohm G, Chen J, Strutz N, Culberson C, Lerche C, Sanguinetti MC. Molecular determinants of KCNQ1 channel block by a benzodiazepine. *Mol Pharmacol* 2003;64(1):70–77.
84. Ackerman MJ, Schroeder JJ, Berry R, *et al.* A novel mutation in KVLQT1 is the molecular basis of inherited long QT syndrome in a near-drowning patient's family. *Pediatr Res* 1998;44(2):148–153.
85. Splawski I, Shen J, Timothy KW, *et al.* Spectrum of mutations in long-QT syndrome genes. KVLQT1, HERG, SCN5A, KCNE1, and KCNE2. *Circulation* 2000;102(10):1178–1185.
86. Abitbol I, Peretz A, Lerche C, Busch AE, Attali B. Stilbenes and fenamates rescue the loss of I(KS) channel function induced by an LQT5 mutation and other IsK mutants. *EMBO J* 1999;18(15):4137–4148.
87. Liu H, Tateyama M, Clancy CE, Abriel H, Kass RS. Channel openings are necessary but not sufficient for use-dependent block of cardiac Na(+) channels by flecainide: Evidence from the analysis of disease-linked mutations. *J Gen Physiol* 2002;120(1):39–51.
88. Abriel H, Wehrens XH, Benhorin J, Kerem B, Kass RS. Molecular pharmacology of the sodium channel mutation D1790G linked to the long-QT syndrome. *Circulation* 2000;102(8):921–925.
89. Judson R, Salisbury BA, Reed CR, Ackerman MJ. Pharmacogenetic issues in thorough QT trials. *Mol Diagn Ther* 2006;10(3):153–162.

45
Mechanisms of Drug-Induced Cardiac Toxicity

Masayasu Hiraoka

Introduction

Drug-induced cardiac toxicity may develop in various functional and structural elements of the heart, but here, the description of cardiac toxicity will be limited to the area of electrical activity. Cardiac toxicity is manifested as proarrhythmia that represents a new development or a worsening of arrhythmias in patients with or without clinical symptoms leading to more severe symptoms such as hemodynamic deterioration, syncope, or sudden death. Manifestations of cardiac toxicity depend not only on high concentrations of drug administration, but also on the types and actions of drugs, the pharmacokinetics, underlying heart disease, genetic considerations, and other intervening conditions for drug actions. As early recognition of proarrhythmia and avoidance of factors exacerbating the clinical symptoms are mandatory for patient care, a precise understanding of the mechanisms and associated conditions involved in the development of cardiac toxicity is of prime importance.

While manifestations of cardiac toxicity have been recognized in clinical cardiology for many years, the first study attracting broad and renewed attention was the report by the Cardiac Arrhythmia Suppression Trial (CAST) Study, which disclosed increased mortality in patients with recent myocardial infarction taking Na^+ channel blockers for treatment of ventricular arrhythmias.[1] The exact reason for this increased mortality resulting from the drugs was not known, but toxic manifestations of Na^+ channel blockers in the presence of an ischemic condition were likely to be involved. Since then many examples of proarrhythmia have been presented for antiarrhythmic drugs as well as for other therapeutic modalities including both cardiac and noncardiac drugs. The examples of drug-induced cardiac toxicity include proarrhythmia caused by drugs with K^+ channel blocking properties for QT prolongation and development of torsade de pointes (TdP), and by antiarrhythmic drugs of Na^+ channel blockers and related compounds for worsening arrhythmia and increased cardiac mortality. A detailed understanding of drug-induced cardiac toxicity has resulted from progress in the fields of cardiac electrophysiology and electropharmacology, as well as clarification of molecular mechanisms for inherited arrhythmic disorders, including long QT syndrome[2,3] and Brugada syndrome.[4,5]

Drug-Induced QT Prolongation and Proarrhythmia

Drug Target for QT Prolongation

While congenital long QT syndrome (LQTS) demonstrates unique electrophysiological and clinical manifestations, gene mutations of ion channels as the pathogenesis of the disease have had a great impact on the mechanism of QT prolongation and the development of TdP associated with the use of drugs. The incidence of congenital LQTS is assumed to be approximately 1/5000 population; however, because of low or incomplete penetrance in the mutation carriers,[6] the actual incidence of QT prolongation and TdP may be much less than that predicted by the number of gene carriers. Drugs with proven QT prolongation and TdP are estimated to comprise approximately 2–3% of all written prescriptions,[7] and, therefore, the incidence of drug-induced TdP must be much higher than TdP in congenital LQTS.

Quinidine is probably the first example of an agent recognized as inducing QT prolongation and proarrhythmia. Soon after its clinical introduction, quinidine was associated with syncope, although there was no delineation of the precise nature of the effect. Later, syncope was proved to be caused by a pause-dependent ventricular tachyarrhythmia, now recognized as TdP.[8,9] Quinidine was then shown to be a potent blocker of the delayed outward K^+ current, especially I_{kr}.[9,10] I_{kr} is now known to be encoded by one of the etiological genes of LQTS, human ether-à-go-go-related gene (*hERG*) (*KCNH2*), and *hERG* has also been shown to be a target for the K^+ channel blocking drugs.[9,11] While many existing and newly developed antiarrhythmic drugs prolong the QT interval, because of a high affinity binding to the hERG channel,[9,11] various cardiac and noncardiac drugs have also been demonstrated to affect the hERG/I_{kr} channel. It is now evident that diverse types of drugs with different chemical structures and pharmacological profiles affect the hERG/I_{kr} channel, causing QT prolongation and development of TdP, as a manifestation of drug toxicity.[9]

The reason why many drugs bind with high affinity to hERG as compared to other K^+ channels has recently been clarified. *hERG (KCNH2)* is a primary pore-forming subunit with six transmembrane spanning regions (S1–S6) composing heteromeric assembly with accessory subunits, *MiRP1 (KCNE2)*.[12,13] The drug-binding sites are mainly located on the S6 region of the main subunit. Key features of the hERG channel protein, absent in other K^+ channels, seem to underlie the basis of inhibition by many structurally unrelated drugs.[14] The hERG (KCNH2) protein lacks proline groups within S6. The lack of proline groups is assumed to facilitate access of drugs to the pore region from the intracellular side of the channel to block the channel current. Two aromatic residues, Tyr-652 and Phe-656, located in the central cavity of the channel (S6) are thought to provide high-affinity drug-binding sites[15]. Two aromatic residues are lacking in other K^+ channels in similar pore regions. The accessory subunit, *MiRP1 (KCNE2)*, also determines the drug sensitivity.[13]

Mechanism of hERG Channel Block and Proarrhythmia

Drug binding to the hERG channel develops in a state-dependent manner similar to Na^+ channel block binding to the Na^+ channel.[16] Drugs bind to the channel at open (O) and/or inactivated (I) channel states and dissociate mainly from the rested (R) state. If drugs with I_{kr}-blocking properties display state-dependent (O/I state) affinity to the channel, tachycardia is expected to promote binding of the drugs causing stronger inhibition of I_{kr}. Conversely, bradycardia would cause less inhibition. When the effects of the K^+ channel blockers on action potential duration (APD) were examined, these drugs demonstrated a prominent APD prolongation at a slow heart rate and the least action at a fast rate. The effects were attributed to a "reverse use dependence" of the blocking action,[17] which is thought to be a major cause of proarrhythmia or toxicity by these drugs. However, since the K^+ channel blockers have been shown to inhibit I_{kr} in a use-dependent manner,[18] and tachycardia activates another K^+ current, I_{ks}, to shorten the APD, reverse use dependence is not a major mechanism of action for these drugs on the hERG channel itself, but it is due to a combined manifestation with the other current activation at rapid rates.[19]

Factors other than APD prolongation in the underlying ventricular myocytes contribute to straightforward QT prolongation. There are heterogeneous cell types in the ventricle with different AP morphologies, mainly attributed to different expressions of ion channels.[20,21] In particular, transmural heterogeneity of APD and AP configurations among epicardial, endocardial, and midmyocardial (M) cells critically influences QT prolongation and T wave morphology.[20] The block of I_{kr} causes more marked APD prolongation in M cells because of less developed I_{ks} than in the other two cell types, leading to increased transmural heterogeneity or disparity of APD and resulting in prominent QT prolongation. In addition, transmural dispersion of APD is modified by adrenergic stimulation, since catecholamine increases the transmural dispersion of repolarization.[22]

Prolongation of APD provides two factors essential for proarrhythmia. Delayed repolarization and prolonged APD may result in early afterdepolarization (EAD), mainly due to the participation of the window L-type Ca^{2+} current ($I_{Ca.}$),[23] and on some occasions by the late I_{Na}[24] or Na^+/Ca^{2+} exchanger current.[25] The EADs are generally believed to develop more easily in Purkinje fibers than in muscle cells, but recent findings have shown that M cell layers can develop EADs as readily as Purkinje fibers.[22] The appearance of EADs causing premature ventricular contractions (PVCs) may be a trigger for the initiation of arrhythmia. At the same time, nonuniform APD prolongation will cause increased dispersion of repolarization among different regions of the ventricle and widening of transmural APD dispersion with slow conduction and block resulting in inhomogeneous excitations. These factors provide the substrate for the development of reentry and the conditions that contribute to the maintenance and perpetuation of arrhythmia.[22,26]

As to the genesis of the unique morphology of TdP in an electrocardiogram (ECG), animal studies suggest that the time-dependent functional arcs of block usually located at the boundary of the M cell and epicardial cell layers appear with a slightly different activation sequence in each succeeding beat allowing reentrant excitations across the ventricular wall.[27,28] In wedge preparations, TdP can readily be elicited by programmed stimulation from the epicardium,[29] whereas programmed stimulation from the endocardium in humans rarely elicits TdP.

Factors Determining Clinical Development of QT Prolongation and Proarrhythmia

Certain drugs with the proven ability to prolong both the APD and QT interval in *in vitro* or animal experiments for some reason do not tend to elicit proarrhythmia in clinical use. On the other hand, some drugs exhibit a high potency for proarrhythmia in patients with similar or even less potent action on prolongation of both the APD and QT interval.[26,30–33] These results imply that toxic manifestations by K^+ channel blockers are not dependent solely on the degree of QT prolongation, but that there are other factors determining development of clinical proarrhythmia. These factors include high doses and routes of drug application, drug action on other channels, age, gender, the presence of organic heart diseases, electrolyte imbalance, pharmacokinetics and pharmakogenetics, silent mutation and polymorphism, etc. (Figure 45–1). Another reason might be the effects of repolarization on dispersion.

While a rapid and high dose of drug application is prone to result in proarrhythmia, drug actions on other channels such as the L-type Ca^{2+}

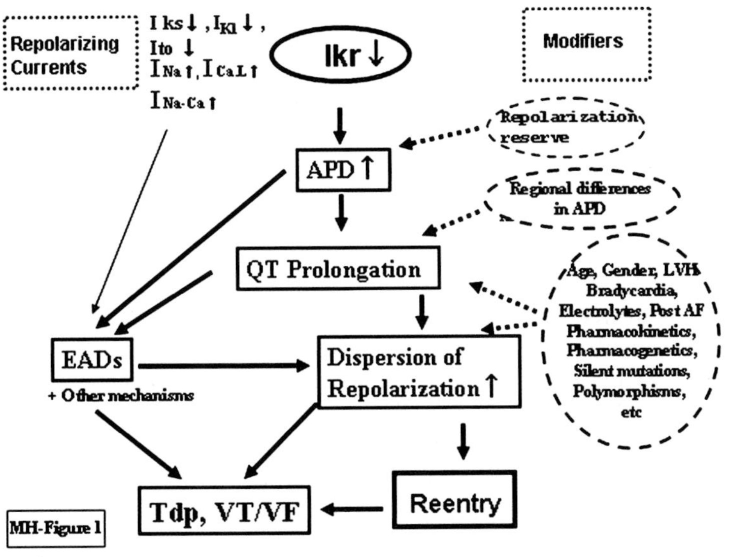

Figure 45–1. Factors modifying the development of QT prolongation and TdP. The main target for QT prolongation is the hERG/I_{Kr} channel and there are many factors involved in the appearance of QT prolongation and TdP (see details in the text).

channel and other K^+ channels may determine the appearance of QT prolongation and TdP. Drugs such as amiodarone also block late I_{Na}, which is more prominent in M cells, and thus may not prolong APD as much compared to more pure K^+ channel blockers. The combined use of potential QT-prolonging drugs may also precipitate the development of toxicity.[34] In a study of 110,000 prescriptions, 22.8% involved taking at least one QT-prolonging drug, 9.4% taking two, and 0.7% taking three; 22% of the patients were over 65 years of age and 74% were women. QT duration is longer in females. The risk of TdP is assumed to be 1.9% in men and 4.1% in women.[35–37] The reason for the female predominance is hormonal influences on QT intervals, but a precise mechanism of hormonal actions on QT intervals and proarrhythmia has not been determined.

Electrolyte imbalance, especially hypokalemia, is an important predisposing condition for the development of QT prolongation and proarrhythmia. Hypokalemia causes APD prolongation due to decreased K^+ conductance, and low external K^+ further modifies the function of the hERG K channel to decrease I_{kr} leading to APD prolongation, since low K^+ accelerates fast inactivation and decreases the ability of K^+ to inhibit Na^+ on the hERG channel.[38–40] Bradycardia is prone to cause QT prolongation and TdP. The conditions after conversion to sinus rhythm from atrial fibrillation are associated with a high incidence in QT prolongation and proarrhythmia without a mechanistic explanation.[41,42] The presence of organic heart disease is also a high risk factor for proarrhythmia, probably due to the fact that hypertrophy and heart failure are associated with prolonged APD due to channel remodeling in the basal condition.[43]

There are four major processes in the pharmacokinetics: absorption, distribution, metabolism, and excretion. Two organs are important for these processes. Hepatic and renal functions are critical for metabolism and excretion of drugs, and impairment of these organs is prone to cause drug retention in plasma. This may explain why elderly persons are susceptible to the development of drug toxicity due to possible impairment in their hepatic and renal functions. In addition, variants of genes in specific drug-metabolizing and drug-transporting molecules may become a critical cause of pharmacogenetically determined adverse drug toxicity.[44] An antihistaminic agent, terfenadine, had been known to prolong the QT interval to a modest degree in animal experiments and in early clinical experience.[45,46] Later, terfenadine was found to cause TdP and sudden cardiac death after the drug was on the market and had been widely used. A later study then disclosed that terfenadine undergoes first pass metabolism in the liver through the enzyme action of CYP3A4 and changes to its active metabolite, which possesses antihistaminic action but no ability for QT prolongation.[47] This is the reason why oral administration of terfenadine does not cause marked QT prolongation but still exhibits the main action. The activity of CYP3A4 varies widely in response to various drugs including macrolide antibiotics, ketoconazol, cimetidine, and amiodarone, which suppress this enzyme function.[47,48] In addition, smoking, hepatic diseases, polymorphism, and grapefruit intake have been proven to inhibit the function of CYP3A4.[49] Therefore, decreased CYP3A4 function associated with these conditions causes a large increase in terfenadine concentration in plasma up to 5–20 times the normal range so that QT prolongation and proarrhythmia as toxic manifestations are readily induced.

Mutations of ion channel genes responsible for LQTS have been implicated as a risk factor, and individuals who are mutation carriers constitute high risk groups for drug-induced QT prolongation and proarrhythmia as shown in several studies in relatively small numbers of patient series. Some of these individuals represent subclinical LQTS with subtle dysfunction showing normal or borderline QT intervals in a basal condition, and display manifest QT prolongation upon exposure to drugs.[50–53] They are assumed to represent a silent mutation or forme fruste LQTS. Some polymorphisms of ion channel genes are also implicated as a cause of drug-induced QT prolongation.[54–57] The polymorphisms in channel genes have been found in *KVLQT1*, *KCNE1*, *KCNE2*, *hERG*, and *SCN5A*. While cases of polymorphisms associated with drug-induced proarrhythmia have been accumulating in the literature, they are mainly found in case presentations and in a small series of population studies, and the actual incidence among large cohorts is not known. Therefore, variants in ion channel genes may be a contributing factor for drug-induced QT prolongation and proarrhythmia, but their actual roles in the general population need to be determined in further studies.

Mechanism of Cardiac Toxicity Induced by Na^+ Channel Blockers

Mechanistic Actions of Na^+ Channel Blockers on the Na^+ Channel

Na^+ channel blockers bind with high affinity to the Na^+ channel, decreasing the density of I_{Na}. The block of I_{Na} by Na^+ channel blockers develops in a voltage- and time-dependent manner and, thus, the block is use or frequency dependent.[17,58] The properties of voltage- and time-dependent blocks indicate that the drugs preferentially bind to open (O) and/or inactivated (I) states of the Na^+ channel (channel state affinity). Depending on channel state affinity, Na^+ channel blockers are divided into two groups: open channel affinity and inactivated channel affinity. Another feature of blocking properties involves the speed of drug binding and unbinding to and from the Na^+ channel (kinetics of the block); in particular, the kinetics of unbinding (dissociation) is an important determinant for inhibitory action and strength of inhibition. Drugs are divided into three groups depending on their dissociation kinetics: fast, intermediate, and slow.[59,60] Slow kinetic drugs show the strongest inhibition among the three groups. Access of drugs to binding sites of the Na^+ channel, another factor in the inhibitory action, is determined by physicochemical properties, such as the charged and uncharged fraction of drugs; these properties determine the mode of access through hydrophilic or hydrophobic pathways.[61]

The cardiac Na^+ channel is encoded by *SCN5A*, a main subunit, and the binding sites of Na^+ channel blockers are thought to be located in S6 of the main subunit.[60] As a result of the Na^+ channel block, there is a decrease in peak current density, changes in voltage dependency, and delayed reactivation of I_{Na}.[59,60] Since I_{Na} forms the upstroke phase of the action potential determining excitability and conduction velocity, decreased I_{Na} causes depressed excitability and slowed conduction and block. Furthermore, postrepolarization refractoriness is widened because of delayed recovery from the I_{Na} inactivation. These actions by Na^+ channel blockers may exert antiarrhythmic effects by decreasing or eliminating abnormal excitations and block of abnormal impulse propagation. With widened postrepolarization refractoriness together with depressed excitability and slowed conduction, tachycardia and short-coupled extrasystolic excitations can be eliminated. On the other hand, the actions of Na^+ channel blockers on I_{Na} tend to suppress excitations and decrease conduction velocity in the basic rhythm leading to bradycardia, P-Q, and QRS widening in the ECG. Further progression of the drug effects results in depressed conduction velocity with the development of one-way block and inhomogeneous impulse propagation; these conditions favor an appearance of reentry. Widening of postrepolarization refractoriness promotes enlargement of the excitable gap, which precipitates macroreentry. These proarrhythmic effects are more prone to develop in injured or pathological regions in a heart with depressed function than in normal hearts, and, therefore, diseased hearts are more susceptible to toxic manifestations by Na^+ channel blockers than healthy hearts. Clinical examples of such toxic manifestations during the treatment of arrhythmias by Na^+ channel blockers are associated with the new development of or the exacerbation of ventricular tachyarrhythmias. In particular, class IC type drugs are known to induce an incessant form of tachycardia, which is one possible reason for the increased mortality in the CAST study from flecainide and encainide used to treat ischemic heart disease.[1] The development of 1:1 atrioventricular (AV) conduction or atrial flutter is also seen, where decreased atrial excitations allow more impulses to AV conduction. The new appearance or increased incidence of premature excitations and tachyarrhythmias, marked sinus bradycardia, sinus arrest, and AV block may also be regarded as toxic manifestations by Na^+ channel blockers.

Mechanism Responsible for Toxic Manifestations of the Na⁺ Channel Block

Since Na^+ channel blockers have access to and from the channel in a state-dependent manner, various factors may contribute to an excess accumulation of drugs that is dependent on the channel state and may promote toxicity (Figure 45–2). The Na^+ channel recycles three states, R, O, and I, at each excitation. The access of Na^+ channel blockers to the Na^+ channel progresses either from the O and/or the I states; dissociation occurs mainly in the R state, but some drugs dissociate from the O state. In addition to dose-dependent access of drugs, increased numbers and rapid excitations (tachycardia) promote drug binding to the channel, especially drugs with open channel affinity. Prolonged APD increases drug binding to the I state of the channel by drugs with inactivated state affinity. Depolarization of the resting membrane potential increases in the I state allowing more binding by drugs with I state affinity. Slowed or decreased dissociation of drugs from the channel is anticipated to cause excess accumulation, leading to toxic manifestations. Tachycardia shortens the diastolic intervals leading to decreased dissociation of drugs during the R state. Some drugs with open channel affinity, however, are trapped in the R state and an excess of drugs from the channel develops during the O state. Therefore, prolongation of diastolic intervals retards rather than promotes dissociation of drugs from the channel in certain types of drugs with properties for R state trapping.

There are modifying factors affecting the channel state-dependent process and influencing drug actions.[59,60] Extracellular ionic concentrations strongly influence the actions of Na^+ channel blockers in various ways. Extracellular Na^+ antagonizes the access or binding of Na^+ channel blockers to the Na^+ channel and, therefore, decreased $[Na^+]_o$ may accelerate the drug effects and manifest toxic actions. In other words, intoxication by Na^+ channel blockers is relieved with the administration of Na^+, such as Na^+-bicarbonate. Increased $[Ca^{2+}]_o$ antagonizes the channel function to decrease I_{Na}. Increased $[K^+]_o$ depolarizes the resting membrane potential resulting in an I-state channel; this leads to increased binding by I-state affinity drugs. A change in pH has an important influence on drug effects. Protonation affects the fractions of charged and uncharged forms of the drugs, leading to altered binding and dissociation from the channel as well as modification of the blocking potency.[61,62] Further, acidosis itself decreases I_{Na}. Therefore, excess accumulation of drug and/or increased blocking actions are anticipated to develop in acidosis. Channel remod-

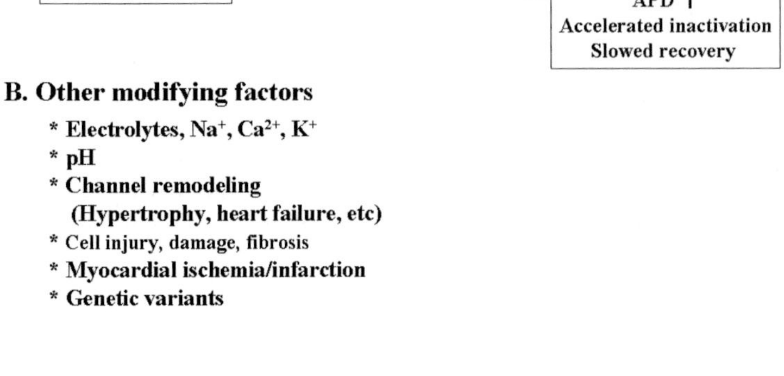

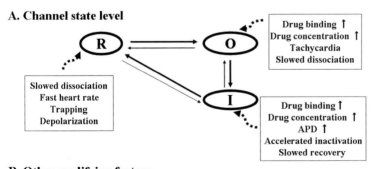

FIGURE 45–2. Factors modifying toxic manifestations by Na^+ channel blockers. (A) Factors influencing the excess accumulation of the drugs at a channel state level. (B) Other modifying factors involved in toxic manifestations of Na^+ channel blockers.

eling in various pathological conditions may influence the drug actions. In atrial fibrillation, Na^+ channel function is decreased. In hypertrophy and heart failure, the remodeling of K^+ and other channels progresses; this may promote the action of Na^+ channel blockers due to altered membrane potential, channel state, and protein expression. These factors may partly explain why patients with organic heart disease are at high risk for the development of proarrhythmia.

Myocardial ischemia/infarction is an important basal condition susceptible to toxic manifestations of Na^+ channel blockers. During acute ischemia and infarction accumulation of $[K^+]_o$ and acidosis develop, together with cell injury, leading to depolarization in the resting membrane potential; these conditions promote decreased I_{Na} and altered AP configuration.[63] Tachycardia and excess catecholamine may modify the drug effects. All these factors tend to accentuate drug actions on the channel. In healing myocardial infarction, fibrosis and patchy necrosis may intervene among normal cell regions at the border of the infarct, where conduction is prone to be slowed and/or inhomogeneous. At these areas, drug actions may manifest an easy induction of slow conduction, inexcitability, one-way block, and reentry, so that drug toxicity is prone to develop. Likewise, cell injury and damage provide susceptible conditions prone to lead to toxic manifestations of the drugs.

An Na^+ channel blocker, propafenone, is eliminated by metabolism through CYP2D6, and in individuals with deficient CYP2D6 activity (poor metabolizers), the parent drug tends to accumulate in the plasma. The poor metabolizers commonly show side effects of propafenone including marked bradycardia due to β blockade, conduction block, new and increased incidences of PVCs, and the development of an incessant form of tachycardia by the Na^+ channel blockade.[64,65] CYP2D6 activity is absent in 7% of whites and African-Americans since they are homozygous for loss of function alleles. CYP2D6 activity is inhibited in the remaining 93% (extensive metabolizers) by drugs such as tricyclic or other antidepressants.[64,65] Therefore, variants of the genes encoding the regulatory protein for drug metabolism may be a factor contributing to the development of toxic manifestations of the drugs.

Na^+ channel blockers are known to unmask the ST elevation of Brugada syndrome[5,66–70] (Figure 45–3). A proposed mechanism for the ST elevation in right precordial leads (V1–V3) in Brugada syndrome is explained by a voltage gradient during AP repolarization between epicardial and endocardial cells in the right ventricular outflow region. A decrease in I_{Na} causes an increased notch at an early phase of repolarization in epicardial cells due to prominent I_{to} and subsequent dome formation at the plateau, but no such changes in endocardial cells; this creates or increases a voltage-gradient-producing/or augmenting ST-segment elevation. Depending on the size of the notch and dome formation, ST-segment elevation is manifested as either a saddleback type or coved type with or without a negative T wave.[5] Sometimes epicardial APs become abortive; the voltage gradient between epicardial and endocardial cells is then further enlarged to manifest a prominent ST elevation merging into a positive T wave ("box-like" ST elevation). When changes in epicardial AP configurations appear in variable degrees depending on the effects of I_{Na} inhibition and changes develop on a beat-by-beat basis, T wave alternans may be observed.[71–73] Delays in excitations of the right ventricular epicardium at or near the final repolarization phase of endocardial APs due to a local conduction delay, possibly as a result of toxic manifestations of the drugs, are another feature of "box-like" ST elevations (Figure 45–4). While the above features of ST elevation in different degrees are associated with the appearance of PVCs and ventricular tachycardias after administration of Na^+ channel blockers, the effects may be considered as toxic manifestations of the drugs. However, when the drugs can induce ST elevation of only the saddleback or coved type without ventricular arrhythmias, the effects may or may not be regarded as a toxic action, unless the drugs are administered for the purpose of unmasking or for the diagnosis of Brugada syndrome. In this situation, ST elevation is frequently associated with a prolonged QRS duration and/or P-Q interval, which indicate an undesirable action of Na^+ channel blockers (see Figure 45–3).

The ST-segment elevation and unmasking effect of Brugada syndrome are produced by maneuvers that are decreased in inward currents of I_{Na} or $I_{Ca.L}$, and are increased in outward K^+ currents.[5]

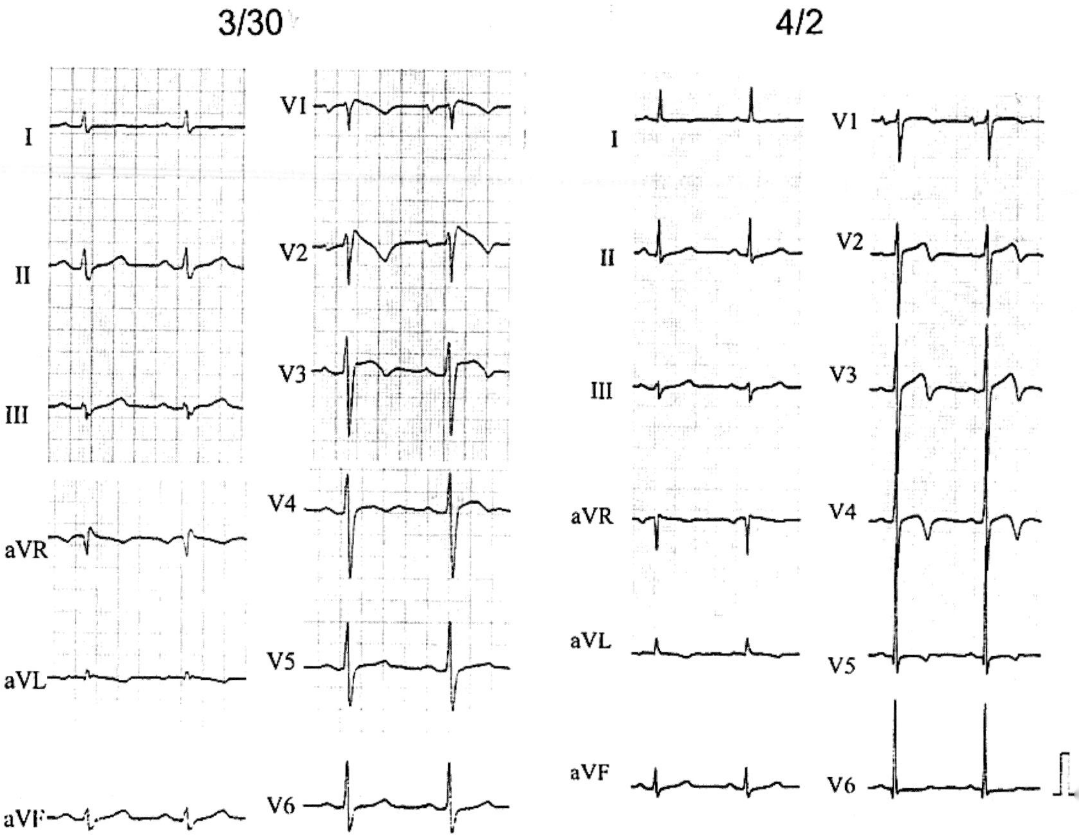

FIGURE 45–3. Manifestation of a Brugada type ST elevation by a class IC agent, pilsicainide. An 82-year-old woman with aortic and mitral valve disease and hypertension was referred to the hospital due to the development of a Brugada-type ECG after taking pilsicainide 150 mg/day for 3 weeks because of paroxysmal atrial fibrillation. She had no previous history of syncope and ventricular tachyarrhythmia. Her family history was negative for sudden cardiac death. Left (3/30): The admission ECG showed a coved-type (Type 1) ST elevation in V1–V3 and prolonged QRS duration to 0.12 sec. Right (4/2): An ECG recorded 4 days after stopping pilsicainide showed an almost normalized ST elevation with terminal T wave inversion in V1–V3; the QRS duration was shortened to 0.08 sec.

Among various Na^+ channel blockers, class IC antiarrhythmic agents (flecainide, propafenone, pilsicainide) are the most potent group of drugs to produce ST elevation, and, therefore, they most effectively unmask Brugada syndrome.[67,68,70,74] At the same time, they carry the strongest potential to induce toxic manifestations among Na^+ channel blockers of other classes. The greatest effect of class IC drugs is due to their strong time- and voltage-dependent block of I_{Na}, and the slow dissociation of the drugs from the Na^+ channel. Class IA agents including ajmaline, procainamide, disopyramide, and cibenzoline have less potent action than class IC agents, since they exhibit less inhibitory potency on I_{Na}, mainly due to their faster dissociation from the Na^+ channel than IC agents.[59,60] They also show variable effects on the K^+ channels including I_{to}. Class IB agents (mexiletine, lidocaine, etc.) are not able to induce ST elevation, especially at a normal or slow heart rate.[7] This lack of effect is due to their rapid dissociation from the Na^+ channel, exerting the channel block only at a fast heart rate.

Various drugs other than Na^+ channel blockers have now been shown to induce ST-segment elevation and unmask the Brugada syndrome.[7

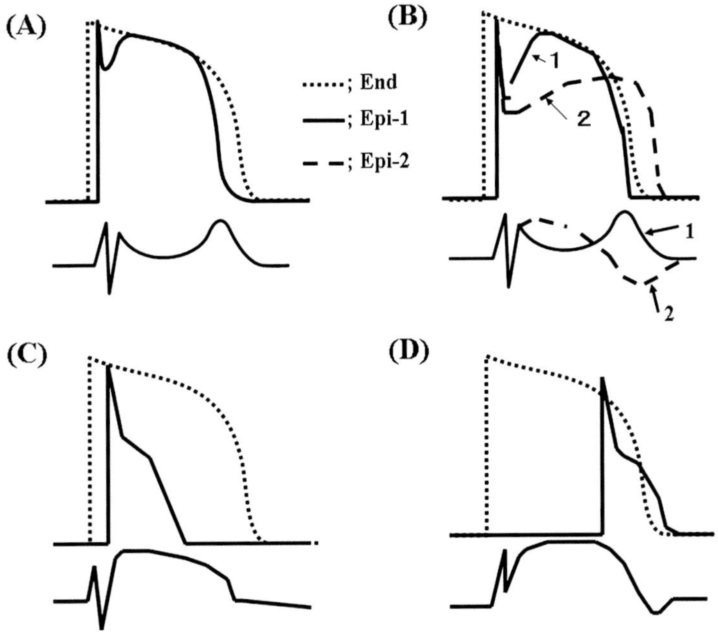

FIGURE 45–4. Various manifestations of ST elevation and T wave changes induced by Na^+ channel blockers in Brugada syndrome. In each panel, epicardial and endocardial action potentials are superimposed at the top and the ECG is shown at the bottom. Solid lines indicate epicardial action potentials and dashed lines are endocardial action potentials. (A) Appearance of junctional ST elevation in a basal condition. (B) The appearance in saddleback (1) and coved-type (2) ST elevation associated with changes in epicardial action potentials. If saddleback and coved types of ST elevation develop at every alternating beat, ST-T alternans appears. (C) Development of "Box-like" ST elevation. (D) Another feature of the development of "Box-like" ST elevation. Conditions in (B) to (D) may manifest as toxic effects of Na^+ channel blockers.

While their administration is usually not intended to unmask the Brugada syndrome, their actions are considered as toxic manifestations due to inhibition of the Na^+ channel and/or the L-type Ca^{2+} channel. Drugs with properties of K^+-channel openers to increase outward currents also unmask the Brugada syndrome.[75]

While gene mutations of *SCN5A* have been identified in various cases of Brugada syndrome, involvement of polymorphisms in drug-induced Brugada syndrome is not known. It has recently been suggested that an *SCN5A* promoter polymorphism common in Asians is associated with conduction abnormality, a higher incidence in Japanese Brugada patients, and high sensitivity to Na^+ channel blockers for conduction parameters in ECGs.[76] The result of this study suggests that genetic polymorphism may have a close association with drug-induced toxic manifestations by Na^+ channel blockers.

Digitalis Intoxication

Digitalis glycosides have been used for many years for the treatment of congestive heart failure and for cardiac arrhythmia, especially for rate control of atrial fibrillation with rapid ventricular responses. Because of the frequent and wide use of digitalis, various side effects and toxic effects have been encountered. Excess digitalis or digitalis toxicity has been known to cause various arrhythmias as well as extracardiac symptoms such as nausea, gastrointestinal irritations, visual abnormalities, and confusion. Digitalis-induced arrhythmias include sinus bradycardia, AV block, premature beats, accelerated ectopic rhythms, and tachycardia arising from the AV junction and the ventricle. Hypokalemia and hypothyroidism are conditions associated with digitalis toxicity.

The main action of digitalis on cardiac cells is exerted through an inhibition of Na^+-K^+-ATPase to suppress Na^+-K^+ pump function. Digitalis intoxication is manifested by decreased Na^+-K^+ pump function resulting in intracellular Ca^{2+} overload through the Na^+-Ca^{2+} exchange mechanism (NCX) after accumulation of $[Na^+]_i$, and by vagotonic action.[77] Excess digitalis induces spontaneous fluctuations of membrane potentials after sinus rhythm or rapid pacing leading to spontaneous and oscillatory depolarizations termed delayed afterdepolarizations (DADs). These reach threshold to induce triggered activity of an ectopic beat, a run of rhythmic activity, or tachycardia.[78] As the underlying ionic mechanism of DADs, a transient inward current (I_{ti}) develops on the basis of intracellular Ca^{2+} overload in association with cyclic Ca^{2+} release from the sarcoplasmic reticulum. The current is carried either through a nonspecific cation channel or an NCX.[79–81] The link between the action of digitalis in causing Ca^{2+} overload and the NCX as a main factor for DAD formation has recently been established by the finding that knockout mice lacking NCX do not develop digitalis intoxication despite excess administration of the drug.[82]

Digitalis, especially digoxin, is excreted primarily from the kidneys and, therefore, digitalis toxicity is prone to develop in subjects with renal dysfunction. Digoxin is a substrate for the drug efflux transporter P-glycoprotein[83] encoded by the gene *MDR1*. *MDR1* is expressed in the kidney and biliary tract where it promotes digoxin efflux, and on the luminal surface of enterocytes in the intestinal tract where it limits digoxin bioavailability. *MDR1* is also present on the endothelial surface of the capillaries of the blood–brain barrier where it limits drug penetration to the central nervous system. Coadministration of quinidine with digoxin is known to increase serum digoxin levels for many years. The mechanism of increased serum digoxin levels by quinidine is explained by the inhibition of P-glycoprotein, reducing renal and biliary excretion and, at the same time, increasing digoxin bioavailability.[84–86] An increase in digoxin concentration leads to local accumulation in the central nervous system through the blood–brain barrier and may produce vagotonic action and noncardiac side effects. An action similar to quinidine is also shared by amiodarone, itraconazole, erythromycin, cyclosporine, and verapamil.[44,87] Therefore, drug interactions are important factors for high-risk pharmacokinetics such as the cardiac toxicity of digitalis.

Summary

Cardiac toxicity as a manifestation of proarrhythmia is caused by cardiac and noncardiac drugs with various pharmacological properties. QT prolongation and TdP are the most frequent and serious manifestations of cardiac toxicity expressed by diverse types of drugs, which mostly have high-affinity binding to the hERG/I_{Kr} channel. The mechanism of high-affinity binding is determined by the channel structure and physicochemical properties of amino acid compositions in the pore region of the hERG channel. In addition, various factors including gender, age, the presence of organic heart disease, pharmakokinetics, pharmacogenetics, and variants of ion channel genes contribute to the manifestation of cardiac toxicity. Proarrhythmia and the unmasking effects of Brugada syndrome are mainly caused by Na^+ channel blockers, depending on the state affinity and the dissociation kinetics from the Na^+ channel as well as the influence of various modifying factors. Digitalis intoxication is manifested by excess drugs causing Ca^{2+} overload in cardiac cells, and the toxicity is frequently manifested through drug interactions by modifying the gene of the regulatory protein, *MDR1*, for the pharmacokinetics of digitalis.

References

1. The Cardiac Arrhythmia Suppression Trial (CAST) Investigator. Preliminary report. Effect of encainide and flecainide on mortality in a randomized trial of arrhythmia suppression after myocardial infarction. *N Engl J Med* 1989;321:406–412.
2. Keating MT, Sanguinetti MC. Molecular and cellular mechanisms of cardiac arrhythmias. *Cell* 2001;104:569–580.

3. Splawski I, *et al.* Spectrum of mutations in long-QT syndrome genes. *KVLQT1, HERG, SCN5A, KCNE1* and *KCNE2*. *Circulation* 2000;102:1178–1185.
4. Brugada P, Brugada J. Right bundle branch block, persistent ST elevation and sudden cardiac death: A distinct clinical and electrocardiographic syndrome: A multicenter study. *J Am Coll Cardiol* 1992;20:1391–1396.
5. Yan GX, Antzelevitch C. Cellular basis for the Brugada syndrome and other mechanisms of arrhythmogenesis associated with ST segment elevation. *Circulation* 1999;100:1660–1666.
6. Priori SG, Napolitano C, Schwartz PJ. Low penetrance in the long-QT syndrome: Clinical impact. *Circulation* 1999;99:529–533.
7. De Ponti F, Poluzzi E, Montanaro N, Ferguson J. QTc and psychotropic drugs. *Lancet* 2000;356:75–76.
8. Selzer A, Wray HW. Quinidine syncope, paroxysmal ventricular fibrillation occurring during treatment of chronic atrial arrhythmias. *Circulation* 1964;30:17–26.
9. Roden DM. Drug-induced prolongation of the QT interval. *N Engl J Med* 2004;350:1013–1022.
10. Hiraoka M, Kawano S, Sawada K. Effects of quinidine on plateau currents of guinea-pig ventricular myocytes. *J Mol Cell Cardiol* 1986;18:1097–1106.
11. Sanguinetti MC, Jiang C, Curran ME, Keating MT. A mechanistic link between an inherited and an acquired cardiac arrhythmia: HERG encodes the I_{kr} potassium channel. Cell 1995;81:299–307.
12. Trudeau MC, Warmke JW, Ganetzky B, Robertson GA. HERG, a human inward rectifier in the voltage-gated potassium channel family. *Science* 1995;269:92–95.
13. Abott GW, Sesti F, Splawski I, *et al.* MiRP1 forms I_{kr} potassium channels with HERG and is associated with cardiac arrhythmia. *Cell* 1999;97:175–187.
14. Mitcheson JS, Chen J, Lin M, Culberson C, Sanguinetti MC. A structural basis for drug-induced long QT syndrome. *Proc Natl Acad Sci USA* 2000;97:12329–12333.
15. Fernandez D, Ghanta A, Kaufman GW, Sanguinettei MC. Physicochemical features of the hERG channel drug binding site. *J Biol Chem* 2004;279:10120–10127.
16. Hondeghem LM, Katzung BG. Time- and voltage-dependent interactions of antiarrhythmic drugs with cardiac sodium channels. *Biochim Biophys Acta* 1977;472:373–398.
17. Hondeghem LM, Snyder DJ. Class III antiarrhythmic agents have a lot of potential but a long way to go. Reduced effectiveness and danger of reverse use dependence. *Circulation* 1990;81:686–690.
18. Carmeliet E. Voltage- and time-dependent block of the delayed K+ current in cardiac myocytes by dofetilide. *J Pharmacol Exp Ther* 1992;262:809–817.
19. Roden DM. Taking the "idio" out of "idiosyncratic", predicting torsades de points. *Pacing Clin Electrophysiol* 1998;21:1029–1034.
20. Antzelevitch C, Sicouri S, Litovsky SH, *et al.* Heterogeneity within the ventricular wall. Electrophysiology and pharmacology of epicardial, endocardial, and M cells. *Circ Res* 1991;69:1427–1449.
21. Nerbonne JM. Molecular basis of functional voltage-gated K^+ channel diversity in the mammalian myocardium. *J Physiol* 2000;525:285–298.
22. Antzelevitch C. Role of transmural dispersion of repolarization in the genesis of drug-induced torsades de pointes. *Heart Rhythm* 2005;2(Suppl. 2):S9–S15.
23. January CT, Liddle JM. Early afterdepolarization: Mechanism of induction and block A role for L-type Ca^{2+} current. *Circ Res* 1989;64:977–990.
24. Hiraoka M, A Sunami, Z Fan, T Sawanobori. Multiple ionic mechanism of early afterdepolarization in isolated ventricular myocytes from guinea-pig hearts. *Ann N.Y. Acad Sci* 1992;644:33–47.
25. Priori SG, Corr PB. Mechanisms underlying early and delayed afterdepolarizations induced by catecholamines. *Am J Physiol* 1990;258:H1796–H1805.
26. Belardinelli L, Antzelevitch C. Assessing predictors of drug-induced torsade de pointes. *Trends Pharmacol Sci* 2003;24:619–625.
27. El-Sherif N, Chinushi M, Caref EB, Restivo M. Electrophysiological mechanism of the characteristic electrocardiographic morphology of torsades de pointes tachyarrhythmias in the long-QT syndrome: Detailed analysis of ventricular tridimensional activation patterns. *Circulation* 1997;96:4392–4399.
28. Akar FG, Yan GX, Antzelevitch C, Rosembaum DS. Unique topographical distribution of M cells underlies reentrant mechanism of torsades de pointes in the long-QT syndrome. *Circulation* 2002;105:1247–1253.
29. Shimizu W, Antzelevitch C. Cellular basis for long QT, transmural dispersion of repolarization, and torsades de pointes in the long QT syndrome. *J Electrocardiol* 1999;32(Suppl.):177–184.
30. Hohnloser SH, Klingenheben T, Singh BN. Amiodarone-associated proarrhythmic effects: A review with special reference to torsade de pointes tachycardia. *Ann Intern Med* 1994;121:529–535.

31. van Opstal JM, Schoenmakers M, Verduyn SC, *et al.* Chronic amiodarone evokes no torsade de points arrhythmias despite QT lengthening in an animal model of acquired long QT syndrome. *Circulation* 2001;104:2722–2727.
32. Milberg P, Eckardt L, Bruns HJ, *et al.* Divergent proarrhythmic potential of macrolide antibiotics despite similar QT prolongation: Fast phase 3 repolarization prevents early afterdepolarizations and torsade de pointes. *J Pharmacol Exp Ther* 2002;303: 218–225.
33. Yang T, Snyders D, Roden DM. Drug block of I(kr): Model systems and relevance to human arrhythmias. *J Cardiovasc Pharmacol* 2001;38:737–744.
34. Curtis LH, Ostbye T, Sendersky V, *et al.* Prescription of QT-prolonging drugs in a cohort of about 5 million outpatients. *Am J Med* 2003;114:135–141.
35. Makkar RR, Promm BS, Steinman RT, *et al.* Female gender as a risk factor for torsades de pointes associated with cardiovascular drugs. *JAMA* 1993; 270:2590–2597.
36. Bednar MM, Harrigan EP, Ruskin JN. Torsades de pointes associated with nonantiarrhythmic drugs and observations on gender and OTc. *Am J Cardiol* 2002;89:1316–1319.
37. Lehmann MH, Hardy S, Archibald D, *et al.* Sex difference in risk of torsade de pointes with d,l-sotalol. *Circulation* 1996;94:2535–2541.
38. Wang S, Morales MJ, Liu S, Strauss HC, Rasmusson RL. Modulation of HERG affinity for E-4031 by $[K^+]_o$ and C-type inactivation. *FEBS Lett* 1997;417: 43–47.
39. Yang T, Snyders DJ, Roden DM. Rapid inactivation determines the rectification and $[K^+]$o dependence of the rapid component of the delayed rectifier K^+ current in cardiac cells. *Circ Res* 1997;80:782–789.
40. Numaguchi H, Johnson JP Jr, Petersen CI, Balser JR. A sensitive mechanism for cation modulation of potassium current. *Nat Neurosci* 2000;3:429–430.
41. Moller M, Torp-Pedersen CT, Kober L. Dofetilide in patients with congestive heart failure and left ventricular dysfunction: Safety aspects and effect on atrial fibrillation. The Danish Investigators of Arrhythmia and Mortality on Dofetilide (DIAMOND) Study Group. *Congest Heart Fail* 2001;7:146–150.
42. Choy AMJ, Darbar D, Dello'Orto S, Roden DM. Increased sensitivity to QT prolonging drug therapy immediately after cardioversion to sinus rhythm. *J Am Coll Cardiol* 1999;34:396–401.
43. Tomaselli GF, Marba E. Electrophysiological remodeling in hypertrophy and heart failure. *Cardiovasc Res* 1999;42:270–283.
44. Roden DM. Proarrhythmia as a pharmacogenomic entity: A critical review and formulation of a unifying hypothesis. *Cardiovasc Res* 2005;67:419–425.
45. Pratt CM, Hertz RP, Ellis BE, *et al.* Risk of developing life-threatening ventricular arrhythmia associated with terfenadine in comparison with over-the-counter antihistamines, ibuprofen and clemastine. *Am J Cardiol* 1994;73:346–352.
46. Hanrahan JP, Choo PW, Carlson W, *et al.* Terfenadine-associated ventricular arrhythmias and QTc interval prolongation. A retrospective cohort comparison with other antihistamines among members of a health maintenance organization. *Ann Epidemiol* 1995;5:201–209.
47. Jurima-Romet M, Crawford K, Cyr T, Inaba T. Terfenadine metabolism in human liver. *Drug Metab Dispos* 1994;22:849–857.
48. Honig PK, Wortham DC, Zamani K, *et al.* Terfenadine-ketoconazole interaction. *JAMA* 1993; 269:1513–1518.
49. Benton RE, Honig PK, Zamani K, *et al.* Grape fruit juice alters terfenadine pharmacokinetics, resulting in prolongation of repolarization on the electrocardiogram. *Clin Pharmacol Ther* 1996;59:383–388.
50. Donger C, Denjoy I, Berther M, *et al.* KVLQT1 C-terminal missense mutation causes of forme fruste long-QT syndrome. *Circulation* 1997;96:2778–2781.
51. Makita N, Horie M, Nakamura T, *et al.* Drug-induced long-QT syndrome associated with subclinical SCN5A mutation. *Circulation* 2002;106: 1269–1274.
52. Kubota T, Shimizu W, Kamakura S, Horie M. Hypokalemia-induced long QT syndrome and underlying novel missense mutation in S2–S5 linker of KCNQ1. *J Cardiovasc Electrophysiol* 2000; 11:1048–1054.
53. Priori SG, Napolitano C. Genetic defects of cardiac ion channels. The hidden substrate for torsades de pointes. *Cardiovasc Drugs Ther* 2002;16:89–92.
54. Sesti F, Abbott GW, Wei J, *et al.* A common polymorphism associated with antibiotic-induced cardiac arrhythmia. *Proc Natl Acad Sci USA* 2000;97: 10613–10618.
55. Splawski I, Timothy KW, Tateyama M, *et al.* Variant of SCN5A sodium channel implicated in risk of cardiac arrhythmia. *Science* 2002;297:1333–1336.
56. Yang P, Kanki H, Drolet B, *et al.* Allelic variants in long QT disease genes in patients with drug associated torsades de pointes. *Circulation* 2002; 105:1943–1948.

57. Paulussen AD, Gilissen RA, Armstrong M, *et al.* Genetic variations of KCNQ1 KCNH2, SCN5A, KCNE1, and KCNE2 in drug-induced long QT syndrome patients. *J Mol Med* 2004;82:182–188.
58. Chen S, Chung MK, Martin D, *et al.* SNP S1103Y in the cardiac sodium channel gene SCN5A is associated with cardiac arrhythmias and sudden cardiac death in a white family. *J Med Genet* 2002;39:913–915.
59. Grant AO, Whalley DW, Wendt DJ. Pharmacology of the cardiac sodium channel. In: Zipes DP, Jalife J, Eds. *Cardiac Electrophysiology*. Philadelphia, PA: W.B. Saunders, 1995:247–259.
60. Balser JR. The cardiac sodium channel: Gating function and molecular pharmacology. *J Mol Cell Cardiol* 2001;33:599–613.
61. Hille B. Local anesthetics: Hydrophilic and hydrophobic pathways for the drug-receptor reaction. *J Gen Physiol* 1977;69:497–515.
62. Sunami A, Fan Z, Hiraoka M, *et al.* Two components of use-dependent block of Na^+ current by disopyramide and lidocaine in guinea pig ventricular myocytes. *Circ Res* 1991;68(3):653–661.
63. Janse MJ, Wit AL. Electrophysiological mechanisms of ventricular arrhythmias resulting from myocardial ischemia and infarction. *Physiol Rev* 1989;69:1049–1169.
64. Siddoway LA, Thompson KAMKT, McAllister CB, Wang T, Wilkinson GR, Roden DM, *et al.* Polymorphism of propafenone metabolism and disposition in man: Clinical and pharmacokinetic consequences. *Circulation* 1987;75:785–791.
65. Lee JT, Kroemer HK, Silberstein DJ, Funck-Brentano C, Lineberry MD, Wood AJ, *et al.* The role of genetically determined polymorphic drug metabolism in the beta-blockade produced by propafenone. *N Engl J Med* 1990;322:1764–1768.
66. Brugada R, Brugada J, Antzelevitch C, *et al.* Sodium channel blockers identify risk for sudden death in patients with ST-segment elevation and right bundle branch block but structurally normal hearts. *Circulation* 2000;101:510–515.
67. Krishnan SC, Josephson ME. ST segment elevation induced by class IC antiarrhythmic agents: Underlying electrophysiologic mechanisms and insights into drug-induced proarrhymia. *J Cardiovasc Electrophysiol* 1998;9:1167–1172.
68. Gasparini M, Priori SG, Mantica M, *et al.* Flecainide test in Brugada syndrome: Reproducible but risky too. *Pacing Clin Electrophysiol* 2003;26:338–341.
69. Rolf S, Bruns HJ, Wichter T, *et al.* The ajmaline challenge in Brugada syndrome: Diagnostic impact, safety, and recommended protocol. *Eur Heart J* 2003;24:1104–1112.
70. Antzelevitch C, Brugada P, Borggrefe M, *et al.* Brugada syndrome. Report of the second consensus conference. *Circulation* 2005;111:659–670.
71. Tada H, Nogami A, Shimizu W, *et al.* ST segment and T wave alternans in a patient with Brugada syndrome. *Pacing Clin Electrophysiol* 2000;23:413–415.
72. Chinishi M, Washizuka T, Okumura H, Aizawa Y. Intravenous administration of class I antiarrhythmic drugs induced T wave alternans in a patient with Brugada syndrome. *J Cardiovasc Electrophysiol* 2001;12:493–495.
73. Nishizaki M, Fujii H, Sakurada H, *et al.* Spontaneous T wave alternans in a patient with Brugada syndrome—Response to intravenous administration of class I antiarrhythmic drug, glucose tolerance test, and atrial pacing. *J Cardiovasc Electrophysiol* 2005;16:217–220.
74. Shimizu W, Antzelevitch C, Suyama K, *et al.* Effect of sodium channel blockers on ST segment, QRS duration, and corrected QT interval in patients with Brugada syndrome. *J Cardiovasc Electrophysiol* 2000;11:1320–1329.
75. Shimizu W. Acquired forms of Brugada syndrome. In: Antzelevitch C, Ed. *The Brugada Syndrome. From Bench to Bedside*. Malden, MA: Blackwell, Futura, 2005:166–177.
76. Bezzina CR, Shimizu W, Yang P, *et al.* Common sodium channel promoter haplotype in asian subjects underlies variability in cardiac conduction. *Circulation* 2006;113:330–332.
77. Smith TW. Digitalis: Mechanisms of action and clinical use. *N Engl J Med* 1988;318:358–365.
78. Ferrier GR. Digitalis arrhythmias: Role of oscillatory afterpotentials. *Prog Cardiovasc Dis* 1977;19:459–474.
79. Kass RS, Tsien RW, Weingart R. Ionic basis of transient inward current induced by strophanthidin in cardiac Purkinje fibres. *J Physiol* 1978;281:209–226.
80. Matsuda H, Noma A, Kurachi Y, *et al.* Transient depolarization and spontaneous voltage fluctuations in isolated single cells from guinea pig ventricle. *Circ Res* 1982;51:142–151.
81. Schlotthauer K, Bers DM. Sarcoplasmic reticulum Ca^{2+} release causes myocyte depolarization. Underlying mechanism and threshold for triggered action potentials. *Circ Res* 2000;87:774–780.
82. Reuter H, Henderson SA, Han T, *et al.* Knockout mice for pharmacological screening: Testing the specificity of Na^+-Ca^{2+} exchanger inhibitors. *Circ Res* 2002;91:90–92.
83. Tanigawa Y, Okamura N, Hirai M, *et al.* Transport of digoxin by human P-glycoprotein expressed in a

porcine kidney epithelial cell line. *J Pharmacol Exp Ther* 1992;263:840–845.

84. Angelin B, Arvidsson A, Dahlqvist R, *et al.* Quinidine reduces biliary clearance of digoxin in man. *Eur J Clin Invest* 1987;17:262–265.
85. De Lannoy IAM, Koren G, Klein J, *et al.* Cyclosporin and quinidine inhibition of renal digoxin excretion: Evidence for luminal secretion of digoxin. *Am J Physiol* 1992;263:F613–F622.
86. Su SF, Huang JD. Inhibition of the intestinal digoxin absorption and exsorption by quinidine. *Drug Metab Dispos* 1996;24:142–147.
87. Fromm MF, Kim RB, Stein CM, Wilkinson GR, Roden DM. Inhibition of P-glycoprotein-mediated drug transport: A unifying mechanism to explain the interaction between digoxin and quinidine. *Circulation* 1999;99:552–557.

46
Acquired (Drug-Induced) Long QT Syndrome

Jeffrey S. Litwin, Robert B. Kleiman, and Ihor Gussak

Introduction

The most common cause of acquired drug-induced long QT syndrome (ADILQTS) in clinical practice is an exposure of the heart to drugs known for their potential to prolong the QT interval. It has long been recognized that most drugs that prolong the duration of the QT interval can cause fatal tachyarrhythmias. However, it took decades to sensitize medical and scientific communities, drug developers, and regulatory authorities to the serious adverse effects of numerous commercially available or investigational cardiovascular and noncardiovascular pharmaceutical agents. The most comprehensive appreciation of the magnitude of drug-induced iatrogenic death took place after the highly publicized withdrawal of the nonsedating antihistamine terfenadine and the gastrointestinal drug cisapride in the late 1990s. Numerous cases of sudden cardiac death (SCD) and life-threatening ventricular tachyarrhythmias, such as torsade de pointes (TdP)—known for its association with prolonged QT interval—induced by those drugs, were reported to the worldwide postmarketing database. As a result, a substantial number of torsadogenic drugs with "QT liability" have been withdrawn from the market over the past decade, in fact, more drugs have been withdrawn for this than for any other reason.[1]

Nevertheless, there are still over 100 therapeutic agents—the vast majority of them noncardiovascular agents—that have been recognized by regulatory agencies for their ability to prolong ventricular repolarization and the QT interval, and to aggravate and/or precipitate malignant ventricular tachyarrhythmias. The vast majority of QT prolonging torsadogenic drugs act through an inhibition of the rapidly activating delayed rectifier potassium channels (I_{Kr}) and, to some extent, the slowly activating delayed rectifier (I_{Ks}). Brief lists of medications known for their association with both QT prolongation and propensity to life-threatening tachyarrhythmias are presented in Tables 46–1 and 46–2, and there are reasonably comprehensive versions—on many web-based sites, including www.qtdrugs.org.

The main objectives of this chapter are the clinical, electrophysiological, and electrocardiographic aspects of ADILQTS, with a special focus on the mechanisms of drug-induced cardiac (arrhythmogenic) toxicity, its clinical manifestation, risk factors, treatment, and prevention of fatal arrhythmias. Acquired arrhythmic syndromes other than ADILQTS will not be discussed in this chapter.

Drug-Induced Cardiovascular Toxicity

Many drugs are known for their toxic effects on the cardiovascular system and many of them have been withdrawn from the market or have been severely restricted to specific indications due to unexpected adverse events, including fatalities. All adverse drugs reactions are undesirable, many of them are unpredictable, and some of them are serious and potentially life-threatening. In general, the majority of serious cardiac adverse events are due to either excessive exposure to the agent or an idiosyncratic drug reaction (this may

TABLE 46–1. Noncardiac drugs associated with QT interval prolongation and propensity to life-threatening tachyarrhythmias.

Macrolide antibiotics	Antipsychotics
Azithromycin	Droperidol
Clarithromycin	Haloperidol
Erythromycin	Mesoridazine
Fluoroquinolones	Pimozide
Ciprofloxacin	Quetiapine
Gatifloxacin	Risperidone
Levofloxacin	Sertindole
Moxifloxacin	Thioridazine
Antidepressants	Chlorpromazine
Amitriptyline	Venlafaxine
Desipramine	
Doxepin	
Fluoxetine	
Imipramine	
Paroxetine	
Sertraline	

occur even at normal doses). An idiosyncratic drug reaction is usually difficult to predict, and it is most commonly caused by unexpected pharmacokinetic and/or pharmacodynamic peculiarities in metabolic pathways and/or drug targets, such as drug absorption, distribution, metabolism, excretion, or drug–drug interaction, especially in genetically predisposed individuals. Even with a normal genotype, drug interactions, coadministration of an agent that is a potent inhibitor of the enzyme system that normally degrades the drug-modulating ion channel function, can result in life-threatening arrhythmias.[2,3] Because of the narrow therapeutic index, these pharmacokinetic interactions are of extreme importance and are of major cardiac safety concern in clinical practice, in research, and in drug development.

Factors predisposing to cardiovascular toxicity and their individual relevance are determined primarily by cardiac diseases and modified by different extracardiac factors and abnormalities, including age, gender, and electrolyte disturbances (Table 46–3), and can vary between different patients, target patient populations, level of disease progression, concomitant diseases, and concurrent drugs. Clinical manifestations of drug-induced cardiovascular toxicity include the following:

1. Cardiac arrhythmias, such as ventricular tachycardia/fibrillation, atrial fibrillation/flutter, increased supraventricular and ventricular ectopic activities, conduction defects, bradycardia, and tachycardia (e.g., terfenadine, cisapride, quinidine, erythromycin, haloperidol).
2. Cardiac failure due to either (a) direct cytotoxic injury to myocytes resulting in loss of contractile function (cardiomyopathies, congestive heart failure) (e.g., adriamycin, cyclophosphamide) or (b) circulatory overload with or without an increase in afterload [e.g., carbenoxolone, fludrocortisone, nonsteroidal anti-inflammatory drugs (NSAIDs)].
3. Hypertension (e.g., sympathomimetics, corticosteroids, NSAIDs).
4. Hypotension (e.g., antihypertensive drugs, diuretics).
5. Myocardial ischemia (e.g., adenosine, amphetamines, β-agonists, calcium antagonists, abrupt withdrawal of β-blockers).
6. Thrombosis and thromboembolic disorders (e.g., COX-2 inhibitors, contraceptives, hormone replacement therapy).
7. Valvular diseases (e.g., ergotamine, fenfluramine-phentermine).

Among these unintended effects, drug-induced cardiac arrhythmogenic toxicity—usually viewed in the context of acquired long QT syndrome—culminating in a fatal event is the most dramatic. We define ADILQTS as a secondary arrhythmogenic cardiac channelopathy that is characterized by a prolonged duration of the electrocardiographic (ECG) QT interval that is associated with life-threatening ventricular tachyarrhythmias, syncope, and SCD. The hallmark of ADILQTS is an abnormally prolonged QT interval (with or without abnormal U waves) that is associated with TdP ventricular tachycardia.

As mentioned earlier, two noncardiac drugs, cisapride and terfenadine, offer good examples of adverse drug–drug and/or drug–food interac-

TABLE 46–2. Antiarrhythmic drugs associated with QT interval prolongation and propensity to life-threatening tachyarrhythmias.

Amiodarone	Flecainide
Azimilide	Ibutilide
Bepridil	Procainamide
Bretylium	Propafenone
Disopyramide	Quinidine
Dofetilide	Tedisamil
D-Sotalol	

TABLE 46–3. predisposing risk factors for ADILQTS.

Cardiac diseases
History of clinically relevant arrhythmias
Coronary artery disease (myocardial ischemia or infarction, aortic stiffness)
Left ventricular hypertrophy
Congestive heart failure
Cardiomyopathies
Hypertension
Peculiar electrocardiographic abnormalities:
Prolonged baseline QTc
Alternans of beat-to-beat QT interval duration
Abnormal U waves
Marked accentuation of U waves after prolonged pause (e.g., after PVC)
Deeply inverted T waves
Notched T waves
Alternans of T waves
Bradycardia, especially in children
Tachycardia
Acute neurological events (intracranial and subarachnoid hemorrhage, stroke, trauma)
Electrolyte disturbances
Metabolic disorders
Diabetes mellitus
Altered nutrition (anorexia nervosa, starvation diets, alcoholism)
Impaired drug elimination (renal or hepatic dysfunction)
Hypoglycemia
Hypothermia
Hypothyroidism
Obesity
Poisoning (arsenic, organophosphates, nerve gas)
Pituitary insufficiency
Female gender
Elderly age (>65)
Abrupt shift in electrolyte balance (e.g., hemodialysis)

tions resulting in serious unintended cardiotoxic arrhythmogenicity, including TdP and SCD. Cisapride was approved for nighttime heartburn in July 1993 and was "withdrawn" from the market in March 2000. This QT-prolonging drug is primarily metabolized by CYP3A4, and when coadministered with any other drug or substance known to inhibit this enzyme (e.g., grapefruit juice, macrolides, ketoconazole, alcohol overdose), it becomes torsadogenic since its blood concentration becomes greatly elevated. Five times, between the time of its approval and January 2000, cisapride's labeling required progressively stronger warnings about life-threatening drug reactions until its removal from the market. The use of cisapride has been associated with 341 reports of cardiac arrhythmias, including 80 reported cases of SCD through December 31, 1999.[4] An analysis of 341 cases of patients on cisapride with QT prolongation and ventricular arrhythmias revealed the following confounding variables:

• CYP3A4 inhibitors	126	(37%)
• Electrolyte imbalance	17	(5%)
• Proarrhythmic drugs	17	(5%)
• Heart failure	29	(8.5%)
• Other cardiac disease	66	(19.4%)
• Cisapride overdose	9	(2.6%)
• No risk factors	38	(11%)

Terfenadine is another classic example of an arrhythmogenic QT-prolonging drug with tremendously increased torsadogenic potential when administered simultaneously with a corresponding enzyme inhibitor. This, the most popular nonsedating antihistamine agent in its time (by 1992, it was the tenth most prescribed medication in the United States), was being considered to change its status to "over-the-counter," but instead was removed from the market due to numerous cases of TdP and SCD that were reported to the worldwide postmarketing database. A "post factum" detailed ECG analysis revealed a linear dose–response relationship with an increase in the QTc interval of 0.28 msec for every 1 mg of terfenadine dosed.[5] Of note, the QTc-prolonging effect was evident only with the parent compound, but not terfenadine's active metabolite. The terfenadine "story" becomes an important case study in better understanding the mechanisms of ADILQTS.

In addition, several drug interactions can cause hypokalemia, a major torsadogenic risk factor. Among the most common "hypokalemic" drugs are diuretics (especially osmotic diuretics), renal toxins (e.g., amphotericin B, gentamicin, toluene), insulin, β-sympathomimetics and glucocorticoids. For example, potassium-wasting diuretics (e.g., loop diuretics and thiazides) can significantly prolong ventricular repolarization and the QT interval and can produce abnormal U waves, another ECG marker for ADILQTS. Drug-induced abnormalities in cardiac conduction are also important, yet are not a subject of this chapter.

Electrocardiographic Indices of Drug-Induced Cardiac Toxicity

A variety of electrophysiological factors determine and modulate the electrocardiographic contour and the duration of ventricular repolarization. Among intrinsic cardiac factors, the most important are as follows:

1. The shape and duration of the action potentials and their transmural heterogeneity.
2. The number of depolarizing cells participating in the generation of the repolarizing currents.
3. The degree of electrotonic transmission and cell-to-cell coupling conductance.
4. The primary asynchrony of the repolarization.
5. The secondary asynchrony of the repolarization due to asynchrony of depolarization.[6]

Extracardiac factors include neurotransmitters, electrolytes, temperature, hormones, age, and gender.

Since both the sensitivity and specificity of a surface resting 12-lead ECG to detect and quantify the changes in ventricular repolarization and their magnitude are limited, the issue of false-negative and false-positive findings is always valid. There is no unique or universal ECG marker of abnormal cardiac repolarization that can detect an arrhythmogenic substrate created by an investigational drug. Therefore, any (even minimal but significant) ECG changes still within the normal range that are induced by any drug should be considered as surrogate markers of drug-induced cardiac toxicity, unless proven otherwise.[6] This is especially relevant for any drug not intended to affect electrophysiological properties of the heart, especially ventricular repolarization.

It has been postulated that an abnormal cardiac repolarization is potentially arrhythmogenic. Furthermore, the most common electrophysiological mechanisms underlying drug-induced malignant ventricular arrhythmias, such as TdP, are those triggered by an abnormal cardiac repolarization, in general, and delayed ventricular repolarization, specifically.

Among ECG indices of ventricular repolarization that could be detected on the surface ECG are those that are associated with the duration of the QT interval and the contour of the ST-T (U) segment. They include the following:

1. The duration of QT interval and its correction for heart rate.
2. The displacement of the ST segment.
3. The morphological pattern of T and U waves.
4. Their combination.

So far, only QT interval duration corrected for the heart rate (QTc) is accepted as a surrogate marker of abnormal (delayed) ventricular repolarization, and the only clinically proven ECG index to link to life-threatening ventricular tachyarrhythmias, such as TdP.[6]

Another pathognomic ECG feature of cardiotoxicity is the appearance of abnormal U waves. The origin of U waves was obscure for many decades, and different hypotheses concerning their origin have been proposed at different times. None of these hypotheses is unique and universal. Also, it appears that the small U waves seen in young and healthy individuals and large or even inverted U waves observed in patients under a variety of abnormal conditions have different origins and different rate dependency. The small "normal" U waves are more prominent at bradycardia, clearly separated from the T waves, and

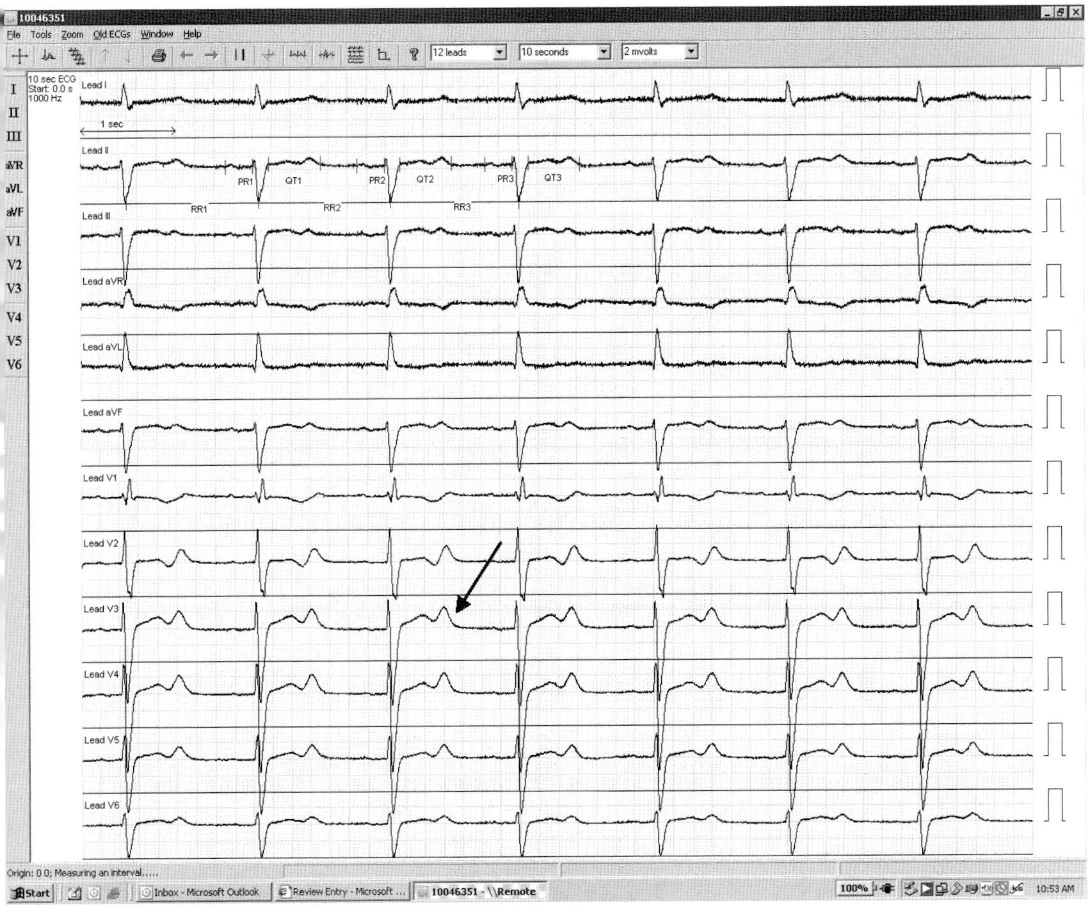

FIGURE 46–1. Abnormal U waves. Note the abnormal (positive) U waves with an amplitude higher than the T wave amplitude within the same leads (best seen in the precordial leads) and also note the presence of left anterior hemiblock.

their magnitude is inversely dependent on the heart rate. Abnormal U waves [commonly defined as either positive U waves with U amplitude ≥ T amplitude within any lead (Figure 46–1), often encroaching on flat T waves or negative U waves in any lead with positive T waves] often "approach" the T waves and even merge with them at higher heart rates (Figure 46–2). Large "abnormal" U waves can be repeatably reproduced in experiments with hypokalemia or certain drug infusions and are associated with drug-induced TdP.

Innovative Electrocardiographic Alternatives to the QT Interval Derivatives

The search for new more sensitive and more specific ECG markers of drug-induced proarrhythmic toxicity has intensified in experimental and clinical research over the past decade, especially after the disappointing failure of interlead QT interval dispersion. Nevertheless, it needs to be emphasized that the clinical validity and prognostic value of any innovative alternatives to QT derivatives must be established and validated clinically.[7] Among them are the following:

1. T_{peak}–T_{end} interval. This particular ECG interval has been proposed as an index of transmural ventricular heterogeneity based on its experimental model of arterially perfused wedge preparation.[8]
2. Nondipolar components of the T wave. This derivative is claimed to reflect localized aberrations of the sequence of intramural repolarization, possibly re-enforced by proximity effects on

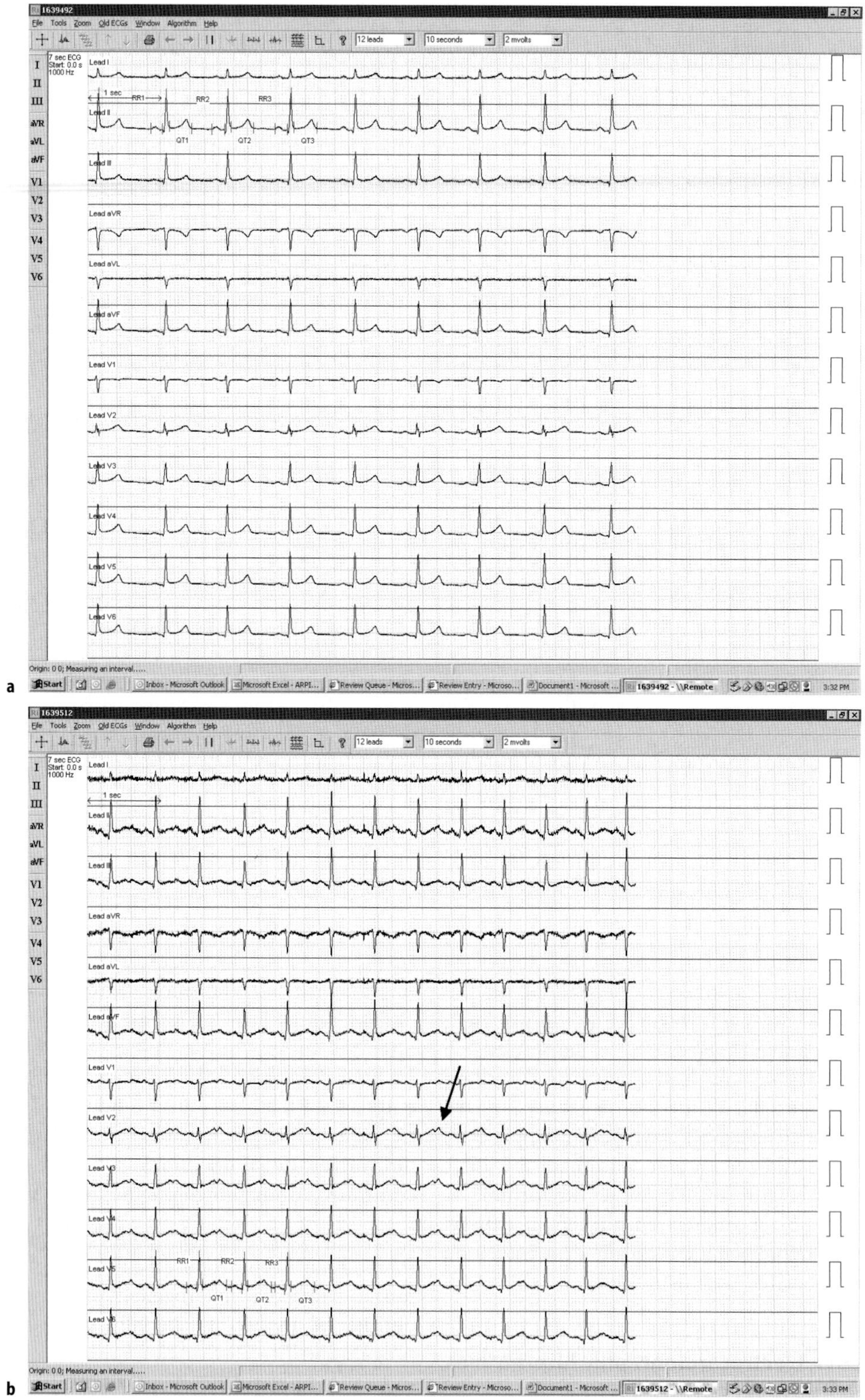

FIGURE 46–2. Development of abnormal U waves. (a) Upper panel: normal ECG. (b) Lower panel: T-U wave fusion.

selective ECG leads. The technical problem in detecting these components is their small magnitude and their high vulnerability to ECG random noise level. Some clinical studies have reported that T wave nondipolar components are a strong ECG predictor of total (but not cardiovascular) mortality.[9] Nevertheless, it remains far from adequately validated and its relationship with the risk of adverse events associated with drug-induced cardiac toxicity remains to be established.

3. T wave morphology changes and T wave complexity. A variable commonly referred to as T wave complexity has become increasingly popular in ECG research. It is derived from principal-component analysis as a ratio of the eigenvalues of the second and the first principal component of the T wave. The interest in T wave morphology has received special attention due to the association between certain T waveform phenotypes and different genotypes in genetically confirmed subjects with hereditary long QT syndrome.[10] However, the variability and the overlap of these T waveform phenotypes are far from negligible.

4. T wave alternans. In the literature, there are many publications that point out that there is substantial evidence associating T wave alternans with malignant arrhythmias in a variety of abnormal clinical conditions. T wave alternans can be quantified by nonspectral and spectral analysis methods. Intriguing is the report from 2002 documenting that increasing complexity of T wave oscillations precedes the onset of ventricular fibrillation.[11,12] Although T wave alternans appears to be one of the more promising of the innovative alternatives for detecting the risk of malignant arrhythmias in conditions of drug-induced QT prolongation, it also will need a continuing series of validation studies.

Acquired Cardiac Channelopathies, Ion Remodeling, and Repolarization Reserve

Many diseases, abnormal conditions, drugs, and their combination can adversely modify cardiac ion channel activity (ionic remodeling) resulting in an abnormal alteration of ion channel function (acquired cardiac channelopathies). The alteration of ion channel function can occur due to the following:

1. Primary alteration in ion channels.
2. Signaling or Ca^{2+} handling proteins.
3. Structural changes in the myocytes or extracellular matrix.
4. Changes in activity of the neurohumoral system.

Depending on the underlying diseases and their stages, the electrophysiological and ionic changes in the heart may vary, which provides a basis for the differences in the pathophysiology of the arrhythmia and variability in response to drugs.

Commonly, ionic remodeling leads to the "silent" reduction in naturally redundant K^+ channels and their normal levels of expression ("cardiac repolarization reserve"), and, therefore, an increased sensitivity of the channel to inhibition, which becomes manifest only after exposure to a K^+ channel blocker that can prolong repolarization.[13,14] For instance, increased sensitivity to I_{Kr} blockade with increased dependence of repolarization on I_{Kr} is a common electrophysiological feature of congestive heart failure, where a reduction in I_{Ks} occurs in the ventricles.[15]

A diminished repolarization reserve, that by itself does not cause symptoms, may potentially lead to fatal arrhythmias in the presence of various drugs.[16] For instance, otherwise innocent polymorphisms in ion channel genes may enhance drug binding and magnify the channel block.[13] The prototype for such polymorphisms may be a mutation in KCNE2 that has been reported to underlie arrhythmias triggered by an antibiotic.[17] Thus, reduction in the repolarizing K^+ current of any cause requires more time to complete ventricular repolarization, resulting in QT prolongation and an elevated risk of TdP and SCD (Figure 46–3).

Abnormal ventricular repolarization induced by drugs is currently best described by ECG parameters reflecting its duration, such as QT interval and its derivative, QT interval corrected (QTc) by the heart rate. The predictive value of the QT parameters to assess the risk of potentially lethal ventricular arrhythmias is substantially higher in patients with drug-induced cardiac toxicity than in patients after myocardial infarction, with ischemic or dilated cardiomyopathy.

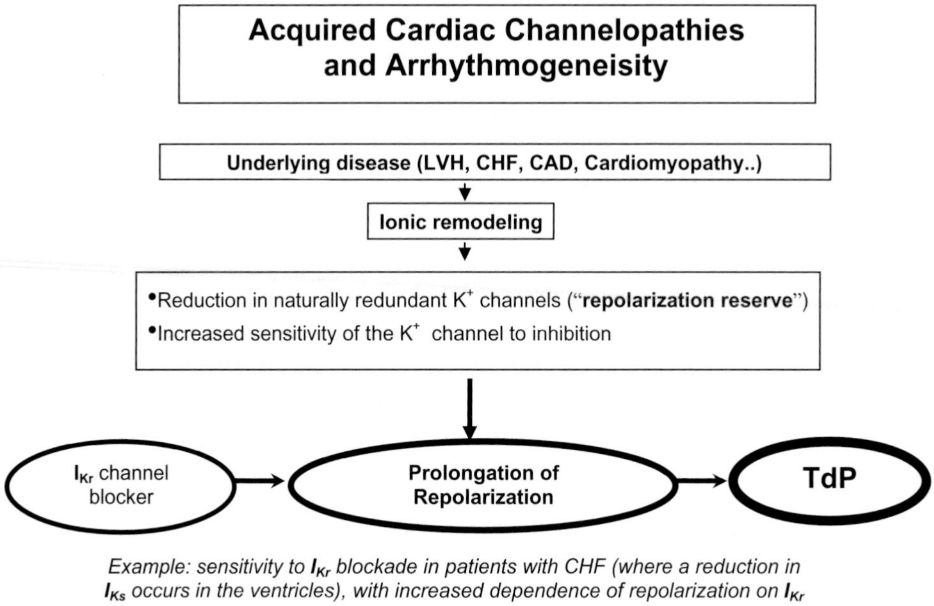

Figure 46–3. Mechanism of drug-induced torsadogenic QT interval prolongation due to a reduction in the repolarizing potassium currents.

Acquired Drug-Induced Long QT Syndrome: Clinical, Electrophysiological, and Electrocardiographic Considerations

Compared to other acquired cardiac channelopathies, the ADILQTS has received most of the attention from regulatory agencies, the scientific and medical communities, and the pharmaceutical industry because of its association with preventable iatrogenic SCD. The arrhythmogenic potential of ADILQTS is primarily determined by the magnitude of adverse effects of drug–drug and drug–food interactions on cardiac repolarization that can be modified by a variety of cardiac and extracardiac diseases and factors. The main mechanism underlying potentially fatal electrical instability due to drug-induced cardiac channelopathies is abnormal (delayed) ventricular repolarization resulting in the prolongation of the electrocardiographic QT interval.

In the past, prolongation of cardiac refractoriness was considered as one of the most desired mechanism of various antiarrhythmics. However, over time, we have learned that in many cases this mechanism can be proarrhythmic. This has resulted in most of the QT-prolonging antiarrhythmic drugs being restricted or contraindicated for the prevention of arrhythmogenic SCD. It is noteworthy, that not all QT-prolonging drugs are proarrhythmic, yet a majority of proarrhythmic drugs that were removed from the market did demonstrate QT prolongation.

In clinical practice, ADILQTS is most commonly associated with QT-prolonging cardiac (antiarrhythmic) agents (Table 46–2). Although, the arrhythmogenic potential of noncardiac drugs in ADILQTS is less malignant compared to ADILQTS associated with antiarrhythmic drugs, many new noncardiac pharmaceutical agents have been withdrawn from the market or severely restricted to specific indications because of clinical concern about rare but unexpected and potentially fatal complications of ADILQTS (Table 46–1). There were 320 well-documented cases of SCD due to noncardiac QT-prolonging drugs in one year in the Netherlands. With a population of 16,407,491 individuals, it can be estimated that the annual mortality rate from the same cause could be as high as 9000 cases in Europe or 6000 cases in the United States.

Regrettably, despite the notion of potentially lethal consequences of ADILQTS, the risk and the risk/benefit ratio of QT-prolonging medications are profoundly underestimated in clinical practice. Based on the patterns of most currently prescribed medications, it appears that clear restrictions, side effects, warnings, and contraindications pertinent to the QT interval-prolonging medications are widely ignored or even disregarded. Unacceptably high rates of prescription of QT-prolonging medications and concomitant therapy with two or more QT-prolonging drugs were found in a retrospective cohort analysis of a large prescription claims database that included 4.8 million patients by Curtis *et al.* from Duke University.[18] The analysis included 50 medications associated with QT-interval prolongation and 26 agents that inhibit hepatic or renal clearance of these medications. They showed that: 22.8% of patients had a prescription for at least one medication associated with QT interval prolongation (47.4% were for erythromycin or clarithromycin and 40% were for antidepressants). Among those patients, 9.4% filled overlapping prescriptions for at least one other QT interval-prolonging medication or for at least one agent that inhibited the medications clearance. Of these patients, 7249 (0.7%) filled overlapping prescriptions for three or more potentially interacting medications.

- Among 103,119 patients who filled two or more prescriptions for medications that may prolong QTc values, 74% were women and 22% were 65 years or older.
- Among 445,668 patients who filled prescriptions for antidepressants associated with QT interval prolongation, 26.9% also filled an overlapping prescription for a potentially interacting medication.

An analysis of the Food and Drug Administration (FDA) safety database from 1969 to 1998 revealed 2194 cases of QT prolongation and TdP. The cases were characterized as follows:

- 61.1% were associated with hospitalization
- 27.9% were life-threatening
- 16.2% were associated with a serious condition
- 9.8% were associated with a fatal outcome
- 61.8% were females and 32.5% were males (5.7% gender unknown)
- Mean (SD) age: 53.9 ± 22.3 years
- 11.7% were associated with drug interactions
- 9.2% were associated with overdoses
- Most common drugs:

Most common drugs:	Cardiac	26.2%
	Central nervous system	21.9%
	Antiinfectives	19.0%
	Antihistamines	11.6%.

Clinical Manifestations, Diagnosis, and Predisposing Risk Factors

Life-threatening arrhythmia with its associated symptoms and complications and SCD are the only clinical manifestations of the ADILQTS. As mentioned earlier, both the drug-induced prolongation of the QT interval and its link to ventricular tachyarrhythmias are required for the diagnosis of ADILQTS. The hallmark of the arrhythmogenic manifestation of ADILQTS is TdP, which like other ventricular tachyarrhythmias could be self-limited or could deteriorate to ventricular fibrillation and SCD; faster and longer TdP is more likely to generate into ventricular fibrillation. In a very conservative estimation, drug-induced TdP generates into ventricular fibrillation in approximately 20% of cases, and results in SCD in 10–17%.[19] However, these statistics should not be construed in a fashion that would lead to an underestimation of the life-threatening potential of TdP, as the statistics are per episode of TdP and TdP can occur multiple times in an affected individual.

The relationship of QT interval duration to risk of TdP is complex rather than linear. Apparently, unexpected abnormal QT prolongation from any cause should be considered of clinical concern. The level of this concern should be higher if QT prolongation (of any magnitude) is caused by a drug, much higher if it is dose dependent, and the highest if it is associated with TdP. In ADILQTS, the risk of TdP depends on (1) the baseline value of QTc and (2) the drug-induced increment in QT duration. Commonly, a QTc longer than 460 msec should merit a clinician's attention, and QTc values exceeding 500 msec often indicate a high risk of arrhythmia in patients receiving a QT-prolonging drug (for more details see Shah[20]).

The incidence of TdP is estimated to be as low as 8.6 cases per 10 million in the general population and it increases up to 40 cases per 10 million in the same population when receiving any medication. The incidence of TdP can be as high as 6.8% or 8.8% in patients treated with sotalol or quinidine, respectively.[21,22]

Some individuals are more prone to the drug-induced QT prolongation and are at higher risk for TdP than others. This would lead to an assessment of how "acquired" the drug-induced QT prolongation is or what the true incidence of latent long QT carriers is. Moss and Schwartz proposed that drug-induced TdP would be more likely observed in subjects with latent forms of congenital LQTS treated with a QT-prolonging drug.[23] The current estimate is that long QT syndrome mutation carriers are present in 1 of 1000–3000 individuals.[24] Evidently, these "asymptomatic" LQTS carriers may become symptomatic when exposed to any QT-prolonging drug. It is noteworthy that 10–15% of patients with drug-associated TdP were positive for known congenital long QT disease.[24] Also, prolonged baseline QT intervals were documented in up to 71% of patients who experience TdP.[25] Furthermore, provocative drug testing challenging repolarization (e.g., an increase in QTc >480 msec after block of I_{Kr} by sotalol infusion) in a highly monitored clinical setting proved to be a conclusive test to discriminate patients with heterogeneous factors predisposing to ADILQTS.

In contrast to congenital LQTS, which can be caused by one of any eight recognized potassium and sodium ion mutations, drugs that cause ADILQTS span many classes and indications, but most of them share one common feature: a decrease or loss of function in the potassium ion channels of the heart due to administration of the potassium current blockers, resulting in a decrease in the effective repolarization current, repolarization reserve, prolongation of cardiac repolarization, QT interval, and the creation of an arrhythmogenic substrate. The main potassium channel of ADILQTS is I_{Kr}, produced by the combination of KCNH2 (commonly called hERG) and KCNE2.

There are two significant questions that need to be addressed: (1) why are hERG channels so readily blocked by so many drugs, and (2) why is blocking of hERG channels so arrhythmogenic? The first question can be explained by the distinctive biochemical peculiarities of hERG channels: (1) a large, funnel-like vestibule that allows many small size molecules (IC_{50} for I_{kr} blockade is less than 10 nM) to enter the channels and block them, and (2) the presence of multiple aromatic residues that provide high-affinity binding sites for a wide range of pharmaceutical agents. The most plausible explanations of arrhythmogenicity of the hERG blockade are (1) enhanced or abnormal impulse formation due to lengthening of the action potential duration associated with the development of early afterdepolarizations and (2) re-entry due to exaggeration of physiological transmural ventricular heterogeneity.

The mechanism of TdP due to hERG blockade is illustrated in Figure 46–4. The next important channel in cardiotoxic channelopathies is another potassium outward current, I_{Ks} (produced by the combination of KCNQ1 and KCNE1). In either case, an acquired reduction in repolarization reserve plays a major role in the arrhythmogenic manifestation of the ADILQTS. If the potassium channels cannot conduct sufficient current to fully repolarize the cell well before the next depolarization step, synchronization of the cells may fail and an arrhythmia can occur.

In addition to arrhythmogenic potentials of potassium currents blockers, there are some common genetic and nongenetic risk factors and preexisting cardiac abnormalities that influence the likelihood of fatal iatrogenic arrhythmias. Among the many genetic risk factors, the most important are (1) the gene mutations of inherited LQTS, and/or (2) a mutation or polymorphism in one of the suspected LQTS-related genes. A list of other predisposing risk factor for ADILQTS is given in Table 46–3. Known trigger factors for TdP include (1) physical exercise or emotional excitements and/or (2) new heart rhythm irregularities (e.g., new onset atrial fibrillation, increased ectopic supraventricular and ventricular activities), especially bradyarrhythmias

The treatment of arrhythmogenic complications of ADILQTS includes withdrawal of the QT-prolonging drug and its metabolic inhibitor,

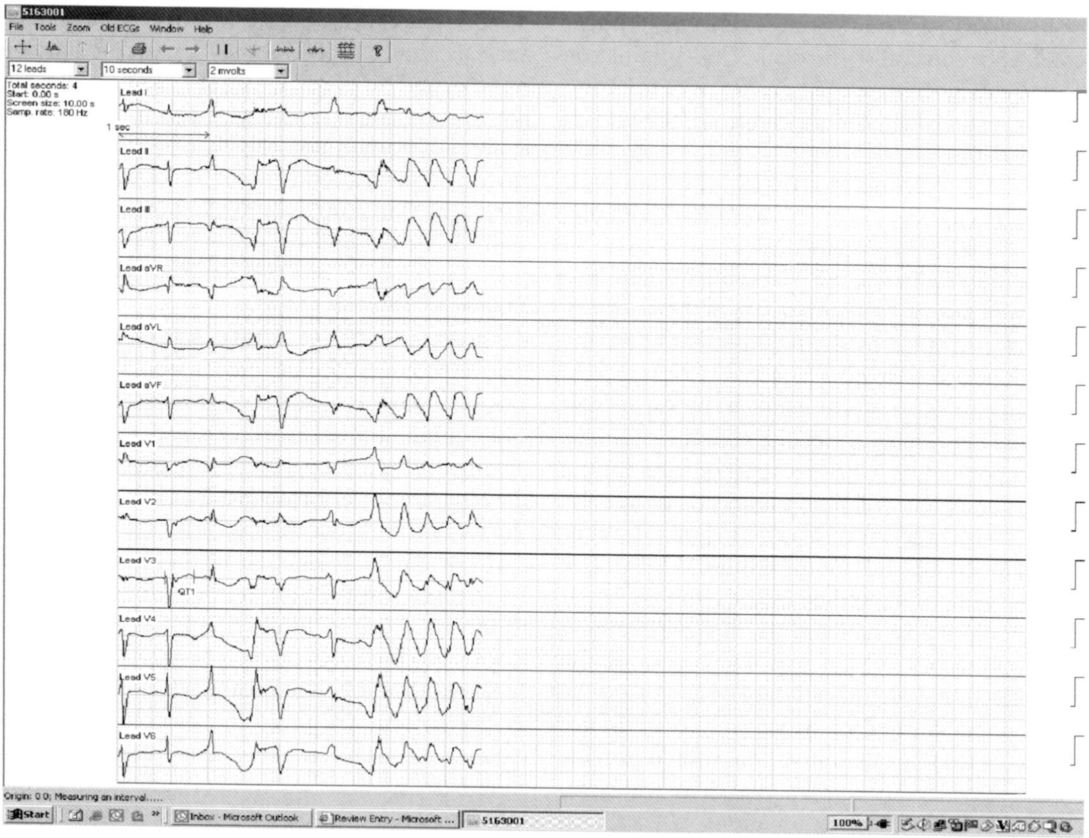

FIGURE 46–4. Development of torsade de pointes ventricular tachycardia in a patient with a prolonged QTc interval. Note the significant repolarization abnormalities (e.g., ST segment depression, T wave inversion) and multifocal premature ventricular complexes.

correction of electrolyte balance (the potassium concentration must not be less than 4 mEq/liter), and administration of magnesium with disregard of its blood serum concentration. Temporary pacing or isoproterenol infusion to prevent bradyarrhythmias is optional.

Acquired Drug-Induced Long QT Syndrome and Its Implication for Clinical Reasearch and Drug Development: Regulatory and Statistical Considerations

The lessons learned by high-profile drug withdrawals, notably of terfenadine and cisapride, and a better understanding of molecular and cellular mechanisms of ADILQTS have important clinical implications for the development of new drugs. In November 2002, the FDA and Health Canada released a new ECG concept paper, which is one in a series of regulatory guidances stemming first from 1996 when the Committee for Proprietary Medicinal Products (CPMP),[26] the United Kingdom FDA equivalent, published its Points to Consider document. Health Canada produced its draft ECG guidance in March 2001. As these guidances[26–28] have progressed, they have become more detailed on how clinical research should be conducted to determine cardiac safety as focused on the QT interval measured by the ECG. The FDA-Health Canada ECG Concept document requires, irrespective of preclinical cardiac findings, a definitive phase I trial for all bioactive agents and even for any agent that is on the market that is brought back for a new indication or for a principal change in target population or dosage. Such a trial must be powered to exclude a 5-msec QTc effect (upper confidence interval = 10 msec). The culmination of these early guidance documents was the completion of the ICH E14 guidance document[29] in October 2005.

To design a definitive QT trial, attention must be given to the sources of QTc duration spontaneous variability. Management of these sources of variability produces a more reliable or definitive set of trial results. The sample size of the definitive QT trial is defined by the requirement of having enough power to detect a 5-msec QTc effect. This generally requires 40–70 subjects per arm (half men and half women). Healthy volunteers are the subject population to use because trying to use the target population will add marked heterogeneity to the study in terms of disease magnitude, concomitant drugs, and comorbidities. A definitive QT trial will be followed by ECG data in the target population in phases II and III, thus determining in a "less definitive" but reasonable manner the ECG effects and identification of "outliers" in the target population of the new agent. The absence of a QTc effect in a definitive trial should provide an increased level of comfort that there will be no QTc effect in the target population.

A definitive QT trial should consist of four arms: a placebo, a positive control (generally moxifloxicin due to its well-documented time-averaged effect of 5–8 msec on QTc), and at least two doses of the new agent to define if there are any dose-related effects. One of the doses should be the standard clinical dose. The other dose selected should be able to cover the expected or theoretical maximum concentration that might occur under the worst circumstance in clinical care. This should account for the coexistence of taking perhaps an extra dose, the presence of metabolic inhibitors, and the presence of renal and/or hepatic dysfunction. A large difference between the supratherapeutic dose and the therapeutic dose is preferable, especially if there is a QT effect of the investigational drug. The regulatory agencies will look at the slope of the QT effect as compared to drug concentration in order to assess the degree of risk to the patient population and to make a determination on what the final labeling for the drug should be.

The primary statistical analysis is based on a time-matched analysis. Individual correction of the QT (QTcI) is the preferred primary method of analysis, but QT correction based on Bazzett (QTcB) and Fredericia (QTcF) should also be done as a secondary analysis. The time-matched analysis is based upon the change from baseline corrected for placebo in the QTcI interval and should be done for each of the time points. The appropriate method to review the data is to subtract the change in QTc on placebo from the change in QTc on drug at the time point with the maximum change in QTc. It is recommended that 12–15 time points be obtained to ensure adequate sampling for a time-matched analysis and a minimum of three ECGs per time point be obtained to reduce variability. It is essential that the laboratory performing the analysis is able to show a moxifloxacin effect of 5–8 msec (time averaged) or a moxifloxicin curve that peaks around 15–20 msec and then diminishes (time matched). Failure to do so is, in effect, an assay sensitivity failure and the trial could be declared invalid.

The outlier or categorical analysis[30] is defined as the determination of the percentage of the patients on each treatment that shows a change from baseline in QTc that is of sufficient magnitude to identify the patients as being at potential risk because of the QTc effect. A specific clinical criterion is a new >500 msec QTc duration or the observation on drug of an abnormal T-U wave often thought to represent an early afterdepolarization that may be a harbinger of TdP. Statistically, a specific change in QTc of >60 msec from baseline in an individual (taken by analyzing the longest QTc duration on any of the several ECG time points on treatment compared with the mean of the baseline ECGs that provide a best point estimate of QTc duration at baseline before treatment) is considered as a specific outlier criterion. An often too-sensitive (too many subjects on placebo will show this effect) criterion is a 30- to 60-msec change from baseline.[31]

References

1. Roden DM. Drug-induced prolongation of the QT interval. *N Engl J Med* 2004;350(10):1013–1022.
2. Legebrve RA, Van Peer A, Woestenborghs R. Influence of itraconazole on the pharmacokinetics and electrocardiographic effect of astemizole. *Br J Clin Pharmacol* 1997;43:319–322.

3. Neuvonen PJ, Kantola T, Kivisto KT. Simvastatin but not pravastatin is very susceptible to interaction with the CYP3A4 inhibitor itraconazole. *Clin Pharmacol Ther* 1998;63:332–341.
4. Wysowski DK, Corken A, Gallo-Torres H, Talarico L, Rodriguez EM. Postmarketing reports of QT prolongation and ventricular arrhythmia in association with cisapride and Food and Drug Administration regulatory actions. *Am J Gastroenterol* 2001;96(6):1698–1703.
5. Morganroth J, Brown AM, Critz S, Crumb WJ, Kunze DL, Lacerda AE, Lopez H. Variability of the QTc interval: Impact on defining drug effect and low-frequency cardiac event. *Am J Cardiol* 1993; 72:26B–32B.
6. Gussak I, Litwin J, Kleiman R, Grisanti S, Morganroth J. Drug-induced cardiac toxicity: Emphasizing the role of electrocardiography in clinical research and drug development. *J Electrocardiol* 2004;37(1):19–24.
7. Rautaharju PM. A farewell to QT dispersion. Are the alternatives any better? *J Electrocardiol* 2005; 38(1):7–9.
8. Yan GX, Antzelevitch C. Cellular basis for the normal T wave and the electrocardiographic manifestations of the long-QT syndrome. *Circulation* 1998;98(18):1928–1936.
9. Zabel M, Malik M, Hnatkova K, Papademetriou V, Pittaras A, Fletcher RD, Franz MR. Analysis of T-wave morphology from the 12-lead electrocardiogram for prediction of long-term prognosis in male US veterans. *Circulation* 2002;105(9):1066–1070.
10. Moss AJ, Zareba W, Benhorin J, Locati EH, Hall WJ, Robinson JL, Schwartz PJ, Towbin JA, Vincent GM, Lehmann MH. ECG T-wave patterns in genetically distinct forms of the hereditary long QT syndrome. *Circulation* 1995;92(10):2929–2934.
11. Nearing BL, Verrier RL. Progressive increases in complexity of T-wave oscillations herald ischemia-induced ventricular fibrillation. *Circ Res* 2002;91(8): 727–732.
12. Nearing BD, Verrier RL. Modified moving average analysis of T-wave alternans to predict ventricular fibrillation with high accuracy. *J Appl Physiol* 2002; 92(2):541–549.
13. Roden DM. Pharmacogenetics and drug-induced arrhythmias. *Cardiovasc Res* 2001;50:224–231.
14. Roden DM, Spooner PM. Inherited long QT syndromes: A paradigm for understanding arrhythmogenesis. *J Cardiovasc Electrophysiol* 1999;10: 1664–1683.
15. Nattel S, Li DS. Ionic remodeling in the heart– pathophysiological significance and new therapeutic opportunities for atrial fibrillation. *Circ Res* 2000;87:440–447.
16. Roden DM, Spooner PM. Inherited long QT syndromes: A paradigm for understanding arrhythmogenesis. *J Cardiovasc Electrophysiol* 1999;10: 1664–1683.
17. Abbott GW, *et al.* MiRP1 forms IKr potassium channels with HERG and is associated with cardiac arrhythmia. *Cell* 1999;97:175–187.
18. Curtis LH, Ostbye T, Sendersky V, Hutchison S, Allen LaPointe NM, Al-Khatib SM, Usdin Yasuda S, Dans PE, Wright A, Califf RM, Woosley RL, Schulman KA. Prescription of QT-prolonging drugs in a cohort of about 5 million outpatients. *Am J Med* 2003;114(2):135–141.
19. Shah RR. Drug-induced prolongation of the QT interval: Why the regulatory concern? *Fundam Clin Pharmacol* 2002;16(2):119–124.
20. Shah RR. Interpretation of clinical ECG data: Understanding the risk from non-antiarrhythmic drugs. In: Morganroth J, Gussak I, Eds. *Cardiac Safety of Noncardiac Drugs: Practical Guidelines for Clinical Research and Drug Development.* Totowa, NJ: Humana Press, 2004:259–301.
21. Bauman JL, Bauernfeind RA, Hoff JV, Strasberg B, Swiryn S, Rosen KM. Torsade de pointes due to quinidine: Observations in 31 patients. *Am Heart J* 1984;107(3):425–430.
22. MacNeil DJ, Davies RO, Deitchman D. Clinical safety profile of sotalol in the treatment of arrhythmias. *Am J Cardiol* 1993;72(4):44A–50A.
23. Moss AJ, Schwartz PJ. Delayed repolarization (QT or QTU prolongation) and malignant ventricular arrhythmias. *Mod Concepts Cardiovasc Dis* 1982; 51(3):85–90.
24. Yang P, Kanki H, Drolet B, Yang T, Wei J, Viswanathan PC, Hohnloser SH, Shimizu W, Schwartz PJ, Stanton M, Murray KT, Norris K, George AL Jr, Roden DM. Allelic variants in long-QT disease genes in patients with drug-associated torsades de pointes. *Circulation* 2002;105(16):1943–1948.
25. Zehender M, Hohnloser S, Just H. QT-interval prolonging drugs: Mechanisms and clinical relevance of their arrhythmogenic hazards. *Cardiovasc Drugs Ther* 1991;5(2):515–530.
26. Committee for Proprietary Medicinal Products (CPMP). Points to consider: The assessment of the potential for QT interval prolongation by non-cardiovascular medicinal products. The European Agency for the Evaluation of Medicinal Products. 17 December 1997.
27. Health Canada: Draft Guidance "Assessment of the QT prolongation potential of non-antiarrhythmic

drugs," March 15, 2001. Available from http://www.hc-sh.gc.ca/hpb-dgps/therapeut/htmleng/guidmain.html.
28. Food and Drug Administration and Health Canada. The clinical evaluation of QT/QTc interval prolongation and proarrhythmic potential for non-antiarrhythmic drugs. 2002 Preliminary Concept paper, November 15. Available from http://www.fda.gov/cder/workshop.htm#upcoming.
29. Guidance for Industry E14 Clinical Evaluation of QT/QTc Interval Prolongation and Proarrhythmic Potential for Non-Antiarrhythmic Drugs. U.S. Department of Health and Human Services Food and Drug Administration Center for Drug Evaluation and Research (CDER), and Center for Biologics Evaluation and Research (CBER). October 2005. http://www.fda.gov/cder/guidance/6922fnl.htm.
30. Morganroth J. A definitive or thorough phase 1 QT ECG trial as a requirement for drug safety assessment. *J Electrocardiol* 2004;37(1):25–29.
31. Pratt CM, Ruberg S, Morganroth J, *et al.* Dose-response relation between terfenadine (Seldane) and the QTc interval on the scalar electrocardiogram: Distinguishing a drug effect from spontaneous variability. *Am Heart J* 1996;131:472.

47
Acquired Form of Brugada Syndrome

Wataru Shimizu

Brugada Syndome

Brugada and Brugada reported in 1992 eight patients with a history of aborted sudden cardiac death due to ventricular fibrillation (VF) and a characteristic electrocardiographic pattern, consisting of right bundle branch block (RBBB) and ST-segment elevation in the right precordial electrocardiogram (ECG) (V1–V3) as a distinct clinical entity.[1–8] The presence of RBBB was thereafter revealed to be not necessary for the diagnosis of Brugada syndrome, although mild to moderate widening of the QRS duration is often observed.[5] Two specific types of ST-segment elevation, coved and saddleback, are observed in this syndrome. The ST-segment elevation is often accentuated and the coved type ST-segment elevation is more frequently recognized just before and after episodes of VF.[9,10] The Brugada Consensus Report in 2002 suggested three patterns of ST-segment elevation in the right precordial ECG.[5] Type 1 is characterized by a coved type ST-segment elevation displaying J wave amplitude or ST-segment elevation of ≥0.2 mV followed by a negative T wave (Figure 47–1A). Type 2 has a saddleback configuration, which has a high take-off ST-segment elevation (≥0.2 mV) followed by a gradually descending ST-segment elevation (remaining ≥0.1 mV above the baseline) and a positive or biphasic T wave (Figure 47–1B). Type 3 has an ST-segment elevation of <0.1 mV of the saddleback, coved type, or both. The second Consensus Report published in 2005, however, emphasized that Type 1 coved ST-segment elevation is required to diagnose Brugada syndrome,[7] because the Type 1 ECG is reported to relate to a higher incidence of VF and sudden cardiac death.[6] Type 2 and Type 3 ST-segment elevation are not diagnostic for the Brugada syndrome. The recordings of V1 and V2 leads at higher (third and second) intercostal spaces increase the sensitivity and the specificity of the ECG diagnosis for detecting the Brugada phenotype (Figure 47–1C),[7,11] and their diagnostic and prognostic values have recently been reported.[12]

Molecular Aspects

In 1998, Chen and co-workers identified the first mutation linked to Brugada syndrome in *SCN5A*, the gene encoding the α subunit of the sodium channel.[13] Antzelevitch and co-workers have recently reported that three probands associated with a Brugada like ST-segment elevation and a short QT interval were linked to mutations in *CACNA1C* (A39V and G490R) or *CACNB2* (S481L), the gene encoding the α1 or β2b subunit of the L-type calcium channel ($I_{Ca\text{-}L}$), respectively.[14] However, approximately tow-thirds of Brugada patients have not been yet genotyped, suggesting the presence of genetic heterogeneity.[8] Other candidate genes for the Brugada phenotype include the genes encoding transient outward current (I_{to}), and delayed rectifier potassium current (I_K), or genes that code for adrenergic receptors, cholinergic receptors, ion-channel-interacting protein, promoters, transcriptional factors, neurotransmitters, or transporters.

Functional analysis employing expression systems was reported in approximately two dozen

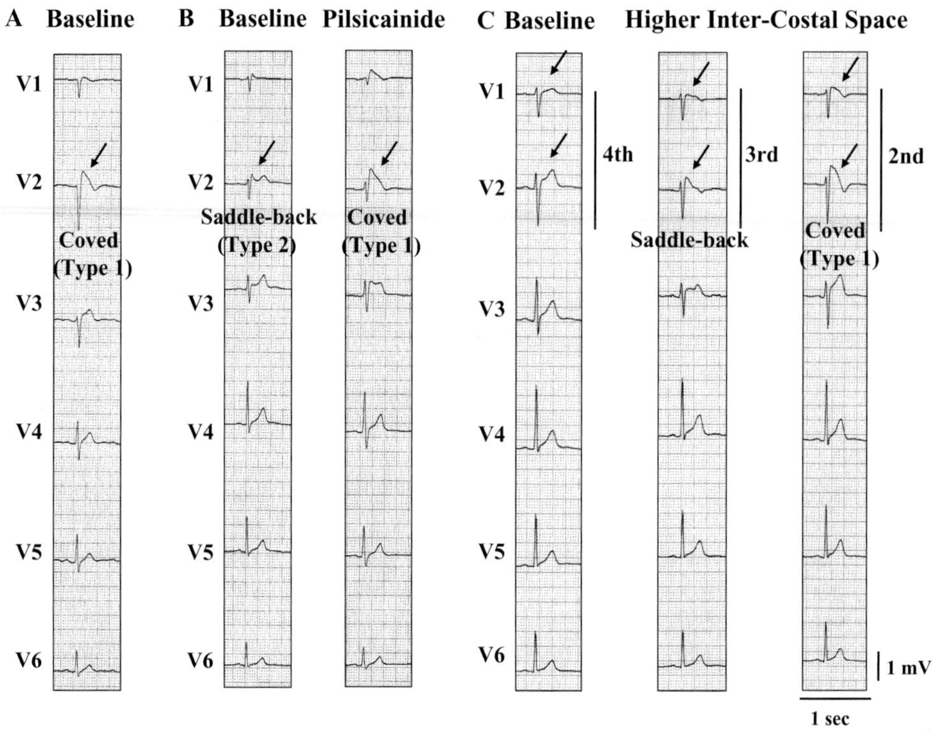

FIGURE 47–1. Type 1 coved ST-segment elevation spontaneously or unmasked by pilsicainide or higher intercostal space recordings of V1 and V2 leads. (A) Spontaneously Type 1 coved ST-segment elevation. (B) Although Type 2 saddleback ST-segment elevation was seen in a V2 lead under baseline conditions, pilsicainide, a class IC drug, unmasked Type 1 coved ST-segment elevation in a V2 lead (arrow). (C) Although no ST-segment elevation was observed at standard (fourth intercostal space) V1 and V2 leads under baseline conditions (arrows), a Type 1 coved ST-segment elevation was recorded at higher (second intercostal space) V1 and V2 leads (arrows).

of the mutations in *SCN5A*, and demonstrated that all of the mutations resulted in "loss of function" of I_{Na} by several mechanisms.[13,15–17] These functional effects include (1) failure of the sodium channel to express, (2) a shift in the voltage and time dependence of I_{Na} activation, inactivation, or reactivation, (3) entry of the sodium channel into an intermediate state of inactivation from which it recovers more slowly, (4) accelerated inactivation of the sodium channel, or (5) trafficking defect.

Cellular Mechanism of Brugada Phenotype

An I_{to}-mediated phase 1 notch of the action potential (AP) has been reported to be greater in the epicardial cells than in the endocardial cells in many species, including humans, by experimental studies.[18] Since the maintenance of the AP dome is determined by the fine balance of currents active at the end of phase 1 of the AP (principally I_{to} and $I_{Ca\text{-}L}$), any agents that cause a net outward shift at the end of phase 1 can increase the magnitude of the AP notch, leading to loss of the AP dome (all-or-none repolarization) in the epicardium, but not in the endocardium, contributing to a significant voltage gradient across the ventricular wall during ventricular activation.[18] The heterogeneous loss of the AP dome in the epicardium was shown to produce premature beats via a mechanism of phase 2 reentry in experimental studies using isolated sheets of canine right ventricle.[19] The Brugada syndrome seems to be a clinical counterpart of the mechanism of all-or-none repolarization in the epicardial cells and phase 2 reentry-induced premature beat between the adjacent epicardial cells.

An experimental model of the Brugada syndrome employing arterially perfused canine right ventricular (RV) wedge preparations provided direct experimental evidence for the cellular mechanism of ST-segment elevation.[20] The I_{to}-mediated AP notch and the loss of the AP dome in the epicardial cells, but not in the endocardial cells, of the right ventricle gives rise to a transmural voltage gradient, producing ST-segment elevation in the ECG (Figure 47–2).[8] In the setting of coved type ST-segment elevation, heterogeneous loss of the AP dome (the coexistence of loss of dome regions and restored dome regions) in the epicardium creates a marked epicardial dispersion of repolarization, giving rise to premature beats due to phase 2 reentry, which sometimes precipitates nonsustained polymorphic ventricular tachycardia (VT) or VF (Figure 47–2).[8]

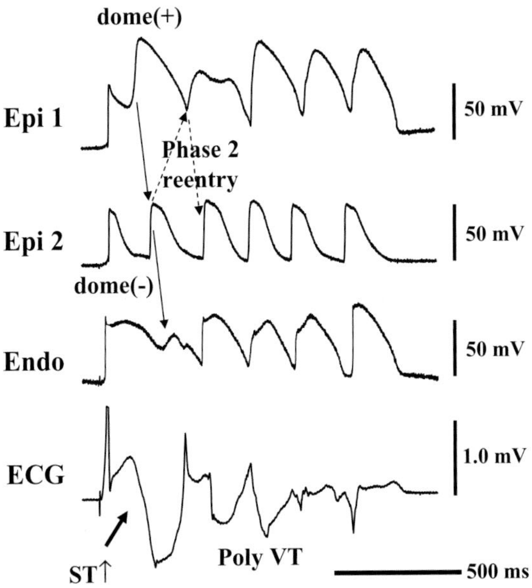

Figure 47–2. Coved ST-segment elevation and phase 2 reentry-induced nonsustained polymorphic ventricular tachycardia (poly VT) in a Brugada model employing an arterially perfused canine right ventricular wedge preparation. Transmembrane action potentials simultaneously recorded from two epicardial (Epi) sites and one endocardial (Endo) site together with a transmural electrocardiogram (ECG) (BCL 2000 msec). Combined administration of terfenadine (5 μM) and pilsicainide (5 μM) causes heterogeneous loss of the action potential dome in the epicardium (restored dome in epicardial site 1, loss of dome in epicardial site 2), giving rise to a coved type Brugada ECG. Electrotonic propagation from the site where the dome is restored (Epi 1) to the site where it is lost (Epi 2) results in development of phase 2 reentry-induced premature beats, triggering poly VT.

Our recently developed high-resolution optical mapping system, which allows us to record transmembrane APs from 256 sites simultaneously, suggested that a steep repolarization gradient between a loss of dome region and a restored dome region in the epicardium is essential to produce phase 2 reentry-induced premature beats, and that mild to moderate conduction delay is required to degenerate the reentrant pathway into VF.[8,21]

Acquired Form of Brugada Syndrome

The ST-segment elevation is well known to be dynamic day-to-day even in the same patient with Brugada syndrome, and to be modulated by several drugs (mainly antiarrhythmic drugs) and autonomic agents.[22] Class IC antiarrhythmic drugs, which are used as a diagnostic tool in latent Brugada syndrome, amplify or unmask the ST-segment elevation most effectively as a result of their strong effect of blocking fast I_{Na}.[23,24] Several drugs and conditions other than IC drugs are reported to induce transient ST-segment elevation like that in Brugada syndrome. Based on the molecular and cellular aspects in Brugada syndrome mentioned above, any interventions that increase outward currents (e.g., I_{to}, adenosine triphosphate-sensitive potassium current [$I_{K\text{-}ATP}$], slow and fast activating components of I_K [I_{Ks}, I_{Kr}]) or decrease inward currents (e.g., $I_{Ca\text{-}L}$, fast I_{Na}) at the end of phase 1 of the AP can accentuate or unmask ST-segment elevation, similar to that found in Brugada syndrome. This is described as an "acquired" form of Brugada syndrome similar to the "acquired" form of long QT syndrome (LQTS) (Table 47–1).

Antiarrhythmic Drugs

Class IC sodium channel blockers (flecainide, propafenone, pilsicainide) produce the most pronounced ST-segment elevation secondary to strong use-dependent blocking of fast I_{Na} due to their slow dissociation from the sodium channels.[23–28] Pilsicainide, a pure class IC drug developed in Japan, is thought to more strongly induce ST-segment elevation than flecainide, which is widely used throughout the world and mildly blocks I_{to}.

TABLE 47–1. Acquired form of Brugada syndrome.

1. Antiarrhythmic drugs
A. Sodium channel blockers
Class IC drugs (flecainide,[23,24,27,28] pilsicainide,[26] propafenone[25])
Class IA drugs (ajmaline,[24,29] procainamide,[22,24] disopyramide,[22,23] cibenzoline[30])
B. Calcium channel blockers
Verapamil[34]
C. β Blockers
Propranolol, etc.
2. Antianginal drugs
A. Calcium channel blockers
Nefedipine, diltiazem, etc.
B. Nitrate
Isosorbide dinitrate, nitroglyceline,[34] etc.
C. Potassium channel openers
Nicorandil, etc.
3. Psychotropic drugs
A. Tricyclic antidepressants
Amitriptyline,[35,36] nortriptyline,[37] desipramine,[38] clomipramine,[39] etc.
B. Tetracyclic antidepressants
Maprotiline,[35] etc.
C. Phenothiazine
Perphenazine,[35] cyamemazine,[36] etc.
D. Selective serotonin reuptake inhibitors
Fluoxetine,[36] etc.
4. Other drugs
A. Histaminic H1 receptor antagonists
Dimenhydrinate,[40] etc.
B. Cocaine intoxication[41]
C. Lithium[42]
5. Hypertestosteronemia[46]
6. Low visceral fat[46]
7. Myocardial ischemia
A. Right ventricular infarction/ischemia[47]
B. Vasospastic angina[48,49]
8. Temperature
A. Hyperthermia (febrile state)[50,51]
B. Hypothermia[53,54]
9. Electrolyte abnormalities
A. Hyperkalemia[55]
B. Hypercalcemia[56]
11. Meal, increaed insulin level[57]
12. Polymorphysims in SCN5A[59]

Class IA sodium channel blockers (ajmaline, procainamide, disopyramide, cibenzoline, etc.), which exhibit less use-dependent block of fast I_{Na} due to faster dissociation of the drug for the sodium channels, are expected to show a weaker ST-segment elevation than class IC drugs.[22–24,29,30] However, the net effects of IA drugs on ST-segment augmentation are influenced by their blocking effect of I_{to} to ameliorate their blocking effect of I_{Na}. Ajmaline is reported to induce or enhance Type 1 ST-segment elevation more frequently than flecainide, a class IC drug, probably due to less inhibition of I_{to} by ajmaline.[29,31] Disopyramide and procainamide show weaker accentuation of the ST-segment elevation due to their smaller effect on fast I_{Na} and mild to moderate action to block I_{to}.[22–24] In contrast, quinidine generally normalizes ST-segment elevation owing to its relatively strong I_{to} blocking effect, and is proposed to be a pharmacological treatment for the Brugada syndrome.[32,33]

Class IB sodium channel blockers (mexiletine, lidocaine, etc.) dissociate from the sodium channel rapidly and therefore block fast I_{Na} principally at rapid rates. At moderate and slow heart rates, class IB drugs have little or no effect on fast I_{Na}, thus are unable to cause ST-segment elevation.[23]

$I_{Ca\text{-}L}$ blockers such as verapamil (Figure 47–3) and β blockers are expected to accentuate ST-segment elevation and possibly to induce VF as a result of inhibiting $I_{Ca\text{-}L}$.[34] Recently, it is reported

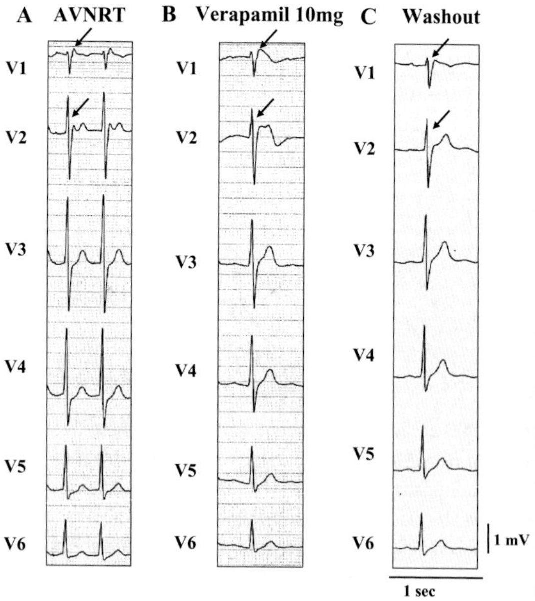

FIGURE 47–3. Acquired form of Brugada syndrome induced by intravenous verapamil in a patient with atrioventricular nodal reentrant tachycardia (AVNRT). During AVNRT (A), intravenous administration of 10 mg verapamil successfully terminated AVNRT, but unmasked Type 1 coved ST-segment elevation in lead V1 and Type 2 saddleback ST-segment elevation in lead V2 (B, arrows). The ST-segment elevation disappeared after washout of verapamil (C).

that vasovagal syncope is accompanied in some patients with Brugada syndrome. β Blockers are often used as a first line of therapy for vasovagal syncope. Therefore, unmasking of Brugada syndrome must always be taken into account in the use of β blockers for vasovagal syncope.

Antianginal Drugs

Calcium antagonists (nefedipine, diltiazem, etc.) and nitrates, which have a blocking action of $I_{Ca\text{-}L}$, are often used as a first line of therapy for ischemic heart diseases. An $I_{K\text{-}ATP}$ opener, nicorandil, is another choice of therapy. These antianginal drugs are expected to provoke ST-segment elevation in patients with the "acquired" form of Brugada syndrome.[7,34]

Psychotropic Drugs

Many psychotropic drugs have been reported to unmask Brugada-like ST-segment elevation. These include tricyclic antidepressants (amitriptyline, nortriptyline, desipramine, clomipramine, etc.), tetracyclic antidepressants (maprotiline, etc.), and phenothiazine (perphenazine, cyamemazine, etc.), most of which block fast I_{Na} usually with overdose (Figure 47–4).[35–39] The selective serotonin reuptake inhibitors (SSRIs), such as fluoxetine, are reported to produce ST-segment elevation, probably as a result of their effect to depress fast I_{Na} and $I_{Ca\text{-}L}$.[36]

Other Drugs

Dimenhydrinate, a sedating, first-generation histaminic H1 receptor antagonist, commonly used as an antiemetic, is reported to produce Brugada-like ST segment elevation.[40] Dimenhydrinate exhibits an anticholinergic action and blocks fast I_{Na}; the latter effect may cause the ST-segment elevation. ST-segment elevation is also reported to be provoked by cocaine intoxication mainly due to its fast I_{Na} blocking effect.[41] More recently, lithium was reported to unmask Brugada ECG.[42]

Hypertestosteronemia and Low Visceral Fat

All of the mutations so far identified in patients with Brugada syndrome display an autosomal dominant mode of transmission. Therefore, males and females are expected to inherit the defective gene equally. However, clinical Brugada phenotype is much more prevalent in males than in females, especially in Asian countries.[43] The male predominance in the Brugada syndrome is at least in part due to intrinsic differences in the ventricular AP between males and females.[44] Recent clinical studies suggested that a male hormone, testosterone, may be attributable to male predominance in patients with Brugada syndrome. Matsuo and co-workers reported two cases of asymptomatic Brugada syndrome, in whom coved type ST-segment elevation disappeared following

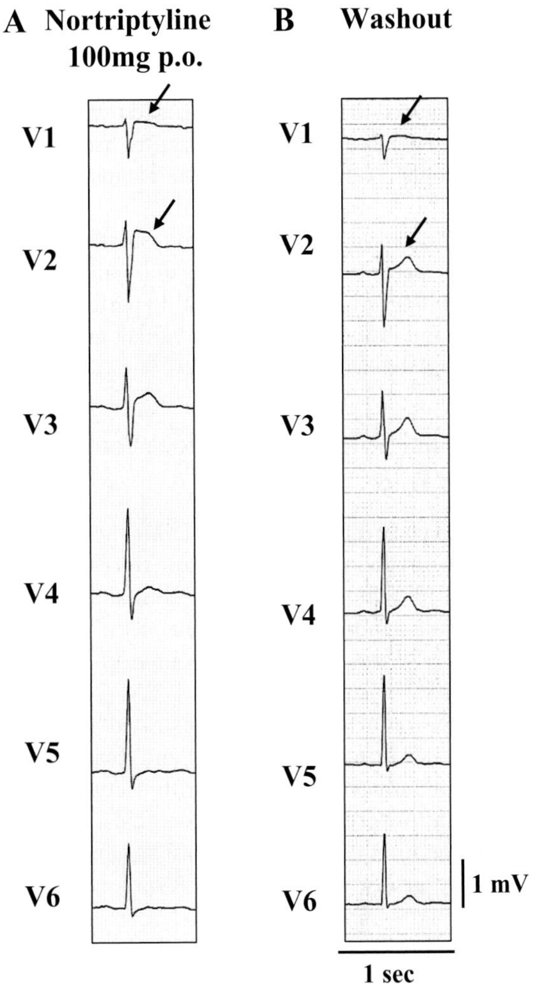

FIGURE 47–4. Tricyclic antidepressant-induced acquired form of Brugada syndrome. Type 1 coved ST-segment elevation was observed in leads V1 and V2 during oral nortriptyline (100 mg/day), a tricyclic antidepressant (A, arrows). The ST-segment elevation disappeared after washout of nortriptyline (B, arrows).

orchiectomy as therapy for prostate cancer,[45] indicating that testosterone may contribute to the Brugada phenotype in these two cases. Our recent data suggested that males with Brugada syndrome were independently and significantly associated with a higher testosterone level and lower body mass index compared to age-matched control males, indicating a critical role of testosterone on the male predominance in Brugada syndrome.[46] These data also suggested that hypertestosteronemia and low visceral fat may be risk factors in provoking the Brugada phenotype.

Myocardial Ischemia in the Right Ventricular Outflow Tract

Acute myocardial infarction (AMI) or acute ischemia involving the RV outflow tract (RVOT) mimics ST-segment elevation similar to that in Brugada syndrome, as a result of the depression of $I_{Ca\text{-}L}$ and the activation of $I_{K\text{-}ATP}$ during ischemia.[47]

Several reports have demonstrated a combination of Brugada syndrome and vasospastic angina or induced vasospasm with acetylcholine (ACh) and/or ergonovine maleate (EM).[48] Along the same lines as the AMI, vasospasm of the coronary artery supplying the RVOT region is expected to produce Brugada-like ST-segment elevation. Noda *et al.* systematically evaluated the frequency of induced coronary spasm and the change of ST-segment elevation with intraright coronary injection of ACh and/or EM in patients with Brugada syndrome.[49] Coronary spasm was induced in 3 (11%) of 27 Brugada patients, suggesting that coronary spasm was not rare in Brugada syndrome. The ST-segment elevation was augmented by 11 (33%) of the 33 right coronary injections [Ach, 6/11 (55%); EM, 5/22 (23%)] without any induction of coronary spasm (Figure 47–5). VF was induced by 3 (9%) of the 33 right coronary injections [Ach, 2/11 (18%); EM, 1/22 (5%)]. These results suggested that mild ischemia and vagal influences act with the substrate responsible for Brugada syndrome to elevate the ST-segment and precipitate VF by decreasing $I_{Ca\text{-}L}$ and activating $I_{K\text{-}ATP}$, and that the congenital and possibly acquired form of Brugada syndrome may place a patient at higher risk for ischemia-related sudden cardiac death.

Temperature: Hyperthermia (Febrile State) and Hypothermia

A number of reports have demonstrated that a febrile state can unmask Brugada-like ST segment

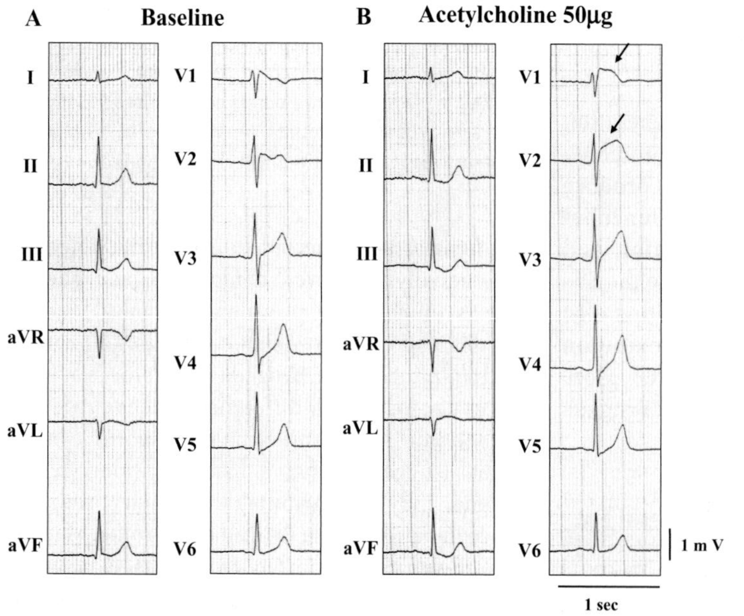

FIGURE 47–5. Type 1 coved ST-segment elevation induced by intraright coronary injection of acetylcholine. A 12 precordial lead electrocardiogram (ECG) under baseline conditions (A) and coronary injection of 50 μg acetylcholine (ACh) into the right coronary artery (B) in a patient with diagnosed Brugada syndrome. Injection of ACh augmented the ST-segment elevation in leads V1 and V2 (B, arrows).

elevation and provoke VF.[50,51] Some functional studies have demonstrated that high temperature (febrile state) reduced I_{Na} in the mutant sodium channel, and was expected to accentuate or unmask Brugada ECG.[52]

On the other hand, a prominent J wave associated with ST-segment elevation mimicking Brugada ECG has long been described as an Osborn wave in hypothermic states due to accidental exposures to cold.[53,54] This is probably due to a low temperature-induced increase of I_{to}.

Electrolyte Abnormalities

Severe hyperkalemia[55] or hypercalcemia[56] is associated with ST-segment elevation in the right precordial leads as in Brugada syndrome.

Meal and Increased Insulin Level

The increased insulin level after meals or the glucose tolerance test is reported to accentuate or unmask the Brugada ECG.[57] This effect may contribute to circadian or day-to-day variation in the degree of ST-segment elevation in this syndrome. Although insulin increases outward current by activating the Na^+/K^+ pump and stimulates $I_{Ca\text{-}L}$, the predominance of the former is thought to contribute to augmentation of the ST-segment elevation.

Polymorphisms

A mutation or polymorphisms in genes responsible for the congenital form of LQTS (LQT1, *KCNQ1*; LQT2, *KCNH2*; LQT3, *SCN5A*) have been identified in some patients with "acquired" forms of LQTS.[58] This naturally suggests that some patients with the "acquired" form of Brugada syndrome may inherit polymorphisms or other mutations in *SCN5A* or other genes. We recently identified a haplotype consisting of six individual DNA polymorphisms within the proximal promoter region of the *SCN5A* gene only in a Japanese population, which reduced transcription of the cardiac sodium channel mRNA.[59] This suggests that individuals carrying these 6 polymorphisms would display mild reduction of I_{Na} and would be candidates of "acquired" form of Brugada syndrome.

Acknowledgments. Dr. W Shimizu was supported by the Uehara Memorial Foundation, Japan Research Foundation for Clinical Pharmacology, Ministry of Education, Culture, Sports, Science and Technology Leading Project for Biosimulation, and health sciences research grants (H18-Research on Human Genome-002) from the Ministry of Health, Labour and Welfare, Japan.

References

1. Brugada P, Brugada J. Right bundle branch block, persistent ST segment elevation and sudden cardiac death: A distinct clinical and electrocardiographic syndrome: A multicenter report. *J Am Coll Cardiol* 1992;20:1391–1396.
2. Brugada J, Brugada R, Brugada P. Right bundle-branch block and ST-segment elevation in leads V_1 through V_3. A marker for sudden death in patients without demonstrable structural heart disease. *Circulation* 1998;97:457–460.
3. Antzelevitch C, Brugada P, Brugada J, Brugada R, Shimizu W, Gussak I, Perez Riera AR. Brugada syndrome. A decade of progress. *Circ Res* 2002;91:1114–1118.
4. Priori SG, Napolitano C, Gasparini M, Pappone C, Della Bella P, Giordano U, Bloise R, Giustetto C, De Nardis R, Grillo M, Ronchetti E, Faggiano G, Nastoli J. Natural history of Brugada syndrome: Insights for risk stratification and management. *Circulation* 2002;105:1342–1347.
5. Wilde AA, Antzelevitch C, Borggrefe M, Brugada J, Brugada R, Brugada P, Corrado D, Hauer RN, Kass RS, Nademanee K, Priori SG, Towbin JA. Proposed diagnostic criteria for the Brugada syndrome: Consensus report. *Circulation* 2002;106:2514–2519.
6. Brugada J, Brugada R, Antzelevitch C, Towbin J, Nademanee K, Brugada P. Long-term follow-up of individuals with the electrocardiographic pattern of right bundle-branch block and ST-segment elevation in precordial leads V1 to V3. *Circulation* 2002;105:73–78.
7. Antzelevitch C, Brugada P, Borggrefe M, Brugada J, Brugada R, Corrado D, Gussak I, Lemarec H, Nademanee K, Perez Riera AR, Shimizu W, Schulze-Bahr E, Tan H, Wilde A. Brugada Syndrome. Report of the Second Consensus Conference. Endorsed by the Heart Rhythm Society and the European Heart Rhythm Association. *Circulation* 2005;111:659–670.
8. Shimizu W, Aiba T, Kamakura S. Mechanisms of disease: Current understanding and future

challenges in Brugada syndrome. *Nat Clin Pract Cardiovasc Med* 2005;2:408–414.

9. Kasanuki H, Ohnishi S, Ohtuka M, Matsuda N, Nirei T, Isogai R, Shoda M, Toyoshima Y, Hosoda S. Idiopathic ventricular fibrillation induced with vagal activity in patients without obvious heart disease. *Circulation* 1997;95:2277–2285.
10. Matsuo K, Shimizu W, Kurita T, Inagaki M, Aihara N, Kamakura S. Dynamic changes of 12-lead electrocardiograms in a patient with Brugada syndrome. *J Cardiovasc Electrophysiol* 1998;9:508–512.
11. Shimizu W, Matsuo K, Takagi M, Tanabe Y, Aiba T, Taguchi A, Suyama K, Kurita T, Aihara N, Kamakura S. Body surface distribution and response to drugs of ST segment elevation in the Brugada syndrome: Clinical implication of 87-leads body surface potential mapping and its application to 12-leads electrocardiograms. *J Cardiovasc Electrophysiol* 2000;11:396–404.
12. Miyamoto K, Yokokawa M, Tanaka K, Nagai T, Okamura H, Noda T, Satomi K, Suyama K, Kurita T, Aihara N, Kamakura S, Shimizu W. Diagnostic and prognostic value of type 1 Brugada electrocardiogram at higher (3rd or 2nd) V1–V2 recording in males with Brugada syndrome. *Am J Cardiol* 2006; 99(1):53–57.
13. Chen Q, Kirsch GE, Zhang D, Brugada R, Brugada J, Brugada P, Potenza D, Moya A, Borggrefe M, Breithardt G, Ortiz-Lopez R, Wang Z, Antzelevitch C, O'Brien RE, Schulze-Bahr E, Keating MT, Towbin JA, Wang Q. Genetic basis and molecular mechanisms for idiopathic ventricular fibrillation. *Nature* 1998;392:293–296.
14. Antzelevitch C, Pollevick GD, Cordeiro JM, Casis O, Sanguinetti MC, Aizawa Y, *et al.* Loss of function mutations in the cardiac calcium channel underlie a new clinical entity characterized by ST segment elevation, short QT intervals and sudden cardiac death. *Circulation* 2007;115:442–449.
15. Makita N, Shirai N, Wang DW, Sasaki K, George AL Jr, Kanno M, Kitabatake A. Cardiac Na(+) channel dysfunction in Brugada syndrome is aggravated by beta(1)-subunit. *Circulation* 2002;101:54–60.
16. Viswanathan PC, Bezzina CR, George AL Jr, Roden DM, Wilde AA, Balser JR. Gating-dependent mechanisms for flecainide action in *SCN5A*-linked arrhythmia syndromes. *Circulation* 2001;104:1200–1205.
17. Baroudi G, Acharfi S, Larouche C, Chahine M. Expression and intracellular localization of an *SCN5A* double mutant R1232W/T1620M implicated in Brugada syndrome. *Circ Res* 2002;90:E11–E16.
18. Litovsky SH, Antzelevitch C. Transient outward current prominent in canine ventricular epicardium but not endocardium. *Circ Res* 1988;62: 116–126.
19. Krishnan SC, Antzelevitch C. Flecainide-induced arrhythmia in canine ventricular epicardium: Phase 2 Reentry? *Circulation* 1993;87:562–5729.
20. Yan GX, Antzelevitch C. Cellular basis for the Brugada syndrome and other mechanisms of arrhythmogenesis associated with ST segment elevation. *Circulation* 1999;100:1660–1666.
21. Aiba T, Shimizu W, Hidaka I, Uemura K, Noda T, Zheng C, Kamiya A, Inagaki M, Sugimachi M, Sunagawa K. Cellular basis for trigger and maintenance of ventricular fibrillation in the Brugada syndrome model: High resolution optical mapping study. *J Am Coll Cardiol* 2006;47:2074–2085.
22. Miyazaki T, Mitamura H, Miyoshi S, Soejima K, Aizawa Y, Ogawa S. Autonomic and antiarrhythmic drug modulation of ST segment elevation in patients with Brugada syndrome. *J Am Coll Cardiol* 1996;27:1061–1070.
23. Shimizu W, Antzelevitch C, Suyama K, Kurita T, Taguchi A, Aihara N, Takaki H, Sunagawa K, Kamakura S. Effect of sodium channel blockers on ST segment, QRS duration, and corrected QT interval in patients with Brugada syndrome. *J Cardiovasc Electrophysiol* 2000;11:1320–1329.
24. Brugada R, Brugada J, Antzelevitch C, Kirsch GE, Potenza D, Towbin JA, Brugada P. Sodium channel blockers identify risk for sudden death in patients with ST-segment elevation and right bundle branch block but structurally normal hearts. *Circulation* 2000;101:510–515.
25. Matana A, Goldner V, Stanic K, Mavric Z, Zaputovic L, Matana Z. Unmasking effect of propafenone on the concealed form of the Brugada phenomenon. *Pacing Clin Electrophysiol* 2000;23: 416–418.
26. Morita H, Morita ST, Nagase S, Banba K, Nishii N, Tani Y, Watanabe A, Nakamura K, Kusano KF, Emori T, Matsubara H, Hina K, Kita T, Ohe T. Ventricular arrhythmia induced by sodium channel blocker in patients with Brugada syndrome. *J Am Coll Cardiol* 2003;42:1624–1631.
27. Gasparini M, Priori SG, Mantica M, Napolitano C, Galimberti P, Ceriotti C, Simonini S. Flecainide test in Brugada syndrome: A reproducible but risky tool. *Pacing Clin Electrophysiol* 2003;26:338–341.
28. Meregalli PG, Ruijter JM, Hofman N, Bezzina CR, Wilde AA, Tan HL. Diagnostic value of flecainide testing in unmasking SCN5A-related Brugada syndrome. *J Cardiovasc Electrophysiol* 2006;17:857–864.
29. Rolf S, Bruns HJ, Wichter T, Kirchhof P, Ribbing M, Wasmer K, Paul M, Breithardt G, Haverkamp

W, Eckardt L. The ajmaline challenge in Brugada syndrome: Diagnostic impact, safety, and recommended protocol. *Eur Heart J* 2003;24:1104–1112.
30. Tada H, Nogami A, Shimizu W, Nakatsugawa M, Naito S, Oshima S, Taniguchi K. ST-segment and T-wave alternans in a patient with Brugada syndrome. *Pacing Clin Electrophysiol* 2000;23:413–415.
31. Wolpert C, Echternach C, Veltmann C, Antzelevitch C, Thomas GP, Spehl S, Streitner F, Kuschyk J, Schimpf R, Haase KK, Borggrefe M. Intravenous drug challenge using flecainide and ajmaline in patients with Brugada syndrome. *Heart Rhythm* 2005;2:254–260.
32. Hermida JS, Denjoy I, Clerc J, Extramiana F, Jarry G, Milliez P, Guicheney P, Di Fusco S, Rey JL, Cauchemez B, Leenhardt A. Hydroquinidine therapy in Brugada syndrome. *J Am Coll Cardiol* 2004; 43:1853–1860.
33. Belhassen B, Glick A, Viskin S. Efficacy of quinidine in high-risk patients with Brugada syndrome. *Circulation* 2004;110:1731–1737.
34. Shimizu W. Acquired forms of Brugada syndrome. In: Antzelevitch C, Ed. *The Brugada Syndrome: From Bench to Bedside*. Oxford, UK: Blackwell Futura, 2004:166–177.
35. Bolognesi R, Tsialtas D, Vasini P, Conti M, Manca C. Abnormal ventricular repolarization mimicking myocardial infarction after heterocyclic antidepressant overdose. *Am J Cardiol* 1997;79:242–245.
36. Rouleau F, Asfar P, Boulet S, Dube L, Dupuis JM, Alquier P, Victor J. Transient ST segment elevation in right precordial leads induced by psychotropic drugs: Relationship to the Brugada syndrome. *J Cardiovasc Electrophysiol* 2001;12:61–65.
37. Tada H, Sticherling C, Oral H, Morady F. Brugada syndrome mimicked by tricyclic antidepressant overdose. *J Cardiovasc Electrophysiol* 2001;12:275.
38. Babaliaros VC, Hurst JW. Tricyclic antidepressants and the Brugada syndrome: An example of Brugada waves appearing after the administration of desipramine. *Clin Cardiol* 2002;25:395–398.
39. Goldgran-Toledano D, Sideris G, Kevorkian JP. Overdose of cyclic antidepressants and the Brugada syndrome. *N Engl J Med* 2002;346:1591–1592.
40. Pastor A, Nunez A, Cantale C, Cosio FG. Asymptomatic Brugada syndrome case unmasked during dimenhydrinate infusion. *J Cardiovasc Electrophysiol* 2001;12:1192–1194.
41. Ortega-Carnicer J, Bertos-Polo J, Gutierrez-Tirado C. Aborted sudden death, transient Brugada pattern, and wide QRS dysrrhythmias after massive cocaine ingestion. *J Electrocardiol* 2001;34:345–349.
42. Darbar D, Yang T, Churchwell K, Wilde AA, Roden DM. Unmasking of Brugada syndrome by lithium. *Circulation* 2005;112:1527–1531.
43. Shimizu W. Editorial comment: Gender difference and drug challenge in Brugada syndrome. *J Cardiovasc Electrophysiol* 2004;15:70–71.
44. Di Diego JM, Cordeiro JM, Goodrow RJ, Fish JM, Zygmunt AC, Perez GJ, Scornik FS, Antzelevitch C. Ionic and cellular basis for the predominance of the Brugada syndrome phenotype in males. *Circulation* 2002;106:2004–2011.
45. Matsuo K, Akahoshi M, Seto S, Yano K. Disappearance of the Brugada-type electrocardiogram after surgical castration: A role for testosterone and an explanation for the male preponderance. *Pacing Clin Electrophysiol* 2003;26:1551–1553.
46. Shimizu W, Matsuo K, Kokubo Y, Satomi K, Kurita T, Noda T, Nagaya N, Suyama K, Aihara N, Kamakura S, Inamoto N, Akahoshi M, Tomoike H. Sex hormone and gender difference. Role of testosterone on male predominance in Brugada syndrome. *J Cardiovasc Electrophysiol* 2007;18:415-421.
47. Kataoka H. Electrocardiographic patterns of the Brugada syndrome in right ventricular infarction/ischemia. *Am J Cardiol* 2000;86:1056.
48. Itoh E, Suzuki K, Tanabe Y. A case of vasospastic angina presenting Brugada-type ECG abnormalities. *Jpn Circ J* 1999;63:493–495.
49. Noda T, Shimizu W, Taguchi A, Satomi K, Suyama K, Kurita T, Aihara N, Kamakura S. ST segment elevation and ventricular fibrillation without coronary spasm by intra coronary injection of acetylcholine and/or ergonovine maleate in patients with Brugada syndrome. *J Am Coll Cardiol* 2002;40:1841–1847.
50. Antzelevitch C, Brugada R. Fever and Brugada syndrome. *Pacing Clin Electrophysiol* 2002;25:1537–1539.
51. Mok NS, Priori SG, Napolitano C, Chan NY, Chahine M, Baroudi G. A newly characterized SCN5A mutation underlying Brugada syndrome unmasked by hyperthermia. *J Cardiovasc Electrophysiol* 2003;14: 407–411.
52. Dumaine R, Towbin J A, Brugada P, Vatta M, Nesterenko DV, Nesterenko VV, Brugada J, Brugada R, Antzelevitch C. Ionic mechanisms responsible for the electrocardiographic phenotype of the Brugada syndrome are temperature dependent. *Circ Res* 1999;85:803–809.
53. Osborn JJ. Experimental hypothermia: Respiratory and blood pH changes in relation to cardiac function. *Am J Physiol* 1953;175:389–398.
54. Noda T, Shimizu W, Tanaka K, Chayama K. Prominent J wave and ST segment elevation: Serial

electrocardiographic changes in accidental hypothermia. *J Cardiovasc Electrophysiol* 2003;14:223.
55. Myers GB. Other QRS-T patterns that may be mistaken for myocardial infarction. IV. Alterations in blood potassium; myocardial ischemia; subepicardial myocarditis; distortion associated with arrhythmias. *Circulation* 1950;2:75–93.
56. Douglas PS, Carmichael KA, Palevsky PM. Exreme hypercalcemia and electrocardiographic changes. *Am J Cardiol* 1984;54:674–675.
57. Nishizaki M, Sakurada H, Ashikaga T, Yamawake N, Fujii H, Arita M, Isobe M, Hiraoka M. Effects of glucose-induced insulin secretion on ST segment elevation in the Brugada syndrome. *J Cardiovasc Electrophysiol* 2003;14:243–249.
58. Donger C, Denjoy I, Berthet M, Neyroud N, Cruaud C, Bennaceur M, Chivoret G, Schwartz K, Coumel P, Guicheney P. *KVLQT1* C-terminal missense mutation causes a forme fruste long-QT syndrome. *Circulation* 1997;96:2778–2781.
59. Bezzina CR, Shimizu W, Yang P, Koopmann TT, Tanck MWT, Miyamoto Y, Kamakura S, Roden DM, Wilde AAM. A common sodium channel promoter haplotype in Asian subjects underlies variability in cardiac conduction. *Circulation* 2006;113:338–344.

Part VI
Treatment Modalities

Treatment Modalities

Mark E. Josephson

The field of cardiac electrophysiology has moved from one of diagnosis and understanding of mechanisms to one of pharmacological and catheter- or surgical-based ablative therapy to treat arrhythmias. This section, Part VI, edited by Shen, Friedman, and Ackerman, discusses the major therapeutic modalities used to treat bradyarrhythmias and tachyarrhythmias as well as the use of electrical therapies to treat heart failure; most importantly, two chapters discuss the morbidity of implantable defibrillators and how to reduce the cost effectiveness of sudden death prevention using these devices.

In terms of the role of antiarrhythmic drugs in the prevention of sudden death, in the past decade and a half it has been demonstrated that standard Class I and Class III antiarrhythmic agents are not as effective in preventing sudden cardiac deaths as implantable cardioverter defibrillators (ICDs). This includes amiodaron, which for many years was touted as being a useful agent to prevent sudden death. This is no way detracts from the potential ability to decrease the incidence as well as the rate of monomorphic ventricular tachycardia, which is not life threatening, but can be hemodynamically debilitating. In addition, antiarrhythmic agents may still be needed to treat other arrhythmias such as atrial fibrillation, which, in and of themselves, may be proarrhythmic. Thus, while the specific use of antiarrhythmic agents in reducing sudden death has been superceded by the use of ICDs, antiarrhythmic agents still may be necessary to slow or prevent non-life-threatening arrhythmias or make them pace-terminatable or ablatable. A major advancement in our understanding of pharmacological agents in preventing sudden cardiac death has been the recognition of the potential role of nonantiarrhythmic agents such as angiotensin-converting enzyme inhibitors (ACEI), antialdosterone agents, and statins. The long and established role of β blockers has been recognized, finally, by the entire cardiology community; they constitute a group of agents that has consistently been of benefit in reducing cardiac sudden death. However, neither the exact mechanism by which β blockers work nor whether all β blockers are the same has yet been established. Both ACEIs and angiotensin receptor blockers have been associated with a reduction of sudden death, as have antialdosterone agents, with particular new interest in eplerenone. These drugs may be antifibrotic, but may have other mechanisms of action. Recent experimental evidence has shown that ACEIs can actually improve cell-to-cell coupling, which may in turn facilitate propagation and be antiarrhythmic in that way. The role of the statins is not clear, but is generally believed to be related to antiinflammatory activity, which may in turn decrease substrate formation. More work is necessary to understand the mechanisms of these agents before a well-defined role in the prevention of sudden cardiac death can be applied. Finally, the interpretation of the results of these drugs as anti-sudden death agents is always in a relative risk-to-hazard ratio methodology. The absolute benefits of all of the drugs are small.

In terms of ICD therapy, it has been established that ICDs prevent sudden death better than drugs. However, we have yet to differentiate between patients in whom the device should be implanted and patients who not only will derive no benefit from implantation but for whom there may be potential morbidity from the device. Implantable defibrillator morbidity is discussed in Chapter 53, but in my opinion appropriate risk stratification to eliminate those patients who do not need a device is important. This relates to the cost effectiveness of the devices and the number of devices that need to be implanted to save one life. In my opinion, in the Primary Prevention Trials there is a marked lack of cost effectiveness of the devices. When actually measured, the cost effectiveness is unacceptable to society. Considering that in an SCDHeft population there is only a 1% per year enhanced survival from sudden cardiac death (1.4% total mortality per year benefit), the majority of patients in whom a device will be implanted will not obtain a significant benefit and will be subjected to the potential morbidity and mortality associated with implantation. A recent study of a Medicare population found a 0.9% mortality (30 days) in patients undergoing ICD implantation and a 10.8% morbidity. It is generally believed that somewhere in the range of 1% of the devices will need to be removed because of infection, and that the second and third implants have two to three times the infection rate. Since many primary prevention devices may lead to repeat implantations, the cost effectiveness will be unacceptable unless patients are restratified. Moreover, the morbidity will far exceed the benefits. If implantation of a device prevents sudden cardiac death in only a small number of patients, the actual number of people receiving inappropriate therapies due to arrhythmias, sensing problems, or lead fractures will exceed those receiving appropriate therapies. Moreover, it is unclear as to whether the devices may in fact be proarrhythmic.

In my opinion the primary goal of therapy should be to prevent the arrhythmia in the first place. Catheter and surgical ablation offer that potential. A significant amount of knowledge is available concerning the arrhythmogenic substrate in coronary artery disease with growing information on noncoronary substrates. Since coronary artery disease with prior infarction is the major substrate for ventricular tachycardia as well as fibrillation, understanding that substrate will lead to the ability to reduce or eliminate ventricular tachycardia and fibrillation. Revascularization is always a primary form of therapy, particularly for ventricular fibrillation associated with small scars and ejection fractions exceeding 45%. In my opinion, surgical intervention for revascularization is probably the best therapy for such patients. When scar formation is extensive, revascularization alone is not useful. However, arrhythmia surgery is extremely valuable in preventing sudden death due to sustained ventricular arrhythmias in patients with prior infarction and ejection fractions less than 40%. My personal experience with surgery for ventricular tachycardia and fibrillation demonstrated an efficacy equal to or exceeding that of ICDs in preventing sudden death or ventricular tachycardia, while at the same time providing revascularization and ventricular remodeling for the patients, resulting in improvement of their heart failure and ischemia. A surgical intervention may provide the best single approach to preventing malignant ventricular arrhythmias in the setting of coronary artery disease. I believe that we should return to the concept that the primary goal of therapy for arrhythmias is to prevent them in the first place. That can be done by preventing the disease process that causes the substrate (i.e., ischemic heart disease) or by destroying or removing the substrate responsible for the arrhythmia (i.e., surgical resection or catheter ablation). Therefore ICD therapy should be considered a safety valve until we better understand the underlying substrate mechanism of arrhythmias so that we can prevent their occurrence.

This section provides all of the current available information on modern electrophysiological therapy for arrhythmias and I believe provides a challenge to all of us to seek the ultimate goal of preventing the problem in the first place.

48
Clinical Role of Antiarrhythmic Drugs in the Prevention of Sudden Death

Hon-Chi Lee

Introduction

Sudden cardiac death is a leading cause of mortality in the United States, but recent studies suggest that its annual incidence is declining. The annual incidence of sudden cardiac death is about 0.55 per 1000 people in North America, accounting for more than 160,000 deaths each year in the United States.[1] In Seattle, there was a 34% decrease in the annual incidence of out-of-hospital cardiac arrest and a 56% decrease in ventricular fibrillation (VF) as the first identified rhythm between 1980 and 2000.[2] This trend corresponds with the declining incidence of cardiovascular disease in this country in the past two decades.[1] Holter monitoring has revealed that more than 75% of sudden cardiac deaths are due to ventricular tachycardia (VT) or VF.[3] A large majority of these patients have underlying structural heart disease including dilated and hypertrophic cardiomyopathies and ischemic heart disease.

The role of antiarrhythmic drugs in the prevention of sudden cardiac death has changed radically in the past 20 years. Once considered the principal modality of treatment, they have now been relegated to being an adjunctive therapy. Despite having lost their prominence in the treatment of lethal ventricular arrhythmias, antiarrhythmic drugs remain widely used, and many high-risk patients for sudden cardiac death take antiarrhythmic drugs. It is therefore important to have an evidence-based understanding of the risks and benefits of antiarrhythmic drugs for use in specific patient groups.

Historical Perspectives

At the advent of the modern electrophysiology (EP) era, the tools available for the treatment of arrhythmias were limited to simple pacemakers, external defibrillators, and antiarrhythmic drugs. Treatment and prevention of sudden cardiac death relied solely on the use of Class IA drugs and lidocaine. Antiarrhythmic drugs were known to suppress ventricular ectopic activities, which were recognized as poor prognostic markers for sudden death in patients with a history of myocardial infarction (MI).[4] With the development of intracardiac recordings and programmed electrical stimulation techniques, EP-guided drug therapy was considered the standard of care in the 1980 s. Class I antiarrhythmic drugs were effective in suppressing VT induced by programmed electrical stimulation in many patients in the EP laboratory, yet long-term follow-up demonstrated that these patients continued to have poor outcomes.[5] The results of the Cardiac Arrhythmia Suppression Trial (**CAST**), however, dealt a death blow to Class I antiarrhythmic drugs and to the hypothesis that suppression of ventricular ectopic activities in post-MI patients would reduce the risk of sudden death. The landscape for prevention of sudden cardiac death has since been completely reshaped (Table 48–1).

Class I Antiarrhythmic Drug Trials

The International Mexiletine and Placebo Antiarrhythmic Coronary Trial (**IMPACT**) was a

Table 48–1. Antiarrhythmic drug trials in patients at high risk of sudden death.[a]

Trial	Number of patients	Patient characteristics	Treatment design	Follow-up duration	Major findings
Class I Antiarrhythmic trials					
IMPACT	630	Recent MI, frequent complex ventricular arrhythmias	Mexiletine vs. placebo	12 months	1. Mexiletine significantly suppressed ventricular arrhythmias 2. Mexiletine trend toward increased mortality (7.6% vs. 4.8% in placebo, p = N.S.)
CAST	1498	6 days to 2 years after MI, PVC >6/h LVEF <55% for MI within 90 days, LVEF <40% for MI greater than 90 days	Placebo vs. encainide vs. flecainide	10 months	Study was prematurely terminated 1. Significant increase in mortality in the encainide/flecainide group (7.7%) vs. placebo (3%), $p = 0.0004$ 2. Significant increase in cardiac arrest in the encainide/flecainide group (4.5%) vs. placebo (1.2%), $p = 0.0004$ 3. Encainide/flecainide was effective in suppressing PVCs
CAST II	1155	Same as CAST	Moricizine vs. placebo	14 days 3 years	1. Exposure phase showed excessive mortality in the moricizine group (2.6% vs. 0.5% in placebo) 2. Study was prematurely terminated; long-term phase showed lack of benefit from treatment with moricizine 3. Moricizine was effective in suppressing PVCs
Class III antiarrhythmic trials					
ESVEM	486	h/o VT/VF, cardiac arrest, or inducible VT/VF	EP- or Holter-guided antiarrhythmic drug therapy (sotalol and Class I drugs)	6 years	1. No difference between EP- and Holter-guided therapies in predicting drug efficacy in preventing death or recurrence of arrhythmia 2. Sotalol was superior to Class I drugs 3. High recurrence of arrhythmia (50.7%) and death (15.5%) among patients in whom drugs were predicted to be effective
SWORD	3121	LVEF ≤40%, recent MI, or remote MI with CHF	*d*-Sotalol vs. placebo	148 days	1. Increased mortality in the *d*-sotalol group (5%) vs. placebo (3.1%) (65% increase in risk, $p = 0.006$ 2. *d*-Sotalol group showed 77% increase in arrhythmia death ($p = 0.008$)
DIAMOND	1510	Within a mean of 3 days of acute MI LVEF ≤35%	Dofetilide vs. placebo	15 months	1. No difference in all-cause mortality, cardiac mortality, or total arrhythmic death between the two groups 2. Dofetilide was significantly more effective than placebo in restoring sinus rhythm in patients with AF, $p = 0.002$
Amiodarone trials					
BASIS	312	h/o MI asymptomatic complex VEA (Lown Class 3 or 4b)	Amiodarone vs. individualized antiarrhythmic drugs (mostly quinidine or mexiletine) vs. no antiarrhythmic drug (control)	1 year	1. Amiodarone group had a significantly higher survival rate ($p < 0.05$) and lower arrhythmia events vs. control ($p < 0.01$) 2. Individualized antiarrhythmic group was not significantly different vs. control

TABLE 48–1. *Continued*

Trial	Number of patients	Patient characteristics	Treatment design	Follow-up duration	Major findings
PAT	613	Postacute MI not eligible for β blocker	Amiodarone vs. placebo	1 year	1. Amiodarone group showed a significant reduction in cardiac death ($p = 0.048$) and in Lown Class 4b VEA ($p < 0.001$) but not in all-cause mortality 2. 30% in the amiodarone group developed adverse effects vs. 10% in the placebo group 3. Substudy showed that amiodarone significantly reduced long-term mortality (9.1% vs. 16.5%, $p < 0.05$) and sudden death (3.4% vs. 8.2%, $p < 0.05$) only in patients with LVEF ≥40%
SSSD	368	10–60 days after acute MI LVEF 20–45%; three or more PVCs/h (pairs or runs)	Amiodarone vs. metoprolol vs. no antiarrhythmic	2.8 years	1. Mortality in the amiodarone group (3.5%) was not different from control (7.7%) but was significantly lower than the metoprolol group (15.4%), $p = 0.006$ 2. Amiodarone significantly reduced PVCs
CASCADE	288	Out-of-hospital VF without Q wave MI, >10 PVCs/h, or inducible VT/VF (mean LEVF 35%, 45% had CHF, 46% had ICD)	Amiodarone vs. Holter- or EP-guided antiarrhythmic (conventional) therapy	6 years	1. Amiodarone group had a significant reduction in combined endpoint of cardiac death, resuscitated VF, or syncopal ICD shocks (47% vs. 60% in control, $p = 0.007$) 2. Amiodarone group had a significant reduction in cardiac and sustained ventricular arrhythmias (59% vs. 80% in control, $p < 0.001$) 3. Overall mortality was high and side effects of therapy were common
EMIAT	1486	5–21 days after MI LVEF <40%	Amiodarone vs. placebo	21 months	1. No difference in all-cause mortality between the two groups 2. Amiodarone group had a 35% risk reduction in arrhythmia deaths
CAMIAT	1202	6–45 days after MI >10 PVCs/h or NSVT	Amiodarone vs. placebo	1.79 years	1. There was no difference in all-cause mortality between the two groups 2. Amiodarone group had a reduced risk of VF or arrhythmic death (3.3% vs. 6% in placebo, $p = 0.016$)
GESICA	516	Advanced chronic CHF, NYHA II–IV, LV systolic dysfunction	Amiodarone vs. placebo	13 months	1. Amiodarone reduced total mortality by 28% ($p = 0.024$) and hospitalization due to CHF by 31% ($p = 0.0024$) compared to placebo 2. Substudy showed that NSVT was an independent risk factor for sudden death ($p < 0.002$) 3. 61% of the patients had dilated cardiomyopathy and Chagas disease
CHF-STAT	674	NYHA class II–IV CHF LVEF ≤40% >10 PVCs/h	Amiodarone vs. placebo	45 months	1. No difference between the two groups in overall mortality and in sudden death 2. Trend favoring amiodarone in reducing mortality in patients with nonischemic cardiomyopathy ($p = 0.07$) 3. Amiodarone significantly improved LV function (LVEF increased by 42%) compared to placebo 4. A substudy showed that amiodarone was more effective in controlling ventricular rate in AF and conversion to sinus rhythm

[a]MI, myocardial infarction; PVC, premature ventricular contraction; N.S., not significant; LVEF, left ventricular ejection fraction; VT/VF, ventricular tachycardia/ventricular fibrillation; h/o, history of; EP, electrophysiology; CHF, congestive heart failure; VEA, ventricular ectopic arrhythmia; ICD, implantable cardioverter defibrillator; NSVT, nonsustained ventricular tachycardia; NYHA, New York Heart Association; LV, left ventricular; AF, atrial fibrillation.

double-blind, placebo-controlled study examining the antiarrhythmic effects of the sustained release form of mexiletine in 630 patients with recently documented MI.[6] The primary endpoint was frequent and complex ventricular arrhythmias based on 24h ambulatory electrocardiographic (ECG) monitoring. The results showed that mexiletine was effective in reducing the occurrence of complex forms of ventricular arrhythmias as well as frequent premature ventricular contractions (PVCs) during the first 4 months following acute MI. Mortality was higher in the mexiletine group (7.6%) than in the placebo group (4.8%), although the difference was not statistically significant.[6,7] These results were a harbinger of what would soon redefine the use of antiarrhythmic drugs in patients at high risk of sudden cardiac death.

CAST was a paradigm-shifting study. It was a multicenter randomized double-blinded study that sought to definitively test the hypothesis that in patients with a history of MI, suppression of ventricular ectopic activities would reduce the risk of sudden cardiac death.[8] The Class IC antiarrhythmic drugs encainide and flecainide were effective in suppressing ventricular ectopies, yet over a follow-up of less than 500 days, patients randomized to take these drugs had a 3-fold increase in mortality compared to patients randomized to control, leading to the premature termination of the trial by the Safety Monitoring Board. The findings were shocking and popularized the concept of proarrhythmia. The revelation that antiarrhythmic drugs could significantly increase mortality has transformed the role of antiarrhythmic drugs in the treatment of arrhythmias and emphasized the need to use mortality and not surrogate markers as the primary endpoint in clinical trials.

CAST II was divided into two blinded randomized phases, an early 14-day exposure phase and a long-term phase, to evaluate the risk and efficacy of moricizine on survival after MI in patients whose ventricular ectopic activities were adequately or partially suppressed by moricizine. The trial was terminated prematurely because treatment with moricizine was associated with excess mortality in the first 14-day period and lacked long-term efficacy compared to placebo.[9]

A major consequence of the CAST results was the dramatic curtailing of the use of Class I antiarrhythmic drugs for treating arrhythmias in patients with structural heart disease. The role of Class III antiarrhythmic drugs, however, was not immediately clear. Hence, drugs like sotalol and amiodarone were evaluated in subsequent clinical trials for their efficacy in the reduction of sudden cardiac death.

Class III Antiarrhythmic Drug Trials

The Electrophysiology Study Versus Electrocardiographic Monitoring (**ESVEM**) trial compared the effectiveness of Holter monitoring plus exercise testing to EP study in predicting antiarrhythmic drug efficacy in preventing sudden cardiac death.[10] A total of 486 patients with a history of VT/VF, cardiac arrest, or syncope with inducible sustained VT/VF were randomized to serial EP-guided or serial Holter-guided antiarrhythmic drug therapy, which included Class I antiarrhythmics and sotalol, but not amiodarone. The results showed that EP study and Holter monitoring had similar accuracy in predicting antiarrhythmic drug efficacy and sotalol was superior to Class I antiarrhythmic drugs in preventing death and the recurrence of arrhythmia.[11] However, over a 6-year follow-up period, 50.7% of the 296 patients receiving the drugs predicted to be effective experienced a recurrence of arrhythmia and 15.5% died. The high rate of recurrence suggests that the effectiveness of these approaches in the treatment and prevention of sudden cardiac death is limited.

Disappointingly, the Survival With Oral *d*-Sotalol (**SWORD**) trial found that *d*-sotalol, which lacks β-adrenergic blocking properties, increased both arrhythmic and total mortality in patients with a history of MI and left ventricular (LV) dysfunction.[12] The Danish Investigation of Arrhythmia and Mortality on Dofetilide (**DIAMOND**) found that dofetilide, another Class III antiarrhythmic drug and an I_{Kr} blocker, did not increase mortality in patients with recent MIs and LV dysfunction.[13] Currently, dofetilide is labeled for treatment of atrial arrhythmias and is deemed safe for use in patients with LV dysfunction.

Amiodarone Trials

The Basel Antiarrhythmic Study of Infarct Survival (**BASIS**) examined the effects of prophylactic antiarrhythmic treatment in patients with persistent asymptomatic complex ventricular arrhythmias after MI.[14] It randomized 312 patients with Lown class 3 or 4b arrhythmia on 24-h ambulatory ECG recordings before hospital discharge. The patients were randomized to individualized antiarrhythmic treatment (mostly quinidine or mexiletine), low-dose amiodarone (200 mg/day), or no antiarrhythmic treatment. During the 1-year follow-up period, patients receiving amiodarone had a significant reduction in mortality ($p < 0.05$) and arrhythmia events ($p < 0.01$) compared to the control group, while there was no difference between the individualized antiarrhythmics and control groups. These results suggest that low-dose amiodarone reduces mortality in the year after MI in patients at high risk for sudden cardiac death. A subsequent report after a mean follow-up of 72 months found that mortality remained significantly lower in the amiodarone group versus the control group with respect to all-cause mortality ($p = 0.03$) and cardiac death ($p = 0.047$).[15]

The Polish Amiodarone Trial (**PAT**) was a multicenter, double-blinded, placebo-controlled study examining the effect of amiodarone on mortality, ventricular arrhythmias, and clinical complications in high-risk post-MI patients ineligible to receive β blockers.[16] In this study, 613 patients were randomized to receive amiodarone or placebo for 1 year. The results showed significant reductions in the amiodarone group for cardiac mortality ($p = 0.048$) and for Lown class 4 ventricular arrhythmias ($p < 0.001$), but not for all-cause mortality. In addition, 30% of the patients who received amiodarone developed adverse effects compared to 10% of those who received placebo. Further analysis showed that most of the benefits from amiodarone were observed in patients with preserved LV function and none in those with left ventricular ejection fraction (LVEF) <40%.[17]

The Spanish Study of Sudden Death (**SSSD**) was a randomized trial to assess the efficacy of amiodarone versus metoprolol or no antiarrhythmic treatment to suppress asymptomatic ventricular ectopic activities in patients who had MI with LVEF of 20–45% and ≥3 PVCs/h in the form of pairs or runs.[18] In this study, 368 patients were randomized to receive amiodarone 200 mg/day, metoprolol 100–200 mg/day, or no antiarrhythmic treatment. After a median follow-up of 2.8 years, mortality in the amiodarone group was not significantly different from that of the untreated control group, but was lower than that in the metoprolol group. Follow-up Holter studies showed that amiodarone and metoprolol were both effective in reducing heart rate, but only amiodarone significantly reduced ventricular ectopic activities ($p < 0.0001$), suggesting that long-term treatment with amiodarone was safe for patients with an LVEF of 20–45% and was effective in suppressing ventricular ectopies.

Amiodarone was the last antiarrhythmic stronghold and was the focus of a number of multicenter clinical trials.[19] The Cardiac Arrest in Seattle: Conventional vs. Amiodarone Drug Evaluation (**CASCADE**)[20] was a randomized study that evaluated survivors of out-of-hospital VF not associated with a Q wave acute MI, who were at high risk of VF recurrence with >10 PVCs/h on Holter and with inducible sustained VT or VF. In this study, 228 patients were randomized to empirical amiodarone or Class I antiarrhythmic drugs guided by EP or Holter studies. The mean LVEF was 35%; 45% of the patients had a history of congestive heart failure (CHF) and 46% had an implantable cardioverter defibrillator (ICD) implantation. Survival free of cardiac death, resuscitated VF, or syncopal defibrillator shocks was significantly better in patients treated with amiodarone than in those treated with other antiarrhythmic drugs (amiodarone 53% vs. conventional arrhythmic 20%, $p < 0.001$), but the overall mortality was relatively high and side effects were common.

The European Myocardial Infarct Amiodarone Trial (**EMIAT**), a multicenter randomized, double-blind placebo-controlled study, found that in survivors of MI with an LVEF ≤ 40% ($n = 1486$), deaths from arrhythmia were reduced by 35% in the amiodarone group ($p = 0.05$ versus placebo group), but there was no difference in all-cause or cardiac mortalities over a mean follow-up of 21 months.[21] Similar to EMIAT, The Canadian

Amiodarone MI Arrhythmia Trial (**CAMIAT**) was a multicenter, randomized, double-blind, placebo-controlled trial that found that in survivors of acute MI with frequent or repetitive PVCs ($n = 1201$), resuscitated VF or arrhythmic death was significantly lower in the amiodarone group ($p = 0.016$ versus placebo group) over a mean follow-up of 1.79 years.[22] The absolute reduction of risk was greatest in patients with CHF or a history of MI. However, all-cause mortality was similar between the two groups. The results of CASCADE, EMIAT, and CAMIAT showed a modest beneficial effect of amiodarone in patients with ischemic heart disease and established that amiodarone does not incur a significant proarrhythmia risk.

Secondary Prevention Trials in Patients with Ischemic Cardiomyopathy: Antiarrhythmic Drugs Versus Implantable Cardioverter Defibrillators

In contrast, in secondary prevention trials that included treatment with ICDs, antiarrhythmic drugs including amiodarone did not measure up to ICDs, which showed a significant improvement in survival for patients at high risk of sudden cardiac death (Table 48–2). The Antiarrhythmic versus Implantable Defibrillators (**AVID**) trial compared the relative efficacy of ICDs and antiarrhythmic drugs in 1016 patients who had survived life-threatening ventricular arrhythmias.[23] Patients were randomized to ICD versus antiarrhythmic drugs; 97% of the patients received amiodarone while the rest received EP-guided sotalol therapy. The trial was terminated prematurely because of a 29% reduction of all-cause mortality in the ICD group.

The Canadian Implantable Defibrillator Study (**CIDS**) was a multicenter randomized study examining the efficacy of ICD versus amiodarone in 658 patients with cardiac arrest, sustained symptomatic VT, and syncope with reduced LV function and inducible VT.[24] The results showed a nonsignificant 20% reduction in all-cause and arrhythmic mortality in the ICD group compared to the amiodarone group, but the results were confounded by significant patient crossover in treatments. A long-term follow-up study showed that after a mean of 5.6 years, 47% of the patients in the amiodarone group died compared to 27% in the ICD group ($p = 0.0213$).[25] In addition, 82% of the patients taking amiodarone developed adverse effects and 50% required discontinuation or reduction of dosage. Hence, the benefit of ICD over amiodarone in this subset of CIDS patients increases with time.

The Cardiac Arrest Study Hamburg (**CASH**) randomized 346 survivors of sudden cardiac death unrelated to MI to ICD or medical therapy consisting of amiodarone, metoprolol, or propafenone.[26] The mean follow-up was 57 months and the propafenone arm was discontinued after an interim analysis showed it had significantly higher all-cause mortality. During long-term follow-up, therapy with an ICD was associated with a nonsignificant reduction of all-cause mortality compared to treatment with amiodarone/metoprolol ($p = 0.081$). Subsequent meta-analysis and subanalysis of the AVID, CIDS, and CASH results[27,28] showed a significant risk reduction in total mortality (25–27% decrease) and arrhythmic death (50–52% decrease) in ICD patients ($p < 0.001$). Patients treated with an ICD in AVID had a maximal survival benefit when the LVEF was 20–34%, suggesting that ICD is the preferential treatment in those with moderately severe LV dysfunction.

Primary Prevention Trials in Patients with Ischemic Cardiomyopathy: Antiarrhythmic Drugs Versus Implantable Cardioverter Defibrillators

Results from the secondary prevention trials firmly established the superiority of ICDs to antiarrhythmic drugs in reducing mortality in patients with ischemic cardiomyopathy who have had life-threatening ventricular arrhythmias. Several large multicenter primary prevention trials followed to examine the efficacy of ICD versus antiarrhythmic drugs in patients with ischemic cardiomyopathy without prior significant ventricular arrhythmia events. The results of these trials further confirmed the dominance of ICD in sudden cardiac prevention in patients with ischemic cardiomyopathy.

The Multicenter Automatic Defibrillator Implantation Trial (**MADIT**) examined whether

TABLE 48–2. Antiarrhythmic drugs versus ICD trials.[a]

Trial	Number of patients	Patient characteristics	Treatment design	Follow-up duration	Major findings
Secondary prevention trials					
AVID	1016	VF or sustained VT with syncope or with LVEF ≤40% or with hemodynamic compromise	ICD vs. antiarrhythmic drug (97% received amiodarone)	18 months	1. Study was stopped prematurely because overall survival was greater for the ICD group (39% reduction in risk for death $p < 0.02$) 2. Subanalysis showed that in patients with LVEF ≥35% ICD therapy had no survival benefit
CIDS	659	VF, cardiac arrest, sustained VT with syncope or with symptoms and LVEF ≤35%, or inducible VT	Amiodarone vs. ICD	36 months 5.6 years	1. ICD group showed a trend toward reduction in all-cause mortality (by 20%) and arrhythmic death (by 32%), but the difference was not statistically significant ($p = 0.14$) 2. Follow-up study showed that the survival benefit of ICD over amiodarone increases with time (27% mortality vs. 47% in the amiodarone group, $p = 0.0213$ 3. Significant patient crossover in treatment; 27% of ICD patients received amiodarone and 21.4% of patients in the amiodarone group received an ICD 4. 82% of patients in the amiodarone group developed side-effects, 50% of whom required discontinuation or dose reduction
CASH	288	Cardiac arrest or symptomatic VT	ICD vs. amiodarone, metoprolol, or propafenone	57 months	1. Propafenone arm was discontinued due to excess mortality 2. ICD group had a nonsignificant reduction in all-cause mortality (by 23%) compared to amiodarone/ metoprolol ($p = 0.08$) 3. ICD group had a significant reduction in risk of sudden death compared to the antiarrhythmic group ($p = 0.005$)
Primary prevention trials					
MADIT	196	h/o MI, NYHA I–IIILVEF <35%, NSVT with inducible nonsuppressible VT	ICD vs. conventional medical therapy (80% on amiodarone)	27 months	1. ICD group had significant reduction in cardiac mortality (12% vs. 27%) and in all-cause mortality (15% vs. 39% in the conventional therapy group, $p = 0.009$) 2. Low level of β blocker used (27% in the ICD group vs. 8% in the medical therapy group) 3. 44% of ICD patients took antiarrhythmics; 23% in the medical therapy group did not take antiarrhythmics

TABLE 48–2. *Continued*

Trial	Number of patients	Patient characteristics	Treatment design	Follow-up duration	Major findings
MUSTT	704	CAD with LVEF ≤40%, NSVT Inducible VT	EP-guided antiarrhythmic or ICD therapy vs. no therapy	39 months	1. EP-guided therapy group had a significant reduction in cardiac death (27% decrease) and total mortality (20% decrease) 2. All benefits in the EP-guided therapy group were due to ICD therapy; sudden death was significantly reduced in ICD patients (9% vs. 37%) as was total mortality (24% vs. 55%) 3. Mortality was higher in the antiarrhythmic group compared with the no therapy group
AMIOVERT	103	Nonischemic dilated cardiomyopathy LVEF ≤35% Asymptomatic NSVT	Amiodarone vs. ICD	2 years	1. Study was stopped early because results were unlikely to show a difference between the two groups 2. Study had unusually low mortality rates
SCD-HeFT	2521	NYHA II–III CHF, LVEF ≤35%	Amiodarone vs. ICD vs. placebo	45 months	1. ICD group had a significant reduction in total mortality vs. control or amiodarone groups ($p = 0.007$) 2. Most of the ICD benefits were due to reduction in arrhythmia death 3. Most of the ICD benefits occurred in those with Class II CHF and not in those with Class III symptoms

[a]ICD, implantable cardioverter defibrillator; VF, ventricular fibrillation; VT, ventricular tachycardia; h/o, history of; MI, myocardial infarction; NSVT, nonsustained ventricular tachycardia; CAD, coronary artery disease; EP, electrophysiology; NYHA, New York Heart Association; CHF, congestive heart failure.

prophylactic ICD therapy, as compared to conventional medical therapy, would improve survival in patients with previous MI, LV dysfunction, and nonsustained VT.[29] In this trial, 196 patients with LVEF ≤ 35% who had a documented episode of asymptomatic nonsustained VT and inducible VT not suppressed by antiarrhythmic drugs (predominantly intravenous procainamide) in the EP study were randomized to receive an ICD or conventional medical therapy (80% on amiodarone). The study was terminated after a mean follow-up of 27 months because the ICD group showed a significant reduction in cardiac mortality (12% versus 27%) and all-cause mortality (15% versus 39%, $p = 0.009$). Notably, 60% of the patients who had ICD implantation received an ICD shock within 2 years after device implantation. However, MADIT was criticized for the relatively low level of β blockers used overall, with a higher level of use in patients with ICD (27% versus 8%); 44% of the patients in the ICD group were taking antiarrhythmic drugs while 23% of the patients in the medical therapy group were not.

The Multicenter Unsustained Tachycardia Trial (**MUSTT**) examined the usefulness of electrophysiological testing for risk stratification in patients with coronary artery disease, LVEF ≤ 40%, and unsustained VT.[30] The study enrolled 2202 patients including 704 with inducible sustained VT who were randomized to therapy or no therapy. Patients assigned to therapy first received antiarrhythmic drugs, but if inducible VT was not suppressed, an ICD would be implanted. Five-year Kaplan–Meier analysis showed the EP-guided therapy group had a 27% reduction in cardiac death and 20% reduction in total mortality. Notably, all the survival benefits occurred in patients who received an ICD. Sudden cardiac death and total mortality were significantly reduced in EP-guided therapy patients who received an ICD versus those who did not, while mortality was higher in patients who received antiarrhythmic drugs (including Class I drugs) than in those who received no therapy. Similar to MADIT, the overall use of β blockers was low and more patients in the no therapy group were taking β blockers than in the ICD or antiarrhythmic groups. The results of MUSTT confirmed that ICD therapy has significant beneficial survival outcomes in high-risk patients with ischemic cardiomyopathy; in contrast, antiarrhythmic drugs did not reduce the risk of sudden death in these patients.

The beneficial effects of ICDs were further substantiated by the results of the Multicenter Automatic Defibrillator Trial II (MADIT II).[31] The study randomized 1232 patients with a history of previous infarct and reduced LVEF of ≤30% to ICD or conventional medical therapy. During an average follow-up of 20 months, there was a 31% reduction in total mortality in the ICD group (14.1% versus 19.8%, $p = 0.016$). These results significantly broadened the clinical indications of ICD therapy, which now included all patients with ischemic cardiomyopathy with reduced LVEF ≤ 30%. The results of the primary prevention trials comparing ICD and antiarrhythmic drugs practically eliminated the latter as a frontline consideration in the prevention of sudden death.

Antiarrhythmic Drug Trials in Patients with Nonischemic Cardiomyopathy and Congestive Heart Failure

In patients with congestive heart failure (CHF), Class I antiarrhythmic drugs were noted to have significant proarrhythmia adverse effects. In the Stroke Prevention in Atrial Fibrillation Study, a randomized clinical trial of 1330 patients, those treated with antiarrhythmic drugs (mostly Class I) had a 2.5-fold increase in cardiac mortality and a 2.6-fold increase in arrhythmia death. The effects were even more pronounced in patients with a history of CHF who received antiarrhythmic drug therapy, with the risk of cardiac death increasing 3.3-fold and arrhythmia death increasing 5.8-fold.[32] In addition, the use of sotalol is frequently avoided in patients with CHF because of its negative inotropic effects. In contrast, amiodarone has a relatively low propensity for proarrhythmic side effects, has a favorable hemodynamics profile, and is usually well tolerated by patients with CHF. Thus, it was the focus of several clinical trials examining its efficacy in reducing mortality in CHF patients.

The Grupo de Estudio de la Sobrevida en la Insuficiencia Cardiac en Argentina (**GESICA**) trial was a multicenter study evaluating the effect of low-dose amiodarone on 2-year mortality in 516 patients with severe heart failure randomized to 300 mg/day amiodarone or to standard therapy.[33] The amiodarone group showed a 28% reduction in total mortality (33.5% versus 41.4%, $p = 0.024$) and a 31% reduction in hospitalization due to worsening heart failure (45.8% versus 58.2%, $p = 0.0024$). The benefits of amiodarone were found in all patients regardless of the presence or absence of nonsustained VT. However, a subsequent substudy reported that during a 2-year follow-up, rates of overall mortality and sudden death were significantly greater in patients who had nonsustained VT in the initial 24-h Holter study than in patients without nonsustained VT.[34] Wide applicability of the results of the GESICA trial is questionable because a high percentage of patients in the study had dilated cardiomyopathy and Chagas disease (61%).

The Congestive Heart Failure Survival Trial of Antiarrhythmic Therapy (**CHF-STAT**) was a double-blinded, placebo-controlled VA COOP study to determine the effectiveness of amiodarone in reducing overall mortality in patients with CHF and asymptomatic ventricular arrhythmias.[35] A total of 674 patients with New York Heart Association (NYHA) Class II–IV symptoms of CHF, LVEF ≤ 40%, and >10 PVCs/h were randomized to receive amiodarone or placebo. After a median follow-up of 45 months, there was no significant difference in overall mortality between the two groups, but there was a trend favoring reduction of mortality by amiodarone in patients with nonischemic cardiomyopathy ($p = 0.07$). Also, amiodarone was significantly more effective in suppressing ventricular arrhythmias and increased the LVEF by 42% at 2 years. Interestingly, a substudy showed that amiodarone was more effective in controlling the ventricular rate in atrial fibrillation and in conversion to sinus rhythm (32% versus 7.7% in the placebo group, $p = 0.002$),[36] resulting in a significantly lower mortality than those who did not convert to sinus rhythm on the drug ($p = 0.04$). Also, patients in sinus rhythm on amiodarone were less likely to develop atrial fibrillation (4.1% versus 8.4%, $p = 0.005$).

The Amiodarone Versus Implantable Cardioverter-Defibrillator Trial (**AMIOVERT**) randomized 103 patients with nonischemic dilated cardiomyopathy, LVEF ≤ 35%, and asymptomatic nonsustained VT to amiodarone or ICD and found no difference in survival between the two groups at 1 or 3 years or in quality of life.[37] There was a trend toward a more beneficial cost profile and improved arrhythmia-free survival with amiodarone therapy ($p = 0.1$). The study, however, was criticized because of the relatively low mortality rate in the two groups, the small number of patients, and the short follow-up.

The Danish Investigations of Arrhythmia and Mortality on Dofetilide in Congestive Heart Failure (**DIAMOND-CHF**) Study examined whether dofetilide affects survival or morbidity among patients with reduced LV function and CHF ($n = 1518$).[38] After a median follow-up of 18 months, overall mortality was similar between placebo (42%) and dofetilide (41%) patients. However, dofetilide was effective in converting atrial fibrillation to sinus rhythm, in maintaining sinus rhythm, and in reducing the risk of hospitalization for worsening CHF. These results suggest that dofetilide is safe to use for control of atrial arrhythmias in patients with CHF but does not confer survival benefits. Importantly, the dofetilide group had a 3.3% incidence of torsade de pointes versus none in the placebo group. Most of these events (76%) occur within the first 3 days of drug treatment, underscoring the importance of initiating dofetilide therapy in the hospital.

The Sudden Cardiac Death in Heart Failure Trial (**SCD-HeFT**) studied 2521 patients with NYHA Class II (70%) or III (30%) CHF and an LVEF ≤ 35% with conventional CHF therapy who were randomized to placebo, amiodarone, or ICD and were followed for a mean period of 45.5 months.[39] The overall risk of death was similar between the placebo (29%) and amiodarone (28%) groups, but was reduced by 23% in the ICD group for both ischemic and nonischemic cardiomyopathy patients (22%, $p = 0.007$). The survival benefit of ICD therapy was entirely due to the reduction in arrhythmia deaths. Compared to placebo, treatment with amiodarone was associated with a 44% increase in mortality in patients with NYHA Class III symptoms ($p = 0.01$), but not in those with Class II symptoms. Results of ICD therapy were also dependent on the severity of CHF. It was found that ICD therapy conferred greater survival benefits in patients with NYHA Class II symptoms. These results further substantiated the benefits of ICD therapy in CHF patients with ischemic and nonischemic cardiomyopathies.

Use of Antiarrhythmic Drugs in the Prevention of Sudden Cardiac Death

With the results from recent primary and secondary prevention trials in patients at high risk for sudden death, ICD has emerged as the superior modality of treatment compared to antiarrhythmic drugs. Class I antiarrhythmic drugs should be avoided in these patients because of proarrhythmia adverse effects, while amiodarone has an overall neutral effect. Thus, ICD therapy is now considered the cornerstone treatment for patients who may be at increased risk of sudden death, though it should not be used indiscriminantly. There are several areas in which antiarrhythmic drugs may play a role in the primary prevention of sudden death.

Ischemic Heart Disease with Moderate Reduction in Left Ventricular Systolic Function

In patients with ischemic heart disease with only moderate reduction in LV function, ICD therapy does not offer survival benefits over amiodarone. Subanalysis of the AVID results showed that in patients with LVEF ≥ 35%, there was no difference in survival between antiarrhythmic-treated and ICD-treated patients.[27,40] These results suggest amiodarone is as efficacious as ICD in the secondary prevention of sudden death in this subset of ischemic heart disease patients. Further subgroup analysis of the AVID cohorts showed that patients who presented with VF, no prior arrhythmia, no cerebrovascular disease, and LVEF ≥ 27% constituted a low-risk subgroup that did not benefit from ICD implantation compared with amiodarone therapy.[41] It is possible that patients with relatively well-preserved LV function are at low risk for sudden death and hence do not significantly benefit from ICD therapy. Another possibility is that antiarrhythmic efficacy increases with improved LV function, as previous studies found that LVEF correlated significantly with antiarrhythmic drug efficacy.[42] Hence, in these patients amiodarone can be used effectively for the prevention of sudden cardiac death.

There are also other subgroups of patients with ischemic heart disease who do not benefit from ICD implantation. First, patients with coronary artery disease, LV dysfunction, and high risk for developing ventricular arrhythmia who have undergone coronary artery bypass grafting surgery do not benefit from prophylactic ICD implantation. The Coronary Artery Bypass Graft (**CABG**) Patch Trial randomly assigned 900 patients with coronary artery disease, LVEF < 36%, and abnormal signal-averaged ECGs to receive an ICD or not (control).[43] After an average follow-up of 32 months, there was no evidence of improved survival in patients with a prophylactic ICD implant. The results from the **CABG-Patch** Trial emphasize the importance of coronary perfusion in the development of life-threatening ventricular arrhythmias and the role of surgical revascularization in the prevention of sudden cardiac death.

Second, patients who have had a recent MI do not benefit from ICD implantation. The Defibrillation in Acute Myocardial Infarction Trial (**DINAMIT**) examined the role of ICDs in 674 patients who were 6–40 days post-MI and who had reduced LV function (LVEF ≤ 35%) and impaired cardiac autonomic function manifested as depressed heart rate variability or elevated average heart rate on Holter monitoring.[44] There was no difference in overall mortality between the ICD group and the control group over a mean follow-up of 30 months. Although ICD therapy was associated with a significant reduction in arrhythmic death (3.6% versus 8.5%, $p = 0.009$), this was offset by an increase in cardiac nonarrhythmic deaths. Recent subanalysis of MADIT II results also confirmed a time dependence of mortality risk and ICD benefit after MI. Mortality risk in patients with ischemic cardiomyopathy increases as a function of time from MI. Implantation of ICD minimized the time-dependent change in mortality in these patients. Hence, the survival benefits associated with ICDs are substantial for remote MI, but nonexistent for recent (<18 months) MI.

Third, patients with coronary artery disease and ischemic cardiomyopathy who have had recent coronary revascularization do not benefit from ICD therapy. A subanalysis of the MADIT II results ($n = 951$) showed that ICD reduced mortality by 36% ($p = 0.01$) and the risk of sudden death by 66% among patients who were enrolled more than 6 months after coronary revascularization, while no such benefits were observed among patients who had ICD implantation in the early postcoronary revascularization period. Percutaneous coronary intervention was more common in the recent (<6 months) revascularization group (55% versus 35%) and CABG was more prevalent in the remote (>6 months) group (65% versus 45%).

Fourth, the results of clinical trials in North America may not be directly applicable to other ethnic populations with different genetic composition. In a retrospective study in Japan, 3258 patients who met MADIT II criteria (Q wave MI ≥ 4 weeks prior and LVEF ≤ 30%) were followed for a mean of 37 months. The overall mortality was 16.9%, comparable to the ICD arm and significantly lower than the control arm in MADIT II.[45] Only 2.2% of the study patients had sudden death. These results suggest that it may not be appropriate to directly apply the MADIT II criteria for ICD implantation to Japanese patients. These concerns should be kept in mind when treating patients with different ethnic and genetic backgrounds.

Hence, in situations in which ICDs do not offer obvious survival benefits, the use of amiodarone can be considered for the management of patients at high risk for sudden death.

Brugada Syndrome

Brugada syndrome is a unique inherited primary electrical disease accounting for 20% of all sudden cardiac deaths in patients with structurally normal hearts.[46] This syndrome with the characteristic right bundle branch block (RBBB) and ST elevations in leads V1–V3 on ECG is thought to be caused by an imbalance between the inward (sodium and L-type calcium currents) and outward currents (mainly the transient outward currents) at the end of phase 1 of the epicardial action potential.[47] Hence, conditions that reduce inward currents (loss-of-function mutations in SCN5A, which encodes the α subunit of the sodium channel, or Class I antiarrhythmic drugs) or enhance the transient outward currents (male gender) would unmask or exacerbate the Brugada phenotype and increase the risk of VF. Indeed, administration of Class I antiarrhythmic drugs is routinely used to unmask the characteristic ECG features to facilitate the diagnosis of Brugada syndrome. Likewise, pharmacotherapies that inhibit the transient outward potassium currents or enhance the L-type Ca^{2+} currents are postulated to be protective and have been the target of several clinical studies.[48] Continuous infusion of isoproterenol, which enhances the Ca^{2+} currents, has been employed to restore normal ECG and to successfully treat electrical storm with frequent episodes of VF in Brugada syndrome patients.[49,50] Cilostazol, an oral phosphodiesterase inhibitor that augments the L-type Ca^{2+} currents through elevation of intracellular cyclic AMP (cAMP), was successfully used to suppress the daily episodes of VF in a patient with Brugada syndrome.[51] The Class IA antiarrhythmic drug quinidine, a specific blocker of the transient outward K^+ currents, caused normalization of ECG in two patients with Brugada syndrome.[52] Furthermore, Belhassen *et al.* studied the effects of quinidine bisulfate on the prevention of inducible and spontaneous VF in 25 Brugada syndrome patients who had inducible VF in baseline EP studies.[53] Quinidine prevented induction of VF in 22 of 25 patients (88%). Of these 25 patients, 16 were treated with quinidine, 6 received ICD therapy, and 3 were treated with both ICD and quinidine. After 6 months to 22.2 years of follow-up, there were no deaths, suggesting quinidine may be a safe alternative to ICD therapy. Similarly, Hermida *et al.* examined the efficacy of hydroquinidine in 35 Brugada syndrome patients, finding that hydroquinidine prevented VT/VF inducibility in 76% of asymptomatic patients who underwent EP-guided therapy.[54] Appropriate ICD shock occurred in 1 of 10 patients who received ICD therapy. In patients who had frequent ICD shocks, hydroquinidine prevented the recurrence of VT/VF in all patients during a mean follow-up period of 14 months. These studies were nonrandomized and had small numbers of patients, but the results suggest that quinidine and hydroquinidine may be effective treatments for preventing sudden death in patients with Brugada syndrome.

Long QT 3 Syndrome

The congenital long QT 3 syndrome (LQT3) is caused by gain-of-function mutations in the cardiac voltage-gated sodium channels that cause the normally rapidly inactivated sodium channels to remain open at depolarized membrane potentials.[55] The non-inactivating sodium currents lead to prolongation of the cardiac action potential, predisposing the heart to develop torsade de pointes. Long QT 3 constitutes about 10% of the long QT genotyped patients. This unique genotype–phenotype correlation provides an opportunity for tailoring genotype-specific therapy. Class I antiarrhythmic drugs, which are sodium channel blockers, are natural choices for treatment of LQT3. In *in vitro* studies of cells expressing SCN5A with LQT3 mutations, mexiletine has been shown to preferentially suppress the late-opening channels.[56] When mexiletine (12–16 mg/kg/day) was given to patients with LQT syndrome, QTc was significantly shortened in LQT3 patients, but not in LQT2 patients.[57] These results suggest that mexiletine may be effective in the treatment of LQT3 patients; however, larger prospective clinical studies are needed.[57]

Flecainide has also been used to treat patients with LQT3. The D1790G mutation in SCN5A produces LQT3 not by promoting sustained inward sodium currents but by a negative shift in the steady-state channel inactivation, thus responding to flecainide but not to Class IB antiarrhythmics like lidocaine and mexiletine. Eight asymptomatic D1790G mutation carriers treated with flecainide (75–150 mg bid) showed 9.5% shortening of QTc ($p = 0.011$), whereas control subjects showed QTc prolongation.[58] Long-term outpatient follow-up for 9–17 months showed no adverse effects from flecainide administration. However, this treatment strategy should be applied with caution because there are overlaps between Brugada syndrome and LQT3. Flecainide administration elicits ECG patterns typical of Brugada syndrome in some LQT3 patients, raising concern about the safety of flecainide therapy in

LQT3 patients without the D1790G mutation.[59] In LQT3 patients with the ΔKPQ mutation, flecainide shortened QTc without any major adverse events,[60,61] suggesting flecainide may be efficacious and safe in these patients. However, larger prospective studies are needed before Class I antiarrhythmic drugs are employed as the primary therapeutic agent in patients with LQT3.

Catecholaminergic Polymorphic Ventricular Tachycardia

Catecholaminergic polymorphic ventricular tachycardia is a rare arrhythmogenic disorder associated with sudden death in children and young adults who have structurally normal hearts and typically present with exercise- or emotion-induced syncope.[62] The hallmark of this disease is the occurrence of bidirectional VT, polymorphic VT, or VF provoked without QT prolongation or Brugada syndrome, reproducible by exercise or exposure to catecholamines.[63] Thirty percent of the patients have a family history of syncope or sudden death.[63] The underlying genetic abnormalities produce defects in Ca^{2+} homeostasis by the sarcoplasmic reticulum (SR). Mutations of the cardiac ryanodine receptor (RyR2), the Ca^{2+} release channel in SR,[64,65] and of calsequestrin, which binds Ca^{2+} and serves as the major Ca^{2+} reservoir in the SR,[66,67] are associated with this condition.

β Blockers have been the treatment of choice and have been shown to be effective in the acute termination of refractory VT/VF.[68] In a 7-year follow-up of 21 patients with catecholaminergic polymorphic VT, all β blockers were effective, but the long-acting ones such as nadolol were preferred.[63] Later reports showed less favorable outcomes with β blocker treatments alone.[64,69] One series showed that β blockers controlled catecholaminergic polymorphic VT in only 41% of the patients while 22% of the patients died during the 6.8-year follow-up.[69] However, most of the patients were taking short-acting propranolol at a dose that was considered too low. Another series showed that even though β blockers were effective in reducing arrhythmias, an ICD may be required in about 30% of the patients because of sustained VT/VF.[64] There is a role for ICD in selected patients with catecholaminergic polymorphic VT, but high-dose long-acting β blockers are still considered the first-line therapy.

Use of Antiarrhythmic Drugs as an Adjunct to Implantable Cardioverter Defibrillator Therapy

At present, ICDs have emerged as the treatment of choice in the prevention of sudden cardiac death for high-risk patients while antiarrhythmics have been relegated to an adjunctive and palliative role. Despite their lackluster record, antiarrhythmic drugs remain widely used in patients who have received ICDs. In fact, in some medical centers, about 40% of the ICD patients also received an antiarrhythmic drug.[70] Hence, antiarrhythmics continue to play an integral role in the management of patients at high risk for sudden cardiac death. There are potential benefits associated with the use of antiarrhythmic drugs in patients with an ICD and these are discussed below.

Prevention of Frequent Implantable Cardioverter Defibrillator Shocks

The major indication for the use of antiarrhythmic drugs is suppression of frequent recurrent VT/VF and reduction of ICD shocks. Even though ICDs are effective in treating VT/VF, ICD recipients are usually at high risk for developing lethal arrhythmias and ICD shocks are expected. Indeed, 50–70% of the patients with ICD implantation for prevention of sudden death received appropriate ICD therapies within the first 2 years after ICD implantation.[71,72] Antiarrhythmic drugs are helpful in reducing the frequency of ICD therapies in the following situations.

Treatment of Electrical Storm

Electrical storm, defined as having three or more episodes of VT or VF within a 24-h period, occurs in 10–20% of the patients who have received an ICD for prevention of VT/VF recurrence. Storms tend to occur months (4–20) after ICD implantation and the number of arrhythmic episodes per storm per patient ranges from 4 to 51.[73–75] Most patients develop syncope or presyncope during electrical storm and require hospitalization.

While some studies have found that electrical storms do not confer increased mortality,[73,74] other studies differ.[75,76] Of the 457 patients (20%) enrolled in the ICD arm of AVID, 90 experienced electrical storms with 86% of the episodes due to VT.[75] The occurrence of electrical storms was associated with a remarkable 5.4-fold increase in risk of mortality in the 3 months following the storm, and most of the patients who died succumbed to cardiac nonsudden causes[75] such as heart failure.[74] Multiple ICD shocks result in elevation in cardiac troponin levels,[77,78] with acute cellular damage, myocardial injury, and fibrosis.[79,80] Hence, it is possible that electrical storm and repetitive ICD shocks may directly contribute to an increase in mortality.

Treatment of electrical storm involves the optimization of β blocker therapy, especially for situations in which storms are triggered by ischemia or heightened sympathetic tone.[73,81] This is usually followed by initiation of antiarrhythmic drugs. The effectiveness of Class I antiarrhythmic drugs is limited,[73] but intravenous amiodarone is efficacious both for acute termination and suppression of recurrent storms.[73,74] Experience from a single tertiary medical center showed that only 12% of patients treated with amiodarone had a recurrence of electrical storm versus 53% in those not treated with amiodarone ($p < 0.001$).[74] Whether amiodarone improves survival in patients with electrical storm is currently unknown, although in patients with electrical storms treated with aggressive use of intravenous amiodarone followed by oral administration, long-term outcomes were similar to patients without storms.[73]

Reduction of Frequent Appropriate Implantable Cardioverter Defibrillator Therapy

Of the 3344 patients in the European Registry of ICD (EURID), 49.5% had ICD interventions and 39.8% had appropriate therapies, while 16.2% had inappropriate therapies during a 1-year follow-up.[82] Of the 1691 hospitalizations, 61.3% were due to VT/VF. Similarly, in the MADIT patients who received an ICD, 60% experienced an ICD shock within 2 years of enrollment.[29] Hence, recurrence of tachyarrhythmias is quite prevalent and suppression of ventricular arrhythmia recurrence is desirable. In addition, antiarrhythmic drugs frequently slow sustained VT, increase hemodynamic tolerance, and enhance the efficacy of antitachycardia pacing to successfully terminate VT.[70] While Class I antiarrhythmic drugs are no longer used routinely in patients with ischemic heart disease, Class III antiarrhythmic drugs do not significantly increase mortality in patients with heart disease and are useful as adjunct therapies in ICD patients.

Sotalol

d,l-Sotalol combines the benefits of nonselective β-adrenergic blockade and Class III antiarrhythmic activities and has been shown to be safe and efficacious as adjunctive drug therapy to prevent ICD shocks. In a prospective study in which 143 patients with a history of VT/VF underwent EP-guided sotalol therapy, sotalol prevented induction of VT/VF in 53 patients who were subsequently treated with sotalol only (330 ± 89 mg/day).[83] The 93 patients in whom sotalol failed to suppress induction of VT/VF underwent ICD implantation and were randomized to also take sotalol (348 ± 78 mg/day, 46 patients) or placebo (47 patients). Over a follow-up period of more than 1 year, 53.2% of the patients in the ICD-only group had VT/VF recurrence versus 28.3% in the sotalol group and 32.6% in the ICD/sotalol group ($p = 0.0013$). Hence, sotalol was effective in preventing recurrence of VT/VF.

In a multicenter double blind, randomized study, 151 patients with ICDs assigned to treatment with sotalol (160–320 mg daily) were compared to 151 matched placebo controls over 12 months.[84] The sotalol group was found to have a significantly lower risk of death from any cause (48% decrease in risk) and of the delivery of first ICD shock for any reason, appropriate (44% decrease) or inappropriate (64% decrease). This reduction in risk of death or delivery of first shock was independent of both ventricular function and the use of β blockers other than sotalol. The mean shocks per year were significantly reduced in the sotalol group (1.43 versus 3.89 in control, $p = 0.008$). However, 27% of the patients assigned to sotalol discontinued the medication because of adverse effects (versus 12% in the placebo group).

Amiodarone

Amiodarone is considered the most efficacious antiarrhythmic drug in the treatment of life-threatening ventricular arrhythmias and in the resuscitation of out-of-the-hospital cardiac arrest patients who have shock-resistant VF.[85] Its role in the reduction of ICD therapy has recently been demonstrated by the results of the Optimal Pharmacological Therapy in Implantable Cardioverter (**OPTIC**) Study, a landmark, multicenter, open label trial. In this study, 412 patients who received ICDs for secondary prevention of spontaneous or inducible VT/VF and with an LVEF ≤ 40% were randomized to treatment for 1 year with amiodarone plus β blocker, sotalol alone, or β blocker alone.[86] The results showed that ICD shocks occurred in 38.5% of patients who received β blocker alone, in 24.3% who received sotalol, and in 10.3% assigned to amiodarone plus β blocker ($p < 0.001$). Amiodarone reduced appropriate shocks by 70% ($p < 0.001$), whereas sotalol had no significant effect. There was a trend for sotalol to reduce ICD shocks compared to β blocker alone, but the difference did not reach statistical significance. It is important to note that patients taking amiodarone had significantly higher adverse pulmonary and thyroid effects as well as symptomatic bradycardia. Discontinuation of the study treatment occurred in 18.2% for amiodarone, 23.5% for sotalol, but only 5.3% for β blocker.

Azimilide

Azimilide is a novel investigational Class III antiarrhythmic that blocks both the rapid (I_{Kr}) and slow (I_{Ks}) components of the delayed rectifier potassium channels. In a double-blind, placebo-controlled, pilot study, 172 patients with ICDs were randomized to receive placebo, 35 mg azimilide, 75 mg azimilide, or 125 mg azimilide.[87] After a mean follow-up of 247–279 days, azimilide was well tolerated and significantly reduced the frequency of appropriate ICD therapies at all administered doses by 69% compared with placebo ($p < 0.00001$).

The results of the pilot study were substantiated by the Shock Inhibition Evaluation with Azimilide (**SHIELD**) Study, a placebo-controlled, double-blind randomized clinical trial that enrolled 633 ICD recipients to determine the effects of azimilide on recurrent symptomatic VT/VF and ICD therapies over 273 days.[88] The total number of ICD shocks plus antitachycardia pacing for symptomatic VTs was significantly reduced by azimilide by 57% at 75 mg and by 43% at 125 mg daily doses. Notably, five patients in the azimilide groups and one patient in the placebo group developed torsade de pointes, and one patient on azimilide developed severe but reversible neutropenia.

Other Antiarrhythmic Drugs

Dofetilide has been examined for its efficacy and safety in the treatment of VT/VF. In a multicenter, double-blind, randomized crossover comparative study of 135 patients with ischemic heart disease and inducible sustained VT, dofetilide was as efficacious as sotalol in preventing the induction of sustained VT by EP study but had fewer adverse effects.[89] Long-term treatment with dofetilide also showed efficacy and safety profiles comparable to sotalol and was deemed a viable alternative.

The use of Class I antiarrhythmic drugs is usually not recommended in patients with ischemic heart disease. Anecdotal and isolated reports exist that suggest the addition of mexiletine to amiodarone may provide additional protection against the recurrence of VT/VF,[90] but overall, the results were discouraging.[73,91] The addition of Class IC antiarrhythmic drugs to amiodarone in patients who failed amiodarone therapy did not show any synergistic effects in suppression of VT/VF, while a high incidence of proarrhythmia effects was noted.[92]

Reduction of Inappropriate Implantable Cardioverter Defibrillator Therapies

Despite advances in modern technology and improvement in features in today's ICDs, inappropriate ICD shocks remain a challenge, occurring in 10–20% of ICD recipients.[82,84,86,88,93] Even though dual-chamber devices significantly reduced inappropriate detection of supraventricular tachycardia (SVT) compared to single-chamber ICDs, it still occurred in 30.9% of the patients, with 24.8% receiving inappropriate ICD therapies.[94] Congestive heart failure,[95] cigarette smoking,[96] a history of SVT,[97] and young age (childhood and adolescence)[98] appear to be risk factors for inappropriate ICD therapies. Also, implantation of an ICD for primary prevention rather than for secondary prevention of VT/VF increases the risk of inappropriate shocks.[99] Implantation of a dual-chamber device lowers the risk of inappropriate ICD detection by 47%,[94] and use of detection enhancement features reduces the risk of inappropriate ICD therapies by 53%.[100] Remote monitoring of ICD from home is also thought to facilitate rapid monitoring of arrhythmias and reduce inappropriate ICD therapies.[101]

Surprisingly, data on the use of antiarrhythmic drugs in the reduction of inappropriate ICD therapies are limited. In the *d,l*-Sotalol Implantable Cardioverter-Defibrillator Study, inappropriate ICD shocks for SVT were reduced 64% in the sotalol group versus the placebo group (p = 0.004).[84] In the OPTIC trial, the annual risk of inappropriate ICD shock was 15.4% in the β blocker group, 9.4% in the sotalol group, but only 3.3% in the β blocker plus amiodarone group.[86] Hence, inappropriate shocks were reduced by 78% in patients taking amiodarone. In the SHIELD trial, there was no difference in inappropriate ICD therapies among patients taking placebo, 75 mg azimilide, or 125 mg azimilide daily.[88]

β Blockers are frequently used for suppression of SVT. They counteract enhanced sympathetic tone, control ventricular rate in atrial fibrillation/atrial flutter, and inhibit the development of reentry for tachycardias involving the AV node. In a subanalysis of MADIT II data, patients who received high dose β blockers showed a significant reduction of risk for VT/VF requiring ICD therapies compared to those who did not receive β blockers, but β blocker therapy did not reduce the frequency of inappropriate ICD therapies.[93] Hence, current data suggest that the two most commonly used antiarrhythmic drugs in patients with ICD implants for suppression of malignant ventricular arrhythmias, amiodarone and sotalol, are also efficacious for suppressing SVT and for reducing the incidence of inappropriate ICD therapies in these patients.

Effects of Antiarrhythmic Drugs on Defibrillation Threshold

An important consideration for the use of antiarrhythmic drugs in patients with ICDs is their effects on defibrillation threshold (DFT). Results from animal studies do not always correlate with human experience.[102,103] Class IA antiarrhythmic drugs do not seem to have a significant effect on DFT in humans.[102–104] In contrast, the Class IB drug lidocaine has been found to consistently increase DFT. In 27 patients undergoing intraoperative testing for ICD, lidocaine increased DFT from a baseline of 14 ± 5 J to 18 ± 7 J ($p < 0.02$) and there was a positive linear correlation between lidocaine plasma concentration and the percent change in defibrillation energy requirement.[104] In a prospective randomized study, the ICD DFT in patients taking 720 mg/day of mexiletine showed no significant change in DFT after a 24-month follow-up.[105,106] However, isolated reports exist that showed the administration of mexiletine could significantly increase DFT rendering failure in defibrillation.[107] More recent reports suggest that mexiletine may have a greater effect in increasing DFT than previously appreciated.[108] The effects of Class IC antiarrhythmic drugs on DFT appear to be variable, with no significant effects or a small increase.[102,103,109]

In contrast, Class III antiarrhythmic drugs, with the exception of amiodarone, have been consistently shown to lower or to have no effect on the DFT.[102,103,110] In a nonrandomized prospective study, 25 patients who received sotalol (average dose 171 ± 58 mg) had significantly lower DFTs compared with 23 concurrent patients, 18 of whom were on amiodarone (5.9 ± 3.4 J versus 16 ± 10 J, $p < 0.01$).[111] These results were further corroborated by a study showing that acute infusion of *d*-sotalol resulted in a 32% decrease in energy required for defibrillation (EC_{50} from 12.4 ± 5.0 J at baseline to 8.4 ± 4.0 J with sotalol, $n = 15$, $p < 0.003$).[112] A novel application of Class III antiarrhythmic drugs for lowering defibrillation energy requirements in patients with marginal DFTs was thus proposed. Indeed, ibutilide and other Class III antiarrhythmic drugs have been used to lower the defibrillation energy requirement for converting atrial fibrillation to sinus rhythm, and they enhance the efficacy of cardioversion.[113,114] Although Class III antiarrhythmic drugs (except amiodarone) are not routinely used with the sole purpose of lowering DFTs, they are sometimes instituted in patients with marginal DFTs when revising the ICD system is not an option.[110] Amiodarone, the most frequently used antiarrhythmic drug in patients with ICDs and the drug of choice for shock resistant out-of-hospital VF,[85] is generally associated with a significant increase in DFT.[102,105,106,110]

However, the issues related to the effects of antiarrhythmic drugs on DFT may have become obsolete and irrelevant in patients with newer generation devices with high output and biphasic defibrillation waveforms. In a retrospective study with 89 patients, those on chronic amiodarone therapy receiving a monophasic ICD had a significantly higher DFT (29 ± 8.8 J, $n = 7$) than patients without antiarrhythmic treatment (19.1 ± 5.1 J, $n = 11$, $p = 0.021$). However, in patients with a biphasic device, DFT was not significantly different between patients on amiodarone (15.3 ± 7.3 J, $n = 22$), sotalol (14.4 ± 7.2 J, $n = 20$), or no antiarrhythmic drug (17 ± 6.1 J, $n = 22$, $p = 0.44$).[83] A substudy of the OPTIC trial examined the DFTs in 94 patients at baseline and again after 8–12 weeks of therapy with β blocker, β blocker plus amiodarone, or sotalol.[115] Patients randomized to β blocker therapy had a significant mean DFT decrease from 8.77 ± 5.15 J at baseline to 7.13 ± 3.43, $n = 29$, $p = 0.027$), but the amiodarone ($n = 35$) and the sotalol ($n = 30$) groups did not have significant DFT changes, suggesting routine DFT reassessment after institution of amiodarone or sotalol may not be necessary. It is, however, important to note that DFTs can be affected by various parameters, including the sympathetic tone and levels of catecholamines,[116] the length of procedure time, left ventricular end-diastolic dimensions,[117] body size,[118] LVEF, NYHA class,[119] and the concomitant administration of other medications.

Other Considerations

Quality of Life

ICD therapy has become the standard treatment for life-threatening arrhythmias and is generally well accepted because of its survival benefits. Also, antiarrhythmic drugs are associated with substantial adverse effects, and ICD therapy may obviate the need for these drugs. However, anxiety and fear of the device are common[120] and ICD firings have a significant adverse impact on device recipients.[121] Studies comparing the quality of life between patients receiving antiarrhythmics and ICDs have only recently been undertaken. Studies on the quality of life 6 months after CABG in the CABG Patch trial showed that ICD negatively affected the patients' perceived and measured quality of life.[122] The difference was mainly due to the negative impact of ICD shocks; there was no difference in quality of life indicators between controls and ICD patients who did not receive ICD shocks.

Quality of life assessment in CIDS patients showed that over 12 months, participants who received an ICD ($n = 86$) had statistically significant better quality of life indicators compared to those who received amiodarone ($n = 92$).[123] However, the quality of life benefits of ICD were lost in patients who have received five or more shocks, indicating a significant negative impact on the quality of life by frequent ICD firings. The AVID quality of life substudy found that ICD and antiarrhythmic drug therapies were associated with similar changes in quality of life among patients who survived at least 1 year ($n = 800$).[124] Overall, 39% of the ICD patients received ICD shocks and the occurrence of any shock compared with those who received no shock during the first year of device implantation was independently associated with significant reductions in mental well being and physical functioning. Psychological and emotional stress from ICD implantation is noted not only in device recipients but also in their family members.[125] Whether the use of antiarrhythmic drugs to suppress ICD firing results in improved quality of life in ICD recipients is presently unknown, but warrants further investigation.

Cost-Effectiveness of Treatment

With the rapid expansion of indications for ICD implantation, the financial implication is enormous and ICD cost-effectiveness will be a critical determinant in future health policymaking.[126,127] It was estimated that device implantation and care of the 55,000–65,000 new MADIT-II eligible patients each year would incur an additional expenditure in excess of $5 billion annually in the United States.[128] Results from AVID showed that the cost-effectiveness ratios (cost per year of life saved by the ICD compared to antiarrhythmic therapy) at 3 years, 6 years, and 12 years were $66,677, $68,000, and $80,000, respectively.[129] Similar analysis from CIDS showed that the cost-effectiveness for ICD compared to amiodarone therapy was Canadian $213,543 per life-year gained over 6.3 years, and extrapolated to be in the range of Canadian $100,000–$150,000 per life-year gained over 12 years.[130] The poor cost-effectiveness of ICD therapy in CIDS is due to the overall lack of efficacy of ICD in improving survival in this cohort of patients.[24]

Results from primary prevention trials also showed that ICD therapy is expensive with varied cost-effectiveness. MADIT reported an incremental cost of $27,000 per life-year saved for ICD therapy, a favorable figure compared to the cost-effectiveness of other cardiac interventions.[131] Similarly, SCD-HeFT reported a cost-effectiveness ratio of $38,389 per life-year saved.[132] A recent report from MADIT II, however, showed an appalling cost effectiveness ratio of $235,000 per year-life saved during the 3.5-year period of the study.[128] With secondary analysis that included projections of survival until 12 years after randomization, the ratio was considerably lower, but was still in the range of $78,600–$114,000. Hence, the economic burden of ICD therapy is substantial, and the cost-effectiveness of therapy must be taken into account in future health care delivery planning. Alternative effective treatments should be further explored.

Potential Adverse Interactions Between Antiarrhythmic Drugs and Implantable Cardioverter Defibrillators

Although antiarrhythmic drugs can be beneficial in the management of patients with an ICD, there are also potential adverse interactions between antiarrhythmic drugs and ICDs. First, amiodarone and certain Class I antiarrhythmic drugs can increase DFT as discussed above. This may lead to failure to defibrillate, rendering the device ineffective. Second, antiarrhythmic drugs can slow VTs excessively to below the cutoff rate for detection, and the VTs may become unrecognized by the device. Third, antiarrhythmic drugs may produce significant sinus bradycardia, especially in patients taking β blockers and other negative chronotropic agents concomitantly. This may result in excessive right ventricular pacing, leading to an increase in generator energy consumption and depletion, as well as inducing deterioration in ventricular function[133] as observed in the Dual Chamber and VVI Implantable Defibrillator (**DAVID**) Trial.[134] Patients with RV pacing greater than 40% of the time have a significantly higher risk of mortality or hospitalization for CHF.[135] The results from DAVID were substantiated by subgroup analysis of MADIT II.[136] Fourth, Class I antiarrhythmic drugs are known to increase pacing threshold.[70] Although this problem is not usually considered clinically important and the almost universal use of steroid-eluting leads has helped to improve capture thresholds, isolated reports suggest that antiarrhythmic drugs may cause failure to pace under certain circumstances.[137–139] Fifth, antiarrhythmic drugs have the potential to increase the incidence of arrhythmia. Class I drugs can be proarrhythmic and Class III drugs can facilitate the development of torsade de pointes.[140] These drugs can also stabilize and organize arrhythmia circuits so that atrial and ventricular arrhythmias can become sustained and incessant; the combined effects of tachycardia slowing and facilitation of AV nodal conduction can result in 1:1 atrial flutter conduction or atrial fibrillation with rapid ventricular response.[140]

Nonantiarrhythmic Drugs

As the role of antiarrhythmic drugs evolves in the management of sudden cardiac death, so has the function of nonantiarrhythmic drugs.[141,142] In fact, the most effective drugs that prevent sudden cardiac death do not have direct effects on the electrophysiological properties of the heart. Some of these medicines are so effective that they should be optimally used in every patient at high risk of sudden cardiac death.

β-Adrenergic blockers are Class II antiarrhythmic drugs according to the Vaughan–Williams classification, but with the exception of sotalol, β blockers do not have membrane active properties. β Blockers are effective in reducing all-cause mortality in patients after an MI with LV dysfunction (CAPRICORN randomized trial[143]), improve survival and prevent sudden death in CHF patients (CIBIS-II,[144] MERIT-HF[145]), and reduce mortality in patients with a history of VT/VF (AVID[146]).

Indeed, β blockers are considered the most effective pharmacological agents in the prevention of sudden cardiac death. Angiotensin-converting enzyme (ACE) inhibitors, which exert a myriad of cellular effects including preventing ventricular remodeling, are effective in reducing total mortality and sudden death in patients who had an acute MI and LV dysfunction (AIRE,[147] TRACE[148]). In CHF patients, administration of spironolactone, an aldosterone receptor blocker, reduced sudden cardiac death, cardiac death, and death from heart failure (RALES[149]). Statins, 3-hydroxy-3-methylglutaryl coenzyme A (HMG-CoA) reductase inhibitors that have significant beneficial effects beyond their hypocholesterolemic properties, reduced total mortality and sudden death in coronary disease and dyslipidemia patients (SSSS,[150] LIPID[151]). Consumption of fatty fish and administration of ω-3 polyunsaturated fatty acids have been shown to reduce the incidence of sudden death.[152,153] These studies strongly suggest that the underlying mechanisms leading to the development of sudden cardiac death are complex. Pharmacological interventions that prevent cardiac remodeling or changes in response to maladaptation in disease states, events that are upstream of sudden death development, are effective in providing better outcomes. In contrast, using antiarrhythmic drugs to block electrical instability that is the end-stage manifestation of advanced disease maladaptation cannot effectively prevent the heart from dying.

Summary

The role of antiarrhythmic drugs for prevention of sudden cardiac death has changed dramatically in the past 20 years. Though antiarrhythmics were once considered first-line therapy for the prevention of sudden death, clinical trials that demonstrated the proarrhythmic effects of Class I antiarrhythmics and others that established the superiority of ICD implantation over amiodarone have driven ICD therapy to supplant antiarrhythmics as the standard of care in patients at high risk for sudden death.

Yet antiarrhythmic drugs have not exhausted their effectiveness. They may confer significant advantages in specific subsets of patients, such as in those with only moderate reductions in LV function, with Brugada syndrome, or with LQT3 syndrome. Moreover, due to the negative impact of ICD shocks and therapies on quality of life, antiarrhythmics remain an important and widely used adjunctive therapy in patients with ICDs. Amiodarone, *d,l*-sotalol, and azimilide may help reduce both appropriate and inappropriate ICD therapies, and β blockers and antiarrhythmics are used to treat electrical storm. Concerns that some antiarrhythmics may increase DFT and render ICD therapy ineffective may be allayed in light of advancements in ICD technology. Nevertheless, further investigation into this and other potential adverse interactions between antiarrhythmics and ICDs is necessary.

References

1. Thom T, Haase N, Rosamond W, Howard VJ, Rumsfeld J, Manolio T, Zheng ZJ, Flegal K, O'Donnell C, Kittner S, Lloyd-Jones D, Goff DC Jr, Hong Y, Adams R, Friday G, Furie K, Gorelick P, Kissela B, Marler J, Meigs J, Roger V, Sidney S, Sorlie P, Steinberger J, Wasserthiel-Smoller S, Wilson M, Wolf P. American Heart Association Statistics C, Stroke Statistics S. Heart disease and stroke statistics—2006 update: A report from the American Heart Association Statistics Committee and Stroke Statistics Subcommittee. *Circulation* 2006;113:e85–151.
2. Cobb LA, Fahrenbruch CE, Olsufka M, Copass MK. Changing incidence of out-of-hospital ventricular fibrillation, 1980–2000. *JAMA* 2002;288: 3008–3013.
3. Bayes de Luna A, Coumel P, Leclercq JF. Ambulatory sudden cardiac death: Mechanisms of production of fatal arrhythmia on the basis of data from 157 cases. *Am Heart J* 1989;117:151–159.
4. Kotler MN, Tabatznik B, Mower MM, Tominaga S. Prognostic significance of ventricular ectopic beats with respect to sudden death in the late postinfarction period. *Circulation* 1973;47:959–966.
5. Steinbeck G, Greene HL. Management of patients with life-threatening sustained ventricular tachyarrhythmias—the role of guided antiarrhythmic drug therapy. *Prog Cardiovasc Dis* 1996;38:419–428.
6. IMPACT. International Mexiletine and Placebo Antiarrhythmic Coronary Trial (IMPACT): II. Results from 24-hour electrocardiograms. IMPACT Research Group. *Eur Heart J* 1986;7:749–759.

7. IMPACT. International Mexiletine and Placebo Antiarrhythmic Coronary Trial: I. Report on arrhythmia and other findings. IMPACT Research Group. *J Am Coll Cardiol* 1984;4:1148–1163.
8. Echt DS, Liebson PR, Mitchell LB, Peters RW, Obias-Manno D, Barker AH, Arensberg D, Baker A, Friedman L, Greene HL. Mortality and morbidity in patients receiving encainide, flecainide, or placebo. The Cardiac Arrhythmia Suppression Trial. *N Engl J Med* 1991;324:781–788.
9. CAST. Effect of the antiarrhythmic agent moricizine on survival after myocardial infarction. The Cardiac Arrhythmia Suppression Trial II Investigators. *N Engl J Med* 1992;327:227–233.
10. Mason JW. A comparison of electrophysiologic testing with Holter monitoring to predict antiarrhythmic-drug efficacy for ventricular tachyarrhythmias. Electrophysiologic Study versus Electrocardiographic Monitoring Investigators. *N Engl J Med* 1993;329:445–451 (see comment).
11. Mason JW. A comparison of seven antiarrhythmic drugs in patients with ventricular tachyarrhythmias. Electrophysiologic Study versus Electrocardiographic Monitoring Investigators. *N Engl J Med* 1993;329:452–458 (see comment).
12. Waldo AL, Camm AJ, deRuyter H, Friedman PL, MacNeil DJ, Pauls JF, Pitt B, Pratt CM, Schwartz PJ, Veltri EP. Effect of d-sotalol on mortality in patients with left ventricular dysfunction after recent and remote myocardial infarction. The SWORD Investigators. Survival With Oral d-Sotalol. *Lancet* 1996;348:7–12.
13. Kober L, Bloch Thomsen PE, Moller M, Torp-Pedersen C, Carlsen J, Sandoe E, Egstrup K, Agner E, Videbaek J, Marchant B, Camm AJ, Danish Investigations of A, Mortality on Dofetilide Study G. Effect of dofetilide in patients with recent myocardial infarction and left-ventricular dysfunction: A randomised trial. *Lancet* 2000;356:2052–2058.
14. Burkart F, Pfisterer M, Kiowski W, Follath F, Burckhardt D. Effect of antiarrhythmic therapy on mortality in survivors of myocardial infarction with asymptomatic complex ventricular arrhythmias: Basel Antiarrhythmic Study of Infarct Survival (BASIS). *J Am Coll Cardiol* 1990;16:1711–1718.
15. Pfisterer ME, Kiowski W, Brunner H, Burckhardt D, Burkart F. Long-term benefit of 1-year amiodarone treatment for persistent complex ventricular arrhythmias after myocardial infarction. *Circulation* 1993;87:309–311.
16. Ceremuzynski L, Kleczar E, Krzeminska-Pakula M, Kuch J, Nartowicz E, Smielak-Korombel J, Dyduszynski A, Maciejewicz J, Zaleska T, Lazarczyk-Kedzia E. Effect of amiodarone on mortality after myocardial infarction: A double-blind, placebo-controlled, pilot study. *J Am Coll Cardiol* 1992;20:1056–1062.
17. Budaj A, Kokowicz P, Smielak-Korombel W, Kuch J, Krzeminska-Pakuoa M, Maciejewicz J, Nartowicz E, Zaleska T, Dyduszynski A, Ceremuzynski L. Lack of effect of amiodarone on survival after extensive infarction. Polish Amiodarone Trial. *Coron Artery Dis* 1996;7:315–319.
18. Navarro-Lopez F, Cosin J, Marrugat J, Guindo J, Bayes de Luna A. Comparison of the effects of amiodarone versus metoprolol on the frequency of ventricular arrhythmias and on mortality after acute myocardial infarction. SSSD Investigators. Spanish Study on Sudden Death. *Am J Cardiol* 1993;72:1243–1248.
19. Naccarelli GV, Wolbrette DL, Patel HM, Luck JC. Amiodarone: Clinical trials. *Curr Opin Cardiol* 2000;15:64–72.
20. Investigators TC. Randomized antiarrhythmic drug therapy in survivors of cardiac arrest (the CASCADE Study). The CASCADE Investigators. *Am J Cardiol* 1993;72:280–287.
21. Julian DG, Camm AJ, Frangin G, Janse MJ, Munoz A, Schwartz PJ, Simon P. Randomised trial of effect of amiodarone on mortality in patients with left-ventricular dysfunction after recent myocardial infarction: EMIAT. European Myocardial Infarct Amiodarone Trial Investigators. *Lancet* 1997;349:667–674.
22. Cairns JA, Connolly SJ, Roberts R, Gent M. Randomised trial of outcome after myocardial infarction in patients with frequent or repetitive ventricular premature depolarisations: CAMIAT. Canadian Amiodarone Myocardial Infarction Arrhythmia Trial Investigators. *Lancet* 1997;349: 675–682.
23. Investigators A. A comparison of antiarrhythmic-drug therapy with implantable defibrillators in patients resuscitated from near-fatal ventricular arrhythmias. The Antiarrhythmics versus Implantable Defibrillators (AVID) Investigators. *N Engl J Med* 1997;337:1576–1583.
24. Connolly SJ, Gent M, Roberts RS, Dorian P, Roy D, Sheldon RS, Mitchell LB, Green MS, Klein GJ, O'Brien B. Canadian implantable defibrillator study (CIDS): A randomized trial of the implantable cardioverter defibrillator against amiodarone. *Circulation* 2000;101:1297–1302.
25. Bokhari F, Newman D, Greene M, Korley V, Mangat I, Dorian P. Long-term comparison of the implantable cardioverter defibrillator versus amiodarone: Eleven-year follow-up of a subset of

patients in the Canadian Implantable Defibrillator Study (CIDS). *Circulation* 2004;110:112–116.
26. Kuck KH, Cappato R, Siebels J, Ruppel R. Randomized comparison of antiarrhythmic drug therapy with implantable defibrillators in patients resuscitated from cardiac arrest: The Cardiac Arrest Study Hamburg (CASH). *Circulation* 2000; 102:748–754.
27. Oseroff O, Retyk E, Bochoeyer A. Subanalyses of secondary prevention implantable cardioverter-defibrillator trials: Antiarrhythmics versus implantable defibrillators (AVID), Canadian Implantable Defibrillator Study (CIDS), and Cardiac Arrest Study Hamburg (CASH). *Curr Opin Cardiol* 2004;19:26–30.
28. Connolly SJ, Hallstrom AP, Cappato R, Schron EB, Kuck KH, Zipes DP, Greene HL, Boczor S, Domanski M, Follmann D, Gent M, Roberts RS. Meta-analysis of the implantable cardioverter defibrillator secondary prevention trials. AVID, CASH and CIDS studies. Antiarrhythmics vs Implantable Defibrillator Study. Cardiac Arrest Study Hamburg. Canadian Implantable Defibrillator Study. *Eur Heart J* 2000;21:2071–2078.
29. Moss AJ, Hall WJ, Cannom DS, Daubert JP, Higgins SL, Klein H, Levine JH, Saksena S, Waldo AL, Wilber D, Brown MW, Heo M. Improved survival with an implanted defibrillator in patients with coronary disease at high risk for ventricular arrhythmia. Multicenter Automatic Defibrillator Implantation Trial Investigators. *N Engl J Med* 1996;335:1933–1940.
30. Buxton AE, Lee KL, Fisher JD, Josephson ME, Prystowsky EN, Hafley G. A randomized study of the prevention of sudden death in patients with coronary artery disease. Multicenter Unsustained Tachycardia Trial Investigators. *N Engl J Med* 1999;341:1882–1890.
31. Moss AJ, Zareba W, Hall WJ, Klein H, Wilber DJ, Cannom DS, Daubert JP, Higgins SL, Brown MW, Andrews ML. Multicenter Automatic Defibrillator Implantation Trial III. Prophylactic implantation of a defibrillator in patients with myocardial infarction and reduced ejection fraction. *N Engl J Med* 2002;346:877–883.
32. Flaker GC, Blackshear JL, McBride R, Kronmal RA, Halperin JL, Hart RG. Antiarrhythmic drug therapy and cardiac mortality in atrial fibrillation. The Stroke Prevention in Atrial Fibrillation Investigators. *J Am Coll Cardiol* 1992;20:527–532.
33. Doval HC, Nul DR, Grancelli HO, Perrone SV, Bortman GR, Curiel R. Randomised trial of low-dose amiodarone in severe congestive heart failure. Grupo de Estudio de la Sobrevida en la Insuficiencia Cardiaca en Argentina (GESICA). *Lancet* 1994;344:493–498.
34. Doval HC, Nul DR, Grancelli HO, Varini SD, Soifer S, Corrado G, Dubner S, Scapin O, Perrone SV. Nonsustained ventricular tachycardia in severe heart failure. Independent marker of increased mortality due to sudden death. GESICA-GEMA Investigators. *Circulation* 1996;94:3198–3203.
35. Singh SN, Fletcher RD, Fisher SG, Singh BN, Lewis HD, Deedwania PC, Massie BM, Colling C, Lazzeri D. Amiodarone in patients with congestive heart failure and asymptomatic ventricular arrhythmia. Survival Trial of Antiarrhythmic Therapy in Congestive Heart Failure. *N Engl J Med* 1995;333:77–82.
36. Deedwania PC, Singh BN, Ellenbogen K, Fisher S, Fletcher R, Singh SN. Spontaneous conversion and maintenance of sinus rhythm by amiodarone in patients with heart failure and atrial fibrillation: Observations from the veterans affairs congestive heart failure survival trial of antiarrhythmic therapy (CHF-STAT). The Department of Veterans Affairs CHF-STAT Investigators. *Circulation* 1998;98:2574–2579.
37. Strickberger SA, Hummel JD, Bartlett TG, Frumin HI, Schuger CD, Beau SL, Bitar C, Morady F, Investigators A. Amiodarone versus implantable cardioverter-defibrillator: Randomized trial in patients with nonischemic dilated cardiomyopathy and asymptomatic nonsustained ventricular tachycardia—AMIOVIRT. *J Am Coll Cardiol* 2003;41:1707–1712.
38. Torp-Pedersen C, Moller M, Bloch-Thomsen PE, Kober L, Sandoe E, Egstrup K, Agner E, Carlsen J, Videbaek J, Marchant B, Camm AJ. Dofetilide in patients with congestive heart failure and left ventricular dysfunction. Danish Investigations of Arrhythmia and Mortality on Dofetilide Study Group. *N Engl J Med* 1999;341:857–865.
39. Bardy GH, Lee KL, Mark DB, Poole JE, Packer DL, Boineau R, Domanski M, Troutman C, Anderson J, Johnson G, McNulty SE, Clapp-Channing N, Davidson-Ray LD, Fraulo ES, Fishbein DP, Luceri RM, Ip JH, Sudden Cardiac Death in Heart Failure Trial I. Amiodarone or an implantable cardioverter-defibrillator for congestive heart failure. *N Engl J Med* 2005;352:225–237.
40. Domanski MJ, Sakseena S, Epstein AE, Hallstrom AP, Brodsky MA, Kim S, Lancaster S, Schron E. Relative effectiveness of the implantable cardioverter-defibrillator and antiarrhythmic drugs in patients with varying degrees of left ventricular dysfunction who have survived malignant ventricular arrhythmias. AVID Investigators.

Antiarrhythmics Versus Implantable Defibrillators. *J Am Coll Cardiol* 1999;34:1090–1095.

41. Hallstrom AP, McAnulty JH, Wilkoff BL, Follmann D, Raitt MH, Carlson MD, Gillis AM, Shih HT, Powell JL, Duff H, Halperin BD. Antiarrhythmics Versus Implantable Defibrillator Trial I. Patients at lower risk of arrhythmia recurrence: A subgroup in whom implantable defibrillators may not offer benefit. Antiarrhythmics Versus Implantable Defibrillator (AVID) Trial Investigators. *J Am Coll Cardiol* 2001;37:1093–1099.
42. Meissner MD, Kay HR, Horowitz LN, Spielman SR, Greenspan AM, Kutalek SP. Relation of acute antiarrhythmic drug efficacy to left ventricular function in coronary artery disease. *Am J Cardiol* 1988;61:1050–1055.
43. Bigger JT Jr. Prophylactic use of implanted cardiac defibrillators in patients at high risk for ventricular arrhythmias after coronary-artery bypass graft surgery. Coronary Artery Bypass Graft (CABG) Patch Trial Investigators. *N Engl J Med* 1997;337: 1569–1575.
44. Hohnloser SH, Kuck KH, Dorian P, Roberts RS, Hampton JR, Hatala R, Fain E, Gent M, Connolly SJ, Investigators D. Prophylactic use of an implantable cardioverter-defibrillator after acute myocardial infarction. *N Engl J Med* 2004;351: 2481–2488.
45. Tanno K, Miyoshi F, Watanabe N, Minoura Y, Kawamura M, Ryu S, Asano T, Kobayashi Y, Katagiri T, Trial MITMADI. Are the MADIT II criteria for ICD implantation appropriate for Japanese patients? *Circ J* 2005;69:19–22.
46. Brugada P, Brugada R, Antzelevitch C, Brugada J. The Brugada syndrome. *Arch Mal Coeur Vaiss* 2005;98:115–122.
47. Shimizu W, Aiba T, Antzelevitch C. Specific therapy based on the genotype and cellular mechanism in inherited cardiac arrhythmias. Long QT syndrome and Brugada syndrome. *Curr Pharm Des* 2005;11:1561–1572.
48. Tsuchiya T. Role of pharmacotherapy in Brugada syndrome. *Indian Pacing Electrophysiol J* 2004;4: 26–32.
49. Tanaka H, Kinoshita O, Uchikawa S, Kasai H, Nakamura M, Izawa A, Yokoseki O, Kitabayashi H, Takahashi W, Yazaki Y, Watanabe N, Imamura H, Kubo K. Successful prevention of recurrent ventricular fibrillation by intravenous isoproterenol in a patient with Brugada syndrome. *Pacing Clin Electrophysiol* 2001;24:1293–1294.
50. Suzuki H, Torigoe K, Numata O, Yazaki S. Infant case with a malignant form of Brugada syndrome. *J Cardiovasc Electrophysiol* 2000;11:1277–1280.
51. Tsuchiya T, Ashikaga K, Honda T, Arita M. Prevention of ventricular fibrillation by cilostazol, an oral phosphodiesterase inhibitor, in a patient with Brugada syndrome. *J Cardiovasc Electrophysiol* 2002;13:698–701.
52. Alings M, Dekker L, Sadee A, Wilde A. Quinidine induced electrocardiographic normalization in two patients with Brugada syndrome. *Pacing Clin Electrophysiol* 2001;24:1420–1422.
53. Belhassen B, Glick A, Viskin S. Efficacy of quinidine in high-risk patients with Brugada syndrome. *Circulation* 2004;110:1731–1737.
54. Hermida JS, Denjoy I, Clerc J, Extramiana F, Jarry G, Milliez P, Guicheney P, Di Fusco S, Rey JL, Cauchemez B, Leenhardt A. Hydroquinidine therapy in Brugada syndrome. *J Am Coll Cardiol* 2004;43:1853–1860.
55. Chiang CE, Roden DM. The long QT syndromes: Genetic basis and clinical implications. *J Am Coll Cardiol* 2000;36:1–12.
56. Wang DW, Yazawa K, Makita N, George AL Jr, Bennett PB. Pharmacological targeting of long QT mutant sodium channels. *J Clin Invest* 1997;99: 1714–1720.
57. Schwartz PJ, Priori SG, Locati EH, Napolitano C, Cantu F, Towbin JA, Keating MT, Hammoude H, Brown AM, Chen LS. Long QT syndrome patients with mutations of the SCN5A and HERG genes have differential responses to Na+ channel blockade and to increases in heart rate. Implications for gene-specific therapy. *Circulation* 1995;92:3381–3386.
58. Benhorin J, Taub R, Goldmit M, Kerem B, Kass RS, Windman I, Medina A. Effects of flecainide in patients with new SCN5A mutation: Mutation-specific therapy for long-QT syndrome? *Circulation* 2000;101:1698–1706.
59. Priori SG, Napolitano C, Schwartz PJ, Bloise R, Crotti L, Ronchetti E. The elusive link between LQT3 and Brugada syndrome: The role of flecainide challenge. *Circulation* 2000;102:945–947.
60. Windle JR, Geletka RC, Moss AJ, Zareba W, Atkins DL. Normalization of ventricular repolarization with flecainide in long QT syndrome patients with SCN5A:DeltaKPQ mutation. *Ann Noninvasive Electrocardiol* 2001;6:153–158.
61. Moss AJ, Windle JR, Hall WJ, Zareba W, Robinson JL, McNitt S, Severski P, Rosero S, Daubert JP, Qi M, Cieciorka M, Manalan AS. Safety and efficacy of flecainide in subjects with long QT-3 syndrome (deltaKPQ mutation): A randomized, double-blind, placebo-controlled clinical trial. *Ann Noninvasive Electrocardiol* 2005;10:59–66.

62. Francis J, Sankar V, Nair VK, Priori SG. Catecholaminergic polymorphic ventricular tachycardia. *Heart Rhythm* 2005;2:550–554.
63. Leenhardt A, Lucet V, Denjoy I, Grau F, Ngoc DD, Coumel P. Catecholaminergic polymorphic ventricular tachycardia in children. A 7-year follow-up of 21 patients. *Circulation* 1995;91:1512–1519.
64. Priori SG, Napolitano C, Memmi M, Colombi B, Drago F, Gasparini M, DeSimone L, Coltorti F, Bloise R, Keegan R, Cruz Filho FE, Vignati G, Benatar A, DeLogu A. Clinical and molecular characterization of patients with catecholaminergic polymorphic ventricular tachycardia. *Circulation* 2002;106:69–74.
65. Laitinen PJ, Brown KM, Piippo K, Swan H, Devaney JM, Brahmbhatt B, Donarum EA, Marino M, Tiso N, Viitasalo M, Toivonen L, Stephan DA, Kontula K. Mutations of the cardiac ryanodine receptor (RyR2) gene in familial polymorphic ventricular tachycardia. *Circulation* 2001;103:485–490.
66. Postma AV, Denjoy I, Hoorntje TM, Lupoglazoff JM, Da Costa A, Sebillon P, Mannens MM, Wilde AA, Guicheney P. Absence of calsequestrin 2 causes severe forms of catecholaminergic polymorphic ventricular tachycardia. *Circ Res* 2002;91: e21–26.
67. Lahat H, Eldar M. Autosomal recessive catecholamine-induced polymorphic ventricular tachycardia. *Isr Med Assoc J* 2002;4:1095–1096.
68. De Rosa G, Delogu AB, Piastra M, Chiaretti A, Bloise R, Priori SG. Catecholaminergic polymorphic ventricular tachycardia: Successful emergency treatment with intravenous propranolol. *Pediatr Emerg Care* 2004;20:175–177.
69. Sumitomo N, Harada K, Nagashima M, Yasuda T, Nakamura Y, Aragaki Y, Saito A, Kurosaki K, Jouo K, Koujiro M, Konishi S, Matsuoka S, Oono T, Hayakawa S, Miura M, Ushinohama H, Shibata T, Niimura I. Catecholaminergic polymorphic ventricular tachycardia: Electrocardiographic characteristics and optimal therapeutic strategies to prevent sudden death. *Heart* 2003;89:66–70.
70. Rajawat YS, Patel VV, Gerstenfeld EP, Nayak H, Marchlinski FE. Advantages and pitfalls of combining device-based and pharmacologic therapies for the treatment of ventricular arrhythmias: Observations from a tertiary referral center. *Pacing Clin Electrophysiol* 2004;27:1670–1681.
71. Zipes DP, Roberts D. Results of the international study of the implantable pacemaker cardioverter-defibrillator. A comparison of epicardial and endocardial lead systems. The Pacemaker-Cardioverter-Defibrillator Investigators. *Circulation* 1995;92:59–65.
72. Block M, Breithardt G. Long-term follow-up and clinical results of implantable cardioverter-defibrillators. In: Zipes DP, Jalife J, Eds. *Cardiac Electrophysiology. From Cell to Bedside,* 2nd ed. Philadelphia, PA: W.B. Saunders Company, 1995:1412–1425.
73. Credner SC, Klingenheben T, Mauss O, Sticherling C, Hohnloser SH. Electrical storm in patients with transvenous implantable cardioverter-defibrillators: Incidence, management and prognostic implications. *J Am Coll Cardiol* 1998;32: 1909–1915.
74. Greene M, Newman D, Geist M, Paquette M, Heng D, Dorian P. Is electrical storm in ICD patients the sign of a dying heart? Outcome of patients with clusters of ventricular tachyarrhythmias. *Europace* 2000;2:263–269.
75. Exner DV, Pinski SL, Wyse DG, Renfroe EG, Follmann D, Gold M, Beckman KJ, Coromilas J, Lancaster S, Hallstrom AP, Defibrillators AIAVI. Electrical storm presages nonsudden death: The antiarrhythmics versus implantable defibrillators (AVID) trial. *Circulation* 2001;103:2066–2071.
76. Villacastin J, Almendral J, Arenal A, Albertos J, Ormaetxe J, Peinado R, Bueno H, Merino JL, Pastor A, Medina O, Tercedor L, Jimenez F, Delcan JL. Incidence and clinical significance of multiple consecutive, appropriate, high-energy discharges in patients with implanted cardioverter-defibrillators. *Circulation* 1996;93:753–762.
77. Joglar JA, Kessler DJ, Welch PJ, Keffer JH, Jessen ME, Hamdan MH, Page RL. Effects of repeated electrical defibrillations on cardiac troponin I levels. *Am J Cardiol* 1999;83:270–272.
78. Hurst TM, Hinrichs M, Breidenbach C, Katz N, Waldecker B. Detection of myocardial injury during transvenous implantation of automatic cardioverter-defibrillators. *J Am Coll Cardiol* 1999; 34:402–408.
79. Singer I, Hutchins GM, Mirowski M, Mower MM, Veltri EP, Guarnieri T, Griffith LS, Watkins L, Juanteguy J, Fisher S. Pathologic findings related to the lead system and repeated defibrillations in patients with the automatic implantable cardioverter-defibrillator. *J Am Coll Cardiol* 1987;10: 382–388.
80. Epstein AE, Kay GN, Plumb VJ, Dailey SM, Anderson PG. Gross and microscopic pathological changes associated with nonthoracotomy implantable defibrillator leads. *Circulation* 1998;98: 1517–1524.
81. Pinter A, Dorian P. Approach to antiarrhythmic therapy in patients with ICDs and frequent activations. *Curr Cardiol Rep* 2005;7:376–381.

82. Gradaus R, Block M, Brachmann J, Breithardt G, Huber HG, Jung W, Kranig W, Mletzko RU, Schoels W, Seidl K, Senges J, Siebels J, Steinbeck G, Stellbrink C, Andresen D, German ER. Mortality, morbidity, and complications in 3344 patients with implantable cardioverter defibrillators: Results from the German ICD Registry EURID. *Pacing Clin Electrophysiol* 2003;26:1511–1518.
83. Kuhlkamp V, Mewis C, Mermi J, Bosch RF, Seipel L. Suppression of sustained ventricular tachyarrhythmias: A comparison of d,l-sotalol with no antiarrhythmic drug treatment. *J Am Coll Cardiol* 1999;33:46–52.
84. Pacifico A, Hohnloser SH, Williams JH, Tao B, Saksena S, Henry PD, Prystowsky EN. Prevention of implantable-defibrillator shocks by treatment with sotalol. d,l-Sotalol Implantable Cardioverter-Defibrillator Study Group. *N Engl J Med* 1999; 340:1855–1862.
85. Dorian P, Cass D, Schwartz B, Cooper R, Gelaznikas R, Barr A. Amiodarone as compared with lidocaine for shock-resistant ventricular fibrillation. *N Engl J Med* 2002;346:884–890.
86. Connolly SJ, Dorian P, Roberts RS, Gent M, Bailin S, Fain ES, Thorpe K, Champagne J, Talajic M, Coutu B, Gronefeld GC, Hohnloser SH. Optimal pharmacological therapy in cardioverter defibrillator patients I. Comparison of beta-blockers, amiodarone plus beta-blockers, or sotalol for prevention of shocks from implantable cardioverter defibrillators: The OPTIC Study: A randomized trial. *JAMA* 2006;295:165–171 (see comment).
87. Singer I, Al-Khalidi H, Niazi I, Tchou P, Simmons T, Henthorn R, Holroyde M, Brum J. Azimilide decreases recurrent ventricular tachyarrhythmias in patients with implantable cardioverter defibrillators. *J Am Coll Cardiol* 2004;43:39–43.
88. Dorian P, Borggrefe M, Al-Khalidi HR, Hohnloser SH, Brum JM, Tatla DS, Brachmann J, Myerburg RJ, Cannom DS, van der Laan M, Holroyde MJ, Singer I, Pratt CM, Investigators SHIEwa. Placebo-controlled, randomized clinical trial of azimilide for prevention of ventricular tachyarrhythmias in patients with an implantable cardioverter defibrillator. *Circulation* 2004;110:3646–3654.
89. Boriani G, Lubinski A, Capucci A, Niederle R, Kornacewicz-Jack Z, Wnuk-Wojnar AM, Borggrefe M, Brachmann J, Biffi M, Butrous GS, Ventricular Arrhythmias Dofetilide I. A multicentre, double-blind randomized crossover comparative study on the efficacy and safety of dofetilide vs sotalol in patients with inducible sustained ventricular tachycardia and ischaemic heart disease. *Eur Heart J* 2001;22:2180–2191.
90. Manolis AG, Katsivas AG, Vassilopoulos C, Tsatiris CG. Electrical storms in an ICD-recipient with 429 delivered appropriate shocks: Therapeutic management with antiarrhythmic drug combination. *J Interv Card Electrophysiol* 2002; 6:91–94.
91. Anderson JL, Karagounis LA, Roskelley M, Osborn JS, Handrahan D. Effect of prophylactic antiarrhythmic therapy on time to implantable cardioverter-defibrillator discharge in patients with ventricular tachyarrhythmias. *Am J Cardiol* 1994;73:683–687.
92. Jung W, Mietzko R, Manz M, Nitsch J, Luderitz B. Efficacy and safety of combination therapy with amiodarone and type 1 agents for treatment of inducible ventricular tachycardia. *Pacing Clin Electrophysiol* 1993;16:778–788.
93. Brodine WN, Tung RT, Lee JK, Hockstad ES, Moss AJ, Zareba W, Hall WJ, Andrews M, McNitt S, Daubert JP, Group M-IR. Effects of beta-blockers on implantable cardioverter defibrillator therapy and survival in the patients with ischemic cardiomyopathy (from the Multicenter Automatic Defibrillator Implantation Trial-II). *Am J Cardiol* 2005;96:691–695.
94. Friedman PA, McClelland RL, Bamlet WR, Acostia H, Kessler DJ, Munger TM, Kavesh NG, Wood M, Daoud E, Massumi A, Schuger CD, Shorofsky S, Wilkoff BL, Glikson M. Dual-chamber versus single-chamber detection enhancements for implantable defibrillator rhythm diagnosis. The Detect Supraventricular Tachycardia Study. *Circulation* 2006;113:2871–2879.
95. Hreybe H, Ezzeddine R, Barrington W, Bazaz R, Jain S, Ngwu O, Saba S. Relation of advanced heart failure symptoms to risk of inappropriate defibrillator shocks. *Am J Cardiol* 2006;97:544–546.
96. Goldenberg I, Moss AJ, McNitt S, Zareba W, Daubert JP, Hall WJ, Andrews ML. Cigarette smoking and the risk of supraventricular and ventricular tachyarrhythmias in high-risk cardiac patients with implantable cardioverter defibrillators. *J Cardiovasc Electrophysiol* 2006;17:1–6.
97. Theuns DA, Klootwijk AP, Simoons ML, Jordaens LJ. Clinical variables predicting inappropriate use of implantable cardioverter-defibrillator in patients with coronary heart disease or nonischemic dilated cardiomyopathy. *Am J Cardiol* 2005;95: 271–274.
98. Korte T, Koditz H, Niehaus M, Paul T, Tebbenjohanns J. High incidence of appropriate and inappropriate ICD therapies in children and adolescents with implantable cardioverter defibrillator. *Pacing Clin Electrophysiol* 2004;27:924–932.

99. Bollmann A, Husser D, Cannom DS. Antiarrhythmic drugs in patients with implantable cardioverter-defibrillators. *Am J Cardiovasc Drugs* 2005; 5:371–378.
100. Dorian P, Philippon F, Thibault B, Kimber S, Sterns L, Greene M, Newman D, Gelaznikas R, Barr A, Investigators A. Randomized controlled study of detection enhancements versus rate-only detection to prevent inappropriate therapy in a dual-chamber implantable cardioverter-defibrillator. *Heart Rhythm* 2004;1:540–547.
101. Res JCJ, Theuns DA, Jordaens L. The role of remote monitoring in the reduction of inappropriate implantable cardioverter defibrillator therapies. *Clin Res Cardiol* 2006;95:III-17–III-21.
102. Page RL. Effects of antiarrhythmic medication on implantable cardioverter-defibrillator function. *Am J Cardiol* 2000;85:1481–1488.
103. Krol RB, Saksena S, Prakash A. Interactions of antiarrhythmic drugs with implantable defibrillator therapy for atrial and ventricular tachyarrhythmias. *Curr Cardiol Rep* 1999;1:282–288.
104. Echt DS, Gremillion ST, Lee JT, Roden DM, Murray KT, Borganelli M, Crawford DM, Stewart JR, Hammon JW. Effects of procainamide and lidocaine on defibrillation energy requirements in patients receiving implantable cardioverter defibrillator devices. *J Cardiovasc Electrophysiol* 1994; 5:752–760.
105. Manz M, Jung W, Luderitz B. Interactions between drugs and devices: Experimental and clinical studies. *Am Heart J* 1994;127:978–984.
106. Jung W, Manz M, Pizzulli L, Pfeiffer D, Luderitz B. Effects of chronic amiodarone therapy on defibrillation threshold. *Am J Cardiol* 1992;70:1023–1027.
107. Crystal E, Ovsyshcher IE, Wagshal AB, Katz A, Ilia R. Mexiletine related chronic defibrillation threshold elevation: Case report and review of the literature. *Pacing Clin Electrophysiol* 2002;25:507–508.
108. Senatore C, Coltorti F, Giordano B, Nocerino P, Stabile G, De Simone A, Caprioli V, Chiariello M. Defibrillation threshold in patients with ICD and concomitant antiarrhythmic drug therapy. *Pacing Clin Electrophysiol* 1999;22:II-803.
109. Qi X, Dorian P. Antiarrhythmic drugs and ventricular defibrillation energy requirements. *Chin Med J* 1999;112:1147–1152.
110. Movsowitz C, Marchlinski FE. Interactions between implantable cardioverter-defibrillators and class III agents. *Am J Cardiol* 1998;82:41I–48I.
111. Dorian P, Newman D. Effect of sotalol on ventricular fibrillation and defibrillation in humans. *Am J Cardiol* 1993;72:72A-79A.
112. Dorian P, Newman D, Sheahan R, Tang A, Green M, Mitchell J. d-Sotalol decreases defibrillation energy requirements in humans: A novel indication for drug therapy. *J Cardiovasc Electrophysiol* 1996;7:952–961.
113. Hayashi M, Tanaka K, Kato T, Morita N, Sato N, Yasutake M, Kobayashi Y, Takano T. Enhancing electrical cardioversion and preventing immediate reinitiation of hemodynamically deleterious atrial fibrillation with class III drug pretreatment. *J Cardiovasc Electrophysiol* 2005;16:740–747.
114. Oral H, Souza JJ, Michaud GF, Knight BP, Goyal R, Strickberger SA, Morady F. Facilitating transthoracic cardioversion of atrial fibrillation with ibutilide pretreatment. *N Engl J Med* 1999;340: 1849–1854.
115. Hohnloser SH, Dorian P, Roberts R, Gent M, Israel CW, Fain E, Champagne J, Connolly SJ. Effect of amiodarone and sotalol on ventricular defibrillation threshold. The Optimal Pharmacological Therapy in Cardioverter Defibrillator Patients (OPTIC) Trial. *Circulation* 2006;114:104–109.
116. Kalus JS, White CM, Caron MF, Guertin D, McBride BF, Kluger J. The impact of catecholamines on defibrillation threshold in patients with implanted cardioverter defibrillators. *Pacing Clin Electrophysiol* 2005;28:1147–1156.
117. Schuger C, Ellenbogen KA, Faddis M, Knight BP, Yong P, Sample R, Investigators VCCCS. Defibrillation energy requirements in an ICD population receiving cardiac resynchronization therapy. *J Cardiovasc Electrophysiol* 2006;17:247–250.
118. Gold MR, Khalighi K, Kavesh NG, Daly B, Peters RW, Shorofsky SR. Clinical predictors of transvenous biphasic defibrillation thresholds. *Am J Cardiol* 1997;79:1623–1627.
119. Shukla HH, Flaker GC, Jayam V, Roberts D. High defibrillation thresholds in transvenous biphasic implantable defibrillators: Clinical predictors and prognostic implications. *Pacing Clin Electrophysiol* 2003;26:44–48.
120. Sola CL, Bostwick JM. Implantable cardioverter-defibrillators, induced anxiety, and quality of life. *Mayo Clinic Proc* 2005;80:232–237.
121. Carroll DL, Hamilton GA. Quality of life in implanted cardioverter defibrillator recipients: The impact of a device shock. *Heart Lung* 2005; 34:169–178.
122. Namerow PB, Firth BR, Heywood GM, Windle JR, Parides MK. Quality-of-life six months after CABG surgery in patients randomized to ICD versus no ICD therapy: Findings from the CABG Patch Trial. *Pacing Clin Electrophysiol* 1999;22: 1305–1313.

123. Irvine J, Dorian P, Baker B, O'Brien BJ, Roberts R, Gent M, Newman D, Connolly SJ. Quality of life in the Canadian Implantable Defibrillator Study (CIDS). *Am Heart J* 2002;144:282–289.
124. Schron EB, Exner DV, Yao Q, Jenkins LS, Steinberg JS, Cook JR, Kutalek SP, Friedman PL, Bubien RS, Page RL, Powell J. Quality of life in the antiarrhythmics versus implantable defibrillators trial: Impact of therapy and influence of adverse symptoms and defibrillator shocks. *Circulation* 2002;105:589–594.
125. Dougherty CM. Psychological reactions and family adjustment in shock versus no shock groups after implantation of internal cardioverter defibrillator. *Heart Lung* 1995;24:281–291.
126. Jauhar S, Slotwiner DJ. The Economics of ICDs. *N Engl J Med* 2004;351:2542–2544.
127. Stevenson LW. Implantable cardioverter-defibrillators for primary prevention of sudden death in heart failure. Are there enough bang for the bucks? *Circulation* 2006;114:101–103.
128. Zwanziger J, Hall WJ, Dick AW, Zhao H, Mushlin AI, Hahn RM, Wang H, Andrews ML, Mooney C, Moss AJ. The cost effectiveness of implantable cardioverter-defibrillators: Results from the Multicenter Automatic Defibrillator Implantation Trial (MADIT)-II. *J Am Coll Cardiol* 2006;47: 2310–2318.
129. Larsen G, Hallstrom A, McAnulty J, Pinski S, Olarte A, Sullivan S, Brodsky M, Powell J, Marchant C, Jennings C, Akiyama T, Investigators A. Cost-effectiveness of the implantable cardioverter-defibrillator versus antiarrhythmic drugs in survivors of serious ventricular tachyarrhythmias: Results of the Antiarrhythmics Versus Implantable Defibrillators (AVID) economic analysis substudy. *Circulation* 2002;105:2049–2057.
130. O'Brien BJ, Connolly SJ, Goeree R, Blackhouse G, Willan A, Yee R, Roberts RS, Gent M. Cost-effectiveness of the implantable cardioverter-defibrillator: Results from the Canadian Implantable Defibrillator Study (CIDS). *Circulation* 2001;103:1416–1421.
131. Mushlin AI, Hall WJ, Zwanziger J, Gajary E, Andrews M, Marron R, Zou KH, Moss AJ. The cost-effectiveness of automatic implantable cardiac defibrillators: Results from MADIT. Multicenter Automatic Defibrillator Implantation Trial. *Circulation* 1998;97:2129–2135.
132. Mark DB, Nelson CL, Anstrom KJ, Al-Khatib SM, Tsiatis AA, Cowper PA, Clapp-Channing NE, Davidson-Ray L, Poole JE, Johnson G, Anderson J, Lee KL, Bardy GH. Cost-effectiveness of defibrillator therapy or amiodarone in chronic stable heart failure. Results from the Sudden Cardiac Death in Heart Failure Trial (SCD-HeFT). *Circulation* 2006;114:135–142.
133. Vernooy K, Verbeek XA, Peschar M, Prinzen FW. Relation between abnormal ventricular impulse conduction and heart failure. *J Interv Cardiol* 2003;16:557–562.
134. Wilkoff BL, Cook JR, Epstein AE, Greene HL, Hallstrom AP, Hsia H, Kutalek SP, Sharma A, Dual C, Investigators VVIIDT. Dual-chamber pacing or ventricular backup pacing in patients with an implantable defibrillator: The Dual Chamber and VVI Implantable Defibrillator (DAVID) Trial. *JAMA* 2002;288:3115–3123.
135. Sharma AD, Rizo-Patron C, Hallstrom AP, O'Neill GP, Rothbart S, Martins JB, Roelke M, Steinberg JS, Greene HL, Investigators D. Percent right ventricular pacing predicts outcomes in the DAVID trial. *Heart Rhythm* 2005;2:830–834.
136. Steinberg JS, Fischer A, Wang P, Schuger C, Daubert J, McNitt S, Andrews M, Brown M, Hall WJ, Zareba W, Moss AJ, Investigators MI. The clinical implications of cumulative right ventricular pacing in the multicenter automatic defibrillator trial II. *J Cardiovasc Electrophysiol* 2005;16: 359–365.
137. Numata T, Abe H, Nagatomo T, Kohshi K, Nakashima Y. Ventricular pacing failure after a single oral dose of pilsicainide in a patient with a permanent pacemaker and paroxysmal atrial fibrillation. *Pacing Clin Electrophysiol* 2000;23: 1436–1438.
138. Kang TS, Yoon YW, Park S, Hong BK, Kim D, Kwon HM, Kim HS. A case of acute ventricular capture threshold rise associated with flecainide acetate. *Yonsei Med J* 2006;47:152–154.
139. Anzawa R, Ishikawa S, Tanaka Y, Okazaki F, Mochizuki S. Atrial pacing failure following termination of atrial fibrillation by acute administration of disopyramide phosphate. *J Interv Card Electrophysiol* 2005;13:51–53.
140. Naccarelli GV, Wolbrette DL, Luck JC. Proarrhythmia. *Med Clin North Am* 2001;85:503–526.
141. Goldberger J, Weinberg KM, Kadish AH. Impact of nontraditional antiarrhythmic drugs on sudden cardiac death. In: Zipes DP, Jalife J, Eds. *Cardiac Electrophysiology. From Cell to Bedside*. Philadelphia, PA: W.B. Saunders, 2004:950–958.
142. Alberte C, Zipes DP. Use of nonantiarrhythmic drugs for prevention of sudden cardiac death. *J Cardiovasc Electrophysiol* 2003;14:S87–95.
143. Dargie HJ. Effect of carvedilol on outcome after myocardial infarction in patients with left-

ventricular dysfunction: The CAPRICORN randomised trial. *Lancet* 2001;357:1385–1390.

144. CIBIS-II IaC. The Cardiac Insufficiency Bisoprolol Study II (CIBIS-II): A randomised trial. *Lancet* 1999;353:9–13 (see comment).
145. MERIT-HF. Effect of metoprolol CR/XL in chronic heart failure: Metoprolol CR/XL Randomised Intervention Trial in Congestive Heart Failure (MERIT-HF). *Lancet* 1999;353:2001–2007.
146. Exner DV, Reiffel JA, Epstein AE, Ledingham R, Reiter MJ, Yao Q, Duff HJ, Follmann D, Schron E, Greene HL, Carlson MD, Brodsky MA, Akiyama T, Baessler C, Anderson JL. Beta-blocker use and survival in patients with ventricular fibrillation or symptomatic ventricular tachycardia: The Antiarrhythmics Versus Implantable Defibrillators (AVID) trial. *J Am Coll Cardiol* 1999;34:325–333.
147. Cleland JG, Erhardt L, Murray G, Hall AS, Ball SG. Effect of ramipril on morbidity and mode of death among survivors of acute myocardial infarction with clinical evidence of heart failure. A report from the AIRE Study Investigators. *Eur Heart J* 1997;18:41–51.
148. Kober L, Torp-Pedersen C, Carlsen JE, Bagger H, Eliasen P, Lyngborg K, Videbaek J, Cole DS, Auclert L, Pauly NC. A clinical trial of the angiotensin-converting-enzyme inhibitor trandolapril in patients with left ventricular dysfunction after myocardial infarction. Trandolapril Cardiac Evaluation (TRACE) Study Group. *N Engl J Med* 1995;333:1670–1676.
149. Pitt B, Zannad F, Remme WJ, Cody R, Castaigne A, Perez A, Palensky J, Wittes J. The effect of spironolactone on morbidity and mortality in patients with severe heart failure. Randomized Aldactone Evaluation Study Investigators. *N Engl J Med* 1999;341:709–717.
150. Anonymous. Randomised trial of cholesterol lowering in 4444 patients with coronary heart disease: The Scandinavian Simvastatin Survival Study (4S). *Lancet* 1994;344:1383–1389.
151. Anonymous. Prevention of cardiovascular events and death with pravastatin in patients with coronary heart disease and a broad range of initial cholesterol levels. The Long-Term Intervention with Pravastatin in Ischaemic Disease (LIPID) Study Group. *N Engl J Med* 1998;339:1349–1357.
152. Kris-Etherton PM, Harris WS, Appel LJ, American Heart Association. Nutrition C. Fish consumption, fish oil, omega-3 fatty acids, and cardiovascular disease. *Circulation* 2002;106:2747–2757.
153. Leaf A, Kang JX, Xiao YF, Billman GE. Clinical prevention of sudden cardiac death by n-3 polyunsaturated fatty acids and mechanism of prevention of arrhythmias by n-3 fish oils. *Circulation* 2003;107:2646–2652.

49
Nonantiarrhythmic Drugs in Sudden Death Prevention

Alan Kadish and Vikram Reddy

Introduction

Mortality from cardiovascular disease has declined in the United States. Despite this, at least 300,000 deaths annually are attributed to sudden cardiac death. As discussed below, the most common mechanism of cardiac death is ventricular fibrillation. Antiarrhythmic drugs that block cardiac ion channels have been shown to be effective in a variety of experimental models, and it was hoped that these drugs would be antiarrhythmic in clinical settings and reduce the incidence of sudden death in susceptible populations. Unfortunately, drugs that block Na^+ or K^+ channels have been ineffective in preventing sudden death and in many cases have been proarrhythmic. In contrast, in a number of studies of patients after myocardial infarction and those with heart failure, other drugs, such as angiotensin-converting enzyme (ACE) inhibitors and β blockers, that are normally not considered traditional antiarrhythmic drugs have been shown to be effective at reducing overall mortality and potentially sudden death mortality in patients with underlying structural heart disease. This chapter will review those drugs and also describe potential pathophysiological mechanisms by which these agents may reduce sudden death (Table 49–1).

Pathophysiology

Although bradycardia or electromechanical dissociation may be more common in patients with advanced congestive heart failure or during prolonged cardiac arrest, evidence suggests that ventricular tachycardia and/or ventricular fibrillation are the major mechanisms of sudden cardiac death. Thus, therapies that lower the occurrence of ventricular tachycardia and ventricular fibrillation may help decrease the incidence of sudden cardiac death. There are also data suggesting that the risk of ventricular tachycardia and ventricular fibrillation varies inversely with left ventricular function. Additionally, left ventricular dilation may be arrhythmogenic by altering cardiac electrophysiological properties through contraction–excitation feedback. Thus, pharmacological agents that alter cardiac hemodynamics may be antiarrhythmic by altering ventricular function and size even if direct antiarrhythmic activity is not present.

Despite extensive research, a coherent pathophysiological scheme for the occurrence of sudden death has not been universally accepted. The majority of patients who experience sudden cardiac death have coronary disease and myocardial ischemia, of whom only a minority of patients have an acute myocardial infarction (MI). Patients with nonischemic cardiomyopathy and other structural heart diseases also have a substantial risk for sudden cardiac death. At present, antiarrhythmic drugs target sodium or potassium channels present throughout the myocardium, and, therefore, are not specific for the arrhythmic mechanism (focal or reentrant) or region. In contrast, if adrenergic surges due to mental or physical stress are a potential contributing factor to the occurrence of sudden cardiac death, then drugs that block these triggers, such as β blockers,

TABLE 49–1. Nonantiarrhythmic drugs.[a]

Class	Drug	Study	Control	Patients	Total N	Total mortality (RR or HR) (95% CI)	SCD (RR or HR) (95% CI)
ACE inhibitors	Ramipril	AIRE[32]	Placebo	Post-MI + CHF	2,006	RR 0.73 (0.60–0.89)	RR 0.70 (0.53–0.92)
	Ramipril	HOPE[37]	Placebo	CV disease of DM + CRF	9,297	RR 0.84 (0.75–0.95)	RR 0.62 (0.41–0.94)[b]
	Captopril	SAVE[79]	Placebo	Post-MI + ↓EF	2,231	RR 0.81 (0.68–0.97)	NS
	Enalapril	CONSENSUS I[38]	Placebo	AMI	6,090	RR 1.10 (0.93–1.29)	NS
	Enalapril	SOLVD-P[39] prevention	Placebo	↓EF	4,228	RR 0.92 (0.79–1.08)	RR 0.93 (0.70–1.22)
	Enalapril	V-Heft II[40]	Hydral/isosorbide	CHF	804	RR 0.72	RR 0.65
	Zofenopril	SMILE[80]	Placebo	AMI	1,556	RR 0.78 (0.52–1.12)	RR 0.37 (0.11–1.02)
	Trandolapril	TRACE[35]	Placebo	Post-MI+ ↓EF	1,749	RR 0.78 (0.67–0.91)	RR 0.76 (0.59–0.98)
ARB	Valsartan	Val-Heft[81]	Placebo	CHF	5,010	RR 1.02 (0.88–1.18) 98% CI	NS
	Losartan	ELITE[45]	Captopril	CHF	722	RR 0.54 (0.31–0.95)	RR 0.36 (0.14–0.97)
	Losartan	ELITE II[46]	Captopril	CHF	3,152	HR 1.13 (0.95–1.35) 95.7% CI	HR 1.30 (1.00–1.69)
	Losartan	LIFE[82]	Atenolol	HTN + LVH	9,193	HR 0.90 (0.78–1.03)	HR 1.91 (0.64–5.72)[c]
	Losartan	OPTIMAAL[47]	Captopril	Post-MI + CHF	5,477	RR 1.13 (0.99–1.28)	RR 1.19 (0.99–1.43)[d]
β-Blockers	Class	1999 Meta- analysis[83]	Placebo	Post-MI	24,974	RR 0.77 (0.69–0.85)	
	Class	Medicare database[9]	Placebo	Post-MI	201,752	RR 0.60 (0.57–0.63)	
	Carvedilol	CAPRICORN[84]	Placebo	Post-MI + ↓EF	1,959	HR 0.77 (0.60–0.98)	HR 0.74 (0.51–1.06)
	Metoprolol	MERIT-HF[23]	Placebo	CHF	3,991	RR 0.66 (0.53–0.81)	RR 0.59 (0.45–0.78)
	Bisoprolol	CIBIS-II[22]	Placebo	CHF	2,657	HR 0.66 (0.54–0.81)	HR 0.56 (0.39–0.80)

[a]ACE, angiotensin-converting enzyme; AMI, acute myocardial infarction; ARB, angiotensin receptor blockers; CHF, congestive heart failure; CI, confidence interval; CRF, cardiac risk factor; CV, cardiovascular; DM, diabetes mellitus; EF, ejection fraction; HR, hazard ratios; HTN, hypertension; LVH, left ventricular hypertension; MI, myocardial infarction; NS, not significant; RR, relative risk; SCD, sudden cardiac death. See text for study abbreviations.

[b]Cardiac arrest.

[c]Resuscitated cardiac arrest.

[d]SCD + resuscitated cardiac arrest.

require fewer physiological assumptions and do not need the specificity required of antiarrhythmic drugs. Therefore, the greater efficacy in preventing sudden cardiac death of nontraditional drugs that act on more global mechanisms of arrhythmia compared to that of drugs that indiscriminantly block ion channels throughout the myocardium is not surprising.

β Blockers

Adrenergic Blocking Drugs

β-Adrenergic blockers (also known as β blockers) have emerged as an important pharmacological agent for both primary and secondary prevention of sudden cardiac death. Steinbeck *et al.*[1]

randomized 115 patients with ventricular tachycardia to one of two treatment approaches: β blocker therapy or electrophysiology testing guided therapy. The 1-year recurrence rate/sudden death rate in the β blocker group exceeded 40%, which was significantly greater than 10% at 1 year in the group treated with an antiarrhythmic drug proven to be efficacious by electrophysiological testing. In both the European Myocardial Infarct Amiodarone Trial (EMIAT)[2] and the Canadian Amiodarone Myocardial Infarction Arrhythmia Trial (CAMIAT),[3] amiodarone therapy produced a greater reduction in mortality in those patients on β blockers.[4] In CAMIAT, there was an 87% reduction in relative risk ($p = 0.008$) related to amiodarone therapy (versus placebo) in patients who were receiving concomitant therapy with β blockers. Most recent implantable cardioverter defibrillator (ICD) trials have shown that even in patients treated with β blockers, ICD can further reduce mortality (SCD-HeFT, DEFINITE).[5,6]

Efficacy of β Blockers after Myocardial Infarction

In 1993, Teo *et al.*[7] published an overview of results from these randomized controlled trials that included more than 50,000 patients. There was a substantial reduction in mortality due to β blocker treatment (relative risk, 0.81; 95% confidence intervals, 0.75–0.87; $p < 0.00001$). The Norwegian Multicenter Study Group[8] demonstrated a survival benefit for at least 6 years after myocardial infarction. The largest report includes over 200,000 patients in the Medicare database.[9] After adjusting for baseline differences, β blocker therapy was associated with a 40% decrease in mortality at 2 years. The benefits of β blocker therapy have withstood the test of time despite the advent of therapies such as thrombolytic therapy,[10] ACE inhibitors,[11–15] and revascularization.[16] In the CAPRICORN study, 1959 patients who had an MI within 3–21 days and an ejection fraction ≤40% were randomly assigned to treatment with either carvedilol ($n = 975$) or placebo ($n = 984$). Although all-cause mortality was not the primary endpoint, after a mean follow-up of 1.3 years, 12% mortality was seen in patients treated with carvedilol and 15% mortality in those treated with placebo (risk reduction, 23%; 95% confidence interval, 2–40%).

In these trials, the doses of β blockers were generally titrated up to doses equivalent to 200 mg of metoprolol or 160 mg of propranolol daily. However, a majority of patients who are treated with β blockers following a myocardial infarction receive ≤50% of the dose found to be effective in the randomized clinical trials.[17,18] In an analysis of the database from the northern California Kaiser Permanente hospitals,[17] low-dose β blocker therapy for myocardial infarction was shown to be beneficial; in addition, the mortality was actually lower in patients receiving low-dose β blockers (25% of the dose used in large-scale clinical trials). In those patients given 1–49% of the dose found to be effective in clinical trials, the long-term mortality was 3.4%, while in those given ≥50% of the dose found to be effective in clinical trials, the mortality was 6.9%; in those not treated with β blockers, the mortality was 18.8%. Similarly, in a study of elderly people receiving low-, standard, and high-dose β blocker therapy after myocardial infarction, there was a 60% reduction in mortality in the low-dose group with similar reductions in the standard and high-dose groups.[19] Finally, in the observational trials[9,20] in the Medicare population, it is unlikely that full-dose β blockers were used in a majority of patients and a marked survival benefit was demonstrated.

Efficacy of β Blockers in Patients with Congestive Heart Failure

β Blockers are also emerging as important agents in the prevention of sudden cardiac death in patients with congestive heart failure.[21] Although this trial was not designed as a mortality trial, carvedilol reduced total mortality by 65%. In the Cardiac Insufficiency Bisoprolol Study II study (CIBIS-II),[22] 2657 patients with Class III or IV congestive heart failure and an ejection fraction less than 35% were randomized either to bisoprolol ($n = 1327$) or to placebo ($n = 1320$). The trial was terminated prematurely because of the significant survival benefit due to bisoprolol. The estimated annual mortality was 8.8% in patients treated with bisoprolol and 13.2% in those receiving placebo (risk reduction 34%; 95% confidence interval 19–46%). Metoprolol has also been demonstrated to improve survival in patients with congestive heart failure.[23,24] In the Metoprolol CR/XL Randomized

Intervention Trial in Congestive Heart Failure (MERIT-HF) trial,[23] 3991 patients with Class II to IV (96% were Class II and III) congestive heart failure (ejection fraction less than 40%) were randomly assigned to treatment with metoprolol (n = 1990) or placebo (n = 2001). The mortality was 7.2% per patient-year of follow-up in the metoprolol group versus 11.0% in the placebo group (relative risk reduction 34%; 95% confidence interval 19–47%).

Efficacy of β Blockers in the Secondary Prevention of Sudden Death

There are some data supporting the efficacy of β blockers in patients known to have ventricular tachyarrhythmias. Hallstrom *et al.*[25] reported an adjusted relative risk reduction of 38% (95% confidence interval 23–50%) related to β blocker therapy in survivors of cardiac arrest. In the Antiarrhythmics Versus Implantable Defibrillators (AVID) registry,[26] 366 patients with hemodynamically significant ventricular tachycardia or ventricular fibrillation did not receive therapy with either amiodarone, sotalol, or an implantable defibrillator. β Blocker use was not controlled in these patients. Approximately 150 of these patients were treated with β blockers. There was an approximately 50% reduction in adjusted relative risk of mortality due to β blocker therapy. Sotalol[27] and, to a greater extent, metoprolol[28] have been shown to reduce the incidence of ventricular tachyarrhythmias in patients with implantable defibrillators. Limited data[29] suggest that β blocker therapy in patients with nonischemic dilated cardiomyopathy and ICDs is associated with a marked reduction in appropriate therapy for ventricular tachyarrhythmias. In a multivariate analysis from this study, β blocker therapy was associated with a 0.15 relative risk (95% confidence intervals 0.05–0.45, $p < 0.0007$) of appropriate ICD therapy.

Renin–Angiotensin–Aldosterone System

Angiotensin-Converting Enzyme Inhibitors

Angiotensin-converting enzyme inhibitors have been extensively studied in patients at risk for sudden cardiac death. Although studies involving ACE inhibitors have shown substantial reductions in total mortality (with risk reductions ranging from 8% to 40%) and/or cardiovascular mortality, very few have shown similar effects with respect to arrhythmic death.

Excluding the postinfarction period, ACE inhibitors have several possible antiarrhythmic actions. A direct antiarrhythmic effect has been reported, but is inconsistent.[30,31] In patients with or without heart failure, hypokalemia has been shown to be an important risk factor for ventricular arrhythmias. Angiotensin-converting enzyme inhibitors can raise serum potassium levels, which may lead to a possible beneficial effect on the myocardial substrate.[32] These results have not been consistent in other studies. However, ACE inhibitors have several direct and indirect effects on the autonomic nervous system that could modify the risk of ventricular arrhythmias.[33] They enhance baroreflex sensitivity, thereby reducing sympathetic and increasing parasympathetic tone. Improvements in hemodynamics may also lead to a decrease in circulating catecholamines. Ventricular remodeling has been shown to have adverse effects on the electrical system of the heart, in ventricular arrhythmias. Angiotensin-converting enzyme inhibitor treatment impedes remodeling and may lead to reductions in ventricular arrhythmias.[34]

The Acute Infarction Ramipril Efficacy Study (AIRE) and the Trandolapril Cardiac Evaluation (TRACE) study have been the only placebo-controlled trials with ACE inhibitors to show significant reductions in sudden cardiac death.[32,35] In the AIRE study, 2006 patients with recent MI and clinical evidence of heart failure were randomly assigned to treatment with ramipril (5 mg daily) or placebo. At 15 months, the ramopril group had 27% reduction in total mortality. There was also a 30% reduction in sudden cardiac death (12.3–8.9%). In the TRACE study, 1749 patients with an acute MI and ejection fraction ≤35% were randomly assigned to treatment with trandolapril or placebo. At follow-up of 24 and 50 months there was a 25% decrease in cardiovascular deaths and a 26% reduction in sudden cardiac death (15.2–12.0%). A meta-analysis of intermediate- or long-term post-MI ACE inhibitor trials (including AIRE and TRACE) involving a total of 15,104 patients showed a trend toward decreased sudden cardiac death in all of the larger trials and an overall reduction in sudden cardiac death with an odds ratio of 0.80 (95% confidence intervals, 0.70–0.92). There were also similar significant reductions in total and cardiovascular mortality.[36]

In the Heart Outcomes Prevention Evaluation (HOPE) study, more than 9000 patients with vascular disease or diabetes mellitus and cardiac risk factor were randomly assigned to treatment with ramipril or placebo.[37] After 5 years, there was a 26% reduction in cardiovascular mortality and a 37% reduction in cardiac arrest. Sudden cardiac death was not specifically studied.

No randomized, controlled trials of an ACE inhibitor versus placebo in patients with chronic heart failure have shown a reduction in sudden cardiac death. The three major trials that have reported results for sudden death are the Cooperative New Scandinavian Enalapril Survival Study (CONSENSUS), the Studies of Left Ventricular Dysfunction (SOLVD)-Treatment, and the SOLVD-Prevention.[38,39] In the Second Veterans Administration Vasodilator-Heart Failure Trial (V-Heft II), 804 men with New York Heart Association (NYHA) Class I or III heart failure were randomly assigned to treatment with enalapril (20 mg daily) or the combination of hydralazine (300 mg daily) and isosorbide dinitrate (160 mg daily).[40] At 2 years, the enalapril group had a 28% reduction in total mortality. This effect was due to a 38% decrease in the incidence of sudden cardiac death. It is possible that the beneficial effect of enalapril was due to an increase in sudden death in the hydralazine–isosorbide arm.

Angiotensin Receptor Blocks

Physiologically active levels of angiotensin II persist despite long-term therapy with ACE inhibitors and may also be formed by non-ACE-dependent pathways. Possible arrhythmogenic mechanisms of angiotensin II include activation of neurohormonal agents (including norepinephrine, aldosterone, and endothelin) as well as increased conduction velocity and shorter refractory periods in cardiac myocytes.[41] Furthermore, unlike ACE inhibitors, angiotensin II receptor blockers (ARBs) do not increase bradykinin levels, which also can increase norepinephrine levels.[42] Elevated catecholamine levels theoretically could result in more ventricular arrhythmias and sudden death. Therefore, direct blockade of angiotensin II receptors might further reduce morbidity and mortality in patients requiring blockade of the renin–angiotensin–aldosterone system. These protective effects of angiotensin II receptor blockade may be questioned by a substudy of the Randomized Aldactone Evaluation Study (RALES) (see later). Patients with congestive heart failure treated with ACE inhibitors and randomly assigned to treatment with spironolactone had significant decreases in sudden death despite significant increases in plasma angiotensin II.[43] Both ARBs as well as ACE inhibitors increase serum potassium levels and many benefit from this potential protective mechanism as well.

Angiotensin II receptor blockers have mostly been compared to ACE inhibitors in several heart failure or hypertension trials. Importantly, a meta-analysis has shown that the overall mortality rates for the two classes are similar.[44] Only one study showed a reduction in sudden death with ARBs compared with ACE inhibitors, and results of larger trials have countered these results. In the Evaluation of Losartan in the Elderly (ELITE) study, 722 patients with Classes II–IV heart failure and ejection fractions ≤40% were randomly assigned to treatment with losartan or captopril.[45] At 48 weeks, the losartan group had a 45% reduction in total mortality. There was also a decrease in the number of deaths attributable to sudden cardiac death (5 vs. 14 patients) with a relative risk reduction of 36%. However, in the much larger ELITE II, 3152 patients (with heart failure and ejection fraction <40%) were again randomly assigned to treatment with losartan or captopril.[46] At 1.5 years, there were strong trends toward reductions in overall mortality and sudden death with captopril compared to losartan. In the Optimal Trial in Myocardial Infarction with the Angiotensin II Antagonist Losartan (OPTIMAAL), losartan and captopril were also studied in patients after MI with heart failure, and favorable results for captopril, similar to those for ELITE II, were obtained.[47] Thus, it appears that both ACE inhibitors and ARBs may reduce mortality and probably sudden death.

Aldosterone Receptor Antagonists

Neurohormonal suppression of the renin-angiotensin-aldosterone system by ACE inhibitors is incomplete. Therefore, aldosterone can continue to exert harmful effects on the cardiovascular system in patients with heart failure. Aldosterone promotes sodium retention, magnesium and potassium wasting, sympathetic activation, parasympathetic inhibition, myocardial and vascular fibrosis, baroreceptor dysfunction, and vascular damage and impairs arterial compliance.

Spironolactone, an aldosterone receptor antagonist and potassium-sparing diuretic, has gained wide acceptance for the treatment of severe congestive heart failure. In the RALES study, 1663 patients with NYHA Class III or IV heart failure and ejection fractions ≤35% were randomly assigned to treatment with spironolactone (25 mg daily) or placebo.[48] After a mean follow-up of 24 months, cardiac death was decreased by 31%. This was due to a 36% decrease in death of progressive heart failure and 29% reduction in sudden cardiac death.

A selective aldosterone blocker Eplerenone was evaluated in the EPHESUS study where 6632 patients who had an ejection fraction of less than 40%, experienced an MI in the last 30 days, and had clinical signs of heart failure were randomly assigned in to Eplerenone treatment or standard treatment groups. The Eplerenone group had a reduction of all-cause mortality by 15% (p = 0.008)[49] and a significant reduction in cardiac deaths (relative risk, 0.83; 95 percent confidence interval, 0.72–0.94; $p = 0.005$).[50]

There are several possible mechanisms for a direct antiarrhythmic effect of spironolactone. One possible explanation is that aldosterone seems to enhance cardiac remodeling. Fibroblasts and inflammatory cells invade the perivascular space of damaged vessels, leading to fibrosis. These changes can have adverse effects on the mechanical function, vasodilatory reserve, and electrical system of the heart.[51] A recent substudy of the RALES trial evaluated serum markers of collagen synthesis, which has been shown to correlate with morphological evidence of cardiac fibrosis.[52] Spironolactone decreased the levels of these markers at 6 months. Several studies have shown that non-potassium-sparing diuretics are associated with an increase in sudden cardiac death and that there is a dose–response curve. One case–control study showed that the risk of primary cardiac arrest was increased with thiazide diuretics and the addition of a potassium-sparing diuretic reduced that risk.[53]

Modulators of Cholesterol and Inflammation

3-Hydroxy-3-methylglutaryl-Coenzyme A Reductase Inhibitors

While the benefit of statin therapy in patients with coronary artery disease has been well established in multiple large-scale randomized clinical trials, only a few studies have focused on their effects on life-threatening ventricular arrhythmias[54–56] or on patients with nonischemic cardiomyopathy.[57–61] A number of nonrandomized clinical studies have demonstrated dramatic reduction in arrhythmic events by statins in patients who have implanted ICDs. In an observational study, De Sutter *et al.*[62] first reported that in patients with coronary artery disease receiving ICDs for secondary prevention of ventricular arrhythmias, treatment with lipid lowering drug therapy (59% statins, 41% fibrates) resulted in a substantial reduction in appropriate shocks (22% in the group treated with lipid lowering drugs and 57% in those not treated). In another observational study in patients with coronary artery disease receiving ICDs, Chiu *et al.*[54] reported that 30% of patients on statins received ICD therapy versus 50% among those who did not receive statin therapy (hazard ratio 0.60). In the AVID trial,[54–56] there was a reported 0.40 reduction in relative hazard (95% confidence interval 0.15–0.58) for recurrence of ventricular tachycardia/fibrillation.

Effects of statins on mortality in patients with coronary disease could be due to lipid lowering or a direct antiarrhythmic effect. However, several small randomized studies[59–61] of 15–108 patients with nonischemic cardiomyopathy revealed that statin therapy was associated with significant improvement in quality of life, exercise capacity, NYHA class, and left ventricular ejection fraction.

Finally, Horwich *et al.*[58] described the outcomes of 551 patients referred to a specialized cardiomyopathy center for heart failure or transplant evaluation; 55% of the patients had a nonischemic cardiomyopathy. Forty-five percent of the total population was treated with statins, but only 22% of those with nonischemic cardiomyopathy. There was a significant improvement in 1-year survival without the need for urgent heart transplantation in patients with nonischemic cardiomyopathy treated with statins. The effect of statin use on time to death or resuscitated cardiac arrest and time to arrhythmic sudden death was evaluated in 458 patients with nonischemic cardiomyopathy in the DEFIbrillators in NonIschemic cardiomyopathy Treatment Evaluation (DEFINITE trial).[6] The effect of statin use on time to first appropriate shock was analyzed only in the 229 patients randomized to ICD therapy. The unadjusted hazard ratio for death among patients on versus those not on statin therapy was 0.22 (95% CI 0.09–0.55; $p = 0.001$). When controlled for statin effects, ICD therapy was associated with improved survival (hazard ratio 0.61; 95% CI 0.38–0.99; $p = 0.04$). There was one arrhythmic sudden death in the 110 patients receiving statin therapy (0.9%) versus 18/348 patients not receiving statins (5.2%; $p = 0.04$). The unadjusted hazard ratio for arrhythmic sudden death among patients on versus those not on statin therapy was 0.16 (95% CI 0.022–1.21; $p = 0.08$).

The mechanism for the effects of statins on arrhythmic sudden death and survival in patients with nonischemic cardiomyopathy remains unclear. An antiischemic effect is plausible as a substantial proportion of patients with nonischemic cardiomyopathy is found to have coronary artery disease at autopsy.[63] However, more recent studies have excluded patients with coronary disease. Statins have been reported to be effective in the prevention of atrial fibrillation suggesting a direct antiarrhythmic effect.[64–66] Finally, as noted previously, the small studies that have found improvements in ejection fraction and exercise capacity related to statin therapy support the notion that statins may have beneficial effects on left ventricular remodeling. Thus, it is most likely that statin therapy exerts multiple beneficial effects in patients with nonischemic cardiomyopathy by its lipid-lowering, antiinflammatory, antioxidant, autonomic effects and/or other effects.[67]

Polyunsaturated Fatty Acids

Important n-3 polyunsaturated fatty acids (PUFAs) include eicosapentaenoic acid, docosahexaenoic acid, and α-linolenic acid. The cardioprotective mechanisms of n-3 PUFAs may include suppression of ventricular arrhythmias, favorable lipid metabolism, a decrease in blood pressure, antiinflammatory actions, platelet stabilization, and anticoagulant effects. Numerous studies have shown an inverse relation between fatty fish intake and coronary heart disease. Data from several trials, however, have pointed to the fact that the predominant effect of PUFAs may be a primary reduction in sudden cardiac death. Experimental evidence in isolated myocytes, animals, and preliminary studies in humans point to a possible direct antiarrhythmic effect of n-3 PUFAs. In canines fed n-3 PUFAs MI models significantly decreased the risk of ischemia-induced ventricular fibrillation.[68] Through their actions on I_{Na} and $I_{Ca,L}$ channels, the n-3 PUFAs cause mild hyperpolarization of the resting membrane potential, resulting in a larger threshold voltage and stimulus and prolonging the refractory period of the cardiac cycle.[69] These properties may explain an enhanced electrical stability in the setting of ischemia and toxins.

Several recent studies have investigated the role of n-3 PUFA in preventing arrhythmic events.[70–73] A recent epidemiological study has shown that Japanese who consume a high intake of n-3 PUFAs had a 3-fold decrease in the risk of myocardial infarction and nonfatal coronary events. However, studies on the antiarrhythmic effect of PUFAs have been less consistent. A randomized trial performed in the United States by Leaf *et al.*[74] in 402 patients with ICDs showed that there was a 28% reduction in the times of the first ICD shock, which was of borderline significance. A more recent larger trial performed in Europe failed to show a substantial decrease in ICD shocks with fish oil supplementation.[70] Differences in fish oil content or the definition of appropriate ICD shocks could have accounted for these differences.

Several prospective cohort studies have shown an association with n-3 PUFAs and sudden cardiac death in patients with and without known coronary disease. In the DART trial, men who recently survived an MI were randomly assigned to one of eight groups of dietary intervention.[75] In the group assigned to receive an increase in fatty fish consumption, at 2 years, there was a 33% relative decrease in deaths due to coronary heart disease, whereas there was a nonsignificant increase in the incidents of nonfatal MI. The mortality benefit was mostly seen in the first 6 months. Similar results were seen in the Lyon Diet Heart study, in which patients randomly assigned to consume a Mediterranean diet, with a high α-linolenic acid content, had a 73% decrease in the combined endpoint of cardiac death and nonfatal MI.[76]

One of the largest trials had the statistical power to look at sudden cardiac death specifically, although not as a primary endpoint. The GISSI-Prevenzione study, a multicenter, open label, randomized trial, tested 11,323 patients with recent infarction.[77] Patients were randomly assigned in a 2×2 factorial design to receive n-3 PUFAs (1 g daily), vitamin E (300 mg daily), both, or neither. All patients received standard care and, in general, ate a Mediterranean diet, with high amounts of fish and olive oil, rather than U.S. diets. Overall, there were 265 sudden deaths: 146 were instantaneous, 103 occurred within 1 h of symptom onset, 10 were documented to be arrhythmic, and 6 were unwitnessed. At an average of 42 months of follow-up, sudden death occurred in 2.7% of control subjects and 2% of patients receiving n-3 PUFAs ($p < 0.001$) and accounted for 59% of the total mortality benefit. Bucher and co-workers[78] conducted a meta-analysis of randomized, controlled trial of n-3 PUFAs in coronary heart disease. In their analysis, total mortality, fatal MI, and sudden death were significantly decreased by n-3 PUFAs, whereas there was a trend toward reduction in nonfatal MI.

Conclusions

In contrast to traditional antiarrhythmic drugs that block sodium or potassium channels, drugs with antiadrenergic effects and neurohormonal effects have been shown to decrease both total and sudden death mortality in patients with underlying structural heart disease.[79–84] There are some lessons that can be learned from the results of drugs trials to decrease sudden death mortality. Life-threatening cardiac arrhythmias that are by nature highly sporadic or at least in part dependent on a complex series of extracardiac influences can be modulated by drugs that modify the adrenergic and the renin–angiotensin–aldosterone systems. In addition, nonspecific drugs whose primary mode of action is on cardiac ion channels are not effective at reducing sudden death. This observation suggests that despite advances in our knowledge of the basic mechanisms for cardiac arrhythmias, our current understanding of the mechanisms of sudden death is not adequate to target specific ion channels to prevent sudden death. Further basic research is needed to more fully understand the mechanisms of sudden death. This could then allow the design of targeted therapies to treat rhythm disturbances.

References

1. Steinbeck G, Andresen D, Bach P, *et al.* A comparison of electrophysiologically guided antiarrhythmic drug therapy with beta-blocker therapy in patients with symptomatic, sustained ventricular tachyarrhythmias. *N Engl J Med* 1992;327:987–992.
2. Julian D, Camm A, Frangin G, *et al.* Randomised trial of effect of amiodarone on mortality in patients with left-ventricular dysfunction after recent myocardial infarction: EMIAT. *Lancet* 1997;349:667–674.
3. Cairns J, Connolly S, Roberts R, Gent M. Randomised trial of outcome after myocardial infarction in patients with frequent or repetitive ventricular premature depolarisations: CAMIAT. *Lancet* 1997;349:675–682.
4. Boutitie F, Boissel J, Connolly S, *et al.* Amiodarone interaction with beta-blockers: Analysis of the merged EMIAT (European Myocardial Infarct Amiodarone Trial) and CAMIAT (Canadian Amiodarone Myocardial Infarction Trial) Databases. Circulation 1999;99:2268–2275.
5. Bardy G, Lee KL, Mark D, *et al.* Amiodarone or an implantable cardioverter- defibrillator for congestive heart failure. *N Engl J Med* 2005;352(3):225–237.
6. Kadish A, Dyer A, Daubert J, *et al.* Prophylactic defibrillator implantation in patients with nonischemic dilated cardiomyopathy. *N Engl J Med* 2004;350:2151–2158.
7. Teo K, Yusuf S, Furberg C. Effects of prophylactic antiarrhythmic drug therapy in acute myocardial

infarction. An overview of results from randomized controlled trials. *JAMA* 1993;270:1589–1595.
8. Pedersen T. Six-year follow-up of the Norwegian Multicenter Study on Timolol after Acute Myocardial Infarction. *N Engl J Med* 1985;313:1055–1058.
9. Gottlieb S, McCarter R, Vogel R. Effect of beta-blockade on mortality among high-risk and low-risk patients after myocardial infarction. *N Engl J Med* 1998;339:489–497.
10. Pfisterer M, Cox J, Granger C, *et al.* Atenolol use and clinical outcomes after thrombolysis for acute myocardial infarction: The GUSTO-I experience. *J Am Coll Cardiol* 1998;32:634–640.
11. Aronow W, Ahn C. Effect of beta blockers on incidence of new coronary events in older persons with prior myocardial infarction and diabetes mellitus. *Am J Cardiol* 2001;87:780–781.
12. Aronow W, Ahn C. Incidence of new coronary events in older persons with prior myocardial infarction and systemic hypertension treated with beta blockers, angiotensin-converting enzyme inhibitors, diuretics, calcium antagonists, and alpha blockers. *Am J Cardiol* 2002;89:1207–1209.
13. O'Rourke R. Beta-adrenergic blocking agents or angiotensin converting enzyme inhibitors, or both, for postinfarction patients with left ventricular dysfunction. *J Am Coll Cardiol* 1997;29(2):237–239.
14. Spargias K, Hall A, Greenwood D, Ball S. Beta blocker treatment and other prognostic variables in patients with clinical evidence of heart failure after acute myocardial infarction: Evidence from the AIRE study. *Heart* 1999;81:25–32.
15. Vantrimpont P, Rouleau J, Wun C, *et al.* Additive beneficial effects of beta-blockers to angiotensin-converting enzyme inhibitors in the survival and ventricular enlargement (SAVE) study. *J Am Coll Cardiol* 1997;29:229–236.
16. Chen J, Radford M, Wang Y, Marciniak T, Krumholz H. Are beta-blockers effective in elderly patients who undergo coronary revascularization after acute myocardial infarction? *Arch Intern Med* 2000;160:947–952.
17. Barron H, Viskin S, Lundstrom R, *et al.* Beta-blocker dosages and mortality after myocardial infarction: Data from a large health maintenance organization. *Arch Intern Med* 1998;158:449–453.
18. Viskin S, Kitzis I, Lev E, *et al.* Treatment with beta-adrenergic blocking agents after myocardial infarction: From randomized trials to clinical practice. *J Am Coll Cardiol* 1995;25:1327–1332.
19. Rochon P, Tu J, Anderson G, *et al.* Rate of heart failure and 1-year survival for older people receiving low-dose beta-blocker therapy after myocardial infarction. *Circulation* 2000;356:639–644.
20. Soumerai S, McLaughlin T, Spiegelman D, Hertzmark E, Thibault G, Goldman L. Adverse outcomes of underuse of b-blockers in elderly survivors of acute myocardial infarction. *JAMA* 1997; 277:115–121.
21. Packer M, Bristow M, Cohn J, *et al.* The effect of carvedilol on morbidity and mortality in patients with chronic heart failure. *N Engl J Med* 1996;334: 1349–1355.
22. Lechat P, Brunhuber K, Hofmann R, *et al.* The cardiac insufficiency bisoprolol study II (CIBIS-II): A randomized trial. *Circulation* 1999;353(9146): 9–13.
23. MERIT-HF Study Group. Effect of metoprolol CR/XL in chronic heart failure: Metoprolol CR/XL randomized intervention trial in congestive heart failure (MERIT-HF). *Circulation* 1999;353(9169): 2001–2007.
24. The RESOLVD Investigators. Effects of metoprolol CR in patients with ischemic and dilated cardiomyopathy: The randomized evaluation of strategies for left ventricular function pilot study. *Circulation* 2000;101(4):378–384.
25. Hallstrom A, Cobb L, Yu B, Weaver W, Fahrehbruch C. An antiarrhythmic drug experience in 941 patients resuscitated from an initial cardiac arrest between 1970 and 1985. *Am J Cardiol* 1991;68:1025–1031.
26. Exner D, Reiffel J, Epstein A, *et al.* Beta-blocker use and survival in patients with ventricular fibrillation or symptomatic ventricular tachycardia: The antiarrhythmics versus implantable defibrillators (AVID) trial. *J Am Coll Cardiol* 1999;34(2):325–333.
27. Pacifico A, Hohnloser S, Williams J, *et al.* Prevention of implantable-defibrillator shocks by treatment with sotalol. *N Engl J Med* 1999;340(24): 1855–1862.
28. Seidl K, Hauer B, Schwick N, Zahn R, Senges J. Comparison of metoprolol and sotalol in preventing ventricular tachyarrhythmias after the implantation of a cardioverter/defibrillator. *Am J Cardiol* 1998;82(6):744–748.
29. Rankovic V, Karha J, Passman R, Kadish A, Goldberger J. Predictors of appropriate implantable cardioverter-defibrillator therapy in patients with idiopathic dilated cardiomyopathy. *Am J Cardiol* 2002;89:1072–1076.
30. Van Gilst W, DeGraeff P, Wesseling H, DeLangen D. Reduction of reperfusion arrhythmia in the ischemic isolated rat heart by angiotensin converting enzyme inhibitors: A comparison of captopril, enalapril, and HOE 498. *J Cardiovasc Pharmacol* 1986;8:722–728.

31. de Langen C, de Graeff P, van Gilst W, Bel K, Kingma J, Wesseling H. Effects of angiotensin II and captopril on inducible sustained ventricular tachycardia two weeks after myocardial infarction in the pig. *J Cardiovasc Pharmacol* 1989;13(2): 186–191.
32. Cleland J, Erhardt L, Murray G, Hall A, Ball S. Effect of ramipril on morbidity and mode of death among survivors of acute myocardial infarction with clinical evidence of heart failure. *Eur Heart J* 1997; 18:41–51.
33. Grassi G, Cattaneo B, Seravalle G, *et al.* Effects of chronic ACE inhibition on sympathetic nerve traffic and baroreflex control of circulation in heart failure. *Circulation* 1997;39:463–470.
34. Pogwizd S. Focal mechanisms underlying ventricular tachycardia during prolonged ischemic cardiomyopathy. *Circulation* 1994;90(3):1441–1458.
35. Kober L, Torp-Pedersen C, Carlsen J, Group FtTCETS. A clinical trial of the angiotensin-converting enzyme inhibitor trandolapril in patients with left ventricular dysfunction after myocardial infarction. *N Engl J Med* 1995;333:1670–1676.
36. Domanski M, Exner D, Borkowf C, Geller N, Rosenberg Y, Pfeffer M. Effect of angiotensin converting enzyme inhibition on sudden cardiac death in patients following acute myocardial infarction: A meta-analysis of randomized clinical trials. *J Am Coll Cardiol* 1999;33:598–604.
37. Yusuf S, Sleight P, Pogue J, *et al.* Effects of an angiotensin-converting-enzyme inhibitor, ramipril, on cardiovascular events in high-risk patients. *N Engl J Med* 2000;342(3):145–153.
38. Group TCTS. Effects of enalapril on mortality in severe congestive heart failure. Results of the Cooperative North Scandinavian Enalapril Survival Study (CONSENSUS). *N Engl J Med* 1987;16(23): 1429–1435.
39. Investigators S. Effect of enalapril on mortality and the development of heart failure in asymptomatic patients with reduced left ventricular ejection fractions. *N Engl J Med* 1992;327(10):685–691.
40. Cohn J, Johnson G, Ziesche S, *et al.* A comparison of enalapril with hydralazine-isosorbide dinitrate in the treatment of chronic congestive heart failure. *N Engl J Med* 1991;325:303–310.
41. Gavras I, Gavras H. The antiarrhythmic potential of angiotensin II antagonism: Experience with losartan. *Am J Hypertens* 2000;13:512–517.
42. Minisi A, Thames M. Distribution of left ventricular sympathetic afferents demonstrated by reflex responses to transmural myocardial ischemia and to intracoronary and epicardial bradykinin. *Circulation* 1993;87(1):240–246.
43. Rousseau M, Gurne O, Duprez D, *et al.* Beneficial neurohormonal profile of spironolactone in severe congestive heart failure: Results from the RALES neurohormonal substudy. *J Am Coll Cardiol* 2002; 40(9):1596–1601.
44. Jong P, Demers C, McKelvie R, Liu P. Angiotensin receptor blockers in heart failure: Meta-analysis of randomized controlled trials. *J Am Coll Cardiol* 2002;39:463–470.
45. Pitt B, Martinez F, Meurers G, *et al.* Randomized trial of losartan vs. captopril in patients ≥ 65 with heart failure (Evaluation of Losartan in the Elderly study, ELITE). *Circulation* 1997;349:747–752.
46. Pitt B, Poole-Wilson P, Segal R, *et al.* Effect of losartan compared with captopril on mortality in patients with symptomatic heart failure: Randomised trial–the Losartan Heart Failure Survival Study ELITE II. *Circulation* 2000;355(9215):1582–1587.
47. Dickstein K, Kjekshus J, Group OSCftOS. Effects of losartan and captopril on mortality and morbidity in high-risk patients after acute myocardial infarction: The OPTIMAAL randomized trial. *Circulation* 2002;360:752–760.
48. Pitt B, Zannad F, Remme W, *et al.* The effect of spironolactone on morbidity and mortality in patients with severe heart failure. *N Engl J Med* 1999;341:709–717.
49. Pitt B, White H, Nicolau J, *et al.* Eplerenone reduces mortality 30 days after randomization following acute myocardial infarction in patients with left ventricular systolic dysfunction and heart failure. *J Am Coll Cardiol* 2005;46(3):425–431.
50. Pitt B, Remme W, Zannad F, *et al.* Eplerenone, a selective aldosterone blocker, in patients with left ventricular dysfunction after myocardial infarction. *N Engl J Med* 2003;348(14):1309–1321.
51. Weber K, Brilla C, Janicki J. Myocardial fibrosis: Functional significance and regulatory factors. *Cardiovasc Res* 1993;27:341–348.
52. Zannad F, Alla F, Dousset B, Perez A, Pitt B. Limitation of excessive extracellular matrix turnover may contribute to survival benefit of spironolactone therapy in patients with congestive heart failure: Insights from the randomized aldactone evaluation study (RALES). *Circulation* 2000;102:2700–2706.
53. Siscovick D, Raghunathan T, Psaty B, *et al.* Diuretic therapy for hypertension and the risk of primary cardiac arrest. *N Engl J Med* 1994;330:1852–1857.
54. Chiu J, Abdelhadi R, Chung M, *et al.* Effect of statin therapy on risk of ventricular arrhythmia among patients with coronary artery disease and an implantable cardioverter-defibrillator. *Am J Cardiol* 2005;95(4):490–491.

55. DeSutter J, Tavernier R, DeBuyzere M, Jordaens L, DeBacker G. Lipid lowering drugs and recurrences of the life-threatening ventricular arrhythmias in high-risk patients. *J Am Coll Cardiol* 2000;36(3): 766–772.
56. Mitchell L, Powell J, Gillis A, Kehl V, Hallstrom A, Investigators A. Are lipid-lowering drugs also antiarrhythmic drugs? An analysis of the antiarrhythmics versus implantable defibrillators (AVID) trial. *J Am Coll Cardiol* 2003;42(1):81–87.
57. Bleske B, Nicklas J, Bard R, *et al.* Neutral effect on markers of heart failure, inflammation, endothelial activation and function, and vagal tone after high-dose HMG-CoA reductase inhibition in non-diabetic patients with non-ischemic cardiomyopathy and average low-density lipoprotein level. *J Am Coll Cardiol* 2006;47(2):338–341.
58. Horwich T, MacLellan W, Fonarow G. Statin therapy is associated with improved survival in ischemic and non-ischemic heart failure. *J Am Coll Cardiol* 2004;43(4):642–648.
59. Laufs U, Wassmann S, Schackmann S, Heeschen C, Bohm M, Nickenig G. Beneficial effects of statins in patients with non-ischemic heart failure. *Z Kardiol* 2004;93(2):103–108.
60. Node K, Fujita M, Kitakaze M, Hori M, Liao J. Short-term statin therapy improves cardiac function and symptoms in patients with idiopathic dilated cardiomyopathy. *Circulation* 2003;108(7): 839–843.
61. Sola S, Mir M, Lerakis S, Tandon N, Khan B. Atorvastatin improves left ventricular systolic function and serum markers of inflammation in nonischemic heart failure. *J Am Coll Cardiol* 2006;47(2):332–337.
62. DeSutter J, Tavernier R, DeBuyzere M, *et al.* Lipid lowering drugs and recurrences of life-threatening ventricular arrhythmias in high-risk patients. *J Am Coll Cardiol* 2000;36:766–772.
63. Uretsky B, Thygesen K, Armstrong P, *et al.* Acute coronary findings at autopsy in heart failure patients with sudden death: Results from the assessment of treatment with lisinopril and survival (ATLAS) trial. *Circulation* 2000;102:611–616.
64. Kumagai K, Nakashima H, Saku K. The HMG-CoA reductase inhibitor atorvastatin prevents atrial fibrillation by inhibiting inflammation in a canine sterile pericarditis model. *Cardiovasc Res* 2004;62: 105–111.
65. Shiroshita-Takeshita A, Schram G, Lavoie J, Nattel S. Effect of simvastatin and antioxidant vitamins on atrial fibrillation promotion by atrial-tachycardia remodeling in dogs. *Circulation* 2004;110:2313–2319.
66. Young-Xu Y, Jabbour S, Goldberg R, *et al.* Usefulness of statin drugs in protecting against atrial fibrillation in patients with coronary artery disease. *Am J Cardiol* 2003;92:1379–1383.
67. Pham M, Oka R, Giacomini J. Statin therapy in heart failure. *Curr Opin Lipidol* 2005;16:630–634.
68. Billman G, Kang J, Leaf A. Prevention of ischemia induced cardiac sudden death by n-3 polyunsaturated fatty acids. *Lipids* 1997;32:1161–1168.
69. Leaf A. The electrophysiological basis for the antiarrhythmic actions of polyunsaturated fatty acids. *Eur Heart J* 2001;3(Suppl. D):D98–D105.
70. Brouwer I, Zock P, Camm A, *et al.* Effect of fish oil on ventricular tachyarrhythmia and death in patients with implantable cardioverter defibrillators. *J Am Coll Cardiol* 2006;295(22):2613–2619.
71. Leaf A, Kang J, Xiao Y, Billman G. Clinical prevention of sudden cardiac death by n-3 polyunsaturated fatty acids and mechanism of prevention of arrhythmias by n-3 fish oils. *Circulation* 2003; 107:2646.
72. McLennan P, Abeywardena M. Membrane basis for fish oil effects on the heart: Linking natural hibernators to prevention of human sudden cardiac death. *J Membr Biol* 2005;206:85–102.
73. Siscovick D, Lemaitre R, Mozaffarian D. The fish story, a diet-heart hypothesis with clinical implications: n-3 poyunsaturated fatty acids, myocardial vulnerability, and sudden death. *Circulation* 2003;107:2632.
74. Leaf A, Albert C, Johnson D, *et al.* Prevention of fatal arrhythmias in high-risk subjects by fish oil n-3 fatty acid intakes. *Circulation* 2005;112(18): 2762–2768.
75. Burr M, Fehily A, Gilbert J, *et al.* Effects of changes in fat, fish, and fiber intakes on death and reinfarction: Diet and reinfarction trial (DART). *Circulation* 1989;ii:757–761.
76. deLorgeril M, Renaud S, Mamelle N, *et al.* Mediterranean alpha linolenic acid-rich diet in secondary prevention of coronary heart disease. *Circulation* 1994;343:1454–1459.
77. Marchioli R, Barzi F, Bomba E, *et al.* Early protection against sudden death by n-3 polyunsaturated fatty acids after myocardial infarction. *Circulation* 2002;105:1997–2003.
78. Bucher H, Hengstler P, Schindler C, Meier G. N-3 polyunsaturated fatty acids in coronary heart disease: A meta-analysis of randomized controlled trials. *Am J Med* 2002 2002;112:298–304.
79. Pfeffer M, Braunwald E, Moye L, *et al.* Effect of captopril on mortality and morbidity in patients with left ventricular dysfunction after myocardial

infarction. Results of the survival and ventricular enlargement trial. The SAVE Investigators. *N Engl J Med* 1992;327(10):669–677.
80. Ambrosioni E, Borghi C, Magnani B. The effect of the angiotensin-converting-enzyme inhibitor zofenopril on mortality and morbidity after anterior myocardial infarction. The Survival of Myocardial Infarction Long-Term Evaluation (SMILE) Study Investigators. *N Engl J Med* 1995;332:80–85.
81. Cohn J, Tognoni G, Investigators VHFT. A randomized trial of the angiotensin-receptor blocker valsartan in chronic heart failure. *N Engl J Med* 2001;345:1667–1675.
82. Dahlof B, Devereux R, Kjeldsen S, *et al.* Cardiovascular morbidity and mortality in the Losartan Intervention For Endpoint reduction in hypertension study (LIFE): A randomised trial against atenolol. *Circulation* 2002;359:995–1003.
83. Freemantle N, Cleland J, Young P, Mason J, Harrison J. Beta blockade after myocardial infarction: Systematic review and meta regression analysis. *BMJ* 1999;318:1730–1737.
84. Dargie HJ. Effect of carvedilol on outcome after myocardial infarction in patients with left-ventricular dysfunction: The CAPRICORN randomised trial. *Circulation* 2001;357(9266):1385–1390.

50 The Implantable Cardioverter Defibrillator: Technical and Clinical Considerations

Bruce L. Wilkoff and Sergio G. Thal

Introduction

The implantable cardioverter defibrillator (ICD) has become the most common device implanted for the treatment of arrhythmia disorders. The enormous technological development of these devices is perhaps the most dramatic progression observed in medicine over the past 30 years. The initial experiments of Mirowski published in 1978 required an external unit developed into epicardial patches; a large abdominal human implantable device was released in 1985, and this yielded to transvenous leads in the early 1990s and smaller pectoral and dual-chamber devices in the late 1990s and ultimately to the combination of cardiac resynchronization devices with defibrillation in the first few years of the new millennium.[1,2]

The aim of this chapter is to review the current ICD indications based on the results of the most recent published trials, comment about the technical aspects involved in the design, implant, and testing of the devices, and present an overview of the follow-up recommendations.

Indications

In 2002, a task force from the North American Society of Pacing and Electrophysiology (NASPE, currently Heart Rhythm Society), the American College of Cardiology, and the American Heart Association delineated most of the current indications for ICD implants.[3] These indications were more recently updated by the Centers for Medicine and Medicaid Services (CMS) guidelines of February 2005, which incorporated the results of randomized clinical trials and widely opened reimbursement as supported by the evidence base (Table 50–1). Initially the use of these devices was restricted to secondary prevention, defined as patients who had experienced a cardiac arrest or who had evidence of sustained VT (VT). The evidence base has expanded over the past several years demonstrating its efficacy as a tool for primary prevention in targeted subgroups of patients at a higher future risk of developing sudden death.

Primary Prevention

The Multicenter Automatic Defibrillator Implantation Trial (MADIT), published in 1996, was the first in demonstrate benefit of ICDs for primary prevention of sudden death in a high-risk group.[4] This trial included patients postmyocardial infarction (MI) (at least 3 weeks), with a low left ventricular ejection fraction (LVEF < 30%) and evidence of nonsustained VT (NSVT). These patients were evaluated during an electrophysiological (EP) study and demonstrated inducible monomorphic sustained VT that was not suppressed with the use of antiarrhythmic medications. Those patients inducible but not suppressible by medications were then randomized to receive antiarrhythmic medications alone or antiarrhythmic medications plus an ICD implant. The study was terminated early due to the significant impact on reduction in sudden death among the patients treated with the ICD. On the same research path, the Multicenter Unsustained Tachycardia Trial

TABLE 50–1. Centers for Medicare and Medicaid Services (CMS) approved indications for ischemic dilated cardiomyopathy implant.[a]

Ischemic dilated cardiomyopathy (ICD) is reasonable and necessary:
1. Patients with IDC, documented prior myocardial infarction (MI), New York Heart Association (NYHA) Class II and III heart failure, and measured left ventricular ejection fraction (LVEF) ≤35%
2. Patients with nonischemic dilated cardiomyopathy (NIDCM) >9 months, NYHA Class II and III heart failure, and measured LVEF ≤35%
3. Patients who meet all current CMS coverage requirements for a cardiac resynchronization therapy (CRT) device and have NYHA Class IV heart failure
ICD is reasonable and necessary for patients with NIDCM >3 months, NYHA Class II or III heart failure, and measured LVEF ≤35% only if the following additional criteria are also met:
1. Patients must not have
Cardiogenic shock or symptomatic hypotension while in a stable baseline rhythm
Had a CABG or PTCA within the past 3 months
Had an acute myocardial infarction within the past 40 days
Clinical symptoms or findings that would make them a candidate for coronary revascularization
Irreversible brain damage from preexisting cerebral disease
Any disease, other than cardiac disease (e.g., cancer, uremia, liver failure), associated with a likelihood of survival less than 1 year
2. Providers must be able to justify the medical necessity of devices other than single-lead devices; this justification should be available in the patient's medical record

[a]CABG, coronary artery bypass grafting; PTCA, percutaneous transluminal coronary angioplasty.

Investigators (MUSTT) reported similar findings.[5] In this trial, patients with coronary artery disease and an LVEF of 40% or less and asymptomatic, unsustained VT were included. The patients underwent EP testing and those with sustained, monomorphic VT induced by any method of stimulation and those with sustained polymorphic VT [including ventricular flutter and ventricular fibrillation (VF)] induced by one or two extrastimuli were randomized to either antiarrhythmic therapy guided by the results of EP testing or no antiarrhythmic therapy. Implantable cardioverter defibrillator therapy was not prespecified, but in 46% of the patients randomized to EP-guided therapy there was no effective antiarrhythmic medication identified and therefore these patients received an ICD as their EP-guided therapy. The investigators concluded that EP-guided antiarrhythmic therapy with implantable defibrillators, but not with antiarrhythmic drugs, reduces the risk of sudden death in this group. Finally, to complete the support for the current indications, the results of the MADIT II trial were published in 2002.[6] In this study patients with previous myocardial infarction and an LVEF ≤ 30% were randomized to receive an ICD or medical treatment. Here, once again, the ICD was shown to decrease the risk of sudden death. It is important to keep in mind that according to the inclusion/exclusion criteria of this study, patients could be included only at least 3 months after any revascularization procedure or 1 month after being admitted for an MI. This is particularly important when we examine the results of the Defibrillator in Acute Myocardial Infarction Trial (DINAMIT) study published in 2004.[7] In this trial an attempt was made to demonstrate that ICD implants immediately after an acute MI were able to significantly modify the survival outcome of patients. The investigators included patients within 6–40 days after an acute MI, with low ventricular ejection fraction (<35%) and abnormal heart rate variability measured during Holter monitoring. The results showed no difference in total mortality between patients treated with ICD compared to those who had not received an ICD. A significant reduction in arrhythmic death was observed in the ICD group, but at the same time a significant increase in nonarrhythmic death was observed in this group. We can at least initially conclude that a prudent waiting time after revascularization or MI would help to target a group that would more likely benefit from ICD therapy.

As described, most of the initial efforts to identify a target population at a higher risk of sudden death were primarily oriented to ischemic patients. But in 2004, the results of the Defibrillators in Non-Ischemic Cardiomyopathy Treatment Evaluation (DEFINITE) trial led physicians to focus attention on patients with a dilated cardiomyopathy of nonischemic origin.[8] This study included patients with a nonischemic dilated cardiomyopathy, symptomatic heart failure, spontaneous premature ventricular contractions (PVCs) (>10/h or NSVT) and poor ventricular function (LVEF < 35%). Patients who met the inclusion criteria were randomized to receive optimal medical therapy [which included angiotensin-converting enzyme (ACE) inhibitors and β blockers] or optimal medical therapy and single-chamber ICD therapy. The primary endpoint of "all-cause mortality" showed a trend toward the benefit of ICD therapy, but it did not achieve statistical significance. As a secondary endpoint, "arrhythmic death" was significantly reduced by ICD therapy. A second larger study of heart failure patients also provides support for ICD therapy of patients with nonischemic dilated cardiomyopathy and evidence of decreased left ventricular function. This study was the Sudden Cardiac Death in Heart Failure Trial (SCD-HeFT) published in May 2005.[9] It included 2521 patients with New York Heart Association (NYHA) Class II or III congestive heart failure (CHF) and an LVEF of 35% or less, and randomized them to receive treatment with optimal medical heart failure therapy alone or together either with amiodarone or a single-lead ICD. This trial concluded that amiodarone has no favorable effect on survival, whereas single-lead, shock-only ICD therapy reduced overall mortality by 23%. This favorable mortality benefit was seen for patients with ischemic and nonischemic cardiomyopathy.

Secondary Prevention

The Antiarrhythmic versus Implantable Defibrillator (AVID) trial was the first randomized trial that prospectively evaluated the use of ICDs in patients with documented spontaneous sustained VT or after resuscitatation from sudden cardiac death.[10] It included patients who had been resuscitated from near-fatal VF or who had undergone cardioversion from sustained VT and patients with VT who also had either syncope or other serious cardiac symptoms, along with an LVEF of 40% or less. It randomized this population to receive medical treatment with a Class III antiarrhythmic agent (primarily amiodarone) or an ICD implant. Its results showed that the ICD group had a significant decreased overall mortality compared with the medical treatment group at 1, 2, and 3 years of follow-up. The Canadian Implantable Defibrillator Study (CIDS) addressed a target population similar to AVID for secondary prevention.[11] It included patients with resuscitated VF or VT, but also included patients with unmonitored syncope if there was inducible sustained VT with programmed stimulation. The patients were randomly assigned to treatment with an ICD or with amiodarone. There was a trend toward reduction of all-cause mortality (20% relative risk reduction) and a statistically significant 33% reduction in arrhythmic mortality with ICD compared to amiodarone therapy. A subsequent subanalysis, published a month after the main trial publication, showed a significant reduction in overall mortality in the highest risk subgroup of the CIDS trial patients. This highest risk group was defined as having at least two of the following: ≥70 years old, an LVEF of ≤35%, or NYHA Class III or IV.[12] Finally, the Cardiac Arrest Study Hamburg (CASH) was published in the same year as the CIDS trial.[13] It included patients who survived a cardiac arrest secondary to documented ventricular arrhythmias, and randomized them to treatment with an ICD or antiarrhythmic drug therapy. It showed that therapy with an ICD was associated with a 23% nonsignificant reduction of all-cause mortality when compared to treatment with amiodarone or metoprolol. The subgroup treated with propaphenone was discontinued early in the study because during an interim analysis it showed a significant increased risk of mortality compared to ICD's.

Technical Aspects of Implantable Cardioverter Defibrillators

Hardware

The current ICDs, developed for thoracic subcutaneous implants, are the results of an amazing evolution since the first experimental implants at the beginning of the 1980s. Initially the size of these devices permitted only abdominal implants. The defibrillation electrodes required patches to be surgically implanted either on the epicardial surface or on the external surface of the pericardium and sometimes a transvenous superior vena cava (SVC) or coronary sinus coil. Sensing electrodes were either epicardial or transvenous, but did not provide bradycardia pacing support or antitachycardia pacing.

Today, the devices available are significantly smaller, 35 cm^3 down from over 200 cm^3 from the initial models, and weigh approximately 40 g. The system implantation avoids open-chest placement of epicardial shocking patches; it employs transvenous combined pacing/shocking leads and the ICD titanium can to provide programmable antibradycardia and antitachycardia pacing support, cardioversion, and defibrillation therapy.

Implantable Cardioverter Defibrillator Generator

The new generators combine the functions of defibrillation with either single-, dual-, or triple-chamber pacemaker stimulation.

The device "case" is made out of titanium and serves to work as an active defibrillation electrode, sometimes programmable off in some ICD models.[14]

The most common battery used today is a lithium silver vanadium cell, providing approximately 18,000 J. Most of the devices contain two of these batteries to power all of the ICD functions including antitachycardia and antibradycardia therapies. The battery voltage can be assessed along with the status of the rest of all ICD activities with a radiofrequency telemetry system that communicates the device data to the external programmer. Each ICD system has a voltage (approximately 2.6 V) at which the system continues to function precisely as programmed, but the system should be electively replaced before the battery is no longer able to guarantee adequate therapy. This voltage reduction sets the elective replacement indicator (ERI); this device sould be able to function properly for 1–3 months. If the battery voltage drops further, the end of life (EOL) indicator is set (approximately 2.2 V) and full capacitor charge times will be prolonged and full shocking voltage may not be achieved. Either immediate device replacement is required at this time or provision must be made for alternative protection through hospitalization or a wearable defibrillator therapy.

To delivery the high energy required for a dc shock, in an appropriate time frame, the devices are provided with capacitors, able to be rapidly charged to 750–800 V in less than 10 sec. The capacitors are discharged over 5–20 msec and deliver up to approximately 35 J of energy less than 15 sec after initiation of tachycardia. As the battery voltage declines over time and depending on the status of the capacitor (due to capacitor deformation) it may take up to 30 sec to fully charge and deliver the defibrillation shock when the device is at EOL status.

The basic ICD lead provides for right ventricular (RV) electrogram detection and pacing through a conventional distal pacemaker electrode and high energy delivery through a right ventricular defibrillation coil. Sensing and capture are established by using the distal pacemaker electrode as the cathode and either by using the RV coil as the anode, termed an integrated bipolar lead, or by providing an anodal ring electrode positioned in between the cathode and the shocking coil. The basic high-energy shock delivery configuration employs the titanium can as one defibrillation electrode and the RV coil as the second electrode. Many ICD leads provide for a second defibrillation coil about 15 cm proximal from the distal electrode. This proximal shock coil is usually combined with the titanium can as a single electrode, and the energy is delivered to and from this electrode to the RV coil electrode. These are non-thoracotomy leads that are inserted through venous access at the subclavian or cephalic vein[15,16] (Figure 50–1). Fixation to the RV myocardium is achieved either by an extendable/retractable helical screw or lodging small tines near the distal electrode of the trabeculations of the muscle. The

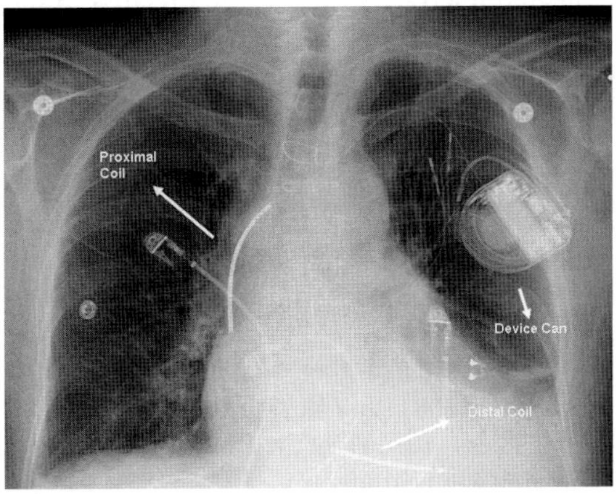

FIGURE 50–1. Chest X-ray of a VVI/ICD. The image corresponds to a chest X-ray from a patient implanted with a VVI/ICD. The ICD lead was inserted through the left subclavian vein and the distal tip of the lead was attached to the right ventricular apex. The arrows show the location of the proximal coil at the superior vena cava and the distal coil at the right ventricle.

development of the device "active can" for ICD shocks makes it possible on some occasions to use leads without a proximal coil and with this avoid future venous complications due to increased venous fibrosis, which could be a potential complication if a future extraction is needed.[17] However, additional defibrillation coils or patches are sometimes required to provide consistent defibrillation efficacy. These electrodes have been placed in the SVC, subclavian vein azygous vein, subcutaneously or submuscularly in the axilla, or posterior to the heart in the subcutaneous tissue.[18–23]

Device Function

Ventricular tachyarrhythmia detection and discrimination from supraventricular tachyarrhythmias are essential aspects of ICD performance. It is necessary to distinguish the absence of rhythm disturbances from the presence of tachycardia or bradycardia. The different models available today use a variety of complex algorithms to be able to differentiate rhythms that require or do not require therapy. These algorithms usually evaluate heart rate, the pattern of atrial and ventricular activation, cycle length stability, suddenness of rhythm initiation, mode of tachycardia initiation, and various aspects of electrogram timing or morphology. The ability to correctly evaluate these variables is directly related to the quality of signals that the device will obtain for evaluation. For this reason the lead should be located at the implant time in a position that provides a good balance between electrogram detection, in the healthiest muscle, and defibrillation efficacy, which has frequently been demonstrated to be best at the RV apex.[24] The amplitude of the signal during sinus rhythm should be able to assure as good as possible detection of an eventual VF. It is estimated that a ventricular activity sensing of at least 5 mV during sinus rhythm predicts that less than 10% of the electrograms during VF events will be undersensed.[25]

Tachyarrhythmia Therapies

Antitachycardia pacing (ATP) is available in almost all current ICD models. It consists of the delivery of ventricular pacing at a faster rate than the tachycardia cycle length. This short burst of impulses will often interrupt the tachycardia circuit and stop the ventricular tachyarrhythmia without a high-energy shock. This can potentially have a significant impact on the patient's quality of life and on device longevity. There are different ways in which this can be delivered including a short burst (constant cycle length of pacing impulses) or a ramp burst in which each subsequent interval is incrementally shorter than the previous one.

One of the problems with this type of therapy is the potential for acceleration of VT cycle length to the VF detection zone. This is observed in approximately 5% of the cases and this rhythm may be more hemodynamically compromising, potentially causing syncope and may require a higher energy to be successfully terminated.[26] Except for this potential problem, antitachycardia-pacing therapy was shown to have a success rate of over 90% for VT rates of less than 200 bpm and over 70% when applied to tachycardias with rates between 200 and 250 bpm when it is empirically programmed at the implantation time.[27] In all cases, if antitachycardia pacing fails, a shock therapy is programmed as the subsequent therapy.

Shock therapy is the electrical shock produced by delivery of 50–800 V stored on the ICD capacitors over 5–20 msec through the defibrillation coils, can, or patches in an attempt to produce a uniform voltage gradient throughout the ventricular myocardium to permit reestablishment of normal ventricular activation and automaticity. The waveform currently in use by almost all the available ICDs is biphasic. This means that the capacitor discharge is divided into two phases. The anode and cathode are switched after several milliseconds to the opposite polarity (Figure 50–2). The clear improvement in defibrillation efficacy of this technique is explained by the "cell membrane burping" theory.[28] This theory established that the function of the first phase of a biphasic shock depolarizes or extends the refractory periods of virtually all ventricular myocytes, and the second phase with opposite polarity is to remove the excess charge from any cells where it remains.[29] Migration from the monophasic truncated exponential capacitor discharge to biphasic waveforms and use of the defibrillator can as an

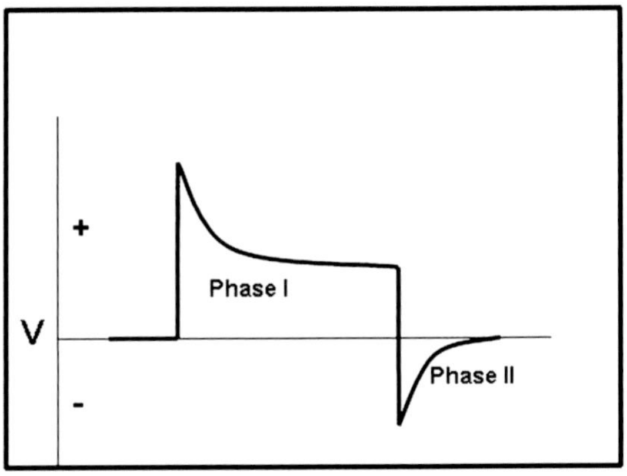

FIGURE 50–2. Biphasic wave shock. Two phases of the biphasic wave currently in use for ICD shocks are shown. Phase I correspond to the initial positive portion and phase II to the final negative deflection. V, voltage; +, positive; –, negative.

electrode in current devices have produced a simplified and more efficient device implantation.

Defibrillation Threshold

As mentioned before, the main objective of a correct device function implies the ability to accurately detect life-threatening ventricular tachyarrhythmias and then to terminate them with a shock. To ensure this correct functioning, VF detection and termination are tested during implantation.

The success of therapy is dependent upon several clinical variables that change with patient status such as electrolytes, metabolic decompensation, hemodynamic condition, and antiarrhythmic medications. Also, the success of a shock is exposed to a probabilistic variance. That is why reproducibility of a successful defibrillation increases the certainty of device performance and is a goal when testing is performed. There are variable data regarding the safety of defibrillation threshold (DFT) testing. Some studies suggested that no adverse effects resulted from multiple DFTs testings, while others suggested that performing these tests could be deleterious or risky for patients. The risk appears to be greater if the baseline ejection fraction is low as is the case for the majority of the patients who receive these devices.[30–33] Despite the poor ventricular function in these patients, unless the patients become compromised with either pulmonary or hemodynamic deterioration during device implantation, fibrillation detection and termination testing can be safely performed and would result in an approximately 1% incidence of an inadequate defibrillation system if omitted.

The initial step for a DFT test is the induction of a VF, most commonly done by delivering a small shock on the T wave through the device. This is more efficient than rapid ventricular pacing and is accomplished by administration of a 200 V shock around 10 msec before the peak of the T wave.[34] The next step is let the device detect the VF and shock cardiovert it. The main objective of the test is to ensure that the implanted device has the ability to deliver a shock capable of terminating VF, the most difficult rhythm to convert. There are many different protocol approaches to perform the test. The simplest one is named the "step-down protocol," which is mainly the reduction of the energy of successives shocks until one fails. The opposite approach would be the "step-up protocol" and the combination of these was one of the most popular classic approaches.

Since defibrillation efficacy is most accurately expressed not as an energy level, but as a percentage of episodes converted at each energy level, it is useful to demonstrate a safety margin. This has been done with multiple techniques, but reproducibility is the most common tool to prove adequacy of the defibrillation configuration. Two successful conversions at 10 J below the maximum output of the device were shown by Strickberger *et al.*, to predict a successful conversion in the clinical setting of about 99.5%.[35] Gold and his colleagues demonstrated that a single successful defibrillation at 14 J stored (11 J delivered) in a 31-J device (27 J delivered) appears to be similarly efficient.[36] However, rarely a practical approach that demonstrates multiple successful conversions at maximal output is the only reasonable alternative, but only after testing of alternative defibrillation configurations, pulse durations, or tilt values.

Telemetry, Diagnostics, and Follow-Up

The basic functional components of an ICD are the battery, capacitor, software and computer processor, and the telemetry coil. Most of the technology of the ICD is in the logic algorithms, but the window into the ICD function and the status of the patient come through the telemetric link and the programmer. On the surface the need for long-term surveillance of defibrillation function is similar to that of pacemakers. However, the seriousness of the underlying condition, sudden cardiac death, the physically and emotionally painful defibrillation shocks, and the increased complexity of the device increase the mandate for regular patient and device follow-up.

The original ICDs had no programmability and no telemetric communication with a programmer, but current device programmability also requires the ability to document the current parameters to interpret the behavior of the device. In addition, multiple self-diagnostic measurements and maintenance behaviors are programmed into the device and provide a unique view into the fitness of the ICD system.

Radiofrequency telemetry uniquely identifies communication of an individual device and a programmer or communicator. Most devices can transmit a signal only over a few inches, but there is now communication over several meters using the frequency spectrum previously dedicated to weather balloons. This extended range has been used to collect full interrogations of the programmed, measured, and event data from the device's memory via home-based interrogators and to transmit those data to an internet-based data center or directly to a physician's office.

The standard for ICD follow-up requires full interrogation of the device at least every 6 months and evaluation of capture and sensing function at yearly intervals. However, the need for more frequent evaluations is dependent on the patient's clinical condition, the age of the ICD, the battery voltage, the condition and function of the leads, and the frequency of ventricular and supraventricular arrhythmias. Remote interrogation of the device can augment formal programming sessions and substitute for situations in which programming or formal threshold testing is not required.

Evaluation of defibrillation efficacy is usually tested only at the time of implantation. There are data that support the concept that defibrillation remains relatively constant over time with a biphasic shock wave configuration.[37–39] For this reason, there is no need for subsequent defibrillation thresholds unless there is evidence of shock failure in the clinical scenario.

Summary

The implantable cardioverter defibrillator has experienced a tremendous evolution since its initial conception to the present. Today, ICD implants are a daily occurrence in the modern EP laboratory instead of the rarer and more complex open chest procedure. The available published data, the result of multiple multicenter clinical trials performed in the past several years and the ones that are currently ongoing, are pushing the manufacturers and the physician community to develop better and safer devices. The present is encouraging and the future is promising with improved technologies and therapy strategies, mostly for heart failure treatment, they will modify the duration and quality of life of our patients.

References

1. Mirowski M, Mower MM, Langer A, Heilman MS, Schreibman J. A chronically implanted system for automatic defibrillation in active conscious dogs. Experimental model for treatment of sudden death from ventricular fibrillation. *Circulation* 1978;58(1):90–94.
2. Device@FDA, U.S. Food and Drug Administration/Center for Devices and Radiological Health, http://www.accessdata.fda.gov/scripts/cdrh/devicesatfda/.
3. Gregoratos G, Abrams J, Epstein AE, Freedman RA, Hayes DL, Hlatky MA, Kerber RE, Naccarelli GV, Schoenfeld MH, Silka MJ, Winters SL. ACC/AHA/NASPE 2002 Guideline Update for Implantation of Cardiac Pacemakers and Antiarrhythmia Devices. A report of the American College of Cardiology/American Heart Association Task Force on Practice Guidelines (ACC/AHA/NASPE Committee on Pacemaker Implantation). *Circulation* 2002;106:2145–2161.
4. Moss AJ, Hall WJ, Cannom DS, Daubert JP, Higgins SL, Klein H, Levine JH, Saksena S, Waldo AL, Wilber D, Brown MW, Heo M. Improved survival with an implanted defibrillator in patients with coronary disease at high risk for ventricular arrhythmia. Multicenter Automatic Defibrillator Implantation Trial Investigators. *N Engl J Med* 1996;335(26):1933–1940.

5. Buxton AE, Lee KL, Fisher JD, Josephson ME, Prystowsky EN, Hafley G. A randomized study of the prevention of sudden death in patients with coronary artery disease. Multicenter Unsustained Tachycardia Trial Investigators. *N Engl J Med* 1999;341(25):1882–1890.
6. Moss AJ, Zareba W, Hall WJ, Klein H, Wilber DJ, Cannom DS, Daubert JP, Higgins SL, Brown MW, Andrews ML; Multicenter Automatic Defibrillator Implantation Trial II Investigators. Prophylactic implantation of a defibrillator in patients with myocardial infarction and reduced ejection fraction. *N Engl J Med* 2002;346(12):877–883.
7. Hohnloser SH, Kuck KH, Dorian P, Roberts RS, Hampton JR, Hatala R, Fain E, Gent M, Connolly SJ; DINAMIT Investigators. Prophylactic use of an implantable cardioverter-defibrillator after acute myocardial infarction. *N Engl J Med* 2004;351(24): 2481–2488.
8. Kadish A, Dyer A, Daubert JP, Quigg R, Estes NA, Anderson KP, Calkins H, Hoch D, Goldberger J, Shalaby A, Sanders WE, Schaechter A, Levine JH; Defibrillators in Non-Ischemic Cardiomyopathy Treatment Evaluation (DEFINITE) Investigators. Prophylactic defibrillator implantation in patients with nonischemic dilated cardiomyopathy. *N Engl J Med* 2004;350(21):2151–2158.
9. Bardy GH, Lee KL, Mark DB, Poole JE, Packer DL, Boineau R, Domanski M, Troutman C, Anderson J, Johnson G, McNulty SE, Clapp-Channing N, Davidson-Ray LD, Fraulo ES, Fishbein DP, Luceri RM, Ip JH; Sudden Cardiac Death in Heart Failure Trial (SCD-HeFT) Investigators. Amiodarone or an implantable cardioverter-defibrillator for congestive heart failure. *N Engl J Med* 2005;352(20): 225–237.
10. A comparison of antiarrhythmic-drug therapy with implantable defibrillators in patients resuscitated from near-fatal ventricular arrhythmias. The Antiarrhythmics versus Implantable Defibrillators (AVID) Investigators. *N Engl J Med* 1997;337(22): 1576–1583.
11. Connolly SJ, Gent M, Roberts RS, Dorian P, Roy D, Sheldon RS, Mitchell LB, Green MS, Klein GJ, O'Brien B. Canadian Implantable Defibrillator Study (CIDS): A randomized trial of the implantable cardioverter defibrillator against amiodarone. *Circulation* 2000;101(11):1297–1302.
12. Sheldon R, Connolly S, Krahn A, Roberts R, Gent M, Gardner M. Identification of patients most likely to benefit from implantable cardioverter-defibrillator therapy: The Canadian Implantable Defibrillator Study. *Circulation* 2000;101(14):1660–1664.
13. Kuck KH, Cappato R, Siebels J, Ruppel R. Randomized comparison of antiarrhythmic drug therapy with implantable defibrillators in patients resuscitated from cardiac arrest: The Cardiac Arrest Study Hamburg (CASH). *Circulation* 2000;102(7):748–754.
14. Wilkoff BL. Implantable cardioverter-defibrillator: Technical aspects. In: Douglas JJ, Zipes P, Eds. *Cardiac Electrophysiology: From Cell to Bedside.* Philadelphia, PA: W.B. Saunders, 2004:970–999.
15. Usui M, Walcott GP, KenKnight BH, Walker RG, Rollins DL, Smith WM, Ideker RE. Influence of malpositioned transvenous leads on defibrillation efficacy with and without a subcutaneous array electrode. *Pacing Clin Electrophysiol* 1995;18(11): 2008–2016.
16. Stajduhar KC, Ott GY, Kron J, McAnulty JH, Oliver RP, Reynolds BT, Adler SW, Halperin BD. Optimal electrode position for transvenous defibrillation: A prospective randomized study. *J Am Coll Cardiol* 1996;27(1):90–94.
17. Bardy GH, Johnson G, Poole JE, Dolack GL, Kudenchuk PJ, Kelso D, Mitchell R, Mehra R, Hofer B. A simplified, single-lead unipolar transvenous cardioversion-defibrillation system. *Circulation* 1993;88(2):543–547.
18. Higgins SL, Alexander DC, Kuypers CJ, Brewster SA. The subcutaneous array: A new lead adjunct for the transvenous ICD to lower defibrillation thresholds. *Pacing Clin Electrophysiol* 1995;18(8):1540–1548.
19. Kettering K, Mewis C, Dornberger V, Vonthein R, Bosch RF, Seipel L, Kuhlkamp V. Long-term experience with subcutaneous ICD leads: A comparison among three different types of subcutaneous leads. *Pacing Clin Electrophysiol* 2004;27(10):1355–1361.
20. Cesario D, Bhargava M, Valderrabano M, Fonarow GC, Wilkoff B, Shivkumar K. Azygos vein lead implantation: A novel adjunctive technique for implantable cardioverter defibrillator placement. *J Cardiovasc Electrophysiol* 2004;15(7):780–783.
21. Markewitz A, Kaulbach H, Mattke S, Dorwarth U, Hoffmann E, Weinhold C, Steinbeck G, Reichart B. The left subclavian vein as an alternative site for implantation of the second defibrillation lead. *Pacing Clin Electrophysiol* 1995;18(3Pt. 1):401–405.
22. Mouchawar GA, Wolsleger WK, Doan PD, Causey JD 3rd, Kroll MW. Does an SVC electrode further reduce DFT in a hot-can ICD system? *Pacing Clin Electrophysiol* 1997;20(1Pt. 2):163–167.
23. Tomassoni G, Newby K, Moredock L, Rembert J, Natale A. Effect of the superior vena cava electrode surface area on defibrillation threshold in different lead systems. *Pacing Clin Electrophysiol* 1998;21 (1Pt. 1):94–99.

24. Fotuhi PC, Keknight BH, Melnick SB, Smith WM, Baumann GF, Ideker RE. Effect of a passive endocardial electrode on defibrillation efficacy of a nonthoracotomy lead system. *J Am Coll Cardiol* 1997; 29(4):825–830.
25. Michelson BI, Iqel DA, Wilkoff BL. Adequacy of implantable cardioverter-defibrillator lead placement for tachyarrhythmia detection by sinus rhythm electrogram amplitude. *Am J Cardiol* 1995;76(16):1162–1166.
26. Schaumann A, von zur Muhlen F, Herse B, Gonska BD, Kreuzer H. Empirical versus tested antitachycardia pacing in implantable cardioverter defibrillators: A prospective study including 200 patients. *Circulation* 1998;97(1):66–74.
27. Wilkoff BL, Ousdigian KT, Sterns LD, Wang ZJ, Wilson RD, Morgan JM; EMPIRIC Trial Investigators. A comparison of empiric to physician-tailored programming of implantable cardioverter-defibrillators: Results from the prospective randomized multicenter EMPIRIC trial. *J Am Coll Cardiol* 2006;48(2):330–339.
28. Kroll MW. A minimal model of the single capacitor biphasic defibrillation waveform. *Pacing Clin Electrophysiol* 1994;17(11Pt. 1):1782–1792.
29. Kroll MW, Efimiv IR, Tchou PJ. Present understanding of shock polarity for internal defibrillation: The obvious and non-obvious clinical implications. *Pacing Clin Electrophysiol* 2006;29(8): 885–891.
30. Poelaert J, Jordaens L, Visser CA, De Clerck C, Herregods L. Transoesophageal echocardiographic evaluation of ventricular function during transvenous defibrillator implantation. *Acta Anaesthesiol Scand* 1996;40(8Pt. 1):913–918.
31. Runsio M, Bergfeldt L, Brodin LA, Ribeiro A, Samuelsson S, Rosenqvist M. Left ventricular function after repeated episodes of ventricular fibrillation and defibrillation assessed by transoesophageal echocardiography. *Eur Heart J* 1997;18(1):124–131.
32. Stoddard MF, Redd RR, Buckingham TA, McBride LR, Labovitz AJ. Effects of electrophysiologic testing of the automatic implantable cardioverter-defibrillator on left ventricular systolic function and diastolic filling. *Am Heart J* 1991;122(3Pt. 1):714–719.
33. Steinbeck G, Dorwarth U, Mattke S, Hoffmann E, Markewitz A, Kaulbach H, Tassani P. Hemodynamic deterioration during ICD implant: Predictors of high-risk patients. *Am Heart J* 1994;127(4Pt. 2):1064–1067.
34. Swerdlow CD, Martin DJ, Kass RM, Davie S, Mandel WJ, Gang ES, Chen PS. The zone of vulnerability to T wave shocks in humans. *J Cardiovasc Electrophysiol* 1997;8(2):145–154.
35. Strickberger SA, Man KC, Souza J, Zivin A, Weiss R, Knight BP, Goyal R, Daoud EG, Morady F. A prospective evaluation of two defibrillation safety margin techniques in patients with low defibrillation energy requirements. *J Cardiovasc Electrophysiol* 1998;9(1):41–46.
36. Gold MR, Breiter D, Leman R, Rashba EJ, Shorofsky SR, Hahn SJ. Safety of a single successful conversion of ventricular fibrillation before the implantation of cardioverter defibrillators. *Pacing Clin Electrophysiol* 2003;26:483–486.
37. Wetherbee JN, Chapman PD, Troup PJ, Veseth-Rogers J, Thakur RK, Almassi GH, Olinger GN. Long-term internal cardiac defibrillation threshold stability. *Pacing Clin Electrophysiol* 1989; 12(3):443–450.
38. Gold MR, Kavesh NG, Peters RW, Shorofsky SR. Biphasic waveforms prevent the chronic rise of defibrillation thresholds with a transvenous lead system. *J Am Coll Cardiol* 1997;30(1):233–236.
39. Tokano T, Pelosi F, Flemming M, Horwood L, Souza JJ, Zivin A, Knight BP, Goyal R, Man KC, Morady F, Strickberger SA. Long-term evaluation of the ventricular defibrillation energy requirement. *J Cardiovasc Electrophysiol* 1998;9(9):916–920.

51
Beyond Sudden Death Prevention: Minimizing Implantable Cardioverter Defibrillator Shocks and Morbidity and Optimizing Efficacy

Michael Glikson, David Luria, Osnat Gurevitz, and Paul A. Friedman

Introduction

Implantable cardioverter defibrillator shocks are the most effective way to immediately terminate life-threatening ventricular arrhythmias. Failed ICD shocks are rare with modern defibrillators. Large database analysis reveals that less than 2% of appropriate ICD therapies fail to terminate ventricular tachycardia or ventricular fibrillation (VT/VF) episodes.[1] Even among ICD recipients who die suddenly, device interrogation demonstrates ineffective shocks as the cause of death in only a minority of cases.[2,3]

Despite their effectiveness, ICD shocks are painful and are associated with significant morbidity, resulting in recurrent hospital admissions, anxiety, depression, and posttraumatic stress disorders.[4,5] In the Antiarrhythmics versus Implantable Defibrillators (AVID) trial, patients who received ICD shocks had a lower quality of life score than those who did not, with reduced physical functioning and mental well being.[6] When ICD shocks fail to terminate a supraventricular or ventricular arrhythmia, or arrhythmia immediately recurs triggering another shock, patients may receive repetitive discharges, an event termed "electrical storm." Electrical storm may occur in up to 10–20% of ICD recipients. The efficacy of β-adrenergic blockade and sedation in the therapy of electrical storm highlights the role of stress and the proarrhythmic effect of shocks themselves in promoting arrhythmia in this extremely stressful situation.[7–11]

While the consistent superiority of ICD therapy over medical therapy in prospective randomized clinical trials has made ICDs the de facto gold standard therapy in preventing sudden cardiac death, minimizing shock delivery is paramount. There are four strategies for minimizing ICD shocks while maintaining their efficacy: (1) programming VT/VF therapies to prevent shock delivery for nonsustained VT, (2) using painless antitachycardia pacing (ATP) instead of shock liberally, (3) preventing VT/VF by means of adjuvant therapies (drugs and/or ablation), and (4) using detection enhancements to prevent inappropriate shocks for SVT. The first part of this chapter will review these strategies in detail. The second section will review minimizing morbidity associated with "recalls," and minimizing morbidity associated with chronic right ventricular (RV) pacing. Proper device programming and postimplant care can profoundly influence the quality of life in ICD recipients.

Minimizing Shocks for Nonsustained Ventricular Arrhythmias

Nonsustained VT (NSVT) is a self-terminating arrhythmia that is usually well tolerated and should not be shocked. In early ICDs, therapy was committed after initial arrhythmia detection, irrespective of arrhythmia termination before charge end ("committed" shocks). In subsequent devices, programmable reconfirmation features enabled

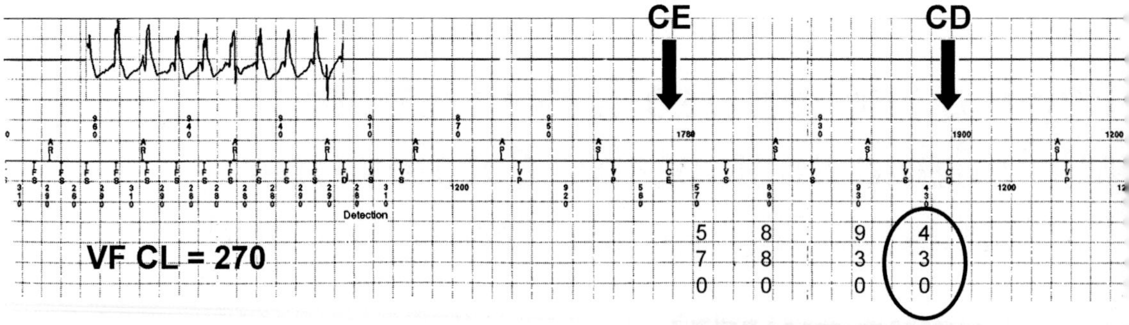

FIGURE 51–1. Shock for nonsustained VT in an old Medtronic device. The case involves a 60-year-old man with ischemic cardiomyopathy and recurrent NSVT who had a Medtronic DDD ICD (GEM DR) implanted. The VT cutoff was programmed at 400 msec. On the night following implantation he received several shocks for nonsustained VTs at a cycle length of 270. Interrogation of one of the episodes is shown here. In old Medtronic devices there is no reconfirmation during charging. When the charge ends (CE+ arrow) there is a 300-msec blanking period; following this even one out of the next four beats that falls within the VTCL+ 60 msec range (= 460 in this case) is considered a reconfirmation of ongoing tachycardia. Unfortunately, the fourth interval here was 430, therefore a shock was delivered (CD+ arrow).

abortion of shock delivery if the arrhythmia terminated prior to the end of charging. Reconfirmation is necessarily "trigger happy" so that even a few intervals shorter (faster) than the VT interval (St. Jude and Guidant) or 60 msec > VT interval (Medtronic) result in shock delivery. Thus, a single ventricular premature complex (VPC) or oversensed complex during the reconfirmation period can result in a shock (Figure 51–1).[12–14] Additionally, this results in a hidden interaction in that the first VF shock is functionally committed if a long VT interval is programmed. The reconfirmation algorithm most commonly applies to the first shock only, making all redected tachyarrhythmias committed.

In the most current ICD models, the sensing channel continues to monitor the rhythm during device charging and is able to recognize arrhythmia termination at any point in time to prevent unnecessary shocks. In older generation Guidant and Biotronik devices the absence of signal on the ventricular channel (i.e., asystole) after VT termination or charge end does not abort device therapy in order to avoid nondetection of fine VF. This necessarily leads to inappropriate shock after termination of nonsustained VT in pacemaker-dependent patients. In newer Biotronik devices, programming of the "fine VF" feature overcomes this limitation; newer Guidant (Boston Scientific CRM) devices no longer shock during asystole, but rather pace. While not an issue with current generation pulse generators, in older models recurrent intractable shocks due to nonsustained VT in a pacemaker-dependent patient may require pulse generator change out (Figure 51–2).

Nonsustained VT that triggers ICD therapy is common.[15] A first line of defense against inappropriate therapy for nonsustained VT or sustained ventricular tachycardia (SVT) is an appropriately long detection interval.[16] Use of a relatively long fast VT detection time (18 of 24 intervals) resulted in a high frequency of fast VT episode termination (34%) before shock delivery in the Painfree Rx II trial without significant detection delay.[17] In patients with frequent and long episodes of nonsustained VF (e.g., long QT syndrome) or rapid VT, the longer detection should be considered. While excessive delays in detection may result in syncope, increased defibrillation threshold, or undersensing of VF, these are rare for VF lasting under 30 sec.

Antitachycardia Pacing

Painless ATP terminates up to 90% of VT episodes,[18–20] with a risk of acceleration requiring shock of 1–5%.[21] Routine electrophysiological testing to tailor ATP is not necessary.[21–25] Noninducibility of VT does not exclude subsequent clinical episodes that are often successfully termi-

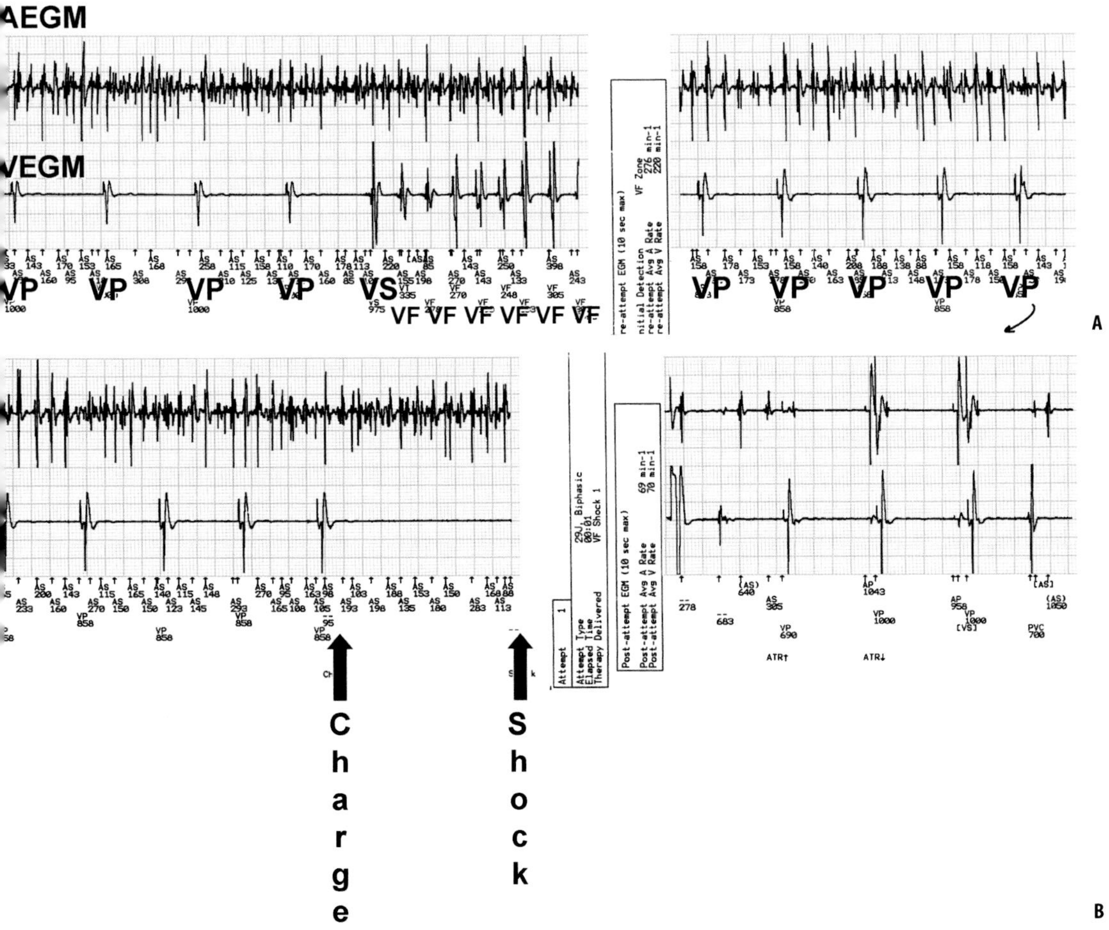

FIGURE 51–2. Shock for nonsustained VT in an old Guidant device. The case involves a 72-year-old man with SSS + VTs with a Prizm DR ICD, admitted with recurrent shocks. The patient is pacing dependent. (A and B) Taken from interrogation of one of the episodes, with an atrial electrogram (EGM) (in AF) on the top channel, a ventricular channel in the middle, and EGMs on the bottom channel. (A) A run of nonsustained fast VT detected in the VF zone; thus charging is initiated. (B) The end of charging (first arrow); the device then attempts to reconfirm VF. When there is no underlying ventricular activity, this device has a safety feature that results in a shock (second arrow). Due to repeated similar episodes the device had to be replaced with a newer model.

nated by ATP. Additionally, programming empiric ATP at implantation is as successful as physician tailored ATP in preventing ICD shocks.[26]

ATP can be delivered as "bursts" (a sequence of pacing pulses delivered at the same cycle length) or "ramps" (the cycle length shortens within the pulse train). The efficacy and safety profile of various ATP algorithms have been extensively studied[18,21,23,27] and can be summarized as follows. (1) Burst and ramp have a similar efficacy. (2) The coupling interval and rate of ATP within the commonly used clinical range of 69–88% of tachycardia cycle length do not significantly affect efficacy. (3) The first ATP attempt is the most effective (up to 80%); in treating slow, relatively stable VTs up to six ATPs may be programmed; in treating faster VTs in the VF zone [heart rate (HR) > 185 bpm] ATP is generally limited to one to two sequences of eight pulses.

Patient and arrhythmia characteristics determine ATP outcomes. The lower the ejection fraction and the faster the VT the lower the likelihood of arrhythmia termination and the higher the risk of acceleration.[17,21,28,29] Sinus tachycardia before VT is associated with diminished ATP efficacy.[30] Medical therapy (β blockers, antiarrhythmic

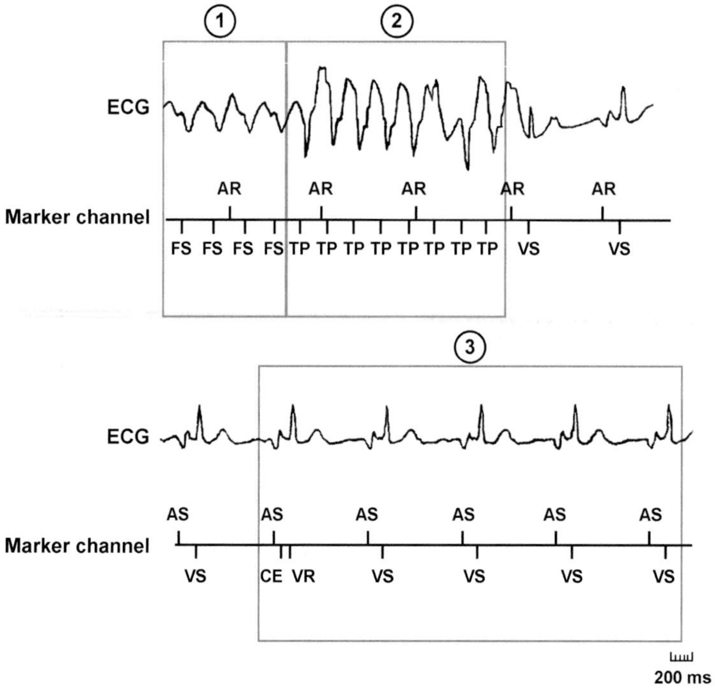

FIGURE 51–3. Antitachycardia pacing during charge in a Medtronic Entrust ICD. (1) The device detects a fast ventricular rate as VF (FS markers then FD marker when VF is detected) and starts charging the capacitors for defibrillation therapy. (2) While charging, the device delivers one sequence of burst ATP therapy (TP markers), which terminates the tachyarrhythmia. (3) After charging is completed (CE marker), the device aborts the defibrillation therapy, because VF is not confirmed. (Courtesy Medtronic Inc.)

drugs) has a synergistic effect with ATP, likely by slowing the VT rate in the case of membrane-active drugs. Antitachycardia pacing is equally effective in ischemic and nonischemic cardiomyopathy.[17,30] Clinical data show that 90% of fast VT (up to 250 bpm) can be successfully terminated by two ATP bursts (eight pulses, 88% of VT cycle length) with a low risk of acceleration (4%) or syncope (2%).[17,29] We routinely program one or two empiric ATP bursts in a fast VT zone (between 200 and 250 bpm), and use additional bursts in slower VT zones in patients with known slow VTs. In devices that support ATP delivery during charge (such as the Medtronic Entrust™) this feature is routinely programmed on (Figure 51–3).

Adjunctive Therapies to Prevent Ventricular Arrhythmias

Antiarrhythmic Drug Therapy

Antiarrhythmic drugs (AAD) are used in up to 50% of ICD recipients to alleviate symptoms of arrhythmia and minimize device shocks.[31,32] The efficacy and safety of various membrane-active drugs in preventing ICD shocks have been the subject of prospective randomized trials.[31,33,34] In one study, sotalol resulted in a 44% relative risk reduction of death or first ICD shock for any reason compared to placebo. Sotalol's effectiveness was similar in patients with moderate and with severe left ventricle dysfunction. The mean frequency of ICD shocks was reduced from 3.9 ± 10.7 in the placebo group to 1.4 ± 3.5 in the sotalol group.[31] However, when compared "head to head" with amiodarone and β blockers in the Optimal Pharmacological Therapy in Implantable Converter (OPTIC) study, sotalol was less effective in preventing ICD shocks than amiodarone, and had only borderline advantage over β blockers alone. After 1 year follow-up, shocks occurred in 38.5% patients treated with β blocker alone, 24.3% of those treated with sotalol and 10% of those receiving amiodarone plus β blocker (Figure 51–4). However, frequent shocks (more than 10 shocks during 1 year or more than two shocks within 24 h) occurred five times less frequently in both sotalol and amiodarone groups compared to β blocker therapy alone.[33] A new agent, azimilide, with potassium channel blocking properties (I_{Kr}

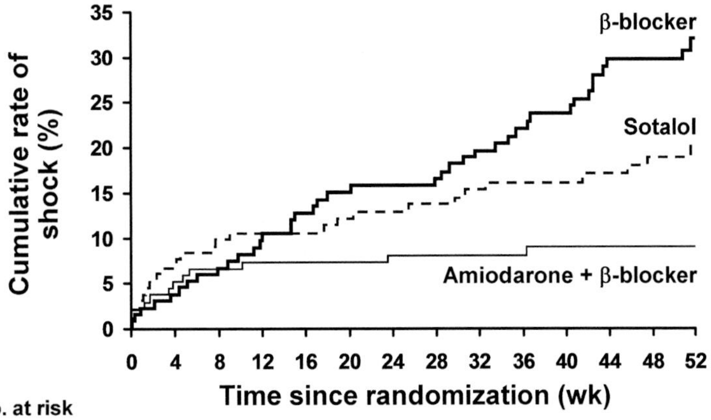

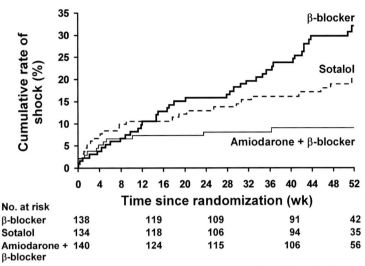

No. at risk					
β-blocker	138	119	109	91	42
Sotalol	134	118	106	94	35
Amiodarone + β-blocker	140	124	115	106	56

Log-rank P<0.001 for amiodarone + β-blocker alone; log-rank P=0.02 for amiodarone + β-blocker vs sotalol alone; log-rank P=0.055 for sotalol vs β-blocker

FIGURE 51–4. Cumulative rate of shocks for the three treatment groups in the OPTIC trial. (Reproduced from Connolly *et al.*,[33] with permission from the American Medical Association.)

and I_{Ks}), reduced total symptomatic ventricular arrhythmia by 50% and reduced hospitalizations. However, the total number of ICD shocks was not affected.[34]

The benefit of membrane-active drugs in preventing shocks must be carefully balanced against the risk of adverse effects. Since most ICD recipients have significant left ventricle dysfunction, they are prone to proarrhythmia and heart failure exacerbation by many agents. Indeed, controlled studies demonstrate a high frequency of AAD discontinuation due to suspected side effects: at 1 year follow-up, sotalol was stopped in about 25% of patients, amiodarone in 18%, and azimilide in 35%.[31,33,34] Of note, torsade de pointes occurred only rarely in these studies and when present was successfully treated by the ICD. Although Class Ic antiarrhythmic drugs (flecainide, propafenone) have not been well tested in ICD patients, they are generally avoided in the setting of left ventricular dysfunction due to their negative inotropy and increased risk of proarrhythmia in that setting.

Drug–device interactions occur when antiarrhythmic drugs affect ICD function. Common effects that must be considered include slowing of the VT rate below the programmed detection rate[35,36] or facilitation of arrhythmia termination by painless ATP, minimizing shock risk.[37] Antiarrhythmic drugs may also modify the defibrillation threshold and thus may facilitate (sotalol) or jeopardize (amiodarone) successful defibrillation.[38–40] While this issue has been the focus of extensive attention in the past, with current technology defibrillation is sufficiently effective that it is of little importance except for the minority of patients with borderline defibrillation function.[41,42]

In summary, the potential complexity of membrane-active drug use in ICD recipients precludes their *routine* use for primary shock prevention in patients receiving prophylactic ICDs. Membrane-active drugs are commonly used in patients with clinical arrhythmia, especially those with recurrent sustained monomorphic VT, which carries a high risk of recurrence and shock.[32,43] When membrane-active drugs are added, the VT detection interval is lengthened by 30–40 msec and defibrillation threshold testing is often performed. Importantly, other commonly used cardiovascular drugs (β blockers, angiotensin-receptor antagonists, statins, diuretics) have little or no effect on ICD function and are routinely used due to their demonstrated mortality benefit across broad populations of cardiovascular disease patients.

Radiofrequency Catheter Ablation of Ventricular Tachycardia

Percutaneous transcatheter ablation of VT/VF has become an important adjuvant therapy in the management of ICD recipients by decreasing shock burden in patients with recurrent VT.[44–49] While originally limited to targeting sustained hemodynamically stable VT,[50,51] innovations in ablation technology have enabled successful ablation of even rapid "unmappable" arrhythmias, resulting in an over 90% reduction of appropriate ICD therapies.[52–54] This progress has been facilitated by the development of advanced three-dimensional mapping systems that permit localization of scar tissue and ablation during sinus rhythm. Consequently, the role of VT ablation has expanded correspondingly from the very symptomatic multidrug-resistant arrhythmias initially treated. Indeed, the role of prophylactic ablation was assessed in the Substart Mapping and Ablation in Sinus Rhythm to Halt Ventricular Tachycardia (SMASH VT) study.[55] This trial randomized patients with old myocardial infarction who had an ICD implanted for VT/VF to "prophylactic" VT ablation or no therapy. Patients in the ablation arm had a 50% reduction in appropriate ICD therapies over 2 years of follow-up. Another novel approach, proposed by Haissaguerre *et al.*, applies ablation to polymorphic VT and VF by targeting the focus that gives rise to triggering premature contractions foci within the Purkinje system.[28] These foci have been shown to be responsible for initiation of the life-threatening arrhythmia after myocardial infarction[43] and in patients with Brugada and long QT syndromes.[56,57]

Although most studies of VT ablation in ICD recipients enrolled patients with ischemic cardiomyopathy, there are now several encouraging reports of successful ablation with diminution of ICD therapies in patients with dilated cardiomyopathy and with arrhythmogenic RV dysplasia.[54,58–60] In these clinical situations, however, ablation procedures are more challenging and might require RV and/or epicardial mapping and ablation.

It needs to be emphasized that most reports on the efficacy and safety of VT ablation in ICD recipients are small observational studies, reflecting the experience of a handful of leading centers. The broad applicability to clinical practice requires further study via randomized controlled multicenter trials. At present, VT ablation typically is reserved for the symptomatic repetitively shocked patient who has failed antiarrhythmic drugs. Ablation techniques have been used successfully to treat electrical storm, albeit at a higher risk of complications and mortality.[11,61,62] The role of ablation is discussed further in this volume, Chapter 56. Rarely, when drugs and ablation fail to prevent multiple ICD discharges during intractable VT/VF storm, cardiac assist devices can be life saving, providing a "bridge" to cardiac transplantation.[63–65]

Minimizing Inappropriate Shocks: Sustained Ventricular Tachycardia Discrimination

Inappropriate therapies delivered for nonventricular arrhythmias have always been the Achilles' heel of ICD therapy.[6,17] The problem affects 8–40% of ICD recipients,[66–70] has a deleterious effect on quality of life, and has a potential for proarrhythmia.[71–73] Supraventricular rhythms, particularly sinus tachycardia and atrial fibrillation (AF), are the most common cause of inappropriate shocks. SVT-VT discriminators are algorithms that are applied for heart rates bounded on the slower end by the VT detection interval and on the faster end by a programmable minimum cycle length, to cover the range of heart rates at which both VT and SVT can occur. Ideally, these algorithms reject supraventricular arrhythmias (i.e., increase the specificity of detection) without affecting the ability to detect VT (sensitivity). In practice, these algorithms are most commonly applied to the "slower VTs" (heart rates 140–190 bpm) for which a small delay in detection to enhance specificity is often acceptable. Time limiters are available in most devices, which override discrimination algorithms to force therapy delivery if arrhythmia persists longer than the programmed time limit. Algorithm specifics vary among manufacturers, but in general terms can be divided based on those requiring only ventricular information (single-chamber algorithms) and those utilizing information from the atria and ventricles to diagnose a rhythm.

Single-Chamber Algorithms

In single-chamber ICDs, algorithms use only ventricular information to distinguish SVT from VT.

They do so by analyzing the patterns of detected ventricular intervals (onset and stability) or by comparison of tachycardia electrogram characteristics to a baseline template (morphology).

Onset

The onset algorithm prevents inappropriate detection of sinus tachycardia by defining VT as a tachycardia with an abrupt onset. This is in contrast to the gradual onset present during sinus tachycardia. Onset has been extensively studied and found to provide a high sensitivity and acceptable specificity.[74,75] Nevertheless, due to its limitations, it is best used in combination with other discriminators.[76–78] Limitations include misdiagnosis of exercise-induced VT (that evolves from sinus tachycardia and thus appears "gradual" in onset) and of SVTs with abrupt onset such as atrial fibrillation (AF) (that are thus classified as VT). Additionally, since this algorithm bases its determination on a single event (arrhythmia onset), it does not get a second chance to "get it right."

Stability

The stability algorithm differentiates VT (stable, regular R-R intervals) from AF ("unstable," variable R-R intervals). Figure 51–5 depicts stability algorithm function. In contrast to onset, stability continually reassesses a tachycardia initially defined as AF (due to interval variability) and rediagnoses it as VT should it become regular. As with the onset algorithm, it is best used in combination with other detection enhancements.[74–77] Ventricular tachycardias with variable cycle length and SVTs with stable intervals defeat this algorithm. Importantly, since R-R intervals in AF are more regular at faster rates, interval stability cannot reliably discriminate AF from VT at rates over 170 bpm.[74,79]

Morphology

Morphology criteria compare the intracardiac QRS recorded during tachycardia to an intracardiac QRS template acquired during sinus rhythm. A tachycardia morphology sufficiently different than the sinus template indicates VT. This technique simulates the clinical approach of electrocardiogram (ECG) arrhythmia diagnosis by visual analysis of the QRS morphology. It necessarily misclassifies rate-related bundle branch block during SVT as VT. Due to electrogram morphology distortions by a delivered shock, morphology is not applied during redection. Used in combination with onset and stability, morphology further improves discrimination function.

Various manufacturers have adopted different approaches to morphology algorithms. The Medtronic Wavelet™[80] algorithm is based on a wavelet transformation of the ECG at baseline and during arrhythmia, which is mathematically compared for fit. Its sensitivity and specificity at nominal settings have been reported as 100% and 78%, respectively.[80] It has replaced an older QRS width-based algorithm that was less reliable.[81] Morphology-based algorithms will likely continue to evolve.

The Guidant Rhythm ID™ morphology algorithm is based on comparing the timing and correlation of rate and shock channel electrograms during arrhythmia and in sinus rhythm. The far-field electrogram, which by its nature has more morphology information due to its use of a wider "antenna" for signal acquisition, is used for morphometric comparison. The sharper near-field rate-sensing signal, with its greater slew, is used to ensure appropriate electrogram alignment. It has been shown to have 99% sensitivity and 97% specificity when used in single-chamber settings in laboratory settings.[82] Its "real life" results were 100% sensitivity for VT/VF and 92% specificity for SVT.[83] Clinical experience with this algorithm is presently limited.

The St. Jude Morphology Discrimination (MD™) algorithm is based on a match score between near-field electrogram complexes during arrhythmia and a near-field template, where the score is derived from differences in the direction and amplitude of the various electrogram deflections. Electrograms are modeled using polygons, facilitating computations. We[76,84,85] and others[86,87] have found it improves the specificity of VT detection, but is best used in combination with other algorithms to avoid a degradation in sensitivity (Figure 51–6).[76,84,85,87] The modes of morphology algorithm failure have been described[16] and are listed in Table 51–1.

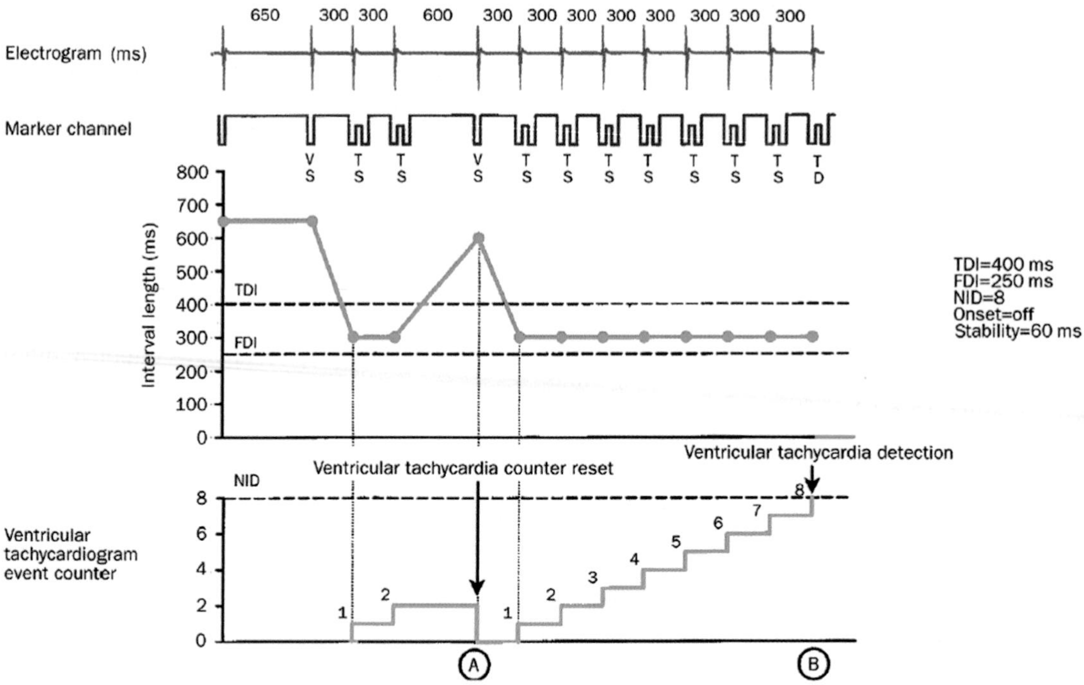

A

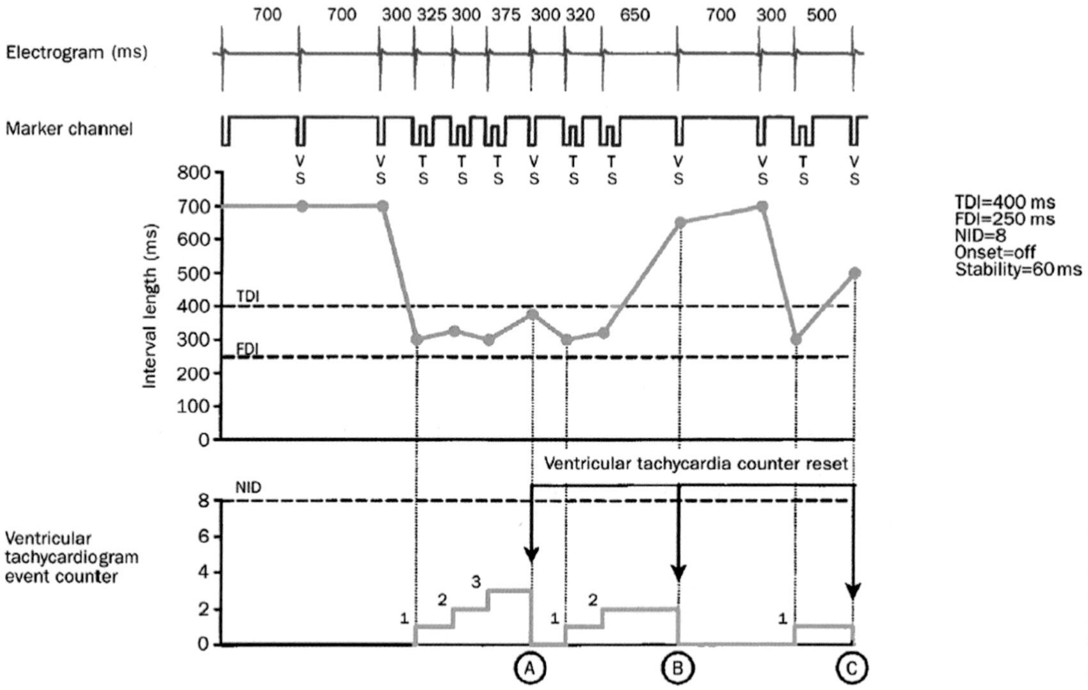

B

FIGURE 51–5. Detection of ventricular tachycardia and stability enhancement. (A) Detection of an episode of tachycardia. Dashed lines show the tachycardia detection interval (TDI) and fibrillation detection interval (FDI). Intervals are labeled as VS in the normal heart rate zone and TS when they are shorter than the TDI. The third electrogram occurs at a cycle length of 300 msec, which is less (faster) than the programmed TDI of 400 msec, incrementing the counter to 1. At point A, the counter is reset to zero by a sensed interval of 600 msec, which is longer than the TDI. At point B, tachycardia is detected, since the eight consecutive intervals that are faster than the TDI mean that the counter reaches the programmed number of intervals to detect tachycardia (NID). Depending upon the type of treatment programmed, antitachycardia pacing or shock delivery would begin at this point. (B) The stability criterion to prevent inappropriate detection of tachycardia for fast atrial fibrillation. Tachycardia counting begins with the first fast interval (300 msec). At point A the counter is reset to zero since the cycle length of 375 msec, although less (faster) than the TDI, is more than 60 msec greater. (Reproduced from Glikson M, Friedman PA. The implantable cardioverter defibrillator. *Lancet* 2001;357:1107–1117.)

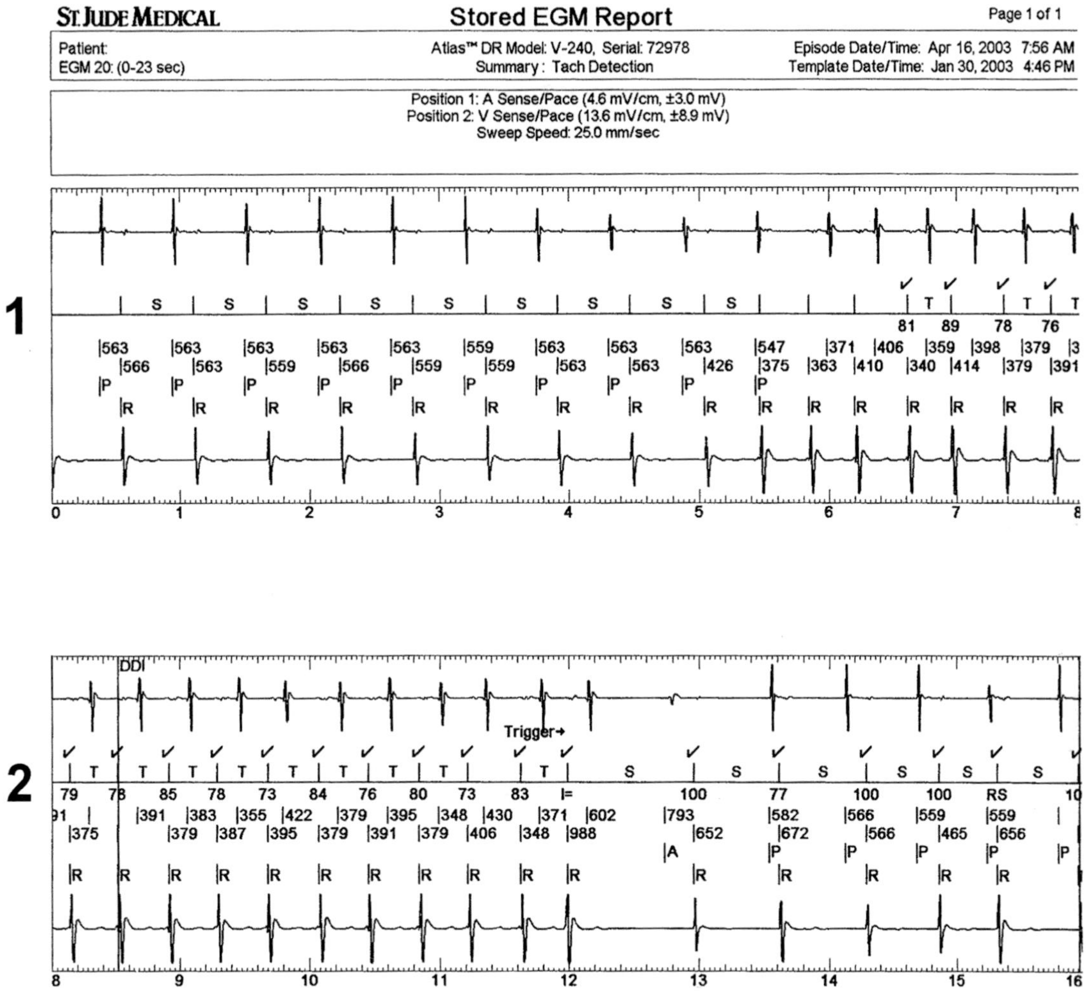

FIGURE 51–6. Morphology algorithm error. An electrogram of an episode of VT. There are two consecutive recordings marked 1 and 2. Each one shows the atrial channel on the top, markers in the middle, and ventricular channel on the bottom. At the end of recording 1 VT starts (VT is clearly diagnosed by its initiation in the ventricle on the top recording). There is a wrong template match that suggests SVT (marked by the V signs above the complexes), therefore therapy is withheld, until the episode terminated spontaneously in the middle of recording 2.

Dual-Chamber Algorithms

Dual-chamber algorithms utilize information collected simultaneously from the atria and ventricles, with the goal of using the additional (atrial) information to improve specificity. They add atrial rate information to standard ventricular only algorithms, or compare the relative timing of atrial and ventricular events during arrhythmia. For example, stability is applied only after the atria are confirmed to be in AF (Guidant) or only when the atrial rate is faster than the ventricular rate (St. Jude). In St. Jude devices, stability has also been fortified by the addition of the atrioventricular (AV) association (AVA) criterion for dual-chamber devices. The AVA algorithm differentiates VT from regular SVT with 2:1 conduction (such as atrial flutter) by recognition of a constant AV interval in the case of regular SVT. When AVA is operational, stable tachycardias with constant AV intervals will not be detected as VT despite their cycle length regularity.

TABLE 51–1. Modes of morphology algorithm failure.

Type of morphology failure	Mechanism	Correction
Inaccurate template	Change in baseline electrogram due to lead maturation or intermittent bundle branch block, or recording of template during abnormal rhythm	Apply automatic template updates or use
Electrogram truncation (clipping)	Recorded electrogram signal exceeds sense amplifier range, altering its morphology	Adjust amplitude scale (Medtronic and SJM) so electrograms are 25–75% of dynamic range available
Alignment errors	Misalignment between tachycardia electrogram and template leads to miscalculation of "match" score	Eliminate clipping and/or change electrogram source (Medtronic), atrially pace at rapid rate to assess sensing (SJM)
Oversensing of pectoral myopotentials	Myopotentials distort the electrogram, altering its morphology	Change the electrogram source; this affects only algorithms utilizing far-field electrograms (Medtronic, SJM)
Rate-related aberrancy	Morphology of electrograms change during sustained ventricular tachycardia due to refractoriness (nonexcitability) of part of the conduction system	If reproducible, record the template during rapid atrial pacing (while aberrancy is present) and turn off autotemplate update; adjust the match score to allow greater variability before defining ventricular tachycardia; turn off morphology
SVT immediately following shocks	Shocks lead to transient distortion of morphology	Morphology is not used for redection

Specific Dual-Chamber Algorithms

The Guidant algorithm uses the principle that an arrhythmia with ventricular rate greater than atrial rate is always VT, and also added AF in the atrium as a condition for operation of the stability criterion. The Medtronic algorithm (PR logic and enhanced PR logic) is based on analyzing the pattern of the timing of atrial and ventricular events to define the arrhythmia mechanism. For example, a tachycardia with 1:1 retrograde atrial conduction and a short VA interval is defined as VT, and other characteristic patterns are used to define various other arrhythmias. Its sensitivity for VT has been reported as 100% with a positive predictive accuracy and specificity for VT just below 80%.[88,89]

The St. Jude algorithm assigns tachycardias to one of three branches based on the relative rates in the atrium and in the ventricle ($V = A$, $V > A$, $V < A$) and then selectively applies detection enhancements (morphology, stability, and onset) in the $V = A$ and $V < A$ branches. If $V > A$, enhancements are not applied, and therapy is immediately delivered, eliminating up to 80% of tachycardias from evaluation and possible algorithm errors. Different combinations of enhancers and logic are programmably applied depending on branch assignment, significantly influencing device performance, resulting in a wide range of sensitivity and specificity results.[84,86,87] We found a sensitivity of 99% and specificity approaching 80% with the "best" nominal combination; performance may be improved when tailored to the individual patient. Similar results were reported with the use of Biotronik SMART[90] and the ELA Parad+ algorithms.[91]

Single Versus Dual-Chamber Algorithms

Intuitively, dual-chamber algorithms, which use atrial and ventricular intracardiac information to diagnose a rhythm, should be superior to single-chamber, ventricular- only detection enhancements. However, early nonrandomized studies and subsequent small randomized trials failed to show any superiority of dual-chamber over single-chamber diagnosis.[66–68] Some employed very early algorithms, which have since been refined; however, the single most common failure mode for dual-chamber algorithms has been atrial sensing malfunction.[66] In a recent carefully designed prospective randomized clinical trial we compared dual-chamber to single-chamber detec-

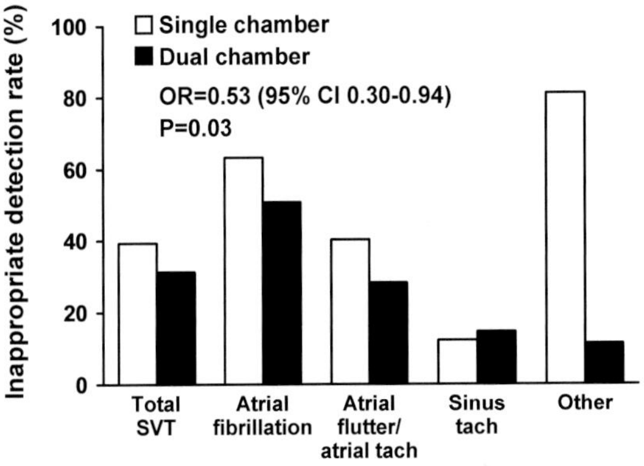

FIGURE 51–7. Results of the detect SVT trial.[93] Rate of inappropriate detection of SVT demonstrating the advantage of dual-chamber over single-chamber detection, with breakdown by arrhythmia subtype [atrial fibrillation, atrial flutter/atrial tachycardia (tach), sinus tachycardia, or other], for subjects with single- or dual-chamber detection. "Other" arrhythmias include atrial tachycardia, junctional tachycardia, AV nodal reentrant tachycardia, and AV reentrant tachycardia. Subtype classification was based on a blinded episode reviewer. The odds ratio (OR) and probability value refer only to the overall comparison of inappropriate detection of SVT. (Reproduced from Friedman *et al.*,[93] with permission, from the American Heart Association.)

tion in 400 recipients of St. Jude dual-chamber ICDs and found that dual-chamber programming of study-specified nominal values significantly reduced inappropriate detection of SVT as VT.[92,93] Careful attention was paid to atrial lead function at implant and during follow-up. We therefore believe that properly programmed dual-chamber ICDs provide better discrimination of SVTs from VTs (Figure 51–7) than single-chamber devices. This advantage may further improve when programming is tailored individually rather than nominally.

Management of Abandoned Leads

Due to lead failure requiring new lead placement,[94,95] or system upgrade from pacemaker to ICD,[96] inactive leads frequently must be left behind or extracted. Either approach may have associated morbidity. Abandoned leads may theoretically shunt current during defibrillation, create "contact" noise affecting new lead function, and promote vascular occlusion. Alternatively, extraction of abandoned leads carries procedural morbidity and mortality.

Evidence for the deleterious effects of abandoned leads on detection has been largely anecdotal.[97] We recently reviewed our experience in a series of 78 ICD recipients with abandoned leads, and found no evidence of electrical interference with detection or defibrillation by the abandoned lead.[98] It has been suggested that the presence of multiple leads contributes to venous occlusion.[99,100] However, this must be balanced against extraction risks, including the thrombogenicity of disrupted endothelium and lead fragments, the laceration of great vessels, and the creation of electrical noise caused by incompletely extracted fragments with disrupted insulation.[100–107] Figure 51–8 demonstrates a case of intractable noise created by a lead damaged during an extraction attempt. The noise inhibited pacing and was falsely detected as VF.

We believe that the decision to abandon or extract leads should be tailored, depending on operator experience and specific clinical circumstance. Leads should be removed if they create noise, if the venous system is blocked, if there is a system-related infection, or if they are easily removed by an experienced operator, particularly in younger patients. Extraction should be avoided in the asymptomatic older patient with no abandoned lead-related complications.

Management of Implantable Cardioverter Defibrillator Recalls and Alerts

Despite their overall high level of reliability, over the years there have been periodic safety alerts and "recalls" of ICDs affecting thousands of patients. Patient concern about ICD recalls and alerts adversely affects quality of life.[108] The number of pacemakers and ICDs affected has increased dramatically since 1995, probably due to increased awareness, greater enforcement of reporting policy, reports by the lay press, and increased device complexity. Malfunction rates for ICDs have recently reached a peak according to a multiregistry meta-analysis[109] and resulted in

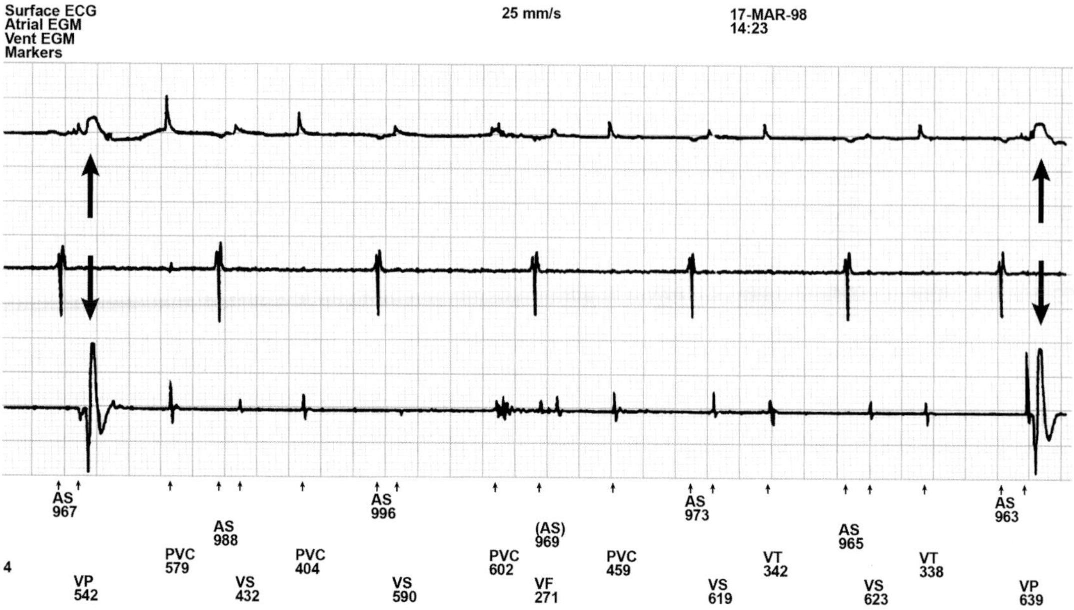

FIGURE 51–8. Noise created by a partially extracted lead. Channels show from top to bottom the surface ECG, the atrial channel with regular sinus activity, the ventricular channel, and the marker channel. Only the complexes marked by arrows represent effective ventricular pacing. All other ventricular events are actually noise signals that inhibit pacing. The noise is strong enough to be seen on the surface ECG as well. (Reproduced from Friedman *et al.*,[102] with permission, from the Futura Publication Company.)

up to 36 replacements per 1000 patient years in its peak during 2001.[110] Such advisories lead to more intensive follow-up and surgical device replacement. They involve tremendous cost to and burden on the health care system and operative morbidity and mortality for patients.[111] The morbidity associated with device replacement is higher than in new implantation procedures and in some "recall" events likely exceeded the morbidity caused by the device malfunctions themselves. A similar phenomenon occurred in the past with the Accufix lead recall, which resulted in more deaths related to extractions than to the injury by the lead malfunction.[112]

Documents published by professional societies provide guidance for the management of device alerts and recalls that aim to detect problems early, to minimize patients' confusion by providing timely and appropriate information, and to avoid unnecessary device replacements.[113,114]

Suggested methods of increasing patient safety while minimizing inconvenience and anxiety include the following:

1. More frequent follow-up of devices that are not replaced.
2. More widespread use of automatic alerts and home monitoring systems for early detection of malfunctions in patients with devices under alert.
3. Efficient, quick, and responsible communication between manufacturers, Physicians, and patients so that relevant information will reach patients through their care givers rather than via mass media.

Recommended measures to decrease unnecessary device replacements include the following:

1. Careful individual risk assessment taking into account not only the probability of intrinsic device failure but also the potential consequences of failure related to current device indication in the individual patient. For instance, a pacemaker-dependent ICD patient with recurrent life-threatening arrhythmia is at much higher risk in the event of device failure than a patient implanted for primary prevention of sudden death. The concept of *current* device indication (as opposed

o original indication for implantation) is important as the clinical condition may have changed since implantation with newly developed arrhythmias or pacemaker dependence.

2. The risks of the replacement operation should also be weighed in the individual patient as should the remaining time to elective replacement of the device.[113] Overall, a risk of malfunction below 1/1000 is considered low when considering replacement in a patient who is not at a special high risk if the device malfunctions.[114]

3. In some specific situations, consideration of alternative noninvasive measures of management, such as reprogramming, frequent monitoring, or daily magnet application, may be applicable.

Given the small risk of device malfunction in most circumstances, the physician must allay patient anxiety and confusion and objectively balance the risk of operation with continued observation. New guidelines are expected in the near future as are new systems for reporting and communication of device failures.

Pacing Morbidity: Minimizing Right Ventricular Pacing

The detrimental role of RV pacing was initially suggested by trials comparing ventricular-based (VVI) and atrial-based (AAI) pacing systems.[115,116] Long-term follow-up demonstrated less AF, less heart failure, and improved survival with atrial pacing compared to ventricular pacing. Subsequently, the Dual Chamber VVI Implantable Defibrillator (DAVID) study demonstrated an increase in composite endpoints of mortality and hospitalization for heart failure in ICD recipients with dual-chamber pacing at 70 bpm as compared to VVI 40 back-up pacing.[117] The frequency of RV pacing was directly correlated with worse outcome in this study.[118] These findings have been supported by analysis of Multicenter Automatic Defibrillator Implantation Trial II (MADIT II) results,[119] by the Multicenter Unsustained Tachycardia Trial (MUSTT),[120] and by other studies.[120,121] Patients with depressed ventricular function are at greater risk for deterioration. Right ventricular pacing induces cardiac dyssynchronization and ventricular remodeling (pacemaker-induced cardiomyopathy) that increase heart failure symptoms.[122,123]

Most ICD recipients have impaired LV function and some degree of heart failure, and are therefore at risk for clinical deterioration by RV pacing. For this reason, efforts should be made to minimize RV pacing in this population. In patients without an indication for pacing, programming the ICD setting to back up low-rate pacing at 40 bpm (VVI 40) seems to be a reasonable solution.[117] In a small subset of patients, chronotropic incompetence and sinus bradycardia aggravated by the use of β blockers and antiarrhythmic drugs may necessitate antibradycardia support. Use of a dual-chamber pacing mode with a long AV delay prevents ventricular pacing when AV conduction is preserved. In this case, potential side effects of pacing with long AV delay need to be considered. These include the following: (1) the long AV delay may permit retrograde ventriculoatrial conduction (due to recovery of AV nodal refractoriness) and increase the risk of pacemaker-mediated tachycardia; (2) prolonged atrial blanking may cause undersensing of AF or flutter, adversely affecting mode switch; (3) the upper pacing and tracking rate is lowered as the AV delay lengthens; and (4) negative hemodynamic consequences of long AV conduction may be poorly tolerated by some patients.

Algorithms have been developed that promote intrinsic AV conduction, while providing ventricular pacing support when needed. The AV Search Hysteresis (Guidant Inc)[124] and Autointrinsic Conduction Search (St. Jude Medical) algorithms are aimed at minimizing ventricular pacing by automatic periodic prolongation of the AV interval to search for intrinsic AV conduction (Figure 51-9). When intrinsic conduction is detected, the AV delay remains prolonged. When a ventricular-paced event occurs at the prolonged AV delay, the AV delay is returned to a shorter physiological AV delay. The limitations of these algorithms are related to their intermittent activation and restriction of the maximal AV interval to predefined maximal values. In addition, all of the potential side effects of DDD programming with a long AV interval can occur, albeit less frequently. A recently published trial demonstrated the utility of AV search hysteresis in significantly decreasing the number of ventricular paced events.[124]

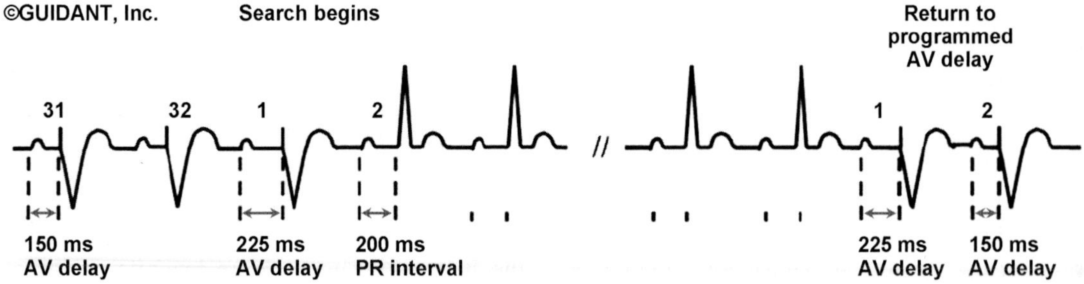

Figure 51–9. Atrioventricular search hysteresis. See the text for explanation. (Reproduced from Olshansky *et al.*,[124] with permission.)

Another approach to minimize unnecessary ventricular pacing is the use of an AAI pacing mode. In some ICD models it can be combined with postshock dual-chamber pacing to allay the concern about postshock conduction abnormalities. However, the risk of unpredictable AV conduction deterioration in ICD patients who frequently required drugs with negative chronotropic effects needs to be considered. For this reason, a novel algorithm [Managed ventricular pacing (MVP) mode, Medtronic] was developed to minimize ventricular pacing. This algorithm provides AAI pacing mode with safety dual-chamber ventricular pacing backup when transient or persistent AV block occurs. During AAI pacing loss of AV conduction in two of four A-A intervals initiates a switch to DDD mode with physiological AV delay (Figure 51–10). A subsequent "conduction check" by inhibition of tracking for one beat allows the detection of return of intrinsic AV conduction, with a switch back of the pacing mode to AAI. Initial clinical experience demonstrated the high efficacy of this algorithm in decreasing ventricular pacing by ICD.[125]

In patients with LV dysfunction and an anticipated high frequency of ventricular pacing, consideration is given to implanting cardiac resynchronization therapy (CRT) defibrillator pacing.[126,127] By pacing both ventricles, CRT mitigates or eliminates the deleterious effects of RV pacing. The role of alternate site RV pacing, para-Hisian pacing, or multisite RV pacing, if any, is not clear.[128] Despite several studies addressing the issue of CRT in patients who need pacing support but who lack a currently accepted CRT indication,[129–131] device selection in this population is not resolved. We favor the use of CRT in patients with ventricular dysfunction who will require significant ventricular pacing. Chapter 54 discusses CRT in detail.

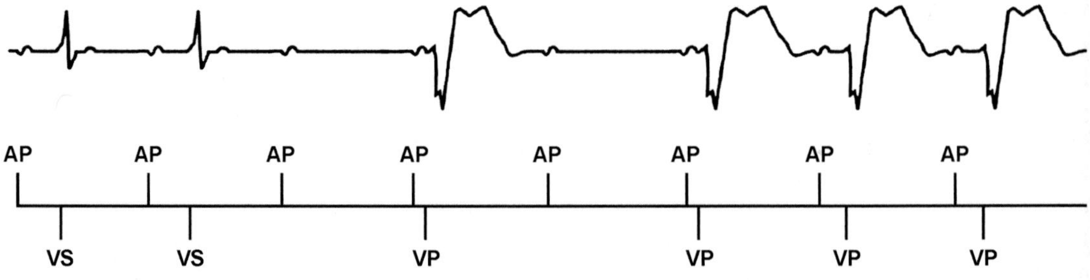

Figure 51–10. Managed ventricular pacing (MVP) mode. Loss of AV conduction triggered a ventricular support beat. After the second nonconducted beat the AAI(R) mode switched to a DDD(R) mode. See the text for explanation. (Courtesy Medtronic, Inc.)

Conclusion

Implantable defibrillators have become the gold standard therapy for preventing death in patients at high risk for sudden death. With careful attention to device programming, device selection, use of adjunctive therapies, and postimplant care, quality as well as length of life are improved.

References

1. Pacifico A, Johnson JW, Stanton MS, *et al.* Comparison of results in two implantable defibrillators. Jewel 7219D Investigators. *Am J Cardiol* 1998;82(7):875–880.
2. Mitchell LB, Pineda EA, Titus JL, Bartosch PM, Benditt DG. Sudden death in patients with implantable cardioverter defibrillators: The importance of post-shock electromechanical dissociation. *J Am Coll Cardiol* 2002;39(8):1323–1328.
3. Pires LA, Hull ML, Nino CL, May LM, Ganji JR. Sudden death in recipients of transvenous implantable cardioverter defibrillator systems: Terminal events, predictors, and potential mechanisms. *J Cardiovasc Electrophysiol* 1999;10(8):1049–1056.
4. Bourke JP, Turkington D, Thomas G, McComb JM, Tynan M. Florid psychopathology in patients receiving shocks from implanted cardioverter-defibrillators. *Heart* 1997;78(6):581–583.
5. Hegel MT, Griegel LE, Black C, Goulden L, Ozahowski T. Anxiety and depression in patients receiving implanted cardioverter-defibrillators: A longitudinal investigation. *Int J Psychiatry Med* 1997;27(1):57–69.
6. Schron EB, Exner DV, Yao Q, *et al.* Quality of life in the Antiarrhythmics versus Implantable Defibrillators trial: Impact of therapy and influence of adverse symptoms and defibrillator shocks. *Circulation* 2002;105(5):589–594.
7. Brigadeau F, Kouakam C, Klug D, *et al.* Clinical predictors and prognostic significance of electrical storm in patients with implantable cardioverter defibrillators. *Eur Heart J* 2006;27(6):700–707.
8. Arya A, Haghjoo M, Dehghani MR, *et al.* Prevalence and predictors of electrical storm in patients with implantable cardioverter-defibrillator. *Am J Cardiol* 2006;97(3):389–392.
9. Gatzoulis KA, Andrikopoulos GK, Apostolopoulos T, *et al.* Electrical storm is an independent predictor of adverse long-term outcome in the era of implantable defibrillator therapy. *Europace* 2005;7(2):184–192.
10. Sears SE Jr, Conti JB. Understanding implantable cardioverter defibrillator shocks and storms: Medical and psychosocial considerations for research and clinical care. *Clin Cardiol* 2003;26(3):107–111.
11. Credner SC, Klingenheben T, Mauss O, Sticherling C, Hohnloser SH. Electrical storm in patients with transvenous implantable cardioverter-defibrillators: Incidence, management and prognostic implications. *J Am Coll Cardiol* 1998;32(7):1909–1915.
12. Hurst TM, Krieglstein H, Tillmanns H, Waldecker B. Inappropriate management of self-terminating ventricular arrhythmias by implantable cardioverter defibrillators despite a specific reconfirmation algorithm: A report of two cases. *Pacing Clin Electrophysiol* 1997;20(5Pt. 1):1328–1331.
13. Mann DE, Kelly PA, Reiter MJ. Inappropriate shock therapy for nonsustained ventricular tachycardia in a dual chamber pacemaker defibrillator. *Pacing Clin Electrophysiol* 1998;21(10):2005–2006.
14. Grimm W, Menz V, Hoffmann J, Maisch B. Failure of third-generation implantable cardioverter defibrillators to abort shock therapy for nonsustained ventricular tachycardia due to shortcomings of the VF confirmation algorithm. *Pacing Clin Electrophysiol* 1998;21(4Pt. 1):722–727.
15. Ellenbogen KA, Levine JH, Berger RD, *et al.* Are implantable cardioverter defibrillator shocks a surrogate for sudden cardiac death in patients with nonischemic cardiomyopathy? *Circulation* 2006;113(6):776–782.
16. Swerdlow CD, Friedman PA. Advanced ICD troubleshooting: Part I. *Pacing Clin Electrophysiol* 2005;28(12):1322–1346.
17. Wathen MS, DeGroot PJ, Sweeney MO, *et al.* Prospective randomized multicenter trial of empirical antitachycardia pacing versus shocks for spontaneous rapid ventricular tachycardia in patients with implantable cardioverter-defibrillators: Pacing Fast Ventricular Tachycardia Reduces Shock Therapies (PainFREE Rx II) Trial results. *Circulation* 2004;110(17):2591–2596.
18. Fries R, Heisel A, Kalweit G, Jung J, Schieffer H. Antitachycardia pacing in patients with implantable cardioverter defibrillators: How many attempts are useful? *Pacing Clin Electrophysiol* 1997;20(1Pt. 2):198–202.
19. Mitchell JD, Lee R, Garan H, Ruskin JN, Torchiana DF, Vlahakes GJ. Experience with an implantable tiered therapy device incorporating

antitachycardia pacing and cardioverter/defibrillator therapy. *J Thorac Cardiovasc Surg* 1993; 105(3):453–462; discussion 62–63.

20. Nasir N Jr, Pacifico A, Doyle TK, Earle NR, Hardage ML, Henry PD. Spontaneous ventricular tachycardia treated by antitachycardia pacing. Cadence Investigators. *Am J Cardiol* 1997;79;820–822.
21. Schaumann A, von zur Muhlen F, Herse B, Gonska BD, Kreuzer H. Empirical versus tested antitachycardia pacing in implantable cardioverter defibrillators: A prospective study including 200 patients. *Circulation* 1998;97(1):66–74.
22. Klein RC, Raitt MH, Wilkoff BL, *et al.* Analysis of implantable cardioverter defibrillator therapy in the Antiarrhythmics Versus Implantable Defibrillators (AVID) Trial. *J Cardiovasc Electrophysiol* 2003;14(9):940–948.
23. Rosenqvist M. Antitachycardia pacing: Which patients and which methods? *Am J Cardiol* 1996; 78(5A):92–97.
24. Wilkoff BL, Ousdigian KT, Sterns LD, Wang ZJ, Wilson RD, Morgan JM. A comparison of empiric to physician-tailored programming of implantable cardioverter-defibrillators: Results from the Prospective Randomized Multicenter EMPIRIC Trial. *J Am Coll Cardiol* 2006;48(2):330–339.
25. Mitra RL, Hsia HH, Hook BG, *et al.* Efficacy of antitachycardia pacing in patients presenting with cardiac arrest. *Pacing Clin Electrophysiol* 1995; 18(11):2035–2040.
26. Wilkoff BL. Can a standardized ICD programming approach match physician tailored programming in preventing shocks post ICD implantation? The Empiric Trial. In: 2005 *Heart Rhythm* Society Scientific Sessions Late Breaking Trials, New Orleans, LA, 2005.
27. Fries R, Heisel A, Nikoloudakis N, Jung J, Schafers HJ, Schieffer H. Antitachycardia pacing in patients with implantable cardioverter-defibrillators: Inverse circadian variation of therapy success and acceleration. *Am J Cardiol* 1997;80(11):1487–1489.
28. Peters RW, Zhang X, Gold MR. Clinical predictors and efficacy of antitachycardia pacing in patients with implantable cardioverter defibrillators: The importance of the patient's sex. *Pacing Clin Electrophysiol* 2001;24(1):70–74.
29. Wathen MS, Sweeney MO, DeGroot PJ, *et al.* Shock reduction using antitachycardia pacing for spontaneous rapid ventricular tachycardia in patients with coronary artery disease. *Circulation* 2001;104(7):796–801.
30. Kouakam C, Lauwerier B, Klug D, *et al.* Effect of elevated heart rate preceding the onset of ventricular tachycardia on antitachycardia pacing effectiveness in patients with implantable cardioverter defibrillators. *Am J Cardiol* 2003;92(1):26–32.
31. Pacifico A, Hohnloser SH, Williams JH, *et al.* Prevention of implantable-defibrillator shocks by treatment with sotalol. d,l-Sotalol Implantable Cardioverter-Defibrillator Study Group. *N Engl J Med* 1999;340(24):1855–1862.
32. Steinberg JS, Martins J, Sadanandan S, *et al.* Antiarrhythmic drug use in the implantable defibrillator arm of the Antiarrhythmics Versus Implantable Defibrillators (AVID) Study. *Am Heart J* 2001;142(3):520–529.
33. Connolly SJ, Dorian P, Roberts RS, *et al.* Comparison of beta-blockers, amiodarone plus beta-blockers, or sotalol for prevention of shocks from implantable cardioverter defibrillators: The OPTIC Study: A randomized trial. *JAMA* 2006; 295(2):165–171.
34. Dorian P, Borggrefe M, Al-Khalidi HR, *et al.* Placebo-controlled, randomized clinical trial of azimilide for prevention of ventricular tachyarrhythmias in patients with an implantable cardioverter defibrillator. *Circulation* 2004;110(24): 3646–3654.
35. Mann DE, Kelly PA, Damle RS, Reiter MJ. Undersensing during ventricular tachyarrhythmias in a third-generation implantable cardioverter defibrillator: Diagnosis using stored electrograms and correction with programming. *Pacing Clin Electrophysiol* 1994;17(9):1525–1530.
36. Bansch D, Castrucci M, Bocker D, Breithardt G, Block M. Ventricular tachycardias above the initially programmed tachycardia detection interval in patients with implantable cardioverter-defibrillators: Incidence, prediction and significance. *J Am Coll Cardiol* 2000;36:557–565.
37. Page RL. Antiarrhythmic drugs for all patients with an ICD? *JAMA* 2006;295(2):211–213.
38. Boriani G, Biffi M, Frabetti L, Maraschi M, Branzi A. High defibrillation threshold at cardioverter defibrillator implantation under amiodarone treatment: Favorable effects of D, L-sotalol. *Heart Lung* 2000;29(6):412–416.
39. Nielsen TD, Hamdan MH, Kowal RC, Barbera SJ, Page RL, Joglar JA. Effect of acute amiodarone loading on energy requirements for biphasic ventricular defibrillation. *Am J Cardiol* 2001;88(4):446–448.
40. Page RL. Effects of antiarrhythmic medication on implantable cardioverter-defibrillator function. *Am J Cardiol* 2000;85(12):1481–1485.
41. Hohnloser SH, Dorian P, Roberts R, *et al.* Optimal pharmacological therapy in cardioverter defibril-

lator patients: Effect of amiodarone and sotalol on ventricular defibrillation threshold: The Optimal Pharmacological Therapy in Cardioverter Defibrillator Patients (OPTIC) Trial. *Circulation* 2006; 114:104–109.
42. Wood MA, Ellenbogen KA. Follow-up defibrillator testing for antiarrhythmic drugs: Probability and uncertainty. *Circulation* 2006;114(2):98–100.
43. Freedberg NA, Hill JN, Fogel RI, Prystowsky EN. Recurrence of symptomatic ventricular arrhythmias in patients with implantable cardioverter defibrillator after the first device therapy: Implications for antiarrhythmic therapy and driving restrictions. CARE Group. *J Am Coll Cardiol* 2001; 37(7):1910–1915.
44. Strickberger SA, Man KC, Daoud EG, *et al.* A prospective evaluation of catheter ablation of ventricular tachycardia as adjuvant therapy in patients with coronary artery disease and an implantable cardioverter-defibrillator. *Circulation* 1997;96(5): 1525–1531.
45. Segal OR, Chow AW, Markides V, Schilling RJ, Peters NS, Davies DW. Long-term results after ablation of infarct-related ventricular tachycardia. *Heart Rhythm* 2005;2(5):474–482.
46. van der Burg AE, de Groot NM, van Erven L, Bootsma M, van der Wall EE, Schalij MJ. Long-term follow-up after radiofrequency catheter ablation of ventricular tachycardia: A successful approach? *J Cardiovasc Electrophysiol* 2002;13(5): 417–423.
47. Della Bella P, De Ponti R, Uriarte JA, *et al.* Catheter ablation and antiarrhythmic drugs for haemodynamically tolerated post-infarction ventricular tachycardia. Long-term outcome in relation to acute electrophysiological findings. *Eur Heart J* 2002;23(5):414–424.
48. Schwartzman D, Jadonath RL, Callans DJ, Gottlieb CD, Marchlinski FE. Radiofrequency catheter ablation for control of frequent ventricular tachycardia with healed myocardial infarction. *Am J Cardiol* 1995;75(4):297–299.
49. Willems S, Borggrefe M, Shenasa M, *et al.* Radiofrequency catheter ablation of ventricular tachycardia following implantation of an automatic cardioverter defibrillator. *Pacing Clin Electrophysiol* 1993;16(8):1684–1692.
50. Morady F, Harvey M, Kalbfleisch SJ, el-Atassi R, Calkins H, Langberg JJ. Radiofrequency catheter ablation of ventricular tachycardia in patients with coronary artery disease. *Circulation* 1993; 87(2):363–372.
51. Stevenson WG, Khan H, Sager P, *et al.* Identification of reentry circuit sites during catheter mapping and radiofrequency ablation of ventricular tachycardia late after myocardial infarction. *Circulation* 1993;88(4Pt. 1):1647–1670.
52. Arenal A, Glez-Torrecilla E, Ortiz M, *et al.* Ablation of electrograms with an isolated, delayed component as treatment of unmappable monomorphic ventricular tachycardias in patients with structural heart disease. *J Am Coll Cardiol* 2003; 41(1):81–92.
53. Bogun F, Good E, Reich S, *et al.* Isolated potentials during sinus rhythm and pace-mapping within scars as guides for ablation of post-infarction ventricular tachycardia. *J Am Coll Cardiol* 2006; 47(10):2013–2019.
54. Marchlinski FE, Callans DJ, Gottlieb CD, Zado E. Linear ablation lesions for control of unmappable ventricular tachycardia in patients with ischemic and nonischemic cardiomyopathy. *Circulation* 2000;101(11):1288–1296.
55. Reddy VY, Neuzil P, Richardson AW, Kralovek SK, Ruskin JN, Josephson ME. Final results from the Substart Mapping & Ablation in Sinus Rhythm to Halt Ventricular Tachycardia (SMASH VT) Trial. In: 17th Annual Scientific Sessions of *Heart Rhythm* Society, Boston, MA, May 17–20, 2006.
56. Haissaguerre M, Extramiana F, Hocini M, *et al.* Mapping and ablation of ventricular fibrillation associated with long-QT and Brugada syndromes. *Circulation* 2003;108(8):925–928.
57. Szumowski L, Sanders P, Walczak F, *et al.* Mapping and ablation of polymorphic ventricular tachycardia after myocardial infarction. *J Am Coll Cardiol* 2004;44(8):1700–1706.
58. Marchlinski FE, Zado E, Dixit S, *et al.* Electroanatomic substrate and outcome of catheter ablative therapy for ventricular tachycardia in setting of right ventricular cardiomyopathy. *Circulation* 2004;110(16):2293–2298.
59. Soejima K, Stevenson WG, Sapp JL, Selwyn AP, Couper G, Epstein LM. Endocardial and epicardial radiofrequency ablation of ventricular tachycardia associated with dilated cardiomyopathy: The importance of low-voltage scars. *J Am Coll Cardiol* 2004;43(10):1834–1842.
60. Verma A, Kilicaslan F, Schweikert RA, *et al.* Short- and long-term success of substrate-based mapping and ablation of ventricular tachycardia in arrhythmogenic right ventricular dysplasia. *Circulation* 2005;111(24):3209–3216.
61. Schreieck J, Zrenner B, Deisenhofer I, Schmitt C. Rescue ablation of electrical storm in patients with ischemic cardiomyopathy: A potential-guided ablation approach by modifying substrate of

intractable, unmappable ventricular tachycardias. *Heart Rhythm* 2005;2(1):10–14.
62. Jordaens LJ, Mekel JM. Electrical storm in the ICD era. *Europace* 2005;7(2):181–183.
63. Kulick DM, Bolman RM 3rd, Salerno CT, Bank AJ, Park SJ. Management of recurrent ventricular tachycardia with ventricular assist device placement. *Ann Thorac Surg* 1998;66(2):571–573.
64. Swartz MT, Lowdermilk GA, McBride LR. Refractory ventricular tachycardia as an indication for ventricular assist device support. *J Thorac Cardiovasc Surg* 1999;118(6):1119–1120.
65. Thomas NJ, Harvey AT. Bridge to recovery with the Abiomed BVS-5000 device in a patient with intractable ventricular tachycardia. *J Thorac Cardiovasc Surg* 1999;117(4):831–832.
66. Kuhlkamp V, Dornberger V, Mewis C, Suchalla R, Bosch RF, Seipel L. Clinical experience with the new detection algorithms for atrial fibrillation of a defibrillator with dual chamber sensing and pacing. *J Cardiovasc Electrophysiol* 1999;10(7):905–915.
67. Deisenhofer I, Kolb C, Ndrepepa G, *et al.* Do current dual chamber cardioverter defibrillators have advantages over conventional single chamber cardioverter defibrillators in reducing inappropriate therapies? A randomized, prospective study. *J Cardiovasc Electrophysiol* 2001;12(2):134–142.
68. Theuns DA, Klootwijk AP, Goedhart DM, Jordaens LJ. Prevention of inappropriate therapy in implantable cardioverter-defibrillators: Results of a prospective, randomized study of tachyarrhythmia detection algorithms. *J Am Coll Cardiol* 2004;44(12):2362–2367.
69. Grimm W, Flores BF, Marchlinski FE. Electrocardiographically documented unnecessary, spontaneous shocks in 241 patients with implantable cardioverter defibrillators. *Pacing Clin Electrophysiol* 1992;15(11Pt. 1):1667–1673.
70. Schmitt C, Montero M, Melichercik J. Significance of supraventricular tachyarrhythmias in patients with implanted pacing cardioverter defibrillators. *Pacing Clin Electrophysiol* 1994;17(3Pt. 1):295–302.
71. Namerow PB, Firth BR, Heywood GM, Windle JR, Parides MK. Quality-of-life six months after CABG surgery in patients randomized to ICD versus no ICD therapy: Findings from the CABG Patch Trial. *Pacing Clin Electrophysiol* 1999;22(9):1305–1313.
72. Pinski SL, Fahy GJ. The proarrhythmic potential of implantable cardioverter-defibrillators. *Circulation* 1995;92(6):1651–1664.
73. Polikaitis A, Arzbaecher R, Bump T, Wilber D. Probability density function revisited: Improved discrimination of VF using a cycle length corrected PDF. *Pacing Clin Electrophysiol* 1997;20(8Pt. 1):1947–1951.
74. Swerdlow CD, Ahern T, Chen PS, *et al.* Underdetection of ventricular tachycardia by algorithms to enhance specificity in a tiered-therapy cardioverter-defibrillator. *J Am Coll Cardiol* 1994;24(2):416–424.
75. Swerdlow CD, Chen PS, Kass RM, Allard JR, Peter CT. Discrimination of ventricular tachycardia from sinus tachycardia and atrial fibrillation in a tiered-therapy cardioverter-defibrillator. *J Am Coll Cardiol* 1994;23(6):1342–1355.
76. Glikson M, Luria D, McClelland RM, *et al.* Mechanisms of device misclassification of arrhythmic episodes in the single chamber arm of the detect SVT trial. *Heart Rhythm* 2006;3(5):S158 (abstract).
77. Barold HS, Newby KH, Tomassoni G, Kearney M, Brandon J, Natale A. Prospective evaluation of new and old criteria to discriminate between supraventricular and ventricular tachycardia in implantable defibrillators. *Pacing Clin Electrophysiol* 1998;21(7):1347–1355.
78. Brugada J, Mont L, Figueiredo M, Valentino M, Matas M, Navarro-Lopez F. Enhanced detection criteria in implantable defibrillators. *J Cardiovasc Electrophysiol* 1998;9(3):261–268.
79. Kettering K, Dornberger V, Lang R, *et al.* Enhanced detection criteria in implantable cardioverter defibrillators: Sensitivity and specificity of the stability algorithm at different heart rates. *Pacing Clin Electrophysiol* 2001;24(9Pt. 1):1325–1333.
80. Swerdlow CD, Brown ML, Lurie K, *et al.* Discrimination of ventricular tachycardia from supraventricular tachycardia by a downloaded wavelet-transform morphology algorithm: A paradigm for development of implantable cardioverter defibrillator detection algorithms. *J Cardiovasc Electrophysiol* 2002;13(5):432–441.
81. Klingenheben T, Sticherling C, Skupin M, Hohnloser SH. Intracardiac QRS electrogram width—an arrhythmia detection feature for implantable cardioverter defibrillators: Exercise induced variation as a base for device programming. *Pacing Clin Electrophysiol* 1998;21(8):1609–1617.
82. Gold MR, Shorofsky SR, Thompson JA, *et al.* Advanced rhythm discrimination for implantable cardioverter defibrillators using electrogram vector timing and correlation. *J Cardiovasc Electrophysiol* 2002;13(11):1092–1097.
83. Lee MA, Corbisiero R, Nabert DR, *et al.* Clinical results of an advanced SVT detection enhancement algorithm. *Pacing Clin Electrophysiol* 2005;28(10):1032–1040.

84. Glikson M, Swerdlow CD, Gurevitz OT, *et al.* Optimal combination of discriminators for differentiating ventricular from supraventricular tachycardia by dual-chamber defibrillators. *J Cardiovasc Electrophysiol* 2005;16(7):732–739.
85. Glikson M, Gurevitz O, Bamlet B, *et al.* Mechanisms of device misclassification of arrhythmic episodes in ICDs with dual chamber enhancements. *Europace* 2006.
86. Bailin SJ, Niebauer M, Tomassoni G, Leman R. Clinical investigation of a new dual-chamber implantable cardioverter defibrillator with improved rhythm discrimination capabilities. *J Cardiovasc Electrophysiol* 2003;14(2):144–149.
87. Boriani G, Biffi M, Dall'Acqua A, *et al.* Rhythm discrimination by rate branch and QRS morphology in dual chamber implantable cardioverter defibrillators. *Pacing Clin Electrophysiol* 2003; 26(1Pt. 2):466–470.
88. Wilkoff BL, Kuhlkamp V, Volosin K, *et al.* Critical analysis of dual-chamber implantable cardioverter-defibrillator arrhythmia detection: Results and technical considerations. *Circulation* 2001; 103(3):381–386.
89. Dijkman B, Wellens HJ. Dual chamber arrhythmia detection in the implantable cardioverter defibrillator. *J Cardiovasc Electrophysiol* 2000;11(10): 1105–1115.
90. Sinha AM, Stellbrink C, Schuchert A, *et al.* Clinical experience with a new detection algorithm for differentiation of supraventricular from ventricular tachycardia in a dual-chamber defibrillator. *J Cardiovasc Electrophysiol* 2004;15(6):646–652.
91. Mletzko R, Anselme F, Klug D, *et al.* Enhanced specificity of a dual chamber ICD arrhythmia detection algorithm by rate stability criteria. *Pacing Clin Electrophysiol* 2004;27(8):1113–1119.
92. Bansch D, Steffgen F, Gronefeld G, *et al.* The 1 + 1 trial: A prospective trial of a dual- versus a single-chamber implantable defibrillator in patients with slow ventricular tachycardias. *Circulation* 2004; 110(9):1022–1029.
93. Friedman PA, McClelland RL, Bamlet WR, *et al.* Dual-chamber versus single-chamber detection enhancements for implantable defibrillator rhythm diagnosis: The detect supraventricular tachycardia study. *Circulation* 2006;113(25):2871–2879.
94. Ellenbogen KA, Wood MA, Shepard RK, *et al.* Detection and management of an implantable cardioverter defibrillator lead failure: Incidence and clinical implications. *J Am Coll Cardiol* 2003; 41(1):73–80.
95. Luria D, Glikson M, Brady PA, *et al.* Predictors and mode of detection of transvenous lead malfunction in implantable defibrillators. *Am J Cardiol* 2001;87(7):901–904.
96. Korley V, Hallet N, Daoust M, Epstein LM. A novel indication for transvenous lead extraction: Upgrading implantable cardioverter defibrillator systems. *J Interv Card Electrophysiol* 2000;4(3): 523–528.
97. Pfitzner P, Trappe HJ. Oversensing in a cardioverter defibrillator system caused by interaction between two endocardial defibrillation leads in the right ventricle. *Pacing Clin Electrophysiol* 1998;21(4Pt. 1):764–768.
98. Martin ML, Glikson M, Hodge DO, *et al.* Do abandoned leads pose risk to implantable defibrillator patients. *J Am Coll Cardiol* 2004:140A (abstract).
99. Suga C, Hayes DL, Hyberger LK, Lloyd MA. Is there an adverse outcome from abandoned pacing leads? *J Interv Card Electrophysiol* 2000;4(3): 493–499.
100. Bracke FA, Meijer A, Van GL. Malfunction of endocardial defibrillator leads and lead extraction: Where do they meet? *Europace* 2002;4(1): 19–24.
101. Lickfett L, Wolpert C, Jung W, *et al.* Inappropriate implantable defibrillator discharge caused by a retained pacemaker lead fragment. *J Interv Card Electrophysiol* 1999;3(2):163–167.
102. Friedman PA, Glikson M, Stanton MS. Defibrillator challenges for the new millennium: The marriage of device and patient-making and maintaining a good match. *J Cardiovasc Electrophysiol* 2000; 11(6):697–709.
103. Epstein LM, Byrd CL, Wilkoff BL, *et al.* Initial experience with larger laser sheaths for the removal of transvenous pacemaker and implantable defibrillator leads. *Circulation* 1999;100(5):516–525.
104. Kantharia BK, Kutalek SP. Extraction of pacemaker and implantable cardioverter defibrillator leads. *Curr Opin Cardiol* 1999;14(1):44–51.
105. Kantharia BK, Padder FA, Pennington JC 3rd, *et al.* Feasibility, safety, and determinants of extraction time of percutaneous extraction of endocardial implantable cardioverter defibrillator leads by intravascular countertraction method. *Am J Cardiol* 2000;85(5):593–597.
106. Le Franc P, Klug D, Jarwe M, *et al.* Extraction of endocardial implantable cardioverter-defibrillator leads. *Am J Cardiol* 1999;84(2):187–191.
107. Meier-Ewert HK, Gray ME, John RM. Endocardial pacemaker or defibrillator leads with infected vegetations: A single-center experience and consequences of transvenous extraction. *Am Heart J* 2003;146(2):339–344.
108. Sneed NV, Finch NJ, Leman RB. The impact of device recall on patients and family members of

patients with automatic implantable cardioverter defibrillators. *Heart Lung* 1994;23(4):317–322.
109. Maisel WH. Pacemaker and ICD generator reliability: Meta-analysis of device registries. *JAMA* 2006;295(16):1929–1934.
110. Maisel WH, Moynahan M, Zuckerman BD, *et al.* Pacemaker and ICD generator malfunctions: Analysis of Food and Drug Administration annual reports. *JAMA* 2006;295(16):1901–1906.
111. Gould PA, Krahn AD. Complications associated with implantable cardioverter-defibrillator replacement in response to device advisories. *JAMA* 2006;295(16):1907–1911.
112. Kawanishi DT, Brinker JA, Reeves R, *et al.* Spontaneous versus extraction related injuries associated with Accufix J-wire atrial pacemaker lead: Tracking changes in patient management. *Pacing Clin Electrophysiol* 1998;21(11Pt. 2):2314–2317.
113. Auricchio A, Gropp M, Ludgate S, Vardas P, Brugada J, Priori SG. European Heart Rhythm Association Guidance Document on cardiac rhythm management product performance. *Europace* 2006;8(5):313–322.
114. Carlson MD. Draft recommendations report by the heart rhythm society task force on device performance policies and guidelines. Washington DC: Heart Rhythm Society, April 26, 2006.
115. Andersen HR, Nielsen JC, Thomsen PE, *et al.* Long-term follow-up of patients from a randomised trial of atrial versus ventricular pacing for sick-sinus syndrome. *Lancet* 1997;350:1210–1216.
116. Rosenqvist M, Brandt J, Schuller H. Long-term pacing in sinus node disease: Effects of stimulation mode on cardiovascular morbidity and mortality. *Am Heart J* 1988;116:16–22.
117. Wilkoff BL, Cook JR, Epstein AE, *et al.* Dual-chamber pacing or ventricular backup pacing in patients with an implantable defibrillator: The Dual Chamber and VVI Implantable Defibrillator (DAVID) Trial. *JAMA* 2002;288(24):3115–3123.
118. Sharma AD, Rizo-Patron C, Hallstrom AP, *et al.* Percent right ventricular pacing predicts outcomes in the DAVID trial. *Heart Rhythm* 2005; 2(8):830–834.
119. Steinberg JS, Fischer A, Wang P, *et al.* The clinical implications of cumulative right ventricular pacing in the multicenter automatic defibrillator trial II. *J Cardiovasc Electrophysiol* 2005;16(4): 359–365.
120. Sweeney MO, Hellkamp AS, Ellenbogen KA, *et al.* Adverse effect of ventricular pacing on heart failure and atrial fibrillation among patients with normal baseline QRS duration in a clinical trial of pacemaker therapy for sinus node dysfunction. *Circulation* 2003;107:2932–2937.
121. Freudenberger RS, Wilson AC, Lawrence-Nelson J, Hare JM, Kostis JB. Permanent pacing is a risk factor for the development of heart failure. *Am J Cardiol* 2005;95:671–674.
122. Nahlawi M, Waligora M, Spies SM, Bonow RO, Kadish AH, Goldberger JJ. Left ventricular function during and after right ventricular pacing. *J Am Coll Cardiol* 2004;44:1883–1888.
123. Sweeney MO, Hellkamp AS. Heart failure during cardiac pacing. *Circulation* 2006;113:2082–2088.
124. Olshansky B, Day J, McGuire M, Hahn S, Brown S, Lerew DR. Reduction of right ventricular pacing in patients with dual-chamber ICDs. *Pacing Clin Electrophysiol* 2006;29(3):237–243.
125. Sweeney MO, Shea JB, Fox V, *et al.* Randomized pilot study of a new atrial-based minimal ventricular pacing mode in dual-chamber implantable cardioverter-defibrillators. *Heart Rhythm* 2004;1:160–167.
126. Leon AR, Greenberg JM, Kanuru N, *et al.* Cardiac resynchronization in patients with congestive heart failure and chronic atrial fibrillation: Effect of upgrading to biventricular pacing after chronic right ventricular pacing. *J Am Coll Cardiol* 2002; 39:1258–1263.
127. Eldadah ZA, Rosen B, Hay I, *et al.* The benefit of upgrading chronically right ventricle-paced heart failure patients to resynchronization therapy demonstrated by strain rate imaging. *Heart Rhythm* 2006;3:435–442.
128. Occhetta E, Bortnik M, Magnani A, *et al.* Prevention of ventricular desynchronization by permanent para-Hisian pacing after atrioventricular node ablation in chronic atrial fibrillation: A crossover, blinded, randomized study versus apical right ventricular pacing. *J Am Coll Cardiol* 2006;47:1938–1945.
129. Brignole M, Gammage M, Puggioni E, *et al.* Comparative assessment of right, left, and biventricular pacing in patients with permanent atrial fibrillation. *Eur Heart J* 2005;26(7):712–722.
130. Doshi RN, Daoud EG, Fellows C, *et al.* Left ventricular-based cardiac stimulation post AV nodal ablation evaluation (The PAVE Study). *J Cardiovasc Electrophysiol* 2005;16:1160–1165.
131. Kindermann M, Hennen B, Jung J, Geisel J, Böhm M, Fröhlig G. Biventricular versus conventional right ventricular stimulation for patients with standard pacing indication and left ventricular dysfunction—the Homburg Biventricular Pacing Evaluation (HOBIPACE). *J Am Coll Cardiol* 2006; 47:1927–1937.

52
Pacing and Cardiac Resynchronization

Robert F. Rea

Introduction

A broadend QRS complex on an electrocardiogram (ECG), often used as a marker of dyssynchronous ventricular activation, has been associated with increased mortality in patients with congestive heart failure (CHF).[1] Pacemaker therapy with right and left ventricular stimulation, which can resynchronize ventricular activation (cardiac resynchronization therapy pacing, CRT-P) improves ejection fraction and CHF symptoms in many patients.[2] Whether CRT-P without automatic defibrillator therapy (CRT-D) reduces sudden cardiac death (SCD) in this high-risk population is less clear. This chapter attempts to address this issue.

Studies of Cardiac Resynchronization Therapy Pacing

The Multisite Stimulation in Cardiomyopathies (MUSTIC)[3] and Multicenter InSync Randomized Clinical Evaluation (MIRACLE)[2] were the first randomized trials to evaluate the effect of CRT-P on signs, symptoms, and physiological parameters in patients with CHF. In each, the maximum follow-up was 6 months. Total mortality was a secondary endpoint in MUSTIC and was analyzed as a combined endpoint along with hospitalization for worsening CHF in MIRACLE. In neither study was an attempt made to distinguish between SCD and other mortality.

In MUSTIC, the duration of active therapy was brief, 3 months, owing to a crossover design. In addition, the number of patients was small, 58. Overall mortality was 7.5% and it was correctly concluded that the study was underpowered to comment on the effect of CRT on mortality. A larger number of patients was studied in MIRACLE (453), with a follow-up of 6 months on active therapy. There was a significant reduction in the combined endpoint of worsening CHF and mortality (Figure 52–1), but conclusions regarding the effect of CRT on mortality alone or sudden death mortality were not advanced. Thus, in these early studies of CRT-P, conclusions regarding the effect on SCD could not be drawn.

The first large-scale study that attempted to discern the effect of CRT-P alone on mortality was the Comparison of Medical Therapy, Pacing, and Defibrillation in Heart Failure (COMPANION).[4] A total of 1520 patients was randomized in a 2:2:1 ratio to CRT-P, CRT-D, or optimal medical therapy and followed for up to 3 years. While the primary endpoint was a composite of death from any cause or hospitalization for any cause (as in MIRACLE), death from any cause was a prespecified secondary endpoint. Thus, CRT-P was associated with a marginally significant 24% reduction in death from any cause ($p = 0.059$). However, CRT-D reduced death from any cause by 36% ($p = 0.003$) (Figure 52–2). Further analysis by cause of death was not carried out. Thus, although CRT-P tended to reduce overall death, COMPANION did not address the effect of CRT-P on SCD. A post hoc substudy of COMPANION

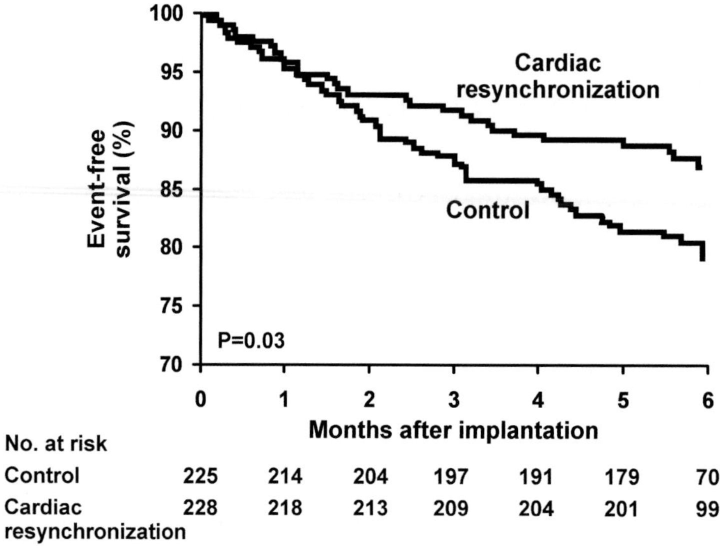

FIGURE 52–1. Kaplan–Meier estimates of the time to death or hospitalization for worsening heart failure in the control and resynchronization groups in MIRACLE. The risk of an event was 40% lower in the resynchronization group (95% confidence interval, 4–63%; $p = 0.03$). (Reprinted with permission.)

subsequently concluded that CRT-D but not CRT-P reduced SCD.[5]

The Cardiac Resynchronization-Heart Failure Trial (CARE-HF)[6] is an important study as it focused on CRT-P alone. Eight hundred and thirteen patients were randomized to receive CRT-P (409) or medical therapy for CHF (404) and were followed for at least 18 months. The primary endpoint was a composite of death from any cause or an unplanned hospitalization for a major cardiovascular event (only the first event in each patient was included in the analysis). The principal secondary endpoint was death from any cause. Importantly, the cause of death was tabulated, though the small number of deaths in each category precluded statistical comparison between treatment groups.

Eighty-two patients assigned to CRT-P died compared to 120 patients assigned to medical therapy for a hazard ratio of 0.64 ($p < 0.002$) (Figure 52–3). The mode of death was classified as sudden in 35% of the CRT-P group (29 of 82) and 32% in the medical therapy group (38 of 120). The study was not powered to address the effect of

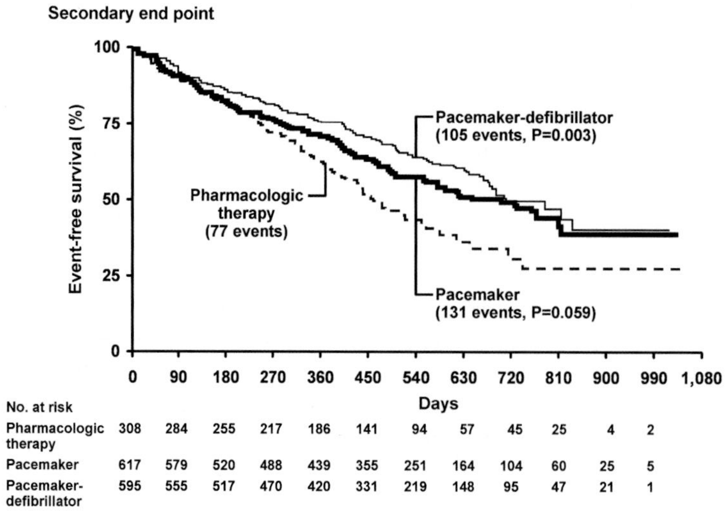

FIGURE 52–2. Kaplan–Meier estimates of the time to the secondary endpoint of death from any cause in COMPANION. The 12-month rates of death from any cause–the secondary endpoint–were 19% in the pharmacological-therapy group, 15% in the pacemaker group, and 12% in the pacemaker-defibrillator group. (Reprinted with permission.)

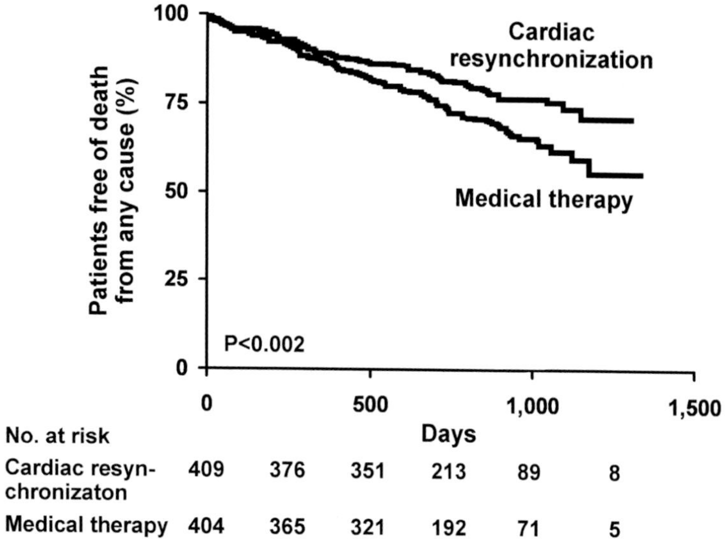

FIGURE 52–3. Kaplan–Meier estimates of the time to the principal secondary outcome in CARE-HF. The primary outcome was death from any cause or an unplanned hospitalization for a major cardiovascular event. The principal secondary outcome was death from any cause. (Reprinted with permission.)

CRT-P on SCD. Given this SCD mortality, however, it is clear that a very large trial might have to be undertaken to determine the effect of CRT-P alone on sudden death mortality.

An extension of CARE-HF in which previously enrolled patients were followed for a mean of 37 months was subsequently published.[7] With longer follow-up the reduction in the risk of SCD and death due to heart failure became statistically significant. Specifically, of 19 sudden deaths that occurred in the extension phase of the trial, 16 occurred in the medical therapy group, bringing the total sudden deaths in the medical therapy arm to 54 (13.4%) and in the CRT arm to 32 (7.8%) (Figure 52–4). This subgroup analysis was not part of the original study plan, nor is it clear that the original study was powered to make this conclusion. However, it is possible that the failure of other studies to demonstrate a significant effect of CRT on SCD is related to the short duration of follow-up.

To address the effect of CRT on ventricular arrhythmias that could precipitate SCD, investigators cleverly used the arrhythmia electrogram

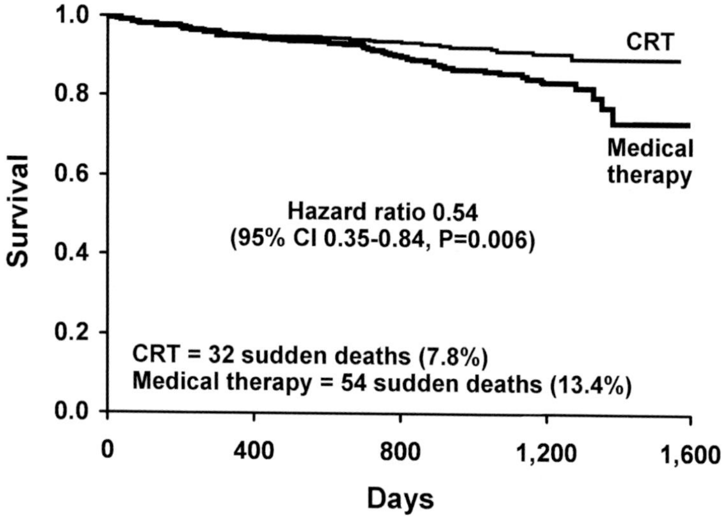

FIGURE 52–4. Kaplan–Meier estimates of the time to sudden death in the CARE-HF extension phase. CRT, cardiac resynchronization therapy. (Reprinted with permission.)

storage capabilities of CRT-D and implantable cardioverter defibrillator (ICD) devices. The frequency of episodes of ventricular tachycardia/ventricular fibrillation (VT/VF) stored in the device memory was compared in patients with CRT on and off. In a post hoc substudy of the VENTAK-CHF trial[8] (which randomized CHF patients with an implanted CRT-D to CRT on or off in 3-month blocks), there was a statistically significant reduction in episodes of VT/VF when CRT was programmed active. This was, however, a very small 32 patient post hoc substudy undertaken over a short period of observation and was likely underpowered to make a definitive conclusion on this issue.

A second small observational study compared the frequency of VT/VF before and after upgrade of a standard ICD to CRT-D. In 18 patients, the frequency of VT, VF, and appropriate ICD shocks over an average of 47 months before and 14 months after upgrade of a standard ICD to CRT-D was compared.[9] There were significantly fewer episodes of VF and appropriate ICD shocks after CRT-D upgrade, though the number of VT episodes was similar. As with the VENTAK-CHF substudy above, the number of patients and events was small and the power of the study to make a definitive conclusion is unclear.

A third study that pooled data from the InSync-ICD[10] and CONTAK CD[11] studies (summarized below) found no effect of CRT on the incidence of polymorphic or monomorphic VT based on a review of stored electrograms in 439 patients randomized to CRT-D compared to 441 patients randomized to ICD alone.[12]

There are experimental data that support the concept that CRT-P might favorably alter the frequency of arrhythmia. First, high-resolution surface ECG recordings made in patients with implanted CRT-P showed a significant reduction in ECG markers of dispersion of ventricular repolarization, an electrophysiological effect that is associated with decreased susceptibility to arrhythmia.[13] This was seen despite epicardial pacing of the left ventricle with the implanted CRT-P, a pacing maneuver associated experimentally with increased transmural heterogeneity of repolarization.[14] Second, simultaneous right and left ventricular programmed stimulation reduced the induction of VT (but not VF) compared to right ventricular stimulation alone in patients with ischemic heart disease.[15] Third, CRT-P was associated with a significant reduction in ambient ventricular ectopy compared to right ventricular pacing in a group of patients with ischemic or nonischemic cardiomyopathy.[16]

Despite these experimental data there are no convincing data to indicate that CRT as it is delivered at the present time reduces the burden of ventricular arrhythmias in patients with CHF.

Studies of Cardiac Resynchronization Therapy Defibrillator

An ICD with CRT-P capability was a logical extension of the stand-alone CRT-P, as most CRT-P candidates also satisfy criteria for prophylactic implantation of an ICD that were subsequently advanced by the Multicenter Automatic Defibrillator Trial II (MADIT II)[17] and the Sudden Cardiac Death in Heart Failure Trial (SCD-HeFT).[18] Clinical trials of CRT-D are difficult to interpret with respect to the independent effect of the CRT-P component on ventricular arrhythmias and sudden death, but it is useful to examine the data from major studies.

The Multicenter InSync ICD Randomized Clinical Evaluation Trial (MIRACLE ICD) was the first randomized trial of CRT-D as compared to ICD therapy alone.[10] Three hundred and sixty-nine patients received a CRT-D implant and were randomized to CRT on or off and followed for 6 months. As in MIRACLE, these were patients with advanced CHF, New York Heart Association (NYHA) function Class III and IV, and an average ejection fraction of 24%. At 6 months, survival was similar in patients randomized to CRT on (92.4%) and CRT off (92.2%). In addition, the frequency with which patients received therapy for ventricular arrhythmias from the device was similar in the two groups. While there were no differences in mortality or detected ventricular arrhythmias in the CRT on and off groups, active CRT did improve the quality of life, NYHA functional class, and maximal oxygen uptake, findings similar to earlier studies of CRT-P in similar patients.

Unlike MIRACLE, COMPANION[4] did not include a direct comparison of CRT-D and ICD therapy, but, rather, emphasized a comparison of CRT-P, CRT-D, and medical therapy alone for advanced CHF. As summarized above, CRT-D had a significantly greater impact on death from any cause (36% reduction, $p = 0.003$) compared to CRT-P (24% reduction, $p = 0.059$). The differences in the combined endpoint of death from or hospitalization for heart failure, however, were less pronounced (CRT-D, 40%, $p < 0.001$; CRT-P, 34%, $p < 0.002$). This again emphasizes the favorable effect of CRT-P on heart failure symptoms and functional status.

CONTAK CD[11] compared CRT-D to ICD therapy alone in a group of 490 patients with documented ventricular arrhythmias, a broadend QRS complex on ECG (>120 msec), and Class II to IV heart failure. Two hundred and forty-five patients were assigned to each group and were followed initially according to a crossover design in which CRT was active in alternate 3-month blocks. Later in the study a parallel design was adopted in which patients in whom CRT was active were compared to those in whom CRT was active during 6 months of follow-up.

Similar to other studies of both CRT-P and CRT-D, in CONTAK CD there were improvements in symptoms and indices of CHF with CRT. There was no effect of CRT, however, on all-cause mortality or the incidence of ventricular arrhythmias logged by the device.

Meta-Analysis of Cardiac Resynchronization Therapy

Meta-analyses, if performed carefully, can provide insights into the effect of therapies not afforded by individual studies. Given the difficulty of understanding the impact of CRT-P and CRT-D on mortality of varying causes, such an analysis was a reasonable undertaking. Bradley and colleagues[19] included CONTAK CD, MIRACLE-ICD, MIRACLE, and MUSTIC in a carefully executed meta-analysis of the effects of CRT (both CRT-P and CRT-D) on death from progressive heart failure. Important to note is that this analysis predated publication of CARE-HF.

Heart failure mortality, the main focus of the study, was reduced by 51% (relative reduction) across all studies. The effect of CRT-P was slightly greater than CRT-D on heart failure mortality, but the confidence intervals were broad and overlapping and statistically nonsignificant (D.J. Bradley, personal communication). In this meta-analysis, however, all-cause mortality was not statistically reduced by either CRT-D or CRT-P. In addition, CRT-D (comprising 1044 patients from CONTAK CD and MIRACLE–ICD) did not reduce the incidence of ventricular arrhythmias.

Why Is It Difficult to Show an Effect of Cardiac Resynchronization Therapy on Sudden Cardiac Death?

Medical therapy, notably β-adrenergic receptor blocking drugs, improves ejection fraction, heart failure symptoms, and heart failure mortality.[20] And the effect of β-adrenergic receptor blocking drugs on heart failure mortality is similar to that observed with CRT.[19]

Unlike medical therapy, CRT involves a surgical procedure with a small but finite mortality and morbidity and a small technical failure rate. Intubation of the coronary sinus os in patients with markedly enlarged hearts can be technically challenging and time consuming and carries a risk of coronary sinus perforation or dissection of up to 6% in major randomized trials.[21] Even when the left ventricular pacing lead is placed successfully, however, dislodgement may occur in 3–8% depending on venous anatomy and the type of lead used[22] and this may require reoperation.

In response to the problem of lead dislodgement, device manufacturers have developed shaped leads for stabilization in coronary vein tributaries. Figure 52–5 shows the chest X-ray of a patient with a straight left ventricular lead in a posterior coronary vein. This lead dislodged during right arm motion and retracted to the region of the coronary sinus os. Figure 52–6 shows a new sigmoid-shaped lead placed in the same vein branch.

Of more concern is the fact that only about two-thirds of patients who undergo CRT implant experience improvement in clinical symptoms.[23] Such a modest clinical response rate might dilute any effect of CRT on SCD. There are several potential explanations for this response rate to CRT.

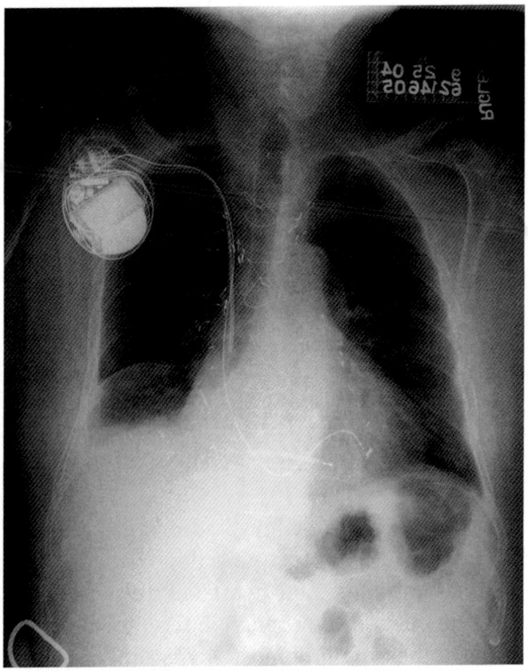

FIGURE 52–5. Posteroanterior chest X-ray of a patient with CRT-D utilizing a straight left ventricular pacing lead in a coronary vein.

First, currently accepted criteria for CRT implant include left ventricular ejection fraction ≤0.35, NYHA functional Class III or IV, and QRS width ≥120 msec.[24] The limitations of QRS duration as a reliable indicator of ventricular dyssynchrony have received substantial attention predominantly from echocardiographers.[25] Sophisticated echocardiographic techniques utilizing tissue Doppler imaging of varying types have been employed to define intraventricular and interventricular dyssynchrony. Some studies have shown a better clinical response in patients with echocardiographically defined dyssynchrony as opposed to prolonged QRS duration.[26] This is an area of intense ongoing investigation and the state of the art is beyond the scope of this chapter.

CARE-HF was the first randomized clinical trial of CRT that used any echocardiographically defined measures of dyssynchrony as a guide to patient selection. Specifically, in patients with a QRS duration of 120–149 msec, two of three additional criteria for ventricular dyssynchrony were required: an aortic preejection delay of more than 140 msec, an interventricular mechanical delay of more than 40 msec, or delayed activation of the posterolateral left ventricular wall.[6] Patients with a QRS duration of ≥150 msec did not have to satisfy these echocardiographic criteria.

Second, placement of the left ventricular pacing lead at the optimal site in the coronary venous system can be technically difficult. Based on early studies with open-chest epicardial pacing and detailed acute hemodynamic assessment, a posterolateral or lateral left ventricular site is generally believed to be most desirable.[27] In a retrospective study from two referral centers with substantial expertise, leads were placed in the preferred region (posterolateral and lateral left ventricle) in 167 of 233 patients (71%). In the remaining 66 patients leads were placed in anterior and anterolateral branches.[28] A significant improvement in mean ejection fraction (19–27%, $p = 0.008$) occurred only in the patients with the lead placed in a lateral or posterolateral site as compared to an anterior or anterolateral site (18–20%, $p = \text{NS}$).

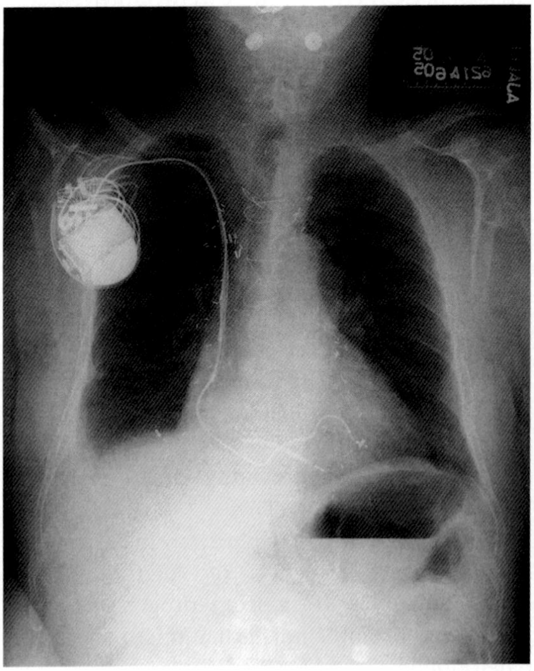

FIGURE 52–6. Posteroanterior chest X-ray of the same patient with CRT-D after replacement of the straight lead with a sigmoid-shaped lead for improved stability.

Third, in the major published trials of CRT reviewed above, right and left ventricular pacing occurred nearly simultaneously. Subsequently, devices were developed that permitted programming of the timing of right and left ventricular pacing (V-V timing). In small studies, echocardiographic stroke volume showed significant increases as the one or the other ventricle was preactivated to varying degrees.[29] The extent to which this improvement in stoke volume measured in the echocardiography laboratory translates into an improved clinical status, however, is unclear. One study showed an improvement in exercise capacity (6 min hall walk) but no effect on NYHA class with optimization of V-V timing.[30]

The Future of Cardiac Resynchronization Therapy

A major challenge for CRT lies in better selection of candidates, as it is clear from echocardiographic studies that a broadened QRS is a weak predictor of dyssynchrony. And in those patients with demonstrable dyssynchrony, it is increasingly clear that targeting the cardiac region with the latest activation for delivery of pacing therapy[31] may lead to improved symptoms and possibly SCD mortality. Such targeting will depend on improved tools for the delivery of pacing leads (endovascular or epicardial) and intraoperative imaging to be as certain as possible that pacing at a particular site has a favorable effect on dyssynchrony. Finally, device-based, automatic optimization of atrioventricular and right-to-left ventricular pacing intervals (available in some current devices) may provide the opportunity for a highly individualized and iteratively adjusted pacing prescription and, it is hoped, improved patient outcomes.

References

1. Balsasseroni S, Opasich C, Gorini M, *et al.* Left bundle-branch block is associated with increased 1-year sudden and total mortality rate in 5517 outpatients with congestive heart failure: A report from the Italian Network on Congestive Heart Failure. *Am Heart J* 2002;143:398–405.
2. Abraham WT, Fisher WG, Smith AL, *et al.* Cardiac resynchronization in chronic heart failure. *N Engl J Med* 2002;346:1845–1853.
3. Cazeau S, Leclercq C, Lavergne T, *et al.* Effects of multisite biventricular pacing in patients with heart failure and intraventricular conduction delay. *N Engl J Med* 2001;344:873–880.
4. Bristow MR, Saxon LA, Boehmer J, *et al.* Cardiac-resynchronization therapy with or without an implantable defibrillator in advanced heart failure. *N Engl J Med* 2004;350:2140–2150.
5. Carson P, Anand I, O'Connor C, *et al.* Mode of death in advanced heart failure. The Comparison of Medical, Pacing and Defibrillation Therapies in Heart Failure (COMPANION) trial. *J Am Coll Cardiol* 2005;46:2329–2334.
6. Cleland JGF, Daubert J-C, Erdmann E, *et al.* The effect of cardiac resynchronization on morbidity and mortality in heart failure. *N Engl J Med* 2005; 352:1539–1549.
7. Cleland JGF, Daubert J-C, Erdmann E, *et al.* Longer-term effects of cardiac resynchronization therapy on mortality in heart failure [the Cardiac Resynchronization-Heart Failure (CARE-HF) trial extension phase]. *Eur Heart J* 2006;27:1928–1932.
8. Higgins SL, Yong P, Scheck D, *et al.* Biventricular pacing diminshes the need for implantable cardioverter therapy. *J Am Coll Cardiol* 2000;36:824–827.
9. Ermis C, Seutter R, Zhu AX, *et al.* Impact of upgrade to cardiac resynchronization therapy on ventricular arrhythmia frequency in patients with implantable cardioverter-defibrillators. *J Am Coll Cardiol* 2005;46:2258–2263.
10. Young JB, Abraham WT, Smith AL, *et al.* Combined cardiac resynchronization and implantable cardioversion defibrillation in advanced chronic heart failure. *JAMA* 2003;289:2685–2694.
11. Higgins SL, Hummel JD, Niazi IK, *et al.* Cardiac resynchronization therapy for the treatment of heart failure in patients with intraventricular conduction delay and malignant ventricular arrhythmias. *J Am Coll Cardiol* 2003;42:1454–1459.
12. McSwain RL, Schwartz RA, DeLurgio DB, *et al.* The impact of cardiac resynchronization therapy on ventricular tachycardia/fibrillation: An analysis from the combined Contak-CD and InSync-ICD studies. *J Cardiovasc Electrophysiol* 2005;16:1168–1171.
13. Berger T, Hanser F, Hintringer F, *et al.* Effects of cardiac resynchronization therapy on ventricular repolarization in patients with congestive heart failure. *J Cardiovasc Electrophysiol* 2005;16:611–617.

14. Fish JM, Di Diego JM, Nesterenko V, *et al.* Epicardial activation of left ventricular wall prolongs QT interval and transmural dispersion of repolarization. Implications for biventricular pacing. *Circulation* 2004;109:2136–2142.
15. Kowal RC, Wasmund SL, Smith ML, *et al.* Biventricular pacing reduces the induction of monomorphic ventricular tachycardia: A potential mechanism for arrhythmia suppression. *Heart Rhythm* 2004;3: 295–300.
16. Walker S, Levy TM, Rex S, *et al.* Usefulness of suppression of ventricular arrhythmias by biventricular pacing in severe heart failure. *Am J Cardiol* 2000;86:231–233.
17. Moss AJ, Zareba W, Hall WJ, *et al.* Prophylactic implantation of a defibrillator in patients with myocardial infarction and a reduced ejection fraction. *N Engl J Med* 2002;346:877–883.
18. Bardy GH, Lee KL, Mark DB, *et al.* Amiodarone or an implantable cardioverter-defibrillator for congestive heart failure. *N Engl J Med* 2005;352:225–237.
19. Bradley DJ, Bradley EA, Baughman KL, *et al.* Cardiac resynchronization and death from progressive heart failure. A meta-analysis of randomized controlled trials. *JAMA* 2003;289:730–740.
20. Anonymous. Effect of metoprolol CR/XL in chronic heart failure: Metoprolol CR/XL randomised intervention trial in congestive heart failure (MERIT-HF). *Lancet* 1999;353:2001–2007.
21. Mehra MR, Greenberg BH. Cardiac resynchronization therapy: Caveat medicus! *J Am Coll Cardiol* 2004;43:1145–1148.
22. Rea RF. New resynchonization lead systems and devices. In: Wang PJ, Ed. *New Arrhythmia Technologies.* Malden, MA: Blackwell Publishing, 2005: 145–153.
23. Pires LA, Abraham WT, Young JB, *et al.* Clinical predictors and timing of New York Heart Association class improvement with cardiac resynchronization therapy in patients with advanced heart failure: Results from the Multicenter InSync randomized clinical evaluation (MIRACLE) and Multicenter InSync ICD randomized clinical evaluation (MIRACLE-ICD) trials. *Am Heart J* 2006;151:837–843.
24. Gregoratos G, Abrams J, Epstein AE, *et al.* ACC/AHA/NASPE 2002 guideline update for implantation of cardiac pacemakers and antiarrhythmia devices: Summary article. *J Am Coll Cardiol* 2002; 40:1703–1719.
25. Bax JJ, Abraham T, Barold SS, *et al.* Cardiac resynchronization therapy. Part 1- Issues before device implantation. *J Am Coll Cardiol* 2005;46:2153–2167.
26. Pitzalis MV, Iacoviello M, Romito R, *et al.* Ventricular asynchrony predicts a better outcome in patients with chronic heart failure receiving cardiac resynchronization therapy. *J Am Coll Cardiol* 2005; 45:65–69.
27. Stellbrink C, Auricchio A, Butter C, *et al.* Pacing therapies in congestive heart failure II study. *Am J Cardiol* 2000;86(9A):138K–143K.
28. Rossillo A, Verma A, Saad EB, *et al.* Impact of coronary sinus lead position on biventricular pacing: Mortality and echocardiographic evaluation during long-term follow-up. *J Cardiovasc Electrophysiol* 2004;15:1120–1125.
29. Sogaard P, Egeblad H, Pedersen AK, *et al.* Sequential versus simultaneous biventricular resynchronization for severe heart failure. Evaluation by tissue Doppler imaging. *Circulation* 2002;106:2078–2084.
30. Leon AR, Abraham WT, Brozena S, *et al.* Cardiac resynchronization with sequential biventricular pacing for the treatment of moderate-to-severe heart failure. *J Am Coll Cardiol* 2005;46:2298–2234.
31. Curtis AB. Cardiac resynchronization 101. If it's not late, pacing it early won't help. *J Am Coll Cardiol* 2005;45:70–71.

53 Device Therapy for Remote Patient Management

Dwight W. Reynolds, Christina M. Murray, and Robin E. Germany

Introduction

It is important that new medical technologies, including those related to the present topic, remote monitoring and management of devices and diseases using implantable devices, provide answers to questions and help solve problems and not simply provide new and expensive "toys." We live in a world in which geographic proximity to advanced medical care is of major importance for those afflicted with many types of illness. And yet, there are vast areas of our world that do not have such proximity, so-called underserved areas. Additionally, even our most advanced medical facilities struggle with volumes of patients and the ability to provide timely care to all who need this care. We are also substantially challenged by the need to collect information about implantable device performance in a meaningful and comprehensive way. Finally, the cost, both in monetary terms and in human aggravation, of traditional in-hospital and in-clinic care using conventional approaches continues to escalate. Remote monitoring and management of chronic and even acute conditions using implanted devices offer substantial answers to each of the major medical issues alluded to above. This chapter will describe what is surely only the beginning forays into this emerging technology and evolving concept.

Remote monitoring of intracardiac devices is a concept that has been reviewed in the literature,[1] but continues to evolve, and, at present, appears to be gaining rather rapid momentum. While technology has allowed remote monitoring of implantable devices, especially pacemakers and more recently implantable cardioverter defibrillators (ICDs), for decades, the ability to acquire more extensive device and patient data using remote monitoring is a phenomenon that began only recently. Twenty years ago we were able, using telephone line communications, to obtain information about heart rates, pacemaker output amplitude and duration, and electrocardiograms (ECGs). Today, using sophisticated but easily available computer linkages, we can obtain remotely almost all information stored in the most sophisticated devices. This includes electrograms and information about remote and recent cardiac arrhythmic and even hemodynamic events. In the not too distant future, it is almost certain that we will be remotely programming devices as the technology advances and professionals and patients (and regulators) become more comfortable in doing so. While much of the focus in this area has been on device monitoring, it is clear that with the evolution of implantable physiological and now chemical sensors, monitoring of chronic and even acute illnesses will be possible. While there is an inevitable concern about the expense of developing and implementing these exciting technologies, it is likely that remote monitoring of implanted devices and diseases will actually reduce the cost of healthcare as fewer hospitalizations and both scheduled and unscheduled outpatient visits occur. There appears to be a substantial opportunity to use remotely acquired device information, logged into computer-based databases, as an adjunct to other device performance surveillance systems.

In this chapter a summary of currently available remote monitoring by several different companies will be discussed. The reader is reminded, again, that because this area is changing rapidly, information here may soon need to be updated.

Current Uses and Goals for the Future

Patient Safety

Patient safety will inevitably drive much of the impetus toward closer monitoring and prompt notifications. Remote monitoring may allow more frequent device checks, with the potential for more timely troubleshooting. The Heart Rhythm Society recommends that manufacturers of devices develop and utilize wireless and remote monitoring technologies for the identification of abnormal device behavior as early as possible. This group has also recently stressed the importance of reducing the underreporting of device malfunction.[2] The American College of Cardiology/American Heart Association/North American Society for Pacing and Electrophysiology (ACC/AHA/NASPE) Guidelines for Implantation of Cardiac Pacemakers and Arrhythmia Devices (1998) recommend close monitoring of devices (specifically ICDs), with frequency of follow-up dictated by the patient's condition. Intervals specified are 1–4 months, with in-office visits supplementing transtelephonic evaluations no less than every 3 months.[3] Current practices have extended the times between follow-up visits.

Benefits Achieved Through Remote Monitoring

There is evidence for the benefit of telephone based remote monitoring in chronically ill patients such as those with advanced heart failure, thereby achieving morbidity and mortality benefits. Although not yet fully evaluated in randomized trials, it is anticipated that the same benefit may be obtained by remote monitoring of parameters measurable by implanted devices.[4] Interventions such as education and nurse telephone calls may reduce hospitalization by increasing disease awareness and compliance, along with therapy changes.[5] A mortality benefit was shown in the randomized, controlled Weight Monitoring in Heart Failure (WHARF) trial, using a scale and symptom response system, with information transmitted via telephone. There was a 56% reduction in mortality ($p < 0.003$) in the monitored group, speculated to be due to facilitated communication of important events to physicians.[6] These benefits have also been seen with a single home visit prior to discharge from the hospital[7] and with a more comprehensive disease management program managed telephonically.[8] A recent European study compared automated telemonitoring (weight, blood pressure, heart rate, and rhythm) with nurse phone calls and usual care and found reduced admission days and mortality in the telemonitored group.[9] Over the course of the 240-day follow-up period, hospital stays were reduced by 6 days in the telemonitored group. Mortality rates were 45% in the usual care group, which was reduced to 27% in the nurse care group and 29% in the telemonitored group ($p = 0.032$).

Integration of Care

The centralized storage of remotely obtained data will permit improvements in integration of care. Information is available for both the heart rhythm specialist as well as the heart failure physician, or any other physician participating in the patient's care. If the observations of remote monitoring trials are correct, it should be possible to improve patient care by accessing this information. This may also facilitate communication regarding important patient care issues between subspecialists who often practice significant distances apart. Remotely obtained data may facilitate a multidisciplinary approach to patient care. It will also allow access to these data by physician extenders, such as physician assistants and nurse practitioners, who can aid in acting promptly on critical data.

Resource Conservation

Resource conservation may be one of the most compelling reasons to pursue remote monitoring. It is estimated that evaluation of remotely obtained data may take as little as 8 min[10] compared to 30 min for a traditional in-office follow-up. Travel costs may be minimized. By reducing the interaction time required, more patients may be served. Time management and cost of follow-up care will be important considerations as the population ages and device indications grow.

Future Uses

As we move to more comprehensive, actually complete, device data availability remotely and as the implanted devices gather increasingly useful physiological information, new goals for remote care will likely emerge, changing the paradigm to one coupling modification of therapy with remote monitoring. It is easy to envision substantially improved clinical algorithms and modifications based on data obtained by this monitoring. Investigationally, using implanted devices, medical modifications have been made based on remote observations, including changes in agents such as β blockers, angiotensin-converting enzyme (ACE) inhibitors, and diuretics.[4] Future standards will almost certainly include remote programming of device settings. Programming to accomplish faster or slower pacing rates and atrioventricular (AV) interval modifications to minimize ventricular pacing could occur. In more technically challenging situations, changes could be made to more complex antitachycardia algorithms such as we do now in-clinic. In the future, home-based care might be possible that would otherwise necessitate hospitalization, with remotely available information such as hemodynamic parameters analogous to those obtained in the setting of a critical care unit.

Novel technologies will incorporate and likely improve on the remote monitoring, making a spectrum of routine to advanced care not only reliable, but possibly financially advantageous for society. This may offer not only benefits with regard to resource conservation, but palliation of end-stage disease.

The History of Monitoring

Transtelephonic Monitoring

The early history of device monitoring began with transtelephonic monitoring (TTM) of early pacemakers in the 1970s.[11] In the early era of pacemaker systems, battery longevity and lead performance were unpredictable. Early telemetry helped ensure patient safety, and provided a level of convenience for patients who were too ill to travel or lived substantial distances from clinics. Transtelephonic transmission was accomplished by connecting electrodes to the patient (wrists, ankles, etc., depending on system design) and to a transmitter, which was then coupled with the mouthpiece of the telephone. The only information available initially was rate determination with a reasonable evaluation of capture and sensing with the device as programmed. Interference artifacts often compromised the recordings obtained. Poor patient understanding of equipment use was also challenging.[12] Electrocardiographic tracings were obtained in regular and magnet modes, and were required to be of 30 sec duration, and a significant part of the medical record.[13] As technology progressed, threshold testing became available via magnet-induced reduction in pacemaker output.

Early Studies Using Transtelephonic Monitoring

Use of these systems became more sophisticated over time. A case report in 1984 described the use of TTM to monitor the use of an early device with antitachycardia therapy.[14] A trial published in 1992 confirmed symptoms of atrial fibrillation (AF) and supraventricular tachycardia (SVT) correlated with data obtained from transtelephonic ECG monitoring. There was significant correlation between symptoms and documented arrhythmia, with 70% of the calls related to symptoms showing paroxysmal supraventricular tachycardia (PSVT) or paroxysmal atrial fibrillation (PAF) attacks.[15] Use of TTM in following ICD patients was described in a report in 1995, in 18 patients, allowing identification of spontaneous arrhythmias and assessment of the success of therapies delivered.[16] The feasibility of this type of monitoring was well established. Expansion of device features and better internet technology led to a greater sophistication for remote monitoring as well.

Current Examples of Remote Monitoring

Over the past several years, with improvement in device telemetry, remote communication, and computer technology, major device manufacturers have developed and implemented increasingly

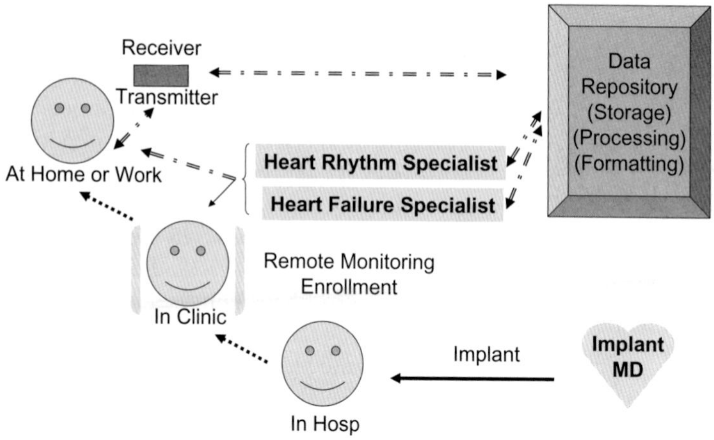

FIGURE 53–1. A schematic representation of a generic remote monitoring program. Other clinicians could be involved either directly or indirectly by receiving the remote monitoring report from the "data repository" or from one of the other clinicians.

sophisticated remote monitoring systems. While each device manufacturer's monitoring systems are restricted to their devices, and there are substantial differences among the systems, all are evolving and are aimed at greater patient safety and satisfaction as well as greater follow-up efficiency. This section explores examples of currently available technology. A general schematic of how most remote monitoring systems work is shown in Figure 53–1. A synopsis of comparative features among the four systems discussed below is contained in Table 53–1.

TABLE 53–1. Comparative features of the four systems.

	Biotronik	Boston Scientific/ Guidant	Medtronic	St. Jude Medical
Name	Home Monitoring™	Latitude™	CareLink™	Housecall Plus™
Remote monitoring connection	Cellular or standard analog telephone line (not digital compatible)	Standard analog telephone line (not digital compatible)	Standard analog telephone line (not digital compatible)	Standard analog telephone line (not digital compatible)
Frequency/ channel bandwidths of wireless components	Medical Implant Communications System (403 MHz); channel bandwidth 100 kHz	FCC license category used by any industrial, consumer, scientific, or medical products (914 MHz)	Medical Implant Communication Service Band (402–405 MHz); multiple channel bandwidth 300 kHz	
Access	Secure internet network; internet access for multiple clinicians	Secure internet network; internet access for multiple clinicians; limited patient access	Secure internet network; internet access for multiple clinicians	Maintained in office or by service providers; no internet access
Data available	Battery voltage, pace and shock impedances, electrograms (EGMs), arrhythmia and therapy data	Complete device data, EGMs, blood pressure, and weight	Complete device data, EGMs, hemodynamic data	Complete device data, EGMs, surface electrocardiogram (ECG)
Alerts	Internet, email, pager, cell phone, or fax	Critical–call to physician and page to local representative Urgent–fax to office and information sent to internet website	Pager or voicemail notification, with patient information to be accessed on the internet	Service center call to clinician
Manufacturer charges	At implant (hospital)	At implant (hospital)	No additional change	Clinic or third party (equipment purchase)

Biotronik

The Biotronik remote monitoring system Home Monitoring™ uses wireless phone technology to transmit patient information, called to a centralized server, via a patient transceiver. Biotronik initially received a license to use the frequency in 2001 for wireless monitoring of pacemakers. In 2002 ICD monitoring followed, with cardiac resynchronization therapy defibrillator (CRT-D) monitoring initiated in 2006. Biotronik remote monitoring is, as of October 2006, in use by approximately 52,000 worldwide patients, with 12,000 of these in the United States.

Home Data Acquisition

Stored data are obtained wirelessly, automatically on a predetermined schedule. A radio frequency transmitter is integrated into the implanted device circuitry, which communicates with the patient transceiver. Data can be acquired by the transceiver at a distance of 2 m from the implanted device. The transmitter is small and can be worn or carried by the patient. The data are transmitted via GSM cellular telephone technology, and can also be used with a standard telephone land-line. Data are transmitted daily at programmed times. Patient-triggered reports can be obtained as well. Transmission (unidirectional) occurs over the Medical Implant Communications System at 403 MHz with a channel bandwidth of 100 kHz. Data are transmitted to the Biotronik Service Center.

Data Obtained

Device-related information obtained at interrogation includes data such as battery voltage and pace and shock impedances. Routine remote device data acquisition using this system has the potential to identify significant events such as lead malfunction with sudden increase in pacing threshold (Figure 53–2). For example, lead fracture, which in this case was the result of patient manipulation (twiddler's syndrome),[17] was identified remotely (Figure 53–3).

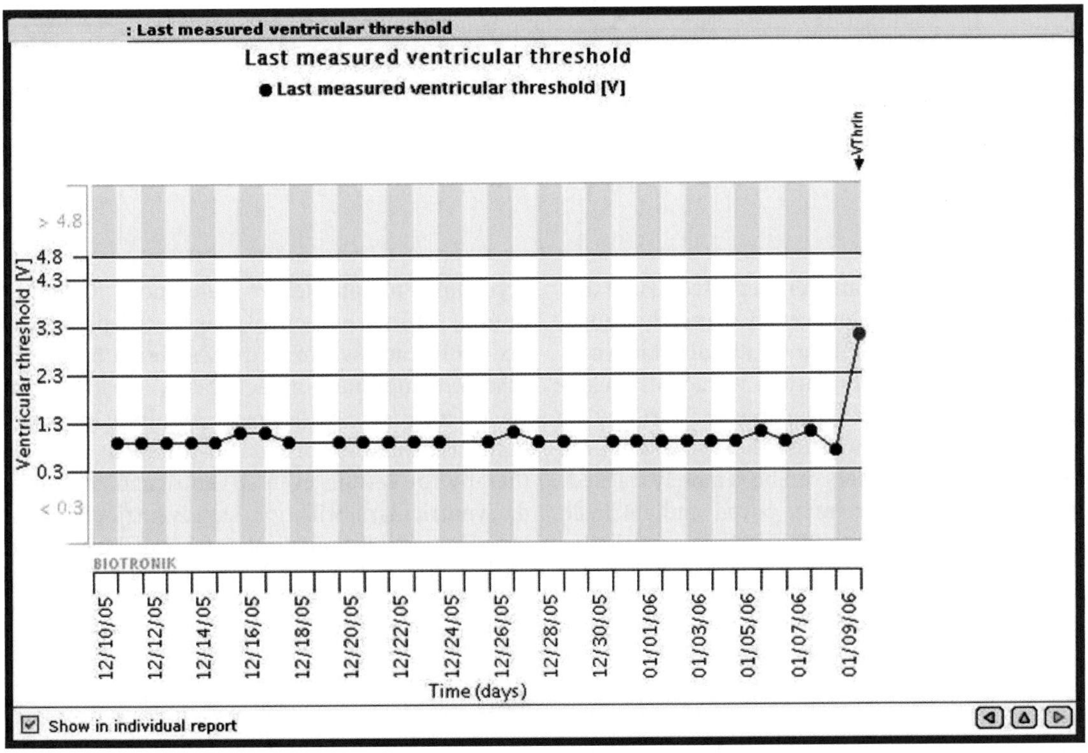

FIGURE 53–2. These data are an example of a remotely acquired report using the Biotronik Home Monitoring™ system. This report shows a sudden increase in pacing threshold. (Courtesy of Biotronik.)

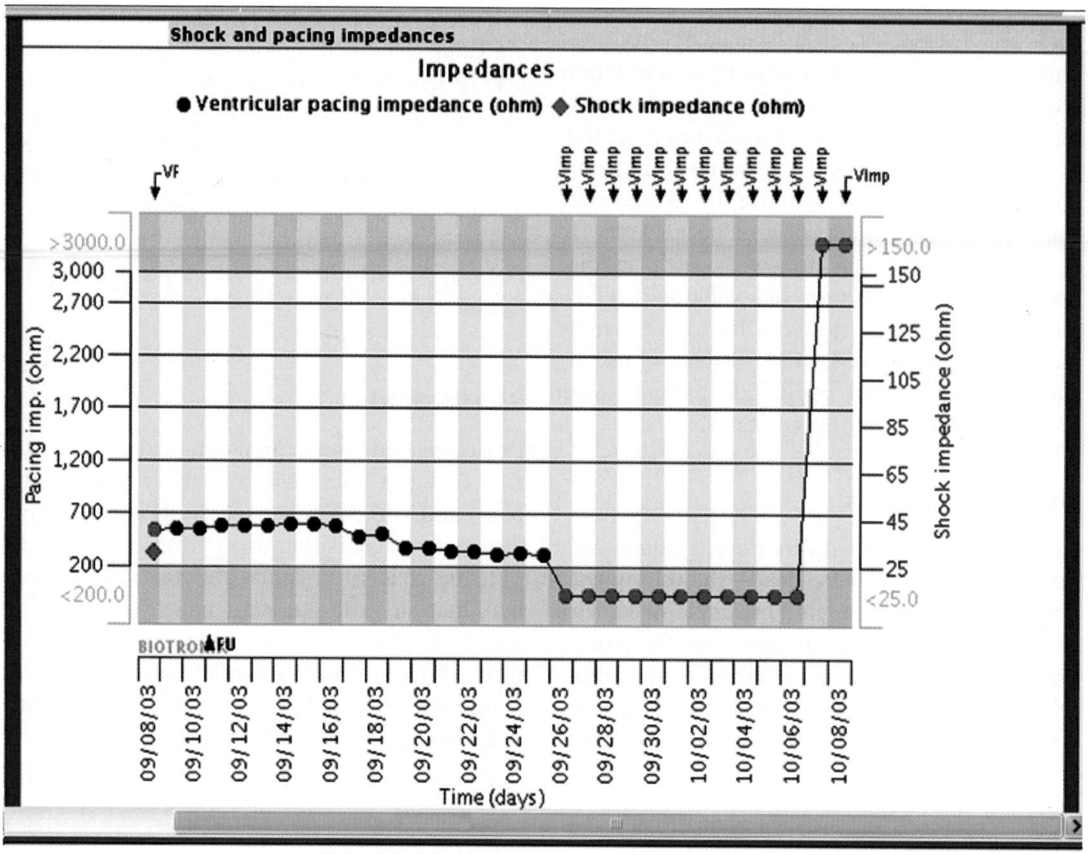

FIGURE 53–3. This is another example of a remotely acquired report of the Biotronik Home Monitoring™ system. This report shows an initial drop in impedance on a pacing lead over a several week period, indicating an insulation breach, followed by a dramatic increase in lead impedance indicating a fracture. This clinically was a result of "twiddler's syndrome." (Courtesy of Biotronik.)

Patient-related parameters reported, using this system, include atrial and ventricular arrhythmias and therapies delivered for ventricular tachycardia and ventricular fibrillation. Intracardiac electrograms (IEGMs) are available for scrutiny of events, to determine whether therapy was appropriate. Other parameters can be remotely tracked, including mean heart rate, paced and intrinsic percentages, percent CRT pacing, ventricular ectopy, and mode switching. Resting heart rate and patient activity level are also available.

Notifications

With the Biotronik System, as with others discussed later, critical patient and device data can be transmitted to physicians. Notification is made according to physician preference, including options of internet, email, pager, cell phone, or fax. Notifications can be patient initiated in the case of symptoms. In such cases, a patient can wave a magnet over the device, resulting in immediate transmission of data. If a patient receives therapy for certain events (ventricular tachycardia, ventricular fibrillation, supraventricular tachycardia, etc.) the medical team can be notified immediately. A physician can choose to be notified of these events within 1 min of the event by one of the methods mentioned above.

Cost

The manufacturer's charge for use of these added features, including the cellular service, is included at the time of device implantation. There are no additional charges for use for the life of the implanted device. The remote monitoring charges by physicians to patients using this and other manufacturers' systems is currently under review and revision.

Boston Scientific/Guidant

The remote monitoring system offered by Boston Scientific, called Latitude™, was introduced to the market in 2006. It is presently in use by approximately 6500 patients. With the newest implantable devices, this technology permits not only remote monitoring but also "wireless" implant and "wireless" in-office follow-up. This is accomplished by a new telemetry system in which the distance between the implanted device and the data acquisition device is substantially increased over earlier versions. There is also optional hardware, a Bluetooth enabled blood pressure cuff and scale, which can be used with the system.

Home Data Acquisition

Remote interrogations can be performed automatically on as much as a daily basis. Frequency and day of the week can be specified and modified. Interim follow-ups can be arranged, even on prespecified dates. Patient-initiated interrogations are also possible (clinician enabled). Scheduling options exist for active monitoring notifications and can be changed according to physician and patient preference (daily or weekly). Data are transmitted from the patient's device to a wireless "communicator," a transceiver, kept in the home. This system currently requires a standard telephone line. Communication occurs via the Industrial, Scientific, Medical band at a frequency of 914 MHz.

Data Obtained

Downloaded information appears on an internet website, maintained on encrypted servers that comply with privacy rules. System information can be followed by multiple physicians. Although the physician-viewed information is the same, schedules, alerts, and notifications can be individualized for different physicians. At the time of data acquisition, critical information is deemed to fall into certain predetermined alert categories ("red" or "yellow"), in addition to standard patient care information.

A report is generated with features designed to assist with heart failure management (Figure 53–4). Arrhythmias including atrial fibrillation, ventricular fibrillation, and ventricular tachycardia are recorded. Weight, blood pressure (if scales and blood pressure cuffs are also included), activity, and heart rate maximum, minimum, and means are available. Autonomic parameters such as heart rate variability (HRV) determinations are incorporated in the report. Weight monitoring, an optional feature, can highlight changes of 5 pounds in 1 week or 2 pounds in a 1- or 2-day period.

The Boston Scientific system offers access to some nontraditional data via remote reporting. Patient quality of life issues can be addressed via self-report questions that may be answered with the home monitor, a function programmable to either "on" or "off." Questions are asked weekly. Symptom queries include fatigue, dizziness, edema, orthopnea, and paroxysmal nocturnal dyspnea (PND) (Figure 53–5). The system also includes the ability to give patient access to limited information via internet access. Patient-available data include dates of recent and scheduled interrogations, weight, blood pressure, battery status, and contact information.

Notifications

The relative importance of information may trigger physician contact, varying from a fax sent to the physician's office to physician and local industry representative calls. If this feature is not enabled, the patient is notified. "Red" events are those that are considered critical to the continuing appropriate operation of the implanted system. Such events include battery end of life, impedance aberrancies, low right ventricular intrinsic (R wave) amplitudes, and high voltage detected on the shock lead during charge. When these criteria are met, the company calls the physician and contacts the local representative. "Yellow" alerts are noted on weekly checks. Alert events include arrhythmic events such as shock delivery, type and timing of tachyarrhythmias, and patient-triggered events. Significant weight

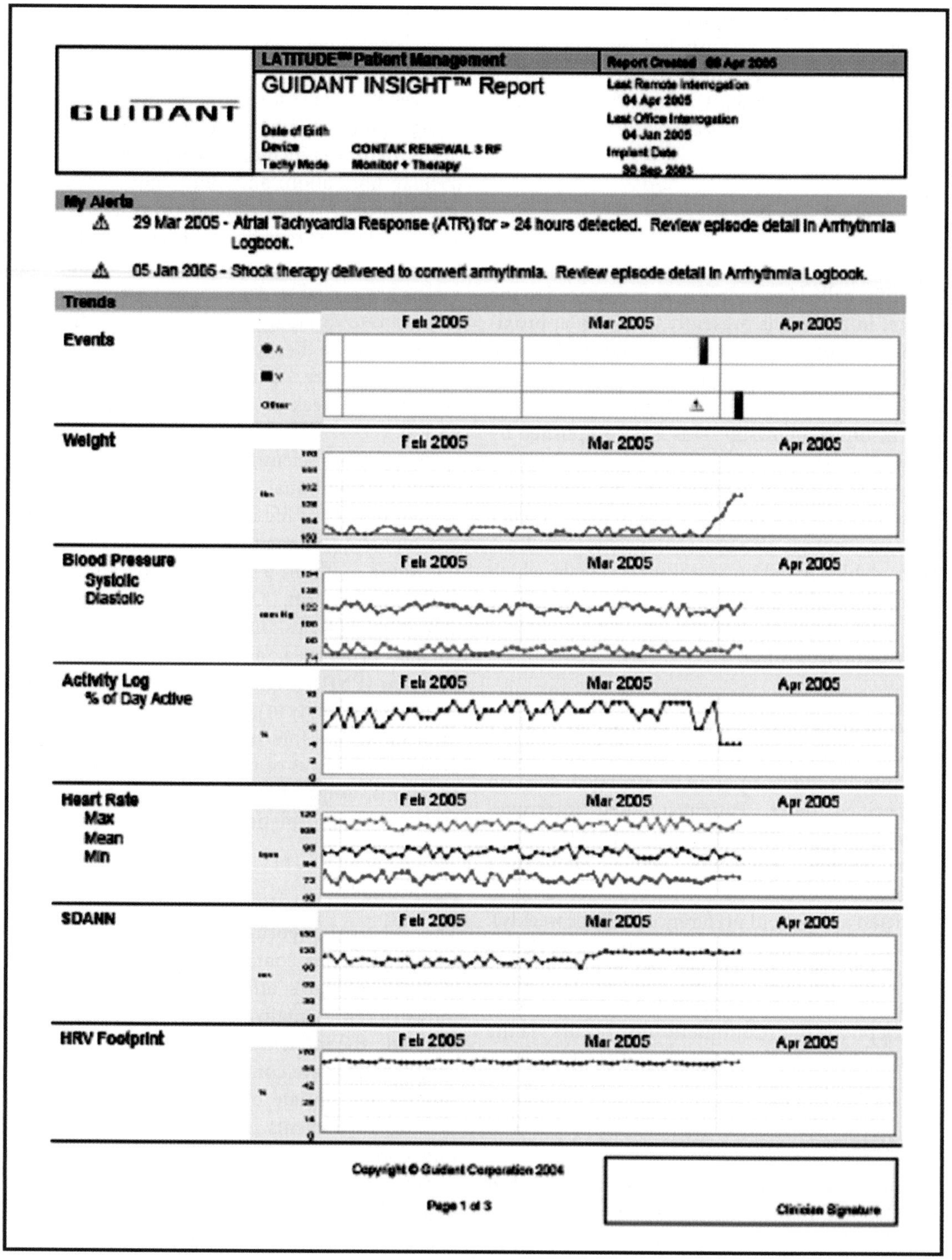

FIGURE 53–4. An example of a heart failure report generated on Boston Scientific's Latitude™ system. Note the inclusion of both blood pressure and weight data. (Courtesy of Boston Scientific.)

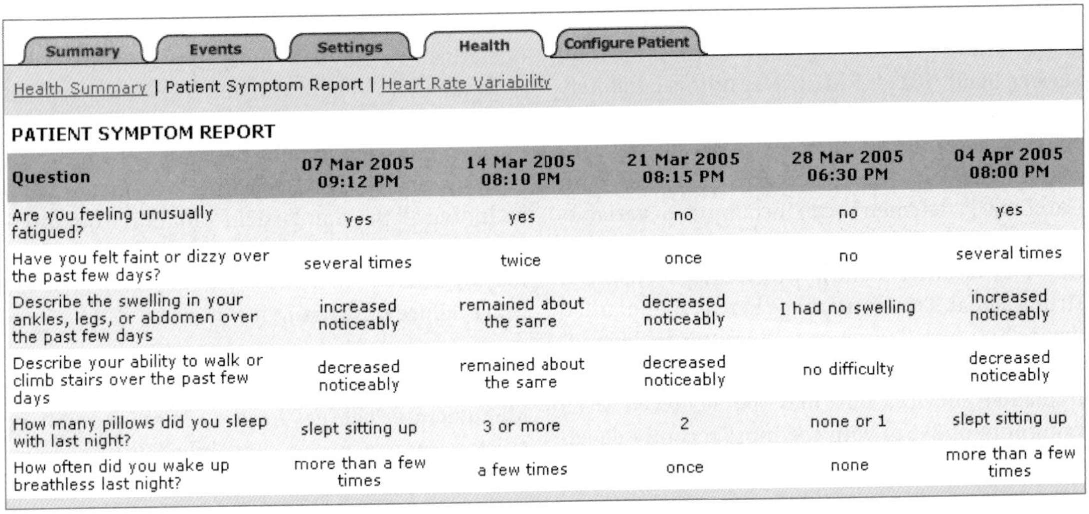

Question	07 Mar 2005 09:12 PM	14 Mar 2005 08:10 PM	21 Mar 2005 08:15 PM	28 Mar 2005 06:30 PM	04 Apr 2005 08:00 PM
Are you feeling unusually fatigued?	yes	yes	no	no	yes
Have you felt faint or dizzy over the past few days?	several times	twice	once	no	several times
Describe the swelling in your ankles, legs, or abdomen over the past few days	increased noticeably	remained about the sarre	decreased noticeably	I had no swelling	increased noticeably
Describe your ability to walk or climb stairs over the past few days	decreased noticeably	remained about the sarre	decreased noticeably	no difficulty	decreased noticeably
How many pillows did you sleep with last night?	slept sitting up	3 or more	2	none or 1	slept sitting up
How often did you wake up breathless last night?	more than a few times	a few times	once	none	more than a few times

FIGURE 53–5. An example of a patient symptoms report generated by the Boston Scientific Latitude™ system. (Courtesy of Boston Scientific.)

changes are noted. Device-specific parameters are noted, including battery status, and lead parameters including intrinsic amplitude and pacing lead impedance. These less critical "yellow" events are noted on the clinician accessible website, and a fax is sent to the physician's office.

Cost

Weight scales and blood pressure cuffs are available as optional components to the Latitude™ system. Manufacturer charges for use of the rest of the system are billed at the time of implant. As previously discussed, physician charges for remote follow-up are currently being reviewed and revised.

Medtronic

The remote monitoring system used by Medtronic called CareLink™ was launched in 2002. Approximately 85,000 patients (involving approximately 1000 clinics) were using the network as of October 2006. Transmission captures device parameters, including diagnostics, and stored episodes of arrhythmia events. A prospective evaluation of the system was completed prior to market release, and demonstrated a high level of physician satisfaction with the system,[18] with 96.5% of physicians reporting that it was either somewhat easy or very easy to use. Patients also found the device easy to use, with 98.1% reporting that the monitor was either somewhat easy or very easy to use. In addition to remote monitoring, Medtronic has recently introduced a new generation of devices that permits "wireless" implant, in-office follow-up, and automated remote follow-up, similar in function to that described with Boston Scientific's Latitude system. These systems, which eliminate a "programming head" from the sterile field at the time of implant, may have the additional advantage of reducing implant time by allowing activities such as pocket closure while doing final programming and interrogation. They also make clinic follow-up more streamlined, potentially. The most important advantage of the "long-distance" telemetry linkages, however, is that it allows automatic remote monitoring to occur, without the need for patients to take specific action to initiate a transmission.

Home Data Acquisition

Just as with the other systems, the monitors (transceivers) used in patient homes are Food and Drug Administration (FDA) approved. These transceivers are portable and can be used outside of the home including internationally, and are patient specific. Downloaded information is stored on a secure internet system that is password protected. Telemetry is transmitted (bidirectionally) on the Medical Implant Communication Service Band, 402–405 MHz. Use of this band may have advantages in the prevention of interference caused by other wireless devices such as cell phones that operate at other frequencies. With CareLink™, telemetry can occur on a variable, "clearest" MICS channel of up to 300 kHz (within the 402–405 MHz band), which helps ensure a strong signal. Telemetry range between implanted device and home receiver-transmitter is dependent on conditions including the model of the implanted device, but may be achieved at a minimum of 2–5 m with the most recently developed implantables. As above, "wireless" technology now allows automated interrogations, in addition to patient-initiated downloads with older devices that do not possess the "long-distance" telemetry of newer implanted devices. Automated relay of information may allow for earlier monitoring of arrhythmias or device-related issues. This automation may also simplify compliance issues for patients and physicians.

Data Obtained

A complete set of stored and real-time device information, just like that obtainable in-clinic, can be obtained at the time of remote interrogation, such as device- and patient-specific information including arrhythmia events data, with electrograms (EGMs) on therapy delivery (Figure 53–6), and specialized heart failure management reports (Figure 53–7). Even hemodynamic information now available from some implanted devices is available remotely. This remote monitoring system has been used with FDA-approved systems[19] and investigational implantable hemodynamic monitors[20–22] as well. The ability to monitor chronic conditions remotely such as heart failure promises to further hasten the development, implementation, and acceptance of this technology.

Notifications

Clinician alerts are initiated by device recognition of preset conditions. The system automatically sends a transmission when an alert is initiated. Alerts may be sent to the clinic or physician, to either voicemail or a pager. Information in the alert includes patient name and date of birth, type of alert, and a phone number to reach the patient.

Data obtained via alerts can be tailored according to physician preference. This allows for ongoing interaction with the system by different types of physicians. Device performance reports including all the standard information from interrogation, or heart failure management reports, may be sent to the heart rhythm specialist, or the heart failure physician, or both.

Cost

Manufacturer charges for the remote monitoring system were recurring, and billed to the clinics where the monitoring takes place but were recently changed to a service provided at no additional charge. Physician billing for these services is being reviewed and revised, and there is significant variability, geographically, in third-party reimbursement for these currently.

St. Jude Medical

The remote monitoring system marketed by St. Jude Medical, Housecall Plus™, was introduced in October 2005, and had 7000 patient enrollments as of October 2006. The system, different than the previous three discussed, utilizes live medical professionals (either in the office of the patient's physician or in service centers) to interface with patients during the transmission process. An early iteration of the system was evaluated in 124 patients, and was found to have a high level of patient satisfaction, along with "safe and successful" monitoring.[23]

Home Data Acquisition

Like the other systems described, data are obtained via a multipart system. The device itself is the first part, the transceiver in the patient's home is the second part, and the receiver is the final part, which may be owned and operated by service centers or by physicians. The home transceiver is equipped with two ECG wristbands, a telemetry wand to place right over the device, and a built-in speakerphone, so patients can speak with the technician assisting with the download process. A standard telephone jack (with land-line) and power outlet are required. After the data are received and formatted, there is PDF export

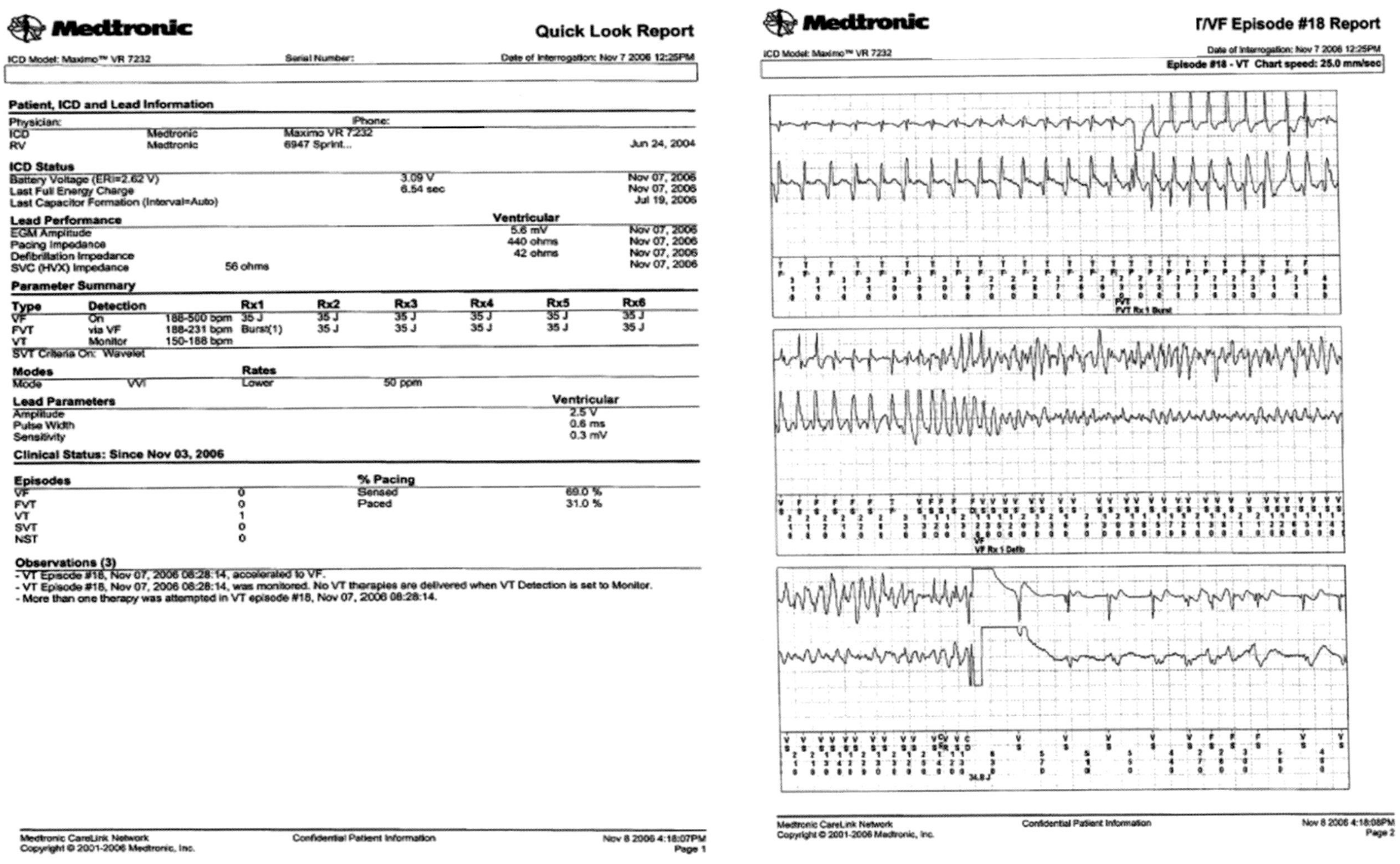

Medtronic **Quick Look Report**

ICD Model: Maximo™ VR 7232 Serial Number: Date of Interrogation: Nov 7 2006 12:25PM

Patient, ICD and Lead Information

Physician:		Phone:	
ICD	Medtronic	Maximo VR 7232	
RV	Medtronic	6947 Sprint...	Jun 24, 2004

ICD Status

Battery Voltage (ERI=2.62 V)	3.09 V	Nov 07, 2006
Last Full Energy Charge	6.54 sec	Nov 07, 2006
Last Capacitor Formation (Interval=Auto)		Jul 19, 2006

Lead Performance

		Ventricular	
EGM Amplitude		5.6 mV	Nov 07, 2006
Pacing Impedance		440 ohms	Nov 07, 2006
Defibrillation Impedance		42 ohms	Nov 07, 2006
SVC (HVX) Impedance	56 ohms		Nov 07, 2006

Parameter Summary

Type	Detection		Rx1	Rx2	Rx3	Rx4	Rx5	Rx6
VF	On	188-500 bpm	35 J	35 J	35 J	35 J	35 J	35 J
FVT	via VF	188-231 bpm	Burst(1)	35 J	35 J	35 J	35 J	35 J
VT	Monitor	150-188 bpm						

SVT Criteria On: Wavelet

Modes **Rates**

Mode	VVI	Lower	50 ppm

Lead Parameters

	Ventricular
Amplitude	2.5 V
Pulse Width	0.6 ms
Sensitivity	0.3 mV

Clinical Status: Since Nov 03, 2006

Episodes		% Pacing	
VF	0	Sensed	69.0 %
FVT	0	Paced	31.0 %
VT	1		
SVT	0		
NST	0		

Observations (3)

- VT Episode #18, Nov 07, 2006 08:28:14, accelerated to VF.
- VT Episode #18, Nov 07, 2006 08:28:14, was monitored. No VT therapies are delivered when VT Detection is set to Monitor.
- More than one therapy was attempted in VT episode #18, Nov 07, 2006 08:28:14.

Medtronic CareLink Network Confidential Patient Information Nov 8 2006 4:18:07PM
Copyright © 2001-2006 Medtronic, Inc. Page 1

Medtronic **T/VF Episode #18 Report**

ICD Model: Maximo™ VR 7232 Date of Interrogation: Nov 7 2006 12:25PM
Episode #18 - VT Chart speed: 25.0 mm/sec

FVT
FVT Rx 1 Burst

VF
VF Rx 1 Defib

34.8 J

Medtronic CareLink Network Confidential Patient Information Nov 8 2006 4:18:08PM
Copyright © 2001-2006 Medtronic, Inc. Page 2

FIGURE 53–6. A Medtronic CareLink™ remote monitoring report on a patient with ventricular tachycardia that was accelerated by antitachycardia pacing resulting in ventricular fibrillation successfully defibrillated with a single internal shock.

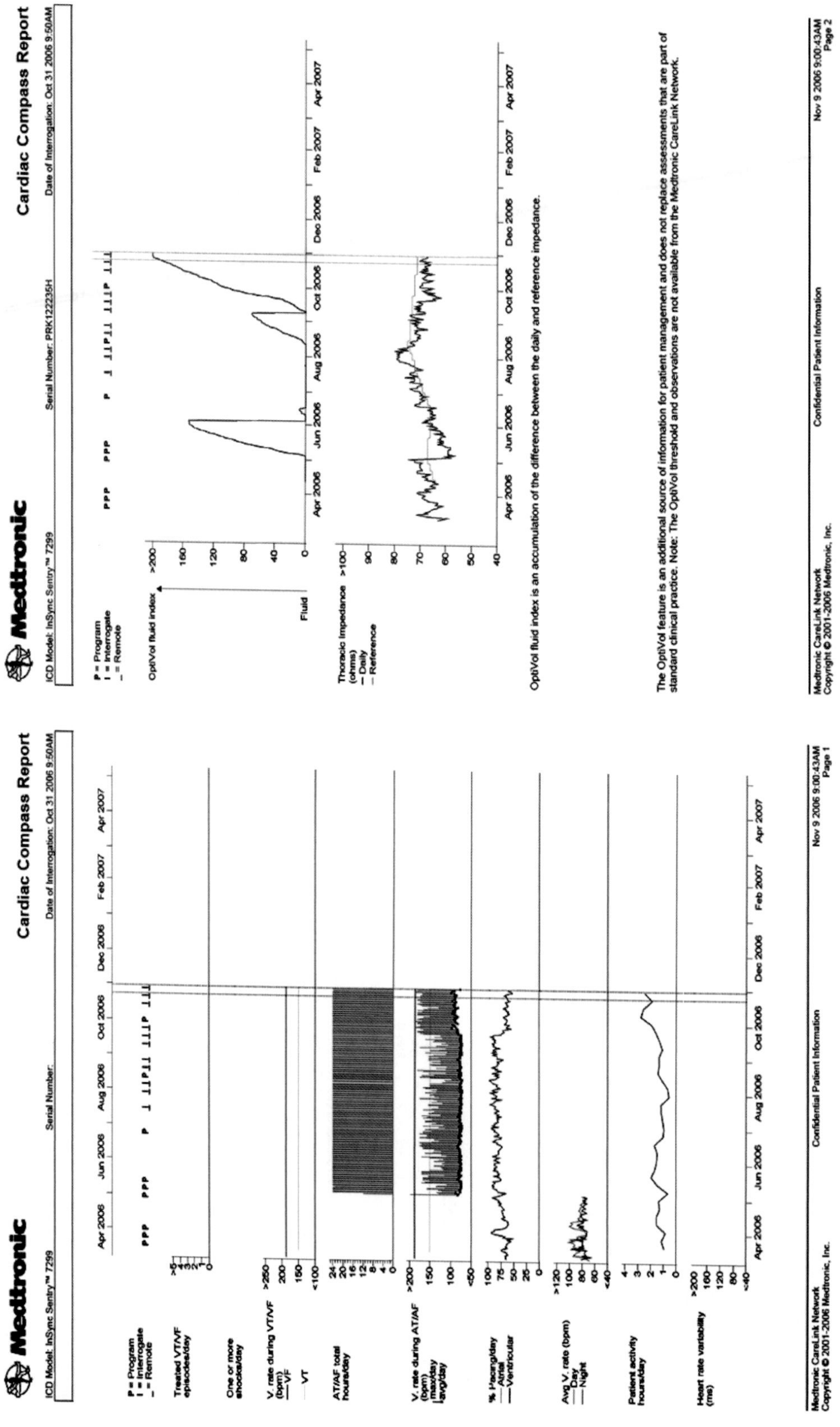

FIGURE 53–7. A Medtronic CareLink™ remote monitoring heart failure report on a patient using OptiVol, a measurement of transthoracic impedance as an indicator of heart failure status.

capability, to capture information for email, in office use such as in an electronic medical record, or other uses. Data can be maintained locally if a physician so chooses (and purchases the necessary equipment), or on servers controlled by service providers, currently the more commonly used approach.

Data Obtained

The data obtained, much like with the other systems discussed, is essentially the same as in-office reports obtained from a standard programmer. There are real time surface EGMs obtained from wristbands, along with stored electrograms from episodes where therapy was indicated and may have been delivered. Device-specific information is assessed, including battery status, thresholds, and impedance measurements, along with other more specific programmed algorithms. Summaries of clinically relevant events may be obtained (Figure 53–8), along with episode-specific EGMs (Figure 53–9). In the service centers, data are evaluated by technicians who have

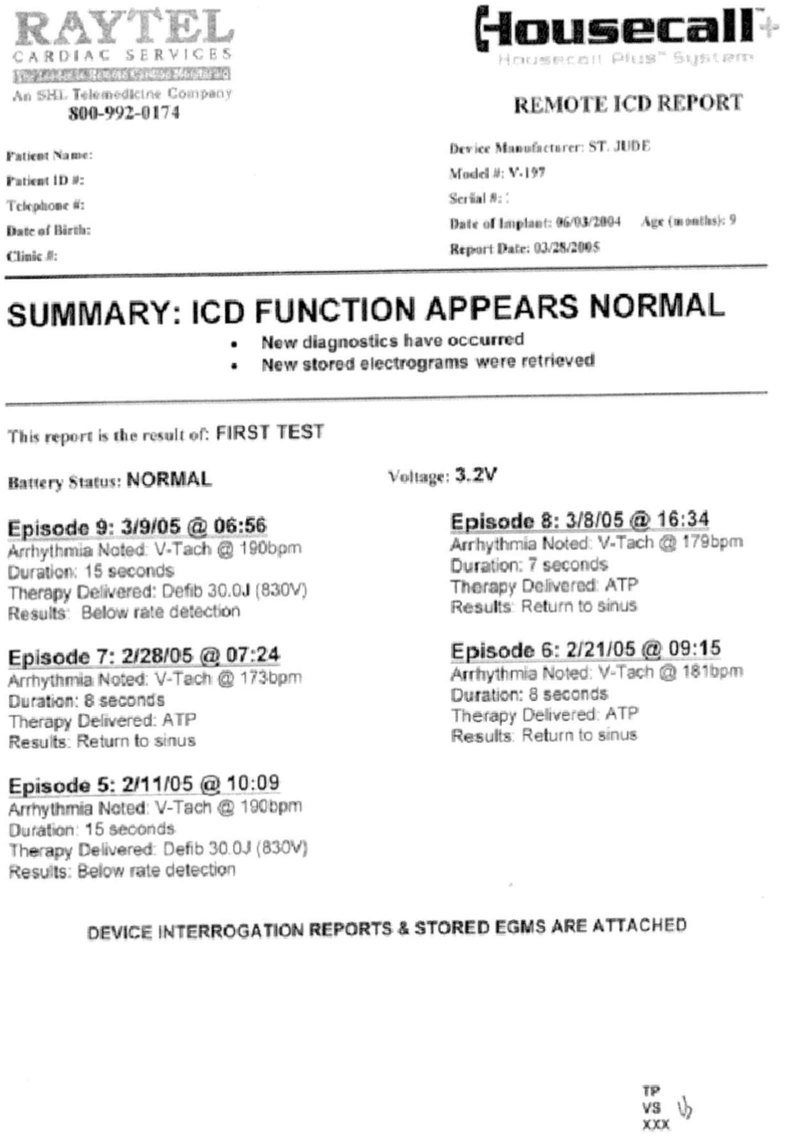
RAYTEL
CARDIAC SERVICES
An SHL Telemedicine Company
800-992-0174

Housecall+
Housecall Plus™ System

REMOTE ICD REPORT

Patient Name:
Patient ID #:
Telephone #:
Date of Birth:
Clinic #:

Device Manufacturer: ST. JUDE
Model #: V-197
Serial #:
Date of Implant: 06/03/2004 Age (months): 9
Report Date: 03/28/2005

SUMMARY: ICD FUNCTION APPEARS NORMAL
- New diagnostics have occurred
- New stored electrograms were retrieved

This report is the result of: FIRST TEST

Battery Status: NORMAL Voltage: 3.2V

Episode 9: 3/9/05 @ 06:56
Arrhythmia Noted: V-Tach @ 190bpm
Duration: 15 seconds
Therapy Delivered: Defib 30.0J (830V)
Results: Below rate detection

Episode 8: 3/8/05 @ 16:34
Arrhythmia Noted: V-Tach @ 179bpm
Duration: 7 seconds
Therapy Delivered: ATP
Results: Return to sinus

Episode 7: 2/28/05 @ 07:24
Arrhythmia Noted: V-Tach @ 173bpm
Duration: 8 seconds
Therapy Delivered: ATP
Results: Return to sinus

Episode 6: 2/21/05 @ 09:15
Arrhythmia Noted: V-Tach @ 181bpm
Duration: 8 seconds
Therapy Delivered: ATP
Results: Return to sinus

Episode 5: 2/11/05 @ 10:09
Arrhythmia Noted: V-Tach @ 190bpm
Duration: 15 seconds
Therapy Delivered: Defib 30.0J (830V)
Results: Below rate detection

DEVICE INTERROGATION REPORTS & STORED EGMS ARE ATTACHED

TP
VS
XXX

FIGURE 53–8. A remote monitoring report from St. Jude Medical's Housecall Plus™ coupled with Raytel service center. (Courtesy of St. Jude Medical.)

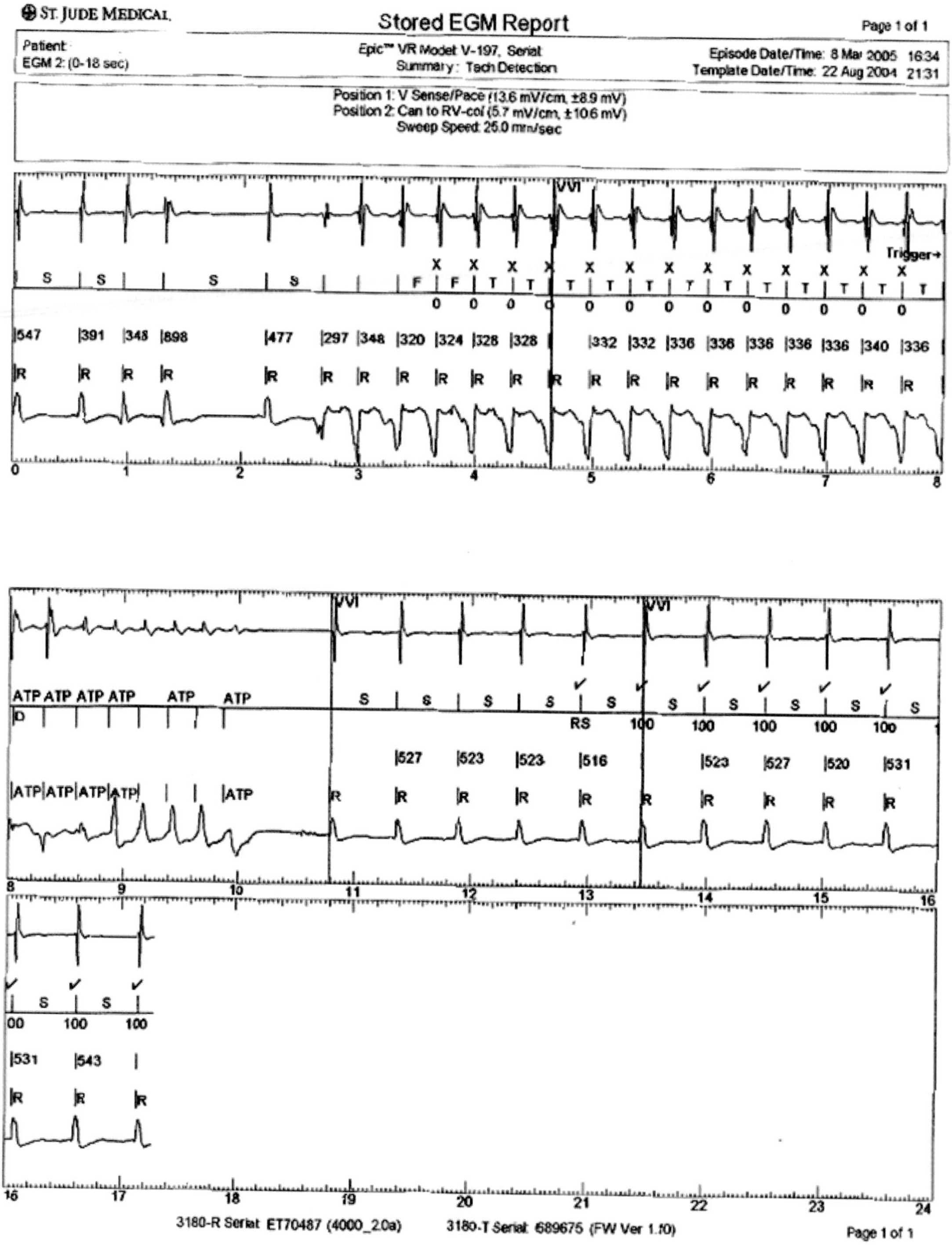

FIGURE 53–9. A St. Jude Housecall Plus™ remote monitoring report showing details of an arrhythmia event (ventricular tachycardia) successfully treated with antitachycardia pacing. (Courtesy of St. Jude Medical.)

become testamurs of NASPExAM (now referred to as IBHRE, International Board of Heart Rhythm Examiners).

Notifications

Critical issues are dealt with initially via the service center (if utilized). The physician may be notified in the case of preselected and customized notification criteria, such as therapy delivery, battery compromise, or impedance changes. Under the physician maintained system, information is received by persons designated by the physician practice.

Cost

There are manufacturer charges for the receiver and the transmitter. Payment structures vary according to whether the equipment is owned or leased, or how service centers are utilized. There are two service centers that can be used with the system, according to practice choice. There are no service fees associated with ongoing use of the system.

Billing for the services provided varies according to the model used, physician-maintained, or by service providers, and involves variable billing of technical and professional fees associated with interrogation.

Challenges

Privacy

One of the challenges for remote monitoring is protection of privacy. Technology has and will no doubt attempt to keep up with federal and international standards for protection of personal information, such as American Health Insurance Portability and Accountability Act (HIPAA), which dictates standards of protection of the privacy of personal health information. While technical challenges such as encryption of data and human challenges such as adequate training of personnel about privacy issues require careful attention, all involved, to date, appear committed to protection of privacy.

Data Management

Management (and formatting for use) of great volumes of data involved in remote monitoring will be problematic. Large volume practices could potentially be challenged with the day-to-day data management of patients with more advanced illness and implanted devices being remotely monitored, such as those typically seen in tertiary care centers. While such data are likely to lead to improved patient care, it is also likely that care pathways will need to be developed in offices specifically to deal with remotely monitored devices and patients. It is probable that large practices will have implanted device remote monitoring "centers" where data will be maintained, formatted, and parceled out to clinicians who can use the information for patient management. Smaller practices may rely solely on manufacturer or other "third-party" entities for data acquisitions, formatting, and management. It is important to point out that centralized data banks may be most important in improved device surveillance and reporting efforts.

Costs and Reimbursement

The direct and indirect costs of this technology will be significant. As has been discussed, direct costs may be billed at the time of implant, or are recurring. There will be further expenses, both direct and indirect, in managing the data (physician time, added staff, etc). At the time of this writing, reimbursement may be obtained in many states, by a variety of insurers for these services. The Centers for Medicare and Medicaid Services (CMS) issued a transmittal (Transmittal 979) in June 2006 authorizing reimbursement for remote monitoring of pacemakers and ICDs using in-office electronic analysis codes. While the initial forays into more sophisticated remote follow-up have targeted ICDs and CRT devices because of reimbursement issues, it is anticipated that over time, virtually all devices including pacemakers will be included.

Limitations

Limitations potentially imposed by this type of care will need to be addressed. Patient care teams will need to ensure that patients feel their care is being enhanced, rather than being compromised, by new technologies. These paradigm changes will likely require time to gain acceptance by the general medical community. Future trials will be designed to validate this approach to patient care and information, and also to investigate the potential economic aspects of remote care. As with any change in care paradigm, concerns will, no doubt, exist about not only the feasibility of the new care style, but also patient acceptance.

Conclusions

It appears that we are on the brink of a new era in healthcare of patients with or at high risk of chronic, and even acute, diseases. Remote monitoring of both implanted devices and chronic illnesses using implanted devices has been developed, technologically, to a point of broad-based utility and availability. Most companies now marketing implantable electronic devices such as pacemakers and defibrillators have developed manufacturer-specific remote monitoring systems. While there are substantial differences in the technology and formatting of the different systems, there are common goals for all of the systems.

Rapid access by patients, even in geographies significantly remote from device and disease expertise, is facilitated by using remote monitoring systems. Patients in need can be more closely monitored using such systems and both the hassles and time for device and disease follow-up can be minimized, potentially at significant financial savings and certainly with improvement in patients' and patients' families peace of mind and sense of well-being. From physicians' perspectives, with what will certainly be dramatic increases in patient volumes as our population ages as well as increases in absolute numbers, the improved efficiencies of remote monitoring will allow better human resource usage by minimizing unnecessary routine (and other) face-to-face visits with patients. It is likely that even hospitalizations can be reduced by remote monitoring systems as more consistent follow-up is done even for patients who otherwise would have difficulty achieving such follow-up because of geographic, physical, or economic restrictions. Remote monitoring and associated data-basing of device performance present as yet untapped opportunities for dramatic improvement in device-performance surveillance.

While the future appears bright for this emerging discipline of remote monitoring, much work needs to be done to further expand what can be monitored remotely, especially in monitoring diseases, as well as other activities that can be accomplished such as remote programming of device function. Additionally, making certain that implementation of these new concepts, technology, and systems is accomplished in economically viable ways is a challenge of utmost importance.

References

1. Schoenfeld MH, Reynolds, DW. Sophisticated remote implantable cardioverter-defibrillator follow-up: A status report. *Pacing Clin Electrophysiol* 2005; 28(3):235–240.
2. Carlson MD, Task Force Chair. Recommendations from the Heart Rhythm Society Task Force on Device Performance Policies and Guidelines. September 2006, www.hrsonline.org.
3. Gregoratos G, Chair. ACC/AHA Guidelines for Implantation of Cardiac Pacemakers and Antiarrhythmia Devices. A report of the American College of Cardiology/American Heart Association Task Force on Practice (Committee on Pacemaker Implantation). *J Am Coll Cardiol* 1998;31(5):1175–1209.
4. Adamson PB, Magalski A, Braunschweig F, *et al.* Ongoing right ventricular hemodynamics in heart failure: Clinical value of measurements derived from an implantable hemodynamic monitor. *J Am Coll Cardiol* 2003;41(4):565–571.
5. Shah NB, Der E, Ruggerio C, *et al.* Prevention of hospitalizations for heart failure with an interactive home monitoring program. *Am Heart J* 1998; 135(3):373–378.
6. Goldberg LR, Piette JD, Walsh MN, *et al.* Randomized trial of a daily electronic home monitoring system in patients with advanced heart failure: The Weight Monitoring in Heart Failure (WHARF) trial. *Am Heart J* 2003:146(4):705–712.
7. Stewart S, Vandenbroeck AJ, Pearson S, *et al.* Prolonged beneficial effects of a home-based intervention on unplanned readmissions and mortality among patients with congestive heart failure. *Arch Intern Med* 1999;159(3):257–261.
8. Galbreath AD, Krasuski RA, Smith B, *et al.* Long-term healthcare and cost outcomes of disease management in a large, randomized, community-based population with heart failure. *Circulation* 2004;110: 3518–3526.

9. Cleland JG, Louis AA, Rigby AS, Janssens U, *et al.* Noninvasive home telemonitoring for patients with heart failure at high risk of recurrent admission and death: The Trans-European Network-Home-Care Management System (TEN-HMS) study. *J Am Coll Cardiol* 2005;45(10):1654–1664.
10. Falk D, Straub K. Practice efficiency improvements resulting from the use of Medtronic CareLink Network remote monitoring system. Fairfield, Iowa: Human Factors International, July 2004.
11. Furman S, Escher DJ. Transtelephone pacemaker monitoring. In: Schaldach M, Furman S, Eds. *Advances in Pacemaker Technology*. Berlin: Springer-Verlag, 1975:177–194.
12. Ellenbogen KA, Kay GN, Wilkoff BL. *Clinical Cardiac Pacing*. Philadelphia, PA: W.B. Saunders, 1995:796–798.
13. Furman S, Hayes DL, Holmes DR. *A Practice of Cardiac Pacing*, 3rd ed. Malden, MA: Futura, 1993: 580–582.
14. Lyons C, Schroeder P, Shankar K, *et al.* Transtelephonic monitoring of a tachycardia-terminating pacemaker. *Pacing Clin Electrophysiol* 1984;7(1): 34–36.
15. Bhandari AK, Anderson JL, Gilbert EM, *et al.* Correlation of symptoms with occurrence of paroxysmal supraventricular tachycardia or atrial fibrillation: A transtelephonic monitoring study. *Am Heart J* 1992;124(2):381–386.
16. Fetter JG, Stanton MS, Benditt DG, *et al.* Transtelephonic monitoring and transmission of stored arrhythmia detection and therapy data from an implantable cardioverter defibrillator. *Pacing Clin Electrophysiol* 1995;18(8):1531–1539.
17. Scholten MF, Thorton AS, Theuns DA, Res J, Jordaens LJ. Twiddlers syndrome detected by home monitoring device. *Pacing Clin Electrophysiol* 2004;5(Suppl. 1):30S–31S.
18. Schoenfeld MH, Comptom SJ, Mead RH, *et al.* Remote monitoring of implantable cardioverter defibrillators: A prospective analysis. *Pacing Clin Electrophysiol* 2004;27(Pt. 1):757–763.
19. Yu CM, Wang L, Chau E, *et al.* Intrathoracic impedance monitoring in patients with heart failure. *Circulation* 2005;112:841–848.
20. Steinhaus D, Reynolds DW, Gadler F, *et al.* Implant experience with an implantable hemodynamic monitor for the management of symptomatic heart failure. *Pacing Clin Electrophysiol* 2005;28:747–753.
21. Magalski A, Adamson P, Gadler F, *et al.* Continuous ambulatory right heart pressure measurements with an implantable hemodynamic monitor: A multicenter, 12-month follow-up study of patients with chronic heart failure. *J Card Fail* 2002;8(2): 63–70.
22. Kjellstrom B, Igel D, Abraham J, *et al.* Transtelephonic monitoring of continuous haemodynamic measurements in heart failure patients. *J Telemed Telecare* 2005;11(5):240–244.
23. Joseph GK, Wilkoff BL, Dresing T, *et al.* Remote interrogation and monitoring of implantable cardioverter defibrillators. *J Interv Card Electrophysiol* 2004;11:161–166.

54 Catheter Ablation of Ventricular Tachycardia and Fibrillation

Frédéric Sacher, Mélèze Hocini, Anders Jönsson, Pierre Jaïs, Dominique Lacroix, Mark D. O'Neill, Yoshihide Takahashi, Nicolas Derval, Antoine Deplagne, Julien Laborderie, Pierre Bordachar, Jacques Clémenty, and Michel Haïssaguerre

Introduction

As in atrial fibrillation (AF), while both triggers and substrate may theoretically be the target of catheter ablation strategies, the presently published literature on catheter ablation of ventricular fibrillation (VF), including isolated case reports, has focused on targeting triggers.[1–11] The large mass of ventricular myocardium, the importance of maintaining normal mechanical ventricular function, and the risk of creating other forms of malignant arrhythmias mean that ablation strategies aimed at substrate modification are not suitable using the currently available technology. However, previous work in AF has shown that both triggers and substrate may share a close structural relationship. The pulmonary veins play an important role in the initiation and maintenance of AF,[12] and recent studies have shed light on their role in the maintenance of AF in some patients. Similarly, several experimental studies demonstrated that Purkinje fibers act as initiators and perpetuators of VF.[13,14] Hence, by ablating an area in which the triggering ectopics are found to originate, an additional effect might be substrate modification if the area is implicated in the maintenance of VF.

This review will focus on mapping and ablation of VF in a variety of clinical substrates as well as mapping and ablation of ventricular tachycardia (VT) in arrhythmogenic right ventricular cardiomyopathy (ARVC).

Mapping and Ablation Procedure

Indication and Timing of the Procedure

To start, we have to emphasize that an implantable cardioverter defibrillator (ICD) remains the first line therapy for patients with primary VF or polymorphic VT. Ablation should be considered in case of multiple episodes of primary VF or polymorphic VT (e.g., not VT degenerating into VF) with no curable underlying condition refractory to pharmacological therapy and with documented frequent ventricular ectopics at the time of the procedure. In some patients, the triggering ventricular ectopics are persistent even after a long absence of VF episodes, and can be mapped easily. However, in most cases of idiopathic VF[5] and/or Purkinje premature ventricular contractions (PVC)-induced VF,[4,5,15] it is likely that the ectopics are episodic, mainly appearing prior to and a few days after the onset of VF or polymorphic VT. This results in a narrow time window whereby mapping and ablation can be performed under optimal conditions, hence the procedure has to be performed within a few days of the VF episodes.

It is of outmost importance that ventricular premature beats (VPBs) are recorded on 12-lead electrocardiograms (ECG) before the procedure. We therefore routinely record a continuous 12-lead ECG immediately after the VF episode, where the electrode position on the skin is marked in

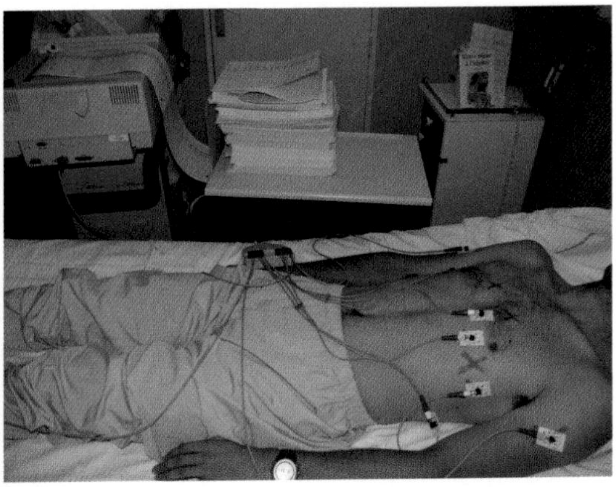

FIGURE 54–1. Continuous 12-lead ECG recording of VPBs. Electrode placements are marked on the skin to allow reproducible recordings. This is important if there is an absence of VPBs during the procedure, where ablation using a pace-mapping technique may be the only remaining alternative. A one night continuous ECG recording is shown on the table.

order to get reproducible recordings and precise localization of the VPBs (Figure 54–1). The latter is of particular value in the absence of VPBs during the procedure, where ablation using a Purkinje pace-mapping technique may be the only remaining alternative.

Electrophysiology Study and Endocardial Mapping

As previously described,[5] the electrophysiology study is performed with 2–4 multielectrode catheters. Surface ECG recordings and bipolar intracardiac electrograms are filtered at 30–500 Hz and recorded simultaneously with a digital polygraph (LabSystem, Bard Electrophysiology, sampling rate 1–4 kHz). High gain amplification (1 mm = 0.1 mV) is used during mapping to clearly identify the Purkinje potential. The VPBs are localized by mapping the earliest electrogram relative to the onset of the ectopic QRS complex. The Purkinje origin is defined by the presence of an initial sharp potential (<10 msec in duration) preceding the larger and slower local ventricular electrogram by <15 msec in sinus rhythm and preceding ventricular activation during ectopy[16] (Figure 54–2). Its absence defines muscular origin.

Radiofrequency Ablation

Ablation is performed with conventional 4-mm tip catheters with a thermocouple, using radiofrequency (RF) energy with a target temperature of 55–60°C and a maximum power of 40–50 W. In case of low power output, an irrigated tip catheter is used with a maximum temperature of 48°C and

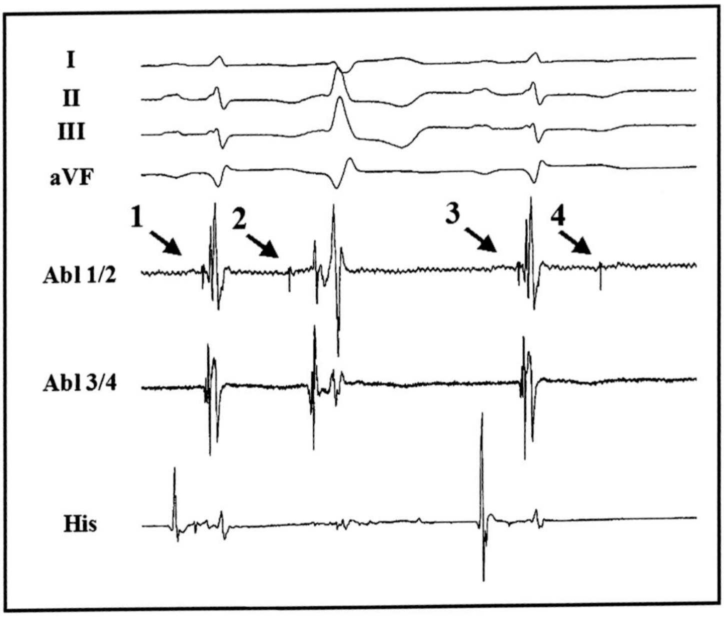

FIGURE 54–2. A distal Purkinje potential (2) precedes local activation during ectopy as well as during sinus rhythm (1 and 3). The second Purkinje discharge (4) is not conducted to the ventricle (conduction block); arrows indicate the Purkinje potential. Abl 1–2, distal ablation catheter; Abl 3–4, proximal ablation catheter.

a power of 30–40 W. The ectopic focus is targeted first, and after abolition of the ectopics, the lesion is extended to cover a larger area around the focus to minimize recurrence. In case of polymorphic VPBs, the most frequent one is targeted and eliminated, and then the second most frequent, etc. In the absence of ectopy during the procedure, provocative maneuvers (pacing and/or pharmacological) are used prior to pace mapping the Purkinje system.

Various Substrates Associated with Ventricular Fibrillation

Idiopathic Ventricular Fibrillation

Clinical Presentation

Thirty-five patients (17 males, mean age 41 ± 14 years) with recurrent episodes of idiopathic VF have been studied. Of these, 17% had a family history of sudden cardiac death (SCD). Patients were studied after having arrhythmic storm, with 9 ± 13 (range 3–50) episodes of VF prior to ablation that persisted despite the use of 3 ± 2 antiarrhythmic agents. The majority of VF episodes occurred during activities of daily living and rarely appeared during sleep. Importantly, none of these patients had arrhythmia during exertion. All patients had frequent VPBs immediately after the VF storm, with 2 ± 1 (range 1–5) different morphologies. The VPBs initiating VF demonstrated a coupling interval to the preceding ventricular complex of 297 ± 42 msec. Importantly, the VPBs triggering VF were also observed to occur independently of VF episodes (Figure 54–3).

Location of Ectopy

The VPBs that were observed to trigger VF had specific morphological features. Most patients demonstrated a positive morphology in V1, suggesting a left ventricular origin. However, in two-thirds of the group, significant morphological variations occurred, especially regarding the limb leads (Figure 54–4). In 30 patients, VPBs were mapped to the left or right Purkinje network, while in five patients they were found to be of right ventricular outflow tract (RVOT) origin. The Purkinje sources were localized to the anterior right ventricle or in a wider region of the lower half of the septum in the left ventricle. In the latter case, VPBs from the ramifications of the anterior and posterior fascicles resulted in an inferior and superior QRS axis, respectively, whereas the origin from the intervening region demonstrated an intermediate axis. In addition, VPBs from the left Purkinje network demonstrated significantly narrower QRS intervals compared with those from the RVOT (128 ± 18 msec versus 145 ± 13 msec). They were polymorphic in 80%, suggesting a different exit or source, while in RVOT they were mainly monomorphic. Several interesting electrophysiological phenomena were observed during intracardiac mapping: different Purkinje to local ventricular myocardial conduction times associated with altering VPBs morphologies; rapid repetitive beats (mean cycle length 221 bpm) demonstrating Purkinje activation, suggesting that this system may drive the onset of VF; and Purkinje to local ventricular myocardial conduction block (Figure 54–2).

At the site of successful ablation, endocardial activity preceded the QRS activation on the surface ECG by 130 ± 19 msec. Ablation resulted in temporary exacerbation of VPBs that, in some cases, were associated with the induction of VF. Ventricular premature beats of different morphologies were progressively eliminated using 13 ± 7 RF energy applications. Electrograms recorded after ablation demonstrated the abolition of the local Purkinje potential and a slight delay in the local ventricular electrogram (Figure 54–5). The fluoroscopic and procedural durations were 51 ± 68 and 189 ± 78 min, respectively. Three patients had recurrent VPBs during their hospital stay and required reablation. All 3 had no ectopy during the initial procedure.

Outcome after Ablation

Patients were followed clinically by Holter-ECG and by routine interrogation of the defibrillator after ablation. All antiarrhythmic therapies were discontinued postablation. Two patients had recurrence of VF and appropriate shocks documented by the device log and one patient had a single presyncope due to polymorphic VT lasting 6 sec without defibrillator discharge. In the remaining patients, Holter recordings showed

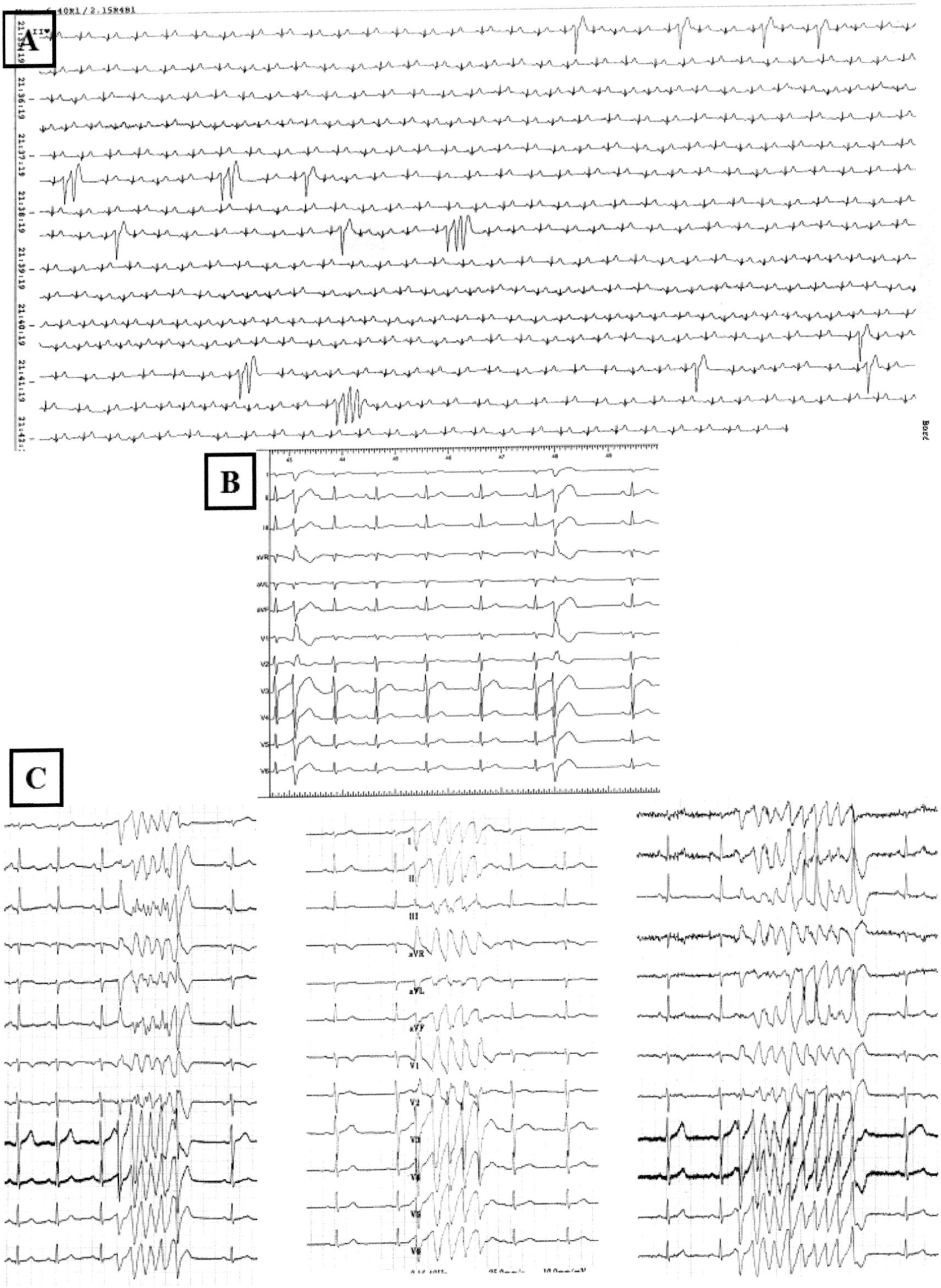

FIGURE 54–3. Examples of ECGs from a 23-year-old female with idiopathic VF. (A) Isolated and short runs of VBPs. (B) The 12-lead ECG morphology of the dominant VBP. (C) Short runs of nonsustained polymorphic VT initiated by three slightly different VPBs, all originating from the Purkinje network.

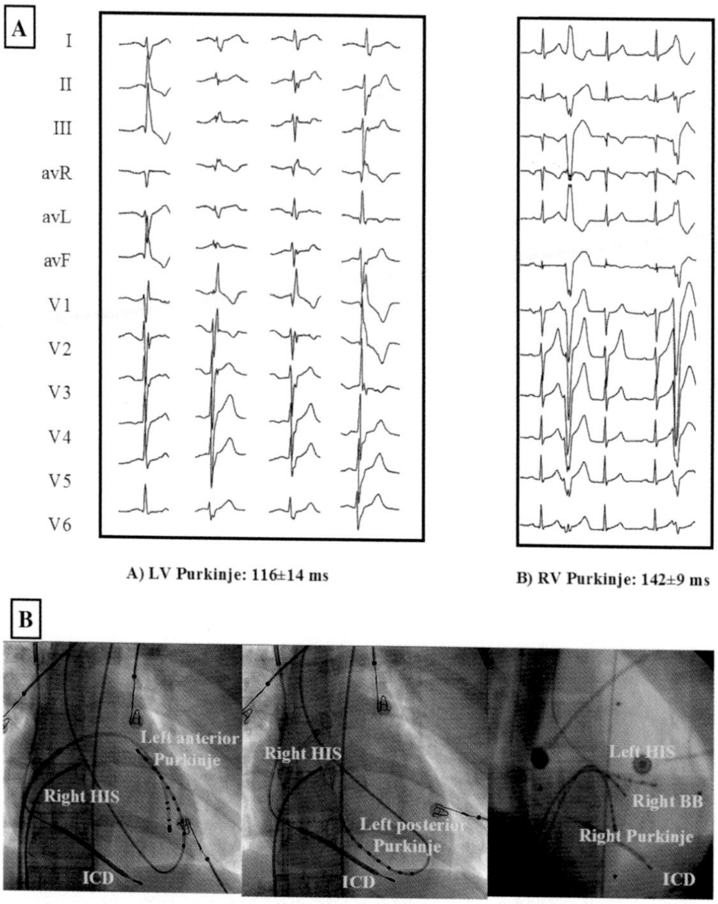

Figure 54–4. (a) A typical 12-lead ECG pattern of ectopic beats originating from the left (A) and right (B) Purkinje network. Left ventricular (LV) Purkinje beats are narrow (116 ± 14 msec) and have a left, right, or intermediate QRS axis. Four different LV Purkinje beats from one patient are shown. Right ventricular (RV) Purkinje beats have a left bundle branch block pattern in V1 and are usually wider (142 ± 0.9 msec). (b) Fluoroscopy images with anteroposterior visualization of catheter positions recording Purkinje potentials. ICD, implantable cardioverter-defibrillator; Right BB, right bundle branch.

infrequent (28 ± 49; range 0–145) isolated VPBs per 24 h (without antiarrhythmic drug). During a follow-up of 48 ± 3 2 months, there was no sudden death, syncope, or recurrence of VF in 86% of patients.

Brugada Syndrome

Clinical Presentation

Various hypotheses have been brought forward with regard to the triggering mechanisms of VF in the Brugada syndrome. A contribution from the autonomic nervous system has been proposed, with vagal stimulation believed to trigger arrhythmia in some patients. Related observations have suggested that the beginning of VT/VF is bradycardia dependent.[17] This could explain the higher incidence of arrhythmia and sudden death at night in this group of patients.

Regardless of the mechanism, it is likely that the actual triggers for VF or polymorphic VT in most cases of the Brugada syndrome are ventricular ectopic beats, most of them monomorphic.[18] In the latter study, 19 patients with the Brugada syndrome and an implanted ICD were followed over a mean duration of 14 months, during which spontaneous VF occurred in 7 (37%), with three having multiple episodes. Analysis of 33 episodes of VF revealed that 22 episodes (67%) were preceded by isolated ventricular ectopic beats, which

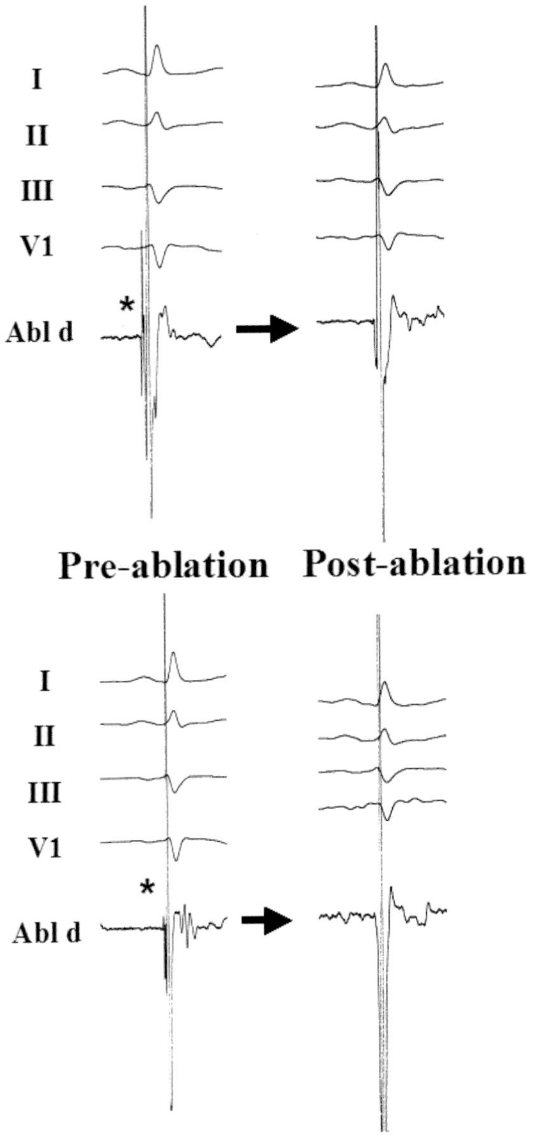

FIGURE 54–5. Radiofrequency applications resulting in abolition of local Purkinje potentials in sinus rhythm. Abl d, distal ablation catheter.

were identical in morphology to the ectopic beats triggering VF. Furthermore, in the three patients with multiple episodes, VFs were always triggered by the same type of VPBs.

Based on this report and on our previous experience with idiopathic VF,[4,5] we devised an ablation strategy where the initial results have been recently published.[7]

To date, we have performed mapping and catheter ablation of VF in six patients with the Brugada syndrome (four males; 38 ± 6 years). All of them had presented with an electrical storm with multiple appropriate ICD shocks (12 ± 9).

Location of Ectopy

Current observations suggest that ectopy arising in the Brugada syndrome are predominantly of RV origin. Chinushi *et al.* described recurrent episodes of VF in a patient with Brugada syndrome initiated by monomorphic ectopics with a left bundle-branch block (LBBB) morphology.[19] This was corroborated by Morita *et al.*,[20] who observed ventricular ectopics in 9 out of 45 patients studied. Eleven ectopic morphologies were observed in these 9 patients, of which 10 were of right ventricular origin (seven RVOT, two septal, and one from the apex).

In our experience, VPBs were monomorphic in four patients. They originated from the RVOT in five (coupling interval: 343 ± 59 msec), from the right septum in two (CI: 280 msec, 320 msec), and from the right ventricular Purkinje network in one (CI: 300 msec). Interestingly, fragmented potentials in RVOT were demonstrated in two patients. The monomorphic RVOT premature beats were first observed at the time of VF in three cases. However, in two patients they were documented 14 and 11 years before they triggered VF, at a time where, notably, no signs of the Brugada phenotype in the 12-lead ECG were seen.

Outcome after Ablation

During a mean follow-up period of 30 ± 15 months, there has been no recurrence of VF as assessed by the ICD recordings, syncope, or SCD in any patient. None used any antiarrhythmic drugs.

Congenital Long QT Syndrome

Clinical Presentation

We have studied four patients with long QT syndrome (LQTS) (two males, aged 37 ± 8 years), three with a history of SCD.[8] All patients presented with documented episodes of polymorphic VT or VF (6 ± 4 episodes of VF or syncope prior to mapping). Medical treatment included β blockers alone or combined with Class IC drugs (three), verapamil (two), and amiodarone (one). The diagnose of LQTS was based on established criteria and was made after the onset of ventricular arrhythmias. No mutations on KVLQT1, hERG, KCNE2, KCNJ2, or SCN5A were found.

All patients were studied within 2 weeks of their arrhythmic storm and had been documented to have frequent VPBs. The triggering role of VPBs in the initiation of VF was observed by ambulatory monitoring or stored electrograms of the defibrillator. Premature beats in the LQTS had a coupling interval of 503 ± 29 msec; they were monomorphic in two patients [one with LBBB-inferior axis typical of RVOT and one with right bundle branch block (RBBB)-superior axis], and polymorphic and repetitive with a positive morphology in lead V1 in two patients; the latter had varying cycle lengths of 280–420 msec with repetitive beats lasting 3–45 beats.

Location of Ectopy

One patient had VPBs originating from the RVOT. Two patients had polymorphic VPBs that originated from the peripheral Purkinje arborization in the left ventricle, including the ramifications of anterior or posterior fascicles, and from the intervening regions. In one patient the premature beats originated from the posterior fascicle. The earliest Purkinje potential preceded the local endocardial muscle activation by a conduction interval of 34 ± 17 msec during the VPBs. Repetitive beats were also preceded by Purkinje activity with a variable delay ranging from 20 to 110 msec (52 ± 24).

Outcome after Ablation

During a mean follow-up period of 24 ± 20 months, there has been no recurrence of VF, syncope, or sudden cardiac death in any patient. One patient died of a noncardiac cause. One patient was maintained on a β blocker and another had a late recurrence of VPBs but declined further procedures.

Andersen–Tawil Syndrome

Clinical Presentation

Andersen–Tawil syndrome (ATS), also called LQT7, is a rare condition consisting of ventricular arrhythmias, potassium-sensitive periodic paralysis, and developmental anomalies. In addition to isolated VPBs, VTs involving a beat-to-beat variability in axis (polymorphic VT), such as bidirectional VT and torsade de pointes, have been described.[21–23]

From initial reports, therapies such as oral potassium supplementation, sodium restriction, spironolactone, and acetazolamide have anecdotally been shown to ameliorate symptoms of weakness,[24] but no therapeutic standards exist to date.

So far we have studied four ATS patients (19 ± 9 years, one male), all with a history of syncope. Bidirectional ventricular tachycardia (n = 2) and frequent polymorphic VPBs (n = 2) were documented prior to the procedure.

Location of Ectopy

Interestingly, rapid atrial pacing as well as isoproterenol and verapamil infusion totally suppressed ventricular arrhythmias; moreover, VT could not be induced by standard programmed stimulation in the right ventricle. We managed to eliminate the most frequent VPB morphologies (four with preceding left Purkinje potential and three without); however, infrequent VPBs were still present at the end of the procedure, as well as bidirectional VT.

Outcome after Ablation

Despite persisting ventricular arrhythmias, all patients remained asymptomatic under β blocker therapy 16 ± 13 months after ablation.

Ventricular Fibrillation Storm following Myocardial Infarction

Clinical Presentation

While VF associated with myocardial infarction is frequently short lived and managed with the use of β blockers with or without amiodarone, patients occasionally present with arrhythmogenic storms that cannot be managed medically (0.0014% of patients[8]). With experimental recognition of the subendocardial Purkinje network surviving during transmural myocardial infarction (MI),[25] some clinical studies have recently evaluated the role of such trigger elimination in the management of VF storms after MI.[8–10] Up to the present we have encountered eight patients (eight males, 63 ± 5 years old), all whom had extensive MI with different localizations and with significant left ventricular dysfunction. All had complete revascularization performed and were considered to be on optimal pharmacological therapy. They presented in the first 2 weeks after myocardial infarction with frequent VPBs triggering VF (50 54 episodes, range: 15–130) and subsequent multiple adequate ICD shocks.

Location of Ectopy

This is a challenging procedure because patients are often hemodynamically unstable and in need of hemodynamic support. Mapping and ablation progressively targeted the most frequent VPB morphology. In all, the origin was located to the Purkinje network bordering the infarct zone, with a coupling interval to the preceding sinus beat of 379 ± 56 msec. In two patients VPBs originated from the Purkinje system *and* the myocardium. These findings are consistent with recently published data, confirming the origin of VPB from the Purkinje arborization at the myocardial scar border zone, with a number of different VPB morphologies varying from one to four (Table 54–1) (maximum 10 in our experience).

Outcome after Ablation

At 28 ± 18 months of VF ablation, seven out of eight patients are free of recurrence. Two presented with monomorphic VT and are being treated with amiodarone. One died of refractory heart failure at 1 week after ablation.

Other Substrates

Mapping and ablation of VF have been reported after aortic valve replacement,[11] with triggering PVCs originating from the left Purkinje network and with cardiac amyloidosis.[26] We performed ablation on a 32-year-old male with idiopathic dilated cardiomyopathy (ejection fraction 45%) with PVCs originating from the right Purkinje network and from the ventricle itself.

Finally, we would like to describe a 15-year-old female with an unclassified primary electrical disease. She was referred to us after having experienced more than 80 ICD appropriate shocks in a short period of time. The 12-lead ECG exhibited a number of interesting features (Figure 54–6). Several VPB morphologies from the left ventricle (with and without Purkinje origin) were mapped and ablated, but VF reoccurred triggered by others VPBs. Quinidine therapy was then initiated and the patient has now remained free of shock for 3 years.

BLE 54–1. Catheter ablation of ventricular fibrillation postmyocardial infarction.[a]

	Number of patients	MI site	PVT after MI	Number of VF episodes prior to ablation	Number of PVC morphology/patient	Distribution of foci	Coupling interval of initiating PVC (msec)	RF time	Success [follow-up (months)]
änsch *t al.*[8]	4	2 anterior 2 inferior	1–7 days	19–60		All in the Purkinje network at the scar border zone	270–400	18 ± 10 applications	100%
larrouche *t al.*[9]	8	3 anteroseptal 2 anterolateral 2 posterolateral 1 lateral	11 ± 5 months	35–89	1	All in the Purkinje network at the scar border zone	195 ± 45	88%	
zumowski *t al.*[10]	5	5 anterior	67 ± 85 4–170 days	2 patients with >30 external defibrillations	2.6 ± 1.1 Purkinje	All in the network at the scar border zone	320–600	19 ± 9 min	100%

, ventricular fibrillation; MI, myocardial infarction; PVT, paroxysmal ventricular tachycardia; PVC, premature ventricular contraction; RF, radiofrequency.

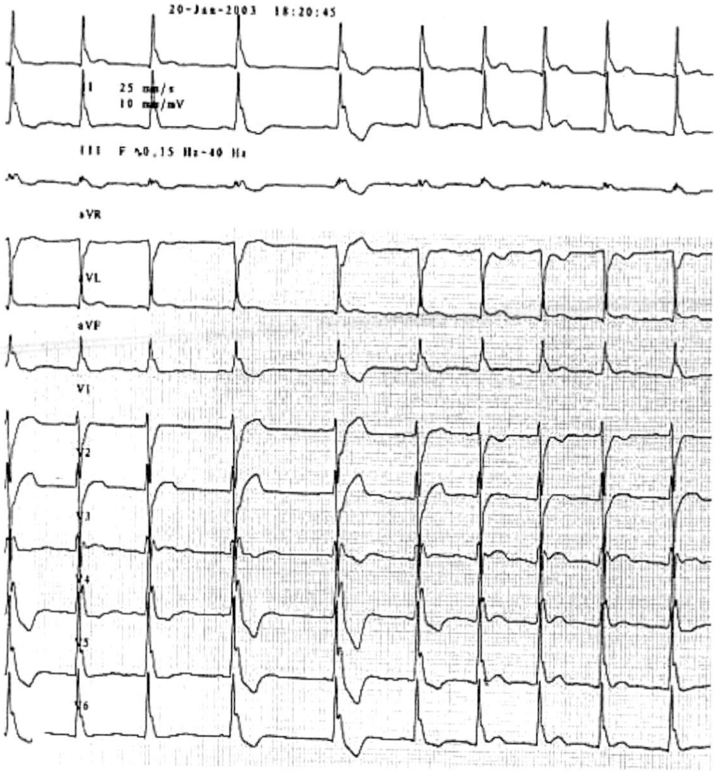

FIGURE 54–6. Twelve-lead ECG from in a 15-year-old female with an unclassified primary electrical disease and multiple ICD shocks. An association between the preceding coupling interval and QRS width was noted. In the fourth and fifth beats with a coupling interval of 840 msec, the QRS interval is 120 msec. The remaining beats on the ECG have a shorter coupling interval accompanied by a shorter QRS duration. The patient's arrhythmias occurred at rest.

Arrhythmogenic Right Ventricular Cardiomyopathy

Clinical Presentation

Arrhythmogenic right ventricular cardiomyopathy is a sporadic or hereditary disease characterized by fibrofatty atrophy of the right ventricular myocardium that could result in right heart failure and/or ventricular arrhythmias. The interventricular septum and the left ventricle may also be involved. VT, due to reentry circuits in areas of abnormal myocardium, is the principal ventricular arrhythmia, but polymorphic VT or VF has also been described.[27,28] Ventricular tachycardias typically demonstrate an LBBB morphology and are easily inducible with programmed stimulation. Critical areas in the tachycardia circuit are frequently situated in the RVOT and in the area around the tricuspid annulus (Figure 54–7).

Mapping and Ablation

Ventricular tachycardia in ARVC shares many of the features observed in postinfarct VT patients. The circuits are composed of zones of abnormal conduction, characterized by low-amplitude abnormal electrograms, with identifiable exit regions to the surrounding myocardium. Targets for ablation previously identified in ischemic VT[29] may also be useful for targeting VT in ARVC.[30,31–34] In patients with hemodynamically well-tolerated VT, conventional activation and entrainment mapping alone or combined with a computerized mapping system are usually applied (Figure 54–8). In case of nonsustained or poorly tolerated VT, linear lesions can be deployed, with the site of ablation guided primarily by pace mapping. These linear lesions typically extended from the most abnormal myocardium, with a signal amplitude <0.5 mV, through the site showing a perfect pace map, further connecting to annular/valvular

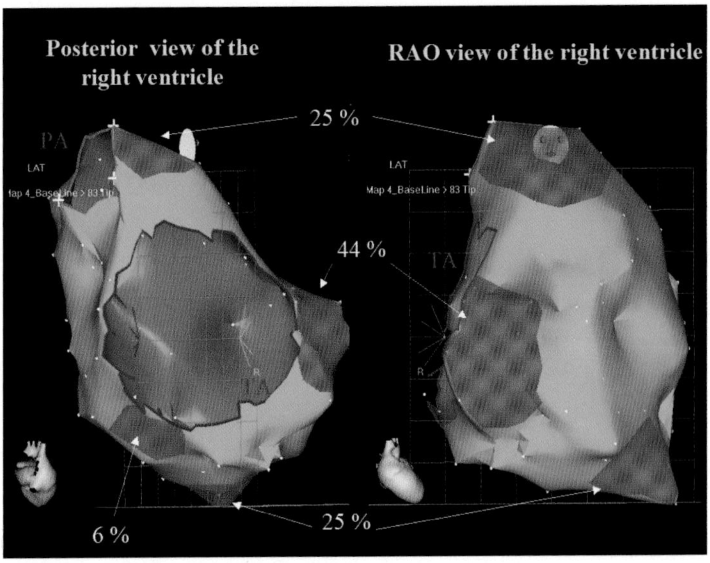

FIGURE 54–7. Localization of VTs successful ablation site in 12 ARVC patients with 16 different VTs. PA, pulmonary annulus; TA, tricuspid annulus; RAO, right oblique anterior. (Courtesy of Pr. Dominique Lacroix, CHRU de Lille, France.)

structures.[35,36] In patients with less extensive perivalvular bipolar voltage abnormalities, a linear lesion can extend across the entire segment of abnormal myocardium[37] (Figure 54–8).

It has recently been reported that epicardial ablation could be performed in ARVC patients in case of failure of endocardial ablation.[38] Interestingly, electroanatomical mapping of the epicardium has shown more extensive areas of low voltage compared to the endocardium, i.e., indicating that the ARVC process starts in the epicardium.

Outcome after Ablation

The clinical experience with catheter ablation of VT related to ARVC is limited (Table 54–2) with acute success varying from 33–80%. Because of the progressive nature of the disease, a substantial recurrence rate of VT can be expected. The place

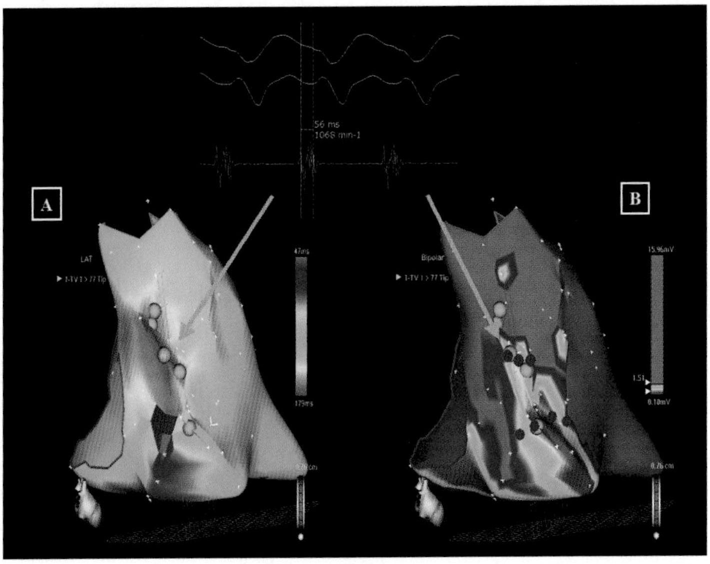

FIGURE 54–8. Mapping of VT in an ARVC patient using an eletroanatomical mapping system (Carto, Biosense Webster). (A) An activation map of the right ventricle during VT; the arrow indicates the site of the earliest ventricular activity. (B) A bipolar voltage map of the same patient. Ablation was performed at the earliest activation site combined with a linear lesion across the entire segment of abnormal myocardium (red circles refer to ablation points). (Courtesy of Pr. Dominique Lacroix, CHRU de Lille, France.)

TABLE 54–2. Catheter ablation of ventricular tachycardia in arrhythmogenic right ventricular cardiomyopathy.[a]

	Patients	ICD prior to ablation	VT ablation approach	Number of VTs/ patient	VTs cycle lengh (msec)	Site of "critical isthmus"	Acute success	Follow-up (months)	Clinical recurrence
Ellison *et al.*[30]	5		Entrainment mapping	3.8		RVOT, tricuspid annulus, apex	44% of inducible VTs	17 (11–24)	0
Della Bella *et al.*[31]	3	2	"Single beat" mapping	1	260 (250–270)		33%	19 (18–20)	
Reithmann *et al.*[32]	5	4	Activation, entrainment, and electroanatomic mapping	1–2	380 (240–520)	RVOT, tricuspid annulus	80%	7 ± 3	40%
O'Donnell *et al.*[33]	17	0	Activation mapping, entrainment mapping, pace-mapping, substrate mapping	1.8 (1–6)	310 (230–420)		41%	58 ± 18	47%
Marchlinski *et al.*[34]	19	14	Activation mapping, entrainment mapping, pace-mapping, substrate mapping			RVOT, tricuspid annulus	74%	27 ± 22	16%
Verma *et al.*[35]	22	18	Pace-mapping, Substrate Mapping	3 ± 2	339 ± 94	RVOT, Tricuspid annulus, Antero and infero apex	82%	37 [25–44]	36%

[a]ICD, implantable cardioverter defibrillator; VT, ventricular tachycardia; ARVC, arrhythmogenic right ventricular cardiomyopathy; RVOT, right ventricular outflow track.

of ablation in ARVC patients is then adjunctive to medical therapy and ICD.

Conclusions

Though catheter ablation of VF is still an emerging technique, the initial experiences with idiopathic VF,[4,5] and later in VF secondary to ischemic heart disease and repolarization disorders,[6–11] provided important insights into the role of focal triggers from the Purkinje system and RVOT in different clinical substrates. In particular, it is eminently applicable to patients having frequent recurrent episodes of VF provided the triggers can be localized by mapping. Reducing the incidence of VF with localized ablation may reduce defibrillation requirement and replacement, but most importantly it will improve the quality of life. Furthermore, in the subset of patient with VF storms, ablation may be the only remaining option for survival. In the setting of ARVC, catheter ablation is an adjunctive option to ICD and medical therapy targeting the critical part of the reentrant circut.

References

1. Aizawa Y, Tamura M, Chinushi M, *et al.* An attempt at electrical catheter ablation of the arrhythmogenic area in idiopathic ventricular fibrillation. *Am Heart J* 1992;95:572–576.
2. Ashida K, Kaji Y, Sasaki Y. Ablation of torsades de pointes after radiofrequency catheter ablation at right ventricular outflow tract. *Int J Cardiol* 1997; 59:171–175.
3. Takatsuki S, Mitamura H, Ogawa S. Catheter ablation of a monofocal premature ventricular complex triggering idiopathic ventricular fibrillation. *Heart* 2001;86:e3.
4. Haissaguerre M, Shah DC, Jais P, *et al.* Role of Purkinje conducting system in triggering of idiopathic ventricular fibrillation. *Lancet* 2002;359:677–678.

5. Haissaguerre M, Shoda M, Jais P, *et al.* Mapping and ablation of idiopathic ventricular fibrillation. *Circulation* 2002;106:962–967.
6. Paul T, Laohakunakorn P, Long B, *et al.* Complete elimination of incessant polymorphic ventricular tachycardia in an infant with MIDAS syndrome: Use of endocardial mapping and radiofrequency catheter ablation. *J Cardiovasc Electrophysiol* 2002; 13:612–615.
7. Haissaguerre M, Extramiana F, Hocini M, *et al.* Mapping and ablation of ventricular fibrillation associated with long-QT and Brugada syndromes. *Circulation* 2003;108:925–928.
8. Bansch D, Oyang F, Antz M, *et al.* Successful catheter ablation of electrical storm after myocardial infarction. *Circulation* 2003;108:3011–3016.
9. Marrouche NF, Verma A, Wazni O, *et al.* Mode of initiation and ablation of ventricular fibrillation storms in patients with ischemic cardiomyopathy. *J Am Coll Cardiol* 2004;43(9):1715–1720.
10. Szumowski L, Sanders P, Walczak F, *et al.* Mapping and ablation of polymorphic ventricular tachycardia after myocardial infarction. *J Am Coll Cardiol* 2004;44(8):1700–1706.
11. Li YG, Gronefeld G, Israel C, *et al.* Catheter ablation of frequently recurring ventricular fibrillation in a patient after aortic valve repair. *J Cardiovasc Electrophysiol* 2004;15:90–93.
12. Haissaguerre M, Sanders P, Hocini M, *et al.* Changes in atrial fibrillation cycle length and inducibility during catheter ablation and their relation to outcome. *Circulation* 2004;109(24):3007–3013.
13. Berenfeld O, Jalife J. Pukinje-muscle reentry as a mechanism of polymorphic ventricular arrhythmias in a 3-dimensional model of the ventricles. *Circ Res* 1998;82:1063–1077.
14. Sasyniuk B, Mendez C. A mechanism for reentry in canine ventricular tissue. *Circ Res* 1971;28:3–15.
15. Sacher F, Victor J, Hocini M, *et al.* Characterization of premature ventricular contraction initiating ventricular fibrillation. *Arch Mal Coeur* 2005;98: 867–873.
16. Nakagawa H, Beckman KJ, McClelland JH, *et al.* Radiofrequency catheter ablation of idiopathic left ventricular tachycardia guided by a Purkinje potential. *Circulation* 1993;88:2607–2617.
17. Kasanuki H, Ohnishi S, Ohtuka M, *et al.* Idiopathic ventricular fibrillation induced with vagal activity in patients without obvious heart disease. *Circulation* 1997;95:2277–2285.
18. Kakishita M, Kurita T, Matsuo K, *et al.* Mode of onset of ventricular fibrillation in patients with Brugada syndrome detected by implantable cardioverter defibrillator therapy. *J Am Coll Cardiol* 2000; 36:1646–1653.
19. Chinushi M, Washizuka T, Chinushi Y, *et al.* Induction of ventricular fibrillation in Brugada syndrome by site-specific right ventricular premature depolarization. *Pacing Clin Electrophysiol* 2002;25:1649–1651.
20. Morita H, Kusano KF, Nagase S, *et al.* Site-specific arrhythmogenesis in patients with Brugada syndrome. *J Cardiovasc Electrophysiol* 2003;14:373–379.
21. Plaster NM, Tawil R, Tristani-Firouzi M, *et al.* Mutations in Kir2.1 cause the developmental and episodic electrical phenotypes of Andersen's syndrome. *Cell* 2001;105:511–519.
22. Zhang L, Benson DW, Tristani-Firouzi M, *et al.* Electrocardiographic features in Andersen-Tawil syndrome patients with KCNJ2 mutations: Characteristic T-U-wave patterns predict the KCNJ2 genotype. *Circulation* 2005;111:2720–2726.
23. Chun TU, Epstein MR, Dick M, *et al.* Polymorphic ventricular tachycardia and KCNJ2 mutations. *Heart Rhythm* 2004;1:235–241.
24. Smith AH,. Fish FA, Kannankeril PJ. Andersen-Tawil syndrome (Review). *Ind Pacing Electrophysiol J* 2006;6(1):32–43.
25. Friedman PL, Stewart JR, Fenoglio JJ Jr, *et al.* Survival of subendocardial Purkinje fibres after extensive myocardial infarction in dogs. *Circ Res* 1973; 33:597–611.
26. Mlcochova H, Saliba WI, Burkhardt DJ, *et al.* Catheter ablation of ventricular fibrillation storm in patients with infiltrative amyloidosis of the heart. *J Cardiovasc Electrophysiol* 2006;17(4):426–430.
27. Bauce B, Nava A, Rampazzo A, *et al.* Familial effort polymorphic ventricular arrhythmias in arrhythmogenic right ventricular cardiomyopathy map to chromosome 1q42–43. *Am J Cardiol* 2000;85:573–579.
28. Leclercq JF, Coumel P. Characteristics, prognosis and treatment of the ventricular arrhythmias of right ventricular dysplasia. *Eur Heart J* 1989; 10(Suppl. D):61–67.
29. Stevenson WG, Friedman PL, Kocovic D, *et al.* Radiofrequency catheter ablation of ventricular tachycardia after myocardial infarction. *Circulation* 1998;98(4):308–314.
30. Ellison KE, Friedman PL, Ganz LI, *et al.* Entrainment mapping and radiofrequency catheter ablation of ventricular tachycardia in right ventricular dysplasia. *J Am Coll Cardiol* 1998;32(3):724–728.
31. Della Bella P, Pappalardo A, Riva S, *et al.* Non-contact mapping to guide catheter ablation of

untolerated ventricular tachycardia. *Eur Heart J* 2002;23(9):742–752.
32. Reithmann C, Hahnefeld A, Remp T, *et al.* Electroanatomic mapping of endocardial right ventricular activation as a guide for catheter ablation in patients with arrhythmogenic right ventricular dysplasia. *Pacing Clin Electrophysiol* 2003;26(6):1308–1316.
33. O'Donnell D, Cox D, Bourke J, *et al.* Clinical and electrophysiological differences between patients with arrhythmogenic right ventricular dysplasia and right ventricular outflow tract tachycardia. *Eur Heart J* 2003;24(9):801–810.
34. Marchlinski FE, Zado E, Dixit S, *et al.* Electroanatomic substrate and outcome of catheter ablative therapy for ventricular tachycardia in setting of right ventricular cardiomyopathy. *Circulation* 2004;110(16):2293–2298.
35. Verma A, Kilicaslan F, Schweikert RA, *et al.* Short- and long-term success of substrate-based mapping and ablation of ventricular tachycardia in arrhythmogenic right ventricular dysplasia. *Circulation* 2005;111(24):3209–3216.
36. Marchlinski FE, Callans DJ, Gottlieb CD, *et al.* Linear ablation lesions for control of unmappable ventricular tachycardia in patients with ischemic and nonischemic cardiomyopathy. *Circulation* 2000;101:1288–1296.
37. Hsia HH, Callans DJ, Marchlinski FE. Characterization of endocardial electrophysiologic substrate in patients with nonischemic cardiomyopathy and monomorphic ventricular tachycardia. *Circulation* 2003;108:704–710.
38. Garcia FC, Sussman JS, Bala R, *et al. Heart Rhythm* 2006;3,1S:S4–S5 (abstract).

55 Surgical Treatment of Atrial Fibrillation

Hartzell V. Schaff

Introduction

In current practice, surgical treatment is rarely used in the management of patients with ventricular tachycardia, although revascularization can eliminate ischemic substrate, and wide subendocardial scar excision with ventricular aneurysmectomy can cure reentrant monomorphic ventricular tachycardia.[1,2] Similarly, catheter-based methods are generally preferred over surgical interruption of supraventricular arrhythmias caused by accessory pathways.[3,4] Atrial fibrillation (AF), however, is commonly encountered in patients having cardiac operations, and there has been considerable progress during the last decade in direct surgical treatment of this arrhythmia. This chapter will focus on indications, techniques, and outcomes of surgical treatment of atrial fibrillation.

Indications

Surgical management of AF is indicated for several patient groups. Operation to ablate AF should be considered for younger patients with limiting symptoms, particularly those who have failed medical treatment or who are intolerant of medications and have failed catheter ablation. A significant number of young patients prefer a curative procedure rather than lifetime treatment with drugs that have bothersome side effects. In addition, there are patients who have medical contraindications to systemic anticoagulation, or a strong personal preference to avoid chronic warfarin therapy.

In addition, there is a small subset of patients who have suffered a thromboembolic stroke while on anticoagulation with warfarin, and these patients should be considered for a Cox-maze procedure because the operation includes removal of the left atrial appendage, and, thus, greatly reduces the risk of left atrial thrombus formation.[5] As will be discussed later, there are select patients with left ventricular (LV) dysfunction who may benefit from surgical treatment of AF in the setting of tachycardia-induced cardiomyopathy.[6] Another group of patients who may benefit from surgical ablation of atrial arrhythmias includes patients with congenital heart disease that results in right atrial dilation. In these patients, we selectively include a right-sided maze procedure at the time of intracardiac repair with incisions limited to the right atrium and interatrial septum.[7]

A large group of patients who may benefit from surgical treatment includes those with valvular heart disease and associated AF who require valve repair or replacement. In these patients, elimination of the arrhythmia allows discontinuation of chronic anticoagulation if the valve is repaired or a bioprosthesis is used.

Techniques

Cox-Maze Procedure

Two modifications of Cox's original operation were made to minimize chronotropic insufficiency and mechanical dysfunction of the left atrium. The original maze I procedure included several incisions around the sinoatrial (SA) node including one that crossed the area immediately anterior to the junction of the superior vena cava (SVC) and right atrium. This lesion led to chronotropic insufficiency during stress and exercise. Further, postoperative left atrial dysfunction appeared to be the result of an interatrial conduction delay due to disruption of conduction through Bachmann's bundle. To address these problems, Cox and his colleagues simplified the procedure by eliminating incisions near the SA node and moving the atrial dome incision so that it was located posterior to the SVC.[8]

Numerous other modifications of the Cox-maze procedure have been proposed, and most of these involve use of alternate energy sources and creation of alternate atrial lesion sets; these new approaches are aimed at simplifying the operation and shortening the time necessary to create atrial ablation lines.[9]

For most patients we continue to prefer the standard "cut and sew" maze operation as described above and have used two technical modifications as shown in Figure 55–1.[10] On the medial aspect of the right atrium, we avoid incision and apply a linear cryolesion from the cut edge of the appendage to the tricuspid valve (Figure 55–2A). This avoids division of the frequently seen branch of the right coronary artery, which supplies the SA node. We have found that the risk of postoperative sinus node dysfunction can be reduced by using a cryolesion instead of an incision in this location.

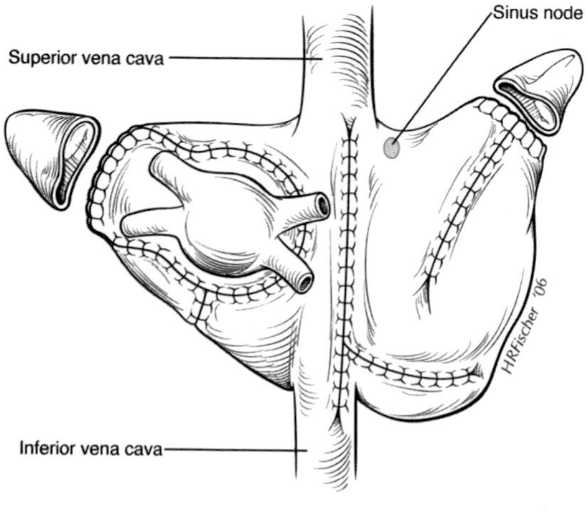

FIGURE 55–1. Posterior view of atrial suture lines in the modified Cox-maze procedure.

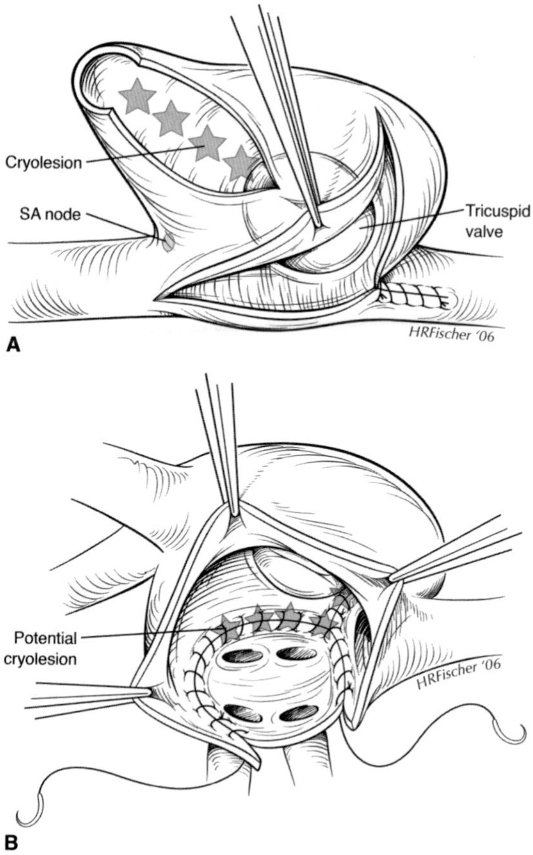

FIGURE 55–2. (A) On the medial aspect of the right atrium, instead of making an incision from the cut edge of the atrial appendage to the tricuspid valve annulus, we prefer linear cryolesions to avoid injury to the arterial blood supply to the sinoatrial node. (B) We routinely include the orifice of the left atrial appendage in closure of the left atrial encircling incision.

In the left atrium, we prefer to extend the incision that encircles the pulmonary veins to the orifice of the left atrial appendage, and then close the orifice transversely as part of the encircling incision. Alternatively, cryolesions can be utilized as part of the lesion encircling the pulmonary veins in order to avoid the conjunction of the encircling suture line and left atrial appendage suture line (Figure 55–2B). The principal advantage of the "cut and sew" technique over other methods is that full-thickness lesions are ensured, particularly around the pulmonary veins. This is particularly important because of the recent recognition that pulmonary venous tissue is the origin of AF in many patients.[11]

Alternate Energy Sources

Alternate energy sources are used by many surgeons to create atrial lesions, and several methods have been described for maze-like procedures in the beating heart on cardiopulmonary bypass. Indeed, some surgeons are attempting "off-pump" ablation of AF by application of various energy sources to the epicardial atrial surface in the beating heart.[12]

The largest clinical experience using alternate energy sources is with radiofrequency (RF) ablation, which employs alternating current to transfer energy to atrial tissue. This technology is widely used in the catheterization laboratory, and several instruments have been developed for intraoperative use; these include rigid unipolar probes with cooled tips, flexible unipolar probes, and bipolar clamps with and without irrigation. Radiofrequency probes can be applied to the endocardial or epicardial surfaces of the atrium in a unipolar configuration. Potential disadvantages of this method are inconsistent depth of injury leading to nontransmural lesions and injury to surrounding mediastinal structures.

Bipolar RF probes configured as clamps minimize the potential for injury to surrounding structures and produce transmural lesions more consistently than unipolar probes. Animal studies suggest a higher rate of success in producing transmural lesions with irrigated delivery of RF when compared to performing ablation without irrigation.[13] This can be attributed to the prevention of char accumulation on the tissue surface due to the cooling effect of the irrigant. The energy is driven deeper into the tissues under these conditions. Both nonirrigated and irrigated RF devices have sensing systems that indicate when transmurality is achieved.

Lesion Sets

The availability of the new technologies has led to numerous alternate lesion sets aimed at elimination of reentrant atrial fibrillation and flutter.[14,15] These lesion sets include bilateral isolation of the pulmonary veins, with either exclusion or excision of the left atrial appendage, and some variation of a connecting incision between the pulmonary vein lesion sets and the mitral valve annulus. Some believe that omission of the connecting incision between the pulmonary vein isolation lesion and the mitral valve annulus leads to increased atrial arrhythmias in the early postoperative period.

Another modification has been termed the minimaze procedure, and essential elements include a pulmonary vein encircling incision, an atrial isthmus lesion to the orifice of the left atrial appendage, and the lateral left atrial incisions without cryolesions.[16] This method is advocated as a simpler approach that does not seem to compromise effectiveness in controlling AF.

Postoperative Management

Protocols for the postoperative management of patients who have undergone a Cox–maze operation vary. For control of arrhythmia some centers utilize antiarrhythmic drugs, such as amiodarone, prophylactically in all patients and maintain this for 3 months. We prefer to use these medications selectively in patients who experience atrial or ventricular arrhythmias during hospitalization. We monitor potassium and magnesium levels and maintain them in the high-normal range. Postoperative AF is treated promptly with amiodarone, and electrical cardioversion is used as needed. If AF occurs early after operation and is treated with amiodarone, we continue the drug for 3 months.

It is important to use diuretics liberally early after operation. Removal of the atrial appendages during the Cox-maze procedure eliminates an important source of atrial natriuretic peptide, and this, along with elevations of aldosterone and antidiuretic hormone early postoperatively, predisposes the patient to fluid retention.[17,18]

We recommend systemic anticoagulation with warfarin for 3 months postoperatively, but there is no consensus on the need for anticoagulation beyond this interval. Some clinicians prefer to continue warfarin believing that the risk of thromboembolism is not reduced sufficiently to avoid systemic anticoagulation. Others argue that if AF is eliminated and ventricular function is normal, the risk of an intracardiac source of thromboemboli from a postoperative patient without a left atrial appendage is very low. Thus, the additional risk and inconvenience of using warfarin are not justified.

Junctional rhythm is common early after operation, but no specific treatment is necessary other than temporary atrial pacing for symptomatic bradycardia; we do not routinely utilize antiarrhythmic medications or stimulants, such as theophylline. Most patients with early junctional rhythm will regain a stable sinus mechanism, and it has been reported that it takes up to 50 weeks for this to occur. Persistent junctional rhythm may reflect sinus node dysfunction, and this will predispose the patient to recurrent arrhythmias and stroke. In these patients, a permanent transvenous pacemaker should be considered.

Outcomes

Outcome of procedures for ablation of AF are influenced by thoroughness of follow-up as well as the method of assessment of cardiac rhythm. The electrocardiogram is a "snap-shot" in time and has limited ability to detect those patients who may have transient atrial arrhythmias in the follow-up period. A better method is the Holter monitor, but widespread use for routine follow-up is not feasible. After clinical evaluation and follow-up of rhythm status are obtained, the second difficulty is in how the results of the analysis are reported. "Rhythm at last follow-up" may underestimate the recurrence rate of atrial arrhythmias in the follow-up period and, thus, overestimate the success of the procedure. Conversely, actuarial methods used to delineate time-related events, such as "freedom from AF," define *any* recurrent arrhythmia as a failure of the procedure, and, thus, may underestimate the actual clinical success. Other factors that contribute to confusion in assessing the results of surgical treatment of AF are viable terminology (intermittent versus paroxysmal, etc.) and differing patient populations (lone paroxysmal AF, AF with mitral valve disease, etc.).

Mayo Clinic Experience

Between March 5, 1993 and January 1, 2003 we performed 443 operations for ablation of AF; 335 patients underwent the standard "cut and sew" Cox-maze procedure and the results of these operations have been analyzed thoroughly. Two hundred and eleven patients (63%) were men, and the median age at operation was 62 years (range, 22–83 years). The duration of preoperative AF ranged from 3 months to 19 years (median, 2.9 years) and was chronic (present continuously >3 months) in 175 (52%) patients and paroxysmal in 160 patients (48%). The arrhythmia was lone paroxysmal in 51 patients (32%) and lone chronic in 29 patients(17%). Prior to surgery, the most common antiarrhythmic medications were digoxin in 188 patients (56%), β blocker (26%), calcium channel blocker (26%), and amiodarone (10%). Fifty-seven percent of patients were taking warfarin preoperatively. Other clinical features included mitral regurgitation in 191 patients (57%), coronary artery disease in 80 (24%), systemic hypertension in 74 (22%), prior cerebrovascular accident or transient ischemic attack in 34 (10%), atrial septal defect in 30 (9%), and diabetes in 10 (3%).

The most frequent concomitant procedures performed at the time of the maze procedure included mitral valve surgery in 198 patients (59%), coronary artery bypass grafting in 64 (19%), atrial septal defect closure in 34 (10%), tricuspid valve surgery in 23 (7%), aortic valve surgery in 13 (4%), and septal myectomy in 7 (2%). For all patients, the mean cross-clamp time was 58 ± 7 min and the mean cardiopulmonary bypass time was 117 ± 7 min. For patients having an isolated maze procedure, the mean cross-clamp time was 49 ± 5 min and the mean total cardiopulmonary bypass time was 102 ± 8 min.

There were three early deaths (0.9%), and new permanent pacemakers were necessary in 33 patients (10%). Two hundred and seventy-nine patients (84%) were dismissed on warfarin anticoagulation. The cardiac rhythm of the 332 early survivors at the time of hospital dismissal was sinus in 212 patients (64%), junctional in 60 (18%), atrial fibrillation (or flutter) in 37 (11%), and paced rhythm in 23 (7%).

Of the 332 early survivors, 23 (7%) have been lost to follow-up beyond initial hospitalization; many were from foreign countries. Late follow-up in 309 patients extends to 10.5 years (median, 3 years). Overall, 226 patients (73%) were free from warfarin anticoagulation. For patients undergoing isolated maze for lone AF, the risk of late stroke was 1.3% (1/68) and freedom from warfarin anticoagulation was 88% (60/68).

Success with the standard Cox-maze procedure has varied from 79% to 99% in published reports. In general, approximately 90% of patients who undergo the Cox-maze operation are free from AF at last follow-up, but as illustrated in our experience, outcomes (success) of the procedure depend on the method of analysis. For example, in our patients, overall freedom from AF is 88% when we used rhythm at last follow-up as the endpoint (Figure 55–3). When outcome is analyzed in a product-limit estimate (Kaplan–Meier), freedom from AF was 76% at 5 years and 51% at 10 years (Figure 55–4). Utilizing a third method of reporting success, freedom from AF at interval contact was 80% at 3 years, 78% at 6 years, and 76% at 9 years. In addition, different subgroups of patients may experience different durability from the Cox-maze procedure, and this represents another variable that affects the reporting of outcomes.

At last follow-up (median, 41 months), 93% of patients with preoperative lone paroxysmal AF were free from their arrhythmia with an actuarial freedom from AF of 90% at 5 years and 64% at 10 years. Patients with preoperative lone chronic AF had 83% freedom from AF at last follow-up (median, 28 months) with an actuarial freedom from AF of 80% at 5 years and 62% at 10 years. The Cox-maze operation is less durable for patients undergoing combined Cox-maze and mitral valve surgery with 70% of patients free from AF at last follow-up (median, 33 months) and an actuarial freedom from AF of 68% at 5 years and 41% at 10 years.

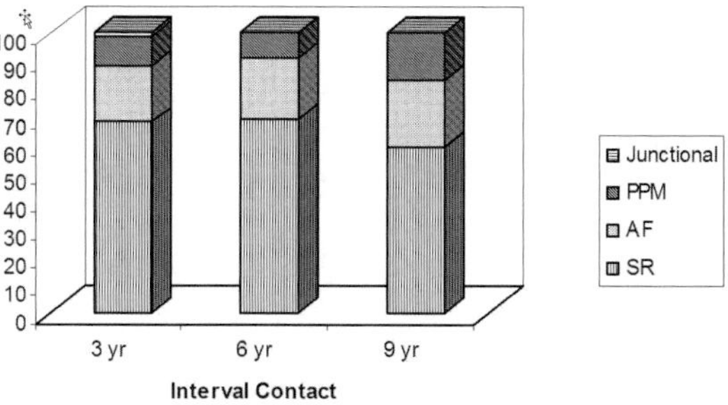

FIGURE 55–3. Electrocardiographic rhythm for patients at interval contact after having undergone a Cox-maze procedure. [From Stulak JM, Sundt TM, III, Dearani JA, *et al.*: Ten-year experience with the Cox-maze procedure for atrial fibrillation: How do we define success? *Ann Thorac Surg* 2007;83(4):1324–1325.]

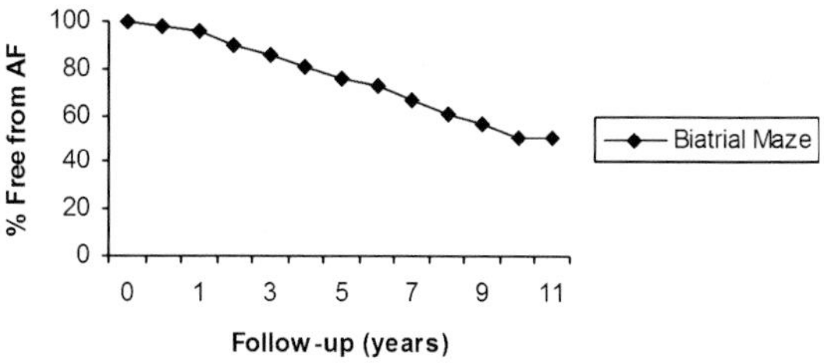

FIGURE 55–4. Kaplan–Meier curve demonstrating the freedom from AF in patients who have undergone a Cox-maze procedure. [From Stulak JM, Sundt TM, III, Dearani JA, *et al.*: Ten-year experience with the Cox-maze procedure for atrial fibrillation: How do we define success? *Ann Thorac Surg* 2007;83(4):1324–1325.]

The Cox-Maze Procedure and Mitral Valve Surgery

A large group of patients to be considered for Cox-maze operation are those with valvular disease and associated AF in whom repair or replacement of the valve with a a bioprosthesis could result in avoidance of both antiarrhythmic medication and chronic anticoagulation with warfarin. Chronic enlargement of the left atrium in these patients creates a substrate for the development of AF, and, consequently, these patients have high rates of failure when AF is treated with drugs or catheter-based ablative techniques.

Because the pulmonary veins provide a trigger for AF in approximately 90% of patients with paroxysmal arrhythmia, pulmonary vein isolation alone would be expected to cure a majority of patients with this type of AF. However, it will fail as an ablative procedure in those 10% of patients in whom the pulmonary veins do not contribute to the substrate for AF. In patients with chronic AF, the goal of treatment shifts from isolating the trigger of the arrhythmia (pulmonary veins in paroxysmal AF) to ablating the macroreentrant pathways responsible for its maintenance. Chronic AF leads to atrial remodeling and the development of macroreentrant pathways that sustain electrical reentry, and, thus, the arrhythmia is not dependent on stimuli from the pulmonary veins, and pulmonary vein isolation may be inadequate treatment. This remodeling is present in a significant portion of patients with mitral valve regurgitation, and especially those who have evidence of left atrial enlargement. Again, in such patients with mitral valve regurgitation and chronic AF, pulmonary vein isolation would not be expected to be as effective as a standard Cox-maze procedure.

Handa *et al.* reported that the Cox-maze operation is a safe adjunct to mitral valve repair for patients with preoperative AF.[19] In this study from our Clinic, the addition of the Cox-maze procedure was particularly useful in patients with chronic AF of more than 3 months duration preoperatively. Freedom from AF was found in 82% of patients who underwent combined maze and mitral valve repair compared to 53% in patients who underwent mitral valve repair alone. Morbidity and mortality were not increased by the addition of the maze procedure, and 75% of patients regained sinus rhythm by last follow-up. In this series, only the omission of the maze procedure and the presence of chronic AF were predictors of the recurrence of arrhythmia.

Some groups advocate only left-sided maze lesions to ablate AF in patients having mitral valve surgery in an attempt to keep morbidity and mortality at a minimum. In our experience, there is little difference in perioperative morbidity and mortality in patients who undergo mitral valve surgery alone and those who had an additional maze procedure, and it is very unlikely that the omission of the right-sided atrial lesions would have decreased the already low complication and death rate that was observed when the biatrial procedure was performed.

Tachycardia-Induced Cardiomyopathy

Surgical treatment of AF should also be considered in patients with tachycardia-induced cardiomyopathy. Rapid heart rate caused by AF can lead to cardiomyopathy, and multiple reports have documented that LV dysfunction caused by supraventricular tachycardia can be cured or improved by conversion to sinus rhythm.[20–22] Furthermore, ventricular dysfunction may resolve with control of tachycardia by the simple ablation of the atrioventricular node and insertion of a pacemaker. A similar improvement in ventricular function has been observed after surgical treatment of AF.[6]

For example, in our series, 99 patients had atrial flutter or fibrillation without associated valvular or congenital heart disease, and 37 (37%) had decreased LV function [ejection fraction (EF) <0.35 in 11 (severe), EF 0.36–0.45 in 8 (moderate), and EF 0.46 to 0.55 in 18 (mild)]. The ages of these 37 patients with AF and LV dysfunction ranged from 35 to 74 years (median, 55 years). Atrial flutter or fibrillation was present for 3 months to 19 years (median, 48 months) preoperatively, and 24 patients (65%) exhibited symptoms of heart failure. Preoperative EF ranged from 0.25 to 0.55 (median, 0.45). At last follow-up (median, 63 months), the Cox-maze procedure eliminated atrial flutter or fibrillation in all but one patient. As shown in Figure 55–5, for all patients, the mean EF improved significantly from 0.439 ± 0.024 to 0.537 ± 0.028 early postoperatively ($p = 0.00006$), and this increase was sustained during follow-up (late postoperative EF, 0.535 ± 0.029; $p = 0.00007$ versus preoperative EF). The most significant improvement in EF was evident in patients with the most severe LV impairment preoperatively (EF <0.35) and those patients who had chronic AF preoperatively. Elimination of AF with the Cox-maze procedure also significantly benefited patients with only moderate preoperative

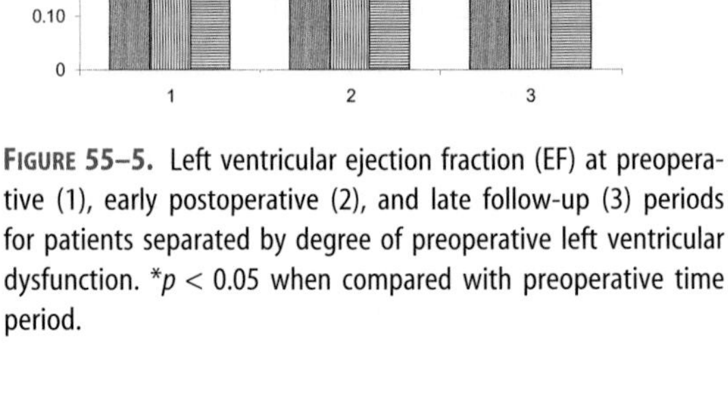

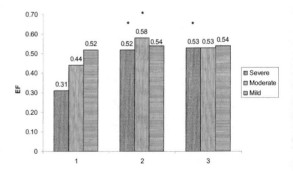

FIGURE 55–5. Left ventricular ejection fraction (EF) at preoperative (1), early postoperative (2), and late follow-up (3) periods for patients separated by degree of preoperative left ventricular dysfunction. *$p < 0.05$ when compared with preoperative time period.

impairment of LV function in the immediate postoperative period. Importantly, improvement in LV function correlated with enhancement of functional status.

Atrial fibrillation impairs hemodynamic function by several mechanisms. First, the arrhythmia results in loss of atrioventricular synchrony and atrial contraction. This may reduce ventricular filling and thereby reduce cardiac output. The consequence of loss of atrial contraction may be especially pronounced in patients with impaired diastolic filling as is seen in the presence of hypertrophied ventricles, restrictive cardiomyopathy, and mitral valve stenosis. Fluctuation in the RR interval changes the diastolic filling interval producing a variable stroke volume. In animals, cardiac output is reduced 15% when ventricular rhythm is irregular compared to a regular rhythm at the same rate.[23]

Second, in addition to these mechanical consequences, AF can lead to tachycardia-induced cardiomyopathy.[24–27] Cardiomyopathy caused by tachycardia is commonly thought to be associated with chronic arrhythmias having rates >120 beats per minute. Our experience suggests that ventricular dysfunction may be associated with resting heart rates considerably lower than this, and, furthermore, paroxysmal AF can lead to ventricular dysfunction.

It is important to identify patients with tachycardia-induced cardiomyopathy because ventricular dysfunction can be reversed by control of the arrhythmia. Improvement in LV function has been documented in patients having cardioversion (medical or electrical) to sinus rhythm and in patients having rate control with ablation of the atrioventricular node coupled with implantation of a transvenous pacemaker.[28,29]

Previously, some surgeons believed that LV dysfunction was a contraindication to the Cox-maze procedure. However, tachycardia-related cardiomyopathy is not uncommon in patients with AF, and our experience suggests that surgical treatment of AF should be considered in select patients with cardiomyopathy, particularly those in whom the onset of tachycardia precedes or is known to coincide with the development of LV dysfunction. Also, it appears that patients with only moderate LV impairment benefit in terms of ventricular function after the procedure.

Atrial Arrhythmias in Congenital Heart Disease

Congenital heart disease (CHD) resulting in right atrial dilation is commonly associated with atrial tachyarrhythmias, particularly AF, and we have used concomitant right-sided modification of the Cox-maze procedure at the time of intracardiac repair to reduce subsequent atrial arrhythmias (Figure 55–6). Because many repairs for CHD in patients with AF are reoperations, the right-sided maze procedure has the advantage of minimizing dissection of adhesions, thus resulting in shorter cardiopulmonary bypass time when compared to the standard biatrial maze procedure. In addition, avoiding suture lines in the left atrium minimizes the risk of bleeding behind the heart where hemostasis can be difficult.

From 1993 to 2002, we have managed 99 patients with a right-sided Cox-maze procedure at the time of repair for congenital heart disease. In these patients, preoperative AF was paroxysmal in more than 80%, and the median preoperative duration of arrhythmia was approximately 3 years. The most common diagnoses were Ebstein's anomaly, isolated atrial septal defect (ASD), and tetralogy of Fallot. At dismissal, approximately 90% were free from AF, with approximately 70% of patients leaving the hospital in sinus rhythm. New pacemakers were necessary in 15 patients, all

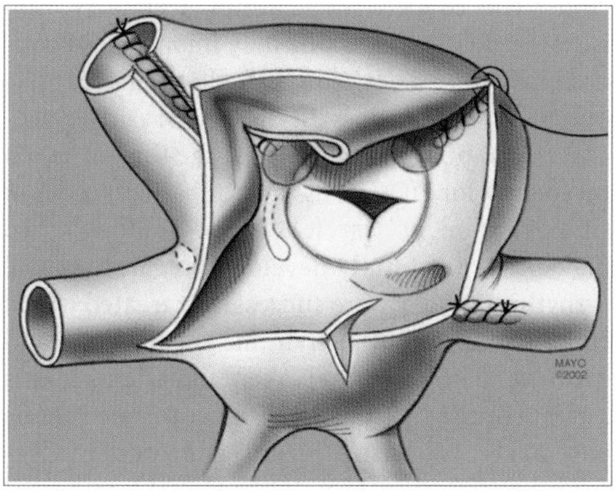

FIGURE 55–6. The right-sided maze procedure includes an incision in the atrial septum and cryolesions placed at the tricuspid valve annulus both anteriorly and inferiorly.

but one for sick sinus syndrome. At a mean follow-up of 33 months, 77% of patients with preoperative chronic arrhythmias were free from AF, and 96% of patients with preoperative paroxysmal arrhythmias were free from AF. The addition of a right-sided maze procedure at the time of repair for congenital heart anomalies causing right atrial enlargement appears to reduce the recurrence of late arrhythmia without increasing morbidity or mortality.

A potential disadvantage of a right-sided maze procedure is that in some patients the left atrium may contribute an additional substrate for AF. Our patients were selected on the basis of right atrial dilation and a normal left atrial size.

Atrial Fibrillation and Hypertrophic Cardiomyopathy

Atrial fibrillation occurs in up to 30% of patients with hypertrophic obstructive cardiomyopathy (HOCM) and can result in profound clinical deterioration due to loss of the atrial component of left ventricular filling. Patients who undergo septal myectomy usually enjoy dramatic relief of symptoms and improved exercise capacity; however, a number of patients will be left with underlying diastolic dysfunction.

There is controversy regarding the usefulness of the Cox-maze procedure in patients with paroxysmal AF and HOCM who undergo septal myectomy. One concern is that although sinus rhythm is restored, atrial incisions may impair atrial contractility, thus decreasing LV filling and cardiac output. Chen *et al.* suggest that the Cox-maze procedure can be safely included at the time of septal myectomy for HOCM, as 80% of patients were in sinus rhythm at last follow-up. Although two patients in their study developed recurrent atrial arrhythmias, they were successfully treated with a combination of antiarrhythmic medications and cardioversion.[30] Twenty percent of patients in this series required a new permanent transvenous pacemaker. We have utilized a concomitant Cox-maze procedure in 11 patients with AF undergoing septal myectomy for HOCM. This combined approach was successful in ablating AF without increasing morbidity or mortality when compared to a maze procedure alone. So, as reported for the combination of various other procedures with the Cox-maze procedure, ablation of AF at the time of septal myectomy for HOCM does not appear to increase operative morbidity beyond what is expected for an isolated maze procedure.

Future Perspectives

New instruments developed to facilitate surgical ablation of AF and the new lesion sets may achieve rates of AF control similar to the traditional "cut and sew" methods. However, equivalency has not yet been proven, and future comparative studies are necessary. Also, there are many unanswered questions regarding the clinical application of the maze operation in conjunction with other cardiac procedures. Is pulmonary vein isolation equally effective as a full Cox-maze procedure for patients with paroxysmal AF and mitral valve disease? Gillinov and colleagues reported that the choice of ablation procedure (full Cox-maze versus pulmonary vein isolation) did not affect the late recurrence of AF or the rate of ablation failure.[15] Perhaps the pathogenesis of AF in patients with mitral valve disease and paroxysmal arrhythmia is different from that of patients with chronic AF in the setting of mitral valve disease and a dilated left atrium.[19] Another unresolved issue is whether concomitant left reduction atrioplasty should be performed at the time of valve repair and maze procedure for patients with AF and a dilated left atria from mitral valve disease. Romano and colleagues[31] have reported an 89% rate of return of sinus rhythm in patients who underwent left atrial reduction combined with a Cox-maze operation. Finally, should a "prophylactic" maze procedure be performed in a patient with preoperative sinus rhythm and a dilated left atrium undergoing surgery for mitral valve disease? The altered atrial tissue in these patients represents an arrhythmogenic substrate, which renders them at high risk (approximately 40%) for the development of postoperative AF even after the mitral valve disease is repaired.[32] Clearly, the risks and benefits should be weighed before an additional procedure is performed, which carries with it the added risk of permanent transvenous pacemaker implantation.

References

1. Cox JL. Cardiac surgery for arrhythmias. *J Cardiovasc Electrophysiol* 2004;15(2):250–262.
2. Lee R, Mitchell JD, Garan H, Ruskin JN, McGovern BA, Buckley MJ, Torchiana DF, Vlahakes GJ. Operation for recurrent ventricular tachycardia. Predictors of short- and long-term efficacy. *J Thorac Cardiovasc Surg* 1994;107(3):732–742.
3. Lowes D, Frank G, Klein J, Manz M. Surgical treatment of the Wolff-Parkinson-White syndrome—experiences in 120 patients. *Eur Heart J* 1993; 14(Suppl. E):99–102.
4. Guiraudon GM, Klein GJ, Sharma AD, Milstein S, McLellan DG. Closed-heart technique for Wolff-Parkinson-White syndrome: Further experience and potential limitations. *Ann Thorac Surg* 1986; 42(6):651–657.
5. Ad N, Cox JL. Stroke prevention as an indication for the Maze procedure in the treatment of atrial fibrillation. *Semin Thorac Cardiovasc Surg* 2000; 12(1):56–62.
6. Stulak JM, Dearani JA, Daly RC, Zehr KJ, Sundt TM 3rd, Schaff HV. Left ventricular dysfunction in atrial fibrillation: Restoration of sinus rhythm by the Cox-maze procedure significantly improves systolic function and functional status. *Ann Thorac Surg* 2006;82(2):494–500.
7. Stulak JM, Dearani JA, Puga FJ, Zehr KJ, Schaff HV, Danielson GK. Right-sided Maze procedure for atrial tachyarrhythmias in congenital heart disease. *Ann Thorac Surg* 2006;81(5):1780–1784.
8. Cox JL, Jaquiss RD, Schuessler RB, Boineau JP. Modification of the maze procedure for atrial flutter and atrial fibrillation. II. Surgical technique of the maze III procedure. *J Thorac Cardiovasc Surg* 1995; 110(2):485–495.
9. Melby SJ, Zierer A, Bailey MS, Cox JL, Lawton JS, Munfakh N, Crabtree TD, Moazami N, Huddleston CB, Moon MR, Damiano RJ Jr. A new era in the surgical treatment of atrial fibrillation: The impact of ablation technology and lesion set on procedural efficacy. *Ann Surg* 2006;244(4):583–592.
10. Schaff HV, Dearani JA, Daly RC, Orszulak TA, Danielson GK. Cox-maze procedure for atrial fibrillation: Mayo Clinic experience. *Semin Thorac Cardiovasc Surg* 2000;12(1):30–37.
11. Haissaguerre M, Jais P, Shah DC, *et al.* Spontaneous initiation of atrial fibrillation by ectopic beats originating in the pulmonary veins. *N Engl J Med* 1998; 339:659–666.
12. Mazzitelli D, Park CH, Park KY, Benetti FJ, Lange R. Epicardial ablation of atrial fibrillation on the beating heart without cardiopulmonary bypass. *Ann Thorac Surg* 2002;73(1):320–321.
13. Hamner CE, Potter DD Jr, Cho KR, Lutterman A, Francischelli D, Sundt TM 3rd, Schaff HV. Irrigated radiofrequency ablation with transmurality feedback reliably produces Cox maze lesions in vivo. *Ann Thorac Surg* 2005;80(6):2263–2270.
14. Sie HT, Beukema WP, Elvan A, Ramdat Misier AR. Long-term results of irrigated radiofrequency modified maze procedure in 200 patients with concomitant cardiac surgery: Six years experience. *Ann Thorac Surg* 2004;77(2):512–516.
15. Gillinov AM, Bhavani S, Blackstone EH, Rajeswaran J, Svensson LG, Navia JL, Pettersson BG, Sabik JF 3rd, Smedira NG, Mihaljevic T, McCarthy PM, Shewchik J, Natale A. Surgery for permanent atrial fibrillation: Impact of patient factors and lesion set. *Ann Thorac Surg* 2006;82(2):502–513.
16. Szalay ZA, Civelek A, Dill T, Klovekorn WP, Kilb I, Bauer EP. Long-term follow-up after the mini-maze procedure. *Ann Thorac Surg* 2004;77(4):1277–1281.
17. Kim KB, Lee CH, Kim CH, Cha YJ. Effect of the Cox maze procedure on the secretion of atrial natriuretic peptide. *J Thorac Cardiovasc Surg* 1998; 115(1):139–146.
18. Albage A, van der Linden J, Bengtsson L, Lindblom D, Kenneback G, Berglund H. Elevations in antidiuretic hormone and aldosterone as possible causes of fluid retention in the maze procedure. *Ann Thorac Surg* 2001;72(1):58–64.
19. Handa N, Schaff HV, Morris JJ, Anderson BJ, Kopecky SL, Enriquez-Sarano M. Outcome of valve repair and the Cox-maze procedure for mitral regurgitation and associated atrial fibrillation. *J Thorac Cardiovasc Surg* 1999;118:628–635.
20. Shibane JS, Wood MA, Jensen DN, Ellenbogen KA, Fitzpatrick AP, Schinman MM. Tachycardia-induced cardiomyopathy: A review of animal models and clinical studies. *J Am Coll Cardiol* 1997; 29(4):709–715.
21. Luschsinger JA, Steinberg JS. Resolution of cardiomyopathy after ablation of atrial flutter. *J Am Coll Cardiol* 1998;32(1):205–210.
22. Redfield MM, Kay GN, Jenkins LS, Jensen DN, Ellenbogen KA. Tachycardia-related cardiomyopathy: A common cause of ventricular dysfunction in patients with atrial fibrillation referred for atrioventricular ablation. *Mayo Clin Proc* 2000;75(8):790–795.
23. Naito M, David D, Michelson EL, Schaffenburg M, Dreifus LS. The hemodynamic consequences of cardiac arrhythmias: Evaluation of the relative roles of abnormal atrioventricular sequencing, irregularity of ventricular rhythm and atrial fibrillation in a canine model. *Am Heart J* 1983;106:284–291.

24. Grogan M, Smith HC, Gersh BJ, Wood DL. Left ventricular dysfunction due to atrial fibrillation in patients initially believed to have idiopathic dilated cardiomyopathy. *Am J Cardiol* 1992; 69:1570–1573.
25. Kessler G, Rosenblatt S, Friedman J, Kaplinsky E. Recurrent dilated cardiomyopathy reversed with conversion of atrial fibrillation. *Am Heart J* 1997; 133:384–386.
26. Packer DL, Brady GH, Worley SJ, *et al.* Tachycardia-induced cardiomyopathy: A reversible form of left ventricular dysfunction. *Am J Cardiol* 1986;57: 563–570.
27. Edner M, Bergfeldt L, *et al.* Prospective study of left ventricular function after radiofrequency ablation of the atrioventricular junction in patients with atrial fibrillation. *Br Heart J* 1995;74:261–267.
28. Kieny JR, Sacrez A, Facello A, *et al.* Increase in radionuclide left ventricular ejection fraction after cardioversion of chronic atrial fibrillation in idiopathic dilated cardiomyopathy. *Eur Heart J* 1992;13: 1290–1295.
29. Van Gelder IC, Crijns HJ, Blanksma PK, *et al.* Time course of hemodynamic changes and improvement of exercise tolerance after cardioversion of chronic atrial fibrillation unassociated with cardiac valve disease. *Am J Cardiol* 1993;72:560–566.
30. Chen MS, McCarthy PM, Lever HM, Smedira NG, Lytle BL. Effectiveness of atrial fibrillation surgery in patients with hypertrophic cardiomyopathy. *Am J Cardiol* 2004;93(3):373–375.
31. Romano MA, Bach DS, Pagani FD, Prager RL, Deeb GM, Bolling SF. Atrial reduction plasty Cox maze procedure: Extended indications for atrial fibrillation surgery. *Ann Thorac Surg* 2004;77(4):1282–1287.
32. Kernis SJ, Nkomo VT, Messika-Zeitoun D, Gersh BJ, Sundt TM 3rd, Ballman KV, Scott CG, Schaff HV, Enriquez-Sarano M. Atrial fibrillation after surgical correction of mitral regurgitation in sinus rhythm: Incidence, outcome, and determinants. *Circulation* 2004;19:1.

Part VII
Risk Stratification and Prevention of Sudden Cardiac Death in Acquired Clinical Conditions

Screening for Risk of Sudden Cardiac Death

John B. Kostis

Sudden cardiac death, primarily sudden arrhythmic death, is a clinical catastrophe that affects unexpectedly many apparently healthy patients as well as patients who have stable cardiovascular disease. It terminates the life of the patient and degrades the quality of life of family and friends. The problem of identifying patients at increased risk for sudden cardiac death is that there is a reciprocal relationship between the risk in different patient subsets and the size of the subset. The size of the subset is an important determinant the number of individuals who will be affected by this unforeseen clinical event. In other words there are many more sudden cardiac deaths among populations at low risk than among those at very high risk. The reason for this is that the size of the population at low risk is much higher than the sizes of populations at high risk (Figure I–1).

Screening strategies must be devised with cost effectiveness in mind because of the reasons discussed above. The cost, in terms of financial expense of screening, cost and adverse effects of potential preventive interventions, follow-up costs and inconvenience, labeling, insurability, and emotional distress, to prevent one sudden cardiac death must be estimated. Cost effectiveness studies "measuring" the dollar cost of the number of deaths prevented or increase in quality adjusted life years have been reported. Most have limitations imposed by the perspective of the analysis, e.g., costs to patients, to the insurance companies, and to society at large, the opportunity cost of employed patients, and especially costs in assuming utilities that have not been explicitly agreed upon. Also, the findings of these analyses pertain to populations with characteristics similar to those in the studies, a caveat that is not always adhered to. The nature of the preventive strategy will affect this calculus. Efficacy and an adverse effect profile are more important in antiarrhythmic drug therapy while complications and financial issues are more relevant for device therapy.

Screening methods that have 100% sensitivity and 100% specificity in predicting sudden cardiac death are not currently available. For this reason, the interplay of sensitivity and specificity of the various screening strategies displayed as receiver–operator characteristic curves should be used in deciding which diagnostic method and what decision criterion (cutoff) of the relevant variable should be used. When the diagnostic screening technique is of low cost and has a low rate of adverse effects, a cutoff of high sensitivity and, necessarily, low specificity can be used. This will result in screening (and potentially treating) a large number of individuals who are not going to suffer sudden cardiac death unnecessarily. This would be acceptable since the intervention is inexpensive and safe. On the other hand, most individuals destined to develop sudden cardiac death will be detected and treated due to the high sensitivity of the test. Alternatively, when the intervention is expensive and carries significant risk and adverse effects, a cutoff criterion of high specificity can be used. The high specificity will ensure that only a small number of persons who will not develop sudden cardiac death will sustain the risk and expense of the intervention. The price of this strategy is that the low sensitivity of the test will leave a significant proportion of those destined to develop sudden cardiac death uncovered (Figure I–2). The relationship of sensitivity to specificity, expressed as a receiver operator characteristic curve (ROC), allows the choice of an appropriate decision criterion, as discussed above, as well as a comparison of the utility of different screening methods. Figure I–2 indicates that among survivors of acute myocardial infarction, the value of the ejection fraction is a better predictor of sudden cardiac death than ambulatory electrocardiography.

The specific screening strategies that may be used in stratifying individuals for the risk of sudden cardiac death is determined in great part by the clinical suspicion in the individual subject. In other words, initial stratification and categorization of patients for risk of sudden cardiac death and the selection of the relevant screening strategy are done on general clinical grounds. The authors of the eight chapters included in Part VII of this volume describe the state of the art in risk stratification and prevention of sudden cardiac death in different patient subsets. Most strategies are based on clinical factors including family history, the pathological substrate for serious arrhythmias such as myocardial hypertrophy, ventricular dilatation, fibrosis, and myofiber disarray; the electrophysiological milieu including the channelopathies, the dynamics of the QT interval, T wave alternans, etc.; and on the presence triggering factors including the autonomic nervous system, ischemia, exercise, transient arrhythmias, etc. A plethora of procedures has been used for each of the factors mentioned above. Also, a combination of variables has been proposed including, in the case of coronary artery disease, low ejection fraction, ventricular ectopic activity, late potentials, and heart rate variability. It must be kept in mind, however, that requiring that two or more tests be positive to classify an individual in a high risk category increases the specificity of the decision criterion (i.e., decreases the number of those not destined to have a cardiac arrest) at the expense of decreasing the sensitivity, i.e., the number of individuals who will sustain sudden cardiac death who are not going to be identified by the combination of tests. In such situations, the additive costs described above must be considered.

Estimation of the marginal improvement of the ROC curves is an important determinant and can be used in comparing the improvement in diagnostic ability with the additional cost and complexity. Genetic screening, whose price is rapidly decreasing with new technologies, may be very useful in identifying patient subsets with channelopathies and hereditary abnormalities of the contractile proteins where the risk may be high and may justify an intervention, especially the presence of a positive family history.

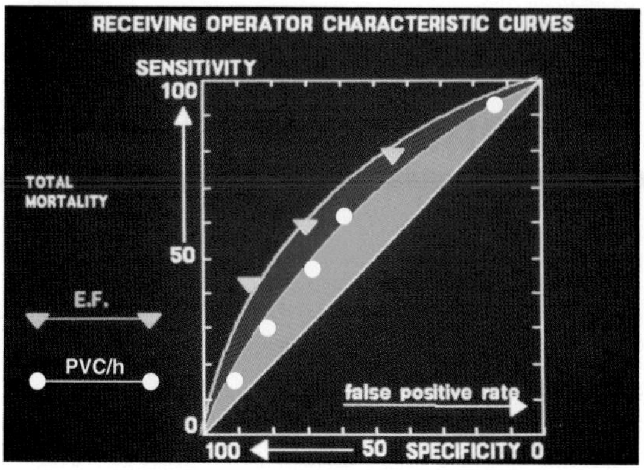

FIGURE I–2. Ejection fraction (E.F.) is a better predictor of sudden cardiac death than ambulatory electrocardiography among survivors of acute myocardial infarction.

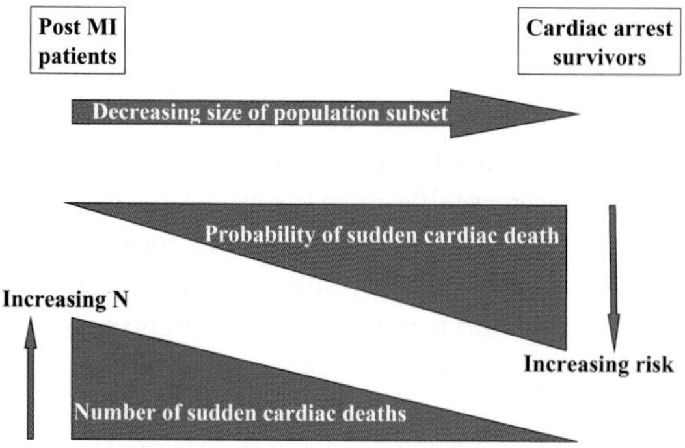

FIGURE I–1. Reciprocal relationship between the risk for sudden cardiac death and the size of the subset.

56
Clinical Trials in Sudden Cardiac Death Prevention: Principles and Endpoints

Andrzej S. Kosinski

Research questions can be approached by means of observational studies, case–control studies, or randomized controlled trials (RCTs). Observational studies are often useful for developing research ideas, but are vulnerable to bias due to an uncontrolled process of treatment assignment. Occasionally, case–control studies may be the only feasible option open to researchers, but such studies are also potentially subject to bias. Randomized controlled trials are currently recognized as the best tool available for definitive comparison of proposed medical therapies, and are pivotal in the practice of evidence based medicine.[1–3] They involve prospective follow-up of patients and compare two or more treatment assignments, one of which is often placebo or a standard treatment. Patients enrolled in an RCT should reflect a well-defined population, selected on the basis of study inclusion and exclusion criteria and enrolled consecutively to avoid the possibility of conscious or unconscious selectiveness in including or excluding patients. The essential feature of RCTs is that they are designed so that treatments are assigned entirely at random, rather than as a result of standard medical care, as would be the case in a prospective observational study.

Randomization produces treatment groups that are comparable with respect to patient characteristics, both recorded and unrecorded, and helps avoid patients' self-selection into treatment groups and investigators' tendencies to advocate a particular treatment, thus avoiding possible biases associated with treatment assignment. In other words, random assignment of patients to a treatment provides a proper experiment, because the decision about the treatment assignment is external to the current knowledge of either the patient or the physician.

Ideally, treatment assignment is unknown both to patients enrolled in the study and to the medical professionals administering the treatment. This approach, known as double-blinding or double-masking, is often not feasible for all treatment arms in trials of sudden cardiac death prevention, because medical devices are commonly used as a treatment or component of treatment. In the Sudden Cardiac Death in Heart Failure Trial (SCD-HeFT),[4] placebo and amiodarone were administered in double-blinded fashion, but assignment to an implantable cardioverter defibrillator (ICD) obviously could not be blinded. Generally, blinding should be utilized whenever possible in designing a clinical trial, and preserved when adjudicating study endpoints.

Randomization in multicenter clinical trials should be stratified by center to ensure that all treatments are utilized in similar proportions at each center. Randomization sequences should not be known to personnel who recruit patients for a study. A telephone call center can be used to verify patient eligibility and provide treatment assignment. For smaller studies, treatment assignment can be provided by an independent statistical center in sealed envelopes; however, this approach is less reliable than using a central call center. It is critical that treatment intervention begin as soon as possible after randomization in order to avoid bias that can arise from events occurring between randomization and initiation of assigned therapy. In other words, randomization assignment should be delayed until the last practical moment before initiation of therapy. For example, in the SCD-HeFT study, patients assigned to drug therapy (amiodarone or placebo) began therapy immediately after randomization. Immediate initiation of the ICD therapy was not feasible, but the time from randomization to ICD implantation was short (median duration was 3 days).[4]

Every effort must be undertaken to minimize the number of patients lost to follow-up before the end of a study (if the endpoint is all-cause mortality, national databases such as the National Death Index can be useful for ascertaining vital status).[5] The potential for biased treatment comparison is substantially greater with increased rates of patient loss to follow-up, because the reason for loss of contact may be related to the outcome under study. Thus, the loss to follow-up of more than a few percent of patients can severely compromise the benefits of randomization. Lack of compliance with a prescribed treatment scheme may also reduce the value of randomization, and substantial effort should be expended to preserve the treatment regimen as described in the protocol.

Randomization is often not to a pure form of a particular treatment, but rather to an initial treatment strategy. Patients assigned to the drug arm of a trial comparing drug and device-based interventions may receive a device during the follow-up, if the physician judges it absolutely necessary according to current practice standards. The primary analysis of such a study should be performed on the basis of the intention-to-treat (ITT) principle, which states that for purposes of primary analysis, patients are considered according to the treatment arm to which they are randomly assigned, regardless of the treatment they actually receive.

An ethical approach to RCTs is mandatory. Study protocols should include detailed descriptions of the research question and study design, and all investigators participating in a multicenter trial must agree to follow the protocol. Furthermore, researchers participating in a clinical trial can offer patients a randomization only when the relative benefit of a particular treatment is not confirmed. This lack of knowledge, or *equipoise*, regarding which treatment is preferable has to be present and fully accepted by all investigators before a trial begins. Otherwise, ethical concerns may arise and patient recruitment is likely to suffer. All proposed studies should be reviewed by *an Institutional* Review Board (IRB) before enrollment begins. Potential subjects need to have an understanding, documented by provision of informed consent, of the nature of the research, including its risks and possible benefits. Patients should also be aware that they have the right to withdraw consent to participate in a study at any time. All RCTs should be overseen by a Data Safety Monitoring Board (DSMB) consisting of experts in the specific field of research and preferably including a biostatistician.[6] Data Safety Monitoring Boards (also known as Data Safety Monitoring Committees [DSMC], Data Monitoring Boards [DMB], Independent Data Monitoring Committees [IDMC], etc.) must be entirely independent of both trial investigators and sponsors. They are charged with monitoring the safety of patients and may recommend early stopping of a trial based either on safety concerns or endpoint related information.

The importance of choosing a clinically relevant primary endpoint (or outcome measure) cannot be overstated. Surrogate measures are often considered in preliminary studies; however, such measures may prove inadequate in RCTs, as occurred in the Cardiac Arrhythmia Suppression Trial (CAST).[7] In this trial, drugs providing suppression of ventricular arrhythmias were found to unexpectedly increase risk of death and sudden death. An endpoint of all-cause mortality may be the most appropriate for the purposes of a definitive clinical trial, and most major clinical trials of ICD therapy have considered overall mortality as the primary endpoint.[8] However, overall mortality may be low, requiring large numbers of patients in order to achieve sufficient statistical power and additional components of the endpoint may be considered, if clinically meaningful (e.g., hospitalizations). Smaller trials of cardiac resynchronization therapy (CRT) considered as primary endpoints one or more of the following nonmortality measures: distance walked in 6 min, exercise capacity as measured be peak oxygen consumption, quality of life score, New York Heart Association (NYHA) class, and/or hospitalization for congestive heart failure (CHF).[8] Choosing the most appropriate primary endpoint is essential for the success and acceptance of a trial, as well as for the progress of clinical practice.

A randomized clinical trial is ultimately a designed statistical experiment. Several key statistical concepts will be reviewed below: type I error, primary endpoint test statistic, treatment effect, statistical power, and sample size.

There is always a possibility that the analysis of study data may show a difference between treatments in a particular trial even when such a difference does not actually exist in the population under study. This mistaken conclusion can result from random variation, because the group of patients enrolled into a particular trial is a random group drawn from the pool of all eligible patients. Such an incorrect conclusion, known as a *type I error*, can have serious consequences, as it may lead to a therapy that in reality is ineffective being mistakenly introduced into medical practice. A 5% chance of such an error is typically considered as the maximum acceptable. In addition, it is always hoped that the new treatment will prove beneficial, it is important to consider a two-sided type I error.

The primary analysis compares the occurrence or value of the primary endpoint across treatment arms by means of a statistical test. The form of the suitable *primary endpoint test statistic* depends on the type of primary outcome and the analysis technique. Outcomes can be continuous (e.g., distance walked in 6 min) or binary (e.g., death). Time-to-death can be informative as well, and time-to-event (survival) analysis is often used when the primary endpoint is death or an event that occurs during follow-up. Although the full statistical analysis plan can be prepared separately, the primary endpoint statistical test and the corresponding test statistic need to be specified in the study protocol.

The magnitude of the hypothesized treatment difference (*treatment effect*) needs to be clinically relevant and should be large enough to have an impact on medical practice if observed in a trial. For example, for all-cause mortality, we may consider a 30% relative reduction in risk of death as the treatment effect we would like to detect. A large treatment effect is easier to detect, and such a trial requires fewer patients than one attempting to detect a small treatment effect. A trial to detect a very small difference between or among treatments can be designed by considering a sufficiently large number of subjects, but such a difference, even if detected, may not matter in medical practice.

Statistical power is the chance of detecting a prespecified treatment effect if such an effect truly exists. Commonly, a definitive clinical trial requires statistical power to be 90% or higher. Power of 80% is occasionally considered if achieving 90% power is not feasible. Small underpowered trials may serve for pilot studies, but low statistical power means that researchers cannot have high confidence that a statistically insignificant result is due to an actual lack of difference between treatments, rather than simply due to a sample size that was insufficient for detection of a clinically meaningful treatment effect.

A sufficient statistical power can be achieved in a trial by considering enough patients or, in other words, considering a large enough *sample size*. Sample size considerations cannot be contemplated before the primary endpoint is defined and the method of analysis (primary endpoint test statistic) is chosen. A clinically relevant magnitude of the treatment effect needs to be considered as well. For a chosen treatment effect, the sample size is commonly calculated by accepting a 5% chance of a type I error (two-sided) and by requiring statistical power to be at least 80% (but preferably 90% or higher). Statistical power for trials in which time-to-event analysis is considered depends on the number of events rather than just the number of patients. Various types of follow-up scenarios can be considered in order to accrue the required number of events. Patients can be followed for the same period of time, or until the last enrolled patient has been followed for a minimum reasonable period of time. In the second scheme, all but the last patient are followed for more than such a minimum time, because enrollment is spread over time. Such a design, incorporating a flexible length of follow-up, may need smaller sample size (fewer patients) to achieve the required statistical power.

Sample size can be often computed using a formula that incorporates treatment effect size, type I error, and statistical power. It is also worthwhile to consider simulations as a means of designing clinical trials, especially in nonstandard situations. Simulations consist of repeated random draws of a fixed-size sample from distributions reflecting the standard treatment and experimental arm endpoints. An example of a nonstandard situation may be a clinical trial in which subjects assigned to one arm receive a drug and those assigned to the other receive a surgical intervention, and it is possible that patients initially randomly assigned to the drug arm will undergo surgery as a consequence of principles guiding best current medical practice. Such an occurrence, sometimes referred to as a "crossover," will lead to departure from the proportional hazards assumption commonly used to compute sample sizes for time-to-event data. The crossover will change event rates in the drug therapy arm when results are analyzed according to the ITT principle, thus affecting the sample size. The timing of such a crossover can also have an impact on the required sample size and can be rather easily explored within the simulations framework. Although formulas for sample size in many nonstandard situations are available under more or less restrictive assumptions, simulations can provide an intuitive and flexible complementary approach to clinical trial design.

It is important to remember that sample size is only an estimate based on assumptions about event rates, effect size, or other summary quantities relevant to a particular trial or primary endpoint. Thus, a range of possible design assumptions needs to be considered, and sample size should be chosen conservatively to be the largest feasible within the range of these assumptions.

There are many other issues to be considered when designing a clinical trial. Secondary endpoints may be of interest and should be prespecified. Subgroup analyses may be planned, although subgroup comparisons will likely lack statistical power. Subgroup analyses should be prespecified in the protocol as much as possible, in order to avoid uncontrolled multiplicity of comparisons. Randomization may be stratified not only by center but also by known risk factors. The ability to pool treatment effects over centers in multicenter clinical trials must be evaluated, especially for trials of medical devices. Interim statistical analyses are commonly done during the course of a trial; such repeated analyses require proper statistical properties.[1] Use of these methods may provide a statistical argument for stopping a clinical trial early due to observed efficacy or a low chance of detecting the predefined treatment effect. Currently, the area of adaptive designs for clinical trials is being actively investigated.[9] These designs may provide benefits; however, they are considered controversial by some researchers.[10]

Conducting a clinical trial is a complex undertaking, particularly when multiple centers are involved. Managing such complexity requires an established infrastructure. Success depends on many individuals understanding and executing their tasks appropriately and timely, following the study protocol, and focusing on details. Training of trial personnel prior to the beginning of a study enrollment is essential, as is accurate evaluation of the timeliness and accuracy of data collection as the trial progresses.

In summary, a properly designed and executed randomized clinical trial requires substantial planning efforts, but such efforts will result in a well-run, ethical experiment with a convincing impact on medical practice.

References

1. Friedman L, Furberg CD, DeMets DL. *Fundamentals of Clinical Trials*, 3rd ed. New York: Springer-Verlag, 1998.
2. Piantadosi S. *Clinical Trials: A Methodologic Perspective*, 2nd ed. Hoboken, NJ: John Wiley & Sons, Inc., 2005.
3. Chow SC, Liu JP. *Design and Analysis of Clinical Trials: Concepts and Methodologies.* Hoboken, NJ: John Wiley & Sons, Inc., 2004.
4. Bardy GH, Lee KL, Mark DB, Poole JE, Packer DL, Boineau R, Domanski M, Troutman C, Anderson J, Johnson G, McNulty SE, Clapp-Channing N, Davidson-Ray LD, Fraulo ES, Fishbein DP, Luceri RM, Ip JH, for the Sudden Cardiac Death in Heart Failure Trial (SCD-HeFT) Investigators. Amiodarone or an implantable cardioverter-defibrillator for congestive heart failure. *N Engl J Med* 2005;352: 225–237.
5. Boyle CA, Decoufle P. National sources of vital status information extent of coverage and possible selectivity in reporting. *Am J Epidemiol* 1990;131:160–168.
6. DeMets DL, Furberg CD, Friedman LM, Eds. *Data Monitoring in Clinical Trials: A Case Studies Approach.* New York: Springer-Verlag, 2006.

7. Echt DS, Liebson PR, Mitchell LB, Peters RW, Obias-Manno D, Barker AH, Arensberg D, Baker A, Friedman L, Greene HL, *et al.* Mortality and morbidity in patients receiving encainide, flecainide, or placebo. The Cardiac Arrhythmia Suppression Trial. *N Engl J Med* 1991;324:781–788.
8. Al-Khatib SM, Sanders GD, Mark DB, Lee KL, Bardy GH, Bigger JT, Buxton AE, Connolly S, Kadish A, Moss A, Feldman AM, Ellenbogen KA, Singh S, Califf RM. Implantable cardioverter defibrillators and cardiac resynchronization therapy in patients with left ventricular dysfunction: Randomized trial evidence through 2004. *Am Heart J* 2005;149:1020–1034.
9. Proschan MA, Lan KKG, Wittes JT. *Statistical Monitoring of Clinical Trials: A Unified Approach.* New York: Springer, 2006.
10. Fleming TR. Standard *versus* adaptive monitoring procedures: A commentary. *Stat Med* 2006;25:3305–3312.

57
Risk Stratification for Sudden Death in Patients with Coronary Artery Disease

Alfred E. Buxton and Lilian Joventino

Introduction

For many years it has been recognized that some persons who survive acute myocardial infarction (MI) remain at considerable risk of mortality, in some cases for years.[1] It has also been recognized that approximately 50% of deaths in survivors of MI occur suddenly and unexpectedly. Since the advent of telemetric electrocardiogram (ECG) monitoring for patients with acute MI in the 1960s, ventricular tachycardia (VT) and fibrillation have been understood to precipitate most cardiac arrests after MI. These events usually occur without any apparent precipitating factor. While we have effective treatment for survivors of cardiac arrest, a minority (2–30%) of arrest victims survive the acute event.[2–7] Thus, there is considerable rationale to attempt primary prevention of cardiac arrest if we are to improve the overall survival of patients with coronary disease.

If we are to carry out primary prevention of sudden death effectively, several requirements must be satisfied. First, the at-risk population must be identified. Second, we must understand mechanisms responsible for sudden death in the population in question. Third, based on our understanding of these mechanisms, practical tests must be developed that identify subpopulations possessing the substrate to support specific arrhythmia mechanisms. Finally, having identified those patients possessing risk factors, effective treatments, preferably specific for each arrhythmia mechanism, must be developed and applied.

The purpose of this chapter is to review the current status of the third factor, risk stratification tests, in patients with coronary heart disease. Tests to identify persons at risk for sudden death have been developed along several lines, and may be classified in different ways. For example, some tests are relatively nonspecific, and identify patients with more advanced disease, thereby placing them at increased risk for nonsudden as well as sudden death. While such tests may be useful in identifying large populations at risk, employment of such tests alone is not likely to be very cost effective, because by their very nature, large numbers of patients will be treated who are not likely to benefit, because their mortality risk may be due primarily to nonarrhythmic mechanisms. One example of such a test is measurement of left ventricular ejection fraction (LVEF), which is an excellent way to identify patients at increased overall mortality risk, but bears no direct relation to arrhythmia mechanisms. Patients with depressed EF are at increased risk for both sudden and nonsudden death, but the risk of sudden death is proportional to the risk for nonsudden death. Thus, a test such as EF may be useful in identifying a high risk population to enroll in a randomized trial to evaluate efficacy of a treatment, in which a large number of events is desirable. On the other hand, tests associated with risk for sudden death that is increased out of proportion to risk for nonsudden death are more likely to bear a cause-and-effect relationship to mechanisms responsible for sudden death, rather than just an association with increased mortality, and therefore may be more cost effective. Examples of the latter would include the signal-averaged ECG and programmed electrical stimulation of the ventricles.

Another way to classify risk stratification tests is to recognize that some identify relatively stable substrates that may cause cardiac arrhythmias by reentrant mechanisms. Examples of these would be the signal-averaged ECG and programmed electrical stimulation performed during electrophysiological studies. T wave alternans may also identify underlying electrophysiological substrates. Other tests have been performed under the presumption that they identify factors that trigger or activate the substrate. Examples of this would be ambulatory ECG monitoring used to recognize frequent ventricular premature depolarizations or episodes of nonsustained VT. The latter tests have not proven to be very helpful. Recognition that the interaction between presumed arrhythmia triggers and the substrate, or the "condition" of the substrate (its ability to be activated), may be modulated by alterations in autonomic nervous system tone led to the development of other tests. The latter include measurement of heart rate variability (HRV) and baroreflex sensitivity (BRS). These tests are thought to measure relative balance between parasympathetic and sympathetic tone.

Some general issues in risk stratification are worth considering before discussion of specific tests. It should be recognized that mechanisms of sudden death are dependent upon a variety of factors. These include the anatomic substrate—the presence, type, and severity of structural heart disease. Even within the common anatomic substrate of ischemic heart disease, mechanisms responsible for sudden death vary, depending on the presence or absence of MI, size of infarct, compensatory responses of noninfarcted ventricular myocardium (such as hypertrophy), as well as coronary artery anatomy that may predispose to recurrent ischemia. Functional alterations, such as development of the syndrome of heart failure, add other mechanisms that may precipitate cardiac arrest, when superimposed on the anatomic substrate. In addition, the fact that coronary disease is a progressive condition means that mechanisms responsible for sudden death in individuals may well evolve over time. The inescapable conclusion is that no one risk stratification test alone will be appropriate for all patients with coronary artery disease. Rather, it is necessary to screen for multiple potential mechanisms of sudden death, and some tests will require repetition at certain time intervals. However, the need to screen for multiple potential mechanisms does not necessarily equate with a need for multiple (expensive) tests. For example, much useful information may be gained from a careful history and physical examination, screening for evidence of heart failure or symptomatic ischemia. In addition, measurement of a variety of risk variables may be accomplished by single tests. For example, a single (extended) exercise test might provide information regarding ischemia, the presence of T wave alternans (TWA), and spontaneous arrhythmias. A 24-h ambulatory monitor may provide information on spontaneous ventricular arrhythmia, TWA, HRV, and heart rate turbulence (HRT). Furthermore, a signal-averaged ECG might be coupled to either of these tests.

The fact that multiple tests have been developed since the 1970s (and continue to be developed) to evaluate risk of sudden death in survivors of MI is testimony to the failure to find one test suitable for all, or even a majority of patients. In addition to the multiplicity of potential mechanisms causing sudden death, we suspect that another source of fault in this area stems from the fact that most (although not all) explorations of this problem have been empiric, following along lines of identifying clinical factors associated with cardiac arrest or sudden death after MI, rather than having as the major focus attempting to understand mechanisms responsible for cardiac arrest and then developing tests that detect the presence of the substrates to support these mechanisms.

In the remainder of this chapter, we will review the various tests that have been developed, discussing their individual strengths and weaknesses. We will group tests into categories, based on whether they are thought to identify the substrate for arrhythmias, triggers, or autonomic dysfunction, recognizing that there is likely to be overlap (i.e., an abnormality in autonomic function might constitute the substrate for some types of arrhythmia), as well as disagreement. Another cautionary note is warranted at this point. Our focus in this chapter is on what we perceive to be primary electrical events precipitating cardiac arrest or sudden death. However, the importance of acute myocardial ischemia as a contributing factor to sudden death cannot be ignored. Multivessel, as opposed to single vessel coronary disease has long been recognized as a marker for patients at increased risk of mortality (though not specifically sudden death). Presumably this recognizes patients having potential for recurrent ischemic events, in contrast to patients with single-vessel disease who may experience a single large MI (that may form a substrate for reentrant VT), but have little potential for recurrent ischemia. Thus, we strongly advocate a search for ischemia in MI survivors, and interventions to correct this whenever possible, prior to evaluation for primary electrical events. Indirect evidence to support the beneficial effects of coronary revascularization were observed in the Coronary Artery Surgery Study, which demonstrated that the major beneficial effect of coronary bypass surgery on overall survival resulted from reduction in sudden death.[8]

In this review, we have been careful to include reports from both the prethrombolytic as well as from more recent periods that include patients treated with thrombolytic therapy or primary angioplasty. The reason for this is that while reperfusion therapy certainly alters the natural history following acute MI, many patients today do not receive this therapy for a variety of reasons. We suspect that a major explanation for differing outcomes in the current era is the widespread, appropriate use of β-adrenergic blocking agents and converting enzyme inhibitors or receptor blockers. It is important to realize that it is possible that patients with differing sets of risk factors may respond differently to these agents, and predictive properties of various risk factors may differ in patients who are treated with β-adrenergic blocking agents.[9] Of note, results from the GISSI trials suggest that clinical variables traditionally associated with increased mortality retain their value in the presence of thrombolytic therapy.[10]

Clinical Factors: Value of the History

Physicians often tend to place more weight on variables that require evaluation by specialized tests. However, it is good to keep in mind the value of factors obtained from a careful history. For example, a history of previous MI has been repeatedly associated with a poorer prognosis.[10–12] It has been recognized since the earliest studies evaluating mortality risk after MI that the presence of congestive heart failure during the initial hospitalization or later is associated with poor long-term prognosis.[10,13,14] The inability to perform an exercise test is also associated with a poorer prognosis.[10,15] One limitation of all clinical variables evaluated to date is lack of specificity for differentiating patients at risk for sudden versus nonsudden death.

Standard 12-Lead Electrocardiogram

The standard ECG is attractive as a potential risk stratification tool because of its universal availability, low cost, and reproducibility. It provides information on ventricular depolarization as well as repolarization. Depolarization abnormalities, such as QRS duration, have been demonstrated to relate to prognosis in both the prethrombolytic as well as postthrombolytic eras.[9,13,14] Studies of patients with recent MI suggested that both right bundle branch block (RBBB) and left bundle branch block (LBBB) are associated with increased risk.[14] A recent study involving predominantly patients with remote (not recent) MI could find no increase in mortality in patients with RBBB, but significantly increased risk in patients with LBBB or nonspecific intraventricular conduction delay (IVCD).[16] None of these analyses has suggested that conduction abnormalities are specifically related to sudden, as opposed to nonsudden death.

Repolarization abnormalities have been used to prognosticate in two ways. First, the magnitude of ST segment deviation after MI has been related to late mortality, as well as risk for recurrent ischemic events.[17,18] This relation has been examined primarily in patients with non-Q wave MI. Repolarization abnormalities have also been examined for their relation to primary arrhythmically mediated sudden death. Most of these analyses have focused on QT dispersion, that is, differences in the measured duration of the QT interval among leads recorded on the standard ECG. The current consensus holds that this technique is not helpful in risk stratification, in part because of methodological difficulties,[19] as well as failure to identify at-risk patients adequately.[20] Other studies have examined measures of the repolarization "gradient" (the angle between depolarization and repolarization)[21] and duration of various components of the T wave.[22] Unfortunately, while theoretically attractive, prospective evaluation of the performance of such measures has been disappointing.[20]

It is well established that myocardial hypertrophy in a variety of settings is linked to increased mortality, both sudden and nonsudden. The standard ECG is certainly not the gold standard for detection of left ventricular hypertrophy (LVH). In light of this, it is interesting that one recent study noted a significant relation between mortality after remote MI and LVH detected on the ECG.[16] This analysis assumes even more interest because the risk of sudden death was increased out of proportion to the increase in total mortality observed in patients with LVH.

Left Ventricular Ejection Fraction

Since the earliest investigations of mortality after MI, abnormalities of left ventricular function have been associated with risk for sudden and nonsudden death.[23] The ejection fraction has repeatedly been one of the most powerful mortality stratifiers in both the prethrombolytic as well as the reperfusion era.[12,24,25] As a result, low EF has been used as a major determinant for inclusion in clinical trials of post-infarction patients evaluating newer therapies, such as implantable cardioverter defibrillators (ICDs).[26–28] However, EF has a number of limitations. First, while low EF is *associated* with increased risk for sudden death, there is no evidence that there is any *causal relationship* between low EF and sudden death (the increase in total mortality parallels the increase in sudden death risk).[29] While EF is obviously a continuous variable, in order to use it in practice (or in the design of clinical trials), it becomes necessary to dichotomize into high- and low-risk groups. Most prospective analyses of EF as a continuous variable show that the breakpoint at which mortality risk begins to increase is 40%.[12] The second problem that results from use of EF as a primary or exclusive risk stratification instrument results from its poor sensitivity, which ranges from 50 to 60% in most studies.[30,31] Thus, low EF is a good tool to identify a high risk population to test the efficacy and safety of an intervention. This utility does not equate with utility to guide therapy in practice, as evidenced by the fact that most sudden deaths occur in patients who are at "lower risk" by virtue of their EF.

Spontaneous Ventricular Ectopy and Nonsustained Ventricular Tachycardia

Multiple studies have demonstrated an adverse prognostic significance attached to frequent ventricular premature complexes (VPCs, usually defined as >10 VPCs per hour on average over a 24-h period) and nonsustained ventricular tachycardia (NSVT) documented after recent (10 days–3 months) MI in both the prethrombolytic and the postreperfusion eras.[25,32–34] The occurrence of NSVT within 1 month of MI more than doubles the risk of subsequent sudden death. Nonsustained ventricular tachycardia detected 3 months to 1 year after MI is also associated with a significantly higher mortality rate.[35,36] Furthermore, frequent VPCs documented 1 year after MI have predicted increased mortality over the subsequent 2 years.[35] Interestingly, while frequent ectopy has remained independent of an adverse prognosis after acute MI, NSVT appears to have lost its independent prognostic significance.[25] It appears that at least part of the explanation for this appears to be the low frequency with which spontaneous NSVT is detected in patients who have received reperfusion therapy.[37] Thus, the sensitivity for prediction of arrhythmic events of spontaneous ventricular arrhythmias on Holter monitoring was only 43% in one comprehensive meta-analysis.[30] The prognostic significance of NSVT has always been tied to left ventricular dysfunction—spontaneous NSVT having adverse prognostic significance only in patients with EF ≤40%. As is the case with clinical variables and EF, the presence of NSVT and frequent VPCs is associated with but is not specifically related to sudden death after MI.

Signal-Averaged Electrocardiography

The signal-averaged electrocardiogram (SAECG) is a method whereby the high-frequency, low-amplitude signals that correlate with local areas of slow, delayed activation after MI may be detected. It was developed as an attempt to specifically detect one of the requisites for reentrant VT (slow conduction). In theory, abnormal results of this test should specifically predict patients at risk for arrhythmic, as opposed to nonarrhythmic mortality. As with all tests, it has limitations. One limitation is the lack of standards for normal SAECG in patients with bundle branch block. Its specificity may be compromised by the fact that not all areas of delayed activation may actually play a role in reentrant tachycardias, and larger MIs, while more likely to give rise to reentrant VT circuits, may also be more likely to result in areas of delayed activation that are merely "dead ends," not able to participate in reentry.[38] In light of the relation of the underlying conduction abnormalities that are represented by the abnormal SAECG to subsequent arrhythmic events, it is noteworthy that the presence and degree of these abnormalities are affected very favorably by thrombolytic therapy and mechanical reperfusion early after acute MI.[39–41] The reduction in frequency of late potentials is directly related to the patency of the infarct-related artery.[42,43]

Multiple studies have examined the prognostic significance of the SAECG alone and in combination with other tests, such as ambulatory electrocardiographic monitoring and measurement of EF after acute MI.[44–48] A majority of the studies have utilized time domain, rather than frequency domain analysis of signals. In these studies, sensitivity has averaged 62% for the prediction of sudden death or spontaneous sustained VT, during follow-up periods of 6–24 months. Its primary benefit in these reports appears to be its ability to identify patients at low risk for developing arrhythmic events, because the reported negative predictive values are in the neighborhood of 95%.[30] The specificity for prediction of sudden death is difficult to determine, as many of the studies report outcomes as sudden death or cardiac arrest grouped together with sustained VT. Furthermore, most reports have not provided the rates of nonsudden cardiac deaths in patients with abnormal SAECG. However, a recent report from the Multicenter UnSustained Tachycardia Trial (MUSTT) did find that the risk for sudden death significantly exceeded the risk of nonsudden death in patients with an abnormal SAECG.[49]

Electrophysiological Testing (Programmed Electrical Stimulation)

Programmed ventricular stimulation was initially developed in the early 1970s as a technique to study mechanisms of monomorphic VT occurring spontaneously after MI. Studies demonstrated that programmed stimulation could reproduce spontaneous sustained monomorphic VT in >90% of patients.[50] The technique was then applied to patients who had been resuscitated form cardiac arrest.[51,52] Cardiac arrest survivors differed from patients presenting with stable sustained VT in a number of respects, including the fact that monomorphic sustained VT was inducible in only 30–40% of cases. Programmed stimulation was then tested as a tool for risk stratification to predict sudden death after MI. The group at Johns Hopkins first reported this, using as an endpoint induction of repetitive ventricular responses.[53] A number of other laboratories then applied programmed stimulation, using induction of sustained VT as the endpoint in most cases.[54–60] Comparison of these studies is difficult because of variations in patient populations, stimulation protocols, and timing of electrophysiological test (5 days to 1.8 months after MI). Monomorphic sustained VT is inducible in 6–30% of patients. Ventricular fibrillation or polymorphic VT is induced in fewer patients. Stimulation protocols utilizing only ≤2 extrastimuli result in lower rates of inducible tachycardias. Patients who have received thrombolytic therapy have lower rates of inducible VT, ranging from 0 to 10% in streptokinase-treated patients versus 12 to 74% in untreated patients.[61,62] Early (day to day, week to week), and long-term (8 months) reproducibility of inducible VT is reported to range from 50% to 80%, and is significantly greater for slower (cycle length >240 msec) induced tachycardias.[63–67]

The prognostic significance of ventricular tachyarrhythmias induced early after MI has varied, in part because of variations in stimulation protocols used and study populations, as well as variable use of pharmacological antiarrhythmic therapy. Protocols limited to ≤2 extrastimuli reported low sensitivity.[59,63] Studies that used ≥3 extrastimuli and follow-up of ≥1 year reported arrhythmic event rates of 25–36% in patients with inducible sustained VT.[60,68] An Australian group reported results in over 1200 patients followed for at least 2 years.[68] They demonstrated that patients with only polymorphic VT (cycle length <230 msec) or induced ventricular fibrillation had no higher risk of arrhythmic events than patients without any induced arrhythmia.[69] The reported negative predictive value of programmed stimulation was approximately 97% in these studies, and the combined sensitivity was approximated 62% for the prediction of major arrhythmic events.[30]

Programmed stimulation was also applied to small numbers of patients with remote (average 3 years after) MI having spontaneous NSVT.[70–73] Sustained VT was inducible in 40–45% of patients studied. The increase in the percent of patients having inducible VT in comparison with those studied early after infarction is noteworthy. Arrhythmic events (sudden death, resuscitated cardiac arrest, or sustained VT) occurred in 12.5–23% of patients with inducible VT after 14–30 months, while only 4–12% of patients without inducible sustained VT experienced events. Almost all events occurred in patients with EF ≤0.40.

These early, small, single center studies provided the rationale for the MUSTT. This large (2202 patients) trial has been the only large-scale prospective evaluation of the utility of programmed stimulation to risk stratify post-MI patients.[74] It demonstrated that patients with inducible sustained VT had significantly increased risk for sudden death and total mortality compared to patients without inducible VT. Of note, the risk for sudden death significantly exceeded the risk for total mortality in patients with inducible VT, supporting the specificity of inducible VT for predicting arrhythmic events. The 2-year risk of sudden death or cardiac arrest in patients without inducible sustained VT was 12%. The freedom from sudden death risk appeared significantly greater with a negative electrophysiological test in patients having an EF of 30–40%, in comparison to patients with an EF <30%.[29]

T Wave Alternans

T wave alternans refers to the variability in morphology or amplitude of repolarization in alternate beats on the surface ECG.[75] This beat-to-beat fluctuation in the T wave amplitude, which can be detected at the microvolt level, has been linked to increased susceptibility for the development of ventricular tachyarrhythmias in patients with coronary artery disease, congestive heart failure, and other cardiac conditions.[76–82]

The standard definition of an abnormal TWA test employing the most commonly used proprietary system is the presence of >1.9 μV of alternans starting at a heart rate <110 beats per minute. The presence of TWA has been highly correlated with the inducibility of ventricular arrhythmias on electrophysiology study (EPS) in patients who have already experienced spontaneous VT.[80] In several observational cohort studies, its positive predictive value has been demonstrated to be as good as or better than other markers of increased risk of arrhythmic death such as EPS, LVEF, SAECG, BRS, and HRV.[76,79,81] A major limitation of most of the studies that have compared the performance of TWA to other tests is the inclusion of patients with multiple types of underlying heart disease (as well as no structural heart disease), and the fact that the majority of patients included in these reports had already experienced symptomatic and/or spontaneous sustained VT or fibrillation. One exception to this is a report from Germany of 107 patients with heart failure, of whom 67 had coronary disease.[78] In his analysis, TWA proved superior to EF, NSVT, BRS, HRV, and SAECG for prediction of arrhythmic events over a mean follow-up of 15 months. Measurement of microvolt T wave alternans has been performed during exercise and during atrial pacing, although one recent study suggested that exercise-induced alternans is superior to pacing-induced alternans in predicting risk of ventricular arrhythmic.[83]

One major limitation of TWA is the large number of indeterminate results, which in some recent studies may exceed the number of positive (abnormal) results. Major reasons for indeterminate results have included the presence of atrial fibrillation, frequent VPCs, and inability to exercise. All of these factors have been associated with adverse outcomes. Initial prospective studies examining the prognostic significance of TWA had difficulty attaining statistically significant results when comparing outcomes of patients with positive versus negative results (excluding those with indeterminate results). Investigators then noted that the prognosis of patients with indeterminate results was often similar to that of patients with positive TWA, and they began combining the patients with positive and indeterminate results for analysis of prognostic significance in comparison to patients with negative results. It is not surprising that indeterminate results appear to have a prognostic significance similar to positive tests. In a recent multicenter study of 549 patients with LVEF ≤40%,[82] the 2-year event rate (nonfatal sustained ventricular tachyarrhythmias or total mortality) was 12.3% for patients with a positive TWA test (162/549), 17.5% for patients with an indeterminate test (198/549), and 2.5% for patients with a negative test (189/549) [Hazard ratio for an abnormal (indeterminate or positive) test result = 6.5]. Note that more patients had indeterminate than positive tests, and the mortality was higher for patients with indeterminate than with positive tests. In several studies, the absence of TWA (negative test) confers a very low risk of sudden death due to its high negative predictive value.[82,84–86] Therefore, the most valuable role of TWA testing in risk stratification may prove to be its ability to identify, out of a group thought to be at high risk of sudden death, patients who are at a particularly low risk of arrhythmic events, and who may therefore not benefit from implantation of an ICD. In a study of patients with coronary disease and an LV EF ≤30%, approximately 30% tested negative for TWA. These patients had a very low risk of sudden cardiac death.[84] In this population, TWA was better than QRS width in identifying patients who are more likely to benefit from implantation of an ICD.

The ideal timing to assess for the presence of TWA has not yet been established. However, early assessment of TWA following an MI does not seem to be helpful. In a prospective study of 379 post-MI patients in whom the presence of TWA was assessed prior to hospital discharge,[87] 56 patients had a positive TWA test. However, over a 14-month follow-up period, 26 patients died, all of who had negative TWA tests.

A large, prospective primary prevention trial (Alternans Before Cardioverter Defibrillator Trial) is ongoing to directly compare the role of TWA to EPS in risk stratifying post-MI patients with decreased left ventricular systolic function and nonsustained VT. Another study (REFINE Trial) will evaluate the utility of TWA in predicting arrhythmic events in patients who have suffered a recent MI and who have varying degrees of left ventricular dysfunction (LVEF ≤50%). At this time, we would conclude that TWA is a promising technique that may aid in risk stratification of some patients with coronary disease. Unfortunately, the majority of studies performed to date have involved patients who have already experienced spontaneous ventricular tachyarrhythmias. Furthermore, most studies used mixed patient populations, including those without structural heart disease, nonischemic cardiomyopathies, as well as coronary disease. Finally, the large number of indeterminate results in each study is problematic, because most reasons for indeterminate results can easily be derived from simple clinical evaluation, without the expense or time involved in performing TWA.

Measures of Abnormalities in Autonomic Nervous System Tone

Heart Rate Variability

Heart rate variability is primarily a reflection of the balance between sympathetic and parasympathetic input to the sinus node. Patients with increased sympathetic tone and decreased parasympathetic tone are at higher risk for both sudden and nonsudden death following an MI. It has been postulated that HRV may be used as a surrogate for autonomic activity in the ventricles and may thus predict risk of arrhythmia and mortality.

Heart rate variability is due to high-frequency (0.15–0.45 Hz) and low-frequency (0.04–0.15 Hz) periodic oscillations in sinus rate.[88] High-frequency oscillations are primarily a result of sinus arrhythmia due to respiratory variation, which is primarily determined by parasympathetic tone. Conversely, sympathetic activity leads to low-frequency oscillations. Both short- and long-term HRV have been studied with regard to mortality risk.

Several methods have been used to assess HRV: time domain measures, frequency domain measures, and nonlinear measures. Common measures available from 24-h ambulatory ECG recording include standard deviation of NN (SDNN) intervals, which may be obtained over a 24-h period or over a few minutes (short-term HRV), SDANN, which is the standard deviation of the average NN intervals for the 288 5-min intervals in a 24-h ECG recording, pNN50, which is the percent NN intervals >50 msec different from the prior interval, rMSSD, which is the root mean square of differences between successive NN intervals, and total power, ultralow-frequency (ULF) power, very low-frequency (VLF) power, low-frequency (LF) power, high-frequency (HF) power, and the ratio of LF/HF.

Short-Term Heart Rate Variability

Short-term HRV (generally assessed over 2–8 min) has been assessed in patients with coronary artery disease and heart failure with regards to their mortality risk. A random sample of 900 patients from a population study of 14,672 men and women without known coronary disease showed that patients whose short-term HRV was severely impaired had an increased risk of mortality.[89] In patients with heart failure, diminished low-frequency power was associated with a 5-fold increase in arrhythmic mortality in multivariate analysis.[90] In the same study, the combination of normal low-frequency oscillations in short-term HRV and the absence of frequent isolated VPCs (<86/h) conferred a very low risk of sudden death (3% compared to 23%). At this time, there are insufficient data to recommend decreased short-term HRV as a risk stratifier of arrhythmic death.

Long-Term Heart Rate Variability

Long-term HRV is assessed on 24-h ambulatory ECG recordings. An increased risk of death in patients with decreased long-term HRV after MI has been reported in several studies.[91–96] A 2- to 5-fold increase in risk has been reported using different methods of evaluating long-term HRV. Multivariate analysis of the ATRAMI study demonstrated a relative risk of 3.2 of increased mortality in patients with decreased HRV, independent of LVEF and ventricular ectopy. In the ATRAMI trial, HRV did not discriminate risk for arrhythmic events as well as BRS. Another large trial designed to evaluate the effects of an antiarrhythmic drug, azimilide, on survival in 3717 patients with decreased left ventricular systolic dysfunction following an MI showed a hazard ratio of 1.46 for increased total mortality in patients with low HRV. However, no significant increase in arrhythmic death was seen.[96] In general, long-term HRV seems to be superior to short-term HRV in predicting risk of total mortality versus arrhythmic death. However, a major limitation of all the HRV evaluations is that there does not seem to be evidence for a causal relationship to sudden death. That is, abnormal HRV is associated with similar increases in risk for sudden and nonsudden death.

Baroreceptor Sensitivity

Baroreflex sensitivity (BRS) reflects the relationship between heart rate (RR intervals) and changes in blood pressure. This relationship is measured after administration of a bolus of phenylephrine. This sympathomimetic agent is a potent direct α receptor stimulant. The increase in blood pressure that accompanies its administration normally produces a reflex slowing of heart rate. Several studies have demonstrated an increased risk of death or ventricular arrhythmias in post-MI patients in whom this response is blunted (<3 msec/mm Hg change).[97,98] These findings were confirmed by the ATRAMI trial, a prospective study of 1284 patients with recent MI over a 21-month follow-up.[93,94] This trial also investigated the prognostic significance of abnormal HRV. In a multivariate analysis, impaired BRS or HRV was associated with a 3.2 and 2.8 relative risk for cardiac mortality, respectively. The relative risk was higher if both autonomic parameters were assessed together or in combination with an LVEF ≤35%. Importantly, in post-MI patients with an LVEF <35%, preserved BRS was associated with a very low risk of cardiac death (3% over a 2-year period). In a fashion similar to a negative TWA test, preserved BRS may be useful in identifying patients who may be at a particularly low risk of cardiac death and who may not benefit from implantation of an ICD. Furthermore, it is very interesting that findings from the ATRAMI study suggest that an abnormally low BRS may identify patients with an LVEF <35% whose risk for arrhythmic death exceeds their risk of total mortality, suggesting a causal relationship with sudden death: the relative risk for arrhythmic events was 6.7 versus a relative risk of 2.8 for total mortality. Further studies are necessary to assess this question prospectively.

Heart Rate Turbulence

Heart rate turbulence (HRT) refers to the change in sinus rate following a VPC. Physiologically, a transient increase in blood pressure is seen after the compensatory pause that follows a VPC. As a result, the sinus rate decreases due to reflex parasympathetic influences, with subsequent return to its baseline level. It is thought that both HRT and BRS are measures of vagal responsiveness. However, unlike BRS, HRT may be assessed from a 24-h ambulatory ECG recording relatively easily without the need for an active intervention (intravenous phenylephrine) to raise blood pressure.

Heart rate turbulence has been characterized by two parameters: the turbulence onset (TO) and the turbulence slope (TS).[99] The TO is "the difference between the mean of the first two sinus RR intervals after a VPC and the last two sinus RR intervals before the VPC divided by the mean of the last two sinus RR intervals before the VPC." The turbulence slope is the "maximum positive slope of a regression line assessed over any sequence of five subsequent sinus rhythm RR intervals within the first 20 sinus rhythm intervals after a VPC." A decreased slope, suggestive of an impaired parasympathetic response, has been associated with an increased risk of mortality.

Schmidt *et al.*[99] showed in patients with coronary artery disease with prior MI that a decreased turbulence slope was associated with a relative mortality risk of 2.7 in the placebo arm of EMIAT (European Myocardial Amiodarone Trial) and of 3.5 for patients entered in the MPIP (Multicenter Post-Infarction Program). Additionally, impaired HRT was associated with a relative mortality risk of 4 in a substudy of the ATRAMI Trial.[100] The relative risk of death doubled when HRT was combined with indices of BRS and HRV. A large, prospective study evaluated a cohort of 1455 post-MI patients with regard to abnormalities of HRT.[101] With a primary endpoint of all-cause mortality over a 22-month follow-up period, patients with an abnormal TO and TS had a hazard ratio of 5.9 (95% CI, 2.9–12.2), which was greater than the hazard ratio of 4.5 (95% CI, 2.6–7.8) from an LVEF ≤30%.

Thus, HRT is a promising predictor of mortality in post-MI patients. Further studies are needed to establish its utility as a risk stratifier for arrhythmic death in patients with coronary disease.

Summary

In spite of the significant differences between the risk stratification tests, it is remarkable that individually, they have all demonstrated fairly similar properties when analyzed in a meta-analysis.[30] While the sensitivity for prediction of arrhythmic events of spontaneous VPCs and NSVT (43%) and HRV (50%) appears lower, the SAECG, EF, and EPS all had sensitivities of approximately 60%. The odds ratio for arrhythmic events ranged from a low of 3.2 (VPCs and NSVT) to 5.1 (EF), 5.7 (SAECG), and 6.3 (HRV), to a high of 8.5 (EPS). Clearly, none of these tests alone displays adequate sensitivity. This is not surprising given the multiplicity of possible mechanisms that may lead to cardiac arrest or sudden death after MI. This leads us to the conclusion that only through the use of multiple tests will we be able to effectively reduce the risk of sudden death after MI. Another good reason to employ multiple tests in each patient is the fact that multiple studies have demonstrated that the prognostic significance of isolated tests is limited, while combining tests results in identification of much higher risk groups.[45,47,94] For example, each of these studies has shown that EF alone, when not associated with other abnormal risk stratification tests, is associated with only a slightly elevated risk of mortality. On the other hand, risk appears to be elevated significantly when two or more risk factors are identified, the degree of elevation depending on the specific risk factor in question.

In conclusion, we hope to have convinced the reader that we have yet to find the ideal risk stratification test. In fact, it is unlikely that there ever will be one ideal test, and testing will have to be individualized. It is likely that combinations of tests will be required to achieve optimum sensitivity and specificity. Because of the progressive nature of coronary artery disease, tests will have to be repeated at intervals. However, the optimal time for initial and repeat testing has not yet been defined. At the present time, most workers in this field agree that a prospective trial seeking to define the optimal risk stratification schema in survivors of MI is desperately needed.

References

1. Graham I, Mulcahy R, Hickey N, O'Neill W, Daly L. Natural history of coronary heart disease: A study of 586 men surviving an initial acute attack. *Am Heart J* 1983;105:249–257.
2. Baum R, Alvarez H, Cobb LA. Survival after resuscitation from out-of-hospital ventricular fibrillation. *Circulation* 1974;50:1231–1235.
3. Becker LB, Han BH, Meyer PM, Wright FA, Rhodes KV, Smith DW, Barrett J. Racial differences in the incidence of cardiac arrest and subsequent survival. The CPR Chicago Project. *N Engl J Med* 1993;329:600–606.
4. Eisenberg MS, Hallstrom A, Bergner L. Long-term survival after out-of-hospital cardiac arrest. *N Engl J Med* 1982;306:1340–1343.
5. Liberthson RR, Nagel EL, Hirschman JC, Nussenfeld SR. Prehospital ventricular defibrillation. Prognosis and follow-up course. *N Engl J Med* 1974;291:317–321.
6. Myerburg RJ, Fenster J, Velez M, Rosenberg D, Lai S, Kurlansky P, Newton S, Knox M, Castellanos A. Impact of community-wide police car deployment of automated external defibrillators on survival from out-of-hospital cardiac arrest. *Circulation* 2002;106:1058–1064.
7. Weaver WD, Hill D, Fahrenbruch CE, Copass MK, Martin JS, Cobb LA, Hallstrom AP. Use of the automatic external defibrillator in the management of out-of-hospital cardiac arrest. *N Engl J Med* 1988;319:661–666.
8. Holmes DRJ, Davis KB, Mock MB, Fisher LD, Gersh BJ, Killip T, Pettinger M, Study PitCAS. The effect of medical and surgical treatment on subsequent sudden cardiac death in patients with coronary artery disease. A report from the Coronary Artery Surgery Study. *Circulation* 1986;73:1254–1263.
9. Huikuri HV, Tapanainen JM, Lindgren K, Raatikainen P, Makikallio TH, Airaksinen KEJ, Myerburg RJ. Prediction of sudden cardiac death after myocardial infarction in the beta-blocking era. *J Am Coll Cardiol* 2003;42:652–658.
10. Tavazzi L, Volpi A. Remarks about postinfarction prognosis in light of the experience with the Gruppo Italiano per lo Studio della Sopravvivenza nell' Infarto Miocardico (GISSI) trials. *Circulation* 1997;95:1341–1345.
11. Madsen EB, Gilpin E, Henning H. Evaluation of prognosis one year after myocardial infarction. *J Am Coll Cardiol* 1983;1:985–993.
12. Rouleau JL, Talajic M, Sussex B, Potvin L, Warnica W, Davies RF, Gardner M, Stewart D, Plante S, Dupuis R, Lauzon C, Ferguson J, Mikes E, Balnozan V, Savard P. Myocardial infarction patients in the 1990s—their risk factors, stratification and survival in Canada: The Canadian Assessment of Myocardial Infarction (CAMI) Study. J Am Coll Cardiol 1996;27:1119–1127.
13. Sanz G, Castaner A, Betriu A, Magrina J, Roig E, Coll S, Pare JC, Navarro-Lopez F. Determinants of prognosis in survivors of myocardial infarction. A prospective clinical angiographic study. *N Engl J Med* 1982;306:1065–1070.
14. Weinberg SL. Natural history six years after acute myocardial infarction. Is there a low risk group? *Chest* 1976;69:23–28.
15. Fioretti P, Brower RW, Simoons ML, ten Katen H, Beelen A, Baardman T, Lubsen J, Hugenholtz PG. Relative value of clinical variables, bicycle ergometry, rest radionuclide ventriculography and 24 hour ambulatory electrocardiographic monitoring at discharge to predict 1 year survival after myocardial infarction. *J Am Coll Cardiol* 1986; 8:40–49.
16. Zimetbaum PJ, Buxton AE, Batsford W, Fisher JD, Hafley GE, Lee KL, O'Toole MF, Page RL, Reynolds M, Josephson ME. Electrocardiographic predictors of arrhythmic death and total mortality in the Multicenter Unsustained Tachycardia Trial. *Circulation* 2004;110:766–769.
17. Schechtman KB, Capone RJ, Kleiger RE, Gibson RS, Schwartz DJ, Roberts R, Young PM, Boden WE, Group DRSR. Risk stratification of patients with non-Q wave myocardial infarction. The critical role of ST segment depression. *Circulation* 1989;80:1148–1158.
18. Cannon CP, McCabe CH, Stone PH, Rogers WJ, Schactman M, Thompson BW, Pearce DJ, Diver DJ, Kells C, Feldman T, Williams M, Gibson RS, Kronenberg MW, Ganz LI, Anderson HV, Braunwald E. The electrocardiogram predicts one-year outcome of patients with unstable angina and non-Q wave myocardial infarction: Results of

the TIMI III registry ECG ancillary study. *J Am Coll Cardiol* 1997;30:133–140.
19. Statters DJ, Malik M, Ward DE, Camm AJ. QT dispersion: Problems of methodology and clinical significance. *J Cardiovasc Electrophysiol* 1994;5:672–685.
20. Zabel M, Klingenheben T, Franz MR, Hohnloser SH. Assessment of QT dispersion for prediction of mortality or arrhythmic events after myocardial infarction: Results of a prospective, long-term follow-up study. *Circulation* 1998;97:2543–2550.
21. Zabel M, Acar B, Klingenheben T, Franz MR, Hohnloser SH, Malik M. Analysis of 12-lead T-wave morphology for risk stratification after myocardial infarction. *Circulation* 2000;102:1252–1257.
22. Savelieva I, Yap YG, Yi G, Guo X, Camm AJ, Malik M. Comparative reproducibility of QT, QT peak, and T peak-T end intervals and dispersion in normal subjects, patients with myocardial infarction, and patients with hypertrophic cardiomyopathy. *Pacing Clin Electrophysiol* 1998;21:2376–2381.
23. Nelson GR, Cohn PF, Gorlin R. Prognosis in medically-treated coronary artery disease. Influence of ejection fraction compared to other parameters. *Circulation* 1975;52:408–412.
24. Schulze RA, Strauss HW, Pitt B. Sudden death in the year following myocardial infarction. Relation to ventricular premature contractions in the late hospital phase and left ventricular ejection fraction. *Am J Med* 1977;62:192–199.
25. Maggioni AP, Zuanetti G, Franzosi MG, Rovelli F, Santoro E, Staszewsky L, Tavazzi L, Tognoni G. Prevalence and prognostic significance of ventricular arrhythmias after acute myocardial infarction in the fibrinolytic era. GISSI-2 results. *Circulation* 1993;87:312–322.
26. Buxton AE, Lee KL, Fisher JD, Josephson ME, Prystowsky EN, Hafley G, the Multicenter Unsustained Tachycardia Trial Investigators. A randomized study of the prevention of sudden death in patients with coronary artery disease. *N Engl J Med* 1999;341:1882–1890.
27. Moss AJ, Zareba W, Hall WJ, Klein H, Wilber DJ, Cannom DS, Daubert JP, Higgins SL, Brown MW, Andrews ML, the Multicenter Automatic Defibrillator Implantation Trial II Investigators. Prophylactic implantation of a defibrillator in patients with myocardial infarction and reduced ejection fraction. *N Engl J Med* 2002;346:877–883.
28. Bardy GH, Lee KL, Mark DB, Poole JE, Packer DL, Boineau R, M. D, Troutman C, Anderson J, Johnson G, McNulty SE, Clapp-Channing N, Davidson-Ray LD, Fraulo ES, Fishbein DP, Luceri RM, Ip JH. Amiodarone or an implantable cardioverter-defibrillator for congestive heart failure. *N Engl J Med* 2005;352:225–237.
29. Buxton A, Hafley G, Lee K, Gold M, Packer D, Lehmann M, Josephson M, Wyse D, Fisher J, Prystowsky E, Talajic M, LA P, the MUSTT Investigators. Relation of ejection fraction and inducible ventricular tachycardia to mode of death in patients with coronary artery disease. *Circulation* 2002;106:2466–2472.
30. Bailey JJ, Berson AS, Handelsman H, Hodges M. Utility of current risk stratification tests for predicting major arrhythmic events after myocardial infarction. *J Am Coll Cardiol* 2001;38:1902–1911.
31. Copie X, Hnatkova K, Staunton A, Fei L, Camm A, Malik M. Predictive power of increased heart rate versus depressed left ventricular ejection fraction and heart rate variability for risk stratification after myocardial infarction. Results of a two-year follow-up study. *J Am Coll Cardiol* 1996;27:270–276.
32. Anderson KP, DeCamilla J, Moss AJ. Clinical significance of ventricular tachycardia (3 beats or longer) detected during ambulatory monitoring after myocardial infarction. *Circulation* 1978;57:890–897.
33. Bigger JT, Weld FM, Rolnitzky LM. Prevalence, characteristics and significance of ventricular tachycardia (three or more complexes) detected with ambulatory electrocardiographic recording in the late hospital phase of acute myocardial infarction. *Am J Cardiol* 1981;48:815–823.
34. Ruberman W, Weinblatt E, Goldberg JD, Frank CW, Shapiro S. Ventricular premature complexes and mortality after myocardial infarction. *N Engl J Med* 1977;297:750–755.
35. Hallstrom AP, Bigger JT, Roden D, Friedman L, Akiyama T, Richardson DW, Rogers WJ, Waldo AL, Pratt CM, Capone RJ, Griffith L, Theroux PA, Barker AH, Woosley RL. Prognostic significance of ventricular premature depolarizations measured 1 year after myocardial infarction in patients with early postinfarction asymptomatic ventricular arrhythmia. *J Am Coll Cardiol* 1992;20:259–264.
36. Tominaga S, Blackburn H, Group CDPR. Prognostic importance of premature beats following myocardial infarction: Experience in the Coronary Drug Project. *JAMA* 1973;223:1116–1124.
37. Hohnloser SH, Klingenheben T, Zabel M, Schopperl M, Mauss O. Prevalence, characteristics and prognostic value during long-term follow-up of nonsustained ventricular tachycardia after myocardial infarction in the thrombolytic era. *J Am Coll Cardiol* 1999;33:1895–1902.

38. Hood MA, Pogwizd SM, Peirick J, Cain ME. Contribution of myocardium responsible for ventricular tachycardia to abnormalities detected by analysis of signal-averaged ECGs. *Circulation* 1992;86:1888–1901.
39. Gang ES, Lew AS, Hong M, Wang FZ, Siebert CA, Peter T. Decreased incidence of ventricular late potentials after successful thrombolytic therapy for acute myocardial infarction. *N Engl J Med* 1989;321:712–716.
40. Pedretti R, Laporta A, Etro MD, Gementi A, Bonelli R, Anza C, Colombo E, Maslowsky F, Santoro F, Caru B. Influence of thrombolysis on signal-averaged electrocardiogram and late arrhythmic events after acute myocardial infarction. *Am J Cardiol* 1992;69:866–872.
41. Zimmermann M, Adamec R, Ciaroni S. Reduction in the frequency of ventricular late potentials after acute myocardial infarction by early thrombolytic therapy. *Am J Cardiol* 1991;67:697–703.
42. Hohnloser SH, Franck P, Klingenheben T, Zabel M, Just H. Open infarct artery, late potentials, and other prognostic factors in patients after acute myocardial infarction in the thrombolytic era. A prospective trial. *Circulation* 1994;90:1747–1756.
43. Vatterott PJ, Hammill SC, Bailey KR, Wiltgen CM, Gersh BJ. Late potentials on signal-averaged electrocardiograms and patency of the infarct-related artery in survivors of acute myocardial infarction. *J Am Coll Cardiol* 1991;17:330–337.
44. Breithardt G, Schwarzmaier J, Borggrefe M, Haerten K, Seipel L. Prognostic significance of late ventricular potentials after acute myocardial infarction. *Eur Heart J* 1983;4:487–495.
45. Gomes JA, Winters SL, Stewart D, Horowitz S, Milner M, Barreca P. A new noninvasive index to predict sustained ventricular tachycardia and sudden death in the first year after myocardial infarction: Based on signal-averaged electrocardiogram, radionuclide ejection fraction and Holter monitoring. *J Am Coll Cardiol* 1987;10:349–357.
46. Steinberg JS, Regan A, Sciacca RR, Bigger JT, Fleiss JL, Salvatore DE, Fosina M, Rolnitzky LM. Predicting arrhythmic events after acute myocardial infarction using the signal-averaged electrocardiogram. *Am J Cardiol* 1992;69:13–21.
47. Kuchar DL, Thorburn CW, Sammel NL. Prediction of serious arrhythmic events after myocardial infarction. Signal-averaged electrocardiogram, Holter monitoring and radionuclide ventriculography. *J Am Coll Cardiol* 1987;9:531–538.
48. El-Sherif N, Denes P, Katz R, Capone R, Mitchell LB, Carlson M, Reynolds-Haertle R. Definition of the best prediction criteria of the time domain signal-averaged electrocardiogram for serious arrhythmic events in the postinfarction period. *J Am Coll Cardiol* 1995;25:908–914.
49. Gomes J, Cain M, Buxton A, Josephson M, Lee K, Hafley G. Prediction of long-term outcomes by signal-averaged electrocardiography in patients with unsustained ventricular tachycardia, coronary artery disease, and left ventricular dysfunction. *Circulation* 2001;104:436–441.
50. Buxton A, Waxman H, Marchlinski F, Untereker W, Waspe L, Josephson M. Role of triple extrastimuli during electrophysiologic study of patients with documented sustained ventricular tachyarrhythmias. *Circulation* 1984;69:532–540.
51. Ruskin J, DiMarco J, Garan H. Out-of-hospital cardiac arrest: Electrophysiologic observations and selection of long-term antiarrhythmic therapy. *N Engl J Med* 1980;303:607–613.
52. Josephson M, Horowitz L, Spielman S, Greenspan A. Electrophysiologic and hemodynamic studies in patients resuscitated from cardiac arrest. *Am J Cardiol* 1980;46:948–955.
53. Greene H, Reid P, Schaeffer A. The repetitive ventricular response in man–a predictor of sudden death. *N Engl J Med* 1978;299:729–734.
54. Hamer A, Vohra J, Hunt D, Sloman G. Prediction of sudden death by electrophysiologic studies in high risk patients surviving acute myocardial infarction. *Am J Cardiol* 1982;50:223–229.
55. Richards D, Cody D, Denniss A, Russell P, Young A, Uther J. Ventricular electrical instability: A predictor of death after myocardial infarction. *Am J Cardiol* 1983;51:75–80.
56. Marchlinski F, Buxton A, Waxman H, Josephson M. Identifying patients at risk of sudden death after myocardial infarction: Value of the response to programmed stimulation, degree of ventricular ectopic activity and severity of left ventricular dysfunction. *Am J Cardiol* 1983;52:1190–1196.
57. Roy D, Marchand E, Theroux P, Waters DD, Pelletier GB, Bourassa MG. Programmed ventricular stimulation in survivors of an acute myocardial infarction. *Circulation* 1985;72:487–494.
58. Waspe L, Seinfeld D, Ferrick A, Kim S, Matos J, Fisher J. Prediction of sudden death and spontaneous ventricular tachycardia in survivors of complicated myocardial infarction: Value of the response to programmed stimulation using a maximum of three ventricular extrastimuli *J Am Coll Cardiol* 1985;5:1292–1301.
59. Bhandari AK, Rose JS, Kotlewski A, Rahimtoola SH, Wu D. Frequency and significance of induced sustained ventricular tachycardia or fibrillation

two weeks after acute myocardial infarction. *Am J Cardiol* 1985;56:737–742.
60. Iesaka Y, Nogami A, Aonuma K, Nitta J, Chun YH, Fujiwara H, Hiraoka M. Prognostic significance of sustained monomorphic ventricular tachycardia induced by programmed ventricular stimulation using up to triple extrastimuli in survivors of acute myocardial infarction. *Am J Cardiol* 1990; 65:1057–1063.
61. Kersschot I, Brugada P, Ramentol M, Zehender M, Waldecker B, Stevenson W, Geibel A, DeZwaan C, Wellens H. Effects of early reperfusion in acute myocardial infarction on arrhythmias induced by programmed stimulation: A prospective, randomized study. *J Am Coll Cardiol* 1986;7:1234–1242.
62. Bourke J, Young A, Richards D, Uther J. Reduction in incidence of inducible ventricular tachycardia after myocardial infarction by treatment with streptokinase during infarct evolution. *J Am Coll Cardiol* 1990;16:1703–1710.
63. Roy D, Marchand E, Theroux P, Waters DD, Pelletier GB, Cartier R, Bourassa MG. Long-term reproducibility and significance of provokable ventricular arrhythmias after myocardial infarction. *J Am Coll Cardiol* 1986;8:32–39.
64. Kuck KH, Costard A, Schluter M, Kunze KP. Significance of timing programmed electrical stimulation after acute myocardial infarction. *J Am Coll Cardiol* 1986;8:1279–1288.
65. Bhandari AK, Au PK, Rose JS, Kotlewski A, Blue S, Rahimtoola SH. Decline in inducibility of sustained ventricular tachycardia from two to twenty weeks after acute myocardial infarction. *Am J Cardiol* 1987;59:284–290.
66. Bhandari AK, Hong R, Kulick D, Petersen R, Rubin JN, Leon C, McIntosh N, Rahimtoola SH. Day to day reproducibility of electrically inducible ventricular arrhythmias in survivors of acute myocardial infarction. *J Am Coll Cardiol* 1990; 15:1075–1081.
67. Nogami A, Aonuma K, Takahashi A, Nitta J, Chun YH, Iesaka Y, Hiroe M, Marumo F. Usefulness of early versus late programmed ventricular stimulation in acute myocardial infarction. *Am J Cardiol* 1991;68:13–20.
68. Bourke JP, Richards DA, Ross DL, Wallace EM, McGuire MA, Uther JB. Routine programmed electrical stimulation in survivors of acute myocardial infarction for prediction of spontaneous ventricular tachyarrhythmias during follow-up: Results, optimal stimulation protocol and cost-effective screening. *J Am Coll Cardiol* 1991;18: 780–788.
69. Bourke J, Richards D, Ross D, McGuire M, Uther J. Does the induction of ventricular flutter or fibrillation at electrophysiologic testing after myocardial infarction have any prognostic significance? *Am J Cardiol* 1995;75:431–435.
70. Gomes JA, Hariman RI, Kang PS, El-Sherif N, Chowdhry I, Lyons J. Programmed electrical stimulation in patients with high-grade ventricular ectopy: Electrophysiologic findings and prognosis for survival. *Circulation* 1984;70:43–51.
71. Buxton AE, Marchlinski FE, Flores BT, Miller JM, Doherty JU, Josephson ME. Nonsustained ventricular tachycardia in patients with coronary artery disease: Role of electrophysiologic study. *Circulation* 1987;75:1178–1185.
72. Klein RC, Machell C. Use of electrophysiologic testing in patients with nonsustained ventricular tachycardia: Prognostic and therapeutic implications. *J Am Coll Cardiol* 1989;14:155–161.
73. Wilber DJ, Olshansky B, Moran JF, Scanlon PJ. Electrophysiological testing and nonsustained ventricular tachycardia. Use and limitations in patients with coronary artery disease and impaired ventricular function. *Circulation* 1990;82:350–358.
74. Buxton AE, Lee KL, DiCarlo L, Gold MR, Greer GS, Prystowsky EN, O'Toole MF, Tang A, Fisher JD, Coromilas J, Talajic M, Hafley G, the Multicenter Unsustained Tachycardia Trial Investigators. Electrophysiologic testing to identify patients with coronary artery disease who are at risk for sudden death. *N Engl J Med* 2000;342:1937–1945.
75. Armoundas AA, Tomaselli GF, Esperer HD. Pathophysiological basis and clinical application of T-wave alternans. *J Am Coll Cardiol* 2002;40: 207–217.
76. Gold MR, Bloomfield DM, Anderson KP, El-Sherif NE, Wilber DJ, Groh WJ, Estes NA 3rd, Kaufman ES, Greenberg ML, Rosenbaum DS. A comparison of T-wave alternans, signal averaged electrocardiography and programmed ventricular stimulation for arrhythmia risk stratification. *J Am Coll Cardiol* 2000;36:2247–2253.
77. Hohnloser SH, Klingenheben T, Bloomfield D, Dabbous O, Cohen RJ. Usefulness of microvolt T-wave alternans for prediction of ventricular tachyarrhythmic events in patients with dilated cardiomyopathy: Results from a prospective observational study. *J Am Coll Cardiol* 2003;41: 2220–2224.
78. Klingenheben T, Zabel M, D'Agostino RB, Cohen RJ, Hohnloser SH. Predictive value of T-wave alternans for arrhythmic events in patients with congestive heart failure. *Lancet* 2000;356:651–652.

79. Rashba EJ, Osman AF, Macmurdy K, Kirk MM, Sarang SE, Peters RW, Shorofsky SR, Gold MR. Enhanced detection of arrhythmia vulnerability using T wave alternans, left ventricular ejection fraction, and programmed ventricular stimulation: A prospective study in subjects with chronic ischemic heart disease. *J Cardiovasc Electrophysiol* 2004;15:170–176.
80. Rosenbaum DS, Jackson LE, Smith JM, Garan H, Ruskin JN, Cohen RJ. Electrical alternans and vulnerability to ventricular arrhythmias. *N Engl J Med* 1994;330:235–241.
81. Tanno K, Ryu S, Watanabe N, Minoura Y, Kawamura M, Asano T, Kobayashi Y, Katagiri T. Microvolt T-wave alternans as a predictor of ventricular tachyarrhythmias: A prospective study using atrial pacing. *Circulation* 2004;109:1854–1858.
82. Bloomfield DM, Bigger JT, Steinman RC, Namerow PB, Parides MK, Curtis AB, Kaufman ES, Davidenko JM, Shinn TS, Fontaine JM. Microvolt T-wave alternans and the risk of death or sustained ventricular arrhythmias in patients with left ventricular dysfunction. *J Am Coll Cardiol* 2006;47:456–463.
83. Rashba EJ, Osman AF, MacMurdy K, Kirk MM, Sarang S, Peters RW, Shorofsky SR, Gold MR. Exercise is superior to pacing for T wave alternans measurement in subjects with chronic coronary artery disease and left ventricular dysfunction. *J Cardiovasc Electrophysiol* 2002;13:845–850.
84. Bloomfield DM, Steinman RC, Namerow PB, Parides M, Davidenko J, Kaufman ES, Shinn T, Curtis A, Fontaine J, Holmes D, Russo A, Tang C, Bigger JT Jr. Microvolt T-wave alternans distinguishes between patients likely and patients not likely to benefit from implanted cardiac defibrillator therapy: A solution to the Multicenter Automatic Defibrillator Implantation Trial (MADIT) II conundrum. *Circulation* 2004;110:1885–1889.
85. Chow T, Kereiakes DJ, Bartone C, Booth T, Schloss EJ, Waller T, Chung ES, Menon S, Nallamothu BK, Chan PS. Prognostic utility of microvolt T-wave alternans in risk stratification of patients with ischemic cardiomyopathy. *J Am Coll Cardiol* 2006;47:1820–1827.
86. Gehi AK, Stein RH, Metz LD, Gomes JA. Microvolt T-wave alternans for the risk stratification of ventricular tachyarrhythmic events: A meta-analysis. *J Am Coll Cardiol* 2005;46:75–82.
87. Tapanainen JM, Still AM, Airaksinen KE, Huikuri HV. Prognostic significance of risk stratifiers of mortality, including T wave alternans, after acute myocardial infarction: Results of a prospective follow-up study. *J Cardiovasc Electrophysiol* 2001;12:645–652.
88. Task Force. Heart rate variability: Standards of measurement, physiological interpretation and clinical use. *Circulation* 1996;93:1043–1065.
89. Dekker JM, Crow RS, Folsom AR, Hannan PJ, Liao D, Swenne CA, Schouten EG. Low heart rate variability in a 2-minute rhythm strip predicts risk of coronary heart disease and mortality from several causes: The ARIC Study. Atherosclerosis Risk In Communities. *Circulation* 2000;102:1239–1244.
90. La Rovere MT, Pinna GD, Maestri R, Mortara A, Capomolla S, Febo O, Ferrari R, Franchini M, Gnemmi M, Opasich C, Riccardi PG, Traversi E, Cobelli F. Short-term heart rate variability strongly predicts sudden cardiac death in chronic heart failure patients. *Circulation* 2003;107:565–570.
91. Kleiger RE, Miller JP, Bigger JT Jr, Moss AJ. Decreased heart rate variability and its association with increased mortality after acute myocardial infarction. *Am J Cardiol* 1987;59:256–262.
92. Tsuji H, Venditti FJ Jr, Manders ES, Evans JC, Larson MG, Feldman CL, Levy D. Reduced heart rate variability and mortality risk in an elderly cohort. The Framingham Heart Study. *Circulation* 1994;90:878–883.
93. La Rovere MT, Bigger JT Jr, Marcus FI, Mortara A, Schwartz PJ. Baroreflex sensitivity and heart-rate variability in prediction of total cardiac mortality after myocardial infarction. ATRAMI (Autonomic Tone and Reflexes After Myocardial Infarction) Investigators. *Lancet* 1998;351:478–484.
94. La Rovere MT, Pinna GD, Hohnloser SH, Marcus FI, Mortara A, Nohara R, Bigger JT Jr, Camm AJ, Schwartz PJ. Baroreflex sensitivity and heart rate Variability in the identification of patients at risk for life-threatening Arrhythmias: Implications for clinical trials. *Circulation* 2001;103:2072–2077.
95. Huikuri HV, Makikallio TH, Peng CK, Goldberger AL, Hintze U, Moller M. Fractal correlation properties of R-R interval dynamics and mortality in patients with depressed left ventricular function after an acute myocardial infarction. *Circulation* 2000;101:47–53.
96. Camm AJ, Pratt CM, Schwartz PJ, Al-Khalidi HR, Spyt MJ, Holroyde MJ, Karam R, Sonnenblick EH, Brum JM. Mortality in patients after a recent myocardial infarction: A randomized, placebo-controlled trial of azimilide using heart rate variability for risk stratification. *Circulation* 2004;109:990–996.

97. Farrell TG, Odemuyiwa O, Bashir Y, Cripps TR, Malik M, Ward DE, Camm AJ. Prognostic value of baroreflex sensitivity testing after acute myocardial infarction. *Br Heart J* 1992;67:129–137.
98. Farrell TG, Paul V, Cripps TR, Malik M, Bennett ED, Ward D, Camm AJ. Baroreflex sensitivity and electrophysiological correlates in patients after acute myocardial infarction. *Circulation* 1991;83: 945–952.
99. Schmidt G, Malik M, Barthel P, Schneider R, Ulm K, Rolnitzky L, Camm AJ, Bigger JT Jr, Schomig A. Heart-rate turbulence after ventricular premature beats as a predictor of mortality after acute myocardial infarction. *Lancet* 1999;353:1390–1396.
100. Ghuran A, Reid F, La Rovere MT, Schmidt G, Bigger JT Jr, Camm AJ, Schwartz PJ, Malik M. Heart rate turbulence-based predictors of fatal and nonfatal cardiac arrest (The Autonomic Tone and Reflexes After Myocardial Infarction substudy). *Am J Cardiol* 2002;89:184–190.
101. Barthel P, Schneider R, Bauer A, Ulm K, Schmitt C, Schomig A, Schmidt G. Risk stratification after acute myocardial infarction by heart rate turbulence. *Circulation* 2003;108:1221–1226.

58
Heart Failure and Sudden Death

Yong-Mei Cha and Win-Kuang Shen

Introduction

The syndrome of congestive heart failure is a clinical manifestation of many cardiac disease processes when cardiovascular compensatory mechanisms are no longer able to maintain homeostasis. Approximately five million people in the United States have heart failure and over 550,000 patients are diagnosed with heart failure for the first time each year.[1] The Framingham heart study reported 62% and 42% 5-year survival rates, respectively, for men and women with newly diagnosed congestive heart failure in the early 1970s.[2] These mortality rates were six to seven times higher than that of the age-matched general population. Of the total mortality, approximately 40–50% were sudden deaths.[3] Trends in the incidence and survival with heart failure among 11,311 subjects in the Framingham heart study during a 50 year interval have been updated.[4] Heart failure occurred in 1075 study participants between 1950 and 1999. The 5-year mortality rate among men declined from 70% in the period from 1950 through 1969 to 59% in the period from 1990 through 1999, whereas the respective rates among woman declined from 57% to 45% (Figure 58–1). Although the relative decline in mortality is encouraging, likely a result of a better understanding of the disease pathophysiology and improvements in medical and device therapy, the growing epidemic of heart failure has been increasingly recognized in the United States and around the globe.

The topic of heart failure and sudden death is very broad. Many specific and related topics are discussed in other chapters of this book. In this chapter, we will provide an overview on the following relevant issues: (1) mode of death in patients with heart failure, (2) arrhythmogenic substrates and triggers of malignant arrhythmias causing sudden death, (3) risk stratification schemes in identifying patients at increased risk of sudden death in heart failure, (4) outcomes from sudden death prevention clinical trials, and (5) a summary of current clinical management in sudden death prevention in heart failure.

Death Mode in Advanced Stage of Heart Failure

Sudden death is often equated with primary arrhythmia events. While ventricular tachyarrhythmias are the most common rhythms associated with unexpected sudden death, bradycardia and other pulseless superventricular rhythms are also common in patients with advanced heart failure.[5] In the Metoprolol CR/XL Randomized Intervention Trial in Congestive Heart Failure (MERIT-HF), a total of 3991 patients with chronic heart failure in New York Heart Association (NYHA) functional Class II–IV and with an ejection fraction of 0.4 or less were randomized to either placebo or Metoprolol CR/XL groups. During a mean follow-up duration of 1 year, total mortality was lower in the Metoprolol group than in the placebo group (7.2% versus 11%). Fifty-eight percent of these deaths were classified as sudden. The study analyzed the total mortality and mode of death in relationship to NYHA functional class at randomization. While the absolute frequency of death is highest in patients with severe symptoms or in NYHA function Class IV (Figure 58–2A), the proportion of sudden death generally decreased with the increasing severity of heart failure, from 60% in Class II or III down to 30% in Class IV heart failure. The proportion of patients who died from pump failure increased from 12% in NYHA Class II to 28% in Class III and up to 56% in Class IV[6] (Figure 58–2B). An implantable cardioverter defibrillator (ICD) provided a unique opportunity to record terminal rhythm at the time of death. Although the frequency of a primary bradycardia-mediated sudden event cannot be assessed in the ICD patient population because of the presence of pacing function in all ICDs, other mechanisms of sudden death were investigated from a nonthoracotomy ICD database.[7] Among 317 patients who died after ICD implantation, 28% were sudden, 49% were nonsudden cardiac, and 27% were noncardiac death. Among the sudden deaths, 29% had postshock electromechanical dissociation (EMD), 25% had ventricular tachycardia/ventricular fibrillation (VT/VF) uncorrected by shocks, 16% had primary EMD, and 13% had recurrent incessant VT/VF despite successful transient termination after shocks. The NYHA functional class was the only independent predictor of postshock EMD. Many patients with end-stage heart failure experience sudden death that is nonetheless expected. Prevention of sudden death in this population may be more effective by focusing on therapies that can modify disease progression.[8,9]

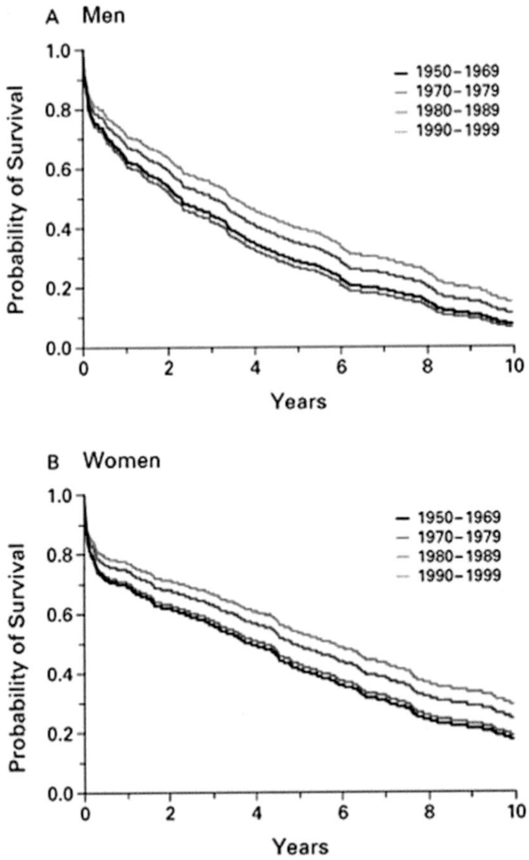

Figure 58–1. Temporal trends in age-adjusted survival after the onset of heart failure among men (A) and women (B). Values were adjusted for age (<55, 55–64, 65–74, 75–84, and ≥85 years). Estimates are shown for subjects who were 65–74 years of age. (Reproduced from Levy *et al.*,[4] with permission from the *New England Journal of Medicine*.)

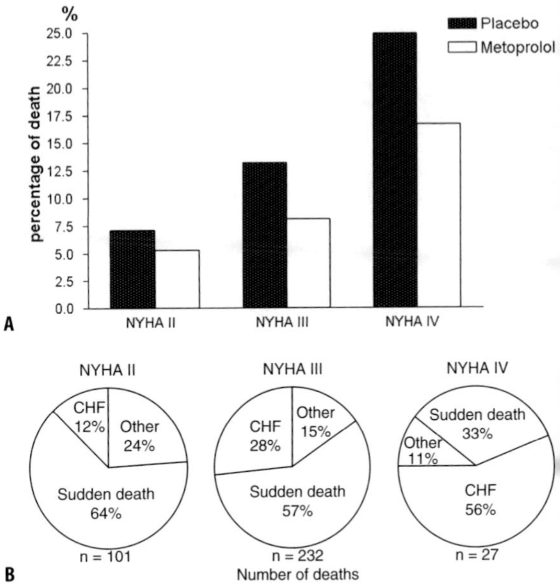

Figure 58–2. (A) Total mortality in relationship to NYHA class in metoprolol and placebo groups from the MERIT-HF trial. (B) Severity of heart failure and mode of death from the MERIT-HF trial. (Reproduced from MERIT-HF trial,[6] with permission from *Lancet*.)

Mechanisms of Sudden Death in Heart Failure

Arrhythmogenic Substrates Predisposing to Sudden Death

Abnormalities in Cellular Electrophysiology

Prolongation of the ventricular action potential has been well documented in both animal models and humans in heart failure. Downregulation of ionic currents I_{to}, I_{Kr}, I_{Ks}, and I_{K1} has been observed from animal or human studies. Despite prolongation of action potential duration and increased dispersion of repolarization, these changes contribute only in part to the genesis of malignant ventricular tachyarrhythmias leading to sudden cardiac death.[10–12] In heart failure, altered calcium handling not only affects ventricular mechanics, but also affects electrophysiological properties. The $I_{Ca\text{-}L}$ density has been reported to be unchanged,[13,14] while the $I_{Ca\text{-}L}$ was decreased in cardiac hypertrophy and severe heart failure primarily from Ca-mediated inactivation of the $I_{Ca\text{-}L}$ current.[15] Spontaneous calcium release from the sarcoplasmic reticulum results in enhanced Na–Ca exchanger current, which likely contributes to the genesis of delayed afterdepolarization (DAD) and DAD-mediated ventricular arrhythmias.[16,17]

Gap Junction

Gap junctions are composed of intercellular channels that permit the transfer of electrical current between neighboring cells. Connexin43 is a principal gap junction protein in the ventricle, playing a critical role in impulse propagation and electrical synchronization between myocytes. To determine transmural connexin43 expression and its relationship to electrophysiological function, Poelzing and Rosenbaum[18] performed a high-resolution transmural optical mapping of the arterially perfused canine preparation to measure the conduction velocity and transmural changes of action potential duration in a pacing-induced heart failure model. The absolute connexin43 expression in failing myocardium, quantified by confocal immunofluorescence, was uniformly reduced by 40%, compared with control. Reduced connexin43 expression in heart failure was associated with a significant reduction in intercellular coupling between transmural muscular layers correlated with reduced conduction velocity. The action potential duration dispersion was greatest in failing myocardium and the largest transmural action potential duration gradient was consistently found in regions exhibiting lowest connexin43 expression. These findings led to the conclusion that reduced connexin43 expression produced uncoupling between transmural muscle layers resulting in a slow conduction and marked dispersion of repolarization between the epicardial and deeper myocardial layers, contributing to an arrhythmia substrate in failing myocardium.

Nerve Spouting and Sympathetic Nerve Activity

Excessive sympathetic activation is one of the mechanisms contributing to the increased mortality and sudden death in heart failure. Ventricular arrhythmia associated with sympathetic activity is often seen in patients with ischemic cardiomyopathy owing to prior myocardial infarction (MI). Following myocardial injury, peripheral nerves undergo Wallerian degeneration, which may be followed by neurilemma cell proliferation and axonal regeneration (nerve sprouting), resulting in sympathetic hyperinnervation.[19] Nerve sprouting activity and sympathetic innervation after MI have been investigated from several experiemental conditions. Meiri used computerized morphometry to quantify the density of nerve fibers that were immunopositive for growth-associated protein 43 (GAP43) or tyrosine hydroxylase (TH) in a mouse model.[20] GAP43 is a protein associated with the axonal growth cone and is upregulated during nerve sprouting. The density of GAP43-positive nerve fibers is a measurement of nerve sprouting activity. In contrast, TH is a measurement of stable sympathetic innervations in the myocardium. There was an acute increase in GAP43 immunoreactive nerve fiber density within 3h, which persisted for 1 week after MI, so was TH-positive nerve fiber density.[21] The magnitude of the increase in TH-positive nerve fiber density, as compared to controls, appeared to be greater in the periinfarct area than in the remote area. In a large animal study, Zhou[22] created MI in dogs by either ligating the coronary artery or by intracoronary balloon inflation. Consistent with findings in the mouse model of MI, GAP43-positive nerve numbers

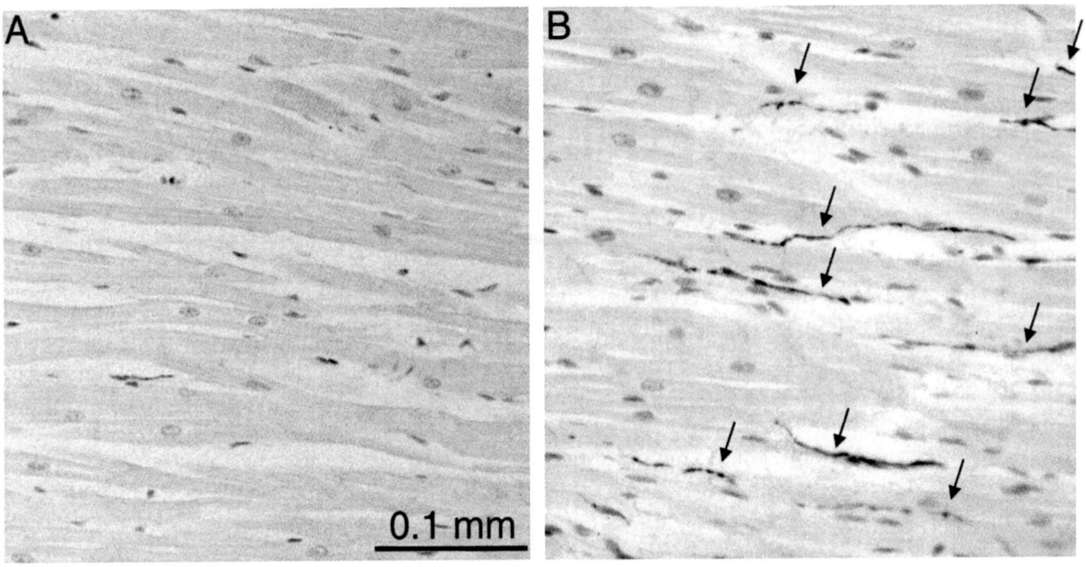

FIGURE 58–3. Nerve sprouting after MI. (A) GAP43 staining of ventricular myocardium from a normal dog. There were no GAP43-positive nerves. (B) The same stain of myocardium 1 week after MI, when abundant GAP43-positive nerves (arrows) were present. (Reproduced from L.S. Chen, S. Zhou, M.C. Fishbein, *et al.*, *J Cardiovasc Electrophysiol* 2007;18:123–127, with permission.)

increased in both infarcted and noninfarcted sites after MI (Figure 58–3). In clinical studies, Cao[23] reported that the nerve density of ventricular myocardium obtained from patients who had a history of cardiac arrhythmia was significantly higher than in patients without arrhythmia who had heart failure and underwent heart transplantation. To determine a causal relationship between sympathetic hyperinnervation and ventricular arrhythmia, a canine MI model was created by ligating the left anterior descending coronary artery, and complete atrioventricular block (AVB) by radiofrequency ablation. Sympathetic nerve sprouting was facilitated by giving a chronic infusion of nerve growth factor (NGF) via osmotic pump[24] to the left stellate ganglion. As compared to control dogs (with MI and AVB), NGF infusion increased sympathetic nerve density 2-fold (33.2 ± 12.1 vs. $16.6 \pm 1.3\,\mu m/mm^2$) and increased the incidence of VT by 10-fold. Four of nine dogs died from documented VF. In a pacing-induced heart failure canine model, an increase of ventricular sympathetic nerve density was also confirmed.[25]

To prove a causal relationship between sympathetic nerve activity and arrhythmogenesis, Jardine recorded cardiac sympathetic nerve activity from sheep by multiple electrodes glued to the left cardiothoracic nerves and found a spontaneous VF episode preceded immediately by a paroxysm of increased cardiac sympathetic nerve activity in one sheep with acute MI.[26] By using implanted radiotransmitters to record long-term continuous (24 h a day and 7 days a week) stellate ganglion nerve activity (SGNA) in dogs, episodes of VT were found to be preceded by an increased SGNA.[27] The evidence from these investigations conveys a consistent message that heterogeneous sympathetic reinnervation (neuronal remodeling) in the diseased myocardium is arrhythmogenic, increasing the propensity for ventricular arrhythmia and sudden death.

Anatomical Alteration of Myocardium

The pathophysiological basis for sustained monomorphic VT due to prior MI is usually reentry. The anatomical substrate for reentry is the interlacing of viable myocardium and scar tissue from prior myocardial damage.[28] The areas of slow conduction in infarct scars serve as the substrate for reentry. The slowly conducting tissue can be identified during endocardial catheter mapping by a fractionated electrogram, mid-diastolic electrograms, and a long delay between the capturing stimulus and QRS complex resulting from the stimulus.[29,30] Spontaneous sustained monomorphic VT is highly reproducible (more than 90%) in the electrophysiology laboratory.[31] The mechanism of sustained monomorphic VT in nonischemic dilated cardiomyopathy is poorly understood and is more diverse. Diffused fibrosis and viable myocardium can produce fractionated and low-amplitude endocardial electrograms compatible with a slow conduction zone seen in the MI and is responsible for sustaining reentry.[32] His-Purkinje system disease is commonly associated with dilated cardiomyopathy. In this setting with differential conduction delays, bundle branch reentry tachycardia, by using the distal His bundle, left and right bundle branches, and ventricular septum as the reentry circuit, is another potential mechanism of monomorphic VT in this subset of patients. Bundle branch reentry can be cured by ablation of the right bundle branch with a success rate of 100%, while ablating the reentry circuit mediated by scarred myocardium has a much lower success rate in general, approximately 50%.[33]

Triggers Responsible for Initiating Ventricular Arrhythmia

Electrolyte Disturbances

Electrolyte disturbances are common in patients with heart failure. Hypokalemia and hypomagnesemia are predisposing factors to ventricular arrhythmia. In the post hoc analysis from the Study of Left Ventricular Dysfunction (SOLVD) registry, a baseline use of nonpotassium-sparing diuretics was independently associated with increased risk of arrhythmic death (relative risk 1.33), where baseline use of potassium-sparing diuretics was not.[34] Hypokalemia shortens the action potential plateau and prolongs the rapid repolarization phase, predisposing myocardium to VT and VF.[35]

Acute Ventricular Dilation

Acute ventricular dilation in the normal heart shortens action potential duration and refractoriness without an apparent effect on conduction velocity, while increasing spontaneous automaticity and triggered activity.[36] Changes in cardiac loading similar to those seen in heart failure have a great tendency to be arrhythmogenic.[37] Among 311 patients in the SOLVD trial, there was a direct correlation between the severity of left ventricular enlargement and diastolic volume and the frequency of ventricular arrhythmia[38] (Figure 58–4). *Myocardial ischemia* alters intracellular oxygen supply and electrocellular homeostasis, resulting in shifting of electrolytes and cellular acidosis. These effects from myocardial ischemia lead to an

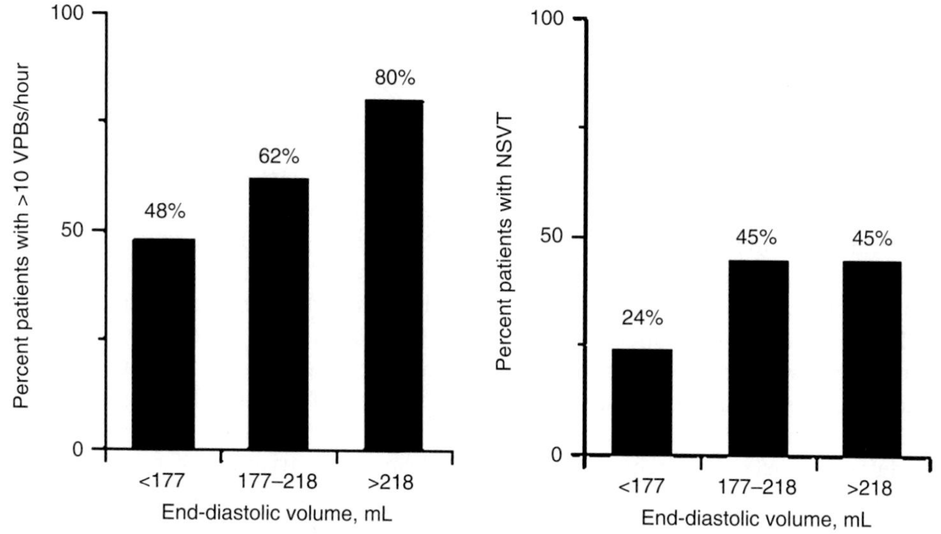

FIGURE 58–4. Correlation between left ventricular end-diastolic volume and ventricular arrhythmia in CHF. The incidence of ventricular premature beats (VPBs) and nonsustained ventricular tachycardia (NSVT) in patients with left ventricular dysfunction increases as the left ventricular size (end-diastolic volume) becomes larger. (Reproduced from Koilpillai,[38] with permission from the *American Journal of Cardiology*.)

impaired electrophysiological milieu predisposing patients to ventricular arrhythmia.[39]

Identifying Patients with Increased Risk of Sudden Death

Many approaches have been developed to detect the presence or propensity of arrhythmogenic substrates that trigger or maintain ventricular arrhythmias in patients with ischemic and nonischemic heart disease. These approaches include, but are not limited to, detection of spontaneous ventricular ectopy, presence or absence of scar or hibernating myocardium, biomarkers, inducibility of sustained ventricular arrhythmias, cardiac function, ventricular conduction delay, inhomogeneity of ventricular repolarization, and fluctuation of autonomic tone. These approaches have been used singly or in combination in a large number of clinical studies. Although many of the risk stratification techniques and approaches have been correlated with increased risks of sudden death in various patient populations, suboptimal predictive values in cardiac patients at large have resulted in a lack of a coherent and dominant strategy in current clinical practice. Many of the techniques and approaches are discussed in detail in other chapters in this book. In the following sections, a few approaches will be highlighted for discussion.

Left Ventricular Ejection Fraction

Left ventricular ejection fraction (LVEF) is the most widely used measure to assess overall prognosis, and in most of the ICD clinical trials for primary sudden death prevention, it has been used, with or without other risk stratifies, as a major inclusion criterion for patient selection. Although the severity of left ventricular dysfunction is a well-known marker of risk, it identifies a broad segment of the heart failure population. The Multicenter Unsustained Tachycardia Trial (MUSTT) identified patients with coronary artery disease and an LVEF of 40% or less. In patients randomized to no antiarrhythmic therapy with inducible VT during electrophysiology testing, the 5-year mortality rate was 48%, yielding an annual mortality rate of approximately 10%.[40] The Sudden Cardiac Death in Heart Failure Trial (ScD-HeFT) showed that patients with an LVEF of 35% or less with New York function Class II or III attributed to either ischemic or nonischemic cardiomyopathy had a mortality rate of 7% in the control group on standard medical therapy. The Multicenter Automatic Defibrillator Trial (MADIT) II study included patients with prior MI and an LVEF less than or equal to 30% with an NYHA function Class I–III. The mortality was 11% in a controlled group.[41] In the Valsartan in Acute Myocardial Infarction Trial (VALIANT), the event rates of sudden death were directly correlated with the degree of ventricular dysfunction during both early and late follow-up.[42]

Noninvasive Testing

Abnormalities of cardiac repolarization are common in heart failure, being closely related to the heterogeneity of depolarization across a diseased left ventricle. Dispersion of the QT interval on the surface electrocardiogram (ECG) was initially reported in high-risk patients, but further perspective studies showed no value in predicting sudden arrhythmic death.[43,44] Beat-to-beat variation in T wave amplitude (TWA) known as microvolt TWA is linked to a susceptibility to ventricular arrhythmias. It was reported as a marker of risk in a few prospective studies in patients with nonischemic and ischemic cardiomyopathy.[45–47] In a study of 107 consecutive patients with heart failure, an LVEF of 0.45 or less, and a positive TWA, the rate of arrhythmic events at 18 months was 21% compared to 0% among those with a negative TWA.[48]

Excessive sympathetic activation in heart failure promotes arrhythmia.[49] Heart rate variability reflects neurohumoral activity and its interaction with the sinus node. Heart rate variability declines proportionally with the severity of heart failure and increased risk of sudden death.[49,50] La-Rovere performed a short-term (8 min recording) study of heart rate variability in patients with chronic heart failure to determine its prognostic value in sudden cardiac death.[50] The study included a derivation sample of 202 consecutive patients in the early 1990s and a validation sample of 242 consecutive patients referred in the late 1990s. Sudden death was predicted by reduced power in the low-frequency heart rate variability spectrum (0.04–0.15 Hz) and 83 or more ventricular premature beats per hour on a 24-h ambulatory Holter recording. This study concluded that reduced short-term (8 min) low-frequency power during controlled breathing is a powerful predictor of sudden death in patients with heart failure that is independent of many other variables[50] (Figure 58–5). One study compared the prognostic value of cardiac iodine-123 metaiodobenzylguanidine (MIBG) imaging to heart rate variability in 65 patients with heart failure. Metaiodobenzylguanidine is a structural analog of the neurotransmitter guanathidine. It is taken up by adrenergic neurons in a manner similar to that of norepinephrine, but it does not undergo intracellular metabolism. Cardiac [^{123}I]MIBG imaging reflects cardiac adrenergic nerve activity. The MIBG heart-to-mediastinum ratio and the washout rate were obtained from MIBG imaging. The time and the frequency domain parameters of heart rate variability were calculated from 24-h Holter recordings. A high washout rate (more than 27%) was the only independent predictor of sudden death. Cardiac events were significantly more frequently observed in patients with both an abnormal washout rate and normalized very low-frequency power (less than 22) than in those with both a normal washout rate and normalized very low-frequency power (54% versus 4%).[51]

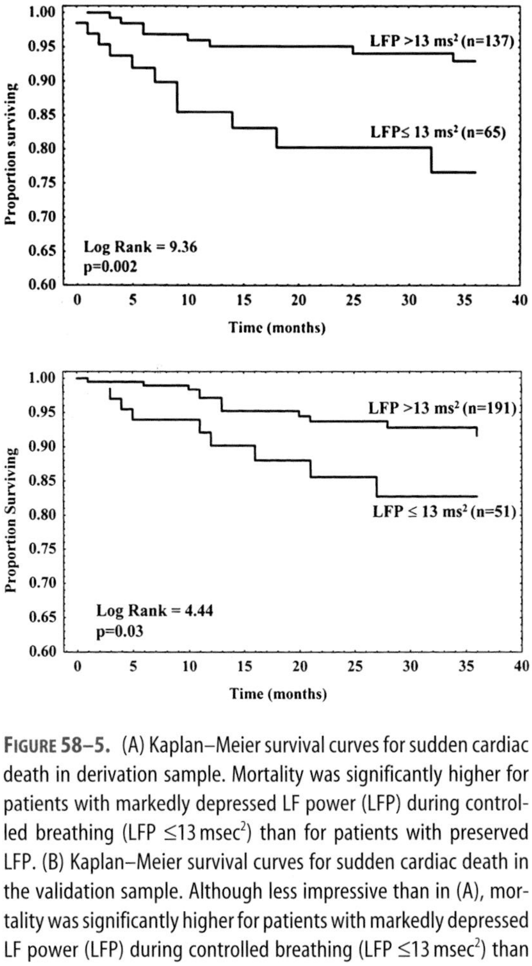

FIGURE 58–5. (A) Kaplan–Meier survival curves for sudden cardiac death in derivation sample. Mortality was significantly higher for patients with markedly depressed LF power (LFP) during controlled breathing (LFP ≤13 msec^2) than for patients with preserved LFP. (B) Kaplan–Meier survival curves for sudden cardiac death in the validation sample. Although less impressive than in (A), mortality was significantly higher for patients with markedly depressed LF power (LFP) during controlled breathing (LFP ≤13 msec^2) than for patients with preserved LFP. (Reproduced from La Rovere *et al.*,[50] with permission from *Circulation.*)

B-type natriuretic peptide (BNP) is produced primarily from the left ventricle in response to a change in myocardial wall stretch or volume load. The plasma concentration of this peptide strongly correlates with the degree of left ventricular systolic function and risk of death. In a study of 452 patients with ischemic or nonischemic cardiomyopathy and an LVEF less than 35%, fewer patients with a level of BNP <130 pg/ml (1%) died, as compared with patients with a BNP >130 pg/ml (18%).[52] A meta-analysis of 19 studies that used BNP to estimate the relative risk of death in heart failure patients concluded that each 100 pg/ml increase in BNP was associated with a 35% increase in the relative risk of death; therefore this is a strong prognostic indicator for heart failure at all stages of disease.[47]

Invasive Electrophysiology Study

Approximately one-third of patients with a prior MI, an LVEF less than or equal to 40%, and spontaneous nonsustained VT have inducible sustained VT, suggesting a 6–9% per year risk of spontaneous sustained VT or sudden death.[40] The utility of electrophysiology testing in sudden death risk stratification in patients with ischemic heart disease is reviewed elsewhere in this book. Electrophysiological testing is not a useful screening tool in nonischemic cardiomyopathy. Fewer than 5% of patients have inducible monomorphic VT in this subset of patients.

Prevention of Sudden Death

Pharmacological Therapy

β Blockers

β Blockers were first advocated for treatment of heart failure in 1975.[53] Results from large clinical trials subsequently showed that three β blockers, including bisoprolol and sustained release metoprolol (selective β_1 receptor blockers), as well as carvedilol (an α_1, β_1, and β_2 receptor blocker), were effective in reducing mortality in patients with chronic heart failure. The positive findings with these three agents, however, should not be considered indicative of a β blocker class effect, as shown by the lack of effectiveness of short acting metoprolol in clinical trials.[54–59] Patients who have been diagnosed with heart failure should be treated with one of these three β blockers. The relative efficacy among these three agents is not known, but available evidence does suggest that β blockers can differ in their effects on survival. In the Carvedilol Or Metoprolol European Trial (Comet), the absolute reduction in mortality over 5 years from carvedilol was 5.7% when compared to immediate-release metoprolol. In addition to the survival benefit, these trials also demonstrated a reduction in heart failure-related hospitalization as well as improvements in NYHA function class and patients' well being. In the MERIT-HF trial, there were fewer sudden deaths in the metoprolol CR/XL group than in the placebo group [RR 0.59 (0.45–0.78), Figure 58–6].[6] Post hoc analysis from the MUSTT trial demonstrated that β blockers were associated with decreased total mortality (5-year mortality was 50% with β blockers versus 66% without β blockers). The mortality benefit associated with β blockers was present in patients with and without inducible tachycardia.[60] However, the rates of arrhythmic death or cardiac arrest were not significantly affected by β blocker therapy.

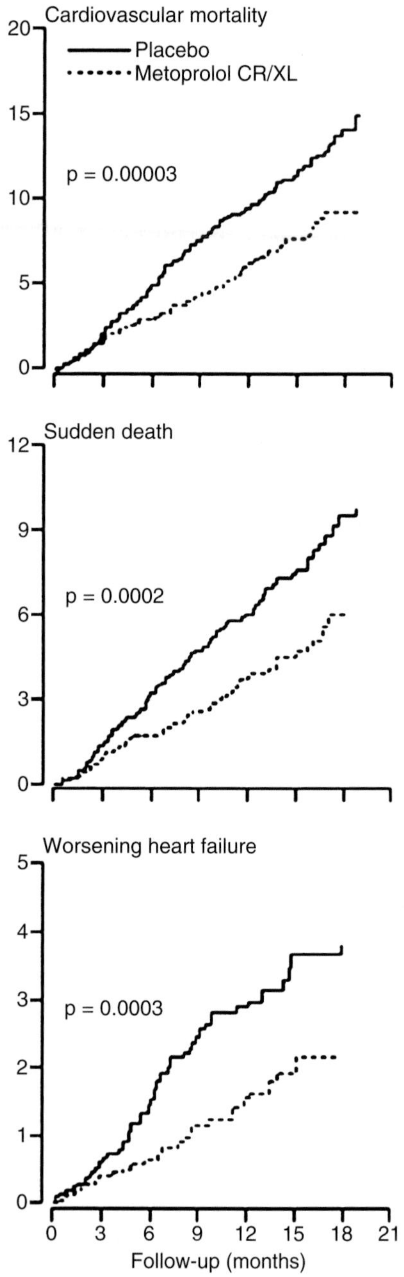

FIGURE 58–6. Kaplan–Meier curves of cumulative percentage of cardiovascular deaths, sudden deaths, and deaths from worsening heart failure. (Reproduced from MERIT-HF Study Group,[6] with permission from *Lancet*.)

Angiotensin-Converting Enzyme Inhibitors and Angiotensin II Receptor Blockers

Angiotensin-converting enzymes (ACEs) and angiotensin II receptor blockers (ARBs) reduce sudden death. The Candesartan in Heart Failure Assessment of Reduction in Mortality and Morbidity (CHARM) program assessed the effect of candesartan on cause-specific mortality in patients enrolled in the CHARM program. This program consisted of three component trials including CHARM-alternative (2028 patients with an LVEF less than or equal to 40%), CHARM-added (2548 patients, an LVEF less than or equal to 40%, already on ACE inhibitors), and CHARM-preserved (3023 patients, an LVEF more than 40%).[61–64] Patients were randomized to candesartan 32 mg once a day or placebo. All three trials were pooled to provide adequate statistical power to evaluate cause-specific mortality. Of all the patients, 8.5% died suddenly and 6.2% died of progressive heart failure. Candesartan reduced both sudden death [hazard ratio (HR) 0.85] and death from worsening heart failure (HR 0.78). This program concluded that cardesartan reduced sudden death and death from worsening heart failure in patients with symptomatic heart failure, although this reduction was more apparent in patients with systolic dysfunction. The mechanisms whereby ARBs reduced the incidence of sudden death in patients with heart failure remain less clear. An overall improvement in hemodynamic status and attenuation of ventricular remodeling may directly and indirectly decrease the propensity to fatal ventricular arrhythmia.[65] Reductions in the incidence of sudden death have been also observed in a trial with ACE inhibitors.[66]

Antiarrhythmic Agents

Amiodarone is a unique antiarrhythmic agent that has Class I, II, III, and IV effects. It has been associated with overall neutral effects on survival when given to patients with a low LVEF and heart failure, although some studies have shown a reduction in sudden death, an increase in LVEF, and a decrease in the incidence of worsening heart failure.[67–73] Despite its side effects of thyroid abnormalities, pulmonary toxicity, hepatotoxicity, neuropathy, and other adverse responses, amiodarone remains the most effective agent to prevent recurrent ventricular tachyarrhythmia, especially in patients who have been receiving frequent ICD therapies. Other pharmacological arrhythmic therapies such as sotalol and mexiletine may be used to suppress recurrent ICD shocks when amiodarone has been ineffective or not tolerated due to side effects. Dofetilide is a Class III antiarrhythmic drug. In the Danish Investigations of Arrhythmia and Mortality on Dofetilide in Congestive Heart Failure (DIAMOND-CHF) study, observed survival was not different between patients randomized to dofetilide or placebo, while atrial fibrillation was significantly less in patients randomized to dofetilide therapy.[74] Although the overall incidence of proarrhythmia appears to be relatively low, clinical use of dofetilide has been limited because of concerns of drug–drug interactions and has been limited in patients with renal insufficiency. Despite a marked suppression of ventricular ectopic activity, the Class 1C antiarrhythmic agents, flecainide and encainide, increased the total and arrhythmic mortality in patients with ischemic heart disease and compromised LVEF.[75] Other Class I antiarrhythmic agents, including quinidine, procainamide, and propafenone, have been poorly studied in patients with ischemic cardiomyopathy. Nevertheless, meta-analysis of existing data consistently showed that Class I agents are associated with a decreased survival in postmyocardial patients.[76]

Implantable Cardioverter Defibrillators

Secondary Prevention

Patients with a previous cardiac arrest or documented sustained ventricular arrhythmias have a high risk of recurrent events. Implantation of an ICD has been shown to reduce mortality in cardiac arrest survivals. Outcomes from secondary sudden prevention trials are summarized in Table 58–1. In the Antiarrhythmic versus Implantable Defibrillators (AVID) study the absolute reduction of mortality was 7% and 11% in 2 and 3 years in patients randomized to the ICD arm compared to the drugs-treated arm.[77] Two other secondary prevention multicenter trials [Canadian Implantable Defibrillator Study (CIDS) and the Cardiac Arrest Study Hamburg (CASH)], with smaller numbers of study patients, also demonstrated a strong trend toward survival benefits among patients who received ICD therapy.[78,79] Clinical data also support the consideration of ICD therapy in patients with chronic heart failure and low ejection fraction who experience syncope of unclear origin.[80] Placement of an ICD is not indicated when ventricular tachyarrhythmias are incessant in patients with progressive and irreversible decompensated heart failure.

TABLE 58–1. Secondary prevention of sudden cardiac death by ICD.[a]

	Patient population	Number	Randomization	Follow-up (months)	Reduction in mortality
AVID,[77] 1997	Survived VT/VF/arrest, VT/syncope, VT/LVEF ≤40%	1016	Antiarrhythmic agents (97% amiodarone) vs. ICD	18	HR 0.66 (0.51–0.85) $p < 0.02$
CASH,[78] 2000	Survived VT/VF/arrest	288	Antiarrhythmic agents (amiodarone, propafenone, metoprolol) vs. ICD	57	HR 0.82 (0.60–1.11) $p = 0.08$
CIDS,[79] 2000	Survived VT/VF/arrest, VT/syncope, VT/LVEF ≤35%	659	Amiodarone vs. ICD	35	HR 0.80 (0.60–1.08) $p = 0.14$

[a]ICD, implantable cardioverter defibrillator; AVID, Antiarrhythmic Vs Implantable Defibrillators; CASH, Cardiac Arrest Study Hamburg; CIDS, Canadian Implantable Defibrillator Study; HR, hazard ratio; VT, ventricular tachycardia; VF, ventricular fibrillation; LVEF, left ventricular ejection fraction.

Primary Prevention

The utility of ICDs in the primary prevention of sudden death in patients without a prior history of life-threatening arrhythmias has been explored in numerous trials. If sustained ventricular tachyarrhythmias can be induced in the electrophysiology laboratory (and not suppressible by procainamide) in patients with a prior MI, an LVEF less than or equal to 35%, and spontaneous nonsustained VT on ambulatory ECG, the absolute risk reduction of total mortality was 23% in an approximate follow-up duration of 2 years.[81] When the inclusion criteria for LVEF were less than or equal to 40%, the incidence of cardiac arrest or death from arrhythmia was 25% among those receiving electrophysiology-guided therapy (half received drug therapy and half received an ICD) and 32% among patients assigned to no antiarrhythmic therapy, yielding an absolute reduction of 7% after 5 years of follow-up. The survival benefit was entirely attributable to the ICD, not to the antiarrhythmic drug therapy.[40]

More recently, the role of ICD in the prevention of primary sudden death was examined in patients with low ejection and heart failure, without risk stratifiers such as spontaneous nonsustained VT on ambulatory ECG or inducible sustained VT during an electrophysiology study. When compared with standard medical therapy in patients with an ejection fraction of less than or equal to 30% after remote MI, ICD decreased the mortality by 5.6% over 20 months.[41] In patients with an ejection fraction of less than 35% and NYHA function Class II–III symptoms of heart failure with either ischemic or nonischemic causes of advanced heart disease, a survival benefit from an ICD was also observed when compared to amiodarone.[69] Outcomes from recent ICD trials for primary prevention of sudden death are shown in Table 58–2. Whereas an ICD is effective in preventing death due to ventricular tachyarrhythmia, frequent shocks from an ICD can lead to a reduced quality of life, whether triggered by appropriately life-threatening arrhythmia or inappropriately by supraventricular tachycardia. In this situation, antiarrhythmic therapy, most often amiodarone and/or catheter-based ablation, can be considered to reduce recurrent ICD discharges. The balance of potential risks and benefits of ICD implantation should be individualized.

A decrease in the incidence of sudden death does not necessarily translate into decreased total mortality, and decreased total mortality does not guarantee a meaningful prolongation of survival with adequate quality. This is particularly important in patients with a poor prognosis due to advanced heart failure. There was no survival benefit observed from ICD implantation within the first year in two of the major trials.[69,41] All ICD primary sudden death prevention trials to date have excluded patients with NYHA Class IV functional status. Consideration of ICD implantation is currently recommended in patients with an ejection fraction less than 35% and mild to moderate symptoms of heart failure without significant comorbid conditions with an anticipated life expectancy extending beyond 1 year.

Cardiac Resynchronization Therapy

Cardiac resynchronization therapy (CRT) is a new therapy that reverses ventricular remodeling and improves ventricular function and symptoms in

TABLE 58–2. Primary prevention of sudden cardiac death by ICD.[a]

	Patient population	LVEF	Number	Randomization	Follow-up (months)	Reduction in mortality
MADIT,[85] 1996	Prior MI, NSVT, inducible VT refractory to procainamide	≤35%	196	Antiarrhythmic agents vs. ICD	27	HR 0.46 (0.26–0.92) $p = 0.009$
CABG-Patch,[86] 1997	All undergo CABG, positive SAECG	≤35%	900	CABG alone vs. CABG plus ICD	32	HR 1.07 (0.81–1.42) $p = 0.64$
MUSTT,[40] 1999	Prior MI/CAD, NSVT, inducible VT	≤40%	704	Antiarrhythmic or ICD vs. conventional therapy	39	HR 0.69 (0.32–0.63) $p < 0.001$
MADIT II,[41] 2002	Prior MI/CAD	≤30%	1232	Conventional therapy vs. ICD	20	HR 0.69 (0.51–0.93) $p = 0.02$
DINAMIT,[87] 2004	Recent MI (<40 days), decrease HRV	≤35%	674	Conventional therapy vs. ICD	39	HR 1.08 (0.76–1.55) $p = 0.66$
DEFINITE,[88] 2004	Nonischemic cardiomyopathy, NSVT, or PVCs	≤36%	458	Conventional therapy vs. ICD	29	HR 0.65 (0.40–1.06) $p = 0.08$
SCD-HeFT,[69] 2005	Ischemic and nonischemic cardiomyopathy, NYHA II–III	≤35%	2521	Conventional therapy vs. amiodarone vs. ICD	45	ICD HR 0.77 (0.62–0.96) $p = 0.007$ Amiodarone HR 1.06 (0.86–1.30) $p = 0.53$

[a]MADIT, Multicenter Automatic Defibrillator Trial; CABG, coronary artery bypass graft; MUSTT, Multicenter Unsustained Tachycardia Trial; DINAMIT, Prophylactic Use of an Implantable Cardioverter-Defibrillator after Acute Myocardial Infarction; DEFINITE, Prophylactic Defibrillator Implantation in Patients with Nonischemic Dilated Cardiomyopathy; SCD-HeFT, Sudden Cardiac Death in Heart Failure Trial; ICD, implantable cardioverter defibrillator; LVEF, left ventricular ejection fraction; NSVT, nonsustained ventricular tachycardia; NYHA, New York Heart Association; MI, myocardial infarction; CAD, coronary artery disease; HRV, heart rate variability; SAECG, signal-averaged electrocardiogram; VT, ventricular tachycardia; HR, hazard ratio; PVC, premature ventricular contractions.

patients with advanced heart failure by using an additional pacing lead that stimulates the lateral wall of the left ventricle to achieve mechanical synchrony between and within the right and left ventricles. Meta-analysis from earlier and smaller randomized trials found that CRT reduces death from progressive heart failure by 51% relative to controls and a trend toward reducing all-cause mortality, but no apparent effect on sudden cardiac death.[82] From a larger study, the Comparison of Medical Therapy, Pacing, And Defibrillation in Chronic Heart Failure (COMPANION) trial found CRT with a pacemaker alone (CRT-P) reduced death from any cause (a secondary endpoint of the trial) by 24% (marginally significant) compared to medical therapy, while CRT with a defibrillator (CRT-D) significantly reduced mortality by 36%.[83] More recently, the Cardiac Resynchronization in Heart Failure Study (CARE-HF) also demonstrated that CRT-P was associated with an absolute 10% reduction in mortality, as compared with the medical-therapy group (20% vs. 30%; HR 0.64). In this study, CRT-P also reduced the interventricular mechanical delay, the end-systolic volume index, and the area of the mitral regurgitation; increased the LVEF; and improved symptoms and quality of life.[84] A positive impact on reduction of sudden death by CRT-P has not been clearly demonstrated by clinical trials at this point.

Summary and Conclusions

Complex interactions reside between cardiac mechanical dysfunction and malignant arrhythmia generation. The cyclical relationship of heart failure and arrhythmogenesis is depicted in Figure 58–7. Sudden death is a common mode of death in patients with advanced heart failure. In patients with heart failure, risk stratification for sudden death should be a routine component of the clinical evaluation. Following determination of underlying heart disease, appropriate and aggressive therapy should be implemented to target the primary disease process in order to modify disease

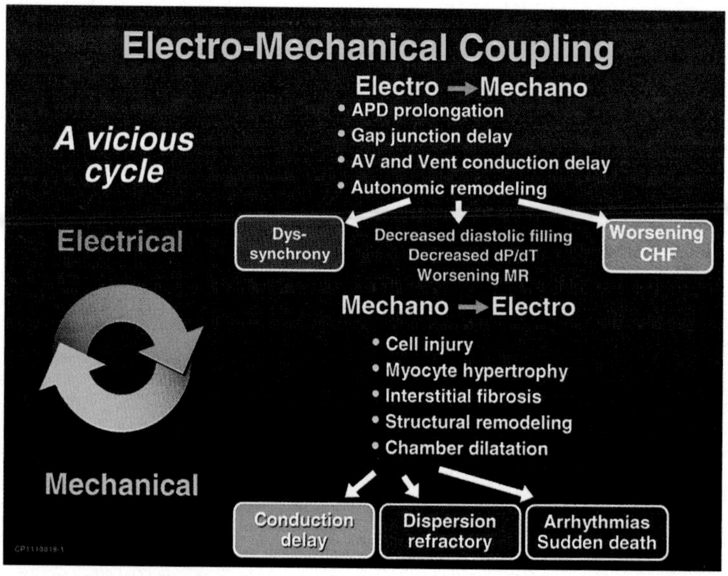

FIGURE 58–7. A vicious cycle of electromechanical coupling in the development of heart failure and sudden death. (Reproduced from MERIT-HF Study Group,[6] with permission from *Lancet*.)

progression, thereby improving symptoms and prognosis. Antiarrhythmic drug therapy is not recommended in any heart failure patient population for prevention of primary sudden death. When an antiarrhythmic drug is needed to treat symptomatic arrhythmias in patients with heart failure, amiodarone usually is the drug of choice, while dofetilide is "safe" when used properly. Among patients with ischemic or nonischemic heart disease and compromised LVEF with mild to moderate heart failure symptoms (NYHA functional Class II–III), clinical evidence supports the recommendation of ICD implantation in patients with an LVEF ≤35%. Although many approaches and techniques are available for sudden death risk stratification, a "dominant" strategy has not been established primarily due to the lack of a strong predictive value either from individual or combinations of various testing modalities. Among patients with very advanced heart failure (Class IV), ICD alone is not recommended. Preliminary data suggest CRT-P or CRT-D may improve survival, in addition to improving functional capacity and symptoms, in selected patients with advanced heart failure. The size of the heart failure patient population will continue to grow as the global population continues to get older and lives longer as a result of advanced medical care. It is expected that sudden death risk stratification techniques will continue to evolve while pharmacological and nonpharmacological therapy for sudden death prevention will continue to be refined.[85–88]

References

1. American Heart Association. 2005 Update.
2. McKee P. The natural history of congestive heart failure: The Framingham study. *N Engl J Med* 1971; 285(26):1441–1446.
3. Kannel W, Plehn J, Cupples L. Cardiac failure and sudden death in the Framingham study. *Am Heart J* 1988;115(4):869–875.
4. Levy D, *et al.* Long-term trends in the incidence of and survival with heart failure. *N Engl J Med* 2002;347(18):1397–1402.
5. Luu M, *et al.* Diverse mechanisms of unexpected cardiac arrest in advanced heart failure. *Circulation* 1989;80:1675–1680.
6. Effect of metoprolol CR/XL in chronic heart failure: Metoprolol CR/XL randomised intervention trial in-congestive heart failure (MERIT-HF). *Lancet* 1999;353(9169):2001–2007.
7. Mitchel L, *et al.* Sudden death in patients with implantable cardioverter defibrillators: The importance of post-shock electromechanical dissociation. *J Am Coll Cardiol* 2002;39(8):1323–1328.
8. Hunt S, *et al.* ACC/AHA guidelines for the evaluation and management of chronic heart failure in the adult: A report of the American College of Cardiology/American Heart Association Task Force on Practice Guidelines (Committee to Revise the 1995 Guidelines for the Evaluation and

studies of epilepsy patients who died suddenly and unexpectedly explored putative risk factors and provided estimates of the frequency of SUDEP.[8–11] Many deaths in earlier studies of patients with epilepsy were attributed to asphyxiation, status epilepticus, or aspiration, but in reality the deaths might have been SUDEP. Interest in SUDEP was renewed during the development of the antiepileptic drugs (AED) when there was concern that subjects in the AED trials had higher rates of sudden death

Incidence of Sudden Unexplained or Unexpected Death in Epilepsy

Many studies have provided the incidence of SUDEP; however, direct comparison between studies is difficult because of differing definitions of SUDEP, varying ascertainment methods, and different source populations. Table 59–1 summarizes the incidence of SUDEP in various studies. Studies of incidence fall into one of several categories.[12]

1. Cases identified through autopsy records.
2. Cases identified from AED prescription registries.
3. Cases identified through clinical trials of AED or devices.
4. Cases identified through hospitals, epilepsy clinics, or centers.
5. Cases identified through community-based cohorts of incident epilepsy cases.

Autopsy-based studies suffer from a referral bias and may overestimate the true incidence of SUDEP because the decision for autopsy is influenced by circumstances surrounding death and a higher proportion of unexplained deaths may be autopsied. In addition, the epilepsy prevalence in the study population is unknown.

Studies of SUDEP in epilepsy referral centers and in AED clinical trials involve persons with high seizure frequency and poor response to AED therapy.[13] The studies are not reflective of the general epilepsy population where an estimated 63% of individuals have well-controlled epilepsy.[14] Table 59–1 shows a trend of increasing SUDEP rates from study cohorts that include persons

Table 59–1. Sudden unexplained or unexpected death in epilepsy rates in the literature, in the order of increasing frequency.

Study	Study population	Number of cases per 1000 person-years
Lahtoo *et al.*, 1999[15]	Population based	0.13
Ficker *et al.*, 1998[16]	Population based	0.35
Leestma *et al.*, 1984[75]	Autopsy cases (retrospective)	0.5–1.9
Tennis *et al.*, 1995[10]	Prescription records in the community	0.5–1.4
Leestma *et al.*, 1989[11]	Autopsy cases (prospective)	0.9–2.7
Walczak *et al.*, 2001[20]	Multicenter referral practice	1.2
Jick *et al.*, 2001[9]	Prescription records in the community	1.3
Langan *et al.*, 1998[76]	Autopsy cases	1.5
Nilsson *et al.*, 1999[21]	Hospital admissions	1.5
Timmings *et al.*, 1993[77]	Epilepsy unit in referral center	2.0
Klenerman *et al.*, 1993[78]	Institutionalized patients	2.1
Derby *et al.*, 1996[79]	Refractory epilepsy population	2.2
Hennessy, *et al.*, 1999[80]	Temporal lobectomy patients	2.2
Nashef *et al.*, 1995[59]	Institutionalized young patients	3.4
Leestma *et al.*, 1997[3]	Drug trial subjects (lamotrigine)	3.5
Racoosin *et al.*, 2001[13]	Antiepileptic drug trials	3.8
Annegers *et al.*, 1998[8]	Vagus nerve stimulator trial	4.5–6.0
Lip *et al.*, 1992[23]	Epilepsy center	4.9
Nashef *et al.*, 1995[82]	Epilepsy center outpatients	5.9
Sperling *et al.*, 1999[58]	Epilepsy surgery patients	7.5
Dasheiff, 1991[83]	Epilepsy surgery candidates	9.3

with well-controlled epilepsy to cohorts with frequent seizures. Thus, the highest SUDEP rate is encountered among epilepsy surgery candidates, whose medically uncontrolled and frequent seizures prompt the consideration of surgery.

Population-based studies are the best studies to estimate the actual incidence of SUDEP. The difficulty of population-based studies arises in collecting data that accurately represent the whole spectrum of all epilepsy patients in the community. Some studies that were alleged to be population based were conducted on cohorts identified from AED prescription rccords.[9,10] In these studies, persons in the community were presumed to have epilepsy if they were taking AED. However, persons taking AED for nonepileptic conditions were most likely included in the study, whereas epilepsy patients who were noncompliant with medications might have been excluded.

The National General Practice Study of Epilepsy in Great Britain found the lowest reported SUDEP rate, which is 1 in about 5000 person-years.[15] This low SUDEP rate may be due to the fact that the study included both patients with active epilepsy and epilepsy in remission. We performed a population-based study of the incidence of SUDEP in Rochester, Minnesota.[16] We found the incidence of SUDEP to be 0.35 per 1000 person-years. The incidence of sudden unexplained death in young nonepileptic adults in Rochester had previously been determined by Shen and colleagues.[17] Our comparison of the incidence rates of sudden unexplained death in epilepsy and in nonepilepsy persons yielded a standard mortality ratio of 23.7 for persons with epilepsy. Thus, the risk for sudden unexplained death in persons with epilepsy markedly exceeds that in the general population by approximately 24 times.

Risk Factors of Sudden Unexplained or Unexpected Death in Epilepsy

Poor seizure control appears to be the most consistent risk factor for SUDEP across several studies reported over the past two decades.[2] The foregoing discussion of SUDEP incidence clearly shows a much higher incidence of SUDEP among persons with poorly controlled epilepsy than among persons with well-controlled epilepsy. Furthermore, it is not uncommon for an epileptic seizure to have occurred near the time of the fatal event. Although it is rare for SUDEP events to have been witnessed, 80% of witnessed SUDEP were associated with a seizure occurrence.[18] Of the many types of epileptic seizures, generalized tonic–clonic seizure ("grand mal" seizure) is the seizure type that is most commonly associated with SUDEP.[11] The risk of SUDEP has been shown to be 14 times greater in persons who had experienced at least one generalized tonic–clonic seizure within the past 3 months than in persons who had not.[19] A collaborative study of three centers in the midwest United States demonstrated that increasing frequency of generalized tonic–clonic seizures is correlated with increasing risk for SUDEP.[20] The same study also disclosed the presence of mental retardation and greater number of AED used as SUDEP risk factors. Although these factors are independent of seizure frequency, they cannot be said to be independent of the severity of the epileptic condition. Seizure frequency may not be the only determinant of the severity of the epileptic condition. Early onset of epilepsy has also been reported to be a risk factor for SUDEP.[21] After adjustment for the factor of seizure frequency, the relative risk of SUDEP when epilepsy began in the period from birth to age 15 years is five times higher than when epilepsy began after age 45 years.

A low AED concentration in the serum is long believed to be a major risk factor for SUDEP. In one series of postmortem examinations of SUDEP, only 10% had serum AED concentrations that were in the therapeutic range.[11] Moreover, epilepsy patients who did not have determinations of their serum AED concentrations within the past 2-year period were found to have a 3.7 times higher SUDEP risk than those who did.[22] However, more recent studies have found no association between low serum AED concentration and occurrence of SUDEP.[20,22] Also, fluctuations in serum AED concentrations do not appear to be associated with increased SUDEP risk.[22] Nonetheless, two studies suggest that recent or frequent adjustments of AED dose elevate the risk for SUDEP.[23] A recent study of AED concentrations in hair samples shows that SUDEP patients had greater variability of the concentrations over time than non-SUDEP epilepsy patients.[24] However, the greater variability in SUDEP may just be a reflection of more frequent AED dose adjustments because of worse seizure control in SUDEP than in non-SUDEP patients.

No single AED has been associated with higher SUDEP risk than other AEDs.[25] Carbamazepine rarely induces bradycardia or complete atrioventricular block.[26] Nilsson and colleagues reported that a high serum carbamazepine concentration is associated with increased risk of SUDEP. The "high"carbamazepine concentrations in that study were observed in only five patients and the concentrations were only slightly elevated.[25] These limitations may explain the wide confidence intervals for the risk ratio determined in the study. More important than the type of AED is the number of AEDs used. After adjustment for seizure frequency, patients taking three AEDs had an eight times greater risk for SUDEP than those taking one AED.[21]

Most reported SUDEP patients are between the age of 20 and 40 years.[2] Whether age is a risk factor for SUDEP is not clear. Sudden deaths in older persons with epilepsy may have been attributed to coronary artery disease without serious consideration of the possibility of SUDEP.

Potential Cardiac Mechanisms in Sudden Unexplained or Unexpected Death in Epilepsy

Because sudden nontraumatic death in the general population is often due to cardiac arrhythmia induced by ischemic heart disease, acute cardiac arrhythmia has often been suspected to be a primary cause of SUDEP. Temporal lobe epilepsy patients were recently reported to have reduced heart rate variability that was more pronounced during nighttime than daytime.[27] This finding is relevant to the fact that most SUDEP events occur at nighttime. However, there was no difference in the nighttime heart rate variability between intractable and well-controlled epilepsy patients. Nonetheless, the finding still raises the possibility that both groups of patients have a background susceptibility to cardiac arrhythmias, but seizure episodes are required to trigger potentially lethal arrhythmias to cause SUDEP.

Some epileptic seizure events are associated with supraventricular tachycardia, bradycardia, asystole, or arrhythmias such as atrioventricular block and ventricular ectopic rhythms.[28–31] These cardiac rhythm abnormalities have been observed in seizures that begin at a number of brain structures, including but not limited to the insular cortex, frontal lobe regions, cingulate gyrus, and the amygdala–hippocampal complex. In the evaluation of patients for epilepsy surgery, sinus tachycardia is a common observation in seizures recorded during video-EEG monitoring; whereas bradycardia is uncommon and asystole is rare. Whereas sinus tachycardia is observed with either focal-onset seizures or primary generalized tonic–clonic seizures, bradycardia and asystole are observed mostly with focal-onset seizures.[32] The rate of electrocardiogram (ECG) abnormalities has been reported to increase with the duration of seizure episode and with the generalized tonic–clonic type of seizure.[33]

A fatal outcome of ictal asystole has rarely been encountered in the epilepsy monitoring unit.[34] The prevalence of ictal or postictal bradycardia or asystole in the epilepsy population is not known. The prevalence of ictal asystole determined in intractable epilepsy patients during videoelectroencephalogram (EEG) monitoring is about 5 in 1200 patients.[29] Implanted loop recordings of ECG over 220,000 h in 20 intractable epilepsy patients detected severe ictal bradycardia or asystole that required permanent cardiac pacing in 21% of the patients.[31] However, only 2.1% percent of all recorded seizures were associated with bradycardia or asystole.

Other studies observed ST-segment depression on the ECG during or following seizures[35] and prolongation of the QT interval with epileptiform EEG discharges.[36] This QT prolongation was noted to be more severe in patients who subsequently developed SUDEP than in those who did not. Animal studies have demonstrated that both ictal and interictal EEG discharges can disrupt autonomic cardiac nerve discharges, consequently predisposing the animal to potentially fatal cardiac arrhythmias.[37]

Autopsy series of SUDEP cases have shown that the heart is heavier than expected for body height, but then similar observations have been made for the lungs and the liver.[11] The severity of abnormalities observed in these organs is not sufficient by themselves to cause sudden death. Fibrotic changes in the deep and subendocardial myocardium have also been described in SUDEP victims. In one prospective study, these fibrotic changes were found in 40% of SUDEP victims versus 6.6% of control specimens.[38] However, another study found no difference in the rate of morphological abnormalities in the conduction system between SUDEP and non-SUDEP autopsy specimens.[39]

Postmortem cardiac investigations into the cause of SUDEP are hampered by low autopsy rates and also the low rate in diagnosing SUDEP cases even when clinical SUDEP criteria are fulfilled.[40] Molecular investigations are rarely performed to determine the role of ion channel defects in SUDEP. The clinician should also be aware that syncopal or seizure attacks induced by primary cardiac arrhythmia have rarely been misdiagnosed as epilepsy.[41] The extent to which this situation contributes to the incidence of SUDEP is not known.

Other Possible Mechanisms in Sudden Unexplained or Unexpected Death in Epilepsy

A frequent autopsy finding in SUDEP is increased lung weight or pulmonary edema.[42] In the clinical practice setting, acute pulmonary edema has been observed following multiple convulsive seizures, or even after a self-limited convulsive seizure. There are rare reports of seizure-related pulmonary edema with fatal consequences.[43,44] Nonconvulsive status epilepticus has also been reported to be associated with adult respiratory distress syndrome.[45] The relevance of pulmonary edema to SUDEP has been doubted because SUDEP is characteristically not preceded by a period of dyspnea. How seizure activity leads to acute pulmonary edema is also undetermined. It has been speculated that seizure induction of adrenergic overdischarge is a possible link between seizure attacks and acute neurogenic pulmonary edema.[46]

There is evidence that respiratory arrest can occur during (ictal apnea) or following seizure activity (postictal apnea) and potentially lead to cardiac arrhythmias.[47–49] Video-EEG monitoring at an epilepsy monitoring unit had documented a near-SUDEP incident in a 20 year-old patient who developed postictal apnea.[49] On-going ECG recording showed normal rhythm following the seizure and asystole did not develop until the respiratory arrest became prolonged. After the patient was revived, evaluation showed no evidence of pulmonary emboli or edema, or airway obstruction. With some of the patient's prior out-of-hospital seizures, first-responders made similar observations that the pulse was still regular even when respiration had already ceased. Although SUDEP and near SUDEP incidents are rarely encountered during video-EEG monitoring, seizure-related apnea (>10 sec) had been observed in 55% of monitored patients and oxyhemoglobin desaturation (<85%) in 35%.[50] The longest apnea duration was 63 sec and the lowest oxyhemoglobin desaturation was 55%. Animal studies support the role of respiratory arrest as an important mechanism in SUDEP. Johnston and colleagues observed in a sheep model of SUDEP that central hypoventilation consistently precedes cardiac arrhythmia.[51,52] Similar observations were made more recently in 75% of audiogenic seizure mice (DBA/2 J strain).[53] Serotonergic mechanisms may play an important role in postical apnea. Whereas normal saline did not protect the mice from respiratory arrest, increasing doses of a serotonin reuptake inhibitor, fluoxetine, was associated with a diminishing incidence of postictal respiratory arrest.[54] The mice became susceptible again to respiratory arrest after the fluoxetine effect had dissipated. Cyproheptadine, an antiserotonergic agent, has the opposite effect on the mice. Mice that were not susceptible to postictal apnea at baseline became susceptible after cyproheptadine was given, and the susceptibility disappeared with the termination of the drug effect. An earlier study showed that a strain of mice altered genetically to be deficient in serotonin receptors develop audiogenic seizures and postictal apnea.[55]

Small studies have noted some differences in baseline measures of autonomic functions between epilepsy patients and control subjects. Some of the differences noted were a higher heart rate at rest and a hypersympathetic response to the Valsalva maneuver and tilt table test.[56] Temporal lobectomy has also been reported to reduce sympathetic cardiovascular modulation and baroreflex sensitivity.[57] The relevance of these observations to SUDEP is still unknown.

Comments Regarding Sudden Unexplained or Unexpected Death in Epilepsy

Because the focus of this book is on sudden cardiac death, the foregoing discussion of the potential mechanisms underlying SUDEP was divided into cardiac and noncardiac mechanisms. It should not be assumed that one mechanism operates in all SUDEP cases. The current state of knowledge is insufficient for us to discount the possibility of the cooccurrence of more than one mechanism in some if not all patients. Such a possibility can arise if seizure activity suppresses brainstem centers for cardiac and for respiratory activities.

The current knowledge regarding SUDEP risk factors and mechanisms is insufficient for developing preventive measures that are practical and reliable in reducing the incidence of SUDEP. Nonetheless, given the strong relationship between seizure control and SUDEP occurrence, a major preventive measure against SUDEP is improvement of seizure control. Compliance with AED intake should be emphasized to patients, and they should be encouraged to strive for the best seizure control possible. When seizures are refractory to AED therapy, patients should be evaluated for epilepsy surgery. Those who became seizure free following epilepsy surgery have a lower risk of SUDEP than those who failed the surgery.[58]

Some investigators have suggested that increased nighttime supervision of patients with poorly controlled epilepsy could potentially prevent SUDEP.[59] The odds ratio for developing SUDEP in these patients was 0.4 when compared with patients who had no supervision.[19] Sudden unexplained or unexpected death in epilepsy often occurs at night without witnesses. The low rate of SUDEP in children with poorly controlled epilepsy may be due to the fact that they are less likely than adults to be in unsupervised settings. Supervision may permit timely detection of seizure occurrence and prompt intervention to interrupt the phenomenon of seizure-related apnea. Anecdotal experience shows that stimulation of the patient, such as repositioning or patting the patient, often induces the resumption of breathing. Provision of oxygen may be needed in some patients. Oxygenation remarkably reduces the risk of death in the audiogenic seizure mouse model of SUDEP.[53] Death due to suffocation from tracheobronchial aspiration of vomitus or from airway obstruction by bed linens is considered accidental death, and hence not SUDEP. Nonetheless, this tragic cause of sudden death can potentially be corrected by supervision. Seventy-one percent of SUDEP patients were found in a prone position.[60] At the current time, constant supervision of intractable epilepsy patients cannot be reasonably expected of family members or caregivers.

Sudden Cardiac Death in Other Neurological Conditions

Sudden death associated with acute neurological disorders such as severe strokes and head trauma has been referred to as neurogenic or cerebrogenic sudden death. Rapid and severe increased intracranial pressure is a frequently suspected event underlying sudden neurogenic death.[61] Intracranial pressure can be increased by lesions outside the cerebral ventricles, or by processes occurring within the ventricular system. An example of the latter is increased intracranial pressure from acute obstruction of the third ventricle by a colloid cyst, which is associated with sudden death in 10% of the cases.[62] Severe increased intracranial pressure can have lethal neuroanatomical and neurochemical consequences. Tentorial and tonsillar herniations directly damage brainstem structures. Extreme increased intracranial pressure may increase autonomic discharges that lead to blood pressure instability and cardiac arrhythmia. Cardiac arrhythmias and ECG repolarization abnormalities occur not infrequently in acute brain disorders, especially in subarachnoid hemorrhage.[63] More common ECG alterations are large peaked T waves ("cerebral T waves"), Q-T interval prolongation, and U waves. Most ECG alterations are transient and unrelated to neurogenic sudden death.

Sudden death also occurs in strokes that are not sufficiently extensive to produce increased intracranial pressure. There is animal and clinical evidence that injury to the insula in these cases is an important factor in the occurrence of potentially lethal cardiovascular instability.[64,65] Intracerebral hemorrhage is also associated with increased cardiac troponin levels, which independently predict in-hospital mortality.[66] Less well understood is the rare occurrence of sudden death in patients with lateral medullary infarction.[67] It is possible that respiratory arrest is the primary complication of this disorder, which then leads to cardiac arrhythmia.

Many patients with myotonic dystrophy or certain forms of mitochondrial encephalomyopathies eventually develop cardiac conduction defects, and sudden cardiac death is not uncommon in those whose illness is moderately or well advanced.[68,69] First-degree heart block is the most common cardiac conduction defect in myotonic dystrophy, and it may precede the presentation of the clinical illness. Conduction abnormalities affecting the His bundle are also common, even in patients without cardiac symptoms. Goodwin and Muntoni have recently reviewed the risk of cardiac involvement in different types of muscular dystrophies.[70] Periodic assessment with ambulatory ECG may benefit patients who have types of muscle dystrophies that are highly associated with potentially fatal cardiac arrhythmias.[71] Such assessments need to be initiated before skeletal muscle involvement becomes severe, because cardiac involvement may occur early in some patients.

Metabolic diseases such as those that affect glycogen storage and lipid metabolism can have associated cardiomyopathies. The topic has been extensively reviewed by Gilbert-Barness.[72] Some mutations, such as those that affect troponin T and B-myosin genes, may carry a higher risk of sudden cardiac death due to conduction defects.

A rare potassium channelopathy, Andersen–Tawil syndrome, which can present as periodic paralysis in the neurological practice, has cardiac conduction defects as one its features. Sudden cardiac death can occur in those with ventricular arrhythmias or long QT syndrome.[73]

Conclusions

The fact that sudden or rapid death does occur in neurological diseases is well known. The cardiac role in causing rapid death is intuitively accepted to be secondary in situations such as massive subarachnoid hemorrhage or stroke, but the exact cardiological mechanisms underlying these rapid neurogenic or cerebrogenic deaths have not been fully elucidated. More intriguing is the phenomenon of SUDEP, a sudden catastrophic condition in which cardiological causative mechanisms have long been suspected but are still unproven. The abruptness of death during normal activities in otherwise healthy individuals compels the consideration of cardiac arrhythmia as the most critical mechanism that leads inexorably to death in SUDEP victims. The understanding and prevention of SUDEP will continue to be hampered by the relatively low incidence of the condition and the declining rate of autopsy investigation of epilepsy-related deaths. Large multicenter studies must continue to investigate vigorously potential SUDEP cases with gross anatomical studies and perhaps with the emerging molecular or genetic markers of sudden cardiac deaths.[74]

References

1. Leestma J. Sudden unexpected death associated with seizures: A pathological review. In: Lathers C, Schraeder P, Eds. *Epilepsy and Sudden Death.* New York: Marcel Dekker, Inc., 1990:61–88.
2. Ficker DM. Sudden unexplained death and injury in epilepsy. *Epilepsia* 2000;41(Suppl. 2):S7–12.
3. Leestma JE, *et al.* Sudden unexplained death in epilepsy: Observations from a large clinical development program. *Epilepsia* 1997;38(1):47–55.
4. Munson JF. Deaths in epilepsy. *Med Rec* 1910;77: 58–62.
5. Krohn E. Causes of death among epileptics. *Epilepsia* 1963;4:315–321.
6. Freytag E, Lindenberg R. 294 medicolegal autopsies on epileptics. *Arch Pathol* 1964;78:274–286.
7. Zielinski JJ. Epilepsy and mortality rate and cause of death. *Epilepsia* 1974;15(2):191–201.
8. Terrence CF Jr, Wisotzkey HM, Perper JA. Unexpected, unexplained death in epileptic patients. *Neurology* 1975;25(6):594–598.
9. Jick SS, *et al.* Idiopathic epilepsy and sudden unexplained death. *Pharmacoepidemiol Drug Saf* 1992;1: 59–64.
10. Tennis P, *et al.* Cohort study of incidence of sudden unexplained death in persons with seizure disorder treated with antiepileptic drugs in Saskatchewan, Canada. *Epilepsia* 1995;36(1):29–36.
11. Leestma J, *et al.* A prospective study on sudden unexpected death in epilepsy. *Ann Neurol* 1989;26: 195–203.

12. Tomson T, *et al.* Sudden unexpected death in epilepsy: A review of incidence and risk factors. *Epilepsia* 2005;46(Suppl. 11):54–61.
13. Racoosin JA, *et al.* Mortality in antiepileptic drug development programs. *Neurology* 2001;56(4):514–519.
14. Kwan P, Brodie MJ. Early identification of refractory epilepsy. *N Engl J Med* 2000;342(5):314–319.
15. Lhatoo SD, *et al.* Sudden unexpected death: A rare event in a large community based prospective cohort with newly diagnosed epilepsy and high remission rates. *J Neurol Neurosurg Psychiatry* 1999;66(5):692–693.
16. Ficker D, *et al.* Population-based study of the incidence of sudden unexplained death in epilepsy. *Neurology* 1998;51:1270–1274.
17. Shen W, *et al.* Sudden unexpected nontraumatic death in 54 young adults: A 30-year population-based study. *Am J Cardiol* 1995;25:699–704.
18. Langan Y, Nashef L, Sander JW. Sudden unexpected death in epilepsy: A series of witnessed deaths. *J Neurol Neurosurg Psychiatry* 2000;68(2):211–213.
19. Langan Y, Nashef L, Sander JW. Case-control study of SUDEP. *Neurology* 2005;64:1131–1133.
20. Walczak T, *et al.* Incidence and risk factors in sudden unexpected death in epilepsy. *Neurology* 2001;56:519–525.
21. Nilsson L, *et al.* Risk factors for sudden unexpected death in epilepsy: A case-control study. *Lancet* 1999;353:888–893.
22. Nilsson L, *et al.* Antiepileptic drug therapy and its management in sudden unexpected death in epilepsy: A case-control study. *Epilepsia* 2001;42(5):667–673.
23. Lip G, Brodie MJ. Sudden death in epilepsy: An avoidable outcome? *J R Med Soc Med* 1992;85:609–611.
24. Williams J, *et al.* Variability of antiepileptic medication taking behaviour in sudden unexplained death in epilepsy: Hair analysis at autopsy. *J Neurol Neurosurg Psychiatry* 2006;77(4):481–484.
25. Walczak T. Do antiepileptic drugs play a role in sudden unexpected death in epilepsy? *Drug Safety* 2003;6(10):673–683.
26. Benassi E, *et al.* Carbamazepine and cardiac conduction disturbances. *Ann Neurol* 1987;22:280–281.
27. Ronkainen E. *et al.* Suppressed circadian heart rate dynamics in temporal lobe epilepsy. *J Neurol Neurosurg Psychiatry* 2005;6(10):1382–1386.
28. Reeves A, *et al.* The ictal bradycardia syndrome. *Epilepsia* 1996;37:983–987.
29. Rocamora R. *et al.* Cardiac asystole in epilepsy: Clinical and neurophysiologic features. *Epilepsia* 2003;44:179–185.
30. Mayer H, *et al.* EKG abnormalities in children and adolescents with symptomatic temporal lobe epilepsy. *Neurology* 2004;63:324–328.
31. Rugg-Gunn F, *et al.* Cardiac arrhythmias in focal epilepsy: A prospective long-term study. *Lancet* 2004;364(9452):2212–2219.
32. Britton J, *et al.* The ictal bradycardia syndrome: Localization and lateralization. *Epilepsia* 2006;47:737–744.
33. Nei M, Ho R, Sperling M. EKG abnormalities during partial seizures in refractory epilepsy. *Epilepsia* 2000;41:542–548.
34. Dasheiff R, Dickinson L. Sudden unexpected death of epileptic patient due to cardiac arrhythmia after seizure. *Arch Neurol* 1986;43:194–196.
35. Tigaran S, *et al.* Evidence of cardiac ischemia during seizures in drug refractory epilepsy patients. *Neurology* 2003;60:492–495.
36. Tavernor SJ, *et al.* Electrocardiograph QT lengthening associated with epileptiform EEG discharges—a role in sudden unexplained death in epilepsy? *Seizure* 1996;5(1):79–83.
37. Lathers C, Schraeder P. Autonomic dysfunction in epilepsy: Characterization of autonomic cardiac neural discharge associated with pentylenetetrazol-induced epileptogenic activity. *Epilepsia* 1982;23:633–647.
38. P-Codrea Tigaran S, *et al.* Sudden unexpected death in epilepsy. Is Death by seizures a cardiac cause? *Am J Forensic Med Pathol* 2005;26:99–105.
39. Opeskin K, Thomas A, Berkovic SF. Does cardiac conduction pathology contribute to sudden unexpected death in epilepsy? *Epilepsy Res* 2000;40(1):17–24.
40. Schraeder P, *et al.* A Nationwide Survey of Coroners and Medical Examiners on Documentation of Sudden Unexpected Death in Epilepsy (SUDEP): Extent of autopsy performance. *Neurology* 2003;60(Suppl. 1):A278.
41. Linzer M, *et al.* Cardiovascular causes of loss of consciousness in patients with presumed epilepsy: A cause of the increased sudden death rate in people with epilepsy? *Am J Med* 1994;96:146–154.
42. Terrence C, Perper J, Rao G. Neurogenic pulmonary edema in sudden unexpected, unexplained death of epileptic patients. *Ann Neurol* 1981;9:458–464.
43. Shanahan W. Acute pulmonary edema as a complication of epileptic seizures. *NY Med J* 1908;54:54–56.
44. Swallow R, Hillier C, Smith P. Sudden unexplained death in epilepsy (SUDEP) following previous seizure-related oedema: Case report and review of possible preventative treatment. *Seizure* 2002;11:446–448.

45. Schraeder P. Adult respiratory distress syndrome (ARDS) associated with nonconvulsive status epilepticus. *Epilepsia* 1987;28:605.
46. Theodore J, Robin E. Speculations on neurogenic pulmonary edema. *Am Rev Respir Dis* 1976;113: 405–411.
47. Coulter D. Partial seizures with apnea and bradycardia. *Arch Neurol* 1984;43:194–196.
48. Bird J, *et al.* Sudden unexplained death in epilepsy: An intracranially monitored case. *Epilepsia* 1996; 38(Suppl. 11):S52–S56.
49. So E, Sam M, Lagerlund T. Postictal central apnea as a cause of SUDEP: Evidence from a near-SUDEP incident. *Epilepsia* 2000;41:1494–1497.
50. Nashef L, *et al.* Apnoea and bradycardia during epileptic seizures: Relation to sudden death in epilepsy. *J Neurol Neurosurg Psychiatry* 1996;60:297–300.
51. Johnston S, *et al.* The role of hypoventillation in a sheep model of epileptic sudden death. *Ann Neurol* 1995;37:531–537.
52. Johnston SC, *et al.* Central apnea and acute cardiac ischemia in a sheep model of epileptic sudden death. *Ann Neurol* 1997;42(4):588–594.
53. Venit E, Shepard B, Seyfried T. Oxygenation prevents sudden death in seizure-prone mice. *Epilepsia* 2004;45:993–996.
54. Tupal S, Faingold C. Evidence supporting a role of serotonin in modulation of sudden death induced by seizures in DBA/2 mice. *Epilepsia* 2006;47:21–26.
55. Heisler L, Chu H, Tecott L. Epilepsy and obesity in serotonin 5-HT2C receptor mutant mice. *Ann NY Acad Sci* 1998;861:74–78.
56. Tinuper P, *et al.* Ictal bradycardia in partial epileptic seizures: Autonomic investigation in three cases and literature review. *Brain* 2001;124(Pt. 12):2361–2371 (see comment).
57. Hilz M, *et al.* Decrease of sympathetic cardiovascular modulation after temporal lobe epilepsy surgery. *Brain* 2002;125:985–995.
58. Sperling M, *et al.* Seizure control and mortality in epilepsy. *Ann Neurol* 1999;46:45–50.
59. Nashef L, *et al.* Sudden death in epilepsy: A study of incidence in a young cohort with epilepsy and learning difficulty. *Epilepsia* 1995;36(12):1187–1194.
60. Kloster R, Engelskjon T. Sudden unexpected death in epilepsy (SUDEP): A clinical perspective and a search for risk factors. *J Neurol Neurosurg Psychiatry* 1999;67:439–444.
61. Black M, Graham DI. Sudden unexplained death in adults caused by intracranial pathology. *J Clin Pathol* 2002;55(1):44–50.
62. Buttner A, *et al.* Colloid cysts of the third ventricle with fatal outcome: A report of two cases and review of the literature. *Int J Legal Med* 1997; 110(5):260–266.
63. Samuels M. Cardiopulmonary aspects of acute neurological diseases. In: Ropper A, Ed. *Neurological and Neurosurgical Intensive Care.* New York: Raven Press, 1993:103–119.
64. Cheung R, Hachinski V. The insula and cerebrogenic sudden death. *Arch Neurol* 2000;57:1685–1688.
65. Abboud H, *et al.* Insular involvement in brain infarction increases risk of cardiac arrhythmia and death. *Ann Neurol* 2006;59:691–699.
66. Hays A, Diringer M. Elevated troponin levels are associated with higher mortality following intracerebral hemorrhage. *Neurology* 2006;66:1330–1334.
67. Jaster J, Porterfield L, Bertorini T. Stroke and cardiac arrest. *Neurology* 1996;41:1357 (letter).
68. Griggs R, *et al.* Cardiac conduction in myotonic dystrophy. *Am J Med* 1975;59:37–42.
69. Santorelli FM, *et al.* Novel mutation in the mitochondrial DNA tRNA glycine gene associated with sudden unexpected death. *Pediatr Neurol* 1996; 15(2):145–149.
70. Goodwin FC, Muntoni F. Cardiac involvement in muscular dystrophies: Molecular mechanisms. *Muscle Nerve* 2005;32(5):577–588.
71. Forsberg H, *et al.* 24-hour electrocardiographic study in myotonic dystrophy. *Cardiology* 1988;75(4): 241–249.
72. Gilbert-Barness E. Metabolic cardiomyopathy and conduction system defects in children. *Ann Clin Lab Sci* 2004;34:15–34.
73. Zhang L. *et al.* Electrocardiographic features in Andersen-Tawil syndrome patients with KCNJ2 mutations: Characteristic T-U-wave patterns predict the KCNJ2 genotype. *Circulation* 2005;111(21): 2720–2726.
74. Ackerman MJ. Cardiac causes of sudden unexpected death in children and their relationship to seizures and syncope: Genetic testing for cardiac electropathies. *Semin Pediatr Neurol* 2005;12(1):52–58.
75. Leestma JE, *et al.* Sudden unexpected death associated with seizures: Analysis of 66 cases. *Epilepsia* 1984;25(1):84–88.
76. Langan Y, Nolan N, Hutchinson M. The incidence of sudden unexpected death in epilepsy (SUDEP) in South Dublin and Wicklow. *Seizure* 1998;7(5): 355–358.
77. Timmings PL. Sudden unexpected death in epilepsy: A local audit. *Seizure* 1993;2(4):287–290.
78. Klenerman P, Sander JW, Shorvon SD. Mortality in patients with epilepsy: A study of patients in long

term residential care. *J Neurol Neurosurg Psychiatry* 1993;56(2):149–152.
79. Derby LE, Tennis P, Jick H. Sudden unexplained death among subjects with refractory epilepsy. *Epilepsia* 1996;37(10):931–935.
80. Hennessy M, *et al*, A study of mortality after temporal lobe epilepsy surgery. *Neurology* 1999;53:1276–1283.
81. Annegers JF, *et al.* Epilepsy, vagal nerve stimulation by the NCP system, mortality, and sudden, unexpected, unexplained death. *Epilepsia* 1998; 39(2):206–212.
82. Nashef L, *et al.* Incidence of sudden unexpected death in an adult outpatient cohort with epilepsy at a tertiary referral centre. *J Neurol Neurosurg Psychiatry* 1995;58(4):462–464.
83. Dasheiff R. Sudden unexpected death in epilepsy: A series from an epilepsy surgery program and speculation on the relationship to sudden cardiac death. *J Clin Neurophysiol* 1991;8:216–222.

60
Obstructive Sleep Apnea and Sudden Death

Apoor S. Gami and Virend K. Somers

Introduction

Obstructive sleep apnea (OSA) is a highly prevalent condition that is associated with a broad range of cardiovascular disease conditions. The pathophysiological events during apneas in patients with OSA cause acute and often profound autonomic, cardiac, and vascular changes during sleep, and may also result in daytime abnormalities of neural circulatory control and cardiovascular structure and function. These changes may contribute to sudden death during sleep and may increase the risk of sudden death during the day. We will review the epidemiology of OSA, the physiology of normal sleep, the distinctive pathophysiology of sleep in patients with OSA, the mechanisms by which OSA may increase the risk of sudden death, and available population data that support such a relationship.

Epidemiology of Obstructive Sleep Apnea

A synthesis of findings from large population-based studies in racially and geographically diverse populations reveals that about 20% of middle-aged adults have at least mild OSA. The OSA syndrome, which consists of not only the physiology but also the symptoms of OSA, is present in about 5% of these populations.[1] The prevalence of OSA increases through the late adult years and plateaus at 20–41% after age 65 years.[1,2] Men are two to three times more likely to have OSA than are women.[1] The condition most strongly associated with and causally related to OSA is obesity.[3] Total body weight, body mass index, and fat distribution all correlate with the presence of OSA, and 40–60% of obese adults have OSA.[1,3] The majority of individuals with OSA are undiagnosed,[4] likely due to the lack of symptoms in people with mild OSA, the ubiquity of its cardinal symptom of sleepiness in others, and the general lack of access to polysomnography to establish the diagnosis. By conservative estimates, over 25 million American adults have OSA.

Physiology of Normal Sleep

Sleep comprises one-fourth to one-third of our lives and generally has been considered a physiologically restorative period. The fact is that sleep consists of dynamic and elaborate physiological processes, many of which impact cardiovascular regulation and function.

A night of sleep usually consists of four or five cycles of rapid eye movement (REM) and non-rapid eye movement (NREM) sleep stages, with REM stages getting progressively longer in later cycles.[5] During NREM sleep, sympathetic neural activity decreases and parasympathetic tone predominates. During REM sleep, a tonic state alternates with multiple periods of phasic activity. The REM stage and its baseline tonic state are periods of high parasympathetic tone, whereas during phasic REM bursts of sympathetic neural activity occur (Figure 60–1).[6] As a result, REM sleep is associated with dynamic fluctuations in autonomic balance. Superimposed upon these changes related to sleep stage, autonomic balance also

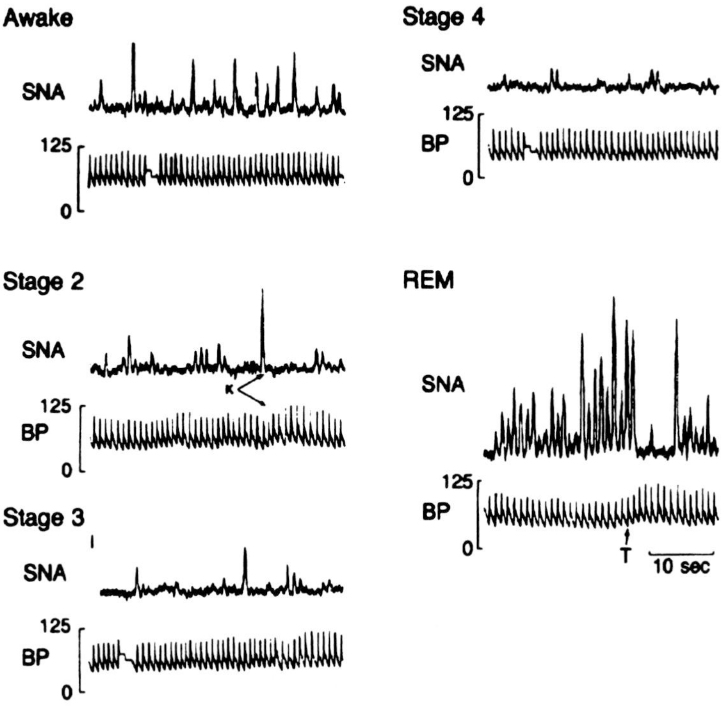

FIGURE 60–1. Recordings of sympathetic nerve activity (SNA) and mean blood pressure (BP) in an individual while awake and during stages 2, 3, 4, and rapid eye movement (REM) sleep. As non-REM sleep deepens (stages 2 through 4), SNA gradually decreases and BP and variability in BP are gradually reduced. Arousal stimuli elicited K complexes on the electroencephalogram (not shown), which were accompanied by increases in SNA and BP (indicated by the arrows, stage 2 sleep). In contrast to the changes during non-REM sleep, heart rate, BP, and BP variability increased during REM sleep, together with a profound increase in both the frequency and the amplitude of SNA. There was a frequent association between REM twitches (momentary periods of restoration of muscle tone, shown by T on the tracing) and abrupt inhibition of SNA and increases in BP. (Reprinted from Somers *et al.*,[6] with permission from the Massachusetts Medical Society.)

exhibits a circadian rhythm. Sympathetic activity is highest during the day and peaks in midmorning, and parasympathetic activity is highest during the night.[7]

The general effect of normal sleep on cardiac electrophysiology is due to the predominance of parasympathetic tone. As a result, normal sleep is associated with decreases in the arterial baroreceptor set point, heart rate, blood pressure, cardiac output, and systemic vascular resistance. This overall cardiovascular "quiescence" during sleep is punctuated by REM sleep-related surges in heart rate and blood pressure to levels similar to wakefulness.[6] Thus, in healthy people, benign nocturnal arrhythmias and conduction disturbances occur due to relative vagotonia. These include sinus bradycardia, marked sinus arrhythmia, sinus pauses, and first-degree and type I second-degree atrioventricular (AV) block.[8] Normal sleep is also associated with delayed cardiac repolarization, as reflected by a prolonged corrected QT interval (QTc) during sleep in healthy individuals.[9,10] Some data suggest that this may be most evident during REM sleep stages in women (Figure 60–2).[11]

Normal sleep is associated with variations in coagulability and vascular function that are also possibly due in part to the predominance of parasympathetic tone during sleep. Compared to the morning awake state, sleep is associated with increased fibrinolytic activity, increased levels of tissue plasminogen activator, decreased blood viscosity, and decreased platelet aggregation, all changes that mitigate pathological coagulation.[12–16] Interestingly, the association of sleep with reduced platelet aggregation seems to be

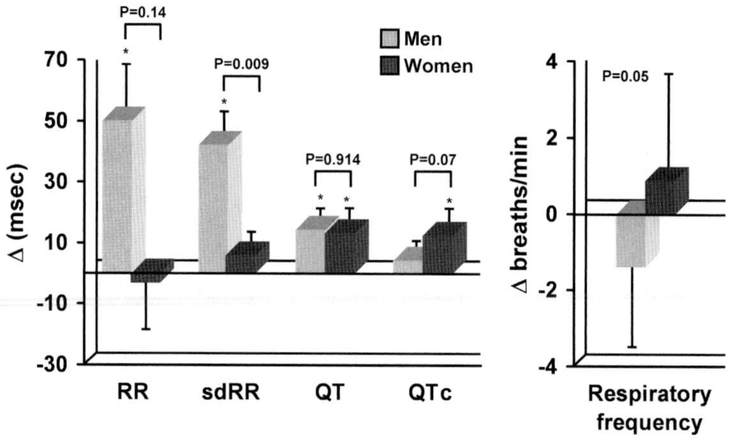

FIGURE 60–2. Electrocardiographic measurements and breathing frequency during wakefulness and rapid eye movement (REM) sleep in men and women. RR interval and RR variability (sdRR) from wakefulness to REM sleep significantly increase in men and remain stable in women. In both men and women, the QT interval increases. The corrected QT interval (QTc) remains stable through sleep in men while it increases significantly during REM sleep in women. Breathing frequency decreases in men and increases in women. Δ, change. *Significant difference between REM and wakefulness within subjects. (Modified from Lanfranchi *et al.*,[11] with permission from Lippincott Williams & Wilkins.)

related specifically to the supine position, as the attenuation of platelet aggregation ceases not with awakening but rather with upright posture in the morning.[17,18] Arterial endothelial function in healthy adults also appears to have a day–night pattern, with better arterial flow-mediated endothelium-dependent vasodilation during the evening compared to the morning.[19] Similarly, in patients with coronary artery disease, both coronary vascular tone and peripheral arterial function have a diurnal variation, with better vascular function evident during the afternoon.[20]

Pathophysiology of Sleep in Obstructive Sleep Apnea

Sleep in individuals with OSA is characterized by transient occlusions of the upper airway, which result in episodes of partial cessation (hypopnea) or complete cessation (apnea) of airflow (Figure 60–3).[21] The patency of the upper airway during inspiration is determined by competition between negative transmural pharyngeal pressures and pharyngeal dilator and abductor muscle tone.[22,23] The dominance of the former results in posterior movement of the tongue and soft palate against the posterior pharyngeal wall, which obstructs airflow.[24] Central nervous system modulation during sleep decreases pharyngeal muscle activity and destabilizes the airway musculature, especially during REM sleep when there is loss of muscle tone, making airway obstruction more likely.[22,25,26] These apneas and hypopneas result in hypoxemia and futile ventilatory efforts, which ultimately activate the central nervous system and produce a transient but usually subconscious arousal to a lighter stage of sleep that allows restoration of airway patency and airflow. Hyperventilation occurs after apneas due to activation of peripheral and central chemoreceptors by the episodic hypoxemia and hypercapnia.[27,28] These series of events can recur hundreds of times during each hour of sleep.[29] The most common measure of the severity of OSA is the apnea–hypopnea index (AHI), which is the average number of obstructive apneic and hypopneic events per hour of sleep. An AHI <5 is considered normal, and an AHI ≥5 is consistent with at least mild OSA physiology and has been associated with the development and progression of cardiovascular diseases.[30,31] Other indices of the severity of OSA that are relevant to cardiovascular outcomes include measures related to the severity or duration of oxygen desaturations during sleep.

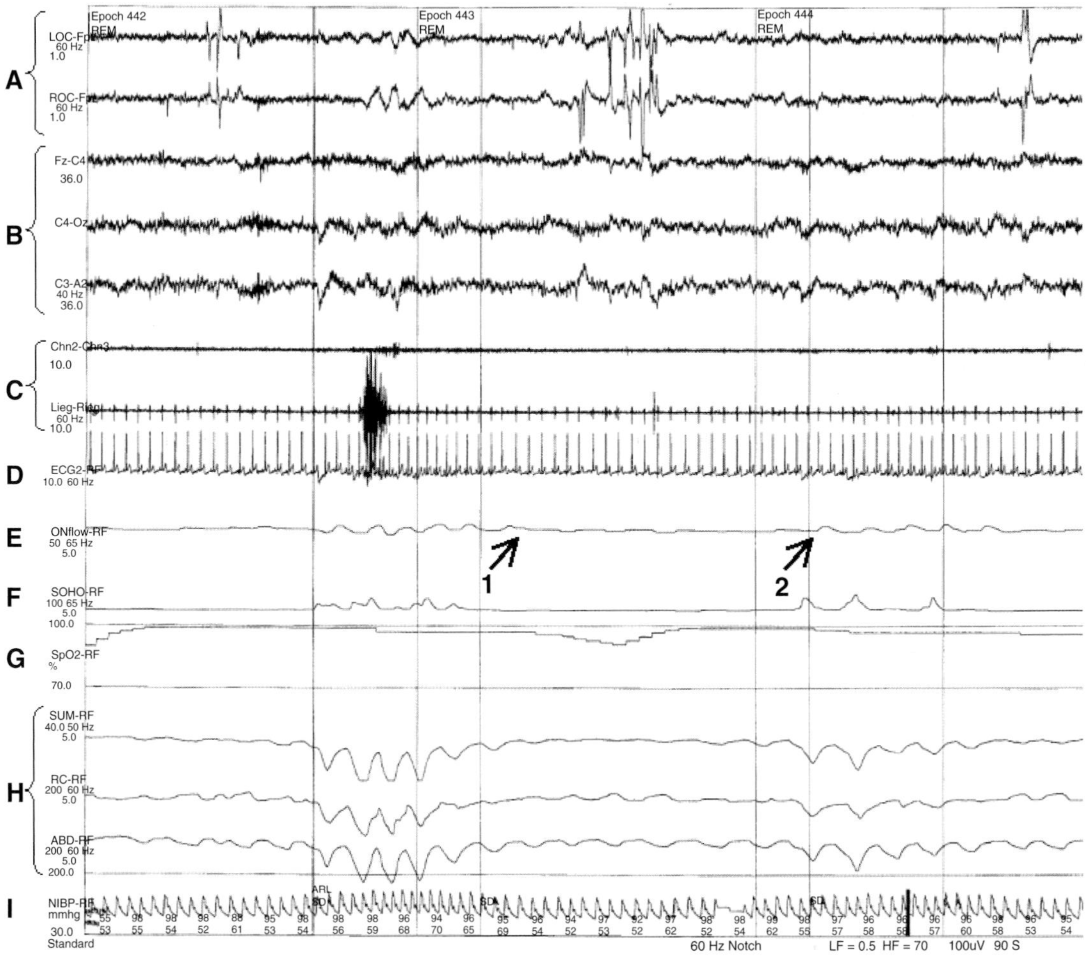

Figure 60–3. Polysomnography recording from a patient with obstructive sleep apnea. The tracing shows the (A) electrooculogram, (B) electroencephalogram, (C) electromyogram, (D) electrocardiogram, (E) measures of airflow, (F) sonogram, (G) oximetry, (H) measures of thoracoabdominal movements, and (I) blood pressure during 90 sec of rapid eye movement (REM) sleep in a subject undergoing an overnight sleep study. Arrow 1 identifies initiation of an obstructive apnea and arrow 2 identifies its termination. (Reprinted from Gami *et al.*,[3] with permission from Elsevier.)

Obstructive Sleep Apnea and Potential Mechanisms of Sudden Death

In contrast to the physiology of normal sleep described earlier, individuals with OSA experience severe perturbations of cardiac regulation *during* sleep, which individually or in concert may increase the risk of sudden death. Obstructive apneic events cause reductions in oxygen saturation and systemic hypoxemia, and in some individuals oxygen saturations can be prolonged and fall below technically measurable levels. It has been shown that these repetitive oxygen desaturations are directly linked to ventricular ectopy in patients with OSA,[32] and this may represent a direct dysrhythmic mechanism linking OSA to nocturnal sudden death.

Hypoxemia, with associated hypercapnia, also causes activation of the chemoreflex,[33,34] which results in marked increases in nocturnal sympathetic drive reflected by vascular sympathetic nerve activity and serum catecholamines.[33,35] This causes repetitive fluctuations and surges in heart rate and blood pressure during sleep.[33] Although the primary cardiac response to hypoxia and apnea is bradycardia (see later), tachycardia is evident at the end of apnea when breathing resumes. This is also the time when the blood pressure peaks are highest. Apneic episodes are thus marked by the simultaneous occurrence of hypoxemia and increased myocardial oxygen demand, due to the increased heart rate and blood pressure caused by sympathetic overdrive. Predictably, this situation can cause nocturnal myocardial ischemia,[36–40] which may induce ventricular dysrhythmias and sudden death in these patients.

Another mechanism for ischemic events and sudden death in patients with OSA may be a paradoxical nocturnal increase in coagulability. Platelet activation and aggregation are increased during sleep in patients with OSA.[41–46] Furthermore, fibrinogen levels are increased[47,48] and fibrinolytic activity is decreased.[42]

Cardiac electrophysiology during sleep in patients with OSA is distinct from that of normal sleep, mostly due to marked nocturnal cardiac autonomic abnormalities. Heart rate variability and the day–night parasympathetic modulation of sinus node activity are attenuated in patients with OSA.[49–53] Obstructive sleep apnea impacts the main autonomic mechanisms mediating heart rate variability, including medullary coupling between respiratory and cardiac vagal neurons, input from the arterial baroreflex, and vagal feedback from pulmonary stretch receptors.[54–56] The latter may be affected by marked fluctuations in negative intrathoracic pressure during obstructive apneas. The duration of ventricular repolarization, represented by the QTc, and the heterogeneity of repolarization, reflected by QTc interval dispersion, are abnormal in patients with OSA (Figure 60–4).[57–61] The increase in QTc dispersion correlates with the severity of OSA, measured by both the AHI and the duration of significant nocturnal hypoxemia.[61]

Significant arrhythmias and conduction abnormalities occur during sleep in OSA patients.[8,32,62–71] A controlled, multicenter study showed that during sleep nonsustained ventricular tachycardia occurred in 5.3% and complex ventricular ectopy occurred in 25% of patients with sleep-disordered breathing (which included OSA as well as central sleep apnea).[72] After adjustment for comorbidities, patients with sleep-disordered breathing had a 3.4-fold risk of nonsustained ventricular tachycardia and a 1.7-fold risk of complex ventricular activity compared to patients with normal sleep. Type 2 second-degree AV block occurred in 2.2% and intraventricular conduction delays occurred in 8.9% of patients with sleep-disordered breathing.[72] Electrophysiology studies in patients with OSA and severe sinus bradycardia or advanced AV block during sleep demonstrated nearly normal sinus node and AV nodal function,[70] which highlights the profound influence of autonomic modulation in these patients.

In addition to ischemia and ventricular tachyarrhythmias, sudden death in patients with OSA may be due to severe bradyarrhythmias. The cessation of airflow and hypoxemia can activate the diving reflex, which simultaneously causes cardiac parasympathetic overdrive and peripheral

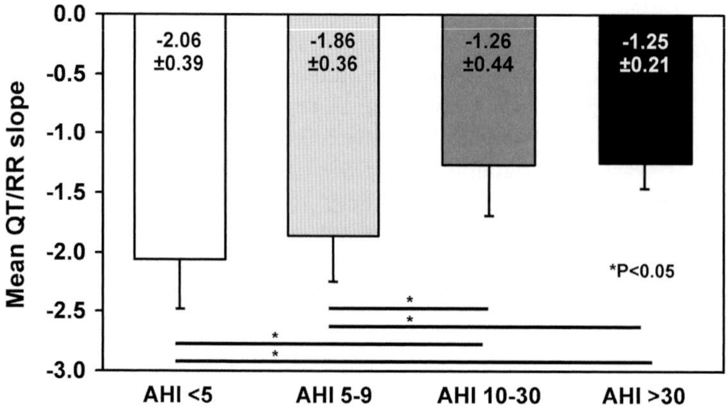

FIGURE 60–4. Alteration of the QT/RR slopes according to the severity of obstructive sleep apnea (OSA). Obstructive sleep apnea leads to abnormal beat-to-beat changes in ventricular repolarization, characterized by a flattened relationship between QT duration and RR intervals at heart rates less than 70 beats per minute. The relationship correlates with the severity of OSA, based on the apnea–hypopnea index (AHI). (Modified from Roche *et al.*,[59] with permission from Blackwell Publishing.)

vasoconstriction in all vascular territories except the brain and heart. The resultant bradyarrhythmias are most frequent during REM sleep, may be severe, and as mentioned above may include sinus arrest and high-degree AV block.[69,72,73] In a series of 239 consecutive patients diagnosed with OSA at one hospital, 7% had profound sinus bradycardia (<30 beats per minute) or advanced atrioventricular block with asystole >2 sec.[71] These severe bradyarrhythmias were limited to patients with an AHI ≥60, representing severe OSA. Sudden deaths due to bradyarrhythmias are well documented,[74–76] and it is conceivable that severe bradyarrhythmias may be causally related to sudden death in patients with OSA.

Obstructive sleep apnea is strongly associated with the occurrence of stroke,[77,78] and stroke itself acutely increases the risk of cardiac dysrhythmias.[79,80] Most patients with strokes are not monitored for cardiac arrhythmias, and it is possible that some sudden deaths in OSA patients are related to strokes that result in malignant arrhythmias.

Other less recognized but potentially important causes of sudden death in patients with OSA are profound cerebral hypoxemia and ineffective arousals due to impaired chemosensitivity. Three illustrative cases of sudden death, one resuscitated and the others fatal, were recently described.[81,82] These patients had polysomnographic monitoring during severe obstructive apneic events that led to profound systemic hypoxemia (oxygen saturation as low as 12%), lack of arousal, and sudden death, evidenced by encephalographic inactivity and cardiopulmonary arrest (Figure 60–5). Electrocardiographic monitoring did not reveal dysrhythmias preceding these events, and autopsy in one patient revealed no significant cardiac structural abnormalities or occlusive coronary artery disease.[81] These cases suggest that OSA may be a direct cause of sudden death. The mechanisms may include severe cerebral and systemic hypoxemia as well as ineffective central arousals during severe apneas due to deranged chemosensitivity.[34,83,84] It is possible that sudden unexplained deaths that historically have been presumptively attributed to cardiac dysrhythmias (due to the lack of structural abnormalities) may in fact be due to the direct effects of OSA in some individuals.

In addition to the acute mechanisms discussed above, OSA has multiple effects on chronic cardiovascular function that may increase the risk of sudden death.[85] A wealth of cross-sectional data have demonstrated a strong association between OSA and chronic systemic hypertension, and prospective epidemiological studies have implicated OSA as an independent risk factor for incident hypertension.[30,31,86,87] OSA is now broadly accepted as a secondary cause of chronic systemic hypertension.[88] In addition, OSA is strongly associated with coronary artery disease. While this might be expected due to the multiple coronary risk factors often present in these patients, cross-sectional and prospective epidemiological studies have shown that the relationship between OSA and coronary artery disease, including incident ischemic events, is independent of major comorbidities such as obesity, diabetes, hypertension, and hyperlipidemia.[89–92] The strong and independent association of OSA with coronary artery disease would be expected to correlate also with a heightened risk of sudden death.

The chronic effects of OSA are also evident in daytime autonomic nervous system activity. Individuals with OSA have significantly increased sympathetic drive during the awake daytime period, reflected by increased catecholamines and sympathetic nerve activity, which is independent of other comorbid conditions, including obesity.[33,54,93–95] This may be due to a carryover from nocturnal autonomic abnormalities and to chronic dysfunction of the peripheral chemoreceptor reflex.[34,96] While the precise interactions between the autonomic nervous system and arrhythmic sudden death remain largely unknown,[97] chronic sympathetic overdrive has been identified as a risk marker for sudden death.[98]

Lastly, OSA is present in a large proportion of patients with heart failure, and it has been implicated in chronic left ventricular dysfunction.[99–103] The treatment of OSA by continuous positive airway pressure causes acute and lasting improvements in ventricular systolic function,[99–101] in one study resulting in an absolute increase of the left ventricular ejection fraction of 9% after 1 month.[103] The contribution of OSA to ventricular dysfunction may be an important contributor to the neurohumoral response and remodeling that produce the myocardial substrate for sudden death,

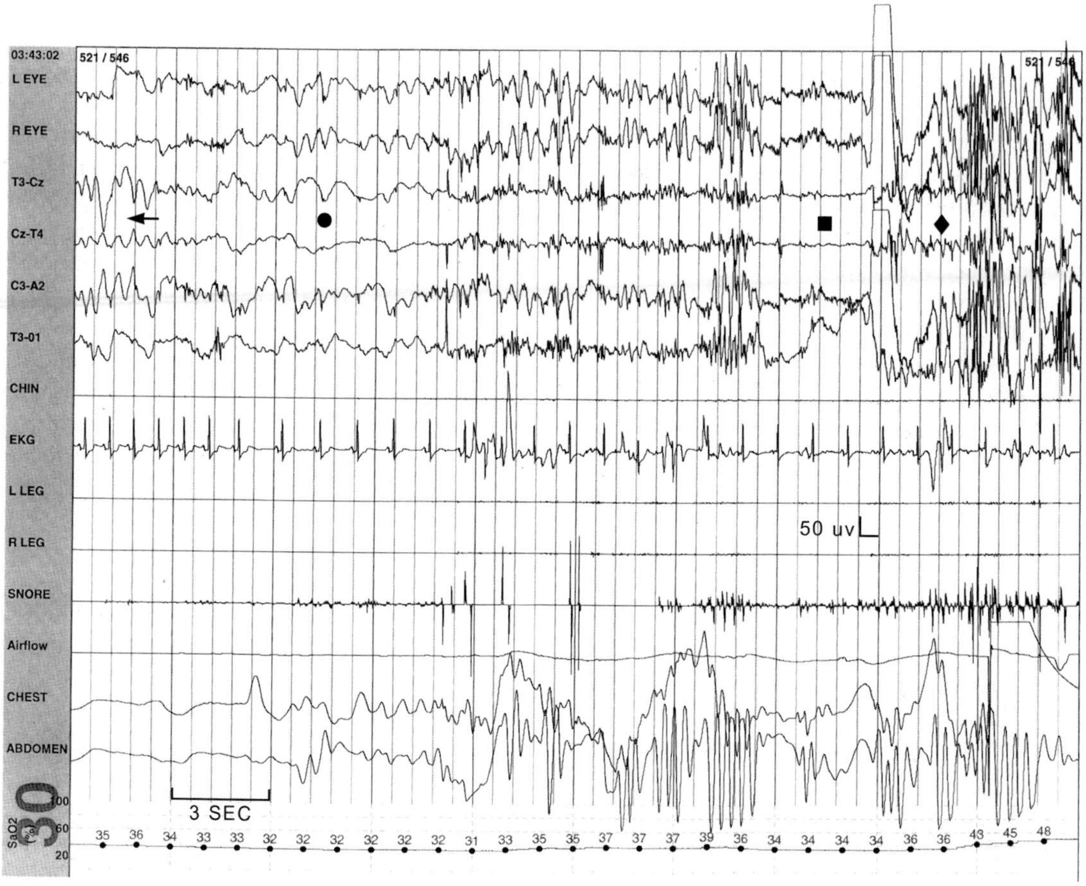

Figure 60–5. Resuscitated sudden death during an obstructive apnea. This patient had a prolonged obstructive apnea, which resulted in a sudden EEG change from a classic REM saw tooth pattern (see arrow) to a poorly organized, diffuse delta slow-wave pattern (see closed circle). This was followed by a general flattening of all activity (see square) that led to attempts to arouse the patient (as evidenced by diffuse movement artifact; see the diamond). Nevertheless, persistent obstruction (see the triangle) necessitated emergent rescue breathing maneuvers. Persistent EEG flattening followed by slowing and eventual recovery of normal waking patterns occurred later (not shown). L, left; R, right; T, temporal; C, central; O, occipital; CHIN, mentalis EMG; L LEG, left anterior tibialis EMG; R LEG, right anterior tibialis EMG; SNORE, snoring microphone; Airflow, nasal airflow; CHEST, thoracic respiratory effort; ABDOMEN, abdominal respiratory effort; SaO_2 (%), oxygen saturation. (Reprinted from Dyken *et al.*,[82] with permission from Lippincott Williams & Wilkins.)

particularly in patients who are already at higher risk, such as those with ischemic or preexisting structural heart disease.

Associations between Obstructive Sleep Apnea and Sudden Death

Not only is OSA associated, sometimes causally, with a number of mechanisms of cardiovascular disease,[85] but OSA is also associated with a heightened risk of cardiovascular disease outcomes. While a number of longitudinal studies assessed the occurrence of cardiac events and mortality in cohorts of patients diagnosed with OSA, most of these studies did not have control groups of patients without OSA for comparison,[104–110] and nearly all did not systematically ascertain sudden death as an outcome.[77,92,104–107] We are aware of only one *controlled* longitudinal study that ascertained the occurrence of sudden death in patients with OSA.[109] Doherty *et al.* followed 168 patients with OSA for an average of 7.5 years. They compared cardiovascular outcomes, including sudden death, in the 107 OSA patients who had continued OSA treatment (with continuous positive airway pressure) with the 61 OSA patients who had discontinued OSA treatment. Sudden unexpected death occurred in four patients (7%) with untreated OSA and in no patients (0%) with treated OSA (there was one arrhythmic death in a treated patient during coronary bypass surgery).[109] This was not a randomized trial of OSA treatment, but these are the only available longitudinal data to date, and they suggest that OSA physiology, when unchecked, is associated with a heightened risk of sudden death.

Additional observations supporting the influence of OSA on the occurrence of sudden death are the strikingly different day–night patterns of sudden death in patients with OSA compared to the general population. In the general population, the risk of sudden death is significantly greater during the second quarter of the day (in the morning hours after waking, i.e., from 6 AM to noon).[111] There is also a significant decrease in the risk of sudden death during the nighttime hours (from midnight to 6 AM).[111] This pattern is likely due to the day–night variation and sleep/wake-related changes in sympathetic activity, baroreflex function, coagulability, vascular function, and cardiac electrophysiology described earlier.

Since many of the putative mechanisms that may link OSA and sudden death occur acutely during sleep, it is intuitive that sudden deaths would be more likely to occur at night in patients with OSA. A Finnish study of 321 men with sudden death provided the first suggestion that this may be true.[112] In the study, Seppala *et al.* obtained snoring histories (as surrogates of OSA) from the cohabitants of the deceased men and found that habitual snorers were more likely to have sudden death in the early morning hours compared to nonsnorers and occasional snorers. This phenomenon was clarified in a recent study of 112 patients who underwent polysomnography to diagnose or exclude OSA prior to having sudden death.[112] Patients with OSA had a significantly increased risk of sudden death during the sleeping hours, from 10 PM to 6 AM, and patients without OSA had a diurnal pattern of sudden death that was similar to that expected in the general population (Figure 60–6). Patients with OSA had a 2.6-fold risk of nocturnal sudden death, and the severity of OSA

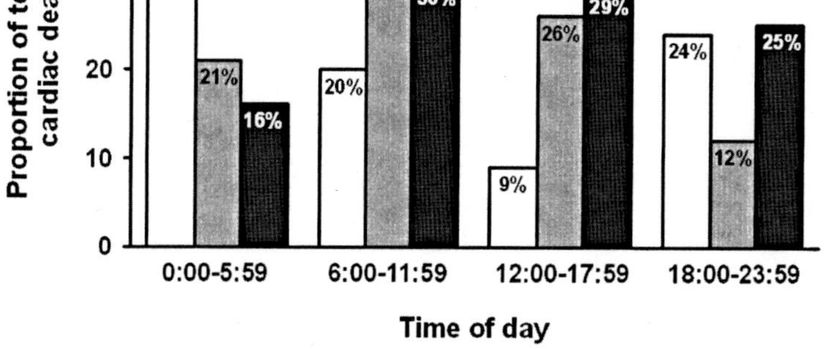

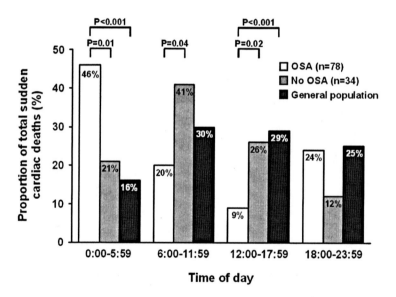

FIGURE 60–6. Day-night pattern of sudden cardiac death (SCD). The frequency of SCD from midnight to 6 AM in individuals with obstructive sleep apnea (OSA) (46%) was significantly higher than that in individuals without OSA (21%) and the general population (16%). The frequency of SCD from 6 AM to noon in individuals with OSA (20%) was significantly lower than that in individuals without OSA (41%) and nonsignificantly lower than that in the general population (30%). The frequency of SCD from noon to 6 PM in individuals with OSA (9%) was significantly lower than that in individuals without OSA (26%) and the general population (29%). The frequency of SCD from 6 PM to midnight was nonsignificantly different between individuals with OSA (24%) and those without OSA (12%) or the general population (25%). (Reprinted from Gami *et al.*, [113] with permission from the Massachusetts Medical Society.)

correlated with the magnitude of this risk.[113] These observational studies suggest that OSA is a risk factor for sudden death, particularly at night. Whether OSA is also associated with an increase in sudden death during the daytime, or whether risk of sudden death in the daytime is relatively decreased, remains to be determined. There is a paucity of data on OSA and sudden death, and definitive longitudinal studies are necessary to clarify this relationship.

Conclusions

Obstructive sleep apnea is a common condition, particularly in individuals with obesity or cardiovascular diseases, and may represent an important modifiable risk factor for sudden death. The unique pathophysiology of OSA creates a nocturnal milieu of mechanisms that may lead to sudden death. These include the effects of hypoxemia, sympathetic drive and autonomic imbalance, baroreflex dysfunction, impaired chemosensitivity, hypercoagulability, and electrophysiological abnormalities. Sudden deaths associated with OSA may be due to acute ischemic events, ventricular tachyarrhythmias, severe bradycardias, strokes, or profound obstructive apneas with ineffective arousals that lead to catastrophic cerebral and systemic hypoxemia. Obstructive sleep apnea increases the likelihood of sudden death during the night, but there are insufficient data regarding the influence of OSA on the overall risk of sudden death. Further research is necessary to clarify these relationships.

References

1. Young T, Peppard PE, Gottlieb DJ. Epidemiology of obstructive sleep apnea: A population health perspective. *Am J Respir Crit Care Med* 2002;165: 1217–1239.
2. Ancoli-Israel S, Kripke DF, Klauber MR, Mason WJ, Fell R, Kaplan O. Sleep-disordered breathing in community-dwelling elderly. *Sleep* 1991;14:486–495.
3. Gami AS, Caples SM, Somers VK. Obesity and obstructive sleep apnea. *Endocrinol Metab Clin North Am* 2003;32:869–894.
4. Young T, Evans L, Finn L, Palta M. Estimation of the clinically diagnosed proportion of sleep apnea syndrome in middle-aged men and women. *Sleep* 1997;20:705–706.
5. Kryger MH, Roth T, Dement WC, Eds. *Principles and Practice of Sleep Medicine*. Philadelphia, PA: Elsevier Saunders, 2005.
6. Somers V, Dyken M, Mark A, Abboud F. Sympathetic-nerve activity during sleep in normal subjects. *N Engl J Med* 1993;328:303–307.
7. Furlan R, Barbic F, Piazza S, Tinelli M, Seghizzi P, Malliani A. Modifications of cardiac autonomic profile associated with a shift schedule of work. *Circulation* 2000;102:1912–1916.
8. Adlakha A, Shepard JW Jr. Cardiac arrhythmias during normal sleep and in obstructive sleep apnea syndrome. *Sleep Med Rev* 1998;2:45–60.
9. Browne KF, Prystowsky E, Heger JJ, Chilson DA, Zipes DP. Prolongation of the Q-T interval in man during sleep. *Am J Cardiol* 1983;52:55–59.
10. Molnar J, Zhang F, Weiss J, Ehlert FA, Rosenthal JE. Diurnal pattern of QTc interval: How long is prolonged? Possible relation to circadian triggers of cardiovascular events. *J Am Coll Cardiol* 1996; 27:76–83.
11. Lanfranchi PA, Shamsuzzaman AS, Ackerman MJ, *et al.* Sex-selective QT prolongation during rapid eye movement sleep. *Circulation* 2002;106:1488–1492.
12. Linsell CR, Lightman SL, Mullen PE, Brown MJ, Causon RC. Circadian rhythms of epinephrine and norepinephrine in man. *J Clin Endocrinol Metab* 1985;60:1210–1215.
13. Tofler GH, Brezinski D, Schafer AI, *et al.* Concurrent morning increase in platelet aggregability and the risk of myocardial infarction and sudden cardiac death. *N Engl J Med* 1987;316:1514–1518.
14. Andreotti F, Davies GJ, Hackett DR, *et al.* Major circadian fluctuations in fibrinolytic factors and possible relevance to time of onset of myocardial infarction, sudden cardiac death and stroke. *Am J Cardiol* 1988;62:635–637.
15. Panza JA, Epstein SE, Quyyumi AA. Circadian variation in vascular tone and its relation to alpha-sympathetic vasoconstrictor activity. *N Engl J Med* 1991;325:986–990.
16. Andreotti F, De Luca L, Renda G, *et al.* Circadianicity of hemostatic function and coronary vasomotion. *Cardiologia* 1999;44(Suppl. 1):245–249.
17. Brezinski DA, Tofler GH, Muller JE, *et al.* Morning increase in platelet aggregability. Association with assumption of the upright posture. *Circulation* 1988;78:35–40.
18. Winther K, Hillegass W, Tofler GH, *et al.* Effects on platelet aggregation and fibrinolytic activity

during upright posture and exercise in healthy men. *Am J Cardiol* 1992;70:1051–1055.
19. Otto ME, Svatikova A, Barretto RB, *et al.* Early morning attenuation of endothelial function in healthy humans. *Circulation* 2004;109:2507–2510.
20. Quyyumi AA, Panza JA, Diodati JG, Lakatos E, Epstein SE. Circadian variation in ischemic threshold. A mechanism underlying the circadian variation in ischemic events. *Circulation* 1992;86:22–28.
21. Guilleminault C, Tilkian A, Dement WC. The sleep apnea syndromes. *Annu Rev Med* 1976;27:465–484.
22. Horner RL. Motor control of the pharyngeal musculature and implications for the pathogenesis of obstructive sleep apnea. *Sleep* 1996;19:827–853.
23. Remmers JE, deGroot WJ, Sauerland EK, Anch AM. Pathogenesis of upper airway occlusion during sleep. *J Appl Physiol* 1978;44:931–938.
24. Suratt PM, Dee P, Atkinson RL, Armstrong P, Wilhoit SC. Fluoroscopic and computed tomographic features of the pharyngeal airway in obstructive sleep apnea. *Am Rev Respir Dis* 1983;127:487–492.
25. Onal E, Lopata M, O'Connor T. Pathogenesis of apneas in hypersomnia-sleep apnea syndrome. *Am Rev Respir Dis* 1982;125:167–174.
26. Onal E, Lopata M. Periodic breathing and the pathogenesis of occlusive sleep apneas. *Am Rev Respir Dis* 1982;126:676–680.
27. Vincken W, Guilleminault C, Silvestri L, Cosio M, Grassino A. Inspiratory muscle activity as a trigger causing the airways to open in obstructive sleep apnea. *Am Rev Respir Dis* 1987;135:372–377.
28. Yasuma F, Kozar LF, Kimoff RJ, Bradley TD, Phillipson EA. Interaction of chemical and mechanical respiratory stimuli in the arousal response to hypoxia in sleeping dogs. *Am Rev Respir Dis* 1991;143:1274–1277.
29. Guilleminault C, Kim YD, Horita M, Tsutumi M, Pelayo R. Power spectral sleep EEG findings in patients with obstructive sleep apnea and upper airway resistance syndromes. *Electroencephalogr Clin Neurophysiol Suppl* 1999;50:113–120.
30. Nieto FJ, Young TB, Lind BK, *et al.* Association of sleep-disordered breathing, sleep apnea, and hypertension in a large community-based study. Sleep Heart Health Study. *JAMA* 2000;283:1829–1836.
31. Peppard PE, Young T, Palta M, Skatrud J. Prospective study of the association between sleep-disordered breathing and hypertension. *N Engl J Med* 2000;342:1378–1384.
32. Shepard JW Jr, Garrison MW, Grither DA, Dolan GF. Relationship of ventricular ectopy to oxyhemoglobin desaturation in patients with obstructive sleep apnea. *Chest* 1985;88:335–340.
33. Somers VK, Dyken ME, Clary MP, Abboud FM. Sympathetic neural mechanisms in obstructive sleep apnea. *J Clin Invest* 1995;96:1897–1904.
34. Narkiewicz K, van de Borne PJ, Pesek CA, Dyken ME, Montano N, Somers VK. Selective potentiation of peripheral chemoreflex sensitivity in obstructive sleep apnea. *Circulation* 1999;99:1183–1189.
35. Jennum P, Wildschiodtz G, Christensen NJ, Schwartz T. Blood pressure, catecholamines, and pancreatic polypeptide in obstructive sleep apnea with and without nasal continuous positive airway pressure (nCPAP) treatment. *Am J Hypertens* 1989;2:847–852.
36. Hanly P, Sasson Z, Zuberi N, Lunn K. ST-segment depression during sleep in obstructive sleep apnea. *Am J Cardiol* 1993;71:1341–1345.
37. Franklin KA, Nilsson JB, Sahlin C, Naslund U. Sleep apnoea and nocturnal angina. *Lancet* 1995;345:1085–1087.
38. Schafer H, Koehler U, Ploch T, Peter JH. Sleep-related myocardial ischemia and sleep structure in patients with obstructive sleep apnea and coronary heart disease. *Chest* 1997;111:387–393.
39. Mooe T, Franklin KA, Wiklund U, Rabben T, Holmstrom K. Sleep-disordered breathing and myocardial ischemia in patients with coronary artery disease. *Chest* 2000;117:1597–1602.
40. Alonso-Fernandez A, Garcia-Rio F, Racionero MA, *et al.* Cardiac rhythm disturbances and ST-segment depression episodes in patients with obstructive sleep apnea-hypopnea syndrome and its mechanisms. *Chest* 2005;127:15–22.
41. Neri Serheri GG, Abbate R, Gensini GF, Galanti G, Paoli G, Laureano R. Platelet aggregation and thromboxane A2 production after adrenergic stimulation in young healthy humans. *Haemostasis* 1982;11:40–48.
42. Rangemark C, Hedner JA, Carlson JT, Gleerup G, Winther K. Platelet function and fibrinolytic activity in hypertensive and normotensive sleep apnea patients. *Sleep* 1995;18:188–194.
43. Bokinsky G, Miller M, Ault K, Husband P, Mitchell J. Spontaneous platelet activation and aggregation during obstructive sleep apnea and its response to therapy with nasal continuous positive airway pressure. A preliminary investigation. *Chest* 1995;108:625–630.
44. Sanner BM, Konermann M, Tepel M, Groetz J, Mummenhoff C, Zidek W. Platelet function in

patients with obstructive sleep apnoea syndrome. *Eur Respir J* 2000;16:648–652.
45. Olson LJ, Olson EJ, Somers VK. Obstructive sleep apnea and platelet activation: Another potential link between sleep-disordered breathing and cardiovascular disease. *Chest* 2004;126:339–341.
46. Hui DS, Ko FW, Fok JP, *et al.* The effects of nasal continuous positive airway pressure on platelet activation in obstructive sleep apnea syndrome. *Chest* 2004;125:1768–1775.
47. Chin K, Ohi M, Kita H, *et al.* Effects of NCPAP therapy on fibrinogen levels in obstructive sleep apnea syndrome. *Am J Respir Crit Care Med* 1996; 153:1972–1976.
48. Wessendorf TE, Thilmann AF, Wang YM, Schreiber A, Konietzko N, Teschler H. Fibrinogen levels and obstructive sleep apnea in ischemic stroke. *Am J Respir Crit Care Med* 2000;162:2039–2042.
49. Keyl C, Lemberger P, Rodig G, Dambacher M, Frey AW. Changes in cardiac autonomic control during nocturnal repetitive oxygen desaturation episodes in patients with coronary artery disease. *J Cardiovasc Risk* 1996;3:221–227.
50. Vanninen E, Tuunainen A, Kansanen M, Uusitupa M, Lansimies E. Cardiac sympathovagal balance during sleep apnea episodes. *Clin Physiol* 1996;16: 209–216.
51. Bauer T, Ewig S, Schafer H, Jelen E, Omran H, Luderitz B. Heart rate variability in patients with sleep-related breathing disorders. *Cardiology* 1996;87:492–496.
52. Shiomi T, Guilleminault C, Sasanabe R, Hirota I, Maekawa M, Kobayashi T. Augmented very low frequency component of heart rate variability during obstructive sleep apnea. *Sleep* 1996;19:370–377.
53. Roche F, Xuong AN, Court-Fortune I, *et al.* Relationship among the severity of sleep apnea syndrome, cardiac arrhythmias, and autonomic imbalance. *Pacing Clin Electrophysiol* 2003;26:669–677.
54. Narkiewicz K, Pesek CA, Kato M, Phillips BG, Davison DE, Somers VK. Baroreflex control of sympathetic nerve activity and heart rate in obstructive sleep apnea. *Hypertension* 1998;32:1039–1043.
55. Bonsignore MR, Parati G, Insalaco G, *et al.* Baroreflex control of heart rate during sleep in severe obstructive sleep apnoea: Effects of acute CPAP. *Eur Respir J* 2006;27:128–135.
56. Jo JA, Blasi A, Valladares E, Juarez R, Baydur A, Khoo MC. Determinants of heart rate variability in obstructive sleep apnea syndrome during wakefulness and sleep. *Am J Physiol Heart Circ Physiol* 2005;288:H1103–H112.
57. Gillis AM, Stoohs R, Guilleminault C. Changes in the QT interval during obstructive sleep apnea. *Sleep* 1991;14:346–350.
58. Roche F, Barthelemy JC, Garet M, Duverney D, Pichot V, Sforza E. Continuous positive airway pressure treatment improves the QT rate dependence adaptation of obstructive sleep apnea patients. *Pacing Clin Electrophysiol* 2005;28:819–825.
59. Roche F, Gaspoz JM, Court-Fortune I, *et al.* Alteration of QT rate dependence reflects cardiac autonomic imbalance in patients with obstructive sleep apnea syndrome. *Pacing Clin Electrophysiol* 2003;26:1446–1453.
60. Dursunoglu D, Dursunoglu N, Evrengul H, *et al.* QT interval dispersion in obstructive sleep apnoea syndrome patients without hypertension. *Eur Respir J* 2005;25:677–681.
61. Nakamura T, Chin K, Hosokawa R, *et al.* Corrected QT dispersion and cardiac sympathetic function in patients with obstructive sleep apnea-hypopnea syndrome. *Chest* 2004;125:2107–2114.
62. Zwillich C, Devlin T, White D, Douglas N, Weil J, Martin R. Bradycardia during sleep apnea. Characteristics and mechanism. *J Clin Invest* 1982;69: 1286–1292.
63. Tilkian AG, Guilleminault C, Schroeder JS, *et al.* Sleep-induced apnea-syndrome: Prevalence of cardiac arrhythmias and their reversal after tracheostomy. *Am J Med* 1977;63:348–358.
64. Guilleminault C, Conolly SJ, Winkle RA. Cardiac arrhythmia and conduction disturbances during sleep in 400 patients with sleep apnea syndrome. *Am J Cardiol* 1983;52:490–494.
65. Fichter J, Bauer D, Arampatzis S, Fries R, Heisel A, Sybrecht GW. Sleep-related breathing disorders are associated with ventricular arrhythmias in patients with an implantable cardioverter-defibrillator. *Chest* 2002;122:558–561.
66. Fries R, Bauer D, Heisel A, *et al.* Clinical significance of sleep-related breathing disorders in patients with implantable cardioverter defibrillators. *Pacing Clin Electrophysiol* 1999;22:223–227.
67. Harbison J, O'Reilly P, McNicholas WT. Cardiac rhythm disturbances in the obstructive sleep apnea syndrome: Effects of nasal continuous positive airway pressure therapy. *Chest* 2000;118:591–595.
68. Koehler U, Fus E, Grimm W, *et al.* Heart block in patients with obstructive sleep apnoea: Pathogenetic factors and effects of treatment. *Eur Respir J* 1998;11:434–439.

69. Koehler U, Becker HF, Grimm W, Heitmann J, Peter JH, Schafer H. Relations among hypoxemia, sleep stage, and bradyarrhythmia during obstructive sleep apnea. *Am Heart J* 2000;139:142–148.
70. Grimm W, Hoffmann J, Menz V, *et al.* Electrophysiologic evaluation of sinus node function and atrioventricular conduction in patients with prolonged ventricular asystole during obstructive sleep apnea. *Am J Cardiol* 1996;77:1310–1314.
71. Becker HF, Koehler U, Stammnitz A, Peter JH. Heart block in patients with sleep apnoea. *Thorax* 1998;53(Suppl. 3):S29–S32.
72. Mehra R, Benjamin EJ, Shahar E, *et al.* Association of nocturnal arrhythmias with sleep-disordered breathing: The Sleep Heart Health Study. *Am J Respir Crit Care Med* 2006;173:910–916.
73. Becker H, Brandenburg U, Peter JH, Von Wichert P. Reversal of sinus arrest and atrioventricular conduction block in patients with sleep apnea during nasal continuous positive airway pressure. *Am J Respir Crit Care Med* 1995;151:215–218.
74. Luu M, Stevenson WG, Stevenson LW, Baron K, Walden J. Diverse mechanisms of unexpected cardiac arrest in advanced heart failure. *Circulation* 1989;80:1675–1680.
75. Kempf FC Jr, Josephson ME. Cardiac arrest recorded on ambulatory electrocardiograms. *Am J Cardiol* 1984;53:1577–1582.
76. Faggiano P, d'Aloia A, Gualeni A, Gardini A, Giordano A. Mechanisms and immediate outcome of in-hospital cardiac arrest in patients with advanced heart failure secondary to ischemic or idiopathic dilated cardiomyopathy. *Am J Cardiol* 2001;87:655–657, A10–A11.
77. Yaggi HK, Concato J, Kernan WN, Lichtman JH, Brass LM, Mohsenin V. Obstructive sleep apnea as a risk factor for stroke and death. *N Engl J Med* 2005;353:2034–2041.
78. Arias MA, Alonso-Fernandez A, Garcia-Rio F. Obstructive sleep apnea as an independent risk factor for stroke and mortality. *Stroke* 2006;37:1150; author reply 1150.
79. Eckardt M, Gerlach L, Welter FL. Prolongation of the frequency-corrected QT dispersion following cerebral strokes with involvement of the insula of Reil. *Eur Neurol* 1999;42:190–193.
80. Oppenheimer S. Cerebrogenic cardiac arrhythmias: Cortical lateralization and clinical significance. *Clin Auton Res* 2006;16:6–11.
81. Pearce S, Saunders P. Obstructive sleep apnoea can directly cause death. *Thorax* 2003;58:369.
82. Dyken ME, Yamada T, Glenn CL, Berger HA. Obstructive sleep apnea associated with cerebral hypoxemia and death. *Neurology* 2004;62:491–493.
83. Hudgel DW, Gordon EA, Thanakitcharu S, Bruce EN. Instability of ventilatory control in patients with obstructive sleep apnea. *Am J Respir Crit Care Med* 1998;158:1142–1149.
84. Garcia-Rio F, Pino JM, Ramirez T, *et al.* Inspiratory neural drive response to hypoxia adequately estimates peripheral chemosensitivity in OSAHS patients. *Eur Respir J* 2002;20:724–732.
85. Shamsuzzaman AS, Gersh BJ, Somers VK. Obstructive sleep apnea: Implications for cardiac and vascular disease. *JAMA* 2003;290:1906–1914.
86. Lavie P, Herer P, Hoffstein V. Obstructive sleep apnoea syndrome as a risk factor for hypertension: Population study. *BMJ* 2000;320:479–482.
87. Peker Y, Hedner J, Norum J, Kraiczi H, Carlson J. Increased incidence of cardiovascular disease in middle-aged men with obstructive sleep apnea: A 7-year follow-up. *Am J Respir Crit Care Med* 2002; 166:159–165.
88. Chobanian AV, Bakris GL, Black HR, *et al.* The Seventh Report of the Joint National Committee on Prevention, Detection, Evaluation, and Treatment of High Blood Pressure: The JNC 7 report. *JAMA* 2003;289:2560–2572.
89. Shahar E, Whitney CW, Redline S, *et al.* Sleep-disordered breathing and cardiovascular disease: Cross-sectional results of the Sleep Heart Health Study. *Am J Respir Crit Care Med* 2001;163:19–25.
90. Mooe T, Franklin KA, Holmstrom K, Rabben T, Wiklund U. Sleep-disordered breathing and coronary artery disease: Long-term prognosis. *Am J Respir Crit Care Med* 2001;164:1910–1913.
91. Peker Y, Hedner J, Kraiczi H, Loth S. Respiratory disturbance index: An independent predictor of mortality in coronary artery disease. *Am J Respir Crit Care Med* 2000;162:81–86.
92. Marin JM, Carrizo SJ, Vicente E, Agusti AG. Long-term cardiovascular outcomes in men with obstructive sleep apnoea-hypopnoea with or without treatment with continuous positive airway pressure: An observational study. *Lancet* 2005;365:1046–1053.
93. Marrone O, Riccobono L, Salvaggio A, Mirabella A, Bonanno A, Bonsignore MR. Catecholamines and blood pressure in obstructive sleep apnea syndrome. *Chest* 1993;103:722–777.
94. Dimsdale JE, Coy T, Ziegler MG, Ancoli-Israel S, Clausen J. The effect of sleep apnea on plasma and urinary catecholamines. *Sleep* 1995;18:377–381.
95. Hedner J, Ejnell H, Sellgren J, Hedner T, Wallin G. Is high and fluctuating muscle nerve sympathetic

activity in the sleep apnea syndrome of pathogenetic importance for the development of hypertension? *J Hypertens* 1988;6:S529–S531.
96. Narkiewicz K, van de Borne P, Montano N, Dyken M, Phillips B, Somers V. Contribution of tonic chemoreflex activation to sympathetic activity and blood pressure in patients with obstructive sleep apnea. *Circulation* 1998;97:943–945.
97. Zipes DP, Rubart M. Neural modulation of cardiac arrhythmias and sudden cardiac death. *Heart Rhythm* 2006;3:108–113.
98. La Rovere MT, Pinna GD, Hohnloser SH, *et al.* Baroreflex sensitivity and heart rate variability in the identification of patients at risk for life-threatening arrhythmias: Implications for clinical trials. *Circulation* 2001;103:2072–2077.
99. Tkacova R, Rankin F, Fitzgerald FS, Floras JS, Bradley TD. Effects of continuous positive airway pressure on obstructive sleep apnea and left ventricular afterload in patients with heart failure. *Circulation* 1998;98:2269–2275.
100. Alchanatis M, Paradellis G, Pini H, Tourkohoriti G, Jordanoglou J. Left ventricular function in patients with obstructive sleep apnoea syndrome before and after treatment with nasal continuous positive airway pressure. *Respiration* 2000;67:367–371.
101. Alchanatis M, Tourkohoriti G, Kosmas EN, *et al.* Evidence for left ventricular dysfunction in patients with obstructive sleep apnoea syndrome. *Eur Respir J* 2002;20:1239–1245.
102. Laaban JP, Pascal-Sebaoun S, Bloch E, Orvoen-Frija E, Oppert JM, Huchon G. Left ventricular systolic dysfunction in patients with obstructive sleep apnea syndrome. *Chest* 2002;122:1133–1138.
103. Kaneko Y, Floras JS, Usui K, *et al.* Cardiovascular effects of continuous positive airway pressure in patients with heart failure and obstructive sleep apnea. *N Engl J Med* 2003;348:1233–1241.
104. Partinen M, Jamieson A, Guilleminault C. Long-term outcome for obstructive sleep apnea syndrome patients. Mortality. *Chest* 1988;94:1200–1204.
105. He J, Kryger MH, Zorick FJ, Conway W, Roth T. Mortality and apnea index in obstructive sleep apnea. Experience in 385 male patients. *Chest* 1988;94:9–14.
106. Koehler U, Wetzig T, Peter JH, Ploch T, Schafer H, Stellwaag M. [Morbidity and mortality in sleep apnea and nocturnal bradyarrhythmia]. *Dtsch Med Wochenschr* 1994;119:1187–1193.
107. Keenan SP, Burt H, Ryan CF, Fleetham JA. Long-term survival of patients with obstructive sleep apnea treated by uvulopalatopharyngoplasty or nasal CPAP. *Chest* 1994;105:155–159.
108. Grimm W, Koehler U, Fus E, *et al.* Outcome of patients with sleep apnea-associated severe bradyarrhythmias after continuous positive airway pressure therapy. *Am J Cardiol* 2000;86:688–692, A9.
109. Doherty LS, Kiely JL, Swan V, McNicholas WT. Long-term effects of nasal continuous positive airway pressure therapy on cardiovascular outcomes in sleep apnea syndrome. *Chest* 2005;127:2076–2084.
110. Campos-Rodriguez F, Pena-Grinan N, Reyes-Nunez N, *et al.* Mortality in obstructive sleep apnea-hypopnea patients treated with positive airway pressure. *Chest* 2005;128:624–633.
111. Cohen MC, Rohtla KM, Lavery CE, Muller JE, Mittleman MA. Meta-analysis of the morning excess of acute myocardial infarction and sudden cardiac death. *Am J Cardiol* 1997;79:1512–1516.
112. Seppala T, Partinen M, Penttila A, Aspholm R, Tiainen E, Kaukianen A. Sudden death and sleeping history among Finnish men. *J Intern Med* 1991;229:23–28.
113. Gami AS, Howard DE, Olson EJ, Somers VK. Day-night pattern of sudden death in obstructive sleep apnea. *N Engl J Med* 2005;352:1206–1214.

61
Sudden Cardiac Death in Athletes

Domenico Corrado, Barry J. Maron, Cristina Basso, Antonio Pelliccia, and Gaetano Thiene

Introduction

Although sudden cardiac death (SCD) during sports is a rare event, it always has a tragic impact on the community because it occurs in apparently healthy individuals and assumes great visibility through the news media, due to the high public profile of competitive athletes.[1–4] For centuries it was a mystery why cardiac arrest should occur in vigorous athletes, who had previously achieved extraordinary exercise performance without complaining of any symptoms. The cause was generally ascribed to myocardial infarction, even though evidence of ischemic myocardial necrosis was rarely reported. It is now clear that the most common mechanism of SCD during sports activity is an abrupt ventricular tachyarrhythmia as a consequence of a wide spectrum of cardiovascular diseases, either acquired or congenital. The culprit diseases are often clinically silent and unlikely to be suspected or diagnosed on the basis of spontaneous symptoms. Systematic preparticipation screening of all subjects embarking in sports activity has the potential to identify those athletes at risk and to reduce mortality. Guidelines for athletic participation have been developed based on the best available information regarding the risks of the underlying cardiovascular condition.

In this chapter we will examine the prevalence, causes, and mechanisms of SCD in the athlete and review the available evidence on systematic preparticipation screening for prevention of fatalities on the athletic field.

Epidemiological Profile of Sudden Cardiac Death in Athletes

The frequency with which SCD occurs during sports activity is fortunately low and varies in the different athlete series reported in the literature. In apparently healthy adults (>35 years of age), joggers, or marathon racers, the estimated rate of sports-related fatalities ranges from 1:15,000 to 1:50,000.[5] In comparison, a significantly lower incidence of fatal events has been reported in young competitive athletes (≤35 years of age). Van Camp *et al.*[6] in a nationally based survey estimated the prevalence of SCD in high school and college athletes in the United States to be 0.4 per 100,000 athletes per year. Maron *et al.*[7] showed the prevalence of SCD in competitive high school athletes (aged 13–19 years, mean 16) from Minnesota to be 0.35 per 100,000 sports participations and 0.46 per 100,000 individual participants per year (0.77 per 100,000 male athletes).

A prospective population-based study in the Veneto Region of Italy reported an incidence of SCD of 2.3 (2.6 in males and 1.1 in females) per 100,000 athletes (aged 12–35 years) per year by all causes and of 2.1 per 100,000 athletes per year by cardiovascular diseases.[8] The reasons for the higher mortality rates found in Italian athletes compared to those reported by Maron *et al.*[7] may include (1) a different study design (prospective vs. retrospective analysis); (2) different underlying pathological substrates, which, in part, reflect differences in ethnic and genetic factors;

(3) participation at a higher level of intensity among Italian competitive athletes; and (4) the higher mean value of the age in our athlete series (mean age 23 years) as compared with U.S. high school and college participants (mean age 16 years). In this regard, it is noteworthy that the development of phenotypic manifestation and arrhythmic substrates of most heart diseases at risk of SCD during sports, including cardiomyopathies, premature coronary artery disease, ion channel diseases (such as Brugada syndrome), and progressive cardiac conduction disease (such as Lenègre disease) is age dependent and occurs during young adulthood.[2,9,10] Therefore, the risk of fatal events in older Italian athletes is expectedly greater and may explain differences from U.S. estimates.

Moreover, in the Veneto region study, athletic field SCD showed a clear gender predilection with striking male predominance (male-to-female ratio of 10:1). This predominance of fatal events in male athletes is consistent with the findings of previous surveys of athletic field deaths and has been explained by the fact that females participate less commonly in competitive sports programs than males.[1–6] Accordingly, the prevalence of sports participation in the female young population in the Veneto region study was only 25% of that of the male individuals.[8] Although the higher incidence of fatal events in male athletes may be related to the higher participation rate of male compared to female athletes in competitive sports, more recent data suggest that male gender may be in itself a risk factor for sports-related SCD. This is likely a consequence of the greater phenotypic expression of cardiomyopathies and the higher prevalence of premature coronary artery risk of sports-related cardiac arrest in males during the competition age range.

Cardiovascular fatalities are most commonly recorded among players of the most popular sports such as basketball and football in the United States and among soccer players in Europe.[1–4] However, it has not been reported that there is a statistically significant higher incidence of SCD in basketball or soccer players compared with athletes participating in all other sports, suggesting that there is not a significant association between specific sports and the risk of cardiovascular events.[8]

Causes of Sudden Cardiac Death in the Athlete

The majority of athletes who die suddenly have underlying structural heart diseases, which provide a substrate for ventricular fibrillation leading to cardiac arrest. As reported in Table 61–1, the causes of SCD reflect the age of the participants. Although atherosclerotic coronary artery disease accounts for the majority of fatalities in adults (aged >35 years),[5,11,12] in younger athletes a broad spectrum of cardiovascular substrates (including congenital and inherited heart disorders) has been reported.[1–4,13–22] Cardiomyopathies have been consistently implicated as the leading cause of sports-related cardiac arrest in the young, with hypertrophic cardiomyopathy accounting for more than one-third of fatal cases in the United States and arrhythmogenic right ventricular cardiomyopathy/dysplasia for approximately one-fourth in the Veneto Region of Italy.[1,2] Other cardiovascular substrates include congenital coronary anomalies, premature atherosclerotic coronary artery disease, myocarditis, dilated cardiomyopathy, mitral valve prolapse, conduction system diseases, and Wolff–Parkinson–White (WPW) syndrome (Figure 61–1).

Coronary Artery Disease

Atherosclerotic coronary artery disease is the major cause of fatal events in athletes over 35 years of age. Most deaths occur with running, jogging, long-distance racing, and other vigorous

Table 61–1. Cardiovascular causes of sudden cardiac death associated with sports.

Age ≥35 years
Coronary artery disease
Age <35 years
Hypertrophic cardiomyopathy
Arrhythmogenic right ventricular cardiomyopathy/dysplasia
Congenital anomalies of coronary arteries
Myocarditis
Aortic rupture
Valvular disease
Preexcitation syndromes and conduction diseases
Ion channel diseases
Congenital heart disease, operated or unoperated

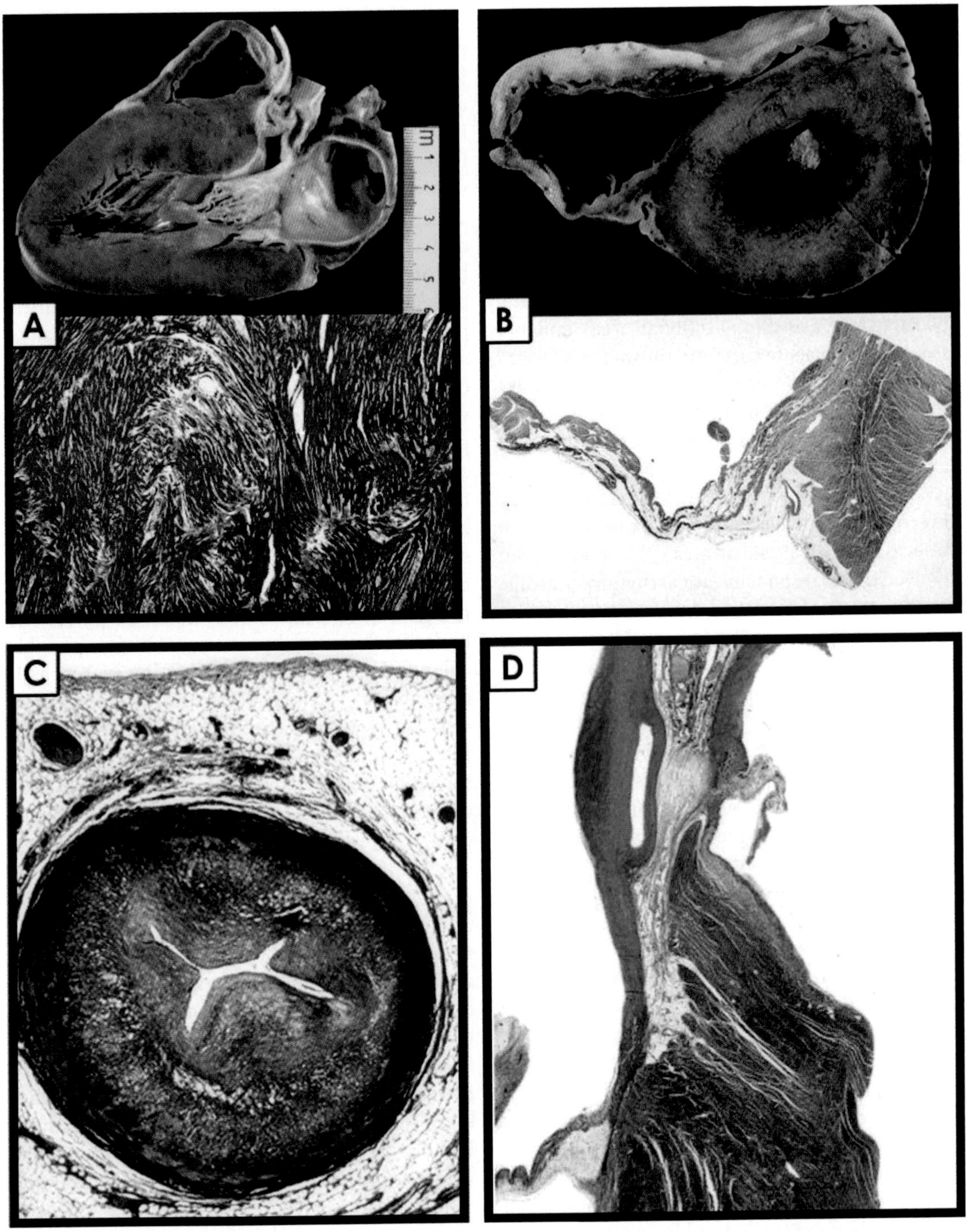

FIGURE 61–1. Leading causes of sudden cardiovascular death in young competitive athletes. (A) Hypertrophic cardiomyopathy: long axis cut of the heart specimen showing asymmetric septal hypertrophy with subaortic bulging and septal endocardial fibrous plaque (top); histology of the interventricular septum revealing typical myocardial disarray with interstitial fibrosis (bottom) (Heidenhain trichrome). (B) Arrhythmogenic right ventricular cardiomyopathy/dysplasia: cross section of the heart specimen with infundibular and inferior subtricuspid aneurysms (top); panoramic histological view of an aneurysm of the inferior wall showing wall thinning with fibrofatty replacement (bottom) (Heidenhain trichrome). (C) Premature coronary artery disease: histology of the proximal tract of the left anterior descending coronary artery showing a fibrous plaque causing severe lumen narrowing (Heidenhain trichrome). (D) Congenital coronary anomaly: panoramic histological view showing the intramural aortic course with a slit-like lumen of the anomalous right coronary artery arising from the left aortic sinus of Valsalva and running between the aorta and the pulmonary trunk (Heidenhain trichrome).

sports such as soccer, tennis, and squash. During exercise, physical and metabolic changes occur, leading to an increased risk of acute coronary complications and life-threatening myocardial ischemia.[23,24] Even in highly conditioned individuals, sudden coronary death may be precipitated by underlying concealed atherosclerotic plaques. At postmortem, pathological findings in SCD victims are consistent with an underlying severe and diffuse atherosclerotic coronary artery disease, with two or more coronary trunks critically obstructed (≥75% cross-sectional area) and are associated with acute coronary thrombosis.[11,12,23,24] In the territory tributary of the culprit coronary artery, the myocardium may show signs of hyperacute myocardial ischemia such as contraction band necrosis, acute myocardial infarction, or myocardial scar due to a healed (often previously unrecognized) myocardial infarction. Based on these pathological substrates, the mechanism involved that is responsible for arrhythmic cardiac arrest consists of ventricular tachycardia/fibrillation related to ventricular scar, acute myocardial ischemia, or both; electrical instability is favored by sympathetic stimulation occurring during physical exertion.

Highly trained athletes, such as marathon runners, are not spared from severe atherosclerotic disease and sudden coronary death. Alarming symptoms suggestive of coronary artery disease and/or coronary risk factors including smoking, hypertension, hypercholesterolemia, and family history of coronary events before 55 years have often been recognized in adults who experienced exercise-induced cardiac arrest. It is thus recommended that a careful history for factors causally related to atherosclerosis or symptoms of coronary artery disease should be taken for athletes older than age 35 years and sports activity undertaken cautiously, particularly in the presence of risk factors. Stress testing may have significant limitations for detecting subjects at risk among the general population, and acute myocardial infarction and sudden coronary death may occur despite a negative exercise test. Education of athletes should be aimed at increasing awareness of warning symptoms such as chest pain, palpitations, or syncope, mostly occurring during physical exercise, and at improving lifestyle for prevention of coronary artery disease.

Coronary atherosclerosis is an important substrate for SCD even in young competitive athletes (≤35 years).[9,31] In these young subjects, coronary artery disease exhibits distinctive characteristics in terms of warning clinical prodromal and pathological features, such as extent, site, and morphology of obstructive atherosclerotic plaques. Young athletes dying of premature coronary artery disease usually had neither risk factors nor a history of angina pectoris and previous myocardial infarction, and SCD is often the first manifestation of the disease. Exercise testing may fail to show myocardial ischemia or arrhythmias. Fatal coronary atherosclerosis is more often a "single-vessel disease" that characteristically affects the proximal left anterior descending coronary artery and is often due to fibrocellular plaques (i.e., fibrous plaques with intimal smooth muscle cell hyperplasia, so-called "accelerated atherosclerosis") and a preserved tunica media in the absence of acute thrombosis[9] (Figure 61–1C). These morphological features have been suggested to underlie abnormal hypervasoreactivity, possibly culminating in cardiac arrest by vasospastic myocardial ischemia. Because of the scarcity of warning symptoms and the limitation of exercise testing, the identification at preparticipation screening of these young athletes with premature coronary atherosclerosis at risk of ischemic cardiac arrest remains a challenge.

Hypertrophic Cardiomyopathy

Hypertrophic cardiomyopathy is a heart muscle disease, usually genetically transmitted, and characterized by a hypertrophied, nondilated left ventricle in the absence of another cardiac or systemic disease capable of producing the magnitude of hypertrophy evident.[32,33] Characteristic morphological and functional cardiac abnormalities include asymmetric left ventricular hypertrophy with disproportionate septal thickening and reduction in left ventricular chamber size with increased myocardial stiffness, which may critically impair diastolic left ventricular and intramural coronary blood filling (Figure 61–1A). Dynamic left ventricular outflow tract obstruction is also demonstrable at rest or with exercise in a large proportion of patients. The histopathological hallmark of hypertrophic cardiomyopathy is myocardial disarray, with a widespread, bizarre, and disordered arrangement of myocytes associated with diffuse interstitial and/or replacement-type fibrosis (Figure 61–1A). Myocardial scarring is an acquired phenomenon, in part related to abnormalities of the intramural coronary arteries, which show dysplasia of the tunica media with luminal narrowing ("small vessel disease").

Hypertrophic cardiomyopathy has been implicated as the principal cause of SCD during sports in the United States.[1] Cardiac arrest in affected athletes has been attributed to ventricular arrhythmias, most likely arising from an electrically unstable myocardial substrate. The observation of acquired myocardial damage, either acute or in the setting of large septal scars, supports the hypothesis that myocardial ischemia intervenes in the natural history of the disease and contributes to the arrhythmogenicity.[19]

Electrocardiogram (ECG) abnormalities such as an increased QRS voltage, pathological "Q" waves, and repolarization changes have been reported in up to 95% of patients with hypertrophic cardiomyopathy.[33] This explains why systematic preparticipation screening of young competitive athletes in Italy by ECG (in addition to history and physical examination) has permitted successful identification of athletes with hypertrophic cardiomyopathy.[14,34]

Arrhythmogenic Right Ventricular Cardiomyopathy/Dysplasia

Arrhythmogenic right ventricular cardiomyopathy/dysplasia is an inherited heart muscle disorder that is characterized pathologically by fibrofatty replacement of right ventricular myocardium.[10,17,35–37] The most frequent clinical manifestations consist of ECG depolarization/repolarization changes mostly localized to right precordial leads, global and/or regional morphological and functional alterations of the right ventricle, and arrhythmias of right ventricular origin that can lead to SCD, especially during physical exercise. The propensity for sudden arrhythmic death during physical exercise is linked to both hemodynamic and neurohumoral factors. Physical exercise may acutely increase right ventricular afterload and cavity enlargement, which in turn, may elicit ventricular arrhythmias by stretching the diseased right ventricular musculature. Alternatively, the hypothesis of "denervation supersensitivity" of the right ventricle to catecholamines has been advanced. Finally, in a subgroup of patients with familial arrhythmogenic right ventricular cardiomyopathy/dysplasia (ARVD2), a cardiac ryanodine receptor (RyR2) missense mutation leading to abnormal calcium release from the sarcoplasmic reticulum during effort has been identified.[38]

The heart of young competitive athletes dying suddenly from arrhythmogenic right ventricular cardiomyopathy/dysplasia demonstrates right ventricular dilation and massive transmural fibrofatty replacement of the right ventricular musculature resulting in aneurysmal dilations of posterobasal, apical, and outflow tract regions, which are potential sources of life-threatening ventricular arrhythmias (Figure 61–1B). These pathological features of the right ventricle allow differential diagnosis with training-induced right ventricular changes ("athlete's heart"), usually consisting of global right ventricular enlargement without wall motion abnormalities.

Arrhythmogenic right ventricular cardiomyopathy/dysplasia has been reported to be the leading cause of sports-related SCD in the Veneto Region of northeastern Italy.[2,8,14] The most likely explanation for this finding is that systematic preparticipation screening of young competitive athletes has changed the natural prevalence of cardiovascular causes of sports-related SCD. In Italy, SCDs due to hypertrophic cardiomyopathy have been largely prevented by identification and disqualification of the affected athletes at preparticipation screening. Therefore, other cardiovascular conditions such as arrhythmogenic right ventricular cardiomyopathy/dysplasia have come to account for a greater proportion of all SCD in Italian athletes.

Early identification of athletes with arrhythmogenic right ventricular cardiomyopathy/dysplasia plays a crucial role in the prevention of SCD during sports. The disease should be suspected in the presence of inverted T waves in right precordial leads.[36,37] Diagnosis relies on visualization of morphofunctional right ventricular abnormalities by current imaging techniques (such as echocardiography, angiography, and cardiac magnetic resonance) and, in selected cases, by histopathological demonstration of fibrofatty substitution at endomyocardial biopsy. It is noteworthy that more than 80% of athletes of the Veneto Region series who died from arrhythmogenic right ventricular cardiomyopathy/dysplasia had a history of syncope, ECG changes, and/or ventricular arrhythmias. Nevertheless, they had not been identified at preparticipation screening because the disease was unrecognized clinically. More recently, with the increased awareness of clinical findings of arrhythmogenic right ventricular cardiomyopathy/dysplasia, more affected athletes are being detected by screening and protected from the risks of athletic competition.

Congenital Coronary Artery Anomaly

An anomalous origin of a coronary artery from the "wrong" coronary sinus is a congenital malformation with a silent clinical course, which may precipitate sudden and unexpected ischemic cardiac arrest in young competitive athletes.[16–18] The most frequent anatomic findings consist of both (left and right) coronary arteries arising either from the right or the left coronary sinus. In both conditions, as the anomalous coronary vessel leaves the aorta, it adopts an acute angle with the aortic wall, and, thus, traverses between the aorta and the pulmonary trunk, often following an aortic intramural course, with a "slit-like" lumen (Figure 61–1D). Fatal myocardial ischemia has been hypothesized to be caused by exercise-induced aortic root expansion, which compresses the anomalous vessel against the pulmonary trunk and increases the acute angulation of the coronary take-off, aggravating the "slit-like" shape of the lumen of the proximal intramural portion of the aberrant coronary vessel. This mechanism of myocardial ischemia is difficult to be reproduced in clinical setting, as shown by the occurrence of negative ECG exercise testing in young athletes who have subsequently died suddenly from the above coronary anomaly.[18]

Other Causes

Myocarditis, either in its acute or healed forms, may provide a myocardial electrical substrate for ventricular arrhythmias and exercise-related SCD.[21–22,38] Life-threatening ventricular arrhythmias in athletes may be due to focal myocarditis, which is clinically silent and difficult to be detected by endomyocardial biopsy.

Spontaneous laceration or dissection of the ascending aorta with rupture into the pericardial cavity and cardiac tamponade is a rare cause of fatal electromechanical dissociation during sports. The basic heart defect is an elastic fragmentation of the aortic tunica media with cystic medial necrosis, which may rarely present as an isolated histological feature, but is more frequently found in association with isthmic coarctation and/or bicuspid aortic valve, or in the setting of Marfan syndrome.

Despite its high prevalence in the general population, mitral valve prolapse is a rare cause of SCD in athletes. The pathogenesis of sudden cardiac arrest remains unresolved. Fatal coronary embolism from atrial platelet deposits and cardiac arrest due to malignant ventricular tachyarrhythmias attributed to "valve friction" have been advanced as possible mechanisms.

Ventricular preexcitation syndrome (WPW syndrome) or progressive cardiac conduction disease (Lenègre disease) may represent an uncommon substrate for exercise-related SCD.[20]

Ion Channel Diseases

Two to five percent of young people and athletes who die suddenly have no evidence of structural heart diseases and the cause of their cardiac arrest is in all likelihood related to a primary electrical heart disease such as inherited cardiac ion channel defects (channelopathies) including long QT syndrome, Brugada syndrome, and cathecholaminergic polymorphic ventricular tachycardia.[22,40–43]

Brugada syndrome is an inherited ion channel disease characterized by a peculiar ECG pattern consisting of right precordial "coved type" ST-segment elevation (both spontaneous or induced by pharmacological sodium channel blockade) in association with arrhythmia-related syncope/cardiac arrest, inducibility at programmed ventricular stimulation, or a familial history of SCD. A cardiac sodium channel gene (SCN5A) mutation has been detected in up to 30% of Brugada syndrome cases. Ventricular fibrillation leading to SCD usually occurs at rest and in many cases at night (during sleep) as a consequence of an increased vagal stimulation and/or withdrawal of sympathetic activity. Enhanced adrenergic drive, such as occurs during sports activity, could have an inhibitory effect and theoretically reduce the risk of SCD. On the other hand, the adaptation of the cardiac autonomic nervous system to systematic training, which results in increased resting vagal tone, or during the postexercise recovery period may enhance the propensity of athletes with Brugada syndrome to die at rest, during sleep, or immediately after effort.[43]

Catecholaminergic ventricular tachycardia is an inherited ion channel disease characterized by exercise-induced polymorphic ventricular tachycardia (most often with the so called "bidirectional" pattern), which can degenerate in ventricular fibrillation. Unlike long QT syndrome and Brugada syndrome, this condition is not associated with abnormalities of basal 12-lead ECG and remains unrecognized unless the athlete undergoes ECG stress testing. A genetically defective ryanodine receptor has been reported to account for an abnormal calcium release from the sarcoplasmic reticulum. Accordingly, the potential arrhythmogenic mechanism is triggered activity due to late afterdepolarizations, which are provoked by intracellular calcium overload and enhanced by adrenergic stimulation such as during sports exercise.

Rarely SCD may be caused either by a nonarrhythmic mechanism such as aortic rupture complicating Marfan syndrome and bicuspid aortic valve or by noncardiac conditions including bronchial asthma and rupture of a cerebral aneurysm.

Trauma-Related Sudden Cardiac Death

Two circumstances in which trauma-related SCD occurs during sports involve blunt, nonpenetrating, and often innocent appearing blows to the precordium or neck.[44,45] Instantaneous death has been reported during ice hockey in which high-velocity blows to the neck by the puck trigger arterial rupture and subarachnoid hemorrhage.[44] The likely mechanism is reflex hyperextension of the head causing vertebral artery dissection at its fixed anchor point within the foramina transversarium.

More commonly, precordial blows may trigger ventricular fibrillation without structural injury to ribs, sternum, or heart itself (commotio cordis).[45,46] These events are more common causes of athletic field deaths than most of the aforementioned cardiovascular diseases. Commotio cordis is most frequently caused by projectiles that are implements of the game and that strike the chest at a broad range of velocities, i.e., hockey pucks or lacrosse balls (up to 90 mph), but more frequently blows with only modest force (e.g., a pitched Little League baseball striking a batter at 30–40 mph), and also by virtue of bodily collision (e.g., a karate blow or two outfielders tracking a baseball).[45]

Based on clinical observations and an experimental animal model (which replicates commotio cordis), the mechanism by which ventricular fibrillation and SCD occur requires a blow directly over the heart, exquisitely timed to within a narrow 10–30 msec window just prior to the T wave peak during the vulnerable phase of repolarization.[46] Basic electrophysiological mechanisms of commotio cordis are largely unresolved, although selective K^+_{ATP} channel activation appears to play a role.[47]

Only about 15% of commotio cordis victims survive, usually associated with timely cardiopulmonary resuscitation and defibrillation.[45] There are reports of both successful and unsuccessful resuscitation with automated external defibrillators.[48,49] Strategies for primary prevention of commotio cordis include innovations in sports equipment design.[50]

Risk of Sudden Cardiac Death During Sports

Death usually occurs either during (80%) or immediately after (20%) athletic activity, suggesting that participation in competitive sports increases the likelihood of cardiac arrest. The risk–benefit ratio of physical exercise differs between adults and young competitive athletes. This may be explained by the different nature of cardiovascular substrates underlying sport-related SCD in the two age groups.

Cardiovascular Risk in Adults

Atherosclerotic coronary artery disease is the most common cause of SCD in adults and elderly exercising subjects. Several epidemiological studies have assessed the relationship between physical exercise and the risk of sudden coronary events in the middle-aged and older population in which physical activity can be regarded as a "two-edged sword."[25,26] The available evidence indicates vigorous exercise acutely increases the incidence rate of both cardiac arrest and acute myocardial infarction in persons who do not exercise regularly. In comparison, epidemiological studies support the concept that habitual sports activity may offer protection over the long term from cardiovascular events.[5,27–29] The relative risk of cardiac arrest or myocardial infarction is greater during exercise than at rest; however, the overall incidence of cardiac arrest, both at rest and during exercise, decreases with increasing exercise levels. Regular exercise prevents the development and progression of atherosclerotic coronary artery disease by favorable effects on lipid metabolism and weight reduction and enhances both coronary artery plaque and myocardial electrical stability.

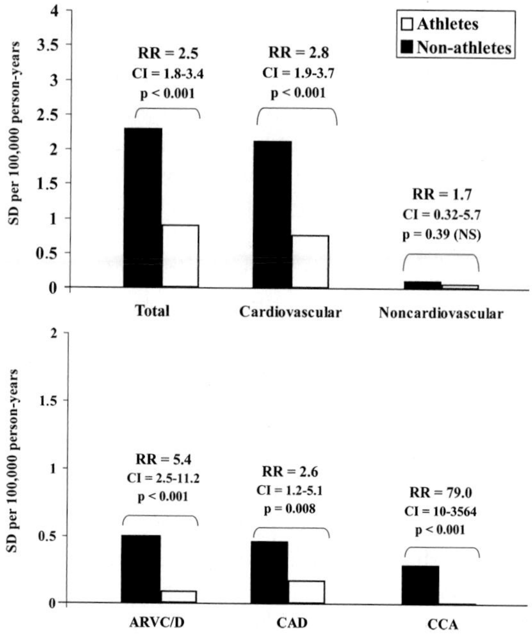

FIGURE 61–2. Incidence and relative risk (RR) of SCD among young athletes and nonathletes from total, cardiovascular, and noncardiovascular causes (top). Incidence and relative risk (RR) of SCD among young athletes and nonathletes from specific cardiovascular causes (bottom). ARVC/D, arrhythmogenic right ventricular cardiomyopathy/dysplasia; CAD, coronary artery disease; CCA, congenital coronary artery anomalies.

Cardiovascular Risk in Young Competitive Athletes

A broad spectrum of cardiovascular substrates (including congenital and inherited heart disorders) may underlie SCD in young competitive athletes (age ≤35 years). An Italian prospective study demonstrated that adolescent and young adults involved in sports activity have a 2.8 greater risk of sudden cardiovascular death than their nonathletic counterparts[8] (Figure 61–2, top). However, sports is not itself the cause of the enhanced mortality, since it triggers cardiac arrest in those athletes who are affected by cardiovascular conditions that predispose to life-threatening ventricular arrhythmias during physical exercise (Figure 61–2, bottom). This reinforces the need for systematic evaluation of adolescent and young individuals embarking in sports activity in order to identify those with potentially lethal cardiovascular diseases and protect them against the increased risk of SCD.

Preparticipation Screening for Prevention of Sudden Cardiac Death

It is a general assumption that if a young athlete is fit enough to participate in competitive sports, then the existence of an underlying disease that may be life-threatening is unlikely and even counterintuitive. Sudden cardiac death during sports is often the first clinical manifestation of cardiovascular disease, because the culprit conditions are usually clinically silent and unlikely to be suspected during life on the basis of spontaneous alarming prodroma. The majority of young athletes who die suddenly show neither a positive family history nor preexistent cardiovascular symptoms. This explains why a screening protocol based solely on the athlete's history and a physical examination, as used in the United States, is of limited value in detecting affected athletes and preventing fatalities.[31] The addition of a

12-lead ECG increases the sensitivity of the screening process for detection of cardiovascular diseases at risk of SCD.

For almost 25 years a systematic preparticipation screening process, based on a 12-lead ECG in addition to a history and physical examination, has been the practice in Italy.[14,44,45] Such a screening strategy has been proven to be effective in the identification of athletes with previously undiagnosed hypertrophic cardiomyopathy. Moreover, during long-term follow-up no deaths were recorded among these disqualified athletes with hypertrophic cardiomyopathy, suggesting that identification and disqualification from competition may potentially improve survival. Furthermore, a subanalysis of Italian data shows that only <25% of young competitive athletes with hypertrophic cardiomyopathy detected at preparticipation screening had a positive family history or an abnormal physical examination; thus, the majority of these athletes would not have been identified by a limited screening protocol without 12-lead ECG. This 3-fold greater number of athletes with hypertrophic cardiomyopathy identified by Italian screening and thereafter disqualified from competitive sports could be expected to result in a corresponding additional number of lives saved compared to other strategies.

In addition, a 12-lead ECG offers the potential to detect asymptomatic athletes with other conditions presenting with ECG abnormalities such as arrhythmogenic right ventricular cardiomyopathy/dysplasia, dilated cardiomyopathy, Lenègre conduction disease, WPW syndrome, long and short QT syndromes, and Brugada syndrome. Overall, these conditions (including hypertrophic cardiomyopathy) account for up to 60% of the SCDs in young competitive athletes.[45] Of note, many of these conditions have been recognized only recently and the impact of their detection at preparticipation screening on mortality will be assessed in the future.

A recent time-trend analysis over 24 years of sudden cardiovascular death in the young screened athletic population versus the unscreened nonathletic population (age range 12–35 years) of the Veneto Region of Italy showed that mortality declined by almost 90% in athletes, but showed no significant change in nonathletes.[46] Mortality reduction in athletes paralleled the implementation of systematic screening in Italy and was predominantly due to fewer cases of SCD from cardiomyopathies over time. The inference of these data is that affected athletes were identified in a timely fashion by preparticipation evaluation and SCD was prevented by their disqualification for competitive sports activity.

The 2005 consensus document of the Study Group of Sports Cardiology of the European Society of Cardiology reinforces the principle of the need for preparticipation medical clearance of all young athletes involved in organized sports programs and recommends the implementation of a common European screening protocol essentially based on a 12-lead ECG for prevention of athletic field sudden cardiovascular death.[45]

Athletic Participation

The ultimate diagnosis of heart muscle diseases may be problematic due to the presence of physiological (and reversible) structural and electrical adaptations of the cardiovascular system to long-term athletic training. This condition, known as "athlete's heart," is characterized by an increase in left ventricular cavity dimension and sometimes wall thickness, which overlaps with cardiomyopathies.[47] An accurate differential diagnosis is crucial because of the potentially adverse outcome associated with cardiomyopathy in an athlete and, on the other hand, the possibility of misdiagnosis of pathological conditions requiring unnecessary disqualifications from sports with financial and psychological consequences.

Diagnostic criteria in favor of physiological hypertrophy are the limited (≤16 mm) thickness and symmetric distribution of left ventricular hypertrophy, as well as the reduction of wall thickness (≥2 mm) after 4–6 weeks of detraining. It is noteworthy that physiological left ventricular hypertrophy is associated with an enlarged (≥55 mm) left ventricular cavity. Abnormalities of left ventricular filling are consistently absent in athletes with physiological left ventricular hypertrophy, but common in hypertrophic cardiomyopathy. A sizable proportion of highly trained athletes shows a substantial increase in right and/or left ventricular cavity dimensions, unavoidably raising the question of differential diagnosis with dilated cardiomyopathy or arrhythmogenic right ventricular cardiomyopathy. Morphological criteria suggesting physiological ventricular enlargement include normal or slightly thickened wall and preserved systolic function without wall motion abnormalities.

Extraordinary advances in molecular genetics during the past two decades have allowed identification of a growing number of defective genes involved in the pathogenesis of cardiomyopathies. It is hoped that in the near future genetic molecular tests will be clinically available for definitive differential diagnosis between heart muscle diseases and athletic training-related physiological changes of the cardiovascular system.

When a definitive cardiovascular condition is identified, athletes are evaluated according to established criteria for eligibility. In this regard, the 16th, 26th, and 36th Bethesda Conferences sponsored by the American College of Cardiology have offered since 1985 consensus recommendations for the disqualification of athletes by taking into account the nature and severity of the cardiovascular disease as well as the type and level of sports training and competition.[48–50] European guidelines have been recently elaborated by the Study Group of Sports Cardiology of the European Society of Cardiology.[51] Both U.S. and European recommendations are based on the concept that intense physical activity (both training and competition) in subjects with a cardiovascular disorder will increase the risk of sudden cardiac death and/or disease progression. Athlete disqualification can be associated with important individual cost in terms of health, contentment, and even future opportunity for professional sports. However, the risk of SCD associated with competitive sports in the setting of known cardiovascular disease is a controllable risk factor, and the devastating impact of even infrequent fatal events in the young athletic population justifies appropriate restriction from competition.[50,52–58]

Early Defibrillation Program

Public access to early defibrillation programs using automated external defibrillators have been successful in improving survival (up to 52%) from out-of-hospital cardiac arrest in many settings including casinos, airlines, and airports.[59–62] These favorable results were obtained in individuals with a mean age >60 years who most likely experienced an ischemic cardiac arrest due to atherosclerotic coronary artery disease. A recent study specifically addressing the effectiveness of early defibrillation occurring during sports performance raised concerns about the benefit of this strategy in the young athletic population with different causes of cardiac arrest, mostly consisting of cardiomyopathies.[63] Despite a witnessed collapse, timely cardiopulmonary resuscitation, and prompt defibrillation in most cases (with an average time from cardiac arrest to defibrillation of 3.1 min), only one of nine athletes in this study survived. In contrast, Maron *et al.*[49] analyzed 128 cases from the United States Commotio Cordis Registry and found an overall survival rate of 46% (19 of 41) in the individuals who received early defibrillation. A plausible explanation for the discrepancy between the two studies is that the majority of athletes in Drezner's study had an underlying structural heart disease and that ventricular tachycardia/fibrillation in the presence of cardiac structural abnormalities may be more resistant to defibrillation (specially if nonimmediate) than arrhythmic cardiac arrest in a structurally normal heart, such as in commotio cordis. Other factors that may decrease the efficacy of defibrillation in athletes include the high catecholamine levels and metabolic changes occurring during strenuous physical exercise and interacting unfavorably with the underlying structural substrate.

In conclusion, the concept of prevention of athletic field SCD by using early automated external defibrillators programs, although promising, is still evolving and further studies are needed to better understand those factors that may affect efficacy of defibrillation and survival in young competitive athletes with structural heart disease who experience an arrhythmic cardiac arrest.

References

1. Maron BJ, Roberts WC, McAllister MA, *et al.* Sudden death in young athletes. *Circulation* 1980; 62:218–229.
2. Corrado D, Thiene G, Nava A, Pennelli N, Rossi L. Sudden death in young competitive athletes:

Clinico-pathologic correlations in 22 cases. *Am J Med* 1990;89:588–596.
3. Maron BJ. Sudden death in young athletes. *N Engl J Med* 2003;349:1064–1075.
4. Corrado D, Basso C, Thiene G. Assay sudden death in young athletes. *Lancet* 2005;366(Suppl. 1):S47–S48.
5. Thompson PD, Funk EJ, Carleton RA, Sturner WQ. Incidence of death during jogging in Rhode Island from 1975 through 1980. *JAMA* 1982;247:2535–2538.
6. Van Camp SP, Bloor CM, Mueller FO, *et al.* Nontraumatic sports death in high school and college athletes. *Med Sci Sports Exerc* 1995;27:641–647.
7. Maron BJ, Gohman TE, Aeppli D. Prevalence of sudden cardiac death during competitive sports activities in Minnesota high school athletes. *J Am Coll Cardiol* 1998;32:1881–1884.
8. Corrado D, Basso C, Rizzoli G, Schiavon M, Thiene G. Does sports activity enhance the risk of sudden death in adolescents and young adults? *J Am Coll Cardiol* 2003;42:1959–1963.
9. Corrado D, Basso C, Poletti A, *et al.* Sudden death in the young: Is coronary thrombosis the major precipitating factor? *Circulation* 1994;90:2315–2323.
10. Thiene G, Nava A, Corrado D, Rossi L, Pennelli N. Right ventricular cardiomyopathy and sudden death in young people. *N Engl J Med* 1988;318:129–133.
11. Burke AP, Farb A, Malcom GT, Liang Y, Smialek JE, Virmani R. Plaque rupture and sudden death related to exertion in men with coronary artery disease. *JAMA* 1999;281:921–926.
12. Giri S, Thompson PD, Kiernan FJ, Clive J, Fram DB, Mitchel JF, Hirst JA, McKay RG, Waters DD. Clinical and angiographic characteristics of exertion-related acute myocardial infarction. *JAMA* 1999;282:1731–1736.
13. Burke AP, Farb A, Virmani R, *et al.* Sports-related and non-sports-related sudden cardiac death in young adults. *Am Heart J* 1991;121:568–575.
14. Corrado D, Basso C, Schiavon M, *et al.* Screening for hypertrophic cardiomyopathy in young athletes. *N Engl J Med* 1998;339:364–369.
15. Corrado D, Thiene G, Cocco P, Frescura C. Nonatherosclerotic coronary artery disease and sudden death in the young. *Br Heart J* 1992;68:601–607.
16. Basso C, Frescura C, Corrado D, *et al.* Congenital heart disease and sudden death in the young. *Hum Pathol* 1995;26:1065–1072.
17. Corrado D, Basso C, Thiene G, *et al.* Spectrum of clinicopathologic manifestations of arrhythmogenic right ventricular cardiomyopathy/dysplasia: A multicenter study. *J Am Coll Cardiol* 1997;30:1512–1520.
18. Basso C, Maron BJ, Corrado D, Thiene G. Clinical profile of congenital coronary artery anomalies with origin from the wrong aortic sinus leading to sudden death in young competitive athletes. *J Am Coll Cardiol* 2000;35:1493–1501.
19. Basso C, Thiene G, Corrado D, Buja GF, Melacini P, Nava A. Hypertrophic cardiomyopathy: Pathologic evidence of ischemic damage in young sudden death victims. *Hum Pathol* 2000;31:988–998.
20. Basso C, Corrado D, Rossi L, Thiene G. Ventricular preexcitation in children and young adults: Atrial myocarditis as a possible trigger of sudden death. *Circulation* 2001;103:269–275.
21. Corrado D, Basso C, Buja G, Nava A, Rossi L, Thiene G. Right bundle branch block, right precordial ST-segment elevation, and sudden death in young people. *Circulation* 2001;103:710–717.
22. Corrado D, Basso C, Thiene G. Sudden cardiac death in young people with apparently normal heart. *Cardiovasc Res* 2001;50:399–408.
23. Waller BF, Roberts WC. Sudden death while running in conditioned runners aged 40 years or over. *Am J Cardiol* 1980;45:1292–1300.
24. Virmani R, Robinowitz M, McAllister HA. Nontraumatic death in joggers. *Am J Med* 1982;72:874–881.
25. Curfman GD. Is exercise beneficial—or hazardous—to your heart? *N Engl J Med* 1993;239:1730–1731.
26. Maron BJ. The paradox of exercise. *N Engl J Med* 2000;343:1409–1411.
27. Siscovick DS, Weiss NS, Fletcher RH, Lasky T. The incidence of primary cardiac arrest during vigorous exercise. *N Engl J Med* 1984;311:874–877.
28. Willich SN, Lewis M, Lowel H, Arntz HR, Schubert F, Schroder R. Physical exertion as a trigger of acute myocardial infarction. Triggers and Mechanisms of Myocardial Infarction Study Group. *N Engl J Med* 1993;329:1684–1690.
29. Mittleman MA, Maclure M, Tofler GH, Sherwood JB, Goldberg RJ, Muller JE. Triggering of acute myocardial infarction by heavy physical exertion. Protection against triggering by regular exertion. Determinants of Myocardial Infarction Onset Study Investigators. *N Engl J Med* 1993;329:1677–1683.
30. Corrado D, Thiene G, Pennelli N. Sudden death as the first manifestation of coronary artery disease in young people (less than or equal to 35 years). *Eur Heart J* 1988;9:139–144.
31. Maron BJ, Shirani J, Poliac LC, Mathenge R, Boberts WC, Mueller FO. Sudden death in young competitive athletes. Clinical, demographics, and pathological profiles. *JAMA* 1996;276:199–204.

32. Maron BJ. Hypertrophic cardiomyopathy: A systematic review. *JAMA* 2002;237:1308–1320.
33. Nistri S, Thiene G, Basso C, Corrado D, Vitolo A, Maron BJ. Screening for hypertrophic cardiomyopathy in a young male military population. *Am J Cardiol* 2003;91:1021–1023.
34. Basso C, Thiene G, Corrado D, *et al.* Arrhythmogenic right ventricular cardiomyopathy. Dysplasia, dystrophy, or myocarditis? *Circulation* 1996; 94:983–991.
35. Corrado D, Fontaine G, Marcus FI, *et al.* Arrhythmogenic right ventricular dysplasia/cardiomyopathy: Need for an international registry. *Circulation* 2000;101:E101–E106.
36. Corrado D, Basso C, Thiene G. Arrhythmogenic right ventricular cardiomyopathy: Diagnosis, prognosis, and treatment. *Heart* 2000;83:588–595.
37. Corrado D, Thiene G. Arrhythmogenic right ventricular cardiomyopathy/dysplasia: Clinical impact of molecular genetic studies. *Circulation* 2006;113: 1634–1637.
38. Basso C, Calabrese F, Corrado D, *et al.* Postmortem diagnosis in sudden cardiac death victims: Macroscopic, microscopic and molecular findings. *Cardiovasc Res* 2001;50:290–300.
39. Basso C, Thiene G, Corrado D, *et al.* Hypertrophic cardiomyopathy and sudden death in the young: Pathologic evidence of myocardial ischemia. *Hum Pathol* 2000;31:988–998.
40. Wilde AA, Antzelevitch C, Borggrefe M, *et al.* Study Group on the Molecular Basis of Arrhythmias of the European Society of Cardiology. Proposed diagnostic criteria for the Brugada syndrome: Consensus report. *Circulation* 2002;106:2514–2519.
41. Maron BJ, Chaitman BR, Ackerman MJ, *et al.* Recommendations for physical activity and recreational sports participation for young patients with genetic cardiovascular diseases. *Circulation* 2004; 109:2807–2816.
42. Corrado D, Pelliccia A, Antzelevitch C, *et al.* ST segment elevation and sudden death in the athlete. In: Antzelevitch C, Brugada P, Eds. *The Brugada Syndrome: From Bench to Bedside.* Malden, MA: Futura Publishing, 2005:119–129.
43. Priori SG, Napolitano C, Memmi M, *et al.* Clinical and molecular characterization of patients with catecholaminergic polymorphic ventricular tachycardia. *Circulation* 2002;106:69–74.
44. Maron BJ, Poliac LC, Ashare AB, Hall WA. Sudden death due to blunt neck blows in amateur hockey players. *JAMA* 2003;290:599–601.
45. Maron BJ, Gohman TE, Kyle SB, Estes NAM, Link MS. Clinical profile and spectrum of commotio cordis. *JAMA* 2002;287:1142–1146.
46. Link MS, Wang PJ, Pandian NG, Bharati S, Udelson JE, Lee M-Y, Vecchiotti MA, VanderBrink BA, Mirra G, Maron BJ, Estes NAM III. An experimental model of sudden death due to low-energy chest-wall impact (commotio cordis). *N Engl J Med* 1998;338:1805–1811.
47. Link MS, Wang PJ, VanderBrink BA, Avelar E, Pandian NG, Maron BJ, Estes NAM III. Selective activation of the K^{+}_{ATP} channel is a mechanism by which sudden death is produced by low energy chest wall impact (commotio cordis). *Circulation* 1999;100:413–418.
48. Strasburger JF, Maron BJ. Commotio cordis. *N Engl J Med* 2002;347:1248.
49. Maron BJ, Wentzel DC, Zenovich AG, Estes NAM 3rd, Link MS. Death in a young athlete due to commotio cordis despite prompt external defibrillation. *Heart Rhythm* 2005;2:991–993.
50. Weinstock J, Maron BJ, Song C, Mane PP, Estes NAM 3rd, Link MS. Failure of commercially available chest wall protectors to prevent sudden cardiac death induced by chest wall blows in an experimental model of commotio cordis. *Pediatrics* 2006;117: 1404–1405 and e656–e662.
51. Pelliccia A, Maron BJ. Preparticipation cardiovascular evaluation of the competitive athlete: Perspectives from the 30-year Italian experience. *Am J Cardiol* 1995;75:827–829.
52. Corrado D, Pelliccia A, Bjornstad HH, Vanhees L, Biffi A, Borjesson M, Panhuyzen-Goedkoop N, Deligiannis A, Solberg E, Dugmore D, Mellwig KP, Assanelli D, Delise P, van-Buuren F, Anastasakis A, Heidbuchel H, Hoffmann E, Fagard R, Priori SG, Basso C, Arbustini E, Blomstrom-Lundqvist C, McKenna WJ, Thiene G. Cardiovascular preparticipation screening of young competitive athletes for prevention of sudden death: Proposal for a common European protocol. Consensus Statement of the Study Group of Sport Cardiology of the Working Group of Cardiac Rehabilitation and Exercise Physiology and the Working Group of Myocardial and Pericardial Diseases of the European Society of Cardiology. *Eur Heart J* 2005;26:516–524.
53. Corrado D, Basso C, Pavei A, Schiavon M, Thiene G. Decline of sudden cardiac death in young competitive athletes after implementation of Italian preparticipation screening. *Circulation* 2005;112: II-604–605.
54. Maron BJ, Pelliccia A, Spirito P. Cardiac disease in young trained athletes. Insights into methods for distinguishing athlete's heart from structural heart disease, with particular emphasis on hypertrophic cardiomyopathy. *Circulation* 1995;91:1596–1601.

55. Mitchell JH, Maron BJ, Epstein SE. 16th Bethesda Conference: Cardiovascular abnormalities in the athlete: Recommendations regarding eligibility for competition. *J Am Coll Cardiol* 1985;6:1186–1232.
56. Maron BJ, Mitchell JH. 26th Bethesda Conference: Recommendations for determining eligibility for competition in athletes with cardiovascular abnormalities. *J Am Coll Cardiol* 1994;24:845–899.
57. Maron BJ, Zipes DP. 36th Bethesda Conference: Recommendations for determining eligibility for competition in athletes with cardiovascular abnormalities. *J Am Coll Cardiol* 2005;45:1373–1375.
58. Pelliccia A, Fagard R, Bjornstad HH, Anastassakis A, Arbustini E, Assanelli D, Biffi A, Borjesson M, Carre F, Corrado D, Delise P, Dorwarth U, Hirth A, Heidbuchel H, Hoffmann E, Mellwig KP, Panhuyzen-Goedkoop N, Pisani A, Solberg EE, van-Buuren F, Vanhees L, Blomstrom-Lundqvist C, Deligiannis A, Dugmore D, Glikson M, Hoff PI, Hoffmann A, Hoffmann E, Horstkotte D, Nordrehaug JE, Oudhof J, McKenna WJ, Penco M, Priori S, Reybrouck T, Senden J, Spataro A, Thiene G. Recommendations for competitive sports participation in athletes with cardiovascular disease: A consensus document from the Study Group of Sports Cardiology of the Working Group of Cardiac Rehabilitation and Exercise Physiology and the Working Group of Myocardial and Pericardial Diseases of the European Society of Cardiology. *Eur Heart J* 2005;26:1422–1445.
59. Hallstrom AP, Ornato JP, Weisfeldt M, Travers A, Christenson J, McBurnie MA, Zalenski R, Becker LB, Schron EB, Proschan M. Public-access defibrillation and survival after out-of-hospital cardiac arrest. *N Engl J Med* 2004;351:637–646.
60. Caffrey SL, Willoughby PJ, Pepe PE, Becker LB. Public use of automated external defibrillators. *N Engl J Med* 2002;347:1242–1247.
61. Page RL, Joglar JA, Kowal RC, Zagrodzky JD, Nelson LL, Ramaswamy K, Barbera SJ, Hamdan MH, McKenas DK. Use of automated external defibrillators by a U.S. airline. *N Engl J Med* 2000;343:1210–1216.
62. Valenzuela TD, Roe DJ, Nichol G, Clark LL, Spaite DW, Hardman RG. Outcomes of rapid defibrillation by security officers after cardiac arrest in casinos. *N Engl J Med* 2000;343:1206–1209.
63. Drezner JA, Rogers KJ. Sudden cardiac arrest in intercollegiate athletes: Detailed analysis and outcomes of resuscitation in nine cases. *Heart Rhythm* 2006;3:755–759.

62
Sudden Cardiac Death in Infancy: Focus on Prolonged Repolarization

Peter J. Schwartz, Marco Stramba-Badiale, Lia Crotti, and Michael J. Ackerman

Introduction

After the first week of life, sudden infant death syndrome (SIDS) is the leading cause of sudden death during the first year of life in the western world and produces devastating psychosocial consequences in the families of the victims.

Sudden infant death syndrome is defined as the sudden unexpected death of any infant prior to his or her first birthday, which is unexpected by history and in which a thorough postmortem examination fails to identify an adequate cause of death. A death scene investigation has been recommended as a requirement for diagnosis.

Despite a large number of theories, mostly focused on abnormalities in the control of respiratory or cardiac function, the causes of SIDS remain unknown. The suggestions over the years that cardiac mechanisms and, specifically, life-threatening arrhythmias[1,2] might account for a significant portion of cases of SIDS have been controversial.

This chapter (1) describes the cardiac QT hypothesis for SIDS according to which some cases of SIDS might be due to ventricular fibrillation associated with prolonged repolarization, (2) summarizes the results of an 18-year-long prospective study with electrocardiogram (ECG) recordings in over 34,000 infants,[3] (3) discusses recent findings[4–9] that provide molecular evidence linking SIDS to cardiac channelopathies such as the congenital long QT syndrome (LQTS) and catecholaminergic polymorphic ventricular tachycardia (CPVT), (4) presents preliminary data on a new prospective study involving 45,000 infants and the main finding of a cost-effectiveness study that analyzes a screening neonatal ECG program in a large European country, and (5) addresses the implications of 30 years of research on LQTS and SIDS.

The QT Hypothesis

Many hypotheses have been proposed to explain SIDS, but none has yet been proven. There is a consensus that SIDS is multifactorial,[2,6] an important concept that implies that a sudden and unexpected death in infancy may stem from many different causes. A logical corollary is that the validity of one mechanism is not negated by the validity of another. Most SIDS cases probably result from an abnormality in either respiratory or cardiac function,[6] or in their neural control, which may be transient in nature but sufficient to initiate a lethal sequence of events.

As to the so-called "apnea hypothesis," its demise came with the large, National Institutes of Health-funded, prospective study Collaborative Home Infant Monitoring Evaluation (CHIME) on over 1000 infants who during the first 6 months of life were observed with home cardiorespiratory monitors for a total of almost 720,000 h of monitoring.[7] The accompanying editorial by Jobe[8] concluded by stating that *"This study justifies a severe curtailing of home monitoring to prevent SIDS."* More details can be found in an earlier review.[10]

As to the cardiac hypothesis, Schwartz considered that in the western world the leading cause of mortality between age 20 and 65 years is sudden cardiac death (SCD), and that the mechanism involved is almost always a lethal arrhythmia, ventricular fibrillation. It would be odd if SCD, and therefore lethal arrhythmias, would not contribute to some unexplained deaths during infancy (i.e., SIDS).

In 1976,[1] Schwartz proposed that some cases of SIDS might have been due to a mechanism similar to that responsible for the sudden death of patients affected by LQTS, a leading cause of autopsy-negative sudden death below age 20 years.[9,11] One such mechanism could be a developmental abnormality in cardiac sympathetic innervation predisposing some infants to lethal arrhythmias in the first year of life.[1] Another possible mechanism could be an LQTS-causing genetic mutation.[9,11] In either case, the only clinically detectable marker might be a prolonged QT interval on the ECG.

Following the editorial[1] by Schwartz in 1976, the hypothesis that QT interval prolongation might play a role in the genesis of SIDS received attention. However, despite some very early support by Maron *et al.*,[12] it was rapidly, and perhaps prematurely, discarded on the basis of a series of apparently negative results.[13–17] The weaknesses in the arguments against a possible role of abnormal cardiac repolarization in the pathogenesis of SIDS have been discussed in detail previously.[2,18]

The Italian Study on Neonatal Electrocardiograms and Sudden Infant Death Syndrome

To test the Schwartz QT-SIDS hypothesis, a prospective study involving 12-lead ECG screening of 3- to 4-day-old infants was designed and was initiated in 1976. Given the low incidence of SIDS (0.5–1.5 per 1000 live births), it was necessary to prospectively collect neonatal ECGs in a very large population and to subsequently follow these infants for 1 year to assess the occurrence of SIDS or deaths from other causes. The results from this 19-year study were published in 1998[3] and are summarized here.

Twelve-lead ECGs were recorded in 34,442 neonates. The QT interval was measured by investigators blinded to the survival status of the infant. Of the 34,442 infants enrolled, 33,034 (96%) completed the 1-year follow-up. Those lost to follow-up were due to change of residence. The mean Bazett's heart rate corrected QT interval (QTc, QT divided by the square root of the RR interval) at 3 or 4 days of life was 400 ± 20 msec, unaffected by gender. The normal and symmetrical distribution of the QTc in our population made the 97.5th percentile value of QTc correspond to 440 msec, two standard deviations above the mean. Consequently, we considered a value greater than 440 msec during the first week of life as a prolonged QTc.

During the 1-year follow-up there were 34 deaths: 24 classified as SIDS and 10 attributed to definite causes. All postmortem examinations of SIDS victims were negative and failed to document an adequate cause of death. No SIDS victim had a family history of LQTS or sudden death. The mean QTc was 435 ± 45 msec in the SIDS group, significantly longer than that of the non-SIDS victims (392 ± 26 msec, $p < 0.05$) and of the cohort alive at 1 year (400 ± 20 msec, $p < 0.01$). Importantly, half of the SIDS victims (12/24) exceeded the 97.5% cutoff value of 440 msec, indicating a strong association between a right-shifted QTc and susceptibility for SIDS. In fact, the odds ratio (OR = 41.3, 95% CI 17.3–98.4) exceeds nearly all of the classic risk factors linked with SIDS, such as prone sleep and cigarette smoke exposure. However, given that 2.5% of healthy infants exceed this cutoff value of 440 msec, screening implications during the first week of life are challenged by the very poor positive predictive value (i.e., <2%). Nonetheless, it is fair to remember that when the event rate is low, positive predictive values for any marker are always poor.

The Molecular Link

Potential Causes for QT Prolongation in Infants

This large prospective study based on more than 34,000 infants demonstrated that QT interval prolongation, on the standard ECG recorded on the third to fourth day of life, is a major risk factor for SIDS.[3] While borderline values and transient QT prolongations do occur in the first week of life, the study provided the first compelling evidence that the observed QT prolongation reflected either a "vulnerable" infant with autonomic dysregulation,[1] drug-induced QT prolongation,[10] acquired QT prolongation secondary to other disease states, or a "vulnerable" infant with a LQTS-predisposing substrate.[19]

The first mechanism is partly based on the fact that an imbalance in cardiac sympathetic innervation with left dominance, experimentally produced by removing the right stellate ganglion, prolongs the QT interval and increases susceptibility to ventricular fibrillation in several conditions, including 3-week-old puppies with normal hearts.[20] The sympathetic innervation of the heart continues to develop after birth and becomes functionally complete by approximately the sixth month of life. The right and left sympathetic nerves may occasionally develop at different rates and lead temporarily to a harmful imbalance.[21] A sudden increase in sympathetic activity, particularly when involving the arrhythmogenic left sided nerves,[21] might easily trigger a lethal arrhythmia in these electrically unstable hearts. The original data with right stellate ganglionectomy[22] have been reproduced by Chen and associates using nerve growth factor injected in the left stellate ganglion.[23] Infants with this type of sympathetic imbalance, either developmental or genetic, would be more vulnerable during the first few months of life and the higher risk for SIDS could be identified by the observation of a prolonged QT interval. This pathogenic mechanism, however, is difficult to prove (or dismiss). Nevertheless, a prolonged QT interval might be a surrogate marker for autonomic dysregulation and the "vulnerable" infant.

The second mechanism relates to the fact that several drugs commonly used in the neonatal period and during infancy may induce QT interval prolongation, as previously discussed.[10] Also, almost half of the neonates born from mothers with autoimmune diseases and positive for the anti-Ro/SSA antibodies show QT interval prolongation,[24] with values of QTc that sometimes exceed 500 msec even in the absence of atrioventricular (AV) conduction abnormalities, the typical manifestation of neonatal lupus syndrome.[25] At variance with congenital heart block, these ventricular repolarization abnormalities are transient and disappear by month 6 of life, concomitantly with the disappearance of the anti-Ro/SSA antibodies.[26] This transient QT prolongation could well predispose some anti-Ro-positive infants to life-threatening arrhythmias. The implications are 2-fold: the presence of asymptomatic autoimmune diseases should be excluded in mothers of neonates showing QT prolongation in the absence of other causes and neonates born from mothers with lupus erythematosus should be followed during the first year of life with repeated ECGs.

As to the possibility that the QT prolongation reflects an infant at risk for SIDS because of congenital LQTS, one potential difficulty in linking LQTS to SIDS is that the latter is not a familial disease. Two concepts are highly relevant here. The first is that "sporadic" cases of LQTS result from *de novo* mutations that, by definition, are not found among the parents. The second is represented by the demonstration of "low penetrance" in LQTS.[19] Low penetrance implies that the clinical diagnosis is often inadequate and that many affected individuals may appear completely normal at clinical examination. In congenital LQTS, the penetrance is estimated at approximately 60%.

Molecular Evidence

Indeed, three independent, anecdotal cases that demonstrate that *de novo* mutations in LQTS genes may manifest as, and be indistinguishable from, typical cases of "near-miss" SIDS or as SIDS itself have been reported.[4,5,27] The first two cases, which represented "proof-of-concept" for the possibility that LQTS could cause events clinically indistinguishable from SIDS, are worth reporting in some detail.

In the first case report, a 7-week-old infant was found cyanotic, apneic, and pulseless by his parents.[4] He was rushed to a nearby hospital while his father was attempting cardiopulmonary resuscitation (CPR). In the emergency room, ventricular fibrillation was recorded (Figure 62–1). Thus, this infant presented as typical "near-miss" for SIDS. After defibrillation, the ECG revealed extreme QT prolongation (QTc 648 msec), LQTS was diagnosed, and therapy was instituted by combining β blockade and the sodium channel

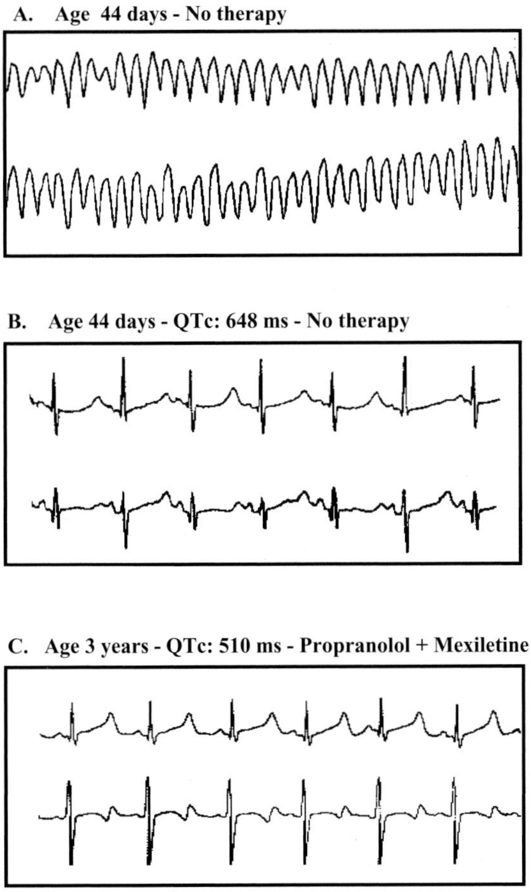

FIGURE 62–1. Electrocardiogram leads II and V2, showing ventricular fibrillation at hospital admission (A); QT interval prolongation observed the same day after restoration of sinus rhythm (B); and ECG recorded at the last follow-up visit (C). (*Modified from* Schwartz *et al.*[4])

blocker mexiletine. A critical point is that the QT interval of both parents was normal, paternity being confirmed. Molecular screening identified a mutation in *SNC5A*, the cardiac sodium channel gene responsible for type 3 LQTS (LQT3).[4] This disease-causing mutation was not present in the mother or in the father, thus establishing that this was a *de novo* mutation. The documentation of ventricular fibrillation at arrival in the emergency room is quite important given the frequent statements such as "*no one has recorded ventricular arrhythmias in infants at risk for SIDS.*"[28] Had the infant died, a certainty without cardioversion, the absence of an ECG, the negative family history, and the parents' normal QT intervals would have prompted the classic labeling of SIDS. Thus, infants who have similar *de novo* mutations, involving one of the ion channels controlling ventricular repolarization, may have a prolonged QT interval at birth. Some of them may die *in utero* because of ventricular fibrillation, and thus become stillbirths,[29] or during the first few months of life, and without an available ECG, these deceased infants would be labeled as victims of SIDS. Others would probably begin to have syncopal episodes or nonfatal cardiac arrests during their childhood and would only then be diagnosed as sporadic cases of LQTS.

In the second case report,[5] a 4-month-old infant was found dead in her crib. A thorough postmortem examination was negative and the diagnosis of SIDS was rendered. When postmortem molecular genetic testing was performed, a missense mutation (KCNQ1–P117L) was identified. Both parents of the victim and her sister had normal QT intervals and no one had the P117L mutation. Paternity was confirmed, once again establishing the presence of a spontaneous, germline mutation (sporadic, *de novo*) in the deceased infant. The same identical mutation is present in one of the LQTS families followed in Pavia (Figure 62–2). This case provided the first evidence that in a child whose death was classified as SIDS, according to current standards, a molecular autopsy made possible the diagnosis of an arrhythmogenic disease, LQTS.

These single case reports provided the "proof-of-concept" evidence linking LQTS and SIDS. These studies provided the first unequivocal demonstration that life-threatening events in infancy and actual unexpected sudden deaths in infancy, with all the characteristics for SIDS or for "near miss" for SIDS, can depend on a *de novo* mutation in one of the LQTS genes, thus escaping recognition in the parents but nevertheless precipitating sudden death due to ventricular fibrillation. Following these case reports, Ackerman and colleagues provided the first genetic epidemiology studies investigating the hypothesis of cardiac channel mutations in SIDS by conducting comprehensive postmortem mutational analysis of the five major long QT disease genes (*KCNQ1*, *KCNH2*, *SCN5A*, *KCNE1*, and *KCNE2*) in a large (n = 93) 2-year, statewide, population-based

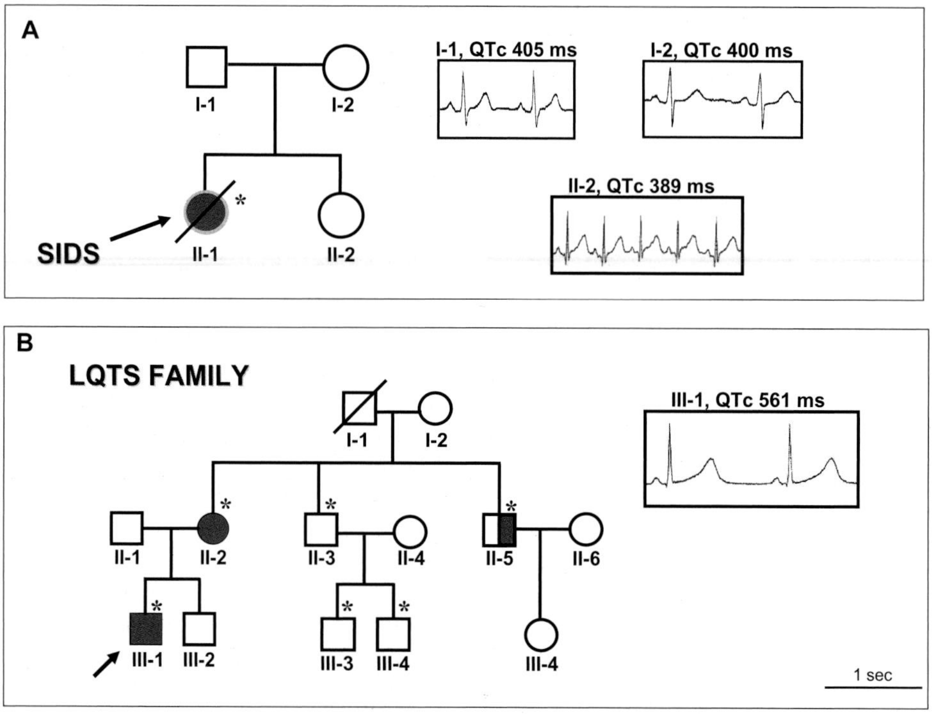

Figure 62–2. Pedigrees and ECG tracings of the two families with the P117L mutation included in the present study. (A) The pedigree of the SIDS family. Electrocardiogram tracings of the parents (I-1 and I-2) and the sister (II-2) of the proband showing a normal QT interval (lead II) are reported on the right. (B) The pedigree of the family with LQT1 due to P117L–KCNQ1. On the left, a lead II ECG recording was obtained in the proband (III-1). Arrows indicate probands. The gray symbol indicates the SIDS victim. Filled symbols represent individuals presenting with syncope and prolonged QT interval. Half-filled symbols represent individuals with QT interval prolongation and no symptoms. Asterisks indicate carriers of the P117L mutation.

cohort of SIDS.[30,31] Notably, genetic testing for these five LQTS-susceptibility genes is now a routine, clinically available diagnostic test. Three of the 58 deceased white infants (5.2%) and 1 of 34 deceased black infants (2.9%) hosted LQTS-causing mutations.

Schwartz and colleagues have independently validated and extended this observation in a much larger cohort of SIDS involving 201 Norwegian infants.[32] Here, the investigators found compelling molecular and functional evidence to implicate LQTS-causing mutations in approximately 9% of cases. Of the 201 SIDS victims, 18 (9%) were carriers of LQTS gene variants with functional effect, and 50% of them had mutations on the sodium channel gene SCN5A.[33] The size of the study population has provided a reliable estimate of the prevalence of mutations in the LQTS genes (at least among Norwegians), as shown by the narrow 95% confidence intervals, which range between 5.4% and 13.8%.

Most recently, Ackerman and colleagues identified putative SIDS-causing mutations in 2/34 black infants involving one of the newest LQTS-susceptibility genes, *CAV3*-encoded caveolin-3.[34,35] In addition, 2 of the 93 infants harbored gain-of-function mutations in the *RyR2*-encoded cardiac ryanodine receptor/calcium release channel, which underlies type 1 CPVT (CPVT1), a heritable channelopathy clinically mimicking LQTS.[36] Thus, derived from this large population-based study in the United States and this large cohort study of Norwegian infants, an estimated 5–15% of SIDS may be due to a primary cardiac channelopathy.

Besides rare, pathogenic LQTS/CPVT-susceptibility mutations, these investigations have also exposed a possible contribution of cardiac channel polymorphisms that may alter "repolarization reserve" and contribute to the makings of the "vulnerable infant" in accordance with the SIDS triple-risk hypothesis that involves (1) an environmental trigger, (2) during a critical developmental period, and (3) in a vulnerable host. Even after excluding the most common channel polymorphisms, KCNH2-K897T, SCN5A-H558R, and KCNE1-G38S, nearly one-third of infants possessed at least one genetic variant noted previously in ethnic-matched reference alleles in one of the five cardiac channel genes.[31,37,38]

Whether or not these channel polymorphisms reduce repolarization reserve and/or facilitate adrenergically mediated cardiac arrhythmias requires further investigation. For example, five of the SIDS victims were positive for KCNH2-R1047L, a polymorphism previously identified as an independent risk factor for drug-induced (dofetilide) torsades.[31,39] In addition, the black-specific sodium channel common polymorphism, SCN5A-S1103Y, appears to be overrepresented among a cohort of 133 black infants and a mexiletine-sensitive increased late sodium current emerges in the setting of acidosis.[40] Indeed, even the most common of single nucleotide polymorphisms (SNPs) in cardiac channels (KCNH2-K897T and SCN5A-H558R) are not necessarily innocent bystanders, having been shown to modulate the properties of other disease-causing mutations.[41–43] In fact, in the Norwegian SIDS study, all seven decedents with mutations/rare variants in *SCN5A* that displayed a modest but definite functional effect were also heterozygous for H558R. Moreover, the allele frequency for H558R was twice as large in this subgroup of SIDS cases compared to controls ($p = 0.02$).

These findings provide conclusive evidence that genetically mediated arrhythmias represent a significant and nondismissible cause of SIDS. Furthermore, given the fact that malignant LQTS is associated with marked QT prolongation, these observations support the concept of widespread neonatal ECG screening and indicate that at least this subset of infants at high risk for sudden death during infancy or beyond can be diagnosed early and that their impending death can probably be prevented, as is the case with most patients affected by LQTS. These implications will be discussed next.

Implications and New Directions

The aforementioned studies carry obvious clinical implications and have forced new investigations. The highly significant association between QT prolongation and occurrence of SIDS unavoidably raises the issue regarding the potential value of routine neonatal ECG screening. This, in turn, requires knowledge on the feasibility and on results that can be expected by such a study and also an accurate estimate of its cost effectiveness. This information has just become available and will be presented in the next sections. A practical issue involves the management of infants found to have significant QT prolongation by such a screening program. Overwhelming data from thousands of LQTS families indicate that treatment with β blockers has reduced mortality below 2%.[44,45] This information is relevant to the prevention not only of early deaths (that would be labeled as SIDS) in newborns with a prolonged QT interval but also of later sudden deaths due to LQTS.

A "Pilot" Study on 45,000 Infants

A requirement made by the Italian Ministry of Health, prior to a final consideration of the implementation of a nationwide neonatal ECG screening program, was the performance of a "large-scale" pilot study with ECGs performed during weeks 3 and 4 of life, as recommended by the guidelines of the European Society of Cardiology.[46]

The study, just completed, enrolled 44,596 infants and constitutes the largest ECG prospective study ever performed in infants. The study involved 16 centers in Italy that transmitted ECG, demographic, and clinical variables to the coordinating centers for analysis. Preliminary data have been presented.[47] A QTc >440 msec was found in 629 (1.4%) infants. Note that this is considerably less than the 2.5% of infants exceeding 440 msec during the first week of life.[3] Of these, 31 (0.7/1000) had a QTc ≥470 msec—the threshold for "marked" QT prolongation—and underwent molecular screening for the LQTS genes. Genotyping has been completed so far in 24/31 and probable LQTS-causing mutations have been identified in 13/24 (54%) including *KCNQ1* ($n = 8$), *KCNH2* ($n = 3$), and *SCN5A* ($n = 2$). Only one of these 13 cases was a *de novo* mutation. In all remaining cases, other family members were found to be affected by LQTS, but had not been previously diagnosed.

These data provide the first estimate of the prevalence of LQTS based on real data. As at least 50% of the infants with QTc ≥470 msec hosted an identifiable LQTS-causing mutation (i.e., 0.35/1000), as some of those with a QTc between 440 and 469 msec are expected to also be affected, and as currently genotyping still misses approximately 25% of patients certainly affected by LQTS, it follows that the prevalence of LQTS is very likely to be between 1/2000 and 1/2500.[48]

Unexpectedly, this "pilot" study also prompted the identification of four cases of two major and life-threatening congenital heart diseases that had escaped recognition during the initial medical visit, including three cases of coarctation of the aorta and one case of anomalous origin of the left coronary artery. Each infant promptly and successfully underwent surgical correction of the defect. This finding has significant implications for the cost effectiveness of a neonatal ECG screening program. The ECG screening was extremely well received by all families, with practically a 100% acceptance. This study proved that such a screening program is feasible and allows early identification of infants affected either by LQTS or by other significant cardiovascular disorders.

Cost-Effectiveness of a Neonatal Electrocardiogram Screening Program

Based on the initial studies linking QT prolongation, LQTS, and SIDS,[3–5] some European countries have begun to consider the possibility of introducing, in their National Health Services, the performance of an ECG during the first month of life in all newborns, as part of a cardiovascular screening program. Should neonatal screening indeed be introduced as part of National Health Services, then hospital cardiologists—most of whom are utterly unfamiliar with neonatal ECGs—would be asked to read these tracings. The European Society of Cardiology has realized the potential implications for European cardiologists and for health care, and has acted accordingly by instituting a Task Force for the creation of guidelines for the interpretation of the neonatal ECG.[46] The Task Force has provided such guidelines, focusing on the most clinically relevant abnormalities, on the ensuing management, and on referral options. As a starting point it was suggested that the number of false positives could be greatly reduced by performing the screening ECG in weeks 3–4 of life and by repeating it when QTc values appear abnormal.

To provide the information necessary for governmental agencies to decide on possible implementation, a formal cost-effectiveness study was performed.[49] It is vital, given the frequent misunderstandings and misquotations, to stress that the objective of such an ECG surveillance program is *not* the identification of infants at risk for SIDS (an unrealistic target), but is instead the *early* identification of infants affected by LQTS, a potentially lethal, highly treatable condition that affects 1 in 2500 infants. Without diagnosis, a few of these infants might die suddenly in the first year of life—and would then almost certainly be labeled as a SIDS victim—or might die later on, as children, teenagers, or young adults. The ultimate objective of early identification is the prevention of sudden death for a significant number of patients with LQTS, irrespective of their age.

The study used Markov process analysis to forecast natural and clinical histories of subjects with or without screening. Monte Carlo simulations were used to simultaneously alter all the uncertain parameters (process-related probabilities and costs) by ±30% to cover for any potential error and for intercountry variability. The main finding was that by screening only for LQTS, the cost per year-of-life saved was 11,740 Euros. When, as it happens in the real world,[48] two congenital heart diseases (coarctation of the aorta and anomalous origin of the left coronary artery) are considered also, then the cost per year-of-life saved was only 7022 Euros. These figures denote a "highly cost-effective" screening program. Traditionally, figures below 50,000 U.S. dollars are deemed "cost effective." In a country such as Italy, with 550,000 new births per year, the cost to screen all infants born would be 11 million Euros per year. This is a very modest cost for saving precious young lives.

Medicolegal Implications

The evidence that neonatal electrocardiography might be useful for the identification of those infants who are at risk for an early arrhythmic death, besides prompting clinical decisions, also carries significant medicolegal implications.

There are two critical points. One is that approximately 10% of future SIDS victims (and probably a larger number of future victims of sudden death in the young) carry LQTS mutations likely to produce repolarization changes identifiable by neonatal electrocardiography[47] and that due to the understanding of the lethal mechanisms involved, there is a high probability of preventing these untimely sudden deaths. The other is the evidence[50,51] that it is possible to make the diagnosis of LQTS even in a dead infant already labeled as SIDS or in a dead youngster, even if an ECG was never made.[4,5,27,50] The very recent study by Tester and Ackerman,[50] who performed molecular analysis and subsequently identified LQTS mutations in 20% of 49 victims of autopsy-negative sudden death, supports the importance of early ECG screening to identify premortem, at-risk individuals affected by LQTS.[51]

The still prevailing concept of the impossibility of identifying infants at truly high and specific risk for SIDS has the undeniable advantage that no one has to be blamed, except a cruel fate. The evidence presented above changes all that. Parents of SIDS victims or, more appropriately, their physicians may now begin to ask for a postmortem molecular genetic test. What will happen when such a molecular autopsy identifies an LQTS-susceptibility mutation and a lethal ventricular arrhythmia as the likely cause of death? The bereaved parents, and their lawyers, will start asking new questions. Indeed, in our opinion, the parents of a newborn child have the right to be informed about the existence of a potentially lethal albeit uncommon cardiovascular disease of which the most malignant forms can be rather easily exposed by a simple ECG and for which very effective and safe therapies are available. It will then be their choice to spend a very small amount of money to determine the presence of this highly unlikely but life-threatening possibility. Without information they would be denied the option. Failure to fully inform families of this possible scenario could, in the very near future, carry medicolegal consequences.

Acknowledgments. These studies on SIDS were partially supported by the National Institutes of Health Grants HL68880 (P.J.S.) and HD42569 (M.J.A.), the CJ Foundation for SIDS (M.J.A.), and by the Italian Ministry of Health research Grants 1999, 2000, and 2001. We are grateful to Pinuccia De Tomasi and David J. Tester for expert editorial support.

References

1. Schwartz PJ. Cardiac sympathetic innervation and the sudden infant death syndrome. A possible pathogenetic link. *Am J Med* 1976;60:167–172.
2. Schwartz PJ. The quest for the mechanism of the sudden infant death syndrome. Doubts and progress. *Circulation* 1987;75:677–683.
3. Schwartz PJ, Stramba-Badiale M, Segantini A, Austoni P, Bosi G, Giorgetti R, Grancini F, Marni ED, Perticone F, Rosti D, Salice P. Prolongation of the QT interval and the sudden infant death syndrome. *N Engl J Med* 1998;338:1709–1714.
4. Schwartz PJ, Priori SG, Dumaine R, Napolitano C, Antzelevitch C, Stramba-Badiale M, Richard TA, Berti MR, Bloise R. A molecular link between the sudden infant death syndrome and the long QT syndrome. *N Engl J Med* 2000;343:262–267.
5. Schwartz PJ, Priori SG, Bloise R, Napolitano C, Ronchetti E, Piccinini A, Goj A, Breithardt G, Schulze-Bahr E, Wedekind H, Nastoli J. Molecular diagnosis in a child with sudden infant death syndrome. *Lancet* 2001;358:1342–1343.
6. Schwartz PJ, Southall DP, Valdes-Dapena M. The sudden infant death syndrome. Cardiac and respiratory mechanisms and interventions. *Ann NY Acad Sci* 1988;533;474.
7. Ramanathan R, Corwin MJ, Hunt CE, Lister G, Tinsley LR, Baird T, Silvestri JM, Crowell DH, Hufford D, Martin RJ, Neuman MR, Weese-Mayer DE, Cupples LA, Peucker M, Willinger M, Keens TG; The Collaborative Home Infant Monitoring Evaluation (CHIME) Study Group. Cardiorespiratory events recorded on home monitors: Comparison of healthy infants with those at increased risk for SIDS. *JAMA* 2001;285:2199–2207.
8. Jobe AH. What do home monitors contribute to the SIDS problem? *JAMA* 2001;285:2244–2245.

9. Schwartz PJ, Priori SG, Napolitano C. Long QT syndrome. In: Zipes DP, Jalife J, Eds. *Cardiac Electrophysiology: From Cell to Bedside,* 3rd ed. Philadelphia, PA: W.B. Saunders, 2000:597–615.
10. Schwartz PJ, Stramba-Badiale M. Prolonged repolarization and sudden infant death syndrome. In: Zipes DP, Jalife J, Eds. *Cardiac Electrophysiology: From Cell to Bedside,* 3rd ed. Philadelphia, PA: W.B. Saunders, 2004:711–719.
11. Priori SG, Barhanin J, Hauer RNW, Haverkamp W, Jongsma HJ, Kleber AG, McKenna WJ, Roden DM, Rudy Y, Schwartz K, Schwartz PJ, Towbin JA, Wilde AM. Genetic and molecular basis of cardiac arrhythmias: Impact on clinical management. Part I and II. *Circulation* 1999;99:518–528, and Part III *Circulation* 1999;99:674–681, and *Eur Heart J* 1999;20:174–195.
12. Maron BJ, Clark CE, Goldstein RE, Epstein SE. Potential role of QT interval prolongation in sudden infant death syndrome. *Circulation* 1976;54:423–430.
13. Kelly DH, Shannon DC, Liberthson R. The role of the QT interval in the sudden infant death syndrome. *Circulation* 1977;55:633–635.
14. Steinschneider A. Sudden infant death syndrome and prolongation of the QT interval. *Am J Dis Child* 1978;132:688–691.
15. Haddad GG, Epstein MAF, Epstein RA, Mazza NR, Mellins RB, Krongrad E. The QT interval in aborted sudden infant death syndrome infants. *Pediatr Res* 1979;13:136–138.
16. Montague TJ, Finley JP, Mukelabai K, Black SA, Rigby SM, Spencer A, Horacek BM. Cardiac rhythm, rate and ventricular repolarization properties in infants at risk for sudden infant death syndrome: Comparison with age- and sex-matched control infants. *Am J Cardiol* 1984;54:301–307.
17. Southall DP, Arrowsmith WA, Stebbens V, Alexander JR. QT interval measurements before sudden infant death syndrome. *Arch Dis Child* 1986;61:327–333.
18. Schwartz PJ, Segantini A. Cardiac innervation, neonatal electrocardiography and SIDS. A key for a novel preventive strategy? *Ann NY Acad Sci* 1988; 533:210–220.
19. Priori SG, Napolitano C, Schwartz PJ. Low penetrance in the long QT syndrome. Clinical impact. *Circulation* 1999;99:529–533.
20. Stramba-Badiale M, Lazzarotti M, Schwartz PJ. Development of cardiac innervation, ventricular fibrillation and sudden infant death syndrome. *Am J Physiol Heart Circ Physiol* 1992;263:H1514–H1522.
21. Schwartz PJ. QT prolongation, sudden death, and sympathetic imbalance: The pendulum swings. *J Cardiovasc Electrophysiol* 2001;12:1074–1077.
22. Schwartz PJ, Snebold NG, Brown AM. Effects of unilateral cardiac sympathetic denervation on the ventricular fibrillation threshold. *Am J Cardiol* 1976;37:1034–1040.
23. Chen PS, Chen LS, Cao JM, Sharifi B, Karagueuzian HS, Fishbein MC: Sympathetic nerve sprouting, electrical remodeling and the mechanisms of sudden cardiac death. *Cardiovasc Res* 2001;50:409–416.
24. Cimaz R, Stramba-Badiale M, Brucato A, Catelli L, Panzeri P, Meroni PL. QT interval prolongation in asymptomatic anti-SSA/Ro-positive infants without congenital heart block. *Arthritis Rheum* 2000;43:1049–1053.
25. Brucato A, Cimaz R, Stramba-Badiale M. Neonatal lupus. *Clin Rev Allergy Immunol* 2002;23:279–299.
26. Cimaz R, Meroni PL, Brucato A, Fesstova VV, Panzeri P, Goulene K, Stramba-Badiale M. Concomitant disappearance of electrocardiographic abnormalities and of acquired maternal autoantibodies during the first year of life in infants who had QT interval prolongation and anti-SSA/Ro positivity without congenital heart block at birth. *Arthritis Rheum* 2003;48:266–268.
27. Christiansen M, Tonder N, Larsen LA, Andersen PS, Simonsen H, Oyen N, Kanters JK, Jacobsen JR, Fosdal I, Wettrell G, Kjeldsen K. Mutations in the HERG K^+-ion channel: A novel link between long QT syndrome and sudden infant death syndrome. *Am J Cardiol* 2005;95:433–434.
28. Guntheroth WG, Spiers PS. Prolongation of the QT interval and the sudden infant death syndrome. *Pediatrics* 1999;103:813–814.
29. Schwartz PJ. Stillbirths, sudden infant deaths, and long QT syndrome. Puzzle or mosaic, the pieces of the jigsaw are being fitted together. *Circulation* 2004;109:2930–2932.
30. Ackerman MJ, Siu BL, Sturner WQ, Tester DJ, Valdivia CR, Makielski JC, Towbin JA. Postmortem molecular analysis of *SCN5A* defects in sudden infant death syndrome. *JAMA* 2001;286:2264–2269.
31. Tester DJ. Ackerman MJ. Sudden infant death syndrome: How significant are the cardiac channelopathies? *Cardiovasc Res* 2005;67:388–396.
32. Crotti L, Arnestad M, Insolia R, Pedrazzini M, Ferrandi C, Rognum T, Schwartz PJ. The role of long QT syndrome in sudden infant death syndrome. *Eur Heart J* 2005;26(Abstr. Suppl.):127.
33. Wang DW, Desai RR, Crotti L, Arnestad M, Insolia R, Pedrazzini M, Ferrandi C, Vege A, Rognum T,

Schwartz PJ, George AL Jr. Cardiac sodium channel dysfunction in sudden infant death syndrome. *Circulation* 2007;115(3):368–376.

34. Vatta M, Ackerman MJ, Ye B, Makielski JC, Ughanze EE, Taylor EW, Tester DJ, Balijepalli RC, Foell JD, Li Z, Kamp TJ, Towbin JA. Mutant caveolin-3 induces persistent late sodium current and is associated with long QT syndrome. *Circulation* 2007; 114(20):2104–2112.
35. Cronk LB, Ye B, Tester DJ, Vatta M, Makielski JC, Ackerman MJ. A novel mechanism for sudden infant death syndrome (SIDS): Persistent late sodium current secondary to mutations in caveolin-3. *Heart Rhythm* 2007;4(2):161–166.
36. Tester DJ, Dura M, Carturan E, Reiken S, Wronska A, Marks AR, Ackerman MJ. A mechanism for sudden infant death syndrome (SIDS): Stress-induced leak via ryanodine receptors. *Heart Rhythm* 2007;4:733–739.
37. Ackerman MJ, Tester DJ, Jones G, Will ML, Burrow CR, Curran ME. Ethnic differences in cardiac potassium channel variants: Implications for genetic susceptibility to sudden cardiac death and genetic testing for congenital long QT syndrome. *Mayo Clin Proc* 2003;78:1479–1487.
38. Ackerman MJ, Splawski I, Makielski JC, Tester DJ, Will ML, Timothy KW, Keating MT, Jones G, Chadha M, Burrow CR, Stephens JC, Xu C, Judson R, Curran ME. Spectrum and prevalence of cardiac sodium channel variants among Black, White, Asian, Hispanic individuals: Implications for arrhythmogenic susceptibility and Brugada/long QT syndrome genetic testing. *Heart Rhythm* 2004;1:600–607.
39. Sun Z, Milos PM, Thompson JF, Lloyd DB, Mank-Seymour A, Richmond J, *et al.* Role of KCNH2 polymorphism (R1047L) in dofetilide-induced torsades de pointes. *J Mol Cell Cardiol* 2004;37: 1031–1039.
40. Plant LD, Bowers PN, Liu Q, Morgan T, Zhang T, State MW, Chen W, Kittles RA, Goldstein SAN. A common cardiac sodium channel variant associated with sudden infant death in African Americans, *SCN5A* S1103Y. *J Clin Invest* 2006;116: 430–435.
41. Crotti L, Lundquist AL, Insolia R, Pedrazzini M, Ferrandi C, De Ferrari GM, Vicentini A, Yang P, Roden DM, George AL Jr, Schwartz PJ: KCNH2-K897T is a genetic modifier of latent congenital long QT syndrome. *Circulation* 2005;112;1251–1258; corrections *Circulation* 2005;112:e295.
42. Ye B, Valdivia CR, Ackerman MJ, Makielski JC. A common human *SCN5A* polymorphism modifies expression of an arrhythmia causing mutation. *Physiol Genomics* 2003;12:187–193.
43. Makielski JC, Ye B, Valdivia CR, Pagel MD, Pu J, Tester DJ, Ackerman MJ. A ubiquitous splice variant and a common polymorphism affect heterologous expression of recombinant human SCN5A heart sodium channels. *Circ Res* 2003;93:821–828.
44. Moss AJ, Zareba W, Hall WJ, Schwartz PJ, Crampton RS, Benhorin J, Vincent GM, Locati EH, Priori SG, Napolitano C, Medina A, Zhang L, Robinson JL, Timothy K, Towbin JA, Andrews ML. Effectiveness and limitations of beta-blocker therapy in congenital long-QT syndrome. *Circulation* 2000;101:616–623.
45. Priori SG, Napolitano C, Schwartz PJ, Grillo M, Bloise R, Ronchetti E, Moncalvo C, Tulipani C, Veia A, Bottelli G, Nastoli J. Association of long QT syndrome loci and cardiac events among patients treated with beta-blockers. *JAMA* 2004;292:1341–1344.
46. Schwartz PJ, Garson A Jr, Paul T, Stramba-Badiale M, Vetter VL, Villain E, Wren C. Guidelines for the interpretation of the neonatal electrocardiogram. A Task Force of the European Society of Cardiology. *Eur Heart J* 2002;23:1329–1344.
47. Goulene K, Stramba-Badiale M, Crotti L, Priori SG, Salice P, Mannarino S, Rosati E, Schwartz PJ. Neonatal electrocardiographic screening of genetic arrhythmogenic disorders and congenital cardiovascular diseases: Prospective data from 31,000 infants. *Eur Heart J* 2005;26(Abstr. Suppl.):214.
48. Crotti L, Stramba-Badiale M, Pedrazzini M, Ferrandi C, Insolia R, Goulene K, Salice P, Mannarino S, Schwartz PJ. Prevalence of the long QT syndrome. *Circulation* 2005;112(Suppl. II):II-660.
49. Quaglini S, Rognoni C, Spazzolini C, Priori SG, Mannarino S, Schwartz PJ. Cost-effectiveness of neonatal ECG screening for the long QT syndrome. *Eur Heart J* 2006;27(15):1824–1832.
50. Tester DJ, Ackerman MJ. Postmortem long QT syndrome genetic testing for sudden unexplained death in the young. *J Am Coll Cardiol* 2006;49(2): 240–246.
51. Schwartz PJ, Crotti L. Can a message from the dead save lives? *J Am Coll Cardiol* 2006;49(2):247–249.

63
Sudden Cardiac Death in Kidney Diseases

Hiie M. Gussak, Mai Ots, and Ihor Gussak

Introduction

Chronic kidney disease (CKD) is a worldwide health problem with increasing incidence, prevalence, morbidity, and mortality.[1–3] The *prevalence* of early stage CKD approaches 20 million (or 10.8% of the U.S. adult population), and has grown by 42% over the past 5 years.[4] The rates of new cases of CKD are more than four times higher in African-Americans and 1.5 times higher in Asians or Pacific Islanders than in whites.[5]

Furthermore, more than a half million Americans have end-stage renal disease (ESRD).[6] The prevalence of ESRD has almost doubled between 1988 and 1997, and is exceptionally high in African-Americans, American Indians, Alaska Natives, diabetic patients, and the elderly. The overall *incidence* of ESRD has increased dramatically over the past decade, from 150 new cases per 1 million population in 1988 to 287 per 1 million in 1997.[7] In 1997, 80,248 new cases of ESRD were reported.[6,8] Also, the incidence of ESRD is especially high in selected populations.[7] The steepest rise in incidence over the past 10 years has been in African-Americans, diabetic patients, and the elderly. Untreated, ESRD is universally fatal, and hospitalization in ESRD patients is very high: on average, 1.41 hospitalizations and 10.8 hospital days per patient per year.[7]

The *mortality* rate in the ESRD population is one of the highest, even when adjusted for age, race, sex, and comorbid conditions.[9,10] The relative risk for cardiovascular death is 10–30 times higher than in the general population.[1] The 30-year-old dialysis patient has the same annual mortality rate as a 75- to 80-year-old individual from the general population.[11] Although the absolute risk for death increased exponentially with decreasing renal function, cardiovascular causes account for at least 40% of deaths in ESRD patients and 20% of these are sudden.[12] Cardiovascular diseases (CVD) are also a significant cause of morbidity and mortality in the chronic dialysis pediatric population.[1,13]

Sudden cardiac death (SCD) is the single largest cause of mortality in dialysis patients.[14–18] The survival of dialysis patients after cardiac arrest is poor, a situation greatly exacerbated by substantially reduced benefits from implantable cardioverter defibrillators in patients with severe renal disease and heart failure.[19] In addition, the effect of statins on the risk of cardiovascular events in advanced CKD is also far less than expected.[20]

The main objectives of this chapter are to elucidate the nature of SCD in the kidney diseases population, describe possible mechanisms, risk factors, and risk stratification, and discuss the prevention of SCD.

Possible Mechanisms

The association between CKD and SCD is accounted for, in part, by higher rates of clinically relevant cardiac arrhythmias. There is a strong and independent relationship between deterioration of the renal function and electrical instability of the heart, including advanced atrioventricular and intraventricular conduction blocks, atrial fibrillation, and life-threatening ventricular tachyarrhythmias. A higher incidence of life-threatening cardiac arrhythmias is associated with a very high prevalence of underlying CVD, particularly, coronary artery disease (CAD), left ventricular hypertrophy (LVH), arterial hypertension, and congestive heart failure (CHF).

In cardiac electrophysiology, CAD, LVH/hypertension, and CHF are known for their strong remodeling of cardiac ion channels[21] resulting in the *acquired cardiac channelopathies* leading to prolonged (or delayed) ventricular repolarization and increased risk of SCD ["disease-associated" acquired long QT syndrome (LQTS)]. Such an adverse modulation of the cardiac electrophysiological matrix is characterized by a progressive reduction of the naturally redundant K^+ channels (diminished "repolarization reserve") and concomitant increase in sensitivity of the remaining K^+ channel to their inhibition. Therefore, administration of any drug that is capable of inhibiting the K^+ channel (predominantly I_{Kr} current) will prolong the time required to complete ventricular repolarization. This results in further prolongation of the electrocardiographic QT interval and elevates the risk for lethal arrhythmias (drug-induced acquired LQTS).

The arrhythmogenic potential of acquired LQTS in renal patients is determined and modified mainly by the following:

1. Electrophysiological remodeling of the heart due to concomitant CVD, chiefly CAD, LVH/hypertension, and CHF.
2. Exposure to multiple (often excessive) proarrhythmic medications and their abnormal excretion or metabolism.

Both forms of acquired LQTS ("disease associated" and drug induced) are among the most important and yet preventable mechanisms of SCD in nephrology. The most common clinical manifestation of acquired LQTS is torsade de points (TdP) polymorphic ventricular tachycardia and SCD. The risk of TdP and SCD will dramatically increase when any QT-prolonging drug is coadministered with any other substance or drug known to inhibit its metabolism (e.g., CYP3A4 inhibitors such as grapefruit juice, macrolides, ketoconazole, and alcohol overdose) or excretion, especially in patients with preexisting abnormal ventricular repolarization (see Chapter 43, this volume, for details). In patients with impaired glomerular filtration, QT-labile drugs with renal excretion can produce an unpredictable increase of the plasma concentration with significant prolongation of the QT interval and development of TdP. To avoid cardiac arrhythmogenic toxicity, the dosage of drugs primarily excreted through the kidneys must be reduced [e.g., antiarrhythmic sotalol can be given as 40 mg after dialysis (every second day), instead of the usual daily dose, 80–120 mg every 12 h].

The short list of noncardiac risk factors for *acquired LQTS in nephrology* includes the following:

1. Impaired drug elimination (e.g., renal or hepatic dysfunction).
2. Electrolyte disturbances (increased K^+, decreased K^+, decreased Mg^{2+}, and increased Ca^{2+}).
3. Acute neurological events (e.g., intracranial and subarachnoid hemorrhage, stroke, trauma) and diabetes mellitus.
4. Altered nutrition (e.g., anorexia nervosa, starvation diets, alcoholism).

Female gender, advanced age, abnormal bradycardia, and tachycardia are among the most common factors predisposing aggravation or initiation of malignant arrhythmias and SCD. In general, females are three times more likely to have an abnormally prolonged QTc interval (corrected by the heart rate QT interval at baseline), and are three times more likely to die from drug-induced TdP. Regrettably, despite the notion of the potentially lethal consequences of drug-induced LQTS, the risk and the risk–benefit ratio of QT-prolonging medications are profoundly underestimated in clinical practice. Based on the patterns of most currently prescribed medications, it appears that clear restrictions, side effects, warnings, and contraindications pertinent to the QT-prolonging medications are widely ignored or even disregarded (see Chapter 43, this volume, for more details).

Sudden Cardiac Death Associated with Hemodialysis

Sudden cardiac death is a devastating complication of hemodialysis (HD). The concomitant presence of CAD, LVH (present in almost 80% patients on HD), CHF, and autonomic dysfunction (with or without diabetes)[22–24] greatly contributes to the SCD in HD patients. Potentially life-threatening ventricular arrhythmias, atrial arrhythmias, and silent myocardial ischemia are often documented on Holter monitor during HD.[25,26] The risk of new onset arrhythmias was shown to increase in patients on peritoneal dialysis (PD), with ventricular arrhythmias increasing from 30% to 43% and supraventricular arrhythmias increasing from 40% to 57% during a mean follow-up period of 20 ± 4 months.[27]

Additional risks for SCD in HD patients during and between HD procedures are associated with sharply fluctuating levels of the following:

1. Electrolytes (chiefly potassium, ionized calcium, and magnesium[28]).
2. Circulating volume and blood pressure. Predialysis and postdialysis blood pressure values have independent associations with mortality.[29]
3. Bicarbonate.[30,31]

These fluctuations are partly driven by the level of potassium and calcium in the dialysate fluid used during previous treatment, and the wide variability in eating habits associated with varying adherence to dietary modifications necessary to control the potassium and calcium phosphate product.[31–34] Each of these factors, particularly in combination, can contribute to a high propensity of developing lethal electrical instability of the heart during and immediately after HD, and link to an irregular distribution of SCD throughout the week due to the intermittent nature of HD.

From the perspective of acquired LQTS, HD is also associated with so-called "paradoxical" QTc prolongation, which many investigators associate with exaggerated risk for the occurrence of fatal arrhythmias during the procedure. The prevailing opinion holds that such a "paradoxical" increment in the QT interval duration is related to the potassium fluxes induced by HD. We studied this electrocardiographic (ECG) phenomenon in ESRD patients and found that the increase in QTc is not a "paradoxical" ECG phenomenon. We discovered that HD-induced QTc prolongation is due to a statistically significant increase in heart rate (secondary to the HD-induced reduction of extracellular fluid) but not in the QT interval, since the absolute value of QT remains unchanged.[35]

As a reminder, QTc is a function of both (1) the heart rate and (2) the absolute value of the QT interval duration. An increase in either parameter will ultimately result in the increase in QTc. Therefore, the impaired adjustment of the prolonged ventricular repolarization to the changes in heart rate, particularly during HD, is evident in ESRD patients.[35]

In our opinion, the direct arrhythmogenic trigger of malignant arrhythmogenicity of HD is related to procedure-induced transient intracellular hypokalemia (and likely hypomagnesemia). Moreover, the sharp (even brief) reduction in the intracellular potassium (and likely magnesium) concentration could be associated with an "aggressiveness" of HD. Of note, the correlation between intracellular and extracellular potassium and magnesium concentrations is pure, and brief "arrhythmogenic" intracellular hypokalemia or hypomagnesemia cannot be detected by measuring the concentration of these ions in the blood serum.

Risk Factors and Risk Stratification

There is a variety of traditional and nontraditional cardiovascular and noncardiovascular risk factors for SCD encountered in CKD patients. Their high prevalence in the CKD population contributes to the enhanced risk for SCD. The knowledge of the major cardiac and noncardiac risk factors can help in the development of strategies to reduce premature morbidity and mortality among CKD patients. Furthermore, there are some important differences among risk factors in CKD patients compared with the general population. In this section we provide a brief summary of the most important risk factors for SCD in the CKD population, particularly in ESRD patients.

Among major factors influencing the high morbidity and mortality of ESRD patients are (1) a high prevalence of concomitant CVD, (2) infection, (3) anemia, (4) hyperparathyroidism, (5) malnutrition, and (6) intrinsic iatrogenic complications of therapies, such as hemodialysis (HD), arteriovenous access thrombosis, electrolyte imbalance, and metabolic abnormalities.

Cardiovascular Risk Factors

The number of cardiovascular risk factors increased with stage of kidney dysfunction.[13] The following most relevant cardiovascular diseases predispose the heart to fatal arrhythmias:

1. Coronary artery disease.
2. Arterial hypertension and left ventricular hypertrophy.
3. Congestive heart failure.
4. Metabolic and uremic cardiomyopathy.
5. Diabetic cardiac autonomic neuropathy.
6. Any combination of the above.

Coronary Artery Disease

There is a high prevalence of atherosclerosis in CKD.[36,37] Atherosclerotic lesions in CKD are characterized by a distinct intima-media thickness and calcification of the coronary arteries. Two major factors contribute to accelerated atherosclerosis of coronary arteries in CKD. They are chronic inflammation and hyperphosphatemia. Hyperphosphatemia and associated secondary hyperparathyroidism result in noncompliant vessels, due to Ca^{2+} deposition in soft tissues and increased vascular calcification with smooth muscle proliferation, known in angiography as the "Spaghetti Syndrome." Not surprisingly, hyperphosphatemia is an independent risk factor for mortality in chronic HD patients: ~40% of them have a serum PO_4 level >6.5 mg/dl.[38]

Approximately 20% of cardiac deaths are attributed to acute myocardial infarction (AMI).[3] Management for acute coronary syndromes in the setting of kidney disease is a paradox: the benefits of current treatment are high, but so are the risks for complications.[39] Furthermore, exacerbation of chronic coronary artery insufficiency—accompanied by intermittent changes in electrolytes, acid–base balance, and volume of circulating fluid—are commonly implicated in the malignant arrhythmias observed during HD.

The U.S. Renal Data System database of 783,171 patients was used to retrospectively examine outcomes of renal transplant recipients hospitalized for a first myocardial infarction (MI) after initiation of renal replacement therapy between the years 1977 and 1996. There were 4250 renal transplant recipients with MI. The in-hospital death rate was 12.8%. Overall, the 2-year cardiac and all-cause mortality rates were 11.8% ± 0.6% and 33.6% ± 0.8%, respectively. The poorest survival after MI occurred in patients with diabetic ESRD, with 2-year cardiac and all-cause mortality rates of 14.9% ± 1.1% and 40.5% ± 1.4%, respectively. The risks for cardiac and all-cause death from MI were 51% ($p = 0.0003$) and 45% fewer ($p < 0.0001$) when compared between the years 1990–1996 and 1977–1984.[15] In addition, patients with CKD and acute coronary syndromes are at high risk for both bleeding and ischemic events. This risk increases with the severity of renal insufficiency.

Arterial Hypertension and Left Ventricular Hypertrophy

Arterial hypertension, one of the most frequent cardiovascular diseases found in CKD patients, is documented in more that 70% of this population before the initiation of hemodialysis.[6] Arterial hypertension is a well-established major risk factor for renal failure and its association with LVH is well established. Left ventricular hypertrophy has also been established as an independent risk factor for adverse cardiovascular events and death. For this reason, considerable attention has been directed toward a better understanding of LVH as a risk factor. As recognition of the risks associated with LVH has grown, investigators have increasingly focused attention on improving methods for the detection of LVH, assessing its effects on cardiac function, defining its relationship with myocardial ischemia and sudden death, evaluating the role of antihypertensive treatment in the regression of LVH, and assessing whether such regression is beneficial in the long term.[40]

Congestive Heart Failure

Heart failure hospitalizations are five times greater in CKD patients and only 30% fewer than those in dialysis patients.[41] The annual mortality from CHF in CKD patients is 13%, and is magnified in the presence of anemia, especially in the elderly population.[16] Diagnosis of CHF may be challenging in dialysis patients because salt and water retention may be treated by ultrafiltration during HD, often leaving other signs and symptoms, such as decreased blood pressure, fatigue, and anorexia, as the only clues to its presence. On the other hand, salt and water retention may reflect inadequate ultrafiltration rather than heart failure, or a combination of both heart failure and inadequate ultrafiltration. Indeed, one of the major causes of inadequate ultrafiltration during dialysis is hypotension, which may be a manifestation of heart failure. Regardless of the cause, heart failure is a powerful risk factor for adverse outcomes in HD patients, which suggests that it is usually a manifestation of advanced CVD.[42]

Metabolic and Uremic Cardiomyopathies

Patients with CKD also have a high prevalence of cardiomyopathy , most commonly metabolic or uremic.[43] The main pathophysiological mechanisms underlying cardiomyopathies are (1) interstitial fibrosis and (2) endothelial dysfunction. Hypertension and arteriosclerosis result in pressure overload and lead to concentric LVH (increased wall-to-lumen ratio), whereas anemia, fluid overload, and arteriovenous fistulas result in volume overload and primarily lead to left ventricular dilation with LVH (a proportional increase in left ventricular mass and diameter). These structural abnormalities may lead to diastolic and systolic dysfunctions. Clinical presentations of cardiomyopathy include heart failure and ischemic heart disease, even in the absence of arterial vascular disease. The incidence of cardiomyopathies is increasing.

Diabetic Cardiac Autonomic Neuropathy

The prevalence of diabetes in the Medicare population increased at a rate of 4.4% per year, reaching 18.9% in the 1999–2000 cohort. Patients with both diabetes and hypertension are 5.9 times more likely to have at least one cardiac condition over those without diabetes or hypertension. The ratio goes to 5.0 times for two cardiac conditions and 4.8 times for three. Patients with renal failure, diabetes, and hypertension are more likely to have heart disease than those only with diabetes or hypertension.[44]

Noncardiovascular Risk Factors

Renal Risk Factors

Both the reduced glomerular filtration rate (GFR) and the proteinuria (albuminuria) appear to be independent risk factors for CVD outcomes, particularly in higher-risk CKD populations. Baseline estimated GFR is linked to worsened outcomes and increased defibrillation thresholds in patients receiving implantable cardioverter defibrillators. Furthermore, preoperative GFR is one of the most powerful predictors of operative mortality and morbidities.[45] Also, the prevalence of LVH is inversely related to the level of GFR.

Other Risk Factors

Increased risk of SCD in CKD patients may also be attributed to anemia, older age, dyslipidemia, hyperhomocysteinemia, oxidant stress, abnormal calcium and phosphorus metabolism, peripheral vascular disease, and the high preponderance of vascular inflammation. Microinflammation is linked to CVD and septicemia and is highly prevalent in HD patients. Septicemia appears to be an important, potentially preventable, cardiovascular risk factor in dialysis patients.[46] Compared with the general population, the incidence of bacterial endocarditis is much greater in long-term HD patients and CKD has been postulated to be an independent host-related risk factor.

Other modified and largely preventable risk factors include unjustified use of multiple medications (polypharmacy), physical inactivity, cigarette smoking, alcoholism, and malnutrition (eating habits with varying adherence to dietary modifications necessary to control the calcium phosphate product).

Summarized, the following clinical variables are most important in the risk stratification of CKD patients:

1. Cardiovascular abnormalities: a history of CAD, CHF, or LVH/hypertension, transient ischemic attacks, low ejection fraction, peripheral vascular diseases, abnormal baseline ECG (especially prolonged QTc interval), and previous shunt thrombosis.
2. Noncardiovascular abnormalities: age >50 years, dialysis duration, dialysis history, insulin-

dependent diabetes, hyperphosphatemia, and body mass index.

Prevention of Sudden Cardiac Death and Future Directions

Cardiovascular disease is the major cause of morbidity, mortality, and SCD in CKD patients. The risk of SCD in CKD, especially in ESRD patients, is very high, and its prevention is of the highest priority. Contrary to earlier expectations and despite decreased overall cardiac mortality in the general population, SCD rates appear to be rising in concert with the escalating global prevalence of CAD and CHF, both major contributors to SCD. The increased prevalence of CVD in patients with renal dysfunction has been attributed, in part, to lack of effective prevention. Regrettably, the most common measures of prevention for SCD used in CVD are much less effective in CKD patients than in the general population. For instance, in patients with severe renal disease and heart failure, benefits from implantable cardioverter defibrillators are minimal or even lacking.[19] In addition, statins appear to have very limited or no effect on the risk of cardiovascular events in advanced CKD.[20]

Nevertheless, many risk factors for SCD in the CKD population are preventable and modifiable. Preventive strategies include meticulous management of electrolytes, baseline treatment for CVD, and, when indicated, implantable cardioverter defibrillators. Among the most important mechanisms for the reduction of mortality are (1) prevention and close monitoring of blood pressure, LVH, CAD, and CHF and (2) avoiding or limiting the use of QT-prolonging drugs. Additionally, underuse of appropriate therapies likely contributes to adverse outcomes.

To reduce the risk of adverse cardiac events associated with HD, the dialysate prescription should be modified in high-risk patients.[47] We also believe that a less aggressive HD procedure with a smaller potassium gradient between dialysate and blood potassium level, longer treatment time, and slower ultrafiltration rates could have a positive impact on procedure-related cardiac mortality. The role of magnesium in HD-related arrhythmogenicity warrants further investigation.[48]

Future research into the mechanisms and prevention of SCD in patients with CKD is warranted.

References

1. Sarnak MJ, Levey AS, Schoolwerth AC, Coresh J, Culleton B, Hamm LL, McCullough PA, Kasiske BL, Kelepouris E, Klag MJ, Parfrey P, Pfeffer M, Raij L, Spinosa DJ, Wilson PW; American Heart Association Councils on Kidney in Cardiovascular Disease, High Blood Pressure Research, Clinical Cardiology, and Epidemiology and Prevention. Kidney disease as a risk factor for development of cardiovascular disease: A statement from the American Heart Association Councils on Kidney in Cardiovascular Disease, High Blood Pressure Research, Clinical Cardiology, and Epidemiology and Prevention. *Hypertension* 2003;42(5):1050–1065.
2. National Institutes of Health, National Institute of Diabetes and Digestive and Kidney Diseases. U.S. Renal Data System, USRDS 1998 Annual Data Report. Bethesda, MD: National Institutes of Health, National Institute of Diabetes and Digestive and Kidney Diseases, 1998. Available at http://www.usrds.org/adr_1998.htm. Accessed September 12, 2003.
3. National Institutes of Health, National Institute of Diabetes and Digestive and Kidney Diseases. U.S. Renal Data System, USRDS 2000 Annual Data Report. Bethesda, MD: National Institutes of Health, National Institute of Diabetes and Digestive and Kidney Diseases, 2000. Available at http://www.usrds.org/atlas_2000.htm. Accessed September 12, 2003.
4. Levey AS, Coresh J, Balk E, Kausz AT, Levin A, Steffes MW, Hogg RJ, Perrone RD, Lau J, Eknoyan G, National Kidney Foundation. National Kidney Foundation practice guidelines for chronic kidney disease: Evaluation, classification, and stratification. *Ann Intern Med* 2003;139(2):137–147.
5. Healthy People 2010, Volume I, Chronic Kidney Disease, National Institutes of Health [http://www.healthypeople.gov/Document/HTML/Volume1/04CKD.htm#_Toc490542780].
6. U.S. Renal Data System (USRDS). 1999 Annual Data Report (ADR). Bethesda, MD: National Institutes of Health (NIH), National Institute of Diabetes and Digestive and Kidney Diseases (NIDDK), April 1999, Appendix, Table A-1.
7. Reikes ST. Trends in end-stage renal disease. Epidemiology, morbidity, and mortality. *Postgrad Med* 2000;108(1):124–126, 129–131, 135–136.

8. U.S. Renal Data System 1999 Annual Data Report: Part II. Incidence and prevalence of ESRD. *Am J Kidney Dis* 1999;34(2 Suppl. 1):S40–S50.
9. Foley RN, Parfrey PS, Sarnak MJ. Clinical epidemiology of cardiovascular disease in chronic renal disease. *Am J Kidney Dis* 1998;32:S112–S119.
10. McCullough PA, Sandberg KR. Chronic kidney disease and sudden death: Strategies for prevention. *Blood Purif* 2004;22(1):136–142.
11. Meyer KB, Levey AS. Controlling the epidemic of cardiovascular disease in chronic renal disease: Report from the National Kidney Foundation Task Force on cardiovascular disease. *J Am Soc Nephrol* 1998;9(12 Suppl.):S31–S42.
12. Developed in Collaboration with the European Heart Rhythm Association and the Heart Rhythm Society, Zipes DP, Camm AJ, Borggrefe M, Buxton AE, Chaitman B, Fromer M, Gregoratos G, Klein G, Moss AJ, Myerburg RJ, Priori SG, Quinones MA, Roden DM, Silka MJ, Tracy C, Smith SC Jr, Jacobs AK, Adams CD, Antman EM, Anderson JL, Hunt SA, Halperin JL, Nishimura R, Ornato JP, Page RL, Riegel B, Priori SG, Blanc JJ, Budaj A, Camm AJ, Dean V, Deckers JW, Despres C, Dickstein K, Lekakis J, McGregor K, Metra M, Morais J, Osterspey A, Tamargo JL, Zamorano JL. ACC/AHA/ESC 2006 Guidelines for Management of Patients with Ventricular Arrhythmias and the Prevention of Sudden Cardiac Death–Executive Summary A Report of the American College of Cardiology/American Heart Association Task Force and the European Society of Cardiology Committee for Practice Guidelines (Writing Committee to Develop Guidelines for Management of Patients with Ventricular Arrhythmias and the Prevention of Sudden Cardiac Death). *J Am Coll Cardiol* 2006;48(5):1064–1108.
13. Foley RN, Wang C, Collins AJ. Cardiovascular risk factor profiles and kidney function stage in the U.S. general population: The NHANES III study. *Mayo Clin Proc* 2005;80(10):1270–1277.
14. Herzog CA. Cardiac arrest in dialysis patients: Approaches to alter an abysmal outcome. *Kidney Int Suppl* 2003;(84):S197–S200.
15. Herzog CA, Ma JZ, Collins AJ. Long-term survival of renal transplant recipients in the United States after acute myocardial infarction. *Am J Kidney Dis* 2000;36(1):145–152.
16. Herzog CA. Cardiac arrest in dialysis patients: Taking a small step. *Semin Dial* 2004;17(3):184–185.
17. Herzog CA, Muster HA, Li S, Collins AJ. Impact of congestive heart failure, chronic kidney disease, and anemia on survival in the Medicare population. *J Card Fail* 2004;10(6):467–472.
18. Herzog CA, Li S, Weinhandl ED, Strief JW, Collins AJ, Gilbertson DT. Survival of dialysis patients after cardiac arrest and the impact of implantable cardioverter defibrillators. *Kidney Int* 2005;68(2): 818–825.
19. Goldenberg I, Moss AJ, McNitt S, Andrews ML, Zareba W, Jackson Hall W, Greenberg H, Case RB. Relationship between renal function, risk of sudden cardiac death, and benefit of the implanted cardiac defibrillator in post myocardial infarction patients with left ventricular dysfunction. Abstract 818-4. *J Am Coll Cardiol* 2006;47(4):19A.
20. Kiberd BA. Atorvastatin has no beneficial effect on cardiovascular outcomes in patients with advanced chronic kidney disease. *Nat Clin Pract Nephrol* 2006;2:354–355.
21. Tomaselli GF, Marban E. Electrophysiological remodeling in hypertrophy and heart failure. *Cardiovasc Res* 1999;42(2):270–222.
22. Collins AJ, Li S, Ma JZ, Herzog C. Cardiovascular disease in end-stage renal disease patients. *Am J Kidney Dis* 2001;38(Suppl. 1):S26–S29.
23. Coresh J, Longenecker JC, Miller ER, Young HJ 3rd, Klag MJ. Epidemiology of cardiovascular risk factors in chronic renal disease. *J Am Soc Nephrol* 1998;9:S24–S30.
24. Foley RN, Parfrey PS, Sarnak MJ. Epidemiology of cardiovascular disease in chronic renal disease. *J Am Soc Nephrol* 1998;9:S16–S23.
25. Narula AS, Jha V, Bali HK, Sakhuja V, Sapru RP. Cardiac arrhythmias and silent myocardial ischemia during hemodialysis. *Ren Fail* 2000;22: 355–368.
26. Ansari N, Manis T, Feinfeld DA. Symptomatic atrial arrhythmias in hemodialysis patients. *Ren Fail* 2001;23:71–76.
27. Renke M, Zegrzda D, Liberek T, Dudziak M, Lichodziejewska-Niemierko M, Kubasik A, Rutkowski B. Interrelationship between cardiac structure and function and incidence of arrhythmia in peritoneal dialysis patients. *Int J Artif Organs* 2001;24:374–379.
28. Foley RN, Parfrey PS, Harnett JD, Kent GM, Hu L, O'Dea R, Murray DC, Barre PE. Hypocalcemia, morbidity, and mortality in end-stage renal disease. *Am J Nephrol* 1996;16:386–393.
29. Foley RN, Herzog CA, Collins AJ, United States Renal Data System. Blood pressure and long-term mortality in United States hemodialysis patients: USRDS Waves 3 and 4 Study. *Kidney Int* 2002; 62(5):1784–1790.
30. Munger MA, Ateshkadi A, Cheung AK, Flaharty KK, Stoddard GJ, Marshall EH. Cardiopulmonary events during hemodialysis: Effects of dialysis

membranes and dialysate buffers. *Am J Kidney Dis* 2000;36:130–139.
31. Saran R, Bragg-Gresham JL, Rayner HC, Goodkin DA, Keen ML, Van Dijk PC, Kurokawa K, Piera L, Saito A, Fukuhara S, Young EW, Held PJ, Port FK. Nonadherence in hemodialysis: Associations with mortality, hospitalization, and practice patterns in the DOPPS. *Kidney Int* 2003;64:254–262.
32. Goodkin DA, Mapes DL, Held PJ. The dialysis outcomes and practice patterns study (DOPPS): How can we improve the care of hemodialysis patients? *Semin Dial* 2001;14:157–159.
33. Goodkin DA, Bragg-Gresham JL, Koenig KG, Wolfe RA, Akiba T, Andreucci VE, Saito A, Rayner HC, Kurokawa K, Port FK, Held PJ, Young EW. Association of comorbid conditions and mortality in hemodialysis patients in Europe, Japan, and the United States: The Dialysis Outcomes and Practice Patterns Study (DOPPS). *J Am Soc Nephrol* 2003; 14:3270–3277.
34. Hecking E, Bragg-Gresham JL, Rayner HC, Pisoni RL, Andreucci VE, Combe C, Greenwood R, McCullough K, Feldman HI, Young EW, Held PJ, Port FK. Haemodialysis prescription, adherence and nutritional indicators in five European countries: Results from the Dialysis Outcomes and Practice Patterns Study (DOPPS). *Nephrol Dial Transplant* 2004;19:100–107.
35. Gussak HM, Gellens ME, Yokoyama Y, Gussak I, Bjerregaard P. Failure of adjustment of QT interval duration to hemodialysis induced changes in heart rate is underlying the prolongation of corrected QT interval duration in end-stage renal disease patients. *J Am Soc Nephrol* 1999;10:281A.
36. Tonelli M, Bohm C, Pandeya S, *et al.* Cardiac risk factors and use of cardioprotective medications in patients with chronic renal insufficiency. *Am J Kidney Dis* 2001;37:484–489.
37. Jungers P, Massy ZA, Khoa TN, *et al.* Incidence and risk factors of atherosclerotic cardiovascular accidents in predialysis chronic renal failure patients: A prospective study. *Nephrol Dial Transplant* 1997; 12:2597–2602.
38. Shoji T, Emoto M, Shinohara K, Kakiya R, Tsujimoto Y, Kishimoto H, Ishimura E, Tabata T, Nishizawa Y. Diabetes mellitus, aortic stiffness, and cardiovascular mortality in end-stage renal disease. *J Am Soc Nephrol* 2001;12(10):2117–2124.
39. Panetta CJ, Herzog CA, Henry TD. Acute coronary syndromes in patients with renal disease: What are the issues? *Curr Cardiol Rep* 2006;8(4): 296–300.
40. Balogun MO, Dunn FG. Left ventricular hypertrophy as a risk factor in hypertension. *Afr J Med Med Sci* 1996;25(3):277–283.
41. Collins AJ, Li S, Gilbertson DT, Liu J, Chen SC, Herzog CA. Chronic kidney disease and cardiovascular disease in the Medicare population. *Kidney Int Suppl* 2003;(87):S24–S31.
42. Harnett JD, Foley RN, Kent GM, *et al.* Congestive heart failure in dialysis patients: Prevalence, incidence, prognosis and risk factors. *Kidney Int* 1995;47:884–890.
43. Foley RN, Parfrey PS, Harnett JD, *et al.* Clinical and echocardiographic disease in patients starting end-stage renal disease therapy. *Kidney Int* 1995;47: 186–192.
44. Xue JL, Frazier ET, Herzog CA, Collins AJ. Association of heart disease with diabetes and hypertension in patients with ESRD. *Am J Kidney Dis* 2005; 45(2):316–323.
45. Cooper WA, O'Brien SM, Thourani VH, Guyton RA, Bridges CR, Szczech LA, Petersen R, Peterson ED. Impact of renal dysfunction on outcomes of coronary artery bypass surgery: Results from the Society of Thoracic Surgeons National Adult Cardiac Database. *Circulation* 2006;113(8):1063–1070.
46. Ishani A, Collins AJ, Herzog CA, Foley RN. Septicemia, access and cardiovascular disease in dialysis patients: The USRDS Wave 2 study. *Kidney Int* 2005;68(1):311–318.
47. Karnik JA, Young BS, Lew NL, Herget M, Dubinsky C, Lazarus JM, Chertow GM. Cardiac arrest and sudden death in dialysis units. *Kidney Int* 2001; 60(1):350–357.
48. Gussak I, Gussak H. Sudden cardiac death in nephrology: Focus on acquired long QT syndrome. Editorial Comments. *Nephrol Dial Transplant* 2007; 22(1):12–14.

Index

E

N

Q

W

X

Z